D1336867

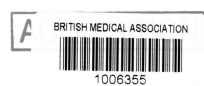

Oxford Textbook of

Cardiothoracic
Anaesthesia

Free personal online access for 12 months

Individual purchasers of this book are also entitled to free personal access to the online edition for 12 months on *Oxford Medicine Online* (www.oxfordmedicine.com). Please refer to the access token card for instructions on token redemption and access.

Online ancillary materials, where available, are noted at the end of the respective chapters in this book. Additionally, *Oxford Medicine Online* allows you to print, save, cite, email, and share content; download high-resolution figures as Microsoft PowerPoint slides; save often-used books, chapters, or searches; annotate; and quickly jump to other chapters or related material on a mobile-optimised platform.

We encourage you to take advantage of these features. If you are interested in ongoing access after the 12-month gift period, please consider an individual subscription or consult with your librarian.

Oxford Textbook of
Cardiothoracic Anaesthesia

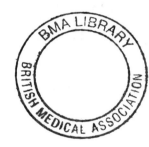

Edited by

R. Peter Alston
Consultant in Anaesthesia, Critical Care and Pain Medicine
Royal Infirmary of Edinburgh
Edinburgh
UK

Paul S. Myles
Professor, Director of the Department of Anaesthesia and Perioperative Medicine
Alfred Hospital and Monash University
Melbourne
Australia

Marco Ranucci
Professor, Head of Clinical Research in the Department of Anesthesia
    and Intensive Care
IRCCS Policlinico San Donato, San Donato Milanese
Milan
Italy

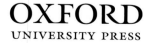

OXFORD
UNIVERSITY PRESS

OXFORD
UNIVERSITY PRESS

Great Clarendon Street, Oxford, OX2 6DP,
United Kingdom

Oxford University Press is a department of the University of Oxford.
It furthers the University's objective of excellence in research, scholarship,
and education by publishing worldwide. Oxford is a registered trade mark of
Oxford University Press in the UK and in certain other countries

First Edition published in 2015
Impression: 1

Published in the United States of America by Oxford University Press
198 Madison Avenue, New York, NY 10016, United States of America

British Library Cataloguing in Publication Data
Data available

Library of Congress Control Number: 2014940088

ISBN 978–0–19–965347–8

Printed in China by
C&C Offset Printing Co. Ltd

Foreword

It is always wise to look ahead, but difficult to look farther than you can see.
Winston Churchill

It is a privilege and great pleasure for me to be asked to write a few words as a Foreword to the *Oxford Textbook of Cardiothoracic Anaesthesia*, which is a new, fine contribution to the ever growing development of this speciality. Like all similar modern textbooks, it contains the recent relevant literature up to 2014 and a gel of the anaesthetic wisdom of many well-known anaesthesiologists, in this field. Many of them have been my associates, who I have enjoyed meeting through the European Association of Cardiothoracic Anaesthesiologists (EACTA) since its establishment in 1986. I congratulate them all for their monumental work.

My long association with cardiac anaesthesia began long before EACTA, in the days when we were only able to carry out two open-heart procedures each week. This was because our only Melrose non-disposable rotating drum oxygenator required to be dismantled, sterilized, and reassembled before being available for a further patient after 48 hours. Successful repair of a regurgitant mitral valve did not come easily in those pioneering days and was associated with a high mortality.

At that time there were no textbooks available for information on how to conduct the anaesthesia for open-heart surgery and we relied on word of mouth and rather limited journal literature. My only sources of information then were from such books as *Synopsis of Anaesthesia* (1947) and *Modern Practice in Anaesthesia* (1954), unsurprisingly with no mention of open-heart surgery. Since then my modest bookshelf tells me that there has been an ever increasing number of books relating to this specific speciality, up-to-date at their time of publication. Journal publications have likewise expanded enormously and the practising anaesthetist may be hard put to find the time to keep abreast of the many aspects of the specialty, let alone the essential skills and knowledge of transoesophageal echocardiography (TOE) and transthoracic echocardiography. This great increase in information reflects the vast amount of knowledge and multiple skills that contemporary anaesthesiologists require to practise cardiothoracic anaesthesia and critical care.

All technical books become dated and the subspecialty of cardiothoracic anaesthesia is no exception. No doubt that there will be further editions of this book. I note that many of the Forewords of previous books have written of the astonishing changes of theory and practice in a very short time, even in 1949. In *Modern Practice in Anaesthesia* (1949), the author wrote 'I think the newer methods (of intravenous barbiturates and curare) will push ether into the background. The administration of ether and chloroform should still be taught for there are times when their use is advisable'. So what can we predict in the faster pace of life nowadays and the exponential rise in the evolution and knowledge of our specialty?

At least this robust volume will not progress to be so large that it follows the prodigious and comprehensive *Oxford English Dictionary*, which may only be available online in future. However, the sources of teaching and knowledge in our speciality will continue to include books and journals (my personal choice), perhaps digitized online, but also from e-learning updates and such facilities as learning the mysteries of TOE from dedicated websites and simulators.

I am sure that both trainees and established cardiothoracic anaesthesiologists will enjoy this latest book. Its contents are also a mine of information useful to the providers of anaesthesia for patients with heart disease requiring non-cardiac surgery, and no doubt other anaesthesiologists will dip into it too.

Dr John Manners

Preface

In comparison with many other areas of medicine, cardiothoracic anaesthesia is a relatively young speciality, underpinned by several historic innovations in a little over 100 years. The first step to overcome was the pneumothorax problem, conquered at the end of the nineteenth century. Other major advances occurred with developments in cardiopulmonary bypass (CPB), lung isolation, intraoperative transoesophageal echocardiography (TOE), and mechanical support for the failing heart. These successes aside, the evolution of cardiothoracic anaesthesia has, at times, wandered down some blind alleys and several misconceptions held back progress. For this reason, and to place contemporary practices in context, we begin in the first chapter with a review of the history of cardiothoracic anaesthesia, including the errors, lest we be condemned to repeat the mistakes of the past.

Editing this book has given us pause for thought in regard to the knowledge and skills, over and above those of a specialist anaesthetist, that are necessary for the subspecialty of cardiothoracic anaesthesia. As a distillation of that thought, this textbook aims to provide the theoretical knowledge required to inform optimum clinical practice. Where possible, this has been done using an evidenced-based approach but not to the detriment of undervaluing extensive clinical experience. Cardiothoracic surgery is now routinely performed around the world and there is a universal need for subspecialty training in cardiothoracic anaesthesia. We are therefore delighted that, in addition to an international editorship, authors of renown from around the world accepted our invitations to write chapters for this textbook.

Whilst in the past too much importance may have been placed on physiological and other surrogate measures rather than true patient-centred outcomes, a sound knowledge of the basic sciences underpinning our speciality remain essential to current practice in cardiothoracic anaesthesia. Additionally, the specific problems in haemostasis and coagulation related to cardiac surgery make this field an optimal playing ground for point-of-care monitoring of the haemostatic system. Therefore, we have included chapters on the relevant anatomy, physiology, pathophysiology, and pharmacology, and consideration is given to inflammation, hypothermia, coagulation, anticoagulation, and transfusion medicine.

Core skills for a cardiothoracic anaesthetist include competency in lung isolation and one-lung ventilation techniques, the ability to invasively monitor the cardiovascular system, and the knowledge and experience to interpret the measurements intra- and postoperatively. In addition, a good theoretical knowledge of CPB,

if not the practical skill to operate the CPB machine, and expertise in the pharmacological and mechanical support of the circulation are essential. In the past, mechanical support was limited to intra-aortic balloon pumps, but increasingly cardiac anaesthesiologists need to know how to use ventricular assist devices, and extracorporeal membrane oxygenation is regaining popularity. For these reasons, chapters that address all these areas have been included in this textbook.

Whilst there are many intraoperative skills that are essential to cardiothoracic anaesthesia, it is also important to appreciate how patients with heart and lung disease are diagnosed. What is even more important is a clear understanding of the factors that must be considered when evaluating whether a patient should be managed surgically, rather than medically. Moreover, cardiothoracic surgery has an associated mortality and comes with adverse events, so knowledge of how to quantify operative risk is also valuable. Therefore, there are chapters in this textbook that cover diagnosis, surgical selection, and risk estimation.

TOE is a hallmark of modern cardiac anaesthesia. Indeed, there are several excellent textbooks devoted solely to this subject. For this reason, although echocardiography images have been used to illustrate anatomy and pathophysiology, we have chosen not to provide a comprehensive overview of TOE in this textbook. Increasingly however, ultrasonic imaging is being applied perioperatively, not only to diagnose and monitor treatment of cardiovascular dysfunction, but also to diagnose other organ dysfunction and to assist the safe insertion of central venous catheters, intra-aortic balloon pumps, tracheostomies, and other procedural interventions. It is for these reasons that we have included a chapter specifically on the use of ultrasound imaging in the critical care unit.

Although surgery has been the mainstay of the treatment of coronary artery, congenital and valvular heart diseases, to their credit and to the benefit of a great many patients, cardiologists have evolved beyond providing diagnostic and pharmacological treatments of heart disease to include interventional therapies. First, there was angioplasty and stenting, and there are now interventions to treat congenital heart disease and to implant prosthetic heart valves. Moreover, cardiologists can treat conduction abnormalities and life threatening arrhythmias with permanent pacemakers and automatic implantable cardioverter-defibrillators. There are also some areas of cardiothoracic anaesthesiology that require extra attention, including: paediatric and adult congenital heart disease, off-pump coronary artery bypass grafting surgery, thoracic aortic surgery, video-assisted thoracoscopic surgery, bronchoscopy, and the management of patients with heart disease undergoing non-cardiac surgery. Chapters in this textbook cover the anaesthetic considerations of each of these procedures.

Cardiothoracic anaesthesia does not end with the transfer of the patient to a critical care area and a continuum of care is required to achieve good outcomes after cardiothoracic surgery. Today, postoperative critical care is a spectrum that varies from immediate tracheal extubation in the operating room and management in an extended recovery room and/or transfer to a high dependency unit, through to elective postoperative care in a cardiothoracic intensive care unit. Fast-track anaesthetic techniques contribute to enhanced recovery after heart surgery and effective pain management techniques, including thoracic epidural and paravertebral analgesia, are essential to postoperative recovery from cardiothoracic surgery and there are also options to reduce the risk of chronic pain. We have therefore included chapters dealing with these and other aspects of the postoperative critical care of patients following cardiothoracic surgery.

The safe delivery of cardiothoracic anaesthesia and critical care requires the anaesthetist to not only have extensive knowledge and skills as described in this textbook, but to consider non-technical skills and team behaviours. The delivery of such complex care needs to be audited and aspects of our practice must be critically examined with randomized controlled trials if cardiothoracic anaesthesiology is to continue to advance. We otherwise risk repeating errors of the past, when techniques and drugs were introduced without proper evaluation, personal and institutional dogma reigned and harmful or otherwise ineffective interventions continued to be used despite evidence to the contrary. Although many of us learnt cardiothoracic anaesthesia in an apprenticeship model, we should improve how we educate and train future generations. Finally, cardiothoracic surgery and anaesthesia need to be delivered in an architecturally designed environment that is conducive to safe, effective care. Hybrid operating suites now have a place, combining interventional cardiology and surgical procedures. For these reasons, we are pleased that this book finishes with chapters on teamwork, training, error, research, audit, and designing a cardiothoracic operating room.

We have enjoyed editing this textbook and are grateful to all the authors who have contributed to it. Our hope is that it will provide both current and future cardiothoracic anaesthesiologists with the theoretical concepts and knowledge to allow them to effectively and safely provide anaesthesia and critical care for patients undergoing cardiothoracic surgery.

R. Peter Alston,
Paul S. Myles,
Marco Ranucci
Editors

Contents

Abbreviations

α_2-PI	α_2-plasmin inhibitor	ASD	atrial septal defect
2DTOE	2-dimensional transoesophageal echocardiography	AT	antithrombin
ABC	Aristotle Basic Complexity score	AT	anaerobic threshold
ABE	actual base excess	AT III	antithrombin III
ABG	arterial blood gas	ATP	adenosine triphosphate
ACC	Aristotle Comprehensive Complexity score	AV	aortic valve
ACCF	American College of Cardiology Foundation	AVA	aortic valve area
ACE	angiotensin converting enzyme	AVR	aortic valve replacement
ACE-I	angiotensin-converting enzyme inhibitor	BART	Blood Conservation Using Antifibrinolytics in a Randomized Trial
ACGME	Accreditation Council for Graduate Medical Education	BB	bronchial blocker
ACLS	advanced cardiac life support	BC	bronchial cuff
ACP	antegrade cerebral perfusion	BI	bronchus intermedius
ACR	American College of Radiology	BMS	bare metal stents
ACS	acute coronary syndrome	BNP	brain natriuretic peptide
ACT	activated clotting time	BPEG	British Pacing and Electrophysiology Group
ADCC	antibody-dependent cell-mediated cytotoxicity	BPF	bronchopleural fistula
ADO	Amplatzer Dust Occluder Device	BRL	black radio-opaque line
AF	atrial fibrillation	BUN	blood urea nitrogen
AHA	American Heart Association	CABG	coronary artery bypass grafting
AICD	automatic implantable cardioverter defibrillator	CAD	coronary artery disease
AKI	acute kidney injury	CARS	compensatory anti-inflammatory response
ALI	acute lung injury	CAVD	complete atrioventricular defects
AMI	acute myocardial infarction	CDC	Centers for Disease Control
ANH	acute normovolaemic haemodilution	CDH	congenital diaphragmatic hernia
ANZICS	Australian and New Zealand Intensive Care Society	CGRP	calcitonin gene-related peptide
		CHD	congenital heart disease
ANZSCTS	Australian and New Zealand Society of Cardiac and Thoracic Surgeons	CHSMPION	Cangrelor versus standard tHerapy to Achieve optimal Management of platelet inhibition
AOR	adjusted odds ratio	CI	confidence interval
AORN	Association of Peri-Operative Registered Nurses	CICM	College of Intensive Care Medicine
APACHE	Acute Physiology and Chronic Health Evaluation	CKMB	creatine kinase-MB
APC	antigen-presenting cell	CMR	cardiac magnetic resonance
APD	Adult Patient Database	CM_RO_2	cerebral metabolic oxygen consumption
APTT	activated partial thromboplastin time	CMV	cytomegalovirus
AR	aortic regurgitation	CO	cardiac output
ARB	Angiotensin receptor blocker	COPD	chronic obstructive pulmonary disease
ARDS	adult respiratory distress syndrome	CRASH	Corticosteroid Randomisation After Significant Head injury
ARVC	arrhythmic right ventricular cardiomyopathy		
AS	aortic stenosis	COX	cyclo-oxygenase
ASA	atrial septal aneurysm	CPB	cardiopulmonary bypass
ASA	acetylsalicylic acid	CPET	cardiopulmonary exercise testing
ASC	adipose tissue-derived mesenchymal stem cell	CPP	coronary perfusion pressure

CPSP	chronic postsurgical pain	FRC	functional residual capacity
CRP	C-reactive protein	FVC	forced vital capacity
CRT	cardiac resynchronization therapy	GABA	gamma-aminobutyric acid
CSF	cerebrospinal fluid	GAG	glycosaminoglycan
CT	computerized tomography	GFR	glomerular filtration rate
CTCA	computed tomography coronary angiography	GUCH	grown-up congenital heart
CUSUM	cumulative sum	GSK-3β	glycogen synthase 3β
CVC	central venous catheter	GTN	glyceryl trinitrate
CVP	central venous pressure	HCM	hypertrophic cardiomyopathy
CXR	chest X-ray	HDU	high dependency unit
CyA	cyclosporin A	HF	heart failure
CYP	cytochrome p450	HFOV	high-frequency oscillatory ventilation
DC	dendritic cell	HFV	high-frequency ventilation
DDAVP	desmopressin (1-desamino-8-D-arginine vasopressin)	HHT	hereditary haemorrhagic telangiectasia
		HIT	heparin-induced thrombocytopenia
DES	drug-eluting stents	HIV	human immunodeficiency virus
DHCA	deep hypothermic circulatory arrest	HK	high molecular weight kininogen
DLCO	diffusing capacity of the lungs for carbon monoxide	HLHS	hypoplastic left heart syndrome
		HOCM	hypertrophic obstructive cardiomyopathy
DLT	double-lumen endobronchial tube	HPV	hypoxic pulmonary vasoconstriction
DLV	differential lung ventilation	HTX	heart transplantation
DM	diabetes mellitus	IABC	intra-aortic balloon counterpulsation
DORV	double-outlet right ventricle	IABP	intra-aortic balloon pump
DOSA	day-of-surgery admission	IARC	Interim Analysis Review Committee
DSE	dobutamine-atropine stress echocardiography	IASP	International Association for the Study of Pain
DVT	deep vein thrombosis		
EACA	epsilon-aminocaproic acid	ICD	implantable cardiac device
EACTA	European Association of Cardiothoracic Anaesthesiologists	ICE	intracardiac echocardiography
		ICU	intensive care unit
EACTS	European Association for Cardio-Thoracic Surgery	IE	infective endocarditis
		IIVS	intact interventricular septum
ECF	extracellular fluid	IL	interleukin
ECG	electrocardiogram	I-MRI	intraoperative magnetic resonance imaging
ECGE	extracorporeal gas exchange		
ECLS	extracorporeal life support	INR	International Normalized Ratio
ECMO	extracorporeal membrane oxygenation	INTERMACS	Interagency Registry for Mechanically Assisted Circulatory Support
EDPVR	end-diastolic pressure–volume relationship		
EEG	electroencephalograph	IPA	inhibition of platelet activity
EF	ejection fraction	IPF	idiopathic pulmonary fibrosis
ENT	ear, nose, and throat	IPPV	intermittent positive pressure ventilation
EPO	erythropoietin	I-R	ischaemia–reperfusion
ERK	extracellular-regulated kinase	I-RI	ischaemia–reperfusion injury
ESC	European Society of Cardiology	ISHLT	International Society of Heart and Lung Transplantation
ESPVR	end-systolic pressure–volume relationship		
ETCO2	end-tidal capnography	ISI	International Sensitivity Index
ETT	endotracheal tube	IU	International unit
EuroSCORE	European System for Cardiac Operative Risk Evaluation	IV	intravenous
		IVC	inferior vena cava
EVLP	ex-vivo lung perfusion	JVP	jugular venous pressure
FCD	functional capillary density	KCCT	kaolin cephalin clotting time
FDA	Food and Drug Administration	LA	left atrium
FDG	^{18}fluoro deoxyglucose	LAD	left anterior descending artery
FEV1	forced expiratory volume in 1 second	LAP	left atrial pressure
FFP	fresh frozen plasma	LAST	left anterior short thoracotomy
FiO2	inspired O_2 fraction	LCA	left coronary artery
FOB	fibreoptic bronchoscope	LCC	left coronary cusp
FOCUS	Flawless Operative Cardiovascular Unified Systems	LCx	left circumflex
		L-DLT	left double-lumen endobronchial tube
Fr	French	LDP	lateral decubitus position

LED	light-emitting diode	PAC	pulmonary artery catheter
LIMA	left internal mammary artery	$PaCO_2$	arterial partial pressure of carbon dioxide
LLL	left lower lobe	PACU	post-anaesthesia care unit
LMWH	low molecular weight heparin	PAD	preoperative autologous donation
Lp(a)	lipoprotein a	PAH	pulmonary arterial hypertension
LPS	lipopolysaccharide	PaO_2	arterial partial pressure of oxygen
LTOC	laryngotracheoesophageal cleft	P_ACO_2	alveolar partial pressure of oxygen
LUL	left upper lobe	PAP	pulmonary artery pressure
LV	left ventricle	PAPVR	partial anomalous pulmonary venous return
LVAD	left ventricular assist device	PAWP	pulmonary artery wedge pressure
LVEDP	left ventricular end-diastolic pressure	PBF	pulmonary blood flow
MAC	minimal alveolar concentration	PCA	patient-controlled analgesia
MAP	mean arterial pressure	PCC	prothrombin complex concentrate
MCS	mechanical circulatory support	PCI	percutaneous coronary intervention
MEP	motor evoked potential	PCWP	pulmonary capillary wedge pressure
METS	multiples of resting energy expenditure	PDA	patent ductus arteriosus
MHC	major histocompatibility complex	PDE	phosphodiesterases
MI	myocardial infarction	PEA	pulseless electrical activity
MIDCAB	minimally invasive direct coronary artery bypass	PEEP	positive end-expiratory pressure
		PET	positron emission tomography
MOF	multiple organ failure	PFO	patent foramen ovale
MPAP	mean pulmonary artery pressure	PG	pressure gradient
MPTP	mitochondrial permeability transition pore	PGD	primary graft dysfunction
MR	mitral regurgitation	PGE	prostaglandin E
MRI	magnetic resonance imaging	PGH	prostaglandin H
MRSA	methicillin-resistant *Staphylococcus aureus*	PGI	prostaglandin I
MS	mitral stenosis	PH	pulmonary hypertension
MSB	main stem bronchus	PI3K	phosphatidyl inositol-3-kinase
MUF	modified ultrafiltration	PKC	protein kinase C
MV	mitral valve	PLATO	PLATelet inhibition and patient Outcomes
MVA	mitral valve area	PLV	protective lung ventilation
MvO_2	myocardial oxygen requirement	PMN	polymorphonuclear
mVSD	muscular ventricular septal defect	PMP	polymethylpentane
MVST	multivessel small thoracotomy	pmVSD	perimembranous ventricular septal defect
NASPE	North American Society of Pacing and Electrophysiology	POC	point-of-care
		PPO	predicted postoperative
NCC	non-coronary cusp	PPPO	post-pneumonectomy pulmonary oedema
NF-κB	nuclear factor kappa b	PPV	pulse pressure variation
NIH	National Institutes of Health	PPVI	percutaneous pulmonary valve implantation
NIRS	near infrared spectroscopy	PR	pulmonary reguritation
NIV	non-invasive ventilation	PT	prothrombin time
NK	natural killer	PV	pulmonary valve
NMB	neuromuscular blockade	PVB	paravertebral block
NMDA	*N*-methyl-D-aspartate	PVC	polyvinyl chloride
NO	nitric oxide	PVD	peripheral vascular disease
NSAID	non-steroidal anti-inflammatory drug	PVR	pulmonary vascular resistance
NSTEMI	non-ST-elevation myocardial infarction	R/F	radiographic and fluoroscopic
NYHA	New York Heart Association	RA	right atrium
OIVI	opioid-induced ventilatory impairment	RACHS	Risk Adjustment in Congenital Heart Surgery
OLV	one lung ventilation		
OPCAB	off-pump coronary artery bypass	RBC	red blood cell
OR	odds ratio	RCA	right coronary artery
OR	operating room	RCC	right coronary cusp
OS	ostium secundum	RCP	retrograde cerebral perfusion
OSCS	oversulfated chondroitin sulphate	RCRI	Revised Cardiac Risk Index
OT	operative tube	RCT	randomized controlled trial
PA	pulmonary artery	R-DLT	right double lumen tube
PA	pulmonary atresia	RE-LY	Randomized Evaluation of Long-term Anticoagulant Therapy
PABC	pulmonary artery balloon catheter		

REMATCH	Randomized Evaluation of Mechanical Assistance for the Treatment of Congestive Heart Failure		T-AT	thrombin–antithrombin complex
			TAVI	transcatheter aortic valve implantation
			TC	tracheal carina
RF	radiofrequency		TEA	thoracic epidural anaesthesia
RFLV	regional functional lung volume		TECAB	totally endoscopic coronary artery bypass
RISK	reperfusion injury risk kinases		TEG	thromboelastography
RLL	right lower lobe		TENS	transcutaneous electrical nerve stimulation
RM	recruitment manoeuvre		TEVAR	thoracic endovascular aneurysm repair
RMM	relative molecular mass		TF	tissue factor
ROS	reactive oxygen species		TFLV	total functional lung volume
RT3DTOE	real-time 3D TOE		TFPI	tissue factor pathway inhibitor
RUL	right upper lobe		TGA	transposition of the great arteries
RV	right ventricle		TGF	transforming growth factor
RVOT	right ventricular outflow tract		Th1	type I helper T cell
RWMA	regional wall motion abnormality		TIVA	total intravenous anaesthesia
SA	sinoatrial		TJC	The Joint Commission
SAE	serious adverse event		TNFR	tumour necrosis factor receptor
SAFE	survivor activating factor enhancement		TNFsr	tumour necrosis factor soluble receptor
SAM	systolic anterior motion		TNF-α	tumour necrosis factor-α
SAM	systemic anterior motion		TOE	transoesophageal echocardiography
SaO_2	arterial oxygen saturation		TOF	tetralogy of Fallot
SAP	systemic arterial pressure		t-PA	tissue plasminogen activator
SBE	standard base excess		TPVB	thoracic paravertebral block
SCA	Society of Cardiovascular Anesthesiologists		TR	tricuspid regurgitation
SCCP	spinal cord perfusion pressure		TRACS	Transfusion Requirements in Cardiac Surgery
SIRS	systemic inflammatory response syndrome		TRALI	transfusion-associated lung injury
SIRS	systemic inflammatory response		TS	tricuspid stenosis
SLT	simple lumen tube		TTE	transthoracic echocardiography
SLV	single lung ventilation		TV	tricuspid valve
SNP	sodium nitroprusside		TV	tidal volume
SPECT	single-photon emission computed tomography		TXA_2	thromboxane a_2
			UFH	unfractionated heparin
SR	sarcoplasmic reticulum		uPA	urokinase plasminogen activator
SSEP	somatosensory evoked potential		uPAR	urokinase plasminogen activator receptor
SSI	surgical site infection		USP	USA Pharmacopeia
STEMI	ST-elevation myocardial infarction		VAD	ventricular assist device
STJ	sinotubular junction		VALI	ventilator-associated lung injury
STS	Society of Thoracic Surgeons		VASP	vasodilator-associated phosphorylation
STS-PROM	STS Predicted Risk of Mortality		VATS	video-assisted thoracoscopic surgery
SV	stroke volume		VF	ventricular fibrillation
SVC	superior vena cava		VHD	valvular heart disease
SVR	systemic vascular resistance		VILI	ventilator-induced lung injury
SVV	stroke volume variation		VKOR	vitamin K epoxide reductase
SWMA	segmental wall motion abnormality		VO_2max	maximum systemic oxygen uptake
TAAA	thoracoabdominal aortic aneurysms		VSD	ventricular septal defect
TACO	transfusion associated circulatory overload		VT	ventricular tachycardia
TAD	transfusion-associated dyspnoea		VTE	venous thromboembolism
TAH	total artificial heart		vWF	von Willebrand factor
TAPVR	total anomalous pulmonary venous return		WHO	World Health Organization

List of Contributors

Sara Jane Allen
Anaesthetist and Intensivist
Department of Cardiothoracic and ORL Anaesthesia and
    Cardiovascular Intensive Care Unit
Auckland City Hospital
Auckland
New Zealand

R. Peter Alston
Consultant in Anaesthesia, Critical Care and Pain Medicine
Royal Infirmary of Edinburgh
Edinburgh
UK

Rubia Baldassarri
Consultant in Cardiothoracic Anaesthesia and Intensive Care
Azienda Ospedaliero Universitaria Pisana
Pisa
Italy

W. Scott Beattie
Professor of Cardiac Anaesthesia
University of Toronto
Toronto
Canada

Jeremy M. Bennett
Assistant Professor
Vanderbilt University Medical Center
Nashville, TN

Jean S. Bussières
Full Clinical Professor of Anaesthesiology
Laval University
Anaesthesiologist
Institut Universitaire de Cardiologie et de
Pneumologie de Québec
Canada

Eleonora Carlesso
Researcher
Università degli Studi di Milano
Milan
Italy

Mario Carminati
Head of Department of Paediatric Cardiology
    and Surgery
San Donato Hospital
Milan
Italy

Anna Cazzaniga
Pediatric Hospital Meyer
Florence
Italy

Cecilia Coccia
Staff Anaesthetist
Regina Ellena National Cancer Institute
Rome
Italy

Lesley Colvin
Consultant and Reader in Pain Medicine
University of Edinburgh
Western General Hospital
Edinburgh
UK

Nicola Curry
Consultant Haematologist
John Radcliffe Hospital
Oxford
UK

Diederik van Dijk
Professor of Intensive Care Medicine
University Medical Center Utrecht
Utrecht
The Netherlands

David J. R. Duthie
Consultant Cardiothoracic Anaesthetist
Leeds General Infirmary
Leeds
UK

Jörg Ender
Director
Heartcenter, University of Leipzig
Leipzig
Germany

Mario Gaudino
Division of Cardiac Surgery
Department of Cardiovascular Sciences
Catholic University
Rome
Italy

Luciano Gattinoni
Professor and Chairman
Fondazione IRCCS Ca' Granda Ospedale Maggiore Policlinico
    di Milano
Milan
Italy

Andy Gaunt
Consultant Anaesthetist
The Royal Brompton and Harefield NHS
    Foundation Trust
Harefield
UK

Donna Greenhalgh
Consultant in Cardiothoracic Anaesthesia & Intensive Care
University Hospital of South Manchester
Manchester
UK

Fabio Guarracino
Head of Department of Anaesthesia and Critical
    Care Medicine
Azienda Ospedaliero Universitaria Pisana
Pisa
Italy

D. Kirk Hamilton
Professor of Architecture
Texas A&M University
College Station
Texas

Neil Hauser
Department of Anaesthesia
Groote Schuur and Red Cross War Memorial Children's Hospitals
University of Cape Town
South Africa

Jane Heggie
Associate Professor and Fellowship Programme Director
University of Toronto
Toronto
Canada

Michael Hiesmayr
Professor and Chairman
Division of Cardiac Thoracic Vascular
Anaesthesia and Intensive Care
Medical University Vienna
Vienna
Austria

Martin G. Hiscock
Cardiologist
The Epworth Hospital
Richmond, Victoria
Australia

Andrew Hilton
Senior Intensivist
Melborune
Australia

Lisen Hockings
Intensivist
School of Public Health and Preventive Medicine
Monash University
The Alfred Hospital
Melbourne
Australia

Michael G. Irwin
Professor and Head
Department of Anaesthesiology
University of Hong Kong
Hong Kong
China

Giuseppe Isgrò
IRCCS Policlinico San Donato
San Donato Milanese
Milan, Italy

Lakshminarasimhan Kuppurao
Consultant Anaesthetist
The Royal Brompton and Harefield NHS
    Foundation Trust
Harefield
UK

Thomas Langer
Research Fellow
Università degli Studi di Milano
Milan
Italy

Madhur Malik
Associate Consultant
Medanta The Medicity
Haryana

Silvana F. Marasco
Acting Director Cardiothoracic Unit
The Alfred Hospital
Melbourne
Australia

Nandor Marczin
Consultant and Senior Lecturer in
    Cardiothoracic Anaesthesia
The Royal Brompton and Harefield
    NHS Foundation Trust
Imperial College London
Harefield
UK

Massimo Massetti
Division of Cardiac Surgery
Department of Cardiovascular Sciences
Catholic University
Rome
Italy

Esther R. McBride
Research Scientist
Antrim
Belfast
UK

William T. McBride
Consultant in Cardiac Anaesthesia and Cardiac Surgical
    Intensive Care
Belfast Trust
Belfast
UK

Desmond P. McGlade
Senior Specialist Anaesthetist
St Vincent's Hospital
Melbourne
Australia

Yatin Mehta
Chairman
Medanta Institute of Critical Care & Anaesthesiology
Medanta The Medicity
Haryana
India

Alan F. Merry
Professor and Head of the School of Medicine
University of Auckland and Specialist Anaesthetist
Auckland City Hospital
Auckland
New Zealand

Angelo Micheletti
Consultant
San Donato Hospital
Milan
Italy

Deirdre Murphy
Head Cardiothoracic ICU
School of Public Health and Preventive Medicine
Monash University
The Alfred Hospital
Melbourne
Australia

Gavin J. Murphy
British Heart Foundation Chair of Cardiac Surgery
University of Leicester
Leicester
UK

Adriaan Myburgh
Consultant Anaesthetist
Department of Anaesthesia
Groote Schuur and Red Cross War Memorial
    Children's Hospitals
University of Cape Town
South Africa

Paul S. Myles
Director of the Department of Anaesthesia and Perioperative
    Medicine
Alfred Hospital and Monash University
Melbourne
Australia

Alastair F. Nimmo
Consultant Anaesthetist
Royal Infirmary of Edinburgh
Edinburgh
UK

Nishith N. Patel
NIHR Lecturer in Cardiac Surgery
Hammersmith Hospital
London
UK

Philip J. Peyton
Associate Professor
Austin Health and University of Melbourne
Melbourne
Australia

Stefan Probst
Senior Consultant
Heartcenter, University of Leipzig
Leipzig
Germany

Thomas H. Ottens
Senior Registrar in Anaesthesiology
University Medical Center Utrecht
Utrecht
The Netherlands

Marco Ranucci
Head of Clinical Research in the Department of Anesthesia and
    Intensive Care
IRCCS Policlinico San Donato,
    San Donato Milanese
Milan
Italy

Giorgio Della Rocca
Professor and Chair of Anesthesia and Intensive Care Medicine
Medical School of the University of Udine
Udine
Italy

Bill Rostenberg
Founding Principal
Architecture for Advanced Medicine
115 Corte Anita
Greenbrae
California

Annie Rousseau
Clinical Professor of Anesthesiology
Laval University
Anesthesiologist and Intensivist
Institut Universitaire de Cardiologie et de
Pneumologie de Québec
Canada

Matthew T. Royds
Consultant Anaesthetist
Royal Infirmary of Edinburgh
Edinburgh
UK

David Royston
Consultant in Cardiothoracic Anaesthesia, Critical Care and Pain
    Management
Royal Brompton and Harefield NHS Foundation Trust
Harefield
UK

Vladimir Saplacan
Cardiac Surgery Department
University Hospital of Caen
Caen
France

Cait P. Searl
Consultant Anaesthetist
Newcastle-upon-Tyne Hospitals NHS Trust
Newcastle
UK

Carlos Scheinkestel
Director ICU and Hyperbaric Medicine
School of Public Health and Preventive Medicine
Monash University
The Alfred Hospital
Melbourne
Australia

David A. Scott
Associate Professor and Director of Anaesthesia
St Vincent's Hospital and University of Melbourne
Melbourne
Australia

Mert Şentürk
Professor Doctor
Istanbul Medical Faculty, Istanbul University
Istanbul
Turkey

Andrew Shaw
Associate Professor
Vanderbilt University Medical Center
Nashville, TN
USA

Andre R. Simon
Consultant Surgeon
The Royal Brompton and Harefield NHS Foundation Trust
Harefield
UK

David Sidebotham
Anaesthetist and Intensivist
Department of Cardiothoracic and ORL Anaesthesia and
    The Cardiovascular
Intensive Care Unit
Auckland City Hospital
Auckland
New Zealand

David Smith
Consultant and Senior Lecturer
Southampton General Hospital
Southampton
UK

Bodil Steen Rasmussen
Professor
Aalborg University Hospital
Aalborg
Denmark

David Story
Chair of Anaesthesia
The University of Melbourne
Melbourne
Australia

Justiaan Swanevelder
Professor and Head
Department of Anaesthesia
Groote Schuur and Red Cross War Memorial
    Children's Hospitals
University of Cape Town
South Africa

Rainer Thell
Cardiothoracic Anaesthetist and Intensivist
Medical University Vienna
Vienna
Austria

Chad Wagner
Associate Professor
Vanderbilt University Medical Center
Nashville, TN

Jennifer M. Weller
Associate Professor and Head of Centre for Medical and Health
    Sciences Education
University of Auckland and Specialist Anaesthetist
Auckland City Hospital
Auckland
New Zealand

Gordon Tin Chun Wong
Clinical Associate Professor
University of Hong Kong
Hong Kong
China

I. Gavin Wright
Consultant Anaesthetist and Intensivist
The Royal Brompton and Harefield NHS Foundation Trust
Harefield
UK

CHAPTER 1

An history of cardiothoracic anaesthesia

R. Peter Alston

Swan–Ganz catheters may be live saving in Atlanta but mostly a nuisance in Houston

Reproduced from Keats AS, 'The Rovenstine Lecture, 1983: Cardiovascular Anesthesia Perceptions and Perspectives', *Anesthesiology*, **60**, 5, pp. 467–474, copyright 1984, with permission from The Journal of the American Society of Anestheiologists, Inc.

Introduction

Starting towards the very end of the nineteenth century, the history of cardiothoracic anaesthesia is brief by comparison with other human endeavours. Before that time surgical trespass into the chest was considered foolhardy and usually fatal. In less than 120 years, cardiothoracic anaesthesia has developed so far that it now allows millions of patients every year to safely undergo surgery not only within the chest but also upon the heart. The history of that development provides the context for our present day practice of cardiothoracic anaesthesia that will described in the following chapters of this textbook. Moreover, reflecting on its history provides pause for thought that aspects of our current accepted practices may turn out to be based on flawed concepts, personal, and institutional biases and the misuse of evidence. Indeed, this has proven to be the case over the history of cardiothoracic anaesthesia and is encapsulated in the quote that opens this chapter, which is taken from Arthur S Keats' Rovenstine Memorial Lecture to the American Society of Anesthesiologists in 1983 (1).

Clearly, enabling surgical treatment of cardiac and thoracic disease was the driver that created the need for a sub-speciality of cardiothoracic anaesthesia. Likewise, cardiopulmonary bypass (CPB) was the keystone that enabled modern cardiac surgery. As the histories of cardiothoracic surgery and CPB have been extensively reviewed elsewhere, this chapter aims to provide an overview of the important historical milestones in the development of cardiothoracic anaesthesia highlighting the successes and some of the blind alleys that were taken along the way (2–4). Some notable advances in cardiac surgery and anaesthesia are presented in Table 1.1.

Management of the open chest

The pneumothorax problem

At the end of the nineteenth century, it had long been recognized that having a large opening into the thorax cavity through the pleura, was incompatible with life. When the pleural space was opened to atmosphere, the ability to generate negative intrathoracic pressure was lost and consequently, so was the ability to breath. Following such an opening in the pleura, vigorous respiratory effort and cyanosis would ensue. Mediastinal swing impaired any attempt at surgery and importantly, could lead to cardiovascular collapse if the pleura was not quickly closed (5). Therefore, the first challenge facing those who wished to allow surgery to be safely undertaken within the chest was 'the pneumothorax problem'.

Animal experiments and early success in humans

Despite physiologists having sustained life by intubating the trachea and applying intermittent positive pressure ventilation (IPPV) at various time over the previous centuries, the technique was very late in being applied to humans (5). In 1887, George Fell in Buffalo described the use of IPPV generated with a bellows administered with a mask or through a tracheostomy tube for treatment of morphine poisoning (6). Subsequently, O'Dwyer, who had experience with tracheal intubation for the treatment of diptheria, modified Fell's technique by using a foot bellows and a tracheal tube, overcoming airway problems associated with masks or the need to perform a tracheostomy (7). Matas, recognizing that the Fell–O'Dwyer apparatus could be the solution to the pneumothorax problem, adapted it for anaesthesia and in 1899, he reported the successful use of the apparatus to allow surgical excision of a chest wall tumour (8). So at the very end of the nineteenth century, Matas had both recognized and demonstrated that tracheal intubation with IPPV was the effective solution to the pneumothorax problem. However, despite being proved effective, this solution was not widely used for thoracic anaesthesia for nearly 40 years (5). In that time, probably because tracheal intubation was an uncommon skill, other solutions to the pneuomthorax problem were sought. Moreover, it was also the great influence of one surgeon Ferdinand Sauerbruch (see figure 1.1) who advocated the use of the positive pressure technique that prevented tracheal

Table 1.1 Important milestones in cardiac anaesthesia

Year	Event	Effect
1899	Tracheal intubation and IPPV	Pneumothorax problem overcome
1916–36	Discovery to production of heparin	Enabled anticoagulation to allow cardiopulmonary bypass (CPB)
1929	Cyclopropane	Facilitated controlled ventilation
1942	Curare introduced	Facilitated controlled ventilation
1952	DLT for thoracic surgery	Simplified lung isolation and one-lung ventilation
1953	CPB	Enabled complex open heart surgery
1956	Halothane introduced	Non-flammable inhalational anaesthetic so safe to use on CPB
1957	Systemic hypothermia on CPB	Organ protection
1972	IABP used to wean from CPB	Mechanical support of the circulation
1969	Morphine 'anaesthesia'	Stable cardiovascular system
1978	High-dose fentanyl 'anaesthesia'	Stable cardiovascular system with less adverse effects than morphine
1979	Pulmonary artery balloon catheter	Measurement of CO, SVR, PAP, PAWP
1980	M-mode TOE	Intra-operative diagnosis and monitoring of CV dysfunction
1982	Fibreoptic bronchoscopy	Confirming position of DLT and bronchial blockers
1987	Aprotinin	First pharmacological agent demonstrated to reduce blood loss and transfusion in heart surgery
1989	TIVA	Stable CV system/ avoided inhalational anaesthesia
1989	Slogoff and Keats demonstrate that outcome from CABG surgery not influenced by anaesthetic agent	End of the era of high-dose opioid 'anaesthesia' and beginning of enhanced receovery

DLT, double-lumen endobronchial tube; IPPV, intermittent positive pressure ventilation, IABP, intra-aortic balloon pump, CO, cardiac output, SVR, systemic vascular resistance, PAP, pulmonary artery pressure, PAWP, pulmonary artery wedge pressure, TIVA, total intravenous anaesthesia, TOE, transoesphageal echocardiography.

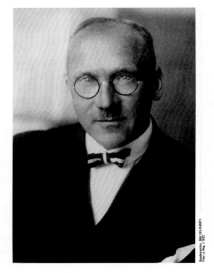

Fig. 1.1 Prof Dr Ferdinand Sauerbruch.
Photograph of Prof Ferdinand Sauerbruch taken in 1938. He pioneered thoracic surgery using negative pressure chambers but his domineering influence on the speciality, held back the solution to the pneumothoracic problem that is tracheal intubation and intermittent positive pressure ventilation, for almost 40 years.

intubation and IPPV being more quickly and widely adopted for thoracic anaesthesia.

Continuous positive pressure

Near the beginning of the twentieth century, Sauerbruch applied the physiologist's principle of maintaining a subatmospheric pressure surrounding the lungs when the chest was opened (9–11). He believed that applying positive pressure to directly to the airways reduced blood flow through the intact lung and consequently, increased the shunting of blood through the collapsed lung, so causing hypoxia and carbon dioxide retention. To keep the lung expanded when the pleura was opened, Sauerbruch operated in a negative pressure chamber keeping patients breathing at atmospheric pressure by excluding their heads from the chamber. However, major drawbacks of this approach were that the equipment was bulky, expensive, and not transportable (5). For these reasons, the alternative approach of raising the pressure in patients airways above atmospheric when the pleura was opened, was adopted by Brauer, using the Tiegal positive pressure apparatus, and by Meyer, using his 'universal differential cabinet' (12,13).

Pendelluft

During this era, the concept of pendelluft or paradoxical respiration was described as the collapsed lung in the open side of the chest becoming smaller during inspiration and larger during expiration (5). The cause of pendelluft was believed to be gas from the collapsed lung passing to the opposite lung during inspiration and then back from the opposite lung into the collapsed lung during expiration (5). This may well have been true during spontaneous ventilation when the pleura was opened and positive airway pressure was applied. However, Maloney dispelled the concept of pendelluft by showing that the paradoxing side increased by its normal volume during inspiration in most situations and that the pattern of carbon dioxide concentration in the bronchus on the paradoxing side was normal throughout the respiratory cycle (14).

Tracheal insufflation

A further improvement in the delivery of positive pressure ventilation that avoided the need to envelope the patient's head, was insufflation of air directly into the trachea using a catheter (15). Surprisingly, this tracheal catheter insufflation technique superseded 'to and fro' respiration through a large tracheal tube by 1909. Meltzer developed 'continuous respiration without respiratory movement' by insufflating a high flow of gas and ether into the trachea through a small tracheal catheter and this followed by insufflation technique allowing spontaneous ventilation (15,16). In 1913, Janeway added 'a little bag, capable of distension' over the tracheal catheter supplying the anaesthetic so as to reduce the wasteful high flow of nitrous oxide required for this technique (17). In addition, he enclosed the reservoir bag in a box that had valves so as to provide true mechanical ventilation once the pleura was opened. This led to the cuffed wide-bore tracheal tube being re-introduced which was a technique popularized by Rowbotham and Magill to deal with facial plastic surgery in 1921, and then by Guedel, using a closed circuit in 1931 (18,19).

Intermittent positive pressure ventilation

When it was confirmed that the insufflation technique resulted in hypercapnia during chest surgery, mechanical ventilation had truly arrived (20). Craaford used the Frenckner Spiropulsator™ while Guedel and Nosworthy simply applied gentle assistance using the rebreathing bag of an anaesthetic (Mapleson C) circuit (20,21). Such techniques produced apnoea, and patients' ventilation could then controlled by hand. However, there had been a gap of well over 30 years since Matas had proposed tracheal intubation and IPPV to overcome the pneumothorax problem.

Saunder's injector

Whilst IPPV was used for intrathoracic surgery, insufflation continued to be used for bronchoscopy under general anaesthesia until 1967 when Sanders introduced the Venturi principle to ventilate patients through the bronchoscope, which remains the standard technique used today (Chapter 34) (22).

Back to the future

As fundamental as tracheal intubation and IPPV is now to the routine anaesthetic management of the open chest, it is possible to undertake cardiac surgery with CPB using thoracic epidural anaesthesia in awake, spontaneously ventilating patients if at least one pleura is intact (23). Moreover, spontaneous ventilation and epidural anaesthesia may prove to be advantageous over IPPV and general anaesthesia in the future surgical treatment of severe lung disease (24).

Lung isolation

The control of secretions during lung surgery was a major anaesthetic problem in the earlier years of thoracic surgery (5). As the incidences of bronchiectasis, lung abscess, empyema, and tuberculosis in patients presenting for thoracic surgery are now far less than in the early years of thoracic anaesthesia, control of secretions is far less important today. However, lung isolation has remained a fundamental technique for thoracic anaesthesia as it facilitates surgical access and increasingly so now, for video-imaged thorascopic surgery.

Spontaneous ventilation and positioning

In the early years of thoracic anaesthesia, a light depth of anaesthesia was used so that the patient would cough and clear their own airway (5). Suction and posturing of the patient in such a way that secretions would not obstruct the airway or contaminate the healthy lung were important. Overholt's approach was to position the patient so that secretions remained in the affected region whereas Parry Brown positioned the patient to allow free drainage (figure 1.2) (25,26).

Bronchial blockers

Magill has previously described the evolution of his bronchus blocker (27). Initially, a suction catheter was placed alongside the tracheal tube. Subsequently, a suction catheter was passed through a t-connector that was attached to the tracheal tube, when suction was required. Lastly, an inflatable cuff was incorporate into suction catheter and this was placed in the bronchus of the diseased lung before tracheal intubation. Vernon Thompson's blocker was a technical improvement on the rubber Magill blocker (28). Crafoord's took a different approach packing the bronchus of the diseased lung with ribbon gauze prior to induction anaesthesia and surgery (20).

Bronchial intubation

A different approach to control secretions was to intubate the bronchus of the sound lung. From Gale and Water's report in 1932, this was performed using a variety of single-lumen bronchial tubes including those of Magill, Macintosh and Leatherdale, Gordon and Green, and others (28,29).

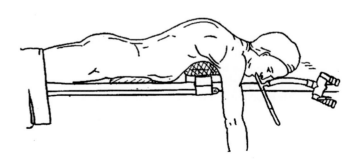

Fig. 1.2 Parry Brown position.
The Parry Brown supine position for a right thoracotomy to allow free drainage of bronchial secretions.
Reproduced from Thorax, Parry Brown, AI., 'Posture in thoracic anaesthesia', 3, 3, pp. 161–65, copyright 1948, with permission from BMJ Publishing Group Ltd.

Double-lumen bronchial tubes

Lung isolation using double-lumen tubes originates from the rigid double-lumen bronchoscope used for differential bronchospirometry that Jacobaeus reported in 1932 (30). A rubber double-lumen tube was developed by Gebauer that was more comfortable for the awake patient under investigation but the size of the lumens was small (31). In 1949, Carlen designed and described a larger diameter double-lumen tube (32). Carlen's double-lumen tube also had a carinal hook to simplify blind placement in the left main bronchus. Bjork described the use of Carlen's double-lumen tube in 1953 for lung resection, and controlled ventilation was delivered using one of the first mechanical ventilators, the Freckner Spiropulsator (33). Over the intervening years, a variety of double-lumen tubes have been developed. In 1962, Robertshaw reported a reusable, red-rubber double-lumen tube that he had designed specifically for thoracic anaesthesia, which became widely used (34). Based around this design, a number of plastic, disposable, double-lumen tubes of varying design were introduced over the years (35). As will be discussed in the next section, the need to confirm their position with bronchoscopy was debated. Robertshaw, working from a time before fibreoptic bronchoscopes were available, was of the opinion that it was unnecessary (34,35).

Bronchoscopy

Whatever approach was used for lung isolation, the introduction of fibreoptic bronchoscopy to aid positioning of double-lumen bronchial tubes or bronchial blockers transformed either technique by simplifying and greatly improving the accuracy of their placement (36,37). Before the development of these instruments, rigid bronchoscopy was the only visual approach to confirm correct placement and was only for anaesthesiologists who were skilled in its use. Unskilled anaesthesiologists had to rely on visual inspection of the chest wall and auscultation to confirm correct placement, and both are unreliable.

Recently, Gosh developed the Papworth BiVent tube, which is a combination of a double-lumen tracheal tube and a bronchial blocker that was designed to have the advantage of ease of tracheal intubation and rapid isolation of either lung without the need for bronchoscopy (38). Time will tell whether this approach will be adopted over standard double-lumen tubes or bronchial blockers and fibreoptic bronchoscopy.

Anaesthetic agents

Over the history of cardiothoracic anaesthesia, every anaesthetic agent that has ever been invented has been used with greater or lesser success (39). Today, a great variety of agents and techniques are used for cardiothoracic anaesthesia. Even in 1983, Keats recognized that this great variation largely reflects personal and institutional biases that have developed without an evidence base that any technique or anaesthetic agent was superior in terms of outcome from cardiothoracic anaesthesia (1).

Agents used in the early years of thoracic anaesthesia

In the early years, ether, chloroform, and nitrous oxide, either alone or in combination, were the mainstays of thoracic anaesthesia (5). Of these anaesthetic agents, only chloroform was suitable for controlled respiration, as cessation of spontaneous ventilation was not easy or safe to induce with either ether or nitrous oxide. Whilst ether was safer than chloroform, it was both inflammable and explosive. Chloroform became the agent of choice for thoracic anaesthesia as it was more potent, easy to administer and not inflammable. Moreover, the respiratory depression and quiet breathing that it caused resulted in less paradoxical movement during continuous positive pressure anaesthesia. However, when Cutler operated on the mitral valve in 1923, the anaesthetic technique was an open ether induction followed by its insufflation into the nasopharynx (40).

Cylcopropane

When cyclopropane was introduced in 1929, it was used for thoracic anaesthesia (41). In 1930, Rovenstine reported the use of cyclopropane for thoracic work, with tracheal intubation but spontaneous respiration (42). Carbon dioxide absorption with the Waters canister made use of cyclopropane, more economical (43). When he described the first successful ligation of a persistent ductus arteriosus in 1938, Gross used cyclopropane (44). Cyclopropane's other advantage was its potency, so the concentration of inspired oxygen could be as high as 85% (45). By 1939, this, along with the ease with which ventilation could be controlled, led to cyclopropane becoming the anaesthetic of choice for thoracic anaesthesiologists (45). The ease of controlling ventilation also facilitated a move back from continuous to IPPV for thoracic anaesthesia, as discussed earlier (5). However, cyclopropane was highly explosive and ignition by diathermy could have serious and even, fatal outcomes (5,45).

Despite cyclopropane's popularity for thoracic anaesthesia, when Blalock reported (in 1945) his first subclavian to left pulmonary artery anastomosis for pulmonary stenosis, the anaesthetic consisted of open ether (46). However, when Harmel and Lamont, Blalock's anaesthesiologists, reported the first 100 cases of Blalock shunts, they used cyclopropane in the majority of cases, with supplementary ether in some (47).

Balanced anaesthetic

Preston (1953) and Brown (1954) described a balanced anaesthetic technique of IV induction with thiopentone, neuromuscular blocker (NMB) with curare, hypnosis with nitrous oxide, and supplementary analgesia with pethidine for closed mitral valvotomy, with complete control of respiration (48,49). Similarly, when Lewis in 1952 successfully closed an atrial septal defect in a 5-year-old girl with the aid of surface cooling and venous inflow occlusion, a thiopentone, curare, intubation sequence was used and this technique was described for surgery with CPB not long afterwards by Parry Brown (50).

At that time, although Nosworthy considered nitrous oxide as a weak anaesthetic, supplements were not always acceptable. Nosworthy always added another drug and thought that the technique should be called nitrous oxide and morphine anaesthesia, and not nitrous oxide anaesthesia alone (51). Wasmouth used only thiopentone and nitrous oxide for patients undergoing mitral valvotomy and regarded the anaesthetic as ideal if the patient experienced no pain or memory of the procedure but responded to the spoken word (40). Wasmouth used a mechanical ventilator and only gave small doses of curare (3 mg) to obtund coughing and to control respiration only if all others means failed.

So, by the late 1950s, the accepted anaesthetic technique was an IV induction agent, nitrous oxide, and oxygen, and NMB supplemented with opioids or volatile anaesthetic agents was firmly established. With some minor deviations, this balanced anaesthetic approach to cardiothoracic anaesthesia was to last until the late 1960s, when a major change occurred.

Anaesthesia and cardiopulmonary bypass

When Kirklin published his account of the use of the Gibbon type bypass machine in 1955, the anaesthetic used was ether (52). It is noteworthy that when Gibbon described his experimental CPB apparatus, using cats, he mentioned the problem of maintaining anaesthesia after going on CPB (53). To overcome this problem, he vaporized ether into the gas supply to the oxygenator, thus establishing in 1937 an inhalational-based anaesthetic technique during CPB, which is still used today albeit with different inhalational agents.

Morphine 'anaesthesia'

One the most profound changes in direction for cardiac anaesthesia occurred towards the end of the 1960s. Edward Lowenstein, who was working at the Massachussetts General Hospital, had observed that administration of large doses of morphine to patients following heart surgery, so that they would tolerate tracheal intubation and mechanical ventilation, usually caused little change in their pulse rate or blood pressure (54). As a result he was first to apply, what was at that time, very high doses of morphine (0.5–3 mg/kg) as the primary and often the sole anaesthetic (54). He also established that in patients with aortic valve disease, that morphine 'anaesthesia' decreased systemic vascular resistance and increased cardiac output (55). Given the prolonged respiratory depression that results from high-dose morphine, the technique would have been impractical before this time as elective postoperative mechanical ventilation was uncommon until the late 1960s. However, he recognized that the technique was not truly anaesthesia, as it did not result in a consistent loss of consciousness but rather a state of profound analgesia. Lowenstein argued that physiological integrity and the provision of good surgical conditions were more important than the patient's awareness of surgery (55).

Despite the problem of awareness and significant cardiovascular drawbacks including bradycardia and hypotension, morphine 'anaesthesia' became a popular technique (39). Attempting to overcome awareness, increasing higher doses of morphine were administered and one group gave up to 11 mg/kg resulting in patients becoming plum coloured and oedematous as a result of histamine release (56). Contemporaneously, it was established that morphine 'anaesthesia' using 2 mg/kg in healthy volunteers could not reliably produce either amnesia or unconsciousness without the addition of 70% nitrous oxide (57).

Opioid 'anaesthesia'

The introduction of coronary artery bypass grafting (CABG) surgery for a relatively fitter group of patients than who had previously undergone cardiac surgery exposed the inability of morphine 'anaesthesia' to 'induce sleep' so driving the development of alternative synthetic opioids (58). Pethidine and alphaprodine proved to be myocardial depressants (59).

Paul janssen

No one person was more successful in developing new opioids for cardiac anaesthesia than Paul Janssen, who was the founder of Janssen Pharmaceutica (60). Janssen and co-workers had noted that pethidine, like morphine, had a piperidine ring, which they believed was responsible for their analgesic properties. Based on that principle, they first developed phenoperidine then fentanyl, sufentanil, alphentanil, and carfentanil (60). All these opioids were both far more potent and caused far less histamine release than morphine, so were far more cardiovascularly stable and could be given in far higher doses. The fentanyl family of opioids, along with the many other anaesthetic agents and analgesics developed by Paul Janssen and his company (table 1.2), made an

Table 1.2 Anaesthetic and analgesic drugs produced by Janssen Pharmaceutica

Trade name	Generic name	Year of synthesis	Year of introduction	Indication
Palfium	dextromoramide	1955	1957	opioid analgesic
Operidine	phenoperidine	1957	1964	opioid analgesic
Haldol	haloperidol	1958	1959	anitpsychotic, neuroleptic, antiemetic
Dipidolor	piritramide	1960	1961	opioid analgesic
Sublimaze	fentanyl	1960	1963	opioid analgesic
Haldol	droperidol	1961	1963	neuroleptic, antiemetic,
Hypnomidate	etomidate	1964	1977	IV anaesthetic
Sufenta	sufentanil	1974	1979	opioid analgesic
Wildnil	carfentanil	1974	1986	veterinary opioid analgesic
Rapafin	alfentanil	1976	1983	opioid analgesic

Some of the anaesthetic and analgesic agents produced by Janssen Pharmaceutica that was founded by Paul Janssen. Many of these agents in particular the opioids, were used for cardiothoracic anaesthesia.
Data from Stanley TH, Egan TD, Van Aken H. A tribute to Dr. Paul A. J. Janssen: entrepreneur extraordinaire, innovative scientist, and significant contributor to anesthesiology. *Anesth Analg* 2008;106:451–62.

immense contribution to the development of cardiac anaesthesia and anaesthesia in general (59,60).

Neurolept anaesthesia

Under the trade Innovar™, fentanyl was first used in combination with droperidol which is a major tranquiliser, for neurolept anaesthesia (39). Some of the stated benefits of neurolept anaesthesia over inhalational techniques included: absence of myocardial depresssion, antifibrillatory and alpha-adrenergic blockade during surgery, sedation, and anti-emesis postoperatively (61). Unfortunately, since its introduction for cardiac anaesthesia 1965, neurolept techniques have failed to ensure anaesthesia (39). Despite this well-reported failure, neurolept techniques were still being used in 2002 with the inevitable consequence of awareness (39).

Fentanyl, sufentanil, and alfentanil

High-dose fentanyl anaesthesia became widely popular just as it was going off-patent, which prompted the development of other members of the fentanyl family (60,62). Sufentanil, which was even more potent, was introduced in 1979; however, like fentanyl, it had a relatively long half-life, so causing prolonged respiratory depression requiring protracted mechanical ventilation. Alfentanil was the next of the family to be introduced; it had a comparatively shorter half-life than fentanyl and sufentanil (60). At the beginning of the 1980s, alfentanil was used alone in high doses for cardiac anaesthesia (63). However, alfentanil came into its own when combined with an IV hypnotic agent to provide total intravenous anaesthesia (TIVA) for cardiothoracic surgery (64).

Outcome research

When the vogue for high-dose opioid anaesthesia was at its height in the 1980s, much of the focus of research was its modify effects on the pathophysiological of surgery and, in particular, the stress response (39). Not until the end of the 1980s did this blind focus on surrogate outcomes get corrected by research examining patient outcome from cardiac anaesthesia. Slogoff and Keats seminal study, established that the choice of primary anaesthetic agent halothane, enflurane, isoflurane, or sufentanil, made no difference to myocardial outcome following CABG surgery (65).

The conclusion that the choice of anaesthetic agent had no bearing on outcome was combined, especially in the USA, with the increasing financial constraints imposed by insurance companies and health maintenance organizations, which led to a drive to earlier recovery from cardiac anaesthesia to reduce the durations of IPPV, critical care, and so costs. These influences combined to drive a paradigm shift in anaesthetic techniques to allow 'fast-track' anaesthetic techniques that was tracheal extubation within 6 hours of the end of surgery. Subsequently, this enhanced recovery has been taken further, as will be discussed in Chapter 27.

Remifentanil

The next major development in opioids occurred in the 1990s with the introduction of the ultra short-acting opioid remifentanil, for cardiac surgery (66,67). Unlike the previous opioids that depended on hepatic metabolism, remifentanil was metabolized by non-specific esterases, and so its half-life was only a few minutes, no matter how long it had been infused IV. The timing of remifentanil's introduction was apt as it was a very suitable agent for TIVA and facilitated 'fast-tracking', both of which were building in popularity through the 1990s (66,67).

Inhalational anaesthetics

Nitrous oxide

Although the use of high-dose opioid anaesthetic techniques became increasingly common from 1970s, inhalational techniques were still being used for cardiac anaesthesia. Whilst ether and then cyclopropane were used in the early years of cardiothoracic anaesthesia, their explosive properties led to the development of new agents (5,45). Nitrous oxide had been infrequently used over the years because the high concentrations required for anaesthesia could lead to hypoxia this was especially so if used during CPB with inefficient oxygenators of the time (68). However, the potential to expand air bubbles became the main reason that nitrous oxide was not used for cardiac surgery during and after CPB (69).

Halogenated hydrocarbons and ethers

Halothane was introduced in the 1950s, and by the 1970s it was widely used for cardiothoracic anaesthesia. For cardiac anaesthesia, it advocated because it caused vasodilation and limited the degree of metabolic acidosis that occurred (70,71). Others argued that it should not be used because it could caused hepatitis, myocardial depression, hypotension, and arrhythmias (39). Methoxyflurane and fluoroxene are other inhalational agents that were introduced after halothane and used for cardiac anaesthesia, but both have failed to stand the test of time (72,73). Methoxyflurane was withdrawn because it caused nephrotoxicity that was dose dependant, whereas fluoroxene was highly flammable and so not suitable for CPB. When enflurane, another halogenated hydrocarbon, was introduced for clinical practice, it also was used for cardiac anaesthesia (74). Until its manufacture at medical grade was discontinued, trichlorethylene had been routinely used for anaesthesia during CPB at Papworth Hospital for many years (75).

As the 1980s progressed, halothane's popularity diminished because of a small but finite risk of causing hepatitis. Isoflurane was the next halogenated ether to be used for cardiac anaesthesia in the 1980s. Initially, there was great concern arising from research in animal models that it might cause coronary steal and thus myocardial ischaemia in patients with coronary artery disease, leading to the recommendation that it should not be used in these patients (76). However, this concern proved misplaced when Slogoff and Keat's outcome study in humans undergoing CABG surgery found no increased incidence of myocardial ischaemia to be associated with isoflurane (65). In addition, isoflurane was found to reduce cerebral metabolic rate leading to the concept that it might be neuroprotective, which set a theme for later inhalational anaesthetics, as discussed later (77).

In the 1990s, sevoflurane and desflurane were the next inhalational anaesthetics to be introduced and used for cardiac surgery (78,79). By this time, as will be discussed later, TIVA was in ascendancy and inhalational techniques were becoming less popular. However, there was a resurgence of interest in inhalational anaesthetics in the 2000s with the possibility that they might confer organ protection and in particular, through preconditioning, reduce myocardial ischaemia. Indeed, a systematic review and meta-analysis indicates that inhalational agents reduces myocardial ischaemia, as measured by troponin, when compared to propofol-based techniques (80).

Xenon

Since the 1990s the noble gas, xenon had attracted increasing interest as a general anaesthetic (81). Like the inhalational anaesthetics, there is the possibility that it may also confer organ protection so it might be an attractive agent for cardiac anaesthesia and in particular, neuroprotection. However, the clinical application of xenon for cardiac anaesthesia has so far been prevented by its extremely high cost compared to other anaesthetic agents and the increased complexity that would be required to administer it during CPB when it might most beneficial.

Awareness resulting from non-administration of inhalational anaesthetics

Unfortunately, even in the 2002, some anaesthesiologists had still failed to learn the lessons of previous years as to the management of anaesthesia during CPB when using an inhalational anaesthetic as the primary agent. One group, using a sevoflurane-based technique, noted a high incidence of awareness and concluded that it was because sevoflurane was not administered during CPB (82). Failure to continue to administer inhalation agents or give an IV anaesthetic agent during CPB was recognized from the earliest days of CPB (39).

Operating room pollution

Increasing concern throughout the 1970s that inhalational anaesthetics might be dangerous for those working in the operating room led to the development of gas-scavenging systems for oxygenators (74). This concern may also have driven a move towards IV-based techniques of anaesthesia, especially during CPB, to avoid contamination of the operating room with inhalational agents; this resulted in the now popular technique of TIVA. Indeed, by the end of the 1980s only a third of anaesthesiologists in the UK were using inhalational anaesthetic during CPB (83).

Intravenous anaesthetics

Barbiturates

From the 1950s onwards, IV agents starting with thiopentone, were used as part of cardiothoracic anaesthesia, most usually as an induction agent in adults (39). In cardiac anaesthesia, they also found favour during CPB (39). In the early years this usage was probably because they avoided the explosive dangers of administering ether or cyclopropane during CPB. However, IV anaesthetics continued to be used during CPB long after the introduction of non-flammable inhalational agents (39,83). In addition, cardiothoracic anaesthesiologists' experience with IV anaesthesia during CPB may in part explain why they were early adopters of TIVA. For examples, when methohexitone was introduced in the 1960s, it was administered as an IV infusion along with phenoperidine and nitrous oxide for cardiac anaesthesia, giving an early form of TIVA (39,84).

In the 1980s, thiopentone found a potential new indication during CPB for heart-valve surgery to reduce neurological deficits albeit at the price of prolonged sedation and increased need for inotropic support (85).

Ketamine

The dissociative anaesthetic ketamine was first used for paediatric cardiac surgery during the 1970s; it remains popular today for IV induction in cyanotic children as it increases systemic vascular resistance and cardiac output without worsening right-to-left shunting (86,87).

Benzodiazepines

In the 1970s, although thiopentone continue to be used during CPB, the variety of IV anaesthetic agents increased (39). Benzodiazipines, most commonly diazepam, were used to induce and maintain anaesthesia (39). In the UK by the end of the 1980s, the great majority of anaesthesiologists were using an IV technique during CPB (83). The benzodiazipines—initially diazepam and lorazepam and then midazolam—were increasingly used during this decade often to confer hypnosis and amnesia to opioid 'anaesthetic' techniques (39). However, they neither ensured lack of awareness or even, intra-operative recall (39).

Althesin, etomidate, and propofol

Three new IV anaesthetic agents—althesin, etomidate, and propofol—were used for cardiac anaesthesia (39). Althesin was administered as an IV infusion during CPB but because of anaphylaxis, the drug was later withdrawn. Etomidate was used for TIVA but failed to gain popularity probably because it was found to cause an increase mortality when used to sedate patients in intensive care units (ICUs) (88).

However, propofol was by far the most important IV agent that was introduced and its use for cardiac anaesthesia as TIVA was reported in 1989 (89). This short-acting IV anaesthetic, along with the availability of smart syringe drivers to administer target controlled infusions of drugs, led to thepopularization of TIVA for cardiac anaesthesia (66,83,89,90). As discussed earlier, combining propofol with the short-acting opioids alfentanil and then remifentanil also contributed to the popularization of TIVA for cardiothoracic anaesthesia to such an extent that it became the most widely used anaesthetic technique used for cardiothoracic anaesthesia by the late 1990s.

Quite why TIVA should have come to dominate cardiothoracic anaesthesia in a little over two decades is worthy of consideration as evidence exists suggesting that some inhalational agents may be associated with a better outcome from CABG surgery than TIVA (91). For cardiac anaesthesia, TIVA obviates the problems of administering inhalational agents into, and scavenging of waste gases from, the oxygenator so as to prevent the recurrent problem of awareness during CPB should they be discontinued (82). For thoracic anaesthesia, TIVA overcomes the difficulty of delivering inhalational agents during bronchoscopy and their limited uptake during one-lung anaesthesia (Chapters 33 and 34). Whilst it has many pragmatic advantages for delivery of cardiothoracic anaesthesia, TIVA is yet another example of a technique which was introduced with no systematic examination of its effect on patient outcome from cardiothoracic surgery.

Neuromuscular blockers

Curare

Introduced into anaesthesia by Griffith in 1942, curare transformed the ability to control ventilation and the use of curare for thoracic anaesthesia was reported by Harroun in 1946 (92,93). Initially, it was not widely accepted as eight years later Wasmouth wrote 'In the opinion of some, curare in anesthesia for cardiac surgery is a toxic agent which makes a poor anesthetic look good' (40).

Suxamethonium

Following on from the use of curare as described earlier, every NMB introduced into clinical practice was applied to cardiothoracic surgery (39). Suxamethonium was used as an IV infusion because of its short duration of action, and was often favoured over curare in the 1960s as resuming spontaneous ventilation at the end of surgery was the normal clinical practice at this time (39).

Steroid based neuromuscular blockers

In the early 1970s, pancuronium started to be favoured over curare as it caused less histamine release and was more cardiovascularly stable (39). Atracurium and vecuronium were introduced in the 1980s and because of their relatively short duration of action were often administered as IV infusions (39,83). Doxacurium and pipercuronium which had durations of action that were similar to pancuronium, were also introduced in the 1980s but have not stood the test of time (39). Indeed, the new NMBs had been specifically developed to have no cardiovascular effects and so revealed the bradycardic effects of high-dose opioids (94). Whilst the new short-acting NMBs found their place in thoracic anaesthesia, pancuronium continued to hold favour for cardiac anaesthesia long beyond the 1980s because its vagolytic effect prevented bradycardia (83). Only the increasing move towards enhanced recovery following cardiac surgery in the 1990s precipitated the decline in use of pancuronium in favour of the shorter-acting NMBs such as rocuronium (95).

Sugammadex

Perhaps the most interesting and important development in the area of NMB in the beginning of the twenty-first century has been the introduction of the first selective relaxant binding agent, sugammadex as reversal agent for rocuronium (96). Compared to neostigmine, sugammadex can more quickly reverse profound NMB from rocuronium (97). Clearly, using this combination of drugs has advantages for patients with minimal respiratory reserve or neuromuscular diseases where any residual paralysis may be precipitate respiratory failure (98).

Regional anaesthesia

The flammability of ether led to an early interest in the use of various spinal, epidural and regional anaesthetic techniques for thoracic surgery to avoid explosions (45). Retention of an active cough reflex was another motivation for avoiding general anaesthesia in favour of regional techniques (5). Diaphragmatic and paradoxical mediastinal movement, as well as coughing, were all problematic and led to the abandonment of regional anaesthesia as the sole anaesthetic. However, there has been a renewed interest in regional anaesthesia as the primary technique for surgical treatment of patients who have severe lung disease (24).

Epidural analgesia for thoracic surgery

Throughout its history, regional techniques in combination with general anaesthesia have played a major role in thoracic anaesthesia (5,99,100). By the 1990s, because it was perceived to deliver a high quality of pain relief, epidural analgesia became the gold standard for postoperative analgesia following thoracic surgery. However, mounting evidence that paravertebral blocks could provide equivalent analgesia with less adverse effects has led to paravertebral replacing epidural analgesia as the gold standard for thoracic anaesthesia (figure 1.3) (101).

Epidural analgesia for cardiac surgery

Whilst regional anaesthesia has long been used for thoracic anaesthesia, it also found favour for cardiac anaesthesia. One of the earliest case series of cardiac surgery reported the use of epidural anaesthesia as part of the general anaesthetic technique in one patient (102). However, epidural anaesthesia came into vogue for cardiac anaesthesia in the 1990s. Initially, this interest was spurred because epidural analgesia was found to reduce catecholamine levels (103). This lead to the hypothesis that ameliorating the stress response to surgery might reduce the incidence of adverse events and in particular, myocardial ischaemia. Whilst epidural analgesia has most commonly been combined with general anaesthesia, some anaesthesiologists have even used epidural anaesthesia without supplementation for cardiac surgery, believing it enhances recovery and improves outcome (23). Increasing concern regarding an increased risk of epidural haematoma because of the pre-operative use of antithrombotic drugs, high doses of heparin used during CPB, and coagulopathy that may arise during surgery, prevented a universal adoption of a combined general and epidural technique. When the potential risk of epidural haematoma became perceived to outweigh the few outcome benefits, enthusiasm for the routine use of epidural analgesia waned midway through the first decade of the 2000s (104). Interestingly, the most recent systematic review and meta-analysis indicates that epidural analgesia is associated with reduced incidences of perioperative acute renal failure, the time on mechanical ventilation, and a composite endpoint of mortality and myocardial infarction in patients undergoing cardiac surgery; so there may be a future resurgence of interest in technique (105).

Monitoring

Although not used in the initial years, invasive monitoring of the cardiovascular system is one of the hallmarks of present day cardiothoracic anaesthesia (Chapter 3). Today, few anaesthesiologists would conceive of undertaking anaesthesia for cardiac surgery without invasive monitoring despite a complete absence of any evidence that they influence patient outcome from cardiothoracic surgery. Two forms of monitoring exemplify this point, and so merit more detailed discussion, because they have greatly influenced cardiac anaesthesia.

Pulmonary artery balloon catheters

In 1970, one of the more invasive and controversial monitoring technique was introduced as the pulmonary artery catheter (PAC) and is popularly known as the Swan–Gantz catheter after two of its pioneers (106). With great rapidity, the technique was widely adopted and in some centres such as the authors, in early 1990s, it was a routine form of monitoring in all patients undergoing heart surgery. However, there was a schism between cardiothoracic anaesthesiologists as PACs were not routinely used by some prominent cardiac surgery centres such as the Texas Heart Institute (1). The PAC is a perfect example of a technology that was adopted because it provided a greater insight into cardiovascular pathophysiology than had previously been available. However, the PAC was introduced into routine practice without any evidence

Urinary retention

Review: Paravertebral block
Comparison: 11 Urinary retention
Outcome: 01 Urinary retention

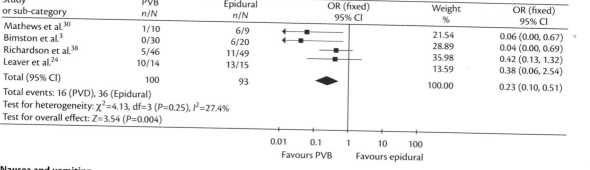

Study or sub-category	PVB n/N	Epidural n/N	OR (fixed) 95% CI	Weight %	OR (fixed) 95% CI
Mathews et al.[30]	1/10	6/9		21.54	0.06 (0.00, 0.67)
Bimston et al.[3]	0/30	6/20		28.89	0.04 (0.00, 0.69)
Richardson et al.[38]	5/46	11/49		35.98	0.42 (0.13, 1.32)
Leaver et al.[24]	10/14	13/15		13.59	0.38 (0.06, 2.54)
Total (95% CI)	100	93		100.00	0.23 (0.10, 0.51)

Total events: 16 (PVD), 36 (Epidural)
Test for heterogeneity: $\chi^2=4.13$, df=3 (P=0.25), $I^2=27.4\%$
Test for overall effect: Z=3.54 (P=0.004)

0.01   0.1   1   10   100
Favours PVB   Favours epidural

Nausea and vomiting

Review: Paravertebral block
Comparison: 12 nausea or vomiting
Outcome: 01 nausea or vomiting

Study or sub-category	PVB n/N	Epidural n/N	OR (fixed) 95% CI	Weight %	OR (fixed) 95% CI
De Cosmo et al.[8]	0/25	2/25		9.95	0.18 (0.01, 4.04)
Perttunen et al.[35]	3/15	5/15		16.24	0.50 (0.10, 2.63)
Bimston et al.[3]	7/30	7/20		26.14	0.57 (0.16, 1.97)
Richardson et al.[38]	2/46	10/49		37.60	0.18 (0.04, 0.86)
Leaver et al.[24]	5/14	4/15		10.08	1.53 (0.31, 7.44)
Total (95% CI)	130	124		100.00	0.47 (0.24, 0.93)

Total events: 17 (PVD), 28 (Epidural)
Test for heterogeneity: $\chi^2=4.04$, df=4 (P=0.40), $I^2=1.1\%$
Test for overall effect: Z=2.17 (P=0.03)

0.01   0.1   1   10   100
Favours PVB   Favours epidural

Hypotension

Review: Paravertebral block
Comparison: 13 Hypotension
Outcome: 01 Hypotension

Study or sub-category	PVB n/N	Epidural n/N	OR (fixed) 95% CI	Weight %	OR (fixed) 95% CI
De Cosmo et al.[8]	0/10	3/25		13.02	0.13 (0.01, 2.58)
Mathews et al.[30]	0/10	6/9		24.65	0.03 (0.00, 0.58)
Bimston et al.[3]	1/30	1/20		4.40	0.66 (0.04, 11.12)
Richardson et al.[38]	0/46	7/49		27.27	0.06 (0.00, 0.10)
Dhole et al.[10]	0/20	1/20		5.55	0.32 (0.01, 0.26)
Leaver et al.[24]	2/14	8/15		25.11	0.15 (0.02, 0.89)
Total (95% CI)	145	138		100.00	0.12 (0.04, 0.34)

Total events: 3 (PVD), 26 (Epidural)
Test for heterogeneity: $\chi^2=2.90$, df=5 (P=0.72), $I^2=0\%$
Test for overall effect: Z=4.01 (P<0.0001)

0.01   0.1   1   10   100
Favours PVB   Favours epidural

Fig. 1.3 Comparison of adverse outcomes from paravertebral block (PVB) and epidural analgesia for thoracic surgery.
Forrest plots showing the meta-analyses comparing adverse effects following paravertebral block and epidural analgesia for thoracic surgery. Compared to epidural analgesia and despite having a comparable quality analgesia, paravertebral block was associated with significantly lower incidences of urinary retention, nausea and vomiting and hypotension. Where OR: odds ratio, 95% CI: 95% confidence intervals.

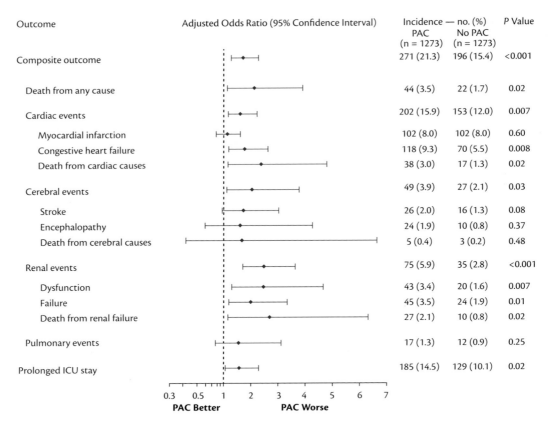

Outcome	Adjusted Odds Ratio (95% Confidence Interval)	Incidence — no. (%)		P Value
		PAC (n = 1273)	No PAC (n = 1273)	
Composite outcome		271 (21.3)	196 (15.4)	<0.001
Death from any cause		44 (3.5)	22 (1.7)	0.02
Cardiac events		202 (15.9)	153 (12.0)	0.007
Myocardial infarction		102 (8.0)	102 (8.0)	0.60
Congestive heart failure		118 (9.3)	70 (5.5)	0.008
Death from cardiac causes		38 (3.0)	17 (1.3)	0.02
Cerebral events		49 (3.9)	27 (2.1)	0.03
Stroke		26 (2.0)	16 (1.3)	0.08
Encephalopathy		24 (1.9)	10 (0.8)	0.37
Death from cerebral causes		5 (0.4)	3 (0.2)	0.48
Renal events		75 (5.9)	35 (2.8)	<0.001
Dysfunction		43 (3.4)	20 (1.6)	0.007
Failure		45 (3.5)	24 (1.9)	0.01
Death from renal failure		27 (2.1)	10 (0.8)	0.02
Pulmonary events		17 (1.3)	12 (0.9)	0.25
Prolonged ICU stay		185 (14.5)	129 (10.1)	0.02

0.3   0.5   1   2   3   4   5   6   7
PAC Better   PAC Worse

Fig. 1.4 Influence of pulmonary artery balloon catheter on outcome from cardiac surgery.
Outcomes of 1273 propensity score matched pairs of patients from an observational study, with pulmonary artery catheter (PAC) and no PAC who underwent cardiac surgery. Mortality and the incidences of congestive heart failure and renal impairment were significantly higher in patients who had a PAC as was the duration of stay in the intensive care unit (ICU). Note that intensive care unit stay is also significantly more often prolonged in patients with PAC monitoring. Adjusted odds ratios (AOR) with 95% confidence intervals and associated P values were calculated from the generalized estimating equations (GENMOD procedure). As discussed in Chapter 43, results from observational studies should be interpreted with caution because of the inherent biases that exist. Furthermore the data was collected from 1996–2000. Reproduced from Schwann NM, Hillel Z, Hoeft A et al., 'Lack of effectiveness of the pulmonary artery catheter in cardiac surgery', *Anesthesia & Analgesia*, 113, 5, pp. 994–1002, copyright 2011, with permission from the International Anaesthesia Research Society

that their use improved patient outcome from cardiac surgery. Even more importantly, PACs were introduced without evidence that they did no harm. Indeed, the findings of a recently published study suggest that the use of PACs in CABG surgery might be associated with a higher mortality and incidence of end-organ damage (figure 1.4) (107). Although this was an observational study, and so low quality evidence with inherent bias (Chapter 43), the findings suggest that the routine use of PACs may not improve outcome from cardiac surgery as was once commonly believed.

Echocardiography

In a little over 20 years, echocardiography has become central to the daily clinical practice of this author and most other cardiothoracic anaesthesiologists. Not only has the ability to undertake and interpret transoephageal echocardiography (TOE) appeared to have improved the care of patients undergoing cardiac surgery, it elevated the status of cardiothoracic anaesthesiologists and beneficially altered their relationship with surgical colleagues. Readers wishing a detailed history of echocardiography and cardiac anaesthesia are referred elsewhere (108).

Without doubt echocardiography has superseded PAC as the standard for monitoring and diagnosing cardiovascular

dysfunction during heart surgery. However, whilst there may be much evidence to guide its use, echocardiography has been widely adopted without high-quality evidence to establish that it improves outcome from cardiac surgery (109). One of the problems for cardiothoracic anaesthesia and medicine in general, is that the regulatory requirements around the world for introducing equipment are generally far less that onerous than for introducing a drug. So we should exert caution introducing any new technologies and recognize that whilst they provide mesmerizing new insights into pathophysiology, new technologies may not only fail to improve outcome but they might make it worse. Maybe in another 20 years, TOE will be shown to adversely affect patient outcome and have been supplanted by a yet unknown technology that provides even better insight into cardiovascular pathophysiology. Let us hope that by then we will have gained the sense to first evaluate new technology to prove it safe and effective before it is introduced into routine clinical practice.

Aprotinin

Over its history, one of the major challenges to the safe delivery of cardiothoracic anaesthesia has been and remains blood loss and transfusion (Chapters 17). One aspect that deserves particular attention is the sorry tale of the use of aprotinin to reduce blood transfusion (110).

Unrecognized efficacy

In 1987, David Royston and colleagues published a landmark paper that reported a small randomized controlled trial (RCT), which found administration of aprotinin during cardiac surgery to be associated with a massive reductions in blood loss and the need for blood transfusion (111). Unsurprisingly, further RCTs were undertaken to confirm these remarkable finding. In fact, far too many were undertaken as by 2002, a further 63 RCTs had been reported (112). Fergusson and colleagues undertook a cumulative meta-analysis of these RCTs demonstrating that the available evidence had clearly established by the twelfth RCT published in June 1992 that aprotinin effectively reduced the need for blood transfusion (112). Despite this strong evidence of aprotinin's efficacy, a further 53 RCTs were needlessly undertaken over the next decade, unethically exposing thousands of patients in the control groups to the risks of increased blood loss and transfusion.

Suspension of aprotinin's licence

As detailed in Chapter 17, major drug regulatory agency around the world suspended the licence for aprotinin in 2007 in response to the publication of three observational studies and one RCT, that suggested aprotinin was associated with adverse outcomes and increased mortality. The most influential of these studies, because it was an RCT, was called the Blood Conservation Using Antifibrinolytics in a Randomized Trial (BART) study and compared aprotinin with the lysine analogues tranexamic acid and aminocaproic acid, in patients undergoing CABG surgery. Surprisingly, because it made the study underpowered, the BART study had been stopped when only about half the planned population had been recruited because of a non-significant increase in mortality associated with aprotinin compared to the lysine analogues. Subsequently, the BART study was published and revealed that aprotinin was associated with a significantly higher mortality than either tranexamic acid or aminocaproic acid (113). Thus, there appeared to be sufficient evidence to justify the drug regulatory agencies around the world to suspend aprotinin's licence. However, this was not the end of the story for aprotinin.

Health canada's review of the bart study

In 2011, Health Canada reviewed and then reanalysed the data from the BART trial finding unexplained major failings in the conduct and analysis of the trial, as are detailed in Chapter 17. In particular, the reanalysis found that mortality in patients who received aprotinin to be no different from the other two drugs. As a consequence, after a period over three years, the suspension of the licence for aprotinin was lifted by Health Canada (114).

Evidence misused

So despite early evidence of efficacy, aprotinin was adopted late into clinical practice. When it did get taken up, aprotinin's licence was suspended as a result of the weak and incorrect evidence that questioned the safety of aprotinin. Thus an effective drug became unavailable for patients for over three years in some countries and maybe for ever in others because of product liability. For cardiothoracic anaesthesia to advance, we need to learn how to use evidence effectively and ethically as well as design, conduct, analyse and report research accurately.

Conclusion

In a little over 100 years, cardiothoracic anaesthesia has gone from being too dangerous to practice to a speciality that safely provides anaesthetic care for millions of patients undergoing cardiothoracic surgery every year. Initially, progress in cardiothoracic anaesthesia was based on an increasing understanding of physiology and pharmacology. Along the way, however, a number of blind alleys were taken such as the failure to apply techniques proven to be effective by physiologists and to learn from past clinical experience. We have also been attracted by shiny advances in equipment, which have led to remarkable insights into cardiovascular pathophysiology yet may not have improved patient outcome. More recently, patient outcome has been used to drive change in practice but even here there has been failings in our use of evidence. Whilst not all aspects of our practice can be rigorously examined, the important ones need to be subjected to RCTs if we are to move forward cardiothoracic anaesthesia into the future. Otherwise, and as Keats recognized in 1983, we will be condemned to repeat the mistakes of our past and one technology or drug will continue to be lifesaving in one centre but merely an irritation in another.

Acknowledgements

The author would like to thank John Manners for access to his notes from a lecture delivered in 1993 and his advice on writing this chapter.

References

1. Keats AS. The Rovenstine Lecture, 1983: cardiovascular anesthesia: perceptions and perspectives. *Anesthesiology* 1984; **60**: 467–74
2. Bosher C, Westaby S. *Landmarks in Cardiac Surgery*: London: Informa Healthcare, 1998
3. Lillehei CW. Historical development of cardiopulmonary bypass in Minnesota. In: Gravlee GP, Davis RF, Stammers AH, Ungerleider RM, editors. *Cardiopulmonary Bypass: Principles and Practice*, 3rd edn. Philadephia, PA, USA: Lippincott Williams & Wilkins, 2008; 3–20
4. Shumacker HB. The birth of an idea and the development of cardiopulmonary bypass. In: Gravlee GP, Davis FA, Stammers AH, Ungerleider RM, editors. *Cardiopulmonary Bypass: Principles and Practice*, Philadephia, PA, USA: Lippincott, Wliiams & Wilkins, 2008; 21–34
5. Mushin WW, Rendall-Baker L. *The Principles of Thoracic Anaesthesia Past and Present*. Oxford: Blackwell Scientific Publications Ltd, 1953
6. Fell GE. Forced respiration in opium poisoning—its possibilities, and the apparatus best adapted to produce it. *Buffalo Med Surg J* 1887; **28**: 145–57
7. O'Dwyer J. Intubation of the larynx. *New York Med J* 1885; **42**: 145–57
8. Matas R. The history and methods of intralaryngeal insufflation for the relief of acute surgical pneumothorax with a description of the latest devices for the purpose. *Trans South Surg Gyne Assoc* 1900; **12**: 52–8
9. Cherian SM, Nicks R, Lord RSA. Ernst Ferdinand Sauerbruch: rise and fall of the pioneer of thoracic surgery. *World J Surg* 2001; **25**: 1012–20
10. Catoca F, Schumacher ED. *Technik der thoraxchirurgie*. Berlin: Verlag von Julius Springer, 1911
11. Sauerbruch EF. Zur pathologie des offenen pneumothorax und die grundlagen meines verfahreas zu seiner ausschaltung. *Mitteilungen aus den Grenzgebieten der Medizin und Chirurgie* 1904; **13**: 399–482

12. Askinson RS, Rushman GB, Lee JA. *A Synopsis of Anaesthesia*. Bristol: Wright, 1973

13. Meyer W. Pneumectomy with the aid of differential air pressure: an experimental study: the new type of apparatus used. *JAMA* 1909; **53**: 1978–87

14. Maloney JV, Jr., Schmutzer KJ, Raschke E. Paradoxical respiration and 'pendelluft'. *J Thorac Cardiovasc Surg* 1961; **41**: 291–8

15. Waters RM, Rovenstine EA, Guedel AE. Endotracheal anesthesia and its historical development. *Anesth Analg* 1933; **12**: 196–203

16. Elsberg CA. III. Clinical experiences with intratracheal insufflation (Meltzer), with remarks upon the value of the method for thoracic surgery. *Ann Surg* 1910; **52**: 23–9

17. Janeway HH. Intratracheal anaesthesia: A. by nitrous oxide and oxygen. B. by nitrous oxide and oxygen under conditions of differential pressure. *Ann Surg* 1913; **58**: 927–33

18. Rowbotham ES, Magill I. Anaesthetics in the plastic surgery of the face and jaws. *Proc R Soc Med* 1921; **14**: 17–27

19. Guedel AE, Waters RM. Endotracheal anesthesia: a new technic. *Ann Otol Rhinol Laryngol* 1931; 40: 1139–45

20. Craaford C. Pulmonary ventilation and anaesthesia in major chest surgery. *J Thorac Surg* 1940; **9**: 237–53

21. Nosworthy MD. Anaesthesia in chest surgery, with special reference to controlled respiration and cyclopropane: (Section of Anaesthetics). *Proc R Soc Med* 1941; **34**: 479–506

22. Sanders RD. Two ventilating attachments for bronchoscopes. *Delaware State Med J* 1967; **39**: 171–75

23. Stritesky M, Semrad M, Kunstyr J, Hajek T, Demes R, Tosovsky J. On-pump cardiac surgery in a conscious patient using a thoracic epidural anesthesia—an ultra fast track method. *Bratisl Lek Listy* 2004; **105**: 51–5

24. Mukaida T, Andou A, Date H, Aoe M, Shimizu N. Thoracoscopic operation for secondary pneumothorax under local and epidural anesthesia in high-risk patients. *Ann Thorac Surg* 1998; **65**: 924–6

25. Overholt RH, Langer L, Szypulski JT, Wilson NJ. Pulmonary resection in the treatment of tuberculosis; present-day technique and results. *J Thorac Surg* 1946; **15**: 384–417

26. Parry Brown AI. Posture in thoracic anaesthesia. *Thorax* 1948; **3**: 161–65

27. Magill IW, Macintosh R, Hewer CL, Nosworthy MD, McConnell WS. Lest we forget. An historic meeting of the Section of Anaesthetics of Royal Society of Medicine on 6 Decemeber 1974. Divynyl ether. *Anaesthesia* 1975; **30**: 630–2

28. White GM. Evolution of endotracheal and endobronchial intubation. *Br J Anaesth* 1960; **32**: 235–46

29. Gale JW, Waters RM. Closed endobronchial anesthesia in thoracic surgery: preliminary report. *J Thorac Surg* 1932; **1**: 432–7

30. Jacobaeus HC, Freckner P, Bjorkman S. Some attempts at determining the volume and function of each lung separately. *Acta Med Scand* 1932; **79**: 174–215

31. Gebauer PW. A catheter for bronchospirometry. *J Thorac Surg* 1939; **8**: 174–215

32. Carlens E. A new flexible double-lumen catheter for bronchospirometry. *J Thorac Surg* 1949; **18**: 742–6

33. Bjork VO, Carlens E, Friberg O. Endobronchial anesthesia. *Anesthesiol* 1953; **14**: 60–72

34. Robertshaw FL. Low resistance double-lumen endobronchial tubes. *Br J Anaesth* 1962; **34**: 576–9

35. Benumof JL. Improving the design and function of double-lumen tubes. *J Cardiothorac Anesth* 1988; **2**: 729–33

36. Shinnick JP, Freedman AP. Bronchofiberscopic placement of a double-lumen endotracheal tube. *Crit Care Med* 1982; **10**: 544–5

37. Ovassapian A. Fibreoptic bronchoscope and double-lumen tracheal tubes. *Anaesthesia* 1983; **38**: 1104

38. Ghosh S, Falter F, Goldsmith K, Arrowsmith JE. The Papworth BiVent tube: a new device for lung isolation. *Anaesthesia* 2008; **63**: 996–1000

39. Alston RP. Anaesthesia and cardiopulmonary bypass: an historical review. *Perfusion* 1992; **7**: 77–88

40. Wasmouth CE. The choice of anesthesia for mitral commissurotomy. *Anesth Analg* 1954; **33**: 115–21

41. Lucas GH, Henderson VE. A new anaesthetic: cyclopropane: a preliminary report. *Can Med Assoc J* 1929; **21**: 173–5

42. Rovenstine EA. Cyclopropane anesthesia in thoracic surgery. *Anesth Analg* 1935; **14**: 270–75

43. Waters RM. Clinical scope and utility of carbon dioxide filtration in inhalation anesthesia. *Anesth Analg* 1924; **3**: 20–22

44. R.E. Gross, Hubbard JP. Surgical ligation of a patent ductus arteriosus. Report of first successful case. *JAMA* 1939; **112**: 729–31

45. Dunlop J. Anesthetic practices in thoracic surgery. *Anesth Analg* 1939; **18**: 301–11

46. Blalock A, Taussig HB. The surgical treatment of malformations of the heart in which there is pulmonary stenosis or pulmonary atresia. *JAMA* 1945; **128**: 189–202

47. Harmel MH, Lamont A. Anesthesia in the surgical treatment of congenital pulmonic stenosis. *Anesthesiol* 1946; **7**: 477–98

48. Preston FS. Anaesthesia for mitral valvotomy. *Br J Anaesth* 1953; **25**: 299–314

49. Brown WM, Reid JE. Anaesthesia for mitral valvotomy. *Anaesthesia* 1954; **9**: 68–73

50. Lewis FJ, Taufic M. Closure of atrial septal defects with the aid of hypothermia; experimental accomplishments and the report of one successful case. *Surgery* 1953; **33**: 52–9

51. Nosworthy MD. Anaesthesia in chest surgery, with special reference to controlled respiration and cyclopropane. *Proc R Soc Med* 1941; **34**: 479–506

52. Kirklin JW, Dushane JW, Patrick RTet al. Intracardiac surgery with the aid of a mechanical pump-oxygenator system (Gibbon type): report of eight cases. *Proc Staff Meet Mayo Clin* 1955; **30**: 201–6

53. Gibbon JH. Artificial maintenance of circulation during experimental occlusion of pulmonary artery. *Arch Surg* 1937; **34**: 1105–31

54. Lowenstein E, Hallowell P, Levine FH, Daggett WM, Austen WG, Laver MB. Cardiovascular response to large doses of intravenous morphine in man. *N Engl J Med* 1969; **281**: 1389–93

55. Lowenstein E. Morphine 'anesthesia'—a perspective. *Anesthesiology* 1971; **35**: 563–5

56. Stanley TH, Gray NH, Stanford W, Armstrong R. The effects of high-dose morphine on fluid and blood requirements in open-heart operations. *Anesthesiology* 1973; **38**: 536–41

57. Wong KC, Martin WE, Hornbein TF, Freund FG, Everett J. The cardiovascular effects of morphine sulfate with oxygen and with nitrous oxide in man. *Anesthesiology* 1973; **38**: 542–9

58. Effler DB, Favaloro RG, Groves LK. Coronary artery surgery utilizing saphenous vein graft techniques. Clinical experience with 224 operations. *J Thorac Cardiovasc Surg* 1970; **59**: 147–54

59. Bovill JG, Sebel PS, Stanley TH. Opioid analgesics in anesthesia: with special reference to their use in cardiovascular anesthesia. *Anesthesiology* 1984; **61**: 731–55

60. Stanley TH, Egan TD, Van Aken H. A tribute to Dr. Paul A. J. Janssen: entrepreneur extraordinaire, innovative scientist, and significant contributor to anesthesiology. *Anesth Analg* 2008; **106**: 451–62

61. Corssen G, Chodoff P, Domino EF, Kahn DR. Neurolept analgesia and anesthesia for open-heart surgery: pharmacologic rationale and clinical experience. *J Thorac Cardiovasc Surg* 1965; **49**: 901–20

62. Stanley TH, Webster LR. Anesthetic requirements and cardiovascular effects of fentanyl-oxygen and fentanyl-diazepam-oxygen anesthesia in man. *Anesth Analg* 1978; **57**: 411–6

63. de Lange S, Stanley TH, Boscoe MJ. Alfentanil-oxygen anaesthesia for coronary artery surgery. *Br J Anaesth* 1981; **53**: 1291–6

64. Gordon PC, Morrell DF, Pamm JD. Total intravenous anesthesia using propofol and alfentanil for coronary artery bypass surgery. *J Cardiothorac Vasc Anesth* 1994; **8**: 284–8

65. Slogoff S, Keats AS. Randomized trial of primary anesthetic agents on outcome of coronary artery bypass operations. *Anesthesiol* 1989; **70**: 179–88

66. Bacon R, Chandrasekan V, Haigh A, Royston BD, Royston D, Sundt T. Early extubation after open-heart surgery with total intravenous anaesthetic technique. *Lancet* 1995; **345**:133–34

67. Duthie DJR, Stevens JJWM, Doyle AR, Baddoo HHK. Remifentanil and coronary artery surgery. *Lancet* 1995; **345**: 649–50

68. Dawson B, Theye RA, Kirklin JW. Halothane in open cardiac operations: a technic for use with extracorporeal circulation. *Anesth Analg* 1960; **39**: 59–63

69. Vandam LD. Anesthesia for operations upon the heart. *Cardiovascular clinics* 1971; **3**: 93–102

70. Norden I. The influence of anaesthetics on systemic vascular resistance during cardiopulmonary bypass. *Scand J Thorac Cardiovasc Surg* 1974; **8**: 81–7

71. Norden I, Norlander O, Rodriguez R. Ventilatory and circulatory effects of anaesthesia and cardiopulmonary bypass. *Acta Anaesthesiol Scand* 1970; **14**: 297–316

72. Pierce JA, Garofalo ML. Anaesthetic management for cardiopulmonary bypass: a review of 200 cases. *Can Anaesth Soc J* 1965; **12**: 179–91

73. Hart SM, Sloan IA, Conn AW. Methoxyflurane in Paediatric Cardiac Surgery. *Can Anaesth Soc J* 1964; **11**: 429–36

74. Muravchick S. Scavenging enflurane from extracorporeal pump oxygenators. *Anesthesiology* 1977; **47**: 468–71

75. Bethune DW, Gill RD, Wheldon DR. The supply of gases and vapours to cardio-pulmonary bypass apparatus. *Anaesthesia* 1976; **31**: 76–7

76. Becker LC. Is isoflurane dangerous for the patient with coronary artery disease? *Anesthesiol* 1987; **66**: 259–61

77. Woodcock TE, Murkin JM, Farrar JK, Tweed WA, Guiraudon GM, McKenzie FN. Pharmacologic EEG suppression during cardiopulmonary bypass: cerebral hemodynamic and metabolic effects of thiopental or isoflurane during hypothermia and normothermia. *Anesthesiology* 1987; **67**: 218–24

78. Parsons RS, Jones RM, Wrigley SR, MacLeod KG, Platt MW. Comparison of desflurane and fentanyl-based anaesthetic techniques for coronary artery bypass surgery. *Br J Anaesth* 1994; **72**: 430–8

79. Searle NR, Martineau RJ, Conzen P, et al. Comparison of sevoflurane/fentanyl and isoflurane/fentanyl during elective coronary artery bypass surgery. Sevoflurane Venture Group. *Can J Anaesth* 1996; **43**: 890–9

80. Landoni G, Biondi-Zoccai GG, Zangrillo A, et al. Desflurane and sevoflurane in cardiac surgery: a meta-analysis of randomized clinical trials. *J Cardiothorac Vasc Anesth* 2007; **21**: 502–11

81. Nunn JF, Halsey MJ. Xenon in anaesthesia. *Lancet* 1990; **336**: 112–3

82. Celebioglu B, Pamuk AG, Aypar U, Pasaoglu I. Use of sevoflurane during cardiopulmonary bypass decreases incidence of awareness. *Eur J Anaesthesiol* 2002; **19**: 283–7

83. Patey R, Alston RP. Anaesthesia and cardiopulmonary bypass. *Perfusion* 1993; **8**: 313–9

84. Vale RJ, Hellewell J. Anaesthesia for open heart surgery. The use of phenoperidine, methohexitone and nitrous oxide. *Anaesthesia* 1966; **21**: 357–62

85. Nussmeier NA, Arlund C, Slogoff S. Neuropsychiatric complications after cardiopulmonary bypass: cerebral protection by a barbiturate. *Anesthesiol* 1986; **64**: 165–70

86. Rachay PA, Hollinger J, Santi A, Nagashima H. Ketamine for padiatric cardiac anesthesia. *Anaesthetist* 1976; **25**: 259–65

87. Wong GL, Morton NS. Total intravenous anesthesia (TIVA) in pediatric cardiac anesthesia. *Paediatr Anaesth* 2011; **21**: 560–6

88. Watt I, Ledingham IM. Mortality amongst multiple trauma patients admitted to an intensive therapy unit. *Anaesthesia* 1984; **39**: 973–81

89. Russell GN, Wright EL, Fox MA, Douglas EJ, Cockshott ID. Propofol-fentanyl anaesthesia for coronary artery surgery and cardiopulmonary bypass. *Anaesthesia* 1989; **44**: 205–8

90. White M, Kenny GN. Intravenous propofol anaesthesia using a computerised infusion system. *Anaesthesia* 1990; **47**: 633–4

91. Bignami E, Biondi-Zoccai G, Landoni G, et al. Volatile anesthetics reduce mortality in cardiac surgery. *J Cardiothorac Vasc Anesth* 2009; **23**: 594–9

92. Griffith HR, Johnson G. The use of curare in general anaesthesia. *Anesthesiology* 1942; **3**: 418–20

93. Harroun P, Hathaway HR. The use of curare in anesthesia for thoracic surgery; preliminary report. *Surg Gynecol Obstet* 1946; **82**: 229–31

94. Starr NJ, Sethna DH, Estafanous FG. Bradycardia and asystole following the rapid administration of sufentanil with vecuronium. *Anesthesiology* 1986; **64**: 521–3

95. McEwin L, Merrick PM, Bevan DR. Residual neuromuscular blockade after cardiac surgery: pancuronium vs rocuronium. *Can J Anaesth* 1997; **44**: 891–5

96. Shields M, Giovannelli M, Mirakhur RK, Moppett I, Adams J, Hermens Y. Org 25969 (sugammadex), a selective relaxant binding agent for antagonism of prolonged rocuronium-induced neuromuscular block. *Br J Anaesth* 2006; **96**: 36–43

97. Abrishami A, Ho J, Wong J, Yin L, Chung F. Sugammadex, a selective reversal medication for preventing postoperative residual neuromuscular blockade. *Cochrane Database Syst Rev* 2009: CD007362.

98. Unterbuchner C, Fink H, Blobner M. The use of sugammadex in a patient with myasthenia gravis. *Anaesthesia* 2010; **65**: 302–5

99. Crawford OB, Ottosen P, Buckingham WW, Brasher CA. Peridural anesthesia in thoracic surgery: a review of 677 cases. *Anesthesiology* 1951; **12**: 73–84

100. Ossipov BK. Local anesthesia in thoracic surgery: 20 years experience with 3265 cases. *Anesth Analg* 1960; **39**: 327–32

101. Davies RG, Myles PS, Graham JM. A comparison of the analgesic efficacy and side-effects of paravertebral vs epidural blockade for thoracotomy—a systematic review and meta-analysis of randomized trials. *Br J Anaesth* 2006; **96**: 418–26

102. Clowes GH, Jr., Neville WE, Hopkins A, Anzola J, Simeone FA. Factors contributing to success or failure in the use of a pump oxygenator for complete by-pass of the heart and lung, experimental and clinical. *Surgery* 1954; **36**: 557–79

103. Stenseth R, Bjella L, Berg EM, Christensen O, Levang OW, Gisvold SE. Thoracic epidural analgesia in aortocoronary bypass surgery. II: Effects on the endocrine metabolic response. *Acta Anaesthesiol Scand* 1994; **38**: 834–9

104. Liu SS, Block BM, Wu CL. Effects of perioperative central neuraxial analgesia on outcome after coronary artery bypass surgery: a meta-analysis. *Anesthesiology* 2004; **101**: 153–61

105. Bignami E, Landoni G, Biondi-Zoccai GG, Boroli F, Messina M, Dedola E, et al. Epidural analgesia improves outcome in cardiac surgery: a meta-analysis of randomized controlled trials. *J Cardiothorac Vasc Anesth* 2010; **24**: 586–97

106. Swan HJC, Ganz W, Forrester J, Marcus H, Diamond G, Chonette D. Catheterization of the heart in man with use of a flow-directed balloon-tipped catheter. *N Engl J Med* 1970; **283**: 447–51

107. Schwann NM, Hillel Z, Hoeft A, Barash P, Mohnle P, Miao Y, et al. Lack of effectiveness of the pulmonary artery catheter in cardiac surgery. *Anesth Analg* 2011; **113**: 994–1002

108. Hessel EA, Klimkina O, Cahalan MK. Evolution of perioperative echocardiography. In: Kaplan JA, Reich DL, Savino JS, editors. *Cardiac Anesthesia; the Echo Era.* Sixth ed. St Louis, Missouri, USA: Elsevier Saunders, 2011; 298–314

109. An updated report by the American Society of Anesthesiologists and the Society of Cardiovascular Anesthesiologists Task Force on Transesophageal Echocardiography. Practice guidelines for perioperative transesophageal echocardiography. *Anesthesiology* 2010; **112**: 1084–96.

110. McMullan V, Alston RP. III. Aprotinin and cardiac surgery: a sorry tale of evidence misused. *Br J Anaesth* 2013; **110**: 675–78

111. Royston D, Taylor KM, Bidstrup BP, Sapsford RN. Effect of aprotinin on need for blood transfusion after repeat open-heart surgery. *Lancet* 1987; **330**: 1289–91

112. Fergusson D, Glass KC, Hutton B, Shapiro S. Randomized controlled trials of aprotinin in cardiac surgery: could clinical equipoise have stopped the bleeding? *Clin Trials* 2005; **2**: 218–29

113. Fergusson DA, Hébert PC, Mazer CD, Fremes S, MacAdams C, Murkin JM, et al. A comparison of aprotinin and lysine analogues in high-risk cardiac surgery. *N Engl J Med* 2008; **358**: 2319–31

114. Health Canada. Health Canada decision of Trasylol. Canada: Health Canada, 2011 http://www.hc-sc.gc.ca/dhp-mps/medeff/res/eap-gce_trasylol-eng.php (accessed 7 May 2014)

CHAPTER 2

Anatomy and pathology of the heart and major vascular system

Neil Hauser, Adriaan Myburgh, and Justiaan Swanevelder

Introduction

The heart and its associated structures form an intricate system that has the primary aim of pumping blood through the lungs and around the body. For this reason, a good knowledge of the normal anatomy is essential to understanding pathology, and the management of patients with cardiovascular disease. Therefore, this chapter will outline the normal anatomy of the heart and its related structures. The pathology of cardiomyopathies, valve abnormalities, infective endocarditis, and cardiac tamponade and finally, cardiac tumours will also be reviewed as will their their effects on the anatomy of the heart. Congenital heart defects will be reviewed in Chapter 21.

The heart

The cardiovascular system is responsible for the transport of oxygen, nutrients, hormones, and vasoactive substances to, and removal of carbon dioxide and metabolic waste products from, the peripheral tissues. The heart is the pump behind this system, acting as a transducer, converting chemical energy into mechanical energy. Any normal heart has three sequential segments: two atrial chambers, two ventricular chambers, and the great vessels.

Each atrial chamber has an appendage, a venous component, a vestibule, and a shared atrial septum. The right-sided atrium (RA) receives desaturated systemic blood, and primes the low pressure right ventricle (RV) to eject blood into the pulmonary circulation for oxygenation. Usually, the left atrium (LA) in turn receives blood from four pulmonary veins, to supply the left ventricle (LV), which is the driving force of cardiac output (CO), pumping oxygenated blood into the high-pressure systemic circulation. However, these four cardiac chambers do not occupy the positions that are implied by their names (1). The RA and RV are located anteriorly to the LA and LV. The RV outflow tract, pulmonary trunk, and pulmonary artery (PA) arise anterior, and to the left of the aortic valve (AV) and aortic trunk, which form the centre of the 'cardiac skeleton'. The AV is wedged between the tricuspid (TV) and mitral valves (MV) with the inlet portion of the RV therefore positioned anteriorly to

the inlet–outlet of the LV. The relative positions of each of the heart valves, as seen on a chest X-ray, are shown in figure 2.1.

From the front of the patient, the cardiac silhouette is trapezoidal in shape, with the RA forming the right heart border and the LV forming the left heart border. Two-thirds of the heart lies to the left of the thoracic midline (figure 2.1), with the long-axis of the heart therefore lying at an angle to the long-axis of the body. The atria are positioned superior and to the right relative to their respective ventricular chambers. The LA is the most posterior cardiac chamber positioned just anterior to the mid-thoracic oesophagus. The RV is situated anteriorly, just behind the sternum. Normal atrial and ventricular chambers have specific morphological characteristics identifying them as either right or left sided chambers (table 2.1). In the setting of congenital malformations such differentiating features may be limited. The appendages of the atria distinguish the morphologically right from morphologically LA,

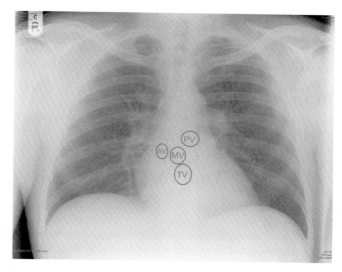

Fig. 2.1 Image of the heart on chest X-ray.
This shows the position of the heart in thorax as seen on a standard posterior anterior chest X-ray. The relative positions of the four primary heart valves are outlined.
AV: aortic valve, MV: mitral valve, TV: tricuspid valve, and PV: pulmonary valve.

Table 2.1 Morphological features of chambers and great arteries

Atriums	Ventricles	Great arteries
Morphologically right triangular, broad-based appendage terminal crest extensive pectinate muscles rim around oval fossa	Morphologically right coarse apical trabeculations with moderator band leaflet of aortic valve attached directly to septum (septal leaflet of tricuspid valve) septomarginal trabeculation	Aorta origin of coronary arteries aortic arch, usually with three arch arteries
Morphologically left tubular, narrow based appendage no terminal crest limited pectinate muscles & valve of oval fossa	Morphologically left fine apical trabeculations smooth upper part of septum (without attachment of mitral valve)	Pulmonary trunk bifurcates into right and left pulmonary arteries
	Morphologically indeterminate very coarse trabeculations no ventricular septum (solitary ventricle)	Common arterial trunk (all three components are present) origin of coronary arteries origin of aortic arch and arch arteries origin of pulmonary trunk or pulmonary arteries
		Solitary arterial trunk origin of coronary arteries origin of aortic arch and arch arteries collateral arteries supply lungs

Reproduced from *Heart*, Ho SY et al., 'Anatomic–echocardiographic correlates: an introduction to normal and congenitally malformed hearts', 86, Supplement 2, pp. ii3–ii11, copyright 2001, with permission from BMJ Publishing Group Ltd.

determining the 'situs' of the heart. Further distinguishing features of the RA include the orifice of the coronary sinus, and a Eustachian valve originating from the inferior vena cava. Normal ventricles comprise three components: an inlet, an outlet and a trabeculated segment with no discrete boundaries between them. The morphology of the RV differs from that of the left and this is important to recognize when dealing with congenital pathology.

The great arteries are distinguished by their branching patterns but this may be more difficult in the setting of congenital abnormalities. The three-leaflet arrangement of semilunar valves is characteristic of the arterial valves.

The venous system

The venous return from the lower body and abdomen travels via the inferior vena cava (IVC), which in the normal human is positioned to the right of the descending thoracic aorta, emptying in to the RA. Even when complex congenital cardiac pathology exists, the IVC will always join to the RA.

Cardiac muscle

The myocardium consists of specialized cardiac myocytes. The striated nature of cardiac muscle cells is due to the structure of the contractile intracellular myofibrils. These myofibrils compromise sarcomere units, consisting of thick and thin filaments, arranged to give the characteristic Z-line, A-band, and I-band striations. The tails of the myosin molecules link to form the thick filaments, leaving the actin binding 'heads' free. Each thick filament is surrounded by six thin filaments composed of a double spiral of actin molecules, in combination with tropomyosin and troponin. The coupling and decoupling interaction that occurs between the myosin heads and actin filaments results in a 'walking' action of the myosin heads along the thin filaments. This actin–myosin coupling and decoupling reaction is the essence of the myocardial contractile process.

Each cardiac muscle cell is surrounded by a sarcolemmal cell membrane. The sarcolemma forms invaginations, called transverse or T-tubules penetrating deep into the cell. A sarcoplasmic reticulum (SR) surrounding each myofibril, acts as a reversible intracellular calcium ion store. In cardiac muscle the individual cells are tightly coupled, by specialized membrane junctions called intercalated discs, into a functional syncytium allowing co-ordinated contractions to occur. Cardiac muscle cells contain great numbers of packed mitochondria and are richly supplied with capillaries to facilitate aerobic metabolism. Ischaemia of sufficient duration rapidly results in cardiac myocyte death.

Ventricles

Both ventricles consist of three components: an inlet portion, a trabeculated apex, and an outlet component. Characteristic of the RV apex is its coarse trabecular nature with one prominent trabeculation called the moderator band, travelling across the cavity. In the LV the trabeculations are characteristically finer in nature. The inlet portion of both ventricles includes the atrioventricular valves. The tricuspid valve (TV) always connects to the

RV and the MV without exception connects to the LV. The LV is cylindrical in shape, while the RV wraps around the left as a ventriculomuscular band. In the LV, the inlet (MV) and outlet (AV) portions are connected by the aorto-mitral continuity. In the RV there is no continuation between the inlet (TV) and the outlet (PV) with the RV infundibulum clearly noticeable as the outflow tract portion.

Myocardial dysfunction

Myocardial dysfunction is most commonly the result of ischaemic, valvular, congenital or hypertensive heart disease. Traditionally abnormal myocardial function, in the absence of these heart diseases and of an unknown cause, has been termed a cardiomyopathy. Increasing knowledge of the aetiology and pathophysiology, together with improved special investigations, led to a Task Force Report being developed in 1995 (2). This report redefined cardiomyopathy as a disease of the myocardium associated with cardiac dysfunction. It recognizes that there is an overlap between ischaemic, valvular, and hypertensive cardiomyopathies, and that the severity of ventricular dysfunction is often disproportionate to the apparent pathology. The report recommended that an aetiologic/pathogenic classification be adapted to describe cardiomyopathies. They also recommend that the classical 'established cardiomyopathy classification' be identified by the dominant pathophysiological and echocardiographic characteristics. These were called dilated-, hypertrophic-, restrictive-, and arrhythmogenic right ventricular cardiomyopathies (table 2.2).

The European Society of Cardiology defines cardiomyopathy as a myocardial disease in which the heart muscle is structurally and functionally abnormal, in the absence of coronary artery disease, hypertension, valvular heart disease, and congenital heart disease sufficient to cause the observed myocardial abnormality (3). Currently, the American Heart Association proposes a more detailed classification taking into account organ involvement, genetics, structural changes, cellular events, and physiological abnormalities.

Dilated cardiomyopathy

A dilated poorly functioning heart is common and can be caused by both acquired or inherited conditions. The classical dilated cardiomyopathy is the commonest form of cardiomyopathy. It presents without specific histological features and in most cases no specific cause is identified (2). The echocardiographic presentation is characterized by impaired systolic function, dilatation of the left or both ventricles, and increased myocardial mass with an often normal wall thickness. Figure 2.2a and b illustrate a dilated LV, in a 3D echocardiographic image obtained from a patient with a dilated cardiomyopathy. Both end-diastolic and end-systolic dimensions are increased, and ejection fraction (EF) and cardiac output (CO) are decreased. Secondary features include mitral regurgitation (MR), atrial dilatation, and often an intracardiac or mural thrombus. A patient with idiopathic dilated cardiomyopathy and associated functional MR that is exacerbated during exercise, has a poor prognosis. In addition, RV dilatation may lead to tricuspid valve regurgitation (TR).

Hypertrophic obstructive cardiomyopathy

Hypertrophic obstructive cardiomyopathy (HOCM) accounts for 50% of all sudden cardiac deaths below the age of 30 years (4) and it is estimated that 60–70% of all patients with hypertrophic cardiomyopathy (HCM) will die suddenly. Syncope is a significant risk factor for sudden death in these patients. Unexplained hypertrophy of a non-dilated ventricle, with a wall thickness exceeding 15 mm is generally considered to be diagnostic. Figure 2.3a and b demonstrate the increased wall mass and resultant left ventricular outflow tract (LVOT) obstruction that is typically associated with HOCM. Most cases are familial, with autosomal dominant inheritance and variable penetration. A variable pattern to the hypertrophy is also seen. Although HOCM can present with concentric, apical or free wall LV hypertrophy, an asymmetric septal hypertrophy is the most common form (60% of cases). On histology, myocyte disorganization and myocardial fibrosis are the hallmarks of this cardiomyopathy. The apical variant is particularly common in Japanese and other Asian populations and is generally considered relatively benign. An under-appreciated subset, in the heterogeneous HCM disease spectrum has left ventricular apical aneurysms, and these are associated with substantial morbidity and mortality (4).

Not all dynamic LVOT obstructions are due to HCM. Any hyperdynamic LV condition, especially with hypovolaemia, can produce systolic anterior motion (SAM) of the MV (5). Aortic stenosis (AS) patients with LV hypertrophy and intravascular volume depletion can present in the postoperative period with LVOT obstruction when given inotropic agents.

Although distinguishing between the athlete's heart and pathological HCM may be difficult, it is important to do. Endurance

Table 2.2 Classification of cardiomyopathies

A. Established cardiomyopathies (of unknown cause)	B. Specific cardiomyopathies (associated with known disorders)	C. Unclassified cardiomyopathies (of unknown cause)
Dilated cardiomyopathy	Ischaemic/valvular/hypertensive cardiomyopathy	Endocardial fibroelastosis (with or without eosinophilia)
Hypertrophic cardiomyopathy	Inflammatory cardiomyopathy	
Restrictive cardiomyopathy	Metabolic cardiomyopathy	
Arrhythmogenic right ventricular cardiomyopathy	General system diseases	
	Muscular dystrophies and neuromuscular disorders	
	Hypersensitivity and toxic reactions	
	Peripartum cardiomyopathy	

Adapted from Richardson P et al., 'Report of the 1995 World Health Organization/International Society and Federation of Cardiology Task Force on the definition and classification of cardiomyopathies', *Circulation*, 93, 5, pp. 841–842, copyright 1996, with permission from American Heart Association and Wolters Kluwer

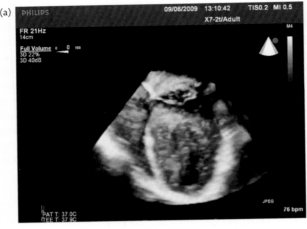
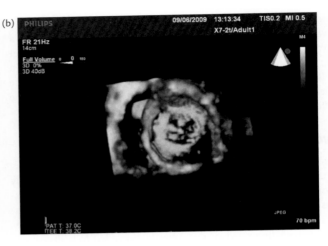

Fig. 2.2 Dilated left ventricle.
(a) 3D echocardiography image illustrating a dilated left ventricle. (b) 3D transoesophageal echocardiography image demonstrating short axis view of a dilated left ventricle. (See also figure in colour plates section)

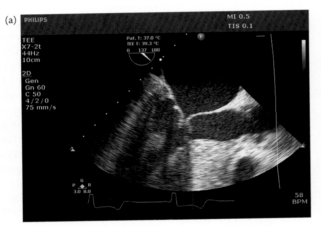
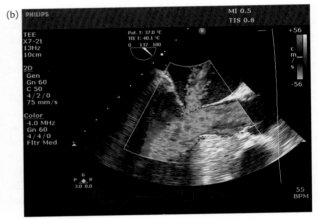

Fig. 2.3 Hypertrophic cardiomyopathy.
(a) 2D Echo image of an obstructed left ventricular outflow tract in a patient with hypertrophic cardiomyopathy. (b) 2D colour flow Doppler image of the same left ventricular outflow tract obstruction demonstrating turbulence during systole, as well as mitral regurgitation. (See also figure in colour plates section)

athletes usually have a physiological increase in LV cavity size, while athletes participating in isometric sports (like weight lifting) will have an increase in LV wall thickness with a smaller cavity. Any asymmetrical hypertrophy or diastolic LV wall thickness of more than 16 mm is considered pathological.

Restrictive cardiomyopathy

Restrictive cardiomyopathy is the least common of the cardiomyopathies and may be associated with infiltrative diseases, storage disorders, and endomyocardial disease, or be idiopathic in nature. Decreased compliance, restricted ventricular filling, and a reduced ventricular diastolic volume are characteristic of restrictive cardiomyopathies. The ventricle is usually a normal size, with or without wall thickness abnormalities.

Endomyocardial fibrosis is the commonest cause of a restrictive cardiomyopathy and is often due to hypereosinophilia that may be caused by parasites, drugs, or malignancy. Amyloidosis is the most common infiltrative restrictive cardiomyopathy and the predominant morphologic feature is increased myocardial wall thickness without dilatation of the LV cavity. Myocardial infiltration from sarcoidosis or haemochromatosis can also progress to a restrictive cardiomyopthay. Pericardial disease is an important differential diagnosis, with effusions and pericardial constriction readily identified on echocardiography.

Arrhythmogenic right ventricular cardiomyopathy

Arrhythmogenic right ventricular cardiomyopathy (ARVC) is a rare but increasingly recognised form of cardiomyopathy, affecting approximately 1 in 5000 individuals. ARVC is characterized by myocardial dysplasia due to progressive fatty infiltration and interstitial fibrosis involving predominantly the RV. The LV is frequently involved, supporting use of the broader term arrhythmogenic cardiomyopathy (6). The fibrofatty infiltrates lead to electrical instability and patients may present with ventricular arrhythmias and sudden death. Due to the autosomal dominant pattern of inheritance screening of relatives is important.

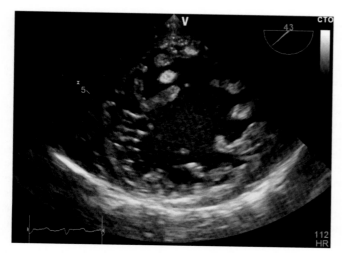

Fig. 2.4 Non-compaction of the left ventricle.
2D transoesophageal echocardiography transgastric view illustrating the two layers typical of a severely trabeculated non-compacted ventricular myocardium.

Non-compaction of the ventricular myocardium

Non-compaction of the ventricle is an uncommon cardiomyopathy, believed to be caused by the arrest of normal endo- and myocardial embryogenesis. The arrested embryogenesis results in a typical layered appearance on echocardiography, as shown in figure 2.4. There are both sporadic and familial cases of LV non-compaction. In familial cases, mode of transmission is autosomal dominant, or rarely, X-linked.

Aortic valve

Aortic valve structural and associated anatomy

The AV consists of a crown-shaped aortic annulus (annulus fibrosa) and three similar semilunar cusps, the right (RCC) and left (LCC) coronary cusps, and the non-coronary cusp (NCC). The leaflets are composed of dense collagen layers, covered by endothelium. The RCC and right sinus of Valsalva are positioned anteriorly and give rise to the right coronary artery (RCA). The left coronary artery (LCA) originates from the LCC and left sinus of Valsalva. The posterior of the three cusps, the NCC, lies adjacent to the interatrial septum. The plane of the AV is oblique to the right posterior side and more inferior to the left anterior side making the origin of the LCA superior to the RCA. Fibrous thickenings, known as nodules of Arantius, may occasionally be seen at the central portion of the free edges of normal leaflets. After years of function valve leaflets may develop a thickening of their edges together with filamentous strands. These small filamentous strands connected to the aortic valve are called Lambl's excrescences and they may appear in the LVOT during diastole, or the aortic side during systole and may be misinterpreted as vegetations. This is usually an incidental finding in elderly patients who are otherwise well.

The sinotubular junction (STJ) connects the root to the proximal ascending aorta. It is circular and thicker than the adjacent sinuses, defining the start of the aorta. The STJ plays an important role in suspending the semilunar AV leaflets. The upper limit diameter of a normal aortic valve annulus and STJ is 2.6 and 3.4 cm respectively. Together with the sinuses of Valsalva and ascending aorta diameters, these measurements are important for surgical planning.

Functional anatomy of the aortic valve

The normal AV area is 2.5–3.5 cm^2. Pressure normally drops by 2–4 mmHg across the valve, assuming a flow velocity of 60–100 cm/s. The opening and closing of the leaflets, inside a normal aortic root, is smooth and symmetrical. During systole in a compliant aorta, root dilatation precedes and aids in the opening of the leaflets. This root dilatation pulls the closed leaflets apart reducing the frictional forces at the commissures. A pressure gradient as low as 2 mmHg is therefore sufficient to open the valve. At maximal leaflet displacement, occurring during early systole, the AV opening is nearly circular but as shown in the normal 3D echocardiographic view figure 2.5, later in systole it becomes triangular in shape. The dynamic echocardiography appearance of the normal valve orifice may therefore be either circular or triangular, depending on whether it is observed in early or late systole (7).

In the normal AV there is no contact between the leaflet body and the aortic wall in the sinuses of Valsalva. If the pressure gradient is increased in a compliant root from 2–8 mmHg, the valve area markedly increases by about 25%. When the CO is increased under certain physiological conditions, for example with exercise, the normal aortic valve copes by increasing dilatation of the compliant root. This effect is absent in a stiff, noncompliant aortic root.

In a stiff, non-compliant aortic root, the valve opening tends to be asymmetric and delayed. The valve opening remains circular and does not become triangular in late systole. There has been speculation that the leaflet wrinkling, inside a non-compliant root, may increase leaflet stresses and may be responsible for earlier calcification. A stiff root seems to function at a maximal efficiency level and is unable to increase the valve area during periods of increased cardiac output. The compliance of the aorta and root also has a very important role in directing coronary blood flow to the myocardium.

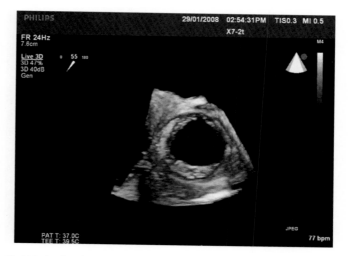

Fig. 2.5 Aortic valve.
3D transoesophageal echocardiography image illustrating the normal triangular shape of the aortic valve in late systole. (See also figure in colour plates section)

Aortic stenosis

Aortic stenosis and sclerosis

AV disease is very common in the developed world, 25% of the population who are over 65 years of age will have aortic sclerosis and 3% of those over 75 years will have severe stenosis. Aortic sclerosis is diagnosed when there is an ejection systolic murmur present in the AV region due to calcification in the ascending aorta, with associated turbulent flow. In this condition there is minor disruption of the AV and minimal obstruction to flow. There may be associated thickening or calcification of one or more leaflets of a tricuspid AV, but in contrast to aortic stenosis (AS), leaflet opening is not restricted much and the velocity through the valve is less than 2.5 m/s. Aortic sclerosis is not innocent and is often antecedent to clinically significant AV stenosis, acting as a marker of increased risk for future cardiovascular events. AS is differentiated from sclerosis by significant restriction of cusp movement and a raised transaortic peak velocity as seen on echocardiography.

Aetiology of aortic stenosis

Calcific degeneration is the most common cause of AS in the elderly adult population (70–90 years old) of the developed world. Degeneration begins with annular and leaflet thickening, which gradually becomes calcified. 2D and 3D echocardiographic images of a calcified AV is shown in Figure 2.6a and b. Although it seems as if most patients with AS start off with aortic sclerosis, the rate of progression is unclear. The RCC is most commonly affected, often fusing with the NCC. These calcified leaflets have decreased mobility and are very echogenic. AS was once viewed as a degenerative disease but is now seen as part of an active inflammatory process resembling atherosclerosis. Inflammation, lipid infiltration, dystrophic calcification, ossification, platelet deposition and endothelial dysfunction have all been observed in both disease processes. In addition, hypercholesterolaemia, lipoprotein a (Lp(a)), smoking, hypertension, and diabetes have all been reported as risk factors common to both. AV disease is also a marker of coronary artery disease.

The congenital bicuspid AV is the most common cardiovascular malformation in humans with an incidence of 1–2%. These patients may present with AS in childhood, or may undergo accelerated calcification of the abnormal AV and present in adulthood when about 50–60 years old. The two leaflets are typically arranged in either a right–left or anterior–posterior orientation, with a variation in coronary arrangement. Figure 2.7 shows a typical bicuspid AV as seen on 2D echocardiography. A pseudo-bicuspid AV (three-leaflet valve with fusion of two of the leaflets) will have similar pathophysiology to a truly bicuspid valve. Patients with the most severely malformed bicuspid valves may require intervention during childhood. The bicuspid AV is also associated with other congenital cardiovascular abnormalities including coarctation of the aorta (50–80%), interruption of the aortic arch (36%), and isolated ventricular septal defect (20%). The high heritability of the bicuspid AV suggests that its determination is almost entirely genetic. Although a non-stenotic bicuspid AV is often considered a benign lesion early in life, it has potential complications including aortic regurgitation, infective endocarditis, aortic dilatation and dissection, resulting in considerable morbidity and mortality later in life. Unicuspid valves are rare but may also be a cause of stenosis.

Although rheumatic heart disease may affect the AV, with leaflet thickening and decreased movement, it preferentially involves the mitral valve. Rheumatic degeneration of the AV thus rarely occurs in isolation. In the rheumatic aortic valve, commissural fusion occurs together with thickening and fibrosis of the leaflet edges, leaving leaflet bodies less affected in the earlier stages.

Progression and clinical features of aortic stenosis

Symptoms alone are not an adequate guide to the management of valvular heart disease and a lack of symptoms does not predict an uncomplicated course. For example, patients with severe AS may remain completely asymptomatic but are at increased risk of sudden death. Once angina, syncope, or heart failure develops, survival is greatly reduced.

About 75% of patients with symptomatic AS will be dead 3 years after the onset of symptoms, unless the AV is replaced. When the

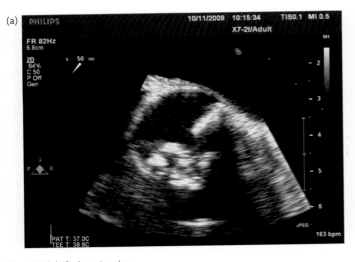
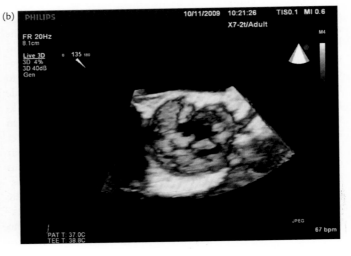

Fig. 2.6 Calcified aortic valve.
(a) 2D echocardiography image of a calcified aortic valve. Bright echogenic area represents increased calcification. (b) 3D echocardiography image clearly illustrating areas of calcification on a stenotic aortic valve. (See also figure in colour plates section)

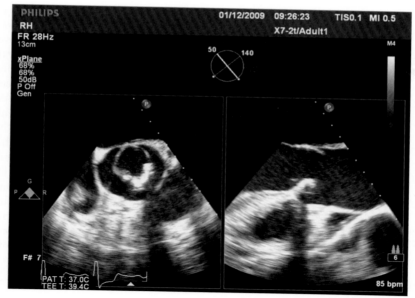

Fig. 2.7 Bicuspid aortic valve.
Orthogonal 2D echocardiography images of a bicuspid aortic valve during systole.

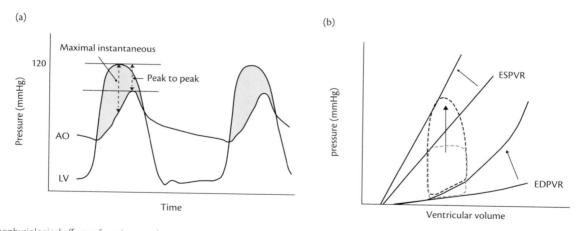

Fig. 2.8 Pathophysiological effects of aortic stenosis.
(a) Cardiac cycle illustrating the pressure drop across a stenotic aortic valve requiring the generation of a higher peak ventricular pressure in order to overcome the decreased aortic valve area. (b) The typical pressure–volume loop of aortic stenosis illustrating increased left ventricular end systolic elastance, impaired compliance, and decreased stroke volume.

peak flow velocity is more than 4.0 m/s, the likelihood of a symptomatic AS patient being alive without a valve replacement in two years is only 21%. In the era of modern echocardiography, it is no longer appropriate to wait for a change in symptoms to guide management. It is important to distinguish the patient with true severe AS from the patient with aortic pseudostenosis, in which the LV is damaged by another process, such as coronary artery disease or cardiomyopathy, and is unable to open a mildly stenotic AV.

The high flow velocity jet of severe AS produces a typical sound. The flow pattern is also helpful, in severe AS the peak will occur during mid-systole, while in more moderate AS it occurs during early systole. Severe AS is defined as a flow velocity greater than 4.5 m/s, a mean pressure gradient (PG) more than 50 mmHg and a peak PG more than 80 mmHg. The mean PG is obtained by accurately tracing the outline of the flow velocity signal.

Due to pressure overload the LV responds to AS with myocardial fibrosis, concentric hypertrophy, and impaired diastolic relaxation. This is followed by systolic LV dilatation, and failure later in the disease process. Figure 2.8a demonstrates the pressure changes occurring during a typical cardiac cycle in AS. The transvalvular PG is only a reliable indicator of severity in the presence of good ventricular function. The PG will decrease if the LV function deteriorates in end stage disease. The typical pressure–volume loop of AS is shown in figure 2.8b.

The effective aortic valve area (AVA) is far less flow dependent than the pressure gradient, and should therefore be the index of choice for quantifying AS in the presence of abnormal flow rate or elevated blood pressure. AS is severe when the AVA is less than 0.8 cm^2. Systemic hypertension can modify the physical

Table 2.3 Types of aortic regurgitation

Type I: Normal appearing cusps with functional aortic annulus dilation	Type II: Cusp prolapse	Type III:
Ia: Distal ascending dilation (sinotubular junction)	Excess of cuspal tissue or commissural disruption	Cusp retraction and thickening
Ib: Proximal (Valsalva sinuses) & sinotubular junction dilation		
Ic: Isolated functional aortic annulus dilation		
Id: Cusp perforation & functional aortic annulus dilation		

Adapted from Khoury G et al., 'Functional classification of aortic root/valve abnormalities and their correlation with etiologies and surgical procedures', *Current Opinion in Cardiology*, 20, 2, pp. 115–121, copyright 2005, with permission from Wolters Kluwer

examination findings in patients with aortic stenosis and this can be misleading when quantifying stenosis severity.

The differential diagnosis of AS includes LVOT obstruction from a subaortic membrane or muscular subaortic stenosis, HOCM, and any form of supravalvular stenosis in the root or aorta.

Aortic regurgitation

Aetiology and classification of aortic regurgitation

Aortic regurgitation (AR) results from a primary valve lesion, an abnormal aortic root and/or ascending aorta, or a combination thereof. Primary valve lesions include calcific or rheumatic AV disease and infective endocarditis. Stenotic AV leaflets often incompletely coapt during diastole, leading to regurgitation. The most common cause of AR in developing countries is rheumatic disease, with clinical presentation in the second or third decade of life. In developed countries it is most frequently due to degenerative (aortic root dilatation) or congenital (bicuspid valve) causes with patients presenting in the fourth to sixth decades of life. The prevalence of AR increases with increasing age.

Although the severity of AR is certainly a consideration, identifying the mechanism of AR by transoesophageal echocardiography (TOE) may help the surgeon to distinguish those AV suitable for repair, from those that are chronic, fixed abnormalities requiring replacement. A functional classification for AR has been described to determine the mechanism of disease and to assist in AV surgical repair procedures (table 2.3) (8). The AV is viewed as a functional unit comprising the annulus, three cusps, sinuses of Valsalva, commissures, and the STJ. Competence of the valve unit depends on the integrity of all its components.

Infective endocarditis (IE) of the AV typically presents with mobile vegetations adherent to a damaged cusp. Vegetations are best visualized on the ventricular side of the valve as it prolapses into the LVOT during diastole. The diagnosis of AV prolapse is made when any part of a leaflet appears in the LVOT, below the level of the aortic annulus. As the endocarditis progresses, the cusps become further damaged resulting in more severe AR. Complications of IE include mycotic aneurysms of the aortic root or perivalvular abscesses. Both are identified relatively easily with TOE. In patients with pure AR, secondary to rheumatic disease, the essential lesion is retraction and thickening of the edges of the cusps with preservation of the hinge mechanism. The haemodynamic lesion may result in progressive aortic annulus dilatation, with worsening of the regurgitation over time.

Although the congenital bicuspid valve usually undergoes premature heavy calcification, a proportion of these patients present with severe regurgitation and pliable cusps. Valve repair may treat some of these patients. The bicuspid AV also predisposes patients to IE, leading to valve destruction and subsequent AR. Another form of congenital AR occurs when the AV is in close proximity to a perimembranous subarterial ventricular septal defect (VSD). In this situation there is usually a degree of prolapse, more commonly in the RCC, due to inadequate fibrous support and in some cases the Venturi effect of the VSD. On current evidence it is very important to repair the VSD and resuspend the prolapsing cusp in order to prevent rapid progression of AR. Quadricuspid AVs are rare, but significant aortic insufficiency is common with this lesion due to an uneven distribution of mechanical stress leading to incomplete cusp coaptation.

Aortic disease and aortic valve regurgitation

A dilated or abnormal aorta and aortic root may be because of hypertension, Marfan syndrome, trauma or aortic dissection. Figure 2.9a and b are 2D echocardiographic images of a dilated aortic root. Aneurysmal dilatation of the ascending aorta can cause AR, via a tethering effect on the cusps, without annular dilatation. Movsowitz and colleagues describe five potential mechanisms of AR in a patient with acute type A aortic dissection (9):

a. Incomplete closure of intrinsically normal leaflets, due to leaflet tethering by a dilated sinotubular junction.

b. A bicuspid aortic valve with associated leaflet prolapse unrelated to the dissection process.

c. Degenerative leaflet thickening resulting in abnormal coaptation.

d. Leaflet prolapse due to disruption of leaflet attachments by a dissection flap that extends below the sinotubular junction and into the aortic root.

e. Prolapse of the dissection flap through intrinsically normal leaflets that disrupts leaflet coaptation.

The first three of these mechanisms (a, b, c), may occur in patients without aortic dissection, while other patients will have more than one mechanism of AR. In aortic dissection the intimal flap prolapsing through the valve (the fifth mechanism), may keep the leaflets in an open position causing severe AR. However, sometimes the flap acts as a valve during diastole, with remarkably little AR even though the leaflets are open. The risk of aortic dissection or rupture increases in patients with a dilated aorta (diameter greater than 5.5 cm). The diameter of the ascending aorta should therefore be assessed routinely and any dilatation needs careful follow up.

Clinical features of aortic regurgitation

On clinical examination the patient with AR will have a characteristic decrescendo diastolic murmur (Austin Flint) and a third heart sound. This is due to an orifice in the valve, which allows regurgitant flow throughout diastole with subsequent rapid filling of the LV. With the increased left ventricular end-diastolic volume (LVEDV), there is an associated increase in the systolic flow across the valve,

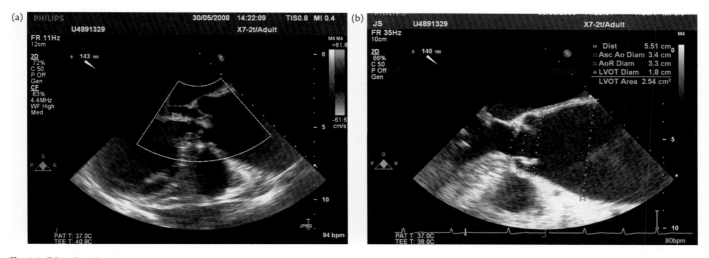

Fig. 2.9 Dilated aortic root.
(a) A 2D colour flow Doppler image illustrating a dilated aortic root and resultant functional aortic regurgitation. (b) A 2D transoesophageal echocardiography image showing increased measurements of a dilated aortic root. (See also figure in colour plates section)

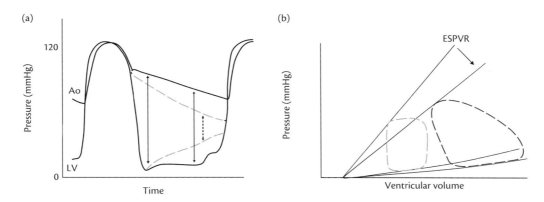

Fig. 2.10 Pathophysiological effects of aortic regurgitation.
(a) Cardiac cycle illustrating the elevated left ventricular diastolic pressures and decreased aortic diastolic pressures associated with aortic regurgitation leading to a decreased coronary perfusion pressure. (b) Illustration of pressure-volume loop with increased end-diastolic left ventricular volume and decreased myocardial end systolic elastance and contractility.

leading to a wide pulse pressure with a collapsing pulse and often an ejection systolic murmur. In AR there is both pressure and volume overload of the LV. The increase in left ventricular end-diastolic pressure (LVEDP) associated with AR is demonstrated on the typical cardiac cycle in figure 2.10a, and the increase in LVEDV can clearly be seen in the pressure-volume loop in figure 2.10b. The mainstay of AR assessment is based on the integration of the information obtained by 2D echocardiography, colour-flow Doppler, and pulsed- and continuous-wave Doppler studies.

Mitral valve

Mitral valve and annular anatomy

The MV is located between the LA and LV allowing unidirectional flow of blood towards the left ventricle (10). An anatomically normal MV taken from a pig heart can be seen in figure 2.11a. It prevents regurgitation of blood back into the LA during ventricular systole and allows unobstructed flow into the LV during diastole, maintaining low LA pressures. The anterior MV leaflet forms part

of the LVOT allowing an unobstructed ejection of blood during systole. The MV complex comprises the anterior (aortic) and posterior (mural) leaflets, the annulus, chordae tendineae, papillary muscles, and left ventricle. The successful functioning of all these structures is integrated to produce a competent MV, as can be seen on 3D echocardiography in figure 2.11b.

The two MV leaflets are separated by two commissures. The anterior leaflet is situated anterior and to the right, attached to the AV. In the normal heart, it occupies one third of the annular circumference and covers the whole valve area during systole. Both the AV and MV annulus contribute to the fibrous skeleton of the heart, connected by this aortomitral continuity. The posterior leaflet occupies the remaining two thirds of the MV annulus and appears much smaller than the anterior leaflet. Although they are similar in surface area the posterior leaflet has less height than the anterior leaflet. The posterior leaflet is subdivided by clefts into three scallops. Adjacent to the anterolateral commissure is P1, with P3 situated in close relation to the posteromedial commissure. Between P1 and P3 is the middle scallop, P2. The

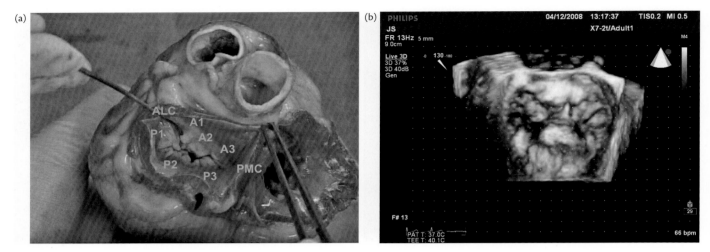

Fig. 2.11 Mitral valve.
(a) Porcine heart illustrating normal arrangement of MV anatomy. (b) 3D echocardiography image of a normal MV, seen en-face from the atrial side. (See also figure in colour plates section)

anterior leaflet is not divided anatomically into scallops but the areas opposing the posterior leaflet scallops are correspondingly referred to as segments A1, A2, and A3. Competent functioning of the MV requires apposition and coaptation of the two leaflets during systole. This occurs along a single semilunar coaptation line, with the commissures at each end of this coaptation line. These commissural areas are situated anterolaterally and posteromedially, in relation to their papillary muscles.

The MV annulus is shaped by lateral extensions of fibroelastic tissue, originating from the left and right fibrous trigones. While the anterior part of the annulus contributes to the fibrous skeleton, the inferolateral part has minimal fibrous support, making it most susceptible to dilatation. The anterior aortomitral fibrous continuity is situated between the two trigones. The mitral annulus is saddle-shaped with the commissural areas more towards the ventricle, and the intertrigonal and inferolateral areas located more towards the LA. The annulus opening is oval shaped with the intercommissural (intertrough) distance greater than the aortic to inferolateral (interpeak) distance. The valve is slightly tilted in the chest, with the anterior part superior to the inferolateral part.

Subvalvular anatomy

The subvalvular apparatus is made up of two papillary muscles, each with multiple chordae tendineae supporting the mitral valve leaflets. The posteromedial papillary muscle is next to the posteromedial commissure and interventricular septum. Unlike the TV, the MV has no direct septal leaflet connection to the interventricular septum. This is an important feature distinguishing the TV and MV in complex congenital pathology. There is usually a single coronary artery supplying blood to the posteromedial papillary muscle. Depending on dominance of the coronary circulation, it can be either a branch from the obtuse marginal artery, or a branch from the posterior descending artery. The anterolateral papillary muscle is found next to the anterolateral commissure and receives blood supply from both the circumflex artery via the first obtuse marginal artery, and from the first marginal artery, which is a branch of the left anterior descending artery. This makes ischaemic dysfunction of the anterolateral papillary muscle less likely.

Primary chordae tendineae connect the papillary muscles to the tips of the mitral valve leaflets. Secondary and tertiary chordae attach to the body and base of the leaflets respectively. During ventricular systole, contraction of the papillary muscles and left ventricle therefore prevents the MV leaflets from prolapsing into the LA. Dysfunction of either the papillary muscles or chordae can therefore cause MV dysfunction by preventing coaptation, either by allowing excessive motion or by restricting leaflet movement. The left ventricular myocardium determines the position of the papillary muscles relative to the mitral coaptation point. Dilatation alters this spatial relation moving the coaptation point deeper into the ventricle, resulting in inadequate coaptation and MV regurgitation. The LA is a continuum of the MV leaflets and annulus and so atrial dilatation can also affect leaflet function.

Mitral stenosis

Aetiology of mitral stenosis

By far the most common cause of mitral stenosis (MS) is rheumatic heart disease. Although the exact pathogenesis of rheumatic carditis is not fully understood, an autoimmune-mediated mechanism following an upper airway streptococcal infection is believed to be the cause. A combination of MS and MR is usually present and pure MS is less common. Disease in the younger age group is the result of a severe initial episode, while MS in the older age group is usually due to a milder initial episode of rheumatic carditis with a gradual progression of leaflet injury. Often the AV and TV are also involved.

Congenital MS may be defined as a developmental abnormality of the mitral leaflets, commissures, annulus, papillary muscles, chordae tendineae, or the immediate supravalvular area producing obstruction to LV inflow. It is usually associated with other left-sided heart defects and isolated congenital MS is very rare. Early recognition and treatment is important to prevent progressive pulmonary hypertension.

Other conditions can produce similar symptoms to that of MS. Partitioning of the LA by a fibromuscular membrane (cor triatriatum sinister or a supramitral membrane) may also result in the patient with severe pulmonary venous congestion. A LA mass,

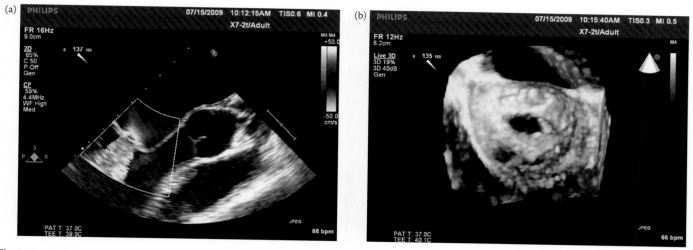

Fig. 2.12 Mitral stenosis.
(a) 2D colour flow Doppler transoesophageal echocardiography image illustrating decreased inflow across a stenotic mitral valve. (b) 3D echocardiography image of a stenotic calcified mitral valve with fused commissures and consequent reduced MV area, seen again from the left atrial side. (See also figure in colour plates section)

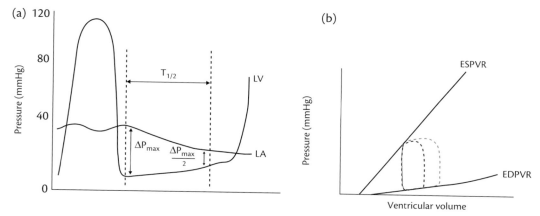

Fig. 2.13 Pathophysiological effects of mitral stenosis.
(a) Cardiac cycle of mitral stenosis illustrating the associated increase of left atrial pressure required in order to overcome the narrowed mitral orifice during diastole.
(b) Pressure-volume loop associated with mitral stenosis with a decreased left ventricular end diastolic volume and stroke volume.

for example a myxoma or thrombus, can prolapse through the MV and cause a mechanical obstruction to LV inflow.

Assessing severity of mitral stenosis

MS is defined as a mitral valve area (MVA) of less than 2 cm^2 (figure 2.12a, b). Severity of MS is categorized according to the MVA as mild 2 cm^2, moderate 1–2 cm^2 or severe/critical <1 cm^2. There are several methods to determine MVA. Each have advantages and disadvantages, and it is best to use more than one technique to confirm the severity of disease. Figure 2.12a shows a method of assessing MS using a colour Doppler flow placed across a stenotic MV. Symptoms typical of left-sided heart failure are usually present: dyspnoea on exertion, orthopnoea, and paroxysmal nocturnal dyspnoea. Haemoptysis, atrial fibrillation, symptoms of pulmonary hypertension, and right-sided failure occur with progressive disease. These symptoms stem from increased LA pressure and a fixed reduced CO, due to inflow obstruction of a small under-filled LV. Figure 2.12b is a 3D echocardiographic image

stenosis of the MV showing how blood flow into the LV from the LA would be impeded by the decreased valve area. The normal MV has a negligible diastolic transvalvular gradient (2–4 mmHg). This gradient increases with a progressive decrease in MVA, but is dependent upon the transvalvular flow rate.

As the severity of MS increases, the time it takes for the pressure between the LA and LV to equalize during diastole increases. The MV pressure half–time is the time in milliseconds that it takes for the peak pressure gradient to decrease by half. In a patient with MS, the peak transmitral pressure gradient is increased and the time it takes to reach half of the initial peak pressure is prolonged and consequently the pressure half-time is increased.

Figure 2.13a shows the pressure changes, in a cardiac cycle that result from MS. The LV pressure–volume relationship loop in MS is small and shifted to the left due to a combination of reduced LV pressure and volume load. The typical pressure–volume loop of MS can be seen in figure 2.13b. Ventricular filling is further reduced by an associated tachycardia or atrial

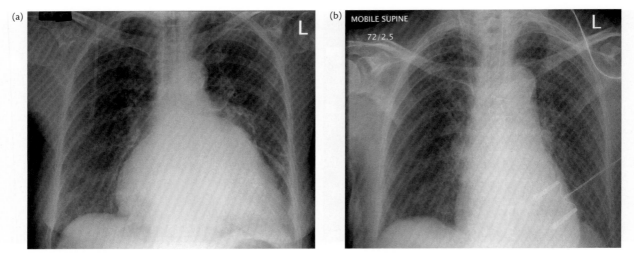

Fig. 2.14 Two chest X-ray images of a patient undergoing MV replacement.
(a) Mitralized heart on posterioanterior chest X-ray prior to surgical repair. (b) The same heart following mitral valve replacement.

fibrillation. Although it is commonly believed that the LV is protected in this condition and is of normal size, its systolic function may be depressed due to myocardial fibrosis and chronic underloading.

In severe MS there will be pulmonary hypertension and right ventricular involvement with some degree of TV regurgitation. The effects on cardiac function in a patient with MS undergoing MV replacement can be dramatic. This is well illustrated by the two chest X-rays in figure 2.14 a and b, one taken pre- and the other postoperatively.

Mitral regurgitation

Classification of mitral regurgitation

Regurgitation of the MV is relatively common in patients undergoing cardiac surgery. MR is either structural or functional, and is classified into three groups (11).

Type i. Dilated annulus with normal leaflet motion, but poor coaptation

Type I occurs in cardiomyopathy or post-myocardial infarction and usually results in a central mitral regurgitant jet. It has been suggested that isolated annular dilatation is a rare cause of structural MR, but an important component of functional MR. Figure 2.15a shows a 2D colour flow Doppler echocardiographic image demonstrating a typical regurgitant jet through the mitral valve.

Type ii. Excessive leaflet motion usually with prolapse and poor apposition

Prolapse is present when any portion of the MV moves above the mitral annulus during systole, while flail is defined as a free leaflet edge and torn chordae tendineae detected in the LA during systole. The MR jet will be eccentric and directed away from the diseased scallop. Type II is typical of the myxomatous degenerative MV. Figure 2.15b shows a 3D echocardiographic image of a typical prolapsing MV leaflet as seen from the LA.

Type iiia. Restricted leaflet motion due to rheumatic commissural fusion or chordal shortening

Type III is found in MR resulting from rheumatic heart disease and usually the jet is directed towards the diseased leaflet.

Type iiib. Restricted leaflet motion due to apical tethering or tenting of the leaflets

This functional MR is secondary to ventricular dilatation. The regurgitant jet is either central in the presence of global LV dysfunction, or occasionally eccentric if there is regional dilatation as for example, due to a LV aneurysm.

The major determinant of MR severity is the effective regurgitant orifice area, which may be fixed as occurs in rheumatic valve disease or MV prolapse or dynamic resulting from ischaemia induced or functional MR. The LA and LV compliance, concomitant AV pathology, and other factors all affect the regurgitant volume. Figure 2.16a illustrates the associated increase in left atrial pressure (LAP) on the cardiac cycle of MR.

Aetiology of mitral regurgitation

Myxomatous degeneration of the valve leaflets with prolapse is the most common cause of MR, with the posterior leaflet (P2–P3 scallops) more frequently involved than the anterior leaflet. If there is anterior leaflet prolapse present, it increases the complexity of the repair procedure. The myxomatous nature of the valve represents a connective tissue defect. The floppy MV with thickened, redundant leaflets, excessive movement, and chronic prolapse produces an increased strain on chordae, often leading to rupture. This MV defect is also associated with an increased risk of endocarditis.

Apart from those patients with rheumatic and myxomatous MV disease, between 10% and 40% of patients with a prior myocardial infarction have MR. Ischaemic MR can present due to several different mechanisms. The leaflets and subvalvular apparatus are typically either normal, in the presence of asymmetric annular dilatation (Type I) (11), or restricted during systole (Type IIIb) (11) due to LV dilatation and chordal tethering. More than one mechanism is often present.

During acute LV ischaemia, coaptation of the MV leaflets is significantly delayed in early systole and is termed 'loitering'. Although papillary muscle dysfunction may contribute to transient MR in patients with intermittent ischaemia, it does not explain the mechanism of functional MR and it has been suggested that the term 'papillary muscle dysfunction' be used

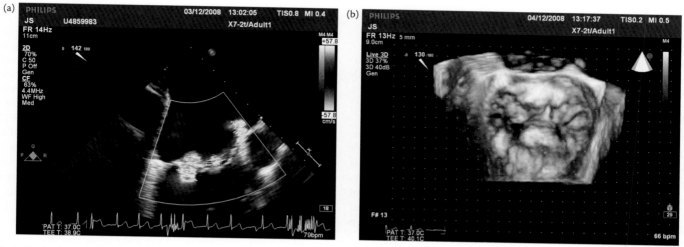

Fig. 2.15 Mitral regurgitation.

(a) 2D colour flow Doppler image of an anteriorly directed eccentric regurgitant jet of mitral regurgitation. (b) 3D echocardiography image of mitral valve posterior leaflet prolapse seen from the atrial side. (See also figure in colour plates section)

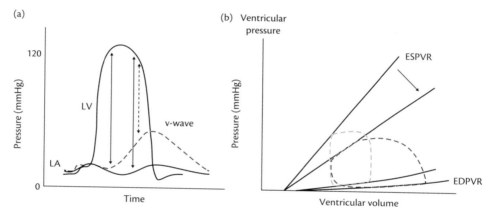

Fig. 2.16 Pathophysiological effects of mitral regurgitation.

(a) Cardiac cycle in mitral regurgitation with increased left atrial pressure during systole. (b) Pressure–volume loop associated with mitral regurgitation illustrating decreased end systolic elastance and contractility, with increased diastolic volumes.

with caution. Ischaemic MR is not only associated with severe symptoms and pulmonary hypertension, but also with a high mortality.

Functional MR occurs as a consequence of LV dilatation despite a structurally normal MV. MR causes pulmonary hypertension and LV volume overload, which in turn potentiates LV remodeling, which is a major determinant of outcome. The pressure–volume loop of MR is seen in figure 2.16b. The posterior part of the annulus is an integral part of the posterior and lateral walls of the LV and it may also dilate if the LV undergoes dilatation. The anterior part of the MV annulus forms part of the fibrous skeleton of the heart and can therefore not increase in dimension. It has, however, been suggested that the intertrigonal distance may increase in dilated cardiomyopathies. A small deformation in MV geometry after a large posterior infarction is sufficient to produce moderate to severe MR. The posteromedial papillary muscle is often displaced away from the anterior part of the annulus leading to restricted leaflet motion. Acute papillary muscle rupture is a catastrophic event and leads to severe MR.

Echocardiography is crucial in revealing features such as vegetations, abscesses and structural damage, such as a perforated leaflet. The echocardiographic presence of vegetations or perivalvular involvement confirms endocarditis, while its absence does not exclude it.

HOCM can lead to an abnormal anterior motion of the anterior leaflet of the MV onto the hypertrophic interventricular septum during systole. This leads to a high-pressure gradient across the LVOT, towards the end of systole. This abnormal motion of the anterior leaflet may lead to poor coaptation of the MV resulting in MR. This cardiac dysfunction is dependent upon LV loading conditions and contractility. Sometimes acute chordal rupture can be seen in a sub group of these patients, with associated severe MR.

Pulmonary valve

Pulmonary stenosis

The vast majority of cases of pulmonary stenosis are congenital in origin. More rarely, pulmonary stenosis may result from either rheumatic heart disease or carcinoid syndrome. Pulmonary stenosis may be anatomically classified as valvular, subvalvular, or supravalvular. The elevated pressure gradient across the stenosed pulmonary valve overloads the RV, resulting in right-sided failure. Long standing pulmonary stenosis can produce infundibular hypertrophy with right ventricular outflow tract obstruction.

Pulmonary regurgitation

Pulmonary regurgitation (PR) is associated with a number of conditions including carcinoid, rheumatic heart disease, connective tissue disorders, trauma and pulmonary embolism. PR is the most common acquired condition affecting the PV. Children undergoing surgery for congenital pulmonary stenosis or Tetralogy of Fallot may have their PV rendered incompetent by the surgical procedure. Long-standing PR results in progressive RV dilatation and volume overload with eventual RV failure.

Tricuspid valve

Tricuspid stenosis

Tricuspid stenosis (TS) is a rare valve lesion, affecting women more frequently than men, and is most commonly due to rheumatic heart disease. Like pulmonary stenosis and PR, TS may also be associated with carcinoid syndrome. Stenosis of the TV results in an increase in RA pressures with resultant signs of right heart failure namely hepatomegaly, ascites, and dependent oedema development. A stenotic TV results in decreased filling of the RV, this becomes particularly relevant once the TV area measures less than 1.5 cm^2.

Tricuspid regurgitation

Dilatation of the RV can result in a functional tricuspid regurgitation (TR). The most likely aetiology for RV dilatation is long standing pulmonary disease with associated pulmonary hypertension requiring increased RV pressure generation, resulting in eventual RV overload and dilatation. TR may also result from primary pathology of the TV, including rheumatic heart disease, IE, carcinoid syndrome or congenital abnormalities of the TV. A perpetuating cycle of TR may develop as chronic TR, resulting in further RV enlargement, and progressive RV systolic dysfunction occuring. The systolic dysfunction results in further RV chamber enlargement with the potential of worsening TR. Due to interventricular dependence, dysfunction of the RV may result in LV dysfunction due to interventricular septal displacement.

Pulmonary artery

The pulmonary trunk gives origin to the main pulmonary artery (PA), branching early into the right and left PAs. Another vessel the ductus arteriosus, which usually closes spontaneously after birth, originates from the pulmonary bifurcation and may be seen in neonates. The normal aortic arch is placed relatively superior to the pulmonary trunk bifurcation with the right PA passing underneath the arch.

Aorta

When the LV contracts the AV opens and blood is ejected into the aorta, the largest systemic artery. The aorta is a conducting vessel supplying oxygenated blood from the heart to the body.

Sections of the aorta

Proximally the aorta starts at the aortic root (as discussed in the section on the AV) and ends distally, at the iliac bifurcation (see Chapter 22). To distinguish the ascending aorta from the pulmonary trunk one needs to look at their branching patterns. The left and right coronary arteries are the only branches originating from the normal ascending aorta, with their ostia in the aortic root immediately distal to the AV. The aorta ascends from the root forming the arch (level T4, angle of Louis), which in normal anatomy has a leftward curve before continuing as the descending thoracic aorta, becoming the abdominal aorta before dividing into the iliac arteries supplying the lower limbs. The root and proximal ascending aorta is inside the pericardial sac, while the arch is extrapericardial in the superior mediastinum.

Branches of the aorta

The 'head vessels' that are the innominate artery and left common carotid artery, and left subclavian artery arise from the arch, in that order (see figure 22.1). The innominate artery, also called the brachiocephalic trunk, gives origin to the right carotid and right subclavian arteries. The isthmus is found immediately after the origin of the left subclavian artery at the beginning of the descending aorta, and is the most common site for congenital aortic coarctation. Because the relatively mobile ascending aorta and arch joins the less mobile descending aorta at the isthmus, it is often also the origin of a traumatic aortic dissection after a blunt deceleration insult. Between T9 and T12 the artery of Adamciewiz is an important branch supplying the spinal cord. Three other thoracic branches originate together from the lower thoracic aorta as the celiac plexus, including the hepatic artery, the splenic artery and the gastric artery.

Wall of the aorta

The aortic wall is composed of three layers: the intima, media, and adventitia. The intima is lined with a thin layer of endothelium, which is in direct contact with the circulation and is considered an additional organ because of its humoral activity. The thicker media layer is made of elastic tissue and is responsible for the aorta's compliance and strength. The collagenous adventitia layer contains a fine blood supply network called vasa vasorum. Aortic dissection most frequently results from an intimal tear with propagation of blood into the media. Intimal tears usually occur in the regions of the aorta subject to the greatest stress and pressure fluctuations (Chapter 22).

Cardiac tamponade

The pericardial sac surrounding the heart consists of two layers, the inner visceral layer adherent to the heart surface, and the outer parietal layer. When excess fluid collects between these two layers it compresses the heart and CO falls due to an inability of the myocardium to contract effectively. This is called cardiac tamponade, and may be present after cardiac surgical intervention or trauma (bloody collection), inflammation, malignancies, cardiac failure (serous clear fluid collection), or infections, such as tuberculosis.

The classical clinical description of cardiac tamponade is Beck's triad, present clinically in approximately 75% of cases, and consisting of hypotension, a raised jugular venous pressure (JVP) with a sharp diastolic collapse (Friedreich's sign), and muffled heart sounds. Other clinical signs include pulsus paradoxus,

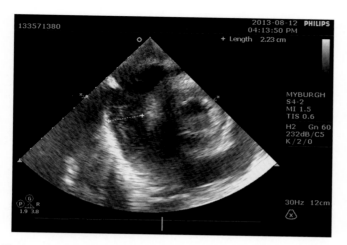

Fig. 2.17 Pericardial effusion.
Transgastric 2D transoesophageal echocardiographic image of a large pericardial effusion resulting in cardiac tamponade.

increased neck vein distension on inspiration (Kussmaul's sign), and dullness to percussion below the angle of the left scapula (Ewart's sign). Patients may complain of a variety of symptoms including chest pain or fullness, shortness of breath, cough, weakness, anorexia, or palpitations.

As cardiac tamponade develops, pressure increases in both the systemic and pulmonary venous systems in order to prevent collapse of the heart chambers. Stroke volume decreases as a result of the pressure changes and a compensatory increase in heart rate attempts to maintain CO. On-going fluid accumulation interferes with ventricular interdependence and filling, which may be clearly seen on echocardiography. Ventricular interdependence is compromised when a change in volume of one side of the heart results in the opposite effect on the other side of the heart and this causes the paradoxical pulse seen.

Investigations

Investigations that aid diagnosis include ECG, chest X-ray, and echocardiography. Echocardiography is the most useful tool for demonstrating the pericardial effusion and associated right-sided collapse seen on diastole, typical of tamponade (12,13). ECG complexes are typically of low voltage and the chest X-ray may show a large globular heart. Figure 2.17 shows a classic 2D echocardiographic image of a patient with cardiac tamponade secondary to a large pericardial effusion.

Treatment

Tamponade is an emergency requiring immediate removal of the effusion compromising the contractility of the heart. The effusion can be tapped via needle, catheter and syringe, or via conventional surgical approach. Re-accumulation can occur and may require pericardial fenestration (12).

Infective endocarditis

Introduction

IE remains a potentially life-threatening disease despite improvements in diagnostic technique, antibiotic therapy, and surgical interventions. Reports on the mortality of IE vary but it may be as high as 40%, with 15–25% mortality during the acute presentation and 30–40% within the first year. Without treatment the mortality of IE is 100%.

Accurate early diagnosis together with prompt planning and intervention gives patients the best chance of survival by limiting the severe complications of the disease (14). Diagnosis remains a challenge despite improvements in the sensitivity and specificity of modalities used.

Classification and pathogenesis of infective endocarditis

IE may be divided into four categories based upon the patient's valve status and history (table 2.4). In order for IE to develop two conditions must exist together: (i) an abnormal endocardium and (ii) infective organisms present in the bloodstream. An abnormality in the vascular endothelium creates areas of turbulence, promoting platelet adhesion and fibrin deposition and the development of a valvular lesion. These valvular lesions are demonstrable on both 2D and 3D echocardiography, as shown by the image of the vegetation affecting a TV in figure 2.18a and b. Infective organisms then infiltrate the thrombus resulting in the development of the characteristic infected thrombus of IE (15).

Diagnosis

The Duke Criteria published in 1994, have been extensively validated for the diagnosis of IE (table 2.5) (16). These criteria incorporate microbiological data and echocardiographic imaging, which together form the cornerstone of diagnosis, along with clinical and pathological information. Culture-negative IE may be due to recent antibiotic administration or due to other conditions such as Libman–Sacks endocarditis.

Definite diagnosis

Pathology or bacteriology of vegetations, major emboli, or intracardiac abscess specimen, or two major criteria, or one major and three minor criteria, or five minor criteria.

Possible diagnosis

One major and one minor criterion, or three minor criteria.

Table 2.4 Classification of infective endocarditis

Native valve infective endocarditis	Prosthetic valve infective endocarditis	Infective endocarditis in intravenous drug abusers	Nosocomial infective endocarditis
Classically associated with congenital heart disease	Subdivided into early and late presentation	Younger patients often no preceding valve disease	Central venous catheters and medical procedures often implicated.

(a)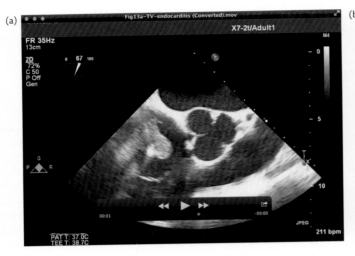

(b)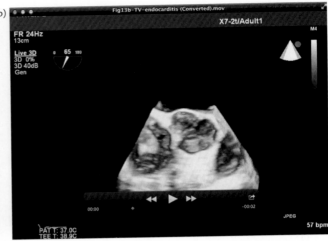

Fig. 2.18 Infective endocarditis.
(a) Large endocarditis vegetation in the right atrium involving the tricuspid valve. (b) 3D echocardiography image clearly demonstrating the same vegetations on the tricuspid valve. (See also figure in colour plates section)

Table 2.5 Duke criteria for diagnosis of infective endocarditis

Major criteria	Minor criteria
Blood culture	*Predisposition*
Positive culture with typical IE organisms	cardiac condition or intravenous drug use, and fever (temperature >38°C)
Persistently positive cultures >12hours part	
Endocardial involvement	*Vascular factors*
Positive IE echo	Major arterial emboli
Oscillating intracardiac mass	Septic pulmonary infarct
Perivalvular abscess	Mycotic aneurysms
Partial/ new dehiscence prosthetic valve	Intracranial haemorrhage
	Conjunctival haemorrhage
	Janeway's lesions
Endocardial involvement	*Immunological factors*
Worsening valvular regurgitation	Glomerulonephritis
	Oslers nodes
	Roth spots
	Rheumatoid factor
	Microbiology
	Positive blood culture not meeting major
	Criteria
	Echocardiography
	Consistent with disease but not meeting
	Major criteria

Reprinted from *The American Journal of Medicine*, **96**, 3, Durack DT et al., 'New criteria for diagnosis of infective endocarditis: utilization of specific echocardiographic findings', pp. 200–209, Copyright 1994, with permission from the Alliance for Academic Internal Medicine and Elsevier

Rejected diagnosis

Firm alternative diagnosis, or resolution of syndrome after less than 4 days of antibiotic therapy, or does not meet the previously mentioned criteria.

Management

Management is generally divided into either medical or surgical management depending on the presentation and underlying pathology. Antimicrobials form the basis of medical therapy and are chosen based on blood culture growth and sensitivity. Antimicrobial therapy is usually 4–6 weeks and response to treatment needs to be monitored on a clinical, cardiological and haematological basis. Surgery is considered necessary if there is extensive valve damage or prosthetic valve endocarditis, persistent infection despite antimicrobial therapy, embolization of vegetation, very large vegetation, perivalvular abscess, positive fungal cultures, or worsening cardiac failure (12).

Cardiac tumours

Primary cardiac tumours are rare, occurring in 0.15% of the population. Patients may have a tumour detected incidentally or present with symptoms relating to interference of normal anatomy by the tumour. Although this may not always be easy to do so, it is important to be able to differentiate anatomically normal structures visible on echo from cardiac tumours of the heart. Primary cardiac tumours originate from any cardiac tissue and are malignant in 25% of cases (17). The most common cardiac malignancies are myxomas, lipomas, and fibro-elastomas. In children the most common cardiac tumour is a rhabdomyoma. The WHO classification system for cardiac tumours (18) is shown in table 2.6.

Atrial myxoma

The most common presentation of a myxoma is a patient complaining of shortness of breath. On auscultation, MV flow murmurs

Table 2.6 WHO cardiac tumour classification

Primary benign tumours

1. Rhabdomyoma

2. Histiocytoid cardiomyopathy (hamartoma of mature cardiac myocytes)

3. Adult cellular rhabdomyoma

4. Cardiac myxoma

5. Papillary fibroelastoma

6. Haemangioma

7. Cardiac fibroma

8. Inflammatory myofibroblastic tumour

9. Lipoma

10. Cystic tumour of the atrioventricular node

Primary malignant tumours

1. Angiosarcoma

2. Epithelioidhemangio endothelioma

3. Malignant pleomorphic fibrous histiocytoma (MFH)/undifferentiated pleomorphic sarcoma

4. Fibrosarcoma and myxoid fibrosarcoma

5. Rhabdomyosarcoma

6. Leiomyosarcoma

7. Synovial sarcoma

8. Liposarcoma

9. Cardiac lymphomas

Travis WT et al., 'Pathology and genetics of tumours of the lung, pleura and heart: World Health Organisation Classification of tumours', IARC; 2004. Reproduced with permission from the World Health Organization

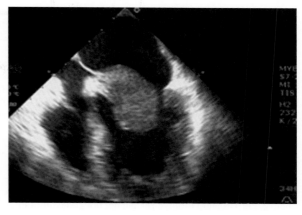

Fig. 2.19 Atrial myxoma.
A transoesophageal echocardiography midoesophageal 4-chamber view of a left atrial myxoma obstructing the mitral valve orifice during diastole.

and a typical diastolic plop may be heard. Myxomas are often benign solitary neoplasms, but multiple masses may occur. Figure 2.19 shows a single atrial myxoma involving the LA obtained with TOE.

Myxomas are pedunculated gelatinous masses projecting into the LA (75%), RA (20%), or elsewhere in the heart (5%). They may contain calcium or be secondarily infected. Proliferation is slow and they may resemble an organized clot on echocardiography imaging. Myxomas arise from undifferentiated cells in the fossa ovalis and are most prevalent in the 30–60-year-old population, with 75% of patients being female. Seven to 10% of cases are familial (autosomal dominant) and these patients may present with multiple myxomas.

Malignancies

Sarcomas are the most common primary malignant tumours of the heart. They can be present as a polyp or infiltrate the myocardium resulting in ventricular obstruction. Angiosarcomas mostly arise from the RA. They are rapidly spreading vascular tumours often extending into the mediastinum. Rhabdomyosarcomas can originate from any chamber and resemble striated muscle. They are

bulky, rapidly growing, and invasive. Pulmonary artery sarcomas are uncommon and remain the subject of case reports. They probably arise from the pulmonary trunk causing non-specific clinical symptoms of dyspnoea, chest pain, and cough. They may be commonly mistaken for other diseases, for example pulmonary embolism, allergy, or infection.

Cardiac lymphomas

Primary cardiac lymphomas account for 1.3% of primary cardiac tumours. They are the most common non-sarcomatous tumours, are usually large B-cell lymphomas, and occur most commonly in the RA. The presenting clinical feature is often that of systemic venous congestion.

Conclusion

Cardiac disease remains problematic in both the developed and developing world, each carrying their own burden and pattern of disease. With the increasing use of transthoracic and transoesophageal echocardiography in the diagnosis and assessment of cardiovascular disease, it is important that the cardiac anaesthetist has knowledge of the spatial origin of normal cardiac anatomy in order to maximize the potential of this technology. In addition, it is also important that they are able identify early acute cardiac pathology so that appropriate life-saving interventions can be employed. Whatever the disease, a good knowledge of normal cardiovascular anatomy allows the cardiac anaesthetist to better understand cardiovascular pathology and to predict its effects on a patient's particular clinical picture.

References

1. Ho SY, McCarthy KP, Josen M, Rigby ML. Anatomic–echocardiographic correlates: an introduction to normal and congenitally malformed hearts. *Heart* 2001; 86 Supplement 2:ii3–ii11

2. Richardson P, McKenna W, Bristow M, et al. Report of the 1995 World Health Organization/International Society and Federation of Cardiology Task Force on the definition and classification of cardiomyopathies. Circulation 1996; **93**: 841–2

3. Elliott P, Andersson B, Arbustini E, et al. Classification of the cardiomyopathies: a position statement from the European Society of Cardiology Working Group on myocardial and pericardial diseases. *Eur Heart J* 2008; **29**: 270–6

4. Maron BJ, Towbin JA, Thiene G, et al. Contemporary definitions and classification of the cardiomyopathies: an American Heart Association Scientific Statement from the Council of Clinical Cardiology, Heart Failure and Transplantation Committee. *Circulation* 2006; **113**: 1807–16

5. Luckie M, Khattar RS. Systolic anterior motion of the mitral valve-beyond hypertrophic cardiomyopathy. *Heart* 2008; 94 (11): 1383–85

6. Basso C, Corrado D, Marcus FI, Nava A, Thiene G. Arrhythmogenic right ventricular cardiomyopathy. *Lancet* 2009; **373**(9671): 1289–300

7. Swanevelder J.. Aortic valve disease. In: Feneck R, Kneeshaw J, Ranucci M eds. *Core Topics in Transesophageal Echocardiography*.. Cambridge, UK: Cambridge University Press, 2010; 73–107

8. Khoury G El, Glineur D, Rubay, J et al. Functional classification of aortic root/ valve abnormalities and their correlation with etiologies and surgical procedures. *Curr Opin Cardiol* 2005; **20**(2): 115–21

9. Movsowitz HD, Levine RA, Hilgenberg AD, Isselbacher EM.Transesophageal echocardiography description of the mechanisms of AR in acute Type A dissection: Implications for AV repair. *J Am Coll Cardiol* 2000; 36(3):884–90

10. Van der Westhuizen J, Swanevelder J. (2010) Mitral valve. In: Mathew JP, Swaminathan M, Ayoub CM, eds. *Clinical Review and Manual of Transesophageal Echocardiography*, 2nd edn. New York: McGraw-Hill Press, 2010; 143–71

11. Carpentier A, Deloche A, Dauptain J, et al. A new reconstructive operation for correction of mitral and tricuspid insufficiency. *J Thorac Cardiovasc Surg* 1971; **61**(1): 1–13

12. Camm AJ. Cardiovascular disease. In: Kumar P & Clarke M, eds. *Clinical Medicine*, 5th edn. London: WB Saunders, 2002; 701–832

13. Nussmeier NA, Hauser MC, Muhammad SF, Grigore AM, Searles BE. Anaesthesia for cardiac surgical procedures. In: Miller R, ed. *Anaesthesia*, 7th edn. London: Churchill Livingstone, 2010; 1889–975

14. Vinay K, Sachin L, Bonnie K, et al. Transthoracic and transesophageal echocardiography for the indication of suspected infective endocarditis: vegetations, blood cultures and imaging. *J Am Soc Echocardiograph* 2010; **23**(4): 396–402

15. Kneeshaw J, Feneck R. Practical issues in transesophageal echocardiography. In: Kneeshaw J, Feneck R, Ranucci M, eds.*Infective Endocarditis*. Chap 18 Section 2. Core Topics in Transesophageal Echocardiography. Cambridge, UK: Cambridge University Press, 2010; 294–309

16. Durack DT, Lukes AS, Bright DK. New criteria for diagnosis of infective endocarditis: utilization of specific echocardiographic findings. *Am J Med* 1994; **96**(3): 200–9

17. Shapiro L: Cardiac tumours: diagnosis and management. *Heart* 2001; **85**(2): 218–22.

18. Burke AP, Veinot JP, Loire R, et al Tumors of the heart. In: Travis WD, Brambilla E, Müller-Hermelink HK, Harris CC, eds. *Tumours of the Lung, Pleura, Thymus and Heart*. Lyon: JARC Press, 2004; 251–88

CHAPTER 3

Cardiovascular physiology, pathophysiology, and monitoring

Philip J. Peyton

Introduction

Anaesthesia for cardiothoracic surgery requires a thorough understanding of the principles of physiology and pathophysiology in both the systemic and pulmonary circulations. Cardiovascular monitoring is central to the safe delivery of cardiothoracic anaesthesia, and these principles and the evolving technologies and options for monitoring are discussed here.

Cardiovascular physiology

Systemic circulation

Comprehensive assessment of the haemodynamic status of a patient requires measurement of both pressure and flow, which then allows calculation of vascular resistance, which is determinant of ventricular afterload:

$$\text{Cardiac output} = (\text{MAP} - \text{CVP})/\text{SVR}$$

where MAP is mean arterial pressure, CVP is central venous pressure and SVR is systemic vascular resistance.

The interrelationship of these variables is depicted in figure 3.1, together with the interventions that can be used to influence each of them in the perioperative setting. Cardiac output, and the adequacy of global tissue perfusion, are dependent on factors influencing both ventricular preload and afterload. Each of these

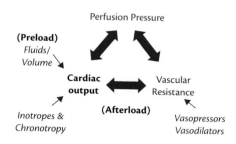

Fig. 3.1 Triad of critical haemodynamic variables.
The triad of critical variables in haemodynamic assessment of the patient and the interventions that are used to manipulate them. The principles are similar in the systemic and pulmonary circulations.

variables is amenable to manipulation independently or in combination to achieve homeostasis, in both the systemic and pulmonary circulations. In the setting of cardiac or pulmonary disease and surgery, factors such as myocardial ischaemia, vascular resistance, and valvular dysfunction can affect left and right ventricular function differently. For this reason, monitoring which provides measurement of critical variables on both systemic and pulmonary circulations is considered mandatory for complex cardiac surgery or patients with critical underlying illness.

Ventricular function

Pressure–volume relationships

The different functional characteristics of the left and right ventricles are indicated by their pressure–volume relationships, as shown in figure 3.2 (1). In contrast to the left ventricle, the thin-walled right ventricle is functionally designed to provide blood flow in a low resistance pulmonary circulation. Diastolic filling and right ventricular output is assisted by the tidal pressure changes that accompany physiological spontaneous breathing, and are less efficient in positive pressure ventilation. The right ventricle accommodates wide variations in venous return in the face of large changes in venous filling pressures, but its output is more afterload dependent than the left ventricle (2). Due to its thicker walled structure and the higher systolic and transmural pressures it generates, coronary perfusion in the left ventricle occurs predominantly during diastole. In contrast, due to its lower systolic pressure, right coronary perfusion occurs during both systole and diastole (figure 3.3) (3).

These differences can provide a particular challenge to the anaesthetist to optimize both left and right side circulations simultaneously. Attempts to alter preload or vascular resistance will generally affect left and right heart circulations in the same direction. For example, attempts to improve coronary perfusion pressure by increasing systemic blood pressure with fluid or vasopressor therapy will increase pulmonary arterial systolic and diastolic pressures as well. Right ventricular myocardial perfusion pressure suffers when right heart diastolic pressures become excessively elevated.

Ventricular interdependence

An important additional factor is ventricular interdependence. Under normal circumstances, with normal physiological

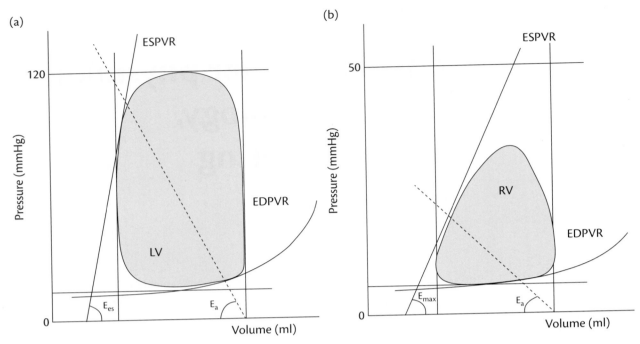

Fig. 3.2 Pressure volume loops for left (a) and right ventricles (b).
Pressure–volume loops for the left (a) and right (b) ventricles. Due to the relatively low pulmonary artery pressure, the isovolumetric contraction phase is very short in the RV. This explains the triangular shape of the RV pressure–volume loop, as opposed to the more rectangular LV loop. The less steep slope of the right ventricular end-diastolic pressure–volume relationship (EDPVR) derives from its higher compliance. The angle of the end-systolic pressure volume relationship (ESPVR) with the volume axis (maximum or E_{max} in the RV; end-systolic or E_{es} in the LV) is an index of ventricular contractility. The arterial elastance (Ea) is a measure of ventricular afterload.
Reproduced from Vandenheuvel MA, Bouchez S, Wouters PF, De Hert SG, 'A pathophysiological approach towards right ventricular function and failure', European Journal of Anaesthesiology, 30, 7, pp. 386–394, copyright 2013, with permission from European Society of Anaesthesiology and Wolters Kluwer Health

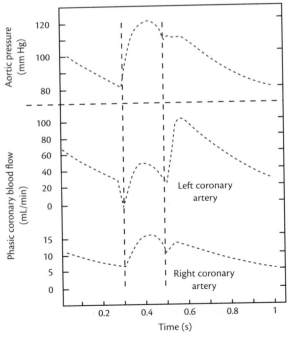

Fig. 3.3 Left and right coronary artery blood flows and their relationship to the cardiac cycle.
This figure was published in Kaplan's Cardiac Anesthesia, 5th edition, Joel A Kaplan et al. (eds), 'Chapter 5: Coronary Physiology and Atherosclerosis', O'Brien RM, Howard JN, p. 97, Copyright Elsevier 2006

propagation of electrical activity throughout the heart, right ventricular systole and ejection are assisted by contraction of the left ventricle and shortening of the thicker interventricular septal wall, which normally bulges into the crescent-shaped right ventricular cavity. Severe global or segmental septal left ventricular dysfunction will impair this, aggravated by the increased right ventricular afterload that accompanies raised left-sided preload. Conversely, severe right ventricular dysfunction and dilatation can impair left ventricular function directly by reverse bulging of the septum, due to the limitation imposed by the pericardium on anterior right ventricle distension ('pericardial restraint'), but which restricts left ventricular filling (figure 3.4). Asynchrony of ventricular contraction, due for example to extrinsic cardiac pacing, interferes further with this process and can reduce the effective stroke volume.

Diastolic function

Diastolic function is a major determinant of overall cardiac function. A substantial proportion of heart failure seen in clinical practice is primarily or partly due to diastolic dysfunction and has similar outcomes to systolic heart failure (5,6). Diastolic myocardial relaxation is an active energy and ATP-consuming process involving calcium return into the sarcoplasmic reticulum of the myocyte. Left ventricular hypertrophy due to hypertension, aortic valve disease, or hypertrophic cardiomyopathy, and ischaemic cardiac scarring or fibrosis, are the commonest associations. Less common causes include infiltrative conditions such as amyloidosis and haemochromatosis, and constrictive pericarditis (table 3.1).

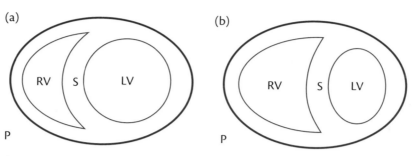

(a)　　　　　　　　　　　　　　　(b)

Fig. 3.4 Movement of the ventricular septum.
Leftward movement of the interventricular septum. (a) Position of the interventricular septum during systole in normal conditions. (b) Dilatation of the right ventricle, which moves the septum over into the cavity of the left ventricle at the end of prolonged right systole. LV, left ventricle; P, pericardium; RV, right ventricle; S, septum. Reproduced from Cecconi M, Johnston E, Rhodes A, 'What role does the right side of the heart play in circulation?', Critical Care, 2006, 10, Suppl 3, pp. S5, with permission from BioMed Central.

Table 3.1 Causes of systolic and diastolic ventricular dysfunction

Diastolic dysfunction	Systolic dysfunction
Hypertrophic heart disease	Ischaemic heart disease
Chronic systemic hypertension	Acute ischaemia
Aortic stenosis or coarctation	Chronic ischaemia
Hypertrophic cardiomyopathy	Valvular heart disease
Mitral or tricuspid stenosis	Hypertensive heart disease
Dilated cardiomyopathy	Left ventricle—systemic hypertension
Myocardial ischaemia	Right ventricle—pulmonary hypertension (see Table 3.2)
Chronic	Idiopathic dilated cardiomyopathy
Acute	Peripartum cardiomyopathy
Constrictive pericarditis	Drugs/ toxins (e.g. doxorubicin, adriamycin, alcohol)
Cardiac tamponade	
Restrictive/ infiltrative/ obliterative cardiomyopathies	Intracardiac shunting
Diabetes	Congenital heart disease
Amyloidosis	High-output cardiac failure
Haemochromatosis	Thyrotoxicosis
Endocardial fibroelastosis	Arteriovenous fistulae
	Paget's disease
	Pregnancy

Figure 3.5 depicts the changes in pressure–volume relationships that accompany left ventricular diastolic dysfunction. In systolic dysfunction, an increase in end diastolic pressure and volume preserves stroke volume despite the reduction in slope of the systolic pressure–volume curve that follows the reduction in contractility. In contrast, in diastolic dysfunction preservation of ventricular filling volume occurs only at the expense of higher filling pressures. The consequence for perioperative management is the requirement for higher left heart preload and filling pressures to maintain an adequate cardiac output and systemic blood pressure. Because increased heart rate is achieved largely through a reduction in diastolic filling time, patients with primary diastolic heart failure are often symptomatic only on exertion.

Pathophysiology of heart failure

The principal causes of systolic and diastolic heart failure are listed in table 3.1. These share some common pathophysiological features and mechanisms. Critical neurohormonal pathways are activated in heart failure. The sympathetic nervous system increases heart rate and contractility, and stimulates renin secretion from the juxtaglomerular apparatus of the kidney. This promotes release of aldosterone, which leads to sodium and water retention. Baroreceptors and osmotic stimuli promote vasopressin release from the hypothalamus, causing water retention via the collecting ducts of the nephron in the kidney. These effects are somewhat counterbalanced by the release of natriuretic peptides by cardiac myocytes in response to myocardial stretching. They promote systemic and pulmonary vasodilation, and sodium and water excretion, and suppression of other neurohormonal pathways.

Overall, these mechanisms increase circulating blood volume and cardiac preload to passively maintain stroke volume via the Frank–Starling relationship (figure 3.6), despite a falling ejection fraction. The slope of the curve is steeper where ventricular preload, estimated by either end-diastolic pressure or end-diastolic volume, is lower. At a point of optimal venous filling pressure, the slope becomes flat. Excessive filling beyond this point is associated in experimental models with ventricular stretch and reduced myocardial contractility. In the failing heart with reduced contractility, the slope is less and the point of optimal filling is pushed to the right. In contrast, in the presence of sympathetic stimulation and increased contractility, the slope is greater.

The failing left ventricle undergoes remodelling, consisting of dilatation and hypertrophy, by hypertrophy and elongation of myocardial cells. Left ventricular dilatation increases wall tension, lowers subendocardial myocardial coronary perfusion pressure and aggravates ischaemia, producing endothelial dysfunction, organ fibrosis, and arrhythmias. Dilation of the left ventricle causes dilatation of the mitral valve annulus and mitral regurgitation, which leads to a vicious circle of worsening cardiac dilatation, deteriorating cardiac output and coronary perfusion, increasing left ventricular filling pressures, and pulmonary congestion and oedema. A similar process ensues on the right side of the heart, with right ventricular overload and dilatation, and tricuspid dilatation and regurgitation, which can lead to progressive

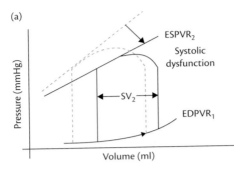 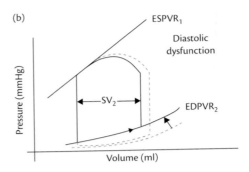

Fig. 3.5 Left ventricular pressure volume relationship in (a) systolic and (b) diastolic dysfunction.
The different pressure volume relationships in systolic and diastolic dysfunction. Normal ventricular filling is depicted by the dashed lines. (a) In patients with systolic dysfunction, a primary abnormality of contractility leads to a decrease in slope of the end-systolic pressure volume relationship (ESPVR) with resultant reduction in stroke volume (SV). Increased ventricular filling improves stroke volume at the expense of higher filling pressures. (b) In patients with diastolic dysfunction, increased ventricular stiffness in diastole is expressed as an increase in the slope of the end-diastolic pressure volume relationship (EDPVR), such that any given filling volume occurs only at the expense of higher filling pressures.
Reproduced from Desai A., 'Current understanding of heart failure with preserved ejection fraction', Current Opinion in Cardiology, 22, 6, pp. 578–585, copyright 2007, with permission from Wolters Kluwer

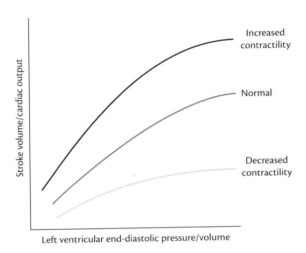

Fig. 3.6 Frank–Starling relationship of left ventricle.
The Frank–Starling relationship between ventricular preload and stroke volume for normal and sympathetically-stimulated hearts and for a heart with reduced contractility.

right heart failure, with hepatic congestion and 'cardiac cirrhosis' as a late sequela.

Pulmonary circulation

The systemic and pulmonary circulations operate in series. Increased awareness of this principle has led to a reappraisal of the critical importance of the right ventricle and pulmonary circulation in haemodynamic status and assessment. In the absence of intracardiac shunting, the pulmonary vascular system conducts the same volumetric blood flow as the systemic circulation

$$\text{Pulmonary blood flow} = (\text{MPAP} - \text{LAP})/\text{PVR}$$

where MPAP is mean pulmonary arterial pressure, LAP is left atrial pressure pressure and PVR is pulmonary vascular resistance. Clinically, LAP is estimated from pulmonary capillary wedge

pressure (PCWP) measurement using a balloon-tipped pulmonary artery catheter. Once floated into position (usually into the right pulmonary artery), balloon inflation leads to pulmonary artery occlusion so that pressure downstream of the occlusion will reflect LAP.

The pulmonary vascular system is a low pressure, low resistance and low volume system, whose primary function is to achieve adequate exchange of respiratory gases across the alveolar–capillary interface. Vital secondary functions of the pulmonary vascular system are to filter particulate matter and microthrombi from the systemic venous return to the heart, and a number of metabolic functions. These include the activity of angiotensin-converting enzyme (ACE) to convert angiotensin I to the potent vasoconstrictor angiotensin II, and to break down the powerful vasodilator bradykinin, as well as prostaglandin formation, serotonin regulation, and adenosine metabolism (8,9). The bronchial arteries from the aorta supply airways down to the terminal bronchioles and promote humidification and warming of respired gases by supplying heat to the airways. The bronchial circulation mixes to some extent with the pulmonary microcirculation and contributes to pulmonary shunt.

Pulmonary blood flow and ventilation

Pulmonary blood flow varies widely across the lung largely due to gravitational hydrostatic factors. Ideal gas exchange is achieved where blood flow and alveolar ventilation are closely matched to each other. This matching of ventilation-perfusion (V/Q) ratios is impaired in patients under a wide variety of conditions, including advancing age, lung disease, and during inhalational anaesthesia (10–15). The continuous gradations of V/Q ratios that exist across the lung can be measured using techniques such as the multiple inert gas elimination technique (16,17), or methods such as photon emission computed tomography using radiolabelled markers in inhaled gas and blood, which provide information about spatial or regional distributions (18). A new approach, which achieves this and can be used at the bedside, is electrical impedance tomography (19–21). Typical V/Q distributions in awake and anaesthetized states in a patient are shown in figure 3.7.

From a practical point of view the degree of scatter or heterogeneity in V/Q ratios across the lung is quantified by simplification of these distributions to a three-compartment model of V/Q

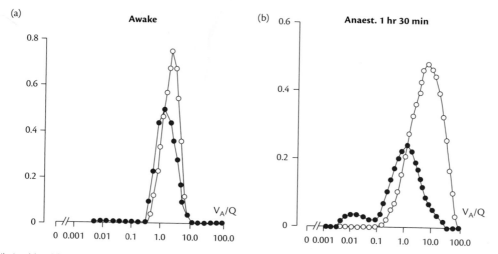

Fig. 3.7 Alveolar ventilation blood flow distribution.
Typical distributions of alveolar ventilation (V_A, hollow circles) and blood flow (Q, solid circles) in awake (a) and anaesthetized (b) states in a patient undergoing surgery under inhalational anaesthesia. The horizontal axis is ventilation/perfusion (V/Q) ratio of each of 25 lung compartments. The vertical axis is the blood flow or ventilation rate to each compartment (L/min). The loss of close matching of ventilation and blood flow and the development of regions of high and low V/Q ratios under inhalational anaesthesia can be seen.

Reproduced from Hedenstierna G, Lundh R, and Johansson H, 'Alveolar Stability during Anesthesia for Reconstructive Vascular Surgery in the Leg', Acta Anaesthesiologica Scandinavica, 27, 1, pp. 26–34, copyright 1983, The Scandinavian Society of Anaesthesiologists, published by Wiley, with permission

scatter. In this model, the contribution of lung units with high and low V/Q ratios to the overall limitation in gas exchange in the lung are summated and expressed as alveolar dead space and shunt respectively, where no gas exchange takes place. The remainder of the lung is considered as an imaginary 'ideal' compartment of uniform V/Q ratio where all gas exchange occurs. These simplified concepts are useful as they lend themselves to calculation using mixing equations requiring readily available measurements of carbon dioxide and oxygen partial pressure or concentration obtained from blood gas and expired gas sampling (table 3.6).

Pulmonary vascular resistance

PVR and the distribution of blood flow are heavily dependent on the degree of lung expansion. Compression or collapse of lung segments will reduce the diameter of intraparenchymal vessels, and shunt blood away from these regions. On the other hand, lung inflation will do the same to pulmonary capillaries. The net effect of varying degrees of lung inflation on overall PVR is depicted in figure 3.8.

Another factor influencing regional PVR and blood flow is hypoxic pulmonary vasoconstriction (HPV). In opposite fashion to the systemic microcirculation, hypoxic lung regions undergo vasoconstriction, to shunt blood away and optimize matching of ventilation and blood flow (figure 3.9). This is driven by the intrinsic specialized response to alveolar hypoxia of pulmonary arterial smooth muscle and endothelial cells, mediated by inhibition of mitochondrial oxidative phosphorylation (22,23). It occurs primarily at the level of the pre-capillary arterioles in response to reduced alveolar oxygen partial pressure. There is a possible influence of reduced oxygen tension in mixed venous blood which also surrounds these vessels, but the effect is unclear (24,25).

There is a progressive increase in vasoconstriction, as PaO_2 falls from 60–100 mmHg to as low as 5 mmHg. HPV is inhibited in a

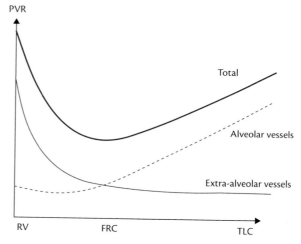

Fig. 3.8 Relationship between lung volume and pulmonary vascular resistance. Where PVR = pulmonary vascular resistance, RV = residual volume, FRC = functional residual capacity, TLC = total lung capacity.

Reproduced from Fischer LG, Van Aken H, and Bürkle H, 'Management of pulmonary hypertension: physiological and pharmacological considerations for anesthesiologists', Anesthesia and Analgesia, 96, 6, pp. 1603–1616, copyright 2003, with permission from International Anesthesia Research Society

dose-dependant manner by inhalational anaesthetics, which contributes toward the increase in V/Q scatter seen in anaesthetized patients. HPV contributes to pulmonary hypertension where generalized hypoxia is present. Other physiological factors that increase pulmonary vascular resistance, pulmonary arterial pressures, and right ventricular workload are hypercapnia, acidosis, catecholamines, and polycythaemia.

During one-lung ventilation for thoracic surgery, the increased pulmonary vascular resistance that follows collapse of the non-ventilated lung, gravitational diversion of blood to the

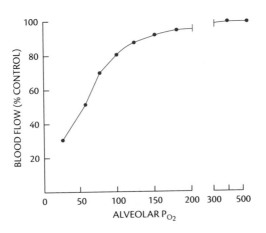

Fig. 3.9 Alveolar blood flow versus oxygen tension in the lung.
The effect of reducing alveolar oxygen tension (PO_2) on pulmonary blood flow in an animal model.
Reproduced from West JB, Respiratory Physiology—The Essentials, Fourth Edition, copyright 1990, with permission from Wolters Kluwer

ventilated lower lung in the lateral decubitus position, and HPV, all contribute to reducing the perfusion of the non-ventilated lung. In general, the upper or operative lung will share a smaller proportion of total pulmonary blood flow than its counterpart, due to the underlying surgical pathology. In combination, these factors limit pulmonary shunting during one-lung ventilation to levels that allow adequate arterial oxygenation in most patients (27,28).

Pulmonary hypertension

Pulmonary arterial hypertension (PAH) is a common condition encountered by the anaesthetist in the setting of cardiac surgery, and is a common co-morbidity in patients presenting with lung disease requiring thoracic surgery. A classification of the causes of pulmonary hypertension is listed in table 3.2 (29).

Pulmonary hypertension associated with left heart disease is reversible in its early stages but PAH becomes fixed with time due to vascular remodelling (30), and less responsive to vasodilator therapy. If progressive it is associated with right ventricular hypertrophy, dilatation and failure, due to the limited capacity

Table 3.2 Classification of the causes of pulmonary hypertension

1. Pulmonary arterial hypertension (PAH)

    Idiopathic PAH

    Familial PAH

    Associated with PAH

        Collagen vascular disease

        Congenital heart disease with systemic-to-pulmonary shunts

        Portal hypertension

        Drugs (e.g. protamine)

        Other—drugs and toxins, HIV infection, thyroid disorders, glycogen storage disease, Gaucher disease, hereditary haemorrhagic telangiectasia, haemoglobinopathies, myeloproliferative disorders, splenectomy

    Associated with significant venous or capillary involvement

        Pulmonary veno-occlusive disease

        Pulmonary capillary haemangiomatosis

        Persistent pulmonary hypertension of the newborn

2. Pulmonary venous hypertension associated with left heart disease

    Left-sided atrial or ventricular heart disease

    Left-sided valvular heart disease

3. Pulmonary hypertension associated with lung diseases and/or hypoxaemia

    Chronic obstructive pulmonary disease

    Interstitial lung disease

    Sleep-disordered breathing, alveolar hypoventilation disorders

    Chronic exposure to high altitude

    Developmental abnormalities

4. Pulmonary hypertension owing to thrombotic and/or embolic disease

    Thromboembolism, air or gas embolism, bone marrow/cement, amniotic fluid embolism

5. Miscellaneous

    Sarcoidosis, histiocytosis X, lymphangiomatosis, compression of pulmonary vessels

Adapted from Venice classification (2003) with additions relevant to perioperative care. Reprinted from *Journal of the American College of Cardiology,* **54**, 1, Simonneau G et al., 'Updated clinical classification of pulmonary hypertension', pp. S43–S54, Copyright 2009, with permission from the American College of Cardiology and Elsevier

of the right ventricle to cope with high afterload. Acute increases in pulmonary arterial pressures can follow pneumonectomy or extensive lung resection (more than 60% of the cross-sectional area of the pulmonary vasculature), which may precipitate right ventricular failure in patients with pre-existing PAH. Proper preoperative assessment of patients presenting for pneumonectomy should identify these patients as unsuitable for surgery.

During cardiac surgery, pulmonary artery pressures can be increased idiosyncratically by protamine administration after cardiopulmonary bypass (CPB) (31,32). CPB itself induces a number of adverse changes leading to endothelial dysfunction in the pulmonary circulation. Ischaemia–reperfusion injury, free radical formation and release of inflammatory mediators, pulmonary leukosequestration, and microemboli accumulation accompany increases in thromboxane and endothelin and reduction in prostacyclin and nitric oxide levels. These factors contribute to increased pulmonary artery pressures, and are worse with prolonged CPB and in the presence of hypoxia, hypercarbia, and acidosis, and the increased catecholamine levels that may occur after CPB.

Management of the failing right ventricle due to increasing pulmonary artery pressures is difficult. Vasodilator therapy may decrease systemic perfusion pressures more than pulmonary pressures, and compromise right ventricular coronary blood flow. Pulmonary vasodilators delivered selectively to the pulmonary circulation still suffer this limitation. Maintenance of systemic blood pressure and right ventricular perfusion pressure is considered to be critical in the successful management of right heart failure (33,34). Perioperative management involves optimization of oxygenation and lung inflation pressures with avoidance of excessive positive end-expiratory pressure, minimisation of hypercapnia, acidosis, hypothermia/shivering, and endogenous or extrinsic catecholamine release (22).

Cardiovascular monitoring

Electrocardiogram

Monitoring of the electrocardiogram (ECG) is non-invasive and continuous ECG monitoring is mandatory according to American Society of Anesthesiologists Standards for Basic Anesthetic Monitoring (35). Arrhythmias are common in cardiac surgery and can occur during manipulation of the heart or mediastinum during lung surgery. Monitoring of ECG changes and ongoing electrical quiescence is essential to ensure the effectiveness of delivery of cardioplegia during cardio-pulmonary bypass and cross-clamping, and subsequent cardioprotection. Monitoring of breakthrough electrical activity during aortic cross clamp in cardiac surgery is also important for this reason.

Patients undergoing cardiac interventions represent a high-risk group for underlying coronary artery disease and coronary ischaemia. An ECG configuration incorporating at least one precordial lead provides more information about regional myocardial ischaemia than does a simple three lead system, and should be routine in this group. The optimal choice of precordial lead placement is the subject of debate, but a large observational study found Lead V_4 was most sensitive to prolonged ischaemia resulting in infarction (36). ST segment analysis with display of trends should be available to help diagnose changes in regional myocardial perfusion. Changes of 0.1 mV (1 mm) or more are considered indicative of significant ischaemia (37).

Systemic arterial pressure

Almost all open intra-thoracic operations, and many endoscopic procedures, warrant invasive arterial blood pressure measurement via an indwelling arterial line. It is mandatory for surgery involving planned or potential CPB where a non-pulsatile circulation makes non-invasive measurement of blood pressure using an oscillotonometric cuff impossible. In addition, invasive arterial pressure monitoring allows frequent sampling of arterial blood for near-patient measurement of blood gas, acid–base, haemoglobin and electrolyte variables (see later), and heparinization, as well as potentially permitting use of less-invasive devices as an alternative for monitoring of ventricular preload and cardiac output.

Invasive arterial blood pressure measurement at multiple sites is required during surgery on the thoracic aorta where the continuity of the arterial tree is likely to be interrupted. Surgery or pathology that may extend beyond the ascending aorta requires separate cannulation and measurement of arterial pressure of both upper limbs. Surgery that involves the distal aortic arch or proximal descending aorta with cross-clamping at this point may include retrograde extracorporeal perfusion via a femoral arterial cannula, and requires additional cannulation of the contralateral femoral artery for measurement of perfusion pressure distal to the cross clamp (38). Simultaneous blood pressure measurement at these multiple sites provides crucial confirmation of the adequacy of perfusion distally from the extracorporeal arterial inflow. For example, equivalence of blood pressure measured in the right upper limb with femoral or left sided pressure confirms adequacy of circulation across the Circle of Willis during cross clamp or exclusion of the aortic arch (39). Discrepancies between pressures measured at two points which are expected to be in continuity suggest the possibility of malperfusion due, for example, to inadvertent perfusion of a false lumen in surgery for aortic dissection (38).

Central venous pressure

CVP provides a measure of right ventricular preload. Elevation of CVP may reflect right heart failure or tricuspid valve disease. The usefulness of a CVP measurement as an index of a patient's global volume status has been shown to be poor (40). Similarly, the correlation of change in CVP with fluid responsiveness, as measured by change in stroke volume or cardiac output in response to a fluid challenge has been shown to be poor (41–43). Insertion of a central venous catheter (CVC) using the internal jugular or subclavian vein nevertheless provides secure and reliable venous access for multiple drug and fluid infusions and is indicated for most major cardiac procedures or surgery in unstable or critically ill patients, particularly where a pulmonary artery catheter is not used. CVCs do, however, have associated complications (table 3.3) (44). Ultrasound guidance for placement of CVCs has been shown in meta-analysis to provide significantly higher success rates with fewer complications (45), and is recommended as the preferred method for insertion in adults and children in elective situations by National Institute for Health and Care Excellence (NICE) Guidelines (46).

Pulse pressure and stroke volume variation

The influence of ventricular preload on stroke volume is defined by the Frank–Starling relationship, and depicted in figure 3.6. The

Table 3.3 Complications of central venous and pulmonary artery catheterization (44)

Central venous catheterization

♦ Vascular trauma including arterial puncture and haematoma

♦ Nerve damage and Horner's syndrome

♦ Pneumothorax, haemothorax, chylothorax, hydrothorax

♦ Air embolism

♦ Catheter or wire shearing, knotting or embolism

♦ Arrhythmias

♦ Atrial or ventricular perforation or trauma to right heart valves

♦ Thromboembolism

♦ Catheter-related sepsis, including endocarditis.

Pulmonary artery catheterization

♦ All of the above, but a higher incidence of arrhythmias including bundle branch block and heart block

♦ Pulmonary artery rupture

♦ Haemoptysis

♦ Pulmonary infarction

Data from Dubensky D, AJC M. Central venous and pulmonary artery catheterization. In: Reich D, editor. Monitoring in Anesthesia and Perioperative Care. New York Cambridge University Press; 2011. p. 67–70.

slope is steeper at low preload, and at a point of optimal venous filling pressure, the slope becomes flat. Cyclical variations in ventricular preload caused by positive pressure ventilation cause synchronous changes in stroke volume due to this relationship. The magnitude of these variations depends on the slope of the Frank-Starling curve at the physiological point occupied by the patient. This pulse pressure variation (PPV) is reflected in the arterial pulse pressure measured via an arterial pressure line or in estimated stroke volume variation (SVV) obtained from devices that provide continuous beat to beat measurement of cardiac output. The variations are greater with low preload, and PPV and SVV have been increasingly used as dynamic markers of volume status. In general, PPV has been shown to be a considerably more reliable predictor of fluid responsiveness than a CVP measurement in ventilated patients (figure 3.10) (42,47). However, PPV and SVV are lower after sternotomy and the relationship between PPV and stroke volume is much weaker during open chest procedures than when the chest is closed (48).

The reliability of PPV or SVV is impaired by low tidal volume (less than 7 ml/kg), poor lung compliance, and arrhythmias (42,43,49,50). Atrial fibrillation makes the method unreliable with current algorithms. The predictive value of PPV is also poorer in patients with increased pulmonary artery pressures (51). A number of studies have attempted to validate a non-invasive equivalent using a finger plethysmographic waveform as a substitute for an invasive pressure trace (42,43,52).

Pulmonary artery catheterization

The pulmonary artery catheter (PAC) is among the most invasive monitoring tools used in clinical anaesthesia practice. The risks associated with placement and use of the PAC (table 3.3) include those associated with central venous cannulation. The additional specific risks of PAC include pulmonary artery rupture, pulmonary infarction, catheter knotting or trauma to right heart structures, thromboembolism and a higher incidence of arrythmias, as well as bundle branch block and heart block (53), and have called into question its use in patient management in critical care. Large observational and prospective case-matched studies have found similar or increased mortality in patients in the intensive care unit where a PAC was used (54,55), and worse outcomes have been found with PAC use after coronary artery surgery (56,57). While this finding has not been replicated in smaller randomized studies, no positive results have been found for outcome benefits of PAC based haemodynamic monitoring either (58) or to assist goal-directed therapy (59) in lower-risk cardiac surgery patients.

While use of the PAC has declined in recent years, its use in cardiac and aortic surgery remains routine in many centres (60,61). Its elective use for perioperative monitoring outside this setting is relatively uncommon, and American Society of Anesthesiologists Practice Guidelines (53) recommend that routine catheterization is generally inappropriate for low- or moderate-risk patients and is reserved for high-risk patients and/or procedures where there is a large chance of fluid changes or haemodynamic disturbances or other factors with high risk of morbidity and mortality, and where placement of the catheter and postoperative intensive care management by appropriately skilled staff is planned (table 3.4) (53). Placement of a PAC is more problematic in surgery involving one-lung anaesthesia, where floating the catheter tip into the operative lung may provide unreliable measurements of pressure and blood flow during lung deflation. Specific placement of the catheter tip into the non-operative lung, particularly where this is the left lung, can be difficult or impossible and is likely to require radiological guidance and confirmation of position using transoesophageal echocardiography (62,63).

Pulmonary circulation pressures

Measurement of pulmonary artery pressures via a PAC provides considerable additional information on the patient's cardiovascular status. PCWP measurement using a balloon-tipped catheter is a direct measurement of left ventricular preload. However, like CVP, PCWP is a static measurement, which has been shown to not predict fluid responsiveness in normal subjects or critically ill patients (64,65). Nevertheless, PCWP provides a more specific indication of left ventricular function than CVP. In high risk cardiac surgery where ventricular function is compromised, differential assessment of left and right heart function and preload assists the optimal choice of volume resuscitation and inotrope and vasodilator use.

PCWP measurement requires floating the catheter tip with balloon inflated into a pulmonary artery branch, until loss of pulse pressure indicates occlusion of the vessel. Left atrial filling pressure is measured at end expiration. The balloon must be deflated in between measurements to minimize the risk of thrombosis or pulmonary infarction, and should not be advanced with the balloon deflated or withdrawn with it inflated to avoid pulmonary artery damage. The catheter should be withdrawn slightly so that the tip sits in a larger branch to minimize the risk of perforation of the pulmonary artery, particularly when initiating CPB when the pulmonary circulation is emptied and the lungs are

Table 3.4 Practice Guidelines for Pulmonary Artery Catheterization, American Society of Anesthesiologists Task Force on Pulmonary Artery Catheterization

(a) Indications

- Patients at high risk (ASA 4 or 5) who have hemodynamic disturbances with a great chance of causing organ dysfunction or death e.g.
  - Significant coronary artery disease
  - Severe left or right ventricular dysfunction
  - Severe pulmonary hypertension
  - High requirement for inotropic or mechanical circulatory support
- Procedures that have a predictably large chance of fluid changes or haemodynamic disturbances or other factors with high risk of morbidity and mortality.
  - Complex cardiac surgery
  - Thoracic aortic surgery
  - Liver transplantation

(b) Contra-indications

- Absolute
  - Tricuspid or pulmonary valve stenosis or prosthesis
  - Right atrial or ventricular mass
  - Tetralogy of Fallot
- Relative
  - Recently placed endocardial pacing/defibrillator wires
  - Unstable ventricular arrythmias
  - Left bundle branch block

Data from ASA Task Force. Practice guidelines for pulmonary artery catheterization: an updated report by the American Society of Anesthesiologists Task Force on Pulmonary Artery Catheterization. *Anesthesiology* 2003; 99(4): 988–1014

allowed to deflate. Pulmonary artery perforation or rupture is a life-threatening complication of PAC use, with a reported incidence of 0.03–1.5% (53). These risks are minimized by avoidance of unnecessary balloon inflation and movement, and satisfactory monitoring of changes in left ventricular preload is usually achievable by tracking of mean or diastolic pulmonary artery pressures instead.

Venous oximetry

Manufacturers have adapted both PACs and CVCs to provide continuous measurement of haemoglobin oxygen saturation in mixed venous (SvO_2) and central venous ($ScvO_2$) blood respectively. These catheters require initial calibration, usually against a venous blood sample processed on a blood gas analyser. There is growing use of central venous and mixed venous oxygen saturations as markers of inadequate tissue oxygenation secondary to factors including decreased cardiac output and anaemia (66). Inadequate tissue oxygen delivery is associated with these venous saturations falling below 70%. Low venous saturations may have both management uses and long term prognostic value (66). Some, however, question the reliability of venous oxygen measurements as targets for goal-directed therapy during anaesthesia and sepsis (67).

Cardiac output measurement

Bolus thermodilution via a PAC is widely recognized as a clinical standard for measurement of pulmonary blood flow (PBF). Multiple boluses of usually 10 mL of either iced or room temperature crystalloid are injected, separated by a brief interval to allow dissipation of the thermal bolus and stabilization of the blood temperature, and then averaged. The reproducibility of the method under stable haemodynamic conditions has been shown to be good (68). Continuous thermodilution catheters deliver a warm thermal bolus signal instead from a heated coil, which sits proximally on the PAC and provides automated measurements that are updated at intervals of approximately one minute under stable conditions. Their accuracy and precision has been shown to be comparable to bolus thermodilution although individual measurements made by each method should not be considered identical or interchangeable (69,70).

Minimally invasive measurement of cardiac output

A number of technologies adapted to perioperative use are available for minimally invasive measurement of cardiac output (71). These include devices that derive stroke volume from interpretation of the pulse pressure waveform using a variety of algorithms, including the pulse contour approach (72). These devices estimate the compliance and resistance characteristics of the arterial tree from a calibration step of some kind. In some devices, this involves an indicator dilution method, such as a transpulmonary bolus thermodilution measurement or a lithium bolus injection and repeat calibration is recommended from time to time. One uncalibrated system uses a proprietary stochastic algorithm based on patient height, weight, age, and the shape of the pulse pressure waveform to estimate initial cardiac output and updates this continually during use (68). These devices deliver beat-to-beat monitoring of cardiac output.

Transthoracic electrical bio-impedance devices derive stroke volume from the changes in the electrical impedance characteristics of the thorax that occur with the changes in thoracic blood volume during the cardiac cycle (71). These systems have evolved to be resistant to interference by surgical diathermy and other sources of electrical interference. Bioreactance is an associated approach which uses phase shifts in oscillating current rather than changes in amplitude. Electrical velocimetry incorporates the cyclical change in conductivity that accompanies the change in orientation of erythrocytes that occurs from systole to diastole and interprets the maximum rate of change of bioimpedance to calculate cardiac output. Most systems use cutaneous electrodes placed on the chest wall, and a newer system uses a probe implanted in a specific endotracheal tube (73). They devices also deliver beat-to-beat monitoring of cardiac output, plus other derived variables such as estimates of extravascular lung water.

Partial carbon dioxide rebreathing is a method which employs the differential Fick principle applied to carbon dioxide elimination by the lungs (74). A brief change in alveolar ventilation is made using an automated partial rebreathing valve which temporarily increases serial deadspace in the breathing system and generates a brief fall in elimination rate and rise in end-tidal partial pressure of carbon dioxide. Its use is largely restricted to ventilated patients but is non-invasive in this group. Its accuracy and precision have been shown to be comparable to thermodilution during cardiac surgery and it has been shown to maintain its accuracy during one lung ventilation, but performs less reliably during spontaneous breathing such as during weaning from ventilatory support in the intensive care unit (75–79).

Table 3.5 Agreement between thermodilution and four generic methods for minimally invasive cardiac output measurement

Method (N studies)	n	Bias (L/min) Mean [+95% CI]	Precision L/min	Percentage error Mean [+ 95% CI]
Pulse contour (n = 24)	714	−0.00 [+ 0.09]	1.22	41.3 [+ 2.7] %
Oesophageal Doppler (n = 2)	57	−0.77 [+ 0.29]	1.07	42.1 [+ 9.9] %
Partial carbon dioxide rebreathing method (n = 8)	167	−0.05 [+ 0.17]	1.12	44.5 [+ 6.0] %
Trans-thoracic electrical bio-impedance (n = 13)	435	−0.10 [+ 0.11]	1.14	42.9 [+ 3.6] %

n = total number of pooled measurements; CIs = confidence intervals.

Percentage error = limits of agreement (1.96 SD)/mean cardiac output.

Precision = one standard deviation (1 SD) of the difference between paired measurements

Reproduced with permission from Peyton PJ and Chong SW, 'Minimally invasive measurement of cardiac output during surgery and critical care: a meta-analysis of accuracy and precision', *Anesthesiology*, 113, 5, pp. 1220–1235, copyright 2010, with permission from The Journal of the American Society of Anestheliologists, Inc.

Oesophageal Doppler devices are commonly used for perioperative stroke volume estimation in non-cardiac surgery but have undergone no validation in adult thoracic surgery to date (80,81). Despite their incompatibility with transoesophageal echocardiography probe placement during cardiac surgery, their use for optimization of haemodynamics in the post-cardiac surgery setting has been investigated (82).

The accuracy of these devices is commonly assessed by comparison with thermodilution. Animal and clinical studies have shown that these generic techniques have similar accuracy and precision to thermodilution in monitoring of cardiac output during unstable haemodynamics when compared to an invasive reference method such as an ultrasonic aortic flow probe (75,83). Their relative accuracy and precision has been compared in a recent meta-analysis using pooled weighted data from published studies in humans and shown to be very similar for all these approaches (table 3.5) (84).

Derived haemodynamic variables

Cardiac output measurement, in combination with arterial and atrial filling pressures, allows calculation of systemic vascular resistance (SVR) and pulmonary vascular resistance (PVR) (figure 3.1). In combination with measurements of oxygenation content of arterial and mixed venous blood, indices of the adequacy of oxygen delivery to body tissues can be calculated (table 3.6). This data allows the most appropriate combination

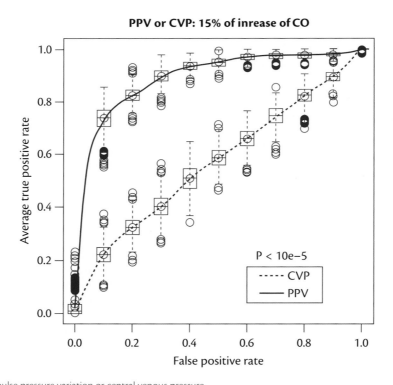

PPV or CVP: 15% of inrease of CO

P < 10e−5

----- CVP
——— PPV

Fig. 3.10 Fluid responsiveness and pulse pressure variation or central venous pressure.
Average receiver operator characteristics (ROC) curves representing the discriminative power of pulse pressure variation (PPV) and central venous pressure (CVP) to predict an increase of more than 15% of cardiac output (CO) after fluid loading.
Reproduced from Cannesson M, et al., 'Assessing the diagnostic accuracy of pulse pressure variations for the prediction of fluid responsiveness: a "gray zone" approach', Anesthesiology, 115, 2, pp. 231–241, copyright 2011, with permission from The Journal of the American Society of Anestheliologists, Inc.

Table 3.6 Derived haemodynamic and metabolic parameters in adults

Variable	Calculation	Reference range
Cardiac output (CO)	$= SV \times HR$	
Cardiac index (CI)	$= CO/BSA$	$2.5–4.0$ L/min/m^2
Stroke volume index (SVI)	$= SV/BSA$	$33–47$ mL/m^2
Systemic vascular resistance (SVR)	$= (MAP – CVP) \times 80/CO$	$80–120$ MPa.sec/m^3
Systemic vascular resistance index (SVRI)	$= (MAP – CVP) \times 80/CI$	$160–240$ MPa.sec/m^3/m^2
Pulmonary vascular resistance (PVR)	$= (MPAP – PCWP) \times 80/CO$	<15 MPa.sec/m^3
Pulmonary vascular resistance index (PVRI)	$= (MPAP – PCWP) \times 80/CI$	<30 MPa.sec/m^3/m^2
Left cardiac work index (LCWI)	$= 0.0136 \times (MAP – PCWP) \times CI$	$3.4–4.2$ kg.m/m^2
Left ventricular stroke work index (LVSWI)	$= 0.0136 \times (MAP – PCWP) \times SVI$	$50–62$ g.m/m^2
Right cardiac work index (RCWI)	$= 0.0136 \times (MPAP – CVP) \times CI$	$0.54–0.66$ kg.m/m^2
Right ventricular stroke work index (RVSWI)	$= 0.0136 \times (MPAP – CVP) \times SVI$	$5–10$ g.m/m^2
Oxygen delivery (DO$_2$)	$= CO \times CaO_2 \times 10$	$950–1150$ mL/min
Oxygen delivery index (DO$_2$I)	$= CO \times CaO_2 \times 10$/m^2	$500–600$ mL/min/m^2
Oxygen consumption (VO$_2$)	$= CO \times (CaO_2 – CvO_2) \times 10$	$200–250$ mL/min
Oxygen consumption index (VO$_2$I)	$= CO \times (CaO_2 – CvO_2) \times 10$/m^2	$102–160$ mL/min/m^2
Oxygen extraction ratio (O$_2$ER)	$= (CaO_2 – CvO_2)/ CaO_2 \times 100$	$22–30\%$
Pulmonary shunt fraction (Qs/Qt)	$= \dfrac{(Cc'O_2 – CaO_2) \times 100}{(Cc'O_2 – CvO_2)}$	$2–8\%$
Lung dead space fraction (VD/VT)	$= 1 – PECO_2/PaCO_2$	
Alveolar dead space fraction	$= 1 – PE'CO_2/PaCO_2$	

SV = Stroke volume; HR = Heart rate; BSA = Body surface area; MAP = Mean systemic arterial blood pressure; CVP = central venous pressure; MPAP = Mean pulmonary arterial pressure; PCWP = Pulmonary capillary wedge pressure; CaO$_2$ = Arterial oxygen content; CvO$_2$ = Mixed venous oxygen content; Cc'O$_2$ = Pulmonary end-capillary oxygen content; PECO$_2$ = Mixed expired carbon dioxide partial pressure; PE'CO$_2$ = End-expired (end-tidal) carbon dioxide partial pressure; PaCO$_2$ = systemic arterial carbon dioxide partial pressure.

Reproduced with kind permission from 'Normal Haemodynamic Parameters and Laboratory Values', Edwards Lifesciences LLC, Irvine, CA, USA.

of vasoconstrictor or vasodilator with volume resuscitation and inotrope to be made, and the responses to therapeutic interventions to be monitored. Devices for continuous measurement of stroke volume or cardiac output provide a ready means for assessing the response of the patient to an intervention such as fluid loading (fluid responsiveness). Where optimization of cardiac output and global organ perfusion is perceived as an important goal of patient management to attempt to improve perioperative outcomes, fluid responsiveness may be the most meaningful index of volume status (41,42,84).

Conclusion

Cardiovascular monitors are fundamental tools that enable us to routinely and safely conduct anaesthesia in patients with cardiac disease who are undergoing surgery within the thorax. However, to use them effectively one must have a sound understanding of the cardiovascular physiology and pathophysiology that they measure. Finally, we should be cautious when adopting new technology for cardiothoracic anaesthesia and first assess its effect on patient outcome, as even if it provides us with deeper insight into cardiovascular pathophysiology, a new monitor may not improve or worse, may adversely affect, patient outcome.

References

1. Vandenheuvel MA, Bouchez S, Wouters PF, De Hert SG. A pathophysiological approach towards right ventricular function and failure. *Eur J Anaesthesiol* 2013; **30**(7): 386–94
2. Johnson B, Adi A, Licina M, et al. Cardiac physiology. In: Kaplan JA, ed. *Kaplan's Cardiac Anesthesia* 5th edn. Philadelphia, PA: Saunders Elsevier, 2007; 84–5
3. O'Brien RM, Howard JN. Coronary physiology and atherosclerosis. In: Kaplan JA, ed. *Kaplan's Cardiac Anesthesia* 5th edn. Philadelphia, PA: Saunders Elsevier, 2007; 97
4. Cecconi M, Johnston E, Rhodes A. What role does the right side of the heart play in circulation? *Critical Care* 2006, **10**(Suppl 3): S5
5. Garg N, Senthilkumar A, Nusair MB, Goyal N, Garg RK, Alpert MA. Heart failure with a normal left ventricular ejection fraction: epidemiology, pathophysiology, diagnosis and management. *Am J Med Sci* 2013 Mar 14. [Epub ahead of print]
6. Gharacholou SM, Scott CG, Takahashi PY, et al. Left ventricular diastolic function and long-term outcomes in patients with normal exercise echocardiographic findings. *Am J Cardiol* 2013 Apr 20. doi: 10.1016/j.amjcard.2013.03.009. [Epub ahead of print]
7. Desai A. Current understanding of heart failure with preserved ejection fraction. *Curr Opin Cardiol* 2007; **22**(6): 578–85
8. Jhaveri RM, Johns RA. Metabolic and hormonal functions of the lung. In: Kaplan JA, Slinger PD, eds. *Thoracic Anesthesia*, 3rd edn. Philadelphia: Elsevier, 2003; 95–120

9. West JB. *Respiratory physiology—the essentials*, 4th edn. Ch 4 Blood flow and metabolism. Baltimore, MD: Williams and Wilkins, 1990

10. Rehder K, Knopp TJ, Sessler AD, Didier EP. Ventilation-perfusion relationship in young healthy awake and anesthetized-paralyzed man. *J Appl Physiol: Respirat Environ Exercise Physiol* 1979; **47**(4): 745–53

11. Bindislev L, Hedenstierna G, Santesson J, Gottlieb I, Carvallhas A. Ventilation-perfusion distribution during inhalation anesthesia. *Acta Anaesth Scand* 1981; **25**: 360–71

12. Hedenstierna G, Lundh R, Johansson H. Alveolar stability during anesthesia for reconstructive vascular surgery in the leg. *Acta Anaesth Scand* 1983; **27**: 26–34

13. Lundh R, Hedenstierna G: Ventilation-perfusion relationships during anesthesia and abdominal surgery. *Acta Anaesth Scand* 1983; **27**: 167–73

14. Lundh RG. Hedenstierna G. Ventilation-perfusion relationships during halothane anesthesia and mechanical ventilation. Effects of varying inspired oxygen concentration. *Acta Anaesth Scand* 1984; **28**: 191–8

15. Dueck R, Young I, Clausen J, Wagner PD. Altered distribution of pulmonary ventilation and blood flow following induction of inhalational anesthesia. *Anesthesiology* 1980; **52**: 113–25

16. Wagner PD, Lavaruso RB, Uhl RR, West JB: Continuous distributions of ventilation-perfusion ratios in normal subjects breathing air and 100% O_2. *J Clin Invest* 1974; **54**: 54–68

17. Wagner PD. The multiple inert gas elimination technique (MIGET). *Intensive Care Med* 2008; **34**: 994–1001

18. Nyrén S, Radell P, Mure M, et al. Inhalation anesthesia increases V/Q regional heterogeneity during spontaneous breathing in healthy subjects. *Anesthesiology.* 2010; **113**(6): 1370–5

19. Steffen Leonhardt S, Lachmann B. Electrical impedance tomography: the holy grail of ventilation and perfusion monitoring? *Intensive Care Med* 2012; **38**: 1917–29

20. Radke OC, Schneider T, Heller A, Koch T. Spontaneous breathing during general anesthesia prevents the ventral redistribution of ventilation as detected by electrical impedance tomography: A randomized trial. *Anesthesiology* 2012; **116**: 1227–34

21. Canet J, Gallart L. The dark side of the lung: unveiling regional lung ventilation with electrical impedance tomography. *Anesthesiology* 2012; **116**: 1186–8

22. Fischer LG, Van Aken H, Bürkle H. Management of pulmonary hypertension: physiological and pharmacological considerations for anesthesiologists. *Anesth Analg* 2003; **96**(6): 1603–16

23. Evans AM, Hardie DG, Peers C, Mahmoud A. Hypoxic pulmonary vasoconstriction: mechanisms of oxygen-sensing. *Curr Opin Anaesthesiol* 2011; **24**(1): 13–20

24. Gal TJ. Anatomy and physiology of the respiratory system and pulmonary circulation. In: Kaplan JA, Slinger PD, eds.*Thoracic Anesthesia*, 3rd edn. Philadelphia: Elsevier, 2003; 68–9

25. Pellett AA, Cairo JM, Levitzky MG. Hypoxemia and hypoxic pulmonary vasoconstriction: autonomic nervous system versus mixed venous PO_2. *Respir Physiol* 1997;**109**(3): 249–60

26. West JB. *Respiratory physiology—the essentials*, 4th edn. Ch 4 Blood Flow and Metabolism. Baltimore, MD: Williams and Wilkins, 1990

27. Benumof JL. One-lung ventilation and hypoxic pulmonary vasoconstriction: Implications for anesthetic management. *Anesth Analg* 1985; **64**: 821–33

28. Karzai W, Schwarzkopf K. Hypoxemia during one-lung ventilation: prediction, prevention, and treatment. *Anesthesiology* 2009; **110**(6): 1402–11

29. Simonneau G, Robbins IM, Beghetti M, et al. Updated clinical classification of pulmonary hypertension. *J Am Coll Cardiol* 2009; **54**: S43–54

30. Stenmark KR, Mecham RP. Cellular and molecular mechanisms of pulmonary vascular remodeling. *Ann Rev Physiol* 1997; **59**: 89–144

31. Lowenstein E, Johnston WE, Lappas DG, et al. Catastrophic pulmonary vasoconstriction associated with protamine reversal of heparin. *Anesthesiology* 1983; **59**: 470–3

32. Conahan TJ, Andrews RW, MacVaugh H. Cardiovascular effects of protamine sulfate in man. *Anesth Analg* 1981; **60**(1): 33–6

33. Vlahakes GJ. Management of pulmonary hypertension and right ventricular failure: another step forward. *Ann Thorac Surg* 1996; **61**: 1051–2

34. Vlahakes GJ, Turley K, Hoffman JI. The pathophysiology of failure in acute right ventricular hypertension: hemodynamic and biochemical correlations. *Circulation* 1981; **63**: 87–95

35. American Society of Anesthesiologists. Standards for Basic Anesthetic Monitoring. 2011 [updated 2011; cited]; Available from: http://www.asahq.org/For-Members/Standards-Guidelines-and-Statements.aspx (accessed 8 May 2014)

36. Landesberg G, Mosseri M, Wolf Y, Vesselov Y, Weissman C. Perioperative myocardial ischemia and infarction: identification by continuous 12-lead electrocardiogram with online ST-segment monitoring. *Anesthesiology* 2002; **96**(2): 264–70

37. Mittnacht A, London M. Electrocardiography. In: Reich D, ed. *Monitoring in Anesthesia and Perioperative Care.* New York: Cambridge University Press, 2011; 39–40

38. Harrington DK, Ranasinghe AM, Shah A, Oelofse T, Bonser RS. Recommendations for haemodynamic and neurological monitoring in repair of acute type A aortic dissection. *Anesthesiol Res Pract* 2011; **2011**: 949034.

39. Merkkola P, Tulla H, Ronkainen A, et al. Incomplete circle of Willis and right axillary artery perfusion. *Ann Thorac Surg* 2006; **82**(1): 74–9

40. Marik PE, Baram M, Vahid B. Does central venous pressure predict fluid responsiveness? A systematic review of the literature and the tale of seven mares. *Chest* 2008; **134**(1): 172–8

41. Marik PE, Rodrigo C. Does the central venous pressure predict fluid responsiveness? An updated meta-analysis and a plea for some common sense. *Crit Care Med* 2013; **41**(7): 1774–81

42. Cannesson M, Le Manach Y, Hofer CK, et al. Assessing the diagnostic accuracy of pulse pressure variations for the prediction of fluid responsiveness: a 'gray zone' approach. *Anesthesiology* 2011; **115**(2): 231–41

43. Cannesson M, Aboy M, Hofer CK, Rehman M. Pulse pressure variation: where are we today? *J Clin Monit Comput.* 2011; **25**(1): 45–56

44. Dubensky D, AJC M. Central venous and pulmonary artery catheterization. In: Reich D, ed. *Monitoring in Anesthesia and Perioperative Care.* New York: Cambridge University Press, 2011; 67–70

45. Keenan SP. Use of ultrasound to place central lines. *J Crit Care* 2002; **17**(2): 126–37.

46. National Institutes for Clinical Excellence. Guidance on the use of ultrasound locating devices for placing central venous catheters. Technology Appraisal Guidance—No. 49. 2002 [updated 2002; cited 10 March, 2011]; Available from: http://www.nice.org.uk/nicemedia/live/11474/32461/32461.pdf (accessed 8 May 2014).

47. Zhang Z, Lu B, Sheng X, Jin N. Accuracy of stroke volume variation in predicting fluid responsiveness: a systematic review and meta-analysis. *J Anesth* 2010; **25**(6): 904–16

48. Rex S, Schalte G, Schroth S, et al. Limitations of arterial pulse pressure variation and left ventricular stroke volume variation in estimating cardiac pre-load during open heart surgery. *Acta Anaesthesiol Scand* 2007; **51**(9): 1258–67

49. Lansdorp B, Lemson J, van Putten MJ, et al. Dynamic indices do not predict volume responsiveness in routine clinical practice. *Br J Anaesth* 2012; **108**(3): 395–401

50. Monnet X, Bleibtreu A, Ferre A, et al. Passive leg-raising and end-expiratory occlusion tests perform better than pulse pressure variation in patients with low respiratory system compliance. *Crit Care Med* 2012; **40**(1): 152–7

51. Wyler von Ballmoos M, Takala J, et al. Pulse-pressure variation and hemodynamic response in patients with elevated pulmonary artery pressure: a clinical study. *Crit Care* 2010; **14**(3): R111

52. Zimmermann M, Feibicke T, Keyl C, et al. Accuracy of stroke volume variation compared with pleth variability index to predict fluid responsiveness in mechanically ventilated patients undergoing major surgery. *Eur J Anaesthesiol* 2011; **27**(6): 555–61

53. ASA Task Force. Practice guidelines for pulmonary artery catheterization: an updated report by the American Society of Anesthesiologists Task Force on Pulmonary Artery Catheterization. *Anesthesiology* 2003; **99**(4): 988–1014

54. Connors AF, Jr., Speroff T, Dawson NV, et al. The effectiveness of right heart catheterization in the initial care of critically ill patients. SUPPORT Investigators. *JAMA* 1996; **276**(11): 889–97

55. Sakr Y, Vincent JL, Reinhart K, et al. Use of the pulmonary artery catheter is not associated with worse outcome in the ICU. *Chest* 2005; **128**(4): 2722–31

56. Ramsey SD, Saint S, Sullivan SD, Dey L, Kelley K, Bowdle A. Clinical and economic effects of pulmonary artery catheterization in non-emergent coronary artery bypass graft surgery. *J Cardiothorac Vasc Anesth* 2000; **14**(2): 113–8

57. Schwann NM, Hillel Z, Hoeft A, et al. Lack of effectiveness of the pulmonary artery catheter in cardiac surgery. *Anesth Analg* 2011; **113**(5): 994–1002

58. Pearson KS, Gomez MN, Moyers JR, Carter JG, Tinker JH. A cost/benefit analysis of randomized invasive monitoring for patients undergoing cardiac surgery. *Anesth Analg* 1989; **69**(3): 336–41

59. Polonen P, Ruokonen E, Hippelainen M, Poyhonen M, Takala J. A prospective, randomized study of goal-oriented hemodynamic therapy in cardiac surgical patients. *Anesth Analg* 2000; **90**(5): 1052–9

60. Wiener RS, Welch HG. Trends in the use of the pulmonary artery catheter in the United States, 1993–2004. *JAMA* 2007; **298**(4): 423–9

61. Jacka MJ, Cohen MM, To T, Devitt JH, Byrick R. The use of and preferences for the transesophageal echocardiogram and pulmonary artery catheter among cardiovascular anesthesiologists. *Anesth Analg* 2002; **94**(5): 1065–71, table of contents

62. Safran D, Journois D, Hubsch JP, Castelain MH, Barrier G. [Continuous monitoring of mixed venous oxygen saturation in anesthesia in pulmonary surgery]. *Ann Fr Anesth Reanim* 1989; **8**(6): 682–7

63. Benumof JL, Saidman LJ, Arkin DB, Diamant M. Where pulmonary arterial catheters go: intrathoracic distribution. *Anesthesiology* 1977; **46**(5): 336–8

64. Kumar A, Anel R, Bunnell E, et al. Pulmonary artery occlusion pressure and central venous pressure fail to predict ventricular filling volume, cardiac performance, or the response to volume infusion in normal subjects. *Crit Care Med* 2004; **32**(3): 691–9

65. Osman D, Ridel C, Ray P, et al. Cardiac filling pressures are not appropriate to predict hemodynamic response to volume challenge. *Crit Care Med* 2007; **35**(1): 64–8

66. van Beest P, Wietasch G, Scheeren T, Spronk P, Kuiper M. Clinical review: use of venous oxygen saturations as a goal—a yet unfinished puzzle. *Crit Care* 2011; **15**(5): 232

67. Della Rocca G, Pompei L. Goal-directed therapy in anesthesia: any clinical impact or just a fashion? *Minerva Anestesiol* 2011; **77**(5): 545–53

68. Peyton PJ, Chong SW. Minimally invasive measurement of cardiac output during surgery and critical care: a meta-analysis of accuracy and precision. *Anesthesiology* 2010; **113**(5): 1220–35

69. Della Rocca G, Costa MG, Pompei L, Coccia C, Pietropaoli P. Continuous and intermittent cardiac output measurement: pulmonary artery catheter versus aortic transpulmonary technique. *Br J Anaesth* 2002; **88**(3): 350–6

70. Bendjelid K, Schutz N, Suter PM, Romand JA. Continuous cardiac output monitoring after cardiopulmonary bypass: a comparison with bolus thermodilution measurement. *Intensive Care Med* 2006; **32**(6): 919–22

71. Funk DJ, Moretti EW, Gan TJ. Minimally invasive cardiac output monitoring in the perioperative setting. *Anesth Analg* 2009; **108**(3): 887–97

72. Montenij LJ, de Waal EE, Buhre WF. Arterial waveform analysis in anesthesia and critical care. *Curr Opin Anaesthesiol* 2011; **24**(6): 651–6

73. Maus TM, Reber B, Banks DA, Berry A, Guerrero E, Manecke GR. Cardiac output determination from endotracheally measured impedance cardiography: clinical evaluation of endotracheal cardiac output monitor. *J Cardiothorac Vasc Anesth* 2011; **25**(5): 770–5

74. Jaffe MB. Partial CO_2 rebreathing cardiac output—operating principles of the NICO system. *J Clin Monit Comput.* 1999; **15**(6): 387–401

75. Botero M, Kirby D, Lobato EB, Staples ED, Gravenstein N. Measurement of cardiac output before and after cardiopulmonary bypass: Comparison among aortic transit-time ultrasound, thermodilution, and noninvasive partial CO2 rebreathing. *J Cardiothorac Vasc Anesth* 2004; **18**(5): 563–72

76. Gueret G, Kiss G, Rossignol B, et al. Cardiac output measurements in off-pump coronary surgery: comparison between NICO and the Swan-Ganz catheter. *Eur J Anaesthesiol* 2006; **23**(10): 848–54

77. Ng JM, Chow MY, Ip-Yam PC, Goh MH, Agasthian T. Evaluation of partial carbon dioxide rebreathing cardiac output measurement during thoracic surgery. *J Cardiothorac Vasc Anesth* 2007; **21**(5): 655–8

78. Tachibana K, Imanaka H, Takeuchi M, Takauchi Y, Miyano H, Nishimura M. Noninvasive cardiac output measurement using partial carbon dioxide rebreathing is less accurate at settings of reduced minute ventilation and when spontaneous breathing is present. *Anesthesiology* 2003; **98**: 830–7

79. Tachibana K, Imanaka H, Miyano H, Takeuchi M, Kumon K, Nishimura M. Effect of ventilatory settings on accuracy of cardiac output measurement using partial CO_2 rebreathing. *Anesthesiology* 2002; **96**: 96–102

80. Schober P, Loer SA, Schwarte LA. Transesophageal Doppler devices: A technical review. *J Clin Monit Comput* 2009; **23**(6): 391–401

81. Schober P, Loer SA, Schwarte LA. Perioperative hemodynamic monitoring with transesophageal Doppler technology. *Anesth Analg* 2009; **109**(2): 340–53

82. McKendry M, McGloin H, Saberi D, Caudwell L, Brady AR, Singer M. Randomised controlled trial assessing the impact of a nurse delivered, flow monitored protocol for optimisation of circulatory status after cardiac surgery. *Br Med J* 2004; **329**(7460): 258

83. Bajorat J, Hofmockel R, Vagts DA, et al. Comparison of invasive and less-invasive techniques of cardiac output measurement under different haemodynamic conditions in a pig model. *Eur J Anaesthesiol* 2006; **23**(1): 23–30

84. Gurgel ST, do Nascimento P, Jr. Maintaining tissue perfusion in high-risk surgical patients: a systematic review of randomized clinical trials. *Anesth Analg* 2011; **112**(6): 1384–91

CHAPTER 4

Thoracic anatomy, physiology, and pathophysiology

David J. R. Duthie

Introduction

Patients presenting for thoracic anaesthesia often look older than their age and commonly have smoking-related co-morbidities and a burden of cancer. Moreover, intrathoracic surgery is a substantial surgical stress, during which the risk of severe haemorrhage is ever-present. After surgery, pain from a thoracotomy wound is often severe. In addition, the shared airway during rigid bronchoscopy and the need for lung isolation and one-lung anaesthesia are technically demanding. For these reasons, a good understanding of the anatomy, physiology, and pathophysiology of the chest provide the foundation for planning and dealing with eventualities that arise during thoracic anaesthesia.

Anatomy

The superior aperture of the thorax is bounded by the first thoracic vertebra, the first ribs and cartilages, and the manubrium sternum. The thorax extends to the inferior aperture comprising the twelfth thoracic vertebra, twelfth and eleventh floating ribs, fused costal cartilages of the seventh to tenth ribs, and the xiphoid cartilage extending into the costal angle. This outlet is at the level of the twelfth thoracic vertebra posteriorly, second lumbar vertebra laterally, and tenth thoracic vertebra anteriorly at the xiphoid cartilage.

Skeleton

The twelve thoracic vertebrae, clavicles, scapulae, ribs and cartilages, sternum, ligaments, intercostal muscles, and tendons form the thoracic wall that is covered by subcutaneous tissue and skin. In deep inspiration, articulation of the curved ribs increases the anteroposterior diameter of the upper thorax, and the transverse diameter of the lower thorax, lowering intrapleural and intrathoracic pressure, allowing air into the lungs.

Between the ribs, the outermost muscle layer, external intercostal muscles pass downwards and forwards from the rib above to the rib below. Deep to them, the internal intercostal muscles pass downwards and backwards. Between internal intercostal muscles and the innermost intercostal muscles lies the neuromuscular bundle just below the rib above, with vein superiorly, then artery, then nerve inferiorly.

The external intercostal muscles and the levatores costarum muscles from transverse processes to the ribs below elevate ribs. The internal intercostal, innermost intercostal, transversus thoracis, subcostales, and serratus posterior muscles depress ribs.

The internal thoracic arteries, that arise from the subclavian arteries and run deep to the transversus thoracis muscle, lateral to the sternum, and the intercostal arteries supply the chest wall. Venous drainage is via intercostal veins, and internal thoracic veins that drain into the brachiocephalic vein.

Lateral to the radiate ligaments of the head of the rib and anterior to the surface of the rib, the sympathetic trunk lies subpleurally where it may be blocked by local anaesthetic drugs to achieve paravertebral regional analgesia.

Diaphragm

The diaphragm has a peripheral muscular attachment to the rim of the thoracic outlet that converges on a 'C' shaped central tendon, concave posteriorly. The diaphragm is pierced by the inferior vena cava and part of the right phrenic nerve at the level of the 8th thoracic vertebra, the oesophagus anterior and posterior vagal trunks at the 10th thoracic vertebra, and the aorta, azygous vein, and thoracic duct, anterior to the body of the 12th thoracic vertebra.

The external intercostal muscles run downwards and anteriorly from a rib to the rib below. The diaphragm and external intercostal muscles contract during quiet inspiration. Elastic recoil of the lungs and chest wall with muscle tone in the abdominal wall achieve expiration. Forced inspiration also uses sternocleidomastoid, trapezius, pectoralis minor, the scalene muscles, and serratus posterior superior to fix and elevate the upper ribs. Forced expiration involves active contraction of the muscles of the abdominal wall, internal intercostal muscles and serratus posterior inferior. The thoracic wall contains the heart, pericardium and great vessels, which are considered elsewhere, and thymus, trachea, lungs, phrenic and vagus nerves, and diaphragm.

Mediastinum

The thymus lies in the superior mediastinum posterior to the sternum and anterior to the left brachiocephalic vein and vena cava and it extends inferiorly to the fibrous pericardium. The trachea enters the thorax at the level of the second thoracic vertebra. It extends into the chest for another two thoracic vertebrae, dividing into left and right main bronchi between fourth and fifth thoracic vertebrae.

Respiratory system

Lungs

The lung parenchyma is invaginated into visceral and parietal pleurae, which are separated by a layer of fluid except where they are continuous around the root of the lung. In health, they weigh 800 g.

Airways

From the nasal cavity and mouth, air passes through the pharynx then larynx at thoracic vertebra T6, 15 cm from the upper teeth. From the larynx, the trachea divides after 10 cm at the main carina into the first division, the right and left main bronchi (figure 4.1). The bronchi then divide successively, branching into lobar, segmental, and subsegmental bronchi until the terminal bronchioles are formed after about 16 divisions. The terminal bronchioles have no alveoli and all the airways above them play no part in gas exchange. These conducting airways comprise the anatomical dead space of 150 mL that must be moved before gas exchange can occur, and occupies part of every tidal volume of 500 mL. Beyond the terminal bronchioles lie respiratory bronchioles, alveolar ducts and blind-ended alveolar sacs formed at about the 23rd generation of airways. At the end of exhalation during quiet respiration the lung is at its functional residual capacity. The volume of air in the alveoli and airways is then about 2.5 L.

From the trachea, Weibel divided up the generations of airways into three bronchi and 12 bronchioles that were conducting airways. Then transitional and respiratory airways included three divisions of respiratory bronchioles, three alveolar ducts, and finally the alveolar sacs at division 23. As the generations of airways divide beyond the terminal bronchioles there is a dramatic increase in cross-sectional area with every further division. The cross sectional area of the trachea is about 2.5 cm^2, rising to 11 800 cm^2 at the alveolae. The increase in the volume of the chest in inspiration has little effect on the forward velocity of air at the respiratory airways. At this level of airway, diffusion becomes the principal form of gas movement to and from the alveoli.

Lung volumes and capacities

There are four lung volumes and combinations of these make lung capacities (figure 4.2). At rest, with the airways open at atmospheric pressure, the volume of air in the lungs and airways is the functional residual capacity (FRC). During quiet breathing, this is increased by the tidal volume. From tidal volume to total lung capacity gives the inspiratory reserve volume. FRC comprises the expiratory reserve volume, the maximum volume that can be exhaled from end quiet expiration, plus the air left in the lungs afterwards, the residual volume. Inspiratory capacity is the sum of tidal volume and inspiratory reserve volume. Vital capacity is total lung capacity less residual volume.

Pulmonary blood vessels

The main pulmonary artery arises beyond the pulmonary valve and divides into left and right main pulmonary arteries underneath the arch of the aorta. Successive divisions through lobar, segmental, and subsegmental branches, until eventually down to capillaries about 9 μm diameter just large enough to permit the passage of a red blood cell. Capillaries encase the alveoli in

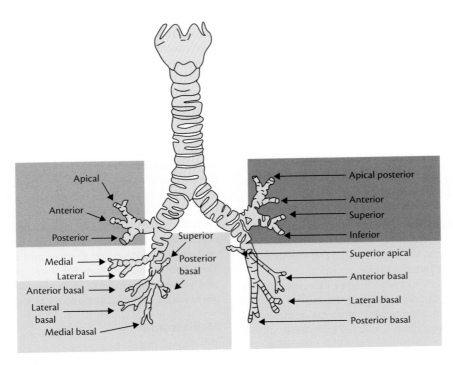

Fig. 4.1 Trachea, bronchi and bronchioles.
This figure was published in Anatomy of the Human Body, H Gray, plate 961, Copyright Elsevier 1918.

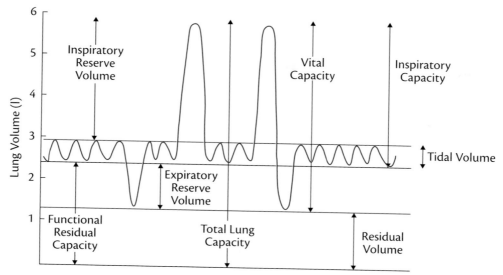

Fig. 4.2 Lung volumes and capacities.

Reproduced from M Harrison, Revision Notes for MCEM Part A, 2011, Figure C.2.1, p. 243, with permission from Oxford University Press

a thin-walled mesh offering a huge surface area for gas exchange between blood and air.

Lung parenchyma

The alveoli are lined by flat Type I epithelial cells and thicker Type II granular pneumocytes that contain lamellar inclusion bodies and secrete surfactant. There are plentiful immunological cells, macrophages, plasma cells, lymphocytes, and mast cells. The lungs are innervated by the vagus nerve and sympathetic nerves.

Physiology

The principal function of the respiratory system is to move air in and out of the lungs and absorb oxygen from and excrete carbon dioxide into air drawn into the alveoli. Gases such as methane and volatile molecules like alcohol may be excreted. The pulmonary circulation can act as a reservoir for blood, which is filtered and some of its contents metabolised as it flows through lung tissue.

Air flow

In health, a tidal volume of air of about 500 mL is inhaled with each breath, 12–15 times per minute. One third is dead space leaving about 5000 mL/min to contribute to gas exchange in the lungs. Every minute, 250 mL of oxygen is absorbed and 200 mL carbon dioxide is excreted. The oxygen is excreted as water. The carbon dioxide is produced from metabolism of substrates. The diaphragm and external intercostal muscles contract, expanding the chest wall. Intrapleural pressure falls as a result and the lungs expand allowing atmospheric pressure to force air through patent airways towards the lung parenchyma. At quiet respiration, a difference of only 3 cmH_2O pressure is required to move a tidal volume of gas.

Air is distributed unequally throughout the lung during inspiration. The intrapleural pressure is more negative at superior parts of the lung than dependent parts. When the chest wall expands, there is a greater change of intrapleural pressure adjacent to

dependent parts. They have a relatively greater increase in volume directing more air to the lung bases when the chest is erect.

Flow within the trachea and large bronchi is turbulent, whereas flow in the narrower but more numerous small bronchi with a greater total cross-sectional area becomes laminar. Gas transport to respiratory bronchi and alveoli is by diffusion.

Exhalation of air during forced expiration is limited when the positive intrathoracic pressure collapses some airways until air from other sites is exhaled, pressure within the lung falls and airways can reopen to allow more gas to leave the chest.

Measurement of inequality of ventilation with the single breath nitrogen test

Breathing air, the subject takes a single vital capacity inspiration of oxygen, then breathes out slowly at less than 0.5 L/s (figure 4.3). Nitrogen concentration in the exhaled gas is measured and plotted against exhaled volume. There is an initial phase of no nitrogen corresponding to dead space. Nitrogen concentration then rises as mixed dead space and alveolar gas are exhaled until there is an alveolar plateau with a nitrogen concentration within about 5%. At the end of expiration, the nitrogen concentration rises until residual volume is reached and no further exhalation is possible.

The rise in concentration of nitrogen at the end indicates the onset of airway closure predominantly at the bases. The volume at which the nitrogen concentration rises is the closing volume. Closing volume plus residual volume is the closing capacity.

The nitrogen concentration rises at the end of expiration when basal lung airways close. Apical regions have a more negative intrapleural pressure and are more expanded at the onset of the single breath of 100% oxygen. The large breath of oxygen is directed therefore more to basal regions than to the apex; so nitrogen concentrations will be less dilute at the apices than the bases. As the airways in the bases close, the apical alveoli with higher nitrogen concentrations continue to empty and the nitrogen concentration measured at the mouth will rise.

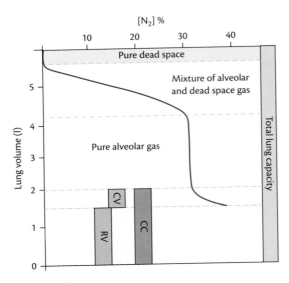

Fig. 4.3 Single breath nitrogen test.
N_2: nitrogen gas, TLC: total lung capacity, CV: closing volume, RV: residual volume; CC: closing capacity
Reproduced from C Spoors and K Kiff, Training in Anaesthesia, 2010, Figure 13.21, p. 335, with permission from Oxford University Press

When closing capacity exceeds FRC, as it can in disease, extremes of age, and obesity, there will be at least part of the respiratory cycle when blood passes through regions with no ventilation. The shunting blood will tend to reduce arterial oxygen haemoglobin saturation.

Lung volumes

Tidal volume, inspiratory reserve volume, and expiratory reserve volume may be measured using a spirometer. Air in the residual volume remains after maximum expiration and cannot be measured by measuring displaced gas volume or integrating the measurement of flow with respect to time.

Residual volume may be calculated by subtracting the expiratory reserve volume from FRC. FRC may be measured by a gas dilution technique using helium that is effectively not absorbed by the lung. Initial volume in the spirometer and concentration of helium are known. With the lung at end expiration, connecting the mouthpiece to the spirometer, then equilibrating gas mixture in spirometer and lung, the final concentration of helium can be measured. The fall in helium concentration is directly proportional to the FRC.

Where C_1 and V_1 are the initial concentration and volume of the helium mixture in the spirometer, and C_2 is the final helium concentration and V_2 the functional residual capacity:

$$C_1 \times V_1 = C_2 \times \left(V_1 + V_2 \right)$$

Rearranging the equation:

$$V_2 = \frac{\left(C_1 - C_2 \right)}{C_2} \times V_1$$

Because the equilibration is not instantaneous, during the test carbon dioxide must be removed by absorption and oxygen supplied at the rate that it is taken up.

A body plesythmograph is another method to calculate FRC. It uses Boyle's law, where at constant temperature, the product of pressure and volume after a change remains constant, to calculate FRC. The subject sits in a box with a known volume. When the subject inspires against a closed airway from FRC, the volume in the box changes (ΔV) with measured changes in the pressure within the box and must be the same as the changes in the volume of the lung.

The pressures at the mouthpiece in the closed airway are measured before and after inspiratory effort. The initial pressure at the mouthpiece times the functional residual capacity is the same as the final pressure times the FRC plus the change in volume, ΔV. Rearranging the equation allows calculation of FRC.

Alveolar ventilation

Tidal volume may be measured at a mouthpiece. Because of the dead space in the airways, only 70% of the tidal volume is able to reach the alveoli, assuming a dead space of 150 mL in a tidal volume of 500 mL. Unless the volume of dead space is known, alveolar ventilation is difficult to calculate from total expired ventilation by subtraction.

Anatomical dead space may be measured by rapid analysis of exhaled gas for nitrogen using Fowler's method. The subject takes a single breath of oxygen 100%, and then breathes air through a mouthpiece that measures volume, and takes a continuous side stream of gas to measure nitrogen concentration. Plots of nitrogen concentration against time and nitrogen concentrations against volume illustrate the phases of ventilation and a plateau when at the end of the breath, mixed alveolar gas that has not been diluted by gas in the dead space is being exhaled. From the mid-point of the nitrogen concentration–volume curve to the abscissa will give the dead space volume.

Physiological dead space is determined by the proportion of gas exchanging parts of the lung to the conducting parts rather than the structural composition of the airways. They are very similar in health, but physiological dead space can be much increased in parenchymal lung disease when lung tissue does not function efficiently exchanging gas. Assumptions are made that the alveolar and arterial partial pressures of carbon dioxide are interchangeable and that a tidal volume is comprised of mixed alveolar and dead space gas.

Assuming that $V_T = V_A + V_D$

where V = volume, F = fraction, T = total, A = alveolar, D = dead space, E = mixed expired

then: $$V_T \times F_{E_{CO_2}} = V_A \times F_{A_{CO_2}}$$

$$V_T \times F_E = \left(V_T - V_D \right) \times F_A$$

so

$$\frac{V_D}{V_T} = \frac{P_{A_{CO_2}} - P_{E_{CO_2}}}{P_{A_{CO_2}}}$$

Alveolar gas concentrations are more difficult to measure than mixed expired gases; so substituting arterial carbon dioxide partial pressures for alveolar carbon dioxide partial pressures gives:

$$\frac{V_D}{V_T} = \frac{P_{a_{CO_2}} - P_{E_{CO_2}}}{P_{a_{CO_2}}}$$

The fraction of a gas is its concentration in a mixture and the partial pressure is proportional to its concentration. Substituting partial pressures for fractions:

$$\frac{V_D}{V_T} = \frac{P_A - F_E}{F_A}$$

During exhalation, the concentration of carbon dioxide at the mouth is about 4%. All this carbon dioxide comes from alveolar gas if you neglect the 0.03% concentration of carbon dioxide in inspired air:

$$\dot{V}_{CO_2} = \dot{V}_A \times F_{A_{CO_2}}$$

Regional variations

All parts of the lung do not receive inhaled gas uniformly. In a subject standing erect, both gas and blood are directed preferentially to the lower zones. Blood is distributed by gravity. The more negative intrapleural pressure at the apices of the lung mean these zones are more expanded at end expiration. When the chest wall expands during inspiration, there is a greater fall in intrapleural pressure at the bases and proportionately greater increase in size and thereby more gas drawn into the bases than the apices during inspiration.

Volume flow and diffusion

The surface area of approximately 500 million alveoli is 50–100 m^2, and the thickness of the epithelial-endothelial layer about 0.3 μm. Oxygen and carbon dioxide cross the alveoli by simple diffusion down gradients of gas partial pressure. The rate of gas flow crossing a membrane is proportional to the area, diffusion constant (D), partial pressure gradient across the membrane ($P_1 - P_2$), and inversely proportional to the thickness by Fick's law.

$$\dot{V} \propto \frac{\text{Area}}{\text{Thickness}} \times D \times (P_1 - P_2)$$

The diffusion constant is proportional to the solubility of a gas and inversely proportional to its relative molecular mass (RMM).

$$\text{Diffusion Constant} (D) \propto \frac{\text{Solubility}}{\sqrt{\text{RMM}}}$$

For oxygen and carbon dioxide, their RMMs are 32 and 44 g/mol, respectively. The square roots of their masses are 5.7 and 6.6 (g/mol)$^{0.5}$. With a greater solubility but little different mass, carbon dioxide diffuses about 20 times more rapidly across the alveoli than oxygen.

The terms Area, Thickness and Diffusion Constant may be combined into a single term called the Diffusing capacity (D$_L$). D$_L$ then becomes a ratio of the amount of gas transferred to the difference in partial pressure across the membrane. For a very soluble gas such as carbon monoxide, the gas capillary partial pressure is very small and may be ignored. D$_L$ then becomes the ratio of the uptake of carbon monoxide, $\dot{V}_{CO}$ to the alveolar partial pressure of the gas ($P_{A_{CO}}$).

$$D_L = \frac{\dot{V}_{CO}}{P_{A_{CO}}} \, \text{mL} \, / \, \text{min} \, / \, \text{mmHg}$$

Impairment of the ability of the alveolus to transfer gases will be accompanied by a fall of the diffusing capacity of carbon monoxide from a normal value of 25 mL/min/mmHg.

In the 0.8 s that it takes a red cell to traverse the pulmonary capillary, there is an inconstant relationship between the amount of gas transferred across the capillary and the pattern of change of partial pressures of gas along the capillary. For an insoluble gas such as nitrous oxide, few molecules of gas cross the capillary into simple solution, but the partial pressures of gas in blood matches that in alveolus rapidly in a hyperbolic course to equilibrium when no further net transfer can take place. Increasing uptake requires more blood to pass through the alveolar capillary and the uptake is said to be *perfusion* limited. For a soluble gas such as carbon monoxide, substantial numbers of molecules may pass into blood from the alveolus and be bound to haemoglobin in the red cell, but the partial pressure of carbon monoxide in blood changes little. It is the transfer of gas across the alveolus that prevents more gas being taken up. Diffusion in this case is said to be *diffusion* limited.

Oxygen has an intermediate time course and pattern. Four molecules of oxygen may be taken up by one molecule of haemoglobin, and the avidity of haemoglobin for oxygen becomes progressively greater, the more molecules of oxygen are taken up. In health, perfusion limits the amount of oxygen that is take up. Blood flow through the lungs is increased during exercise in order to take up more oxygen for anaerobic metabolism. In parenchymal lung disease, changes to the alveolar wall may impede the transfer of oxygen. Slowed diffusion may prevent the partial pressure of oxygen in blood equilibrating with the partial pressure of oxygen in the alveolus and the uptake of oxygen can become diffusion limited.

At rest there is a minimum requirement for 250 mL of oxygen to be taken up and to excrete 200 mL of carbon dioxide each minute. This is achieved with a minute volume of 5000mL mL air. Gas requirements increase during exercise and disease and will limit endurance exercise. A maximum oxygen uptake of 35–40mL mL/kg/min is a measure of maximum aerobic capacity.

Blood flow

The pulmonary circulation begins where the main pulmonary artery arises from the right ventricle and contains mixed venous blood with an oxyhaemoglobin saturation with oxygen of about 75%. Pulmonary arteries divide successively adjacent to the airways until they form an interconnected mesh of capillaries covering the alveoli, presenting a large surface for exchange between alveolar gas. The capillaries drain into tributaries of pulmonary veins that eventually form the four pulmonary veins that deliver oxygenated blood into the back of the left atrium.

Pulmonary blood flow can be estimated from the oxygen uptake into the body using the Fick principle. The amount of oxygen taken up by the body is equal to the difference in content between pulmonary vein and artery multiplied by pulmonary blood flow.

$$\dot{V}_{O_2} = \dot{Q}\left(Ca_{O_2} - C\bar{v}_{O_2}\right), \quad \text{or} \quad \dot{Q} = \frac{\dot{V}_{O_2}}{Ca_{O_2} - C\bar{v}_{O_2}}$$

where $\dot{Q}$ is the pulmonary blood flow, $\dot{V}_{O_2}$ is the systemic oxygen uptake in mass per unit time, Ca and Cv the content of oxygen in pulmonary arteries and veins in mass per unit volume, giving flow in volume per unit time. Care must be paid to the units.

Modern ventilators measure oxygen concentrations in inspired and expired limbs and gas flows. Arterial and mixed-venous blood oxygen contents may be calculated from the saturation of haemoglobin with oxygen and the dissolved blood concentrations of oxygen in blood samples from peripheral artery and pulmonary artery catheters. This will allow a calculation of pulmonary blood flow to be made. The accuracy of the measurements and the assumptions that are necessary mean that the values obtained will illustrate the principles involved rather than be a reliable measure to guide clinical decisions.

Mean arterial pressure in the systemic circulation is about seven times that in the pulmonary circulation. The left and right atrial pressures are very similar, being about 5 and 2 mmHg respectively, but the maximum pressure in the systemic circulation is about five times that in the lung. The pulmonary circulation receives the entire cardiac output and has only to perfuse the lungs for gas exchange that can be achieved in a low-pressure high-flow system at roughly the same level as the right ventricle. Pulmonary capillaries are closely applied to alveoli that can be at atmospheric pressure at end expiration. The pressure between blood within the vessel and surrounding tissues is the transmural pressure.

The systemic circulation has to overcome differences in hydrostatic pressure from head to foot in the erect position and provide a driving pressure in the renal circulation, to achieve filtration from glomerulus to Bowman's capsule. The relationship between flow, pressure and resistance pertains in both circulations, but by *distending* arteries in use and *recruiting* more arteries in the pulmonary circulation when cardiac output is increased, the pulmonary artery pressures need not rise as much as expected were vascular resistance unchanged. The same mechanisms are employed by the lungs to act as a reservoir for blood when blood is redistributed from other parts of the body, for example after a change in position or cessation of exercise.

Because the pulmonary circulation operates at lower pressure, the pulmonary artery walls are thinner and contain less smooth muscle than systemic arteries. The lower pressures mean that gravity has a noticeable difference in the distribution of blood within the pulmonary circulation, more blood being directed to dependent parts of the lung. The parts are dependent changes with the position of the body. In the erect position, the pressure in the apices of the lung may be less than atmospheric pressure. Capillaries there will collapse and there will be no flow. The apices will still be ventilated, rendering them part of the dead space of the lung. Inferior to the apices there can be zones where during the respiratory cycle, alveolar pressure lies between end capillary arterial and venous pressures. Then, blood flow will be intermittent, occurring when alveolar pressure is less than capillary venous pressure.

The low pressures in the pulmonary circulation also render the circulation affected by the changes in intrapleural pressure caused by expansion and elastic recoil of the chest wall. Changes in pressure are conducted through the surrounding lung parenchyma. They increase the diameter of pulmonary vessels in inspiration and reduce them in expiration. These changes are most marked in the thinnest vessels closest to the alveoli. The relationship between lung volume and blood flow is non-linear. At extremes of vital capacity, the vessels are either compressed or stretched by the surrounding lung parenchyma, narrowing their diameter. Nearer functional residual capacity, the external influences are less and vessel diameter larger.

Matching perfusion to ventilation

Perfusion with no ventilation, that is a shunt, in a region of the lung causes de-oxygenated blood to pass through the lungs without the opportunity for gas exchange. This de-oxygenated blood mixes with oxygenated blood in the left side of the heart reducing the oxygen content of the blood and causing hypoxaemia. In health some bronchial artery blood and blood in the left ventricle draining directly into the cavity by thebesian veins will constitute a small shunt. A lung lobe with pneumonia or collapse, pulmonary arteriovenous fistulae, and congenital heart disease with right to left shunt will cause pathological shunt.

The proportion of blood that is shunting may be calculated by assuming that the oxygen content in arterial blood $\dot{Q}T \times Ca_{O_2}$ is made up of blood that either still has the oxygen content of mixed venous blood $\dot{Q}S \times Ca_{O_2}$, or is oxygenated fully, end alveolar capillary blood $\left(\left(\dot{Q}T - \dot{Q}S\right) \times CC'_{O_2}\right)$.

$$\dot{Q}T \times Ca_{O_2} = \dot{Q}S \times C\bar{v}_{O_2} + \left(\dot{Q}T - \dot{Q}S\right) \times CC'_{O_2}$$

From which:

$$\frac{\dot{Q}S}{\dot{Q}T} = \frac{CC'_{O_2} - Ca_{O_2}}{CC'_{O_2} - C\bar{v}_{O_2}}$$

Arterial oxygen content is taken from a peripheral artery, mixed venous blood is taken from a pulmonary artery catheter and end capillary blood oxygen content is derived from a calculation of the alveolar oxygen partial pressure related to the oxygen dissociation curve. These assumptions will not hold if there is a problem with diffusion across the alveolar-capillary membrane. Increasing the inspired oxygen concentration can only improve the content of end capillary blood. This may be sufficient to control hypoxaemia, but will not affect the content of blood that shunts past the alveoli.

In practice, there is a gradation of effect from regions of the lung that are ventilated but not perfused high $\dot{V}A/\dot{Q}$, alveolar dead space, to regions of the lung that are perfused but not ventilated, shunt low $\dot{V}A/\dot{Q}$. The sum of these effects in different units produces the total oxygen content of the systemic arterial blood.

Global hypoventilation of the lung, for example as caused by opioids or anaesthetic agents, reduces minute alveolar ventilation.

As carbon dioxide production is unaffected, the alveolar concentration of carbon dioxide rises at the expense of alveolar oxygen concentration, with resulting hypoxaemia if the inspired oxygen concentration is unchanged.

$$PA_{CO_2} \propto \frac{\dot{V}_{CO_2}}{\dot{V}A}$$

Capillary flow

The entire cardiac output passes through the pulmonary capillaries making it ideally placed to filter small blood thrombi and trap air bubbles before they can reach the brain or other vital organs. Oxygen by facemask will increase the inspired and therefore alveolar oxygen concentrations improving and possibly correcting hypoxaemia according the simplified alveolar air equation:

$$PA_{O_2} = PI_{O_2} - \frac{PA_{CO_2}}{R} + F$$

where F is a constant, about 0.3 kPa, and R is the respiratory quotient: 0.8 on a mixed diet. The rate of change of alveolar concentrations depends on the change in ventilation and the body stores of the gases. Considerably more carbon dioxide is stored in the body in the form of bicarbonate than oxygen, which is being consumed continually by tissues.

Regional gas exchange

Gravity has a greater effect on blood than gas flow. Blood flow and ventilation are both greater in the lower lobes than the upper lobes when standing erect because gravity diverts more blood to the bases and the less negative intrapleural pressure at the bases changes more when the chest wall expands reducing intrapleural pressure and generating the force to move gas from the atmosphere into the lungs. However, the regional influence of gravity on blood flow is greater than the regional effect of intrapleural pressure on lung ventilation.

At the lung apices, $VA/\dot{Q}$ is above 3. The ratio falls to unity at the level of the third rib. Because blood flow exceeds ventilation at the bases, the ratio reduces further to 0.6. Lying supine, the same changes distinguish the anterior from posterior segments of the lung. The distance in height anteroposteriorly is less than with the lung erect; so the influence of gravity is reduced as a consequence, with less change in VA/Q ratios.

Lying on the side during thoracic surgery for lung resection, there is the advantage that about 10% more blood is directed to the dependent ventilated lung. So, if the right lung receives 55% of pulmonary blood flow when erect then it receives 65% in the right lateral position. Similarly the left lung receives 55% of pulmonary blood flow in the left lateral position. This helps ameliorate hypoxia due to one-lung ventilation.

Carbon dioxide

The 20 times greater solubility of carbon dioxide than oxygen, and the near-linear carbon dioxide dissociation curve and, mean that alveolar gas diffusion problems are less likely to affect arterial carbon dioxide tensions, and increasing ventilation may overcome ventilation perfusion mismatch effects on carbon dioxide

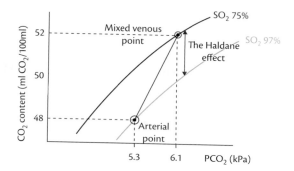

Fig. 4.4 Carbon dioxide dissociation curve.
CO_2: carbon dioxide and $PaCO_2$: carbon dioxide tension (kPa); SO_2; oxygen saturation
Reproduced from C Spoors and K Kiff, Training in Anaesthesia, 2010, Figure 13.37, p. 357, with permission from Oxford University Press

(figure 4.4). The increased ventilation may restore carbon dioxide tension, but will likely increase dead space by ventilating already under-perfused alveoli and increasing the work of breathing.

Capillary flow

It takes about 0.8 s for a red cell to traverse a pulmonary capillary. The influence on alveolar blood flow by cardiac output and gravity is further affected by local factors. A protective mechanism exists to reduce deoxygenated blood shunting past non-ventilating alveoli by diverting blood elsewhere, hypoxic pulmonary vasoconstriction. The oxygen tension in alveolar gas determines the response in arterioles supplying that segment of lung, possibly by a direct effect on vascular smooth muscle.

Parenchymal fluid in the lung

Although the pulmonary circulation pressures in the lung are low, there has to be a hydrostatic pressure driving blood across the pulmonary capillaries. This will tend to expel liquid from the circulation into the tissues. Conventional teaching has it that the difference in colloid oncotic pressure within the blood and tissues acts to oppose this net flow of liquid with the residual liquid in the tissues being drained by the lymphatics in perivascular spaces.

An alternative explanation proposes that the glycocalyx influences the retention of liquid within the circulation. The glycocalyx is a covering of transmembrane and membrane bound molecules of heparan sulphate and syndecan-1 that combine with plasma proteins and dissolved glycosaminoglycans to retain part of the intravascular plasma volume stationary against the endothelium. With a frond-like appearance of a sea anemone against the endothelial wall, this combination of molecules and plasma presents a barrier to permeability across the endothelium. Loss of this barrier leads to an increase in capillary permeability and oedema, with subsequent inflammation and infection.

Metabolic and hormonal functions of the lungs

Receiving the whole cardiac output and having a low pressure, the lungs present a very large surface area of endothelium to the blood that has the opportunity to filter blood and gases returning to the heart from the systemic circulation, and metabolize molecules in solution before they are propelled to the brain and vital organs.

Angiogensin-converting enzyme (ACE) resides in the capillary endothelial cells and promotes metabolism to convert the little active polypeptide angiotensin I to the more potent vasoconstrictor angiotensin II in the lung. Bradykinin, serotonin, some catecholamines, prostaglandins, and leukotrienes may undergo similar transformation. Antagonising this transformation by enzyme inhibitors to prevent activation during the passage of substrates through the lung in solution, is used to control hypertension. Uptake and metabolism also inactivates vasoactive drugs such as serotonin, bradykinin, and noradrenaline.

The proper functioning of the lung requires metabolism to produce phospholipid-derived surfactant to line the alveoli, preventing their collapse and mucopolysaccharide containing mucus to trap particles and be wafted by cilia into the main airways to be coughed up. Proteins such as collagen and elastin are generated within the lung to provide structure and elasticity within the lung parenchyma.

Oxygen molecules have to be conducted to the mitochondria in cells to participate in the electron transport chain. A low inspired fraction of oxygen, inadequate mass transfer of gas into and out of the alveoli, impaired transport across the alveolar capillary membrane, reduced blood supply to the lung, and perfusion from the right ventricle to left atrium that does not pass lung that is taking part in gas exchange, shunt, will all produce hypoxaemia in blood in the left atrium and systemic circulation and reduce the supply of oxygen to the tissues of the body.

Inadequate ventilation

Loss of parenchymal lung tissue, depression of the spontaneous drive in ventilation by disease or drugs, damage to the integrity and function of the chest wall, and increased resistance to the flow of gas by narrowing of the airways or increased density of inspired gas will all reduce the ability of the lungs to move gas into and out of the alveoli.

With this fall of alveolar ventilation comes a rise in alveolar fraction of carbon dioxide and a consequent rise in arterial carbon dioxide tension, because less carbon dioxide can be excreted whilst the production of carbon dioxide is unchanged.

$$F_{A_{CO_2}} \propto \frac{\dot{V}_{CO_2}}{\dot{V}_A}$$

The alveolar gas equation describes the relationship between the fall in alveolar oxygen tension and rise in alveolar carbon dioxide tension. It involves the respiratory quotient, R, that is the ratio between the minute volume of production of carbon dioxide and uptake of oxygen. R is 1 for a purely carbohydrate diet and about 0.8 with a mixed diet.

$$PA_{O_2} = PI_{O_2} - \frac{PA_{CO_2}}{R} + F$$

F is a constant and is small in comparison to the other terms. It is often ignored. Alveolar carbon dioxide tensions, are difficult to measure; so arterial carbon dioxide partial pressures are substituted usually assuming that there is little difference between the two. Increasing the inspired oxygen tension, PI, will increase the alveolar oxygen tension without needing to change the alveolar ventilation, and this may be sufficient in clinical practice.

Gradient across the alveolar capillary membrane

In health, there is a small gradient in oxygen tension across the alveolar capillary membrane from alveolus to capillary. This can be increased in disease.

Shunt

Mixed venous blood that is not oxygenated or deoxygenated blood that drains into the left side of the heart contribute to reducing the oxygenation of arterial blood by 'shunt.' Blood from the bronchial arteries that drains into the pulmonary venous system and Thebesian veins that drain blood from the coronary circulation directly into the cavity of the left ventricle contribute to shunt in health. Cyanotic congenital heart disease (Chapter 22), pulmonary arteriovenous fistulae and perfusion of consolidated or collapsed lung will all cause hypoxaemia by shunt.

The magnitude of shunt may be calculated from the flow and oxygen content of blood in different parts of the pulmonary and systemic circulations.

Oxygen dissolved in plasma

Oxygen will pass into solution in plasma according to Henry's law where the amount dissolved is proportional to the partial pressure of oxygen in the alveoli. The solubility coefficient of oxygen in plasma at body temperature is 0.23 mL/L/kPa. In health this amounts to oxygen 0.3 mL per 100 mL blood in solution, substantially less than 20 mL/100mL carried by blood, including oxyhaemoglobin.

Haemoglobin

The compound haemoglobin is contained within red blood cells. Haemoglobin A has a central iron containing porphyrin surrounded by four polypeptide chains, two alpha and two beta chains. Each polypeptide chain can combine reversibly with an oxygen molecule to make oxyhaemoglobin.

The avidity with which haemoglobin takes up oxygen is increased with each oxygen molecule that is combined, giving rise to the oxygen dissociation curve when oxygen saturation is plotted against partial pressure of oxygen of the blood. The amount of oxygen that blood carries increases rapidly to 7 kPa, when the curve flattens off.

The saturation of haemoglobin is the ratio of the amount of oxygen combined with haemoglobin to the maximum capacity of oxygen carriage expressed as a percentage.

$$\text{Haemoglobin oxygen saturation} = \frac{\text{Oxygen in combination with haemoglobin}}{\text{Maximum amount of oxygen that can be combined}} \times 100$$

Above a haemoglobin saturation of 94%, increasing the oxygen saturation to 100% carries proportionately much less additional oxygen than the same increase at lower saturations.

The maximum amount of oxygen that may be carried by haemoglobin is proportional to the amount of haemoglobin in grams of haemoglobin per 100 mL blood, and the percentage saturation of haemoglobin. The constant of proportionality, Hüfner's constant, is 1.39, but lesser values around 1.34 may be used to take account of methaemoglobin and carboxyhaemoglobin.

$$\text{Haemoglobin oxygen capacity} = \left(1.39 \times [\text{Hb}] \times \frac{\text{Saturation}}{100}\right)$$

Oxygen dissociation curve

The shape of the oxygen dissociation curve is affected by conditions within the blood (figure 4.5). Increased 2,3-diphosphoglycerate that is produced during red cell metabolism, and acidaemia and high temperature that are found in exercising muscle, shift the curve to the right reducing the oxygen carrying capacity of haemoglobin and releasing oxygen to the tissues. Conversely, a lack of 2,3-diphosphoglycerate that occurs in stored blood, alkalaemia and cold shift the curve to the left making haemoglobin more avid for oxygen. The PO_2 at which 50% of haemoglobin is saturated is known as the P_{50} and has a normal value of 3.6 kPa.

Carbon dioxide

Unlike oxygen, a small proportion of carbon dioxide is carried in the blood in combination with proteins. Carbon dioxide is carried principally as bicarbonate, but also dissolved in solution in plasma. Carbon dioxide is about 20 times more soluble than oxygen in water, a property that limits the alveolar arterial difference in carbon dioxide compared to oxygen. Arterial blood has about 5% of carbon dioxide carried in solution.

Carbonic acid is formed by the combination of carbon dioxide and water. This is slow in solution, but the enzyme carbonic anhydrase catalyses the reaction within the red blood cell. Carbonic acid then dissociates into bicarbonate and hydrogen ions.

$$CO_2 + H_2O \underset{}{\overset{CA}{\rightleftharpoons}} H_2CO_3 \rightleftharpoons H^+ + CO_3^-$$

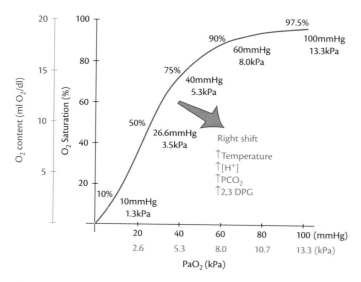

The bicarbonate ions diffuse down a concentration gradient across the red cell membrane into the plasma. The red cell membrane is less permeable to hydrogen ions; so chloride ions shift into the red cell to maintain electrical equilibrium.

Carbon dioxide is produced in the tissues where haemoglobin delivers its oxygen and becomes reduced. Reduced haemoglobin is less acid and better able to accept hydrogen ions than oxygenated haemoglobin. Hydrogen ions are taken up onto the reduced haemoglobin enhancing the ability of deoxygenated blood to carry carbon dioxide as described by the Haldane effect. The reverse process happens in pulmonary capillaries when haemoglobin is oxygenated, hydrogen ions are displaced and carbon dioxide liberated to be excreted into the alveoli.

Similarly, reduced haemoglobin is better able to carry about 30% of carbon dioxide bound to terminal amine groups and form carbamino-haemoglobin than oxygenated haemoglobin that carries 10% of carbon dioxide as carbaminohaemoglobin, that is for the same $PaCO_2$, reduced haemoglobin carries more carbon dioxide than oxygenated haemoglobin. The process is reversed in the pulmonary capillary enhancing the transport and excretion of carbon dioxide.

Acid–base

Hydrogen ions generated during the electron transport system in mitochondria combine with oxygen ions from inhaled oxygen to form 'metabolic water' molecules that amount to about 400 mL. The oxygen and carbon atoms in carbon dioxide that are exhaled from the lung derive from carbohydrates and other substrates that are metabolized for energy. The excretion of carbon dioxide from the lung eliminates about 100 times the equivalent of fixed acids that the kidneys remove. Pulmonary disease can affect profoundly the acid–base status and alterations in ventilation may compensate for metabolic acidosis and alkalosis.

Retention of carbon dioxide gives respiratory acidosis and hyperventilation a respiratory alkalosis. Retention and excretion of bicarbonate by the kidney may compensate for these two changes respectively to avoid or limit acidaemia and alkalaemia.

Mechanism of ventilation

Normal ventilation

Skeletal muscle provides mechanical forces to move gases cyclically into and out of the lung. During quiet respiration inspiration is active, and expiration is passive and over a longer period than inspiration. The apex of the dome-shaped diaphragm descends as it contracts and the rib cage widens at the costal margins increasing the volume of the chest axially and horizontally. Abdominal contents are displaced inferiorly and anteriorly during inspiration.

The external intercostal muscles run diagonally downwards and forwards. Internal intercostal muscles run downwards and backwards. External intercostal muscles lift and move forward the ribs during active inspiration. Internal intercostal muscles have the opposite effect and are utilised during exercise or respiratory difficulty.

Accessory muscles

Accessory muscles of respiration are the scalene muscles, sternocleidomastoids, abdominal wall muscles, and muscles in the head

Fig. 4.5 Oxygen dissociation curve.
2,3-DPG: 2,3 diphosphoglycerate, O_2: oxygen, [H$^+$]: hydrogen ion concentration, PCO_2: carbon dioxide tension
Reproduced from C Spoors and K Kiff, Training in Anaesthesia, 2010, Figure 13.34, p. 357, with permission from Oxford University Press

and neck. These muscles are active during exercise, hyperventilation, and coughing.

Relationship between gas flow and respiratory movements

There is resistance to gas flow through the airways, the elastic forces of the chest wall, and viscous forces of the lung tissues to overcome. The response to muscle activity is non-linear. Little gas is moved at the limits of each breath and more during mid inspiration and mid expiration giving a sigmoid shaped relationship between muscle contraction and movement of gas. Some energy overcoming forces in inspiration is returned during expiration, but energy is lost moving gas and as heat. The difference between the two parts of the ventilation cycle is represented by hysteresis.

For a given intrapleural pressure, the volume of the lung is larger during expiration than during inspiration. This obtains whether the lung is inflated by expanding the surrounding pleura as happens during spontaneous ventilation or by positive pressure into the airways as happens during mechanical ventilation.

Compliance

The slope of the pressure–volume curve gives the compliance.

$$\text{Compliance} = \frac{\text{change in volume}\left(\Delta V\right)}{\text{change in pressure}\left(\Delta P\right)}\text{mL/cmH}_2\text{O}$$

Normal values are around 200 mL/cmH$_2$O. With the chest erect, lung segments in the lower lobes are on the steep, more compliant, mid part of the pressure volume curve, whereas the apices, being more expanded at functional residual capacity by the more negative intrapleural pressure at the apices, are at the upper, flatter part of the curve and less compliant (figure 4.6). During inspiration, proportionately more gas is directed to the lower parts of the lung as a result, matching ventilation to the greater blood flow to the bases on account of gravity.

Compliance of the lung is determined both by the composition of elastic and collagen fibres within the parenchyma and the phospholipid surfactant within the alveoli. Surfactant is produced by the type II epithelial cells within the alveolus and reduces the surface tension, stabilizing the alveoli against collapse and increasing the compliance of the lung, and reducing the transudation of fluid from the parenchyma into the alveolar spaces.

Airway resistance

Gas flow is turbulent as it passes through the trachea, becoming laminar in the smaller airways. Although turbulent flow offers more resistant than laminar flow, flow becomes dependent on the fourth power of the radius of the airway. However, as the airways branch, the sum of the cross sectional areas of each division increases, and from terminal bronchioles, gas moves by diffusion rather than periodic ventilation. Medium-sized bronchi at about generation five offer the greatest resistance to airflow. The smooth muscle within their walls can constrict these airways to reduce gas flow in response to parasympathetic stimulation, but are amenable to treatment by β-adrenergic agonists to dilate the airways.

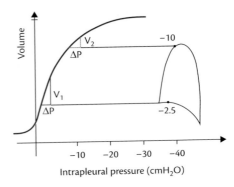

Fig. 4.6 Sigmoid shape of the changes in lung volume in response to more negative intrapleural pressure during expansion of the chest wall.
The apex, with a more negative pressure at functional reserve capacity, does not expand as much as the base for the same change in intrapleural pressure
Reproduced from C Spoors and K Kiff, Training in Anaesthesia, 2010, Figure 13.14, p. 343, with permission from Oxford University Press

Airway compression during forced expiration

During inspiration, negative pressures within the pleurae develop when the chest wall expands. The pressure transmitted to the alveoli is negative, elastic forces tend to keep airways open and air is forced into the lung by ambient pressures. In expiration the chest wall exerts positive pressures within the pleurae that are transmitted to the alveoli. Air is forced out of the lung down the airways with a consequent pressure gradient from the alveolus along the airway towards the trachea as resistance to airflow is overcome. At a point when the alveolar pressure less the pressure drop down the airway is less than the positive pressure in the pleura, the airway is compressed and no further expiration is possible until the pleural pressure falls. Expiratory flow is limited by this mechanism and cannot be increased by greater voluntary expiratory effort.

In disease, if there is greater resistance to airflow within the airways or less elastic tissue within the lung to distend the airways and keep them open, the airway compression during expiration is more likely.

Energy of breathing

About 65% of the energy expended to oxygenate blood is taken up by overcoming elastic forces. This is released as heat. Additional work has to be expended to overcome viscous forces comprising airway (28%) and tissue (7%) resistance. A proportion of energy expended is recovered during expiration. At rest during quiet respiration, the work expended during ventilation consumes less than 5% of the systemic oxygen uptake. During exercise and disease this fraction is increased, limiting the efficiency of breathing and oxygen available for other processes.

Regulation of ventilation

The brainstem centres regulating ventilation are found in the pons and medulla. The pneumotaxic centre in the upper pons inhibits inspiration, regulating volume and rate of ventilation. The apneustic centre in the lower pons promotes activity in the medullary respiratory centre stimulating inspiration. The medullary respiratory centre lies beneath the floor of the fourth ventricle of the brain. Cells in the dorsal aspect are associated with inspiration.

Cells in the ventral aspect are associated with expiration. The dorsal inspiratory cells are inactive, then spontaneous depolarisations are associated with contractions of inspiratory muscles, primarily via the phrenic nerve to the diaphragm, and inspiration begins. Expiration in quiet breathing is passive, but electrical activity is evident in the ventral aspect during forced expiration or exercise.

Voluntary hyperventilation and hypoventilation are possible, but the urge to breathe becomes strong when there is hypercarbia or hypoxia. Exercise, emotion, and fear all influence the pattern of breathing via the brainstem centres.

Central chemoreceptors

Brain chemoreceptors are found on the ventral surface of the brain in the medulla. They respond to the hydrogen ion concentration in extracellular fluid that is affected by carbon dioxide diffusing through the blood–brain barrier from the circulation. An increase in arterial carbon dioxide tension leads to an increase in cerebrospinal fluid (CSF) hydrogen ions that stimulate breathing to correct the change. Cerebrospinal pH is 7.32, less than arterial pH and with less protein than plasma in CSF is not as well buffered as plasma.

Peripheral chemoreceptors

At the bifurcation of the common carotid arteries and on the arch of the aorta, peripheral chemoreceptors in the aortic bodies respond to changes in arterial pH and oxygen and carbon dioxide tensions. Despite a high metabolic rate, they receive a very high blood flow and effectively measure arterial tensions. A low arterial oxygen tension stimulates ventilation. An increase in arterial carbon dioxide tension generates a rapid response to increase ventilation. The carotid bodies are also the principal site of response to a fall in arterial pH.

Neural reflexes

There are reflexes mediated by nerve pathways that moderate breathing. Irritation of the bronchial mucosa can stimulate coughing and provoke bronchoconstriction. Stretching the lung slows ventilation, whereas deflation initiates inspiration. Pulmonary oedema and exercise are associated with an increased breathing rate that is not always explained by a response to the requirement for oxygen or the excretion of carbon dioxide. Pain and emotion can alter similarly the pattern of breathing.

Pulmonary function tests

Ventilation

A forced expiration from total lung volume empties the airways of the vital capacity of gas rapidly initially and then more slowly as the volume of gas in the lung decreases towards residual volume. The volume of gas exhaled in the first second is the forced expiratory volume (FEV_1). In health the FEV_1 is about 4 L and the forced vital capacity (FVC) 5 L, giving a ratio ($FEV_1\%$) of FEV_1:FVC of 80%.

In obstructive diseases, the $FEV_1\%$ is reduced (figure 4.7). Both FEV_1 and FVC are reduced in restrictive diseases but the $FEV_1\%$ may be normal or even increased (figure 4.7).

Forced expiration may be plotted as volume against time in spirometry and flow against volume in a flow volume curve. The

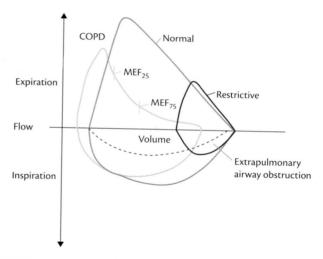

Fig. 4.7 Lung volume time relationship in obstructive airways disease and restrictive airways disease.
COPD: chronic obstructive pulmonary disease; MEF_{25} and MEF_{75}: maximum expiratory flow at 25% and 75% of forced vital capacity.
Reproduced from C Spoors and K Kiff, Training in Anaesthesia, 2010, Figure 13.28, p. 353, with permission from Oxford University Press.

average flow over the middle half of expiration, the forced expiratory flow rate, $FEF_{25–75\%}$, gives results that change in the same way that $FEV_1\%$ does.

Tests of expiratory flow are reduced when there is obstruction to airflow or a reduction in the elastic properties of the lung. In obstructive diseases the lung is likely to be enlarged, but expiration cannot empty the lung because compression by the chest wall collapses airways, trapping gas. Rough guides indicate that FEV_1 of 800–1000 mL is required for an effective cough.

Mucus and cilia

Goblet cells in the respiratory epithelium secrete mucus that is wafted up the trachea-bronchial tree by ciliated epithelial cells into the pharynx where it is swallowed. Coughing also expels collections of mucus from the larger airways. There are no cilia in the alveoli, but particles have to be less than 300 μm to reach the alveoli and once there they can be phagocytosed by macrophages, and then the cells drained in blood or by the lymphatics.

Oxygen toxicity

Breathing oxygen 100% for over 24 hours is associated with retrosternal discomfort, exacerbated by deep inspiration, and a fall in tidal volume. The fall in tidal volume is due to absorption atelectasis. Small mammals will develop pulmonary oedema after days of breathing oxygen 100%. If supplemental oxygen sustains the arterial PaO_2 above 18 kPa in premature babies, they may become blind due to retrolental fibroplasia.

Pathophysiology

During thoracic surgery, the patient is anaesthetized in the lateral position with the lung collapsed in the superior chest, which is open or penetrated by ports for video-assisted thoracoscopic surgery (VATS) procedures.

Open chest

The open chest abolishes the close approximation of the visceral to parietal pleura with a pleural pressure negative to the atmosphere. During spontaneous ventilation, the chest wall expands, and pleural pressure falls around the inferior or dependent lung and it expands with the chest wall. There is no such expansion in the superior lung that is surrounded by atmospheric pressure, whose gas contents empty into the dependent lung. During expiration, the elastic recoil of the chest wall expresses increases pleural pressure, forcing gas out of the dependent lung. Some gas is exhaled and some is directed to the superior lung still surrounded by atmospheric pressure. The paradoxical ventilation of the superior lung prevents fresh gas containing oxygen from participating in gas exchange in the still functioning dependent lung. Mechanical ventilation of both lungs with positive pressure ventilation restores synchronous expansion and deflation of both lungs.

Flail chest, with multiple adjacent ribs fractured in two or more places, combines loss of integrity of the chest wall with damage to underlying lung from the transfer of energy to the chest sufficient to fracture ribs. Stabilization of the chest wall and control of pain from the rib fractures will still require supportive management until the lung has had time to heal.

One-lung ventilation

Isolating one lung to permit surgery on that lung, or that side of the chest, immediately introduces a shunt of about 50% and more if it is the right lung that is isolated than the left. Positioning the patient laterally with the ventilated lung dependent reduces the shunt because more blood flows to the dependent lung under the effects of gravity. Maintaining the ventilated lung expanded with appropriate tidal volumes and using positive end expiratory pressure (PEEP) avoids further shunt. Avoiding over-expanding the lung will avoid generating dead space when alveolar pressure exceeds pulmonary artery venous or even arterial pressures.

The collapsed lung has less blood flow than expected because of mechanical effects. Hypoxic pulmonary vasoconstriction plays an inconsistent role during anaesthesia without the differences seen between intravenous and volatile anaesthetic agents in the laboratory. Should it be difficult to control hypoxaemia during one-lung anaesthesia, clamping the main or lobar pulmonary artery in the operative site may control the shunt to acceptable systemic oxygen concentrations.

An inspired oxygen concentration of 50% at the onset of one lung anaesthesia may need to be adjusted up or down in the light of measurements of arterial blood gases. Oxygen introduced down to the main bronchus by a catheter may overcome hypoxia by diffusion down a concentration gradient to alveoli that remain expanded. A PEEP of 5 cmH$_2$O sustained by oxygen passed into reservoir bag held open using a variable aperture valve may expand more alveoli, but the expanded lung may interfere with access to the operative site.

Further limitation of hypoxaemia is possible by maintaining cardiac output. Avoiding a fall in the mixed venous haemoglobin oxygen saturation by avoiding low cardiac output will return better-oxygenated blood to the right atrium. Better-oxygenated blood in the blood that does shunt through the collapsed lung will limit the subsequent fall in systemic arterial haemoglobin oxygen saturation when blood from the lungs is mixed in the left atrium.

Bronchoconstriction

Increased reactivity of bronchial smooth muscle, inflammation and excessive secretions all contribute to bronchoconstriction in asthma. Parenchymal oedema and excess secretions accompany rapid respiration rate, hyperinflation of the lungs, obstruction to airflow, and a prolonged expiratory phase from an increased capillary permeability.

Bronchiectasis

Bronchiectasis is characterized by chronic inflammation and infection leading to a persistent widening of the bronchi with an associated productive cough. There is airflow obstruction and a progressive decline in lung function.

Airway obstruction

Principal airways such as the trachea and main bronchi may be obstructed within the lumen, in the wall or by external compression. Foreign bodies, secretions, and blood may block an airway; bronchial tumours and tracheomalacia disrupt the wall itself; and trauma, parenchymal tumours, lymph nodes, the thyroid, and haematomas can compress the wall and lumen. There is no response to bronchodilators, stridor if the obstruction is above the thoracic inlet and prolonged expiration if the obstruction is within the chest. The flow–volume curve is fixed and small and eventually hypoventilation causes hypoxaemia and hypercapnia.

Tracheomalacia is an uncommon complication following thyroidectomy for goitre. Collapse of the unsupported airway may resolve if the trachea is kept patent by an endotracheal tube. Persisting weakness of the wall may involve tracheostomy and multiple procedures to reconstruct the airway. Vocal cord paralysis is another cause of airway obstruction after thyroidectomy. Bilateral vocal cord paralysis leaves vocal cords that approximate when air flows through the glottic chink causing obstruction that requires tracheostomy.

Bronchial obstruction can leave a fully functioning trachea and opposite lung. The distal lobe or lung may collapse and cause hypoxaemia with blood shunting through non-ventilated parenchyma. Retention of secretions and infection in the collapsed lung further worsens the hypoxaemia.

Mild haemoptysis may have transient pathophysiological effects, but can be the first symptom of a bronchial tumour. Massive haemoptysis can lead to exsanguination and airway obstruction.

Acute lung injury

Acute lung injury leading to adult respiratory distress syndrome (ARDS) demonstrates alveolar epithelial damage, capillary leak and protein rich pulmonary oedema caused by neutrophils, inflammatory mediators, abnormal coagulation and fibrinolysis, high inspired oxygen concentrations, and the effects of mechanical ventilation. These changes produce hypoxaemia, decreased lung compliance and bilateral diffuse infiltrates on the chest radiograph. There is subsequent increased pulmonary vascular resistance then fibrosis within the lung following the initial inflammation.

A pulmonary artery occlusion pressure of less than 18 mmHg is used to exclude left heart failure as the cause. The ratio of arterial oxygen tension to inspired concentration of oxygen (PaO$_2$:FiO$_2$) is less than 40 in acute lung injury falling to less than 26.7 in established ARDS.

Lung injury following thoracic surgery

Lung resection still carries an appreciable mortality. Acute lung injury in the remaining lung tissue is an important contributor. Excessive lung inflation and repeated collapse and expansion of alveoli during mechanical ventilation are associated with lung injury, but protective ventilation with small tidal volumes of 6 mL/kg with PEEP to keep the alveoli distended has not produced an improvement in outcome. A common feature is extravascular lung water in the affected parenchyma. Attention has moved from interruption of lymphatic drainage being responsible, to disruption of interstitial proteoglycans and intravascular glycocalyx increasing microvascular permeability. Pulmonary hypertension and right heart overload may develop as the microvasculature in affected lung tissue is compressed, further worsening prognosis.

Pleural effusions

Fluid in the pleural space restricts movement of the chest and reduces air entry on that side. A distinction between exudates from inflammation and malignancy, and transudates from heart or live failure may be made by measuring lactate dehydrogenase and protein concentrations in the pleural aspirate. Subsequent infection of the fluid, often from underlying pneumonia may loculate the effusion or generate an empyema.

Trauma to the skeleton of the chest wall or disease or trauma to its vessels may result in blood collecting in the pleural space to give a haemothorax. A volume of blood greater than 1500 mL is termed a massive haemothorax.

Pneumothorax

Rupture of a bleb on the lung surface, needle puncture, or trauma, and gas forced at pressure down the airways can introduce air into the pleural space. The negative pressure in the pleural space is lost and the lung can collapse away from the chest wall producing a pneumothorax. The rib cage is expanded and diaphragm depressed. There can be symptoms of pain and breathlessness, and signs of reduced chest movements and air entry on the affected side. Small pockets of air will be absorbed spontaneously. Chest drainage with an underwater seal will accelerate the absorption.

A massive open pneumothorax with spontaneous ventilation will have gas transferring from lung to lung during the breathing cycle reducing the amount of oxygen that can be inhaled with each breath. The chest wall defect has to be closed with a flap valve or drain and underwater seal to restore synchronous expansion and collapse of both lungs during respiration.

When expansion of the chest wall increases the size of the pneumothorax and air cannot then escape the size and pressure of the gas in the pleura increases generating a tension pneumothorax. The functioning lung is then compressed requiring emergency decompression of the affected side to produce a simple pneumothorax that may then be drained.

Pleural tumours

A thickened, rigid, contracted pleura from fibrosis or reactive changes to tumours such as mesothelioma can result in restrictive functional impairment of respiratory function.

Mediastinal tumours

Tumours within the mediastinum can vary greatly in origin, position, size, and cardiorespiratory influence from small and unobtrusive to life-threatening. Breathlessness, cough, hoarseness, and syncope may form part of the presentation. The tumour may be concealed within the mediastinal shadow on plain chest radiograph, but be defined better on computed tomography of the chest.

Mediastinal mass syndrome may obstruct airways and impede blood flow within the chest. The patient may be satisfactory at rest leaning forward, for example, but can decompensate when laid flat. Anaesthesia and muscle relaxation can remove respiratory reserve. The chest cavity is reduced by 500–1000 mL when the diaphragm is paralysed and abdominal contents move cephalad. Loss of bronchial muscle tone compromises airway patency further. Spontaneous ventilation in the erect patient matches ventilation and perfusion better than mechanical ventilation in a paralysed patient. The change may be the difference between satisfactory oxygenation and decompensation. Air trapping may develop behind airway obstruction within the chest cavity, decreasing gas exchange.

The major blood vessels may suffer external compression. The pulmonary arteries are protected by the neighbouring aorta and trachea, but when compressed may generate right heart failure. The superior vena cava has little pressure within the lumen and an exposed course making it susceptible to external compression, reducing venous return to the heart and engorging the upper half of the body.

External radiotherapy, chemotherapy, and intravascular and airway stents may be used to ameliorate the external compression that mediastinal masses can produce. In severe cases, femoral access for cardiopulmonary bypass can sustain life whilst an intrathoracic mass is resected.

Mediastinitis

Inflammation of the mediastinum is most likely after surgical intervention, but may follow trauma, oesophageal rupture, descending infection from the head and neck, and be associated with neoplasms. Mortality is most likely with neoplasms and least likely following trauma. As well as the features of deep wound and systemic infection, an anterior defect in the integrity of the chest wall impedes effective mechanical activity. Excision of tissue affected by osteomyelitis and closure of the defect with omentum, muscle, or skin flaps may be required to restore effective ventilation by expansion of the chest wall.

Pulmonary embolus

Pulmonary thromboembolus generates dead space by occluding the pulmonary artery supplying lung that continues to be ventilated. Tachypnoea, tachycardia, hypoxaemia, and hypocarbia are early signs in significant pulmonary embolus. Initial hypoxaemia stimulates increases in breathing rate and cardiac output in an attempt to restore delivery of oxygen to the tissues. More substantial pulmonary emboli may cause sudden death or cause the right ventricle to fail. The right side of the heart is distended and contracts poorly, with an enlarged right atrium and electrographic changes of right axis deviation, S waves in lead I, and Q waves and inverted T waves in lead III.

Sternal abnormalities

Apart from the cosmetic appearance, pectus excavatum compresses lung tissue, displaces the heart and may restrict cardiac output, limiting exercise capacity. Following repair appearance and aerobic exercise capacity are improved. There is little change in cardiac index, but respiratory function tests and cardiorespiratory exercise testing demonstrate improvements.

Kyphoscoliosis

Progressive untreated curvature of the spine, especially when the spine above the 10th thoracic vertebra is involved causes a worsening restrictive respiratory defect. As lung function deteriorates, cor pulmonale develops.

Conclusion

A thorough understanding of the anatomy of the chest, physiology and pathophysiology of respiration and diseases of the chest allows cardiothoracic anaesthesiologists to manage patients safely during and after the severe trespass of cardiothoracic surgery.

Further reading

Agur AMR, Dalley AFI. *Grant's Atlas of Anatomy*. 13th ed. Philadelphia: Walters Kluwer, Lippincott Williams & Wilkins, 2013. 853 p

Bakowitz M, Bruns B, McCunn M. Acute lung injury and the acute respiratory distress syndrome in the injured patient. *Scand J Trauma Resusc Emerg Med* 2012; **20**: 54

Barrett KE, Barman S.M.; Biotano S, Brooks HL. *Ganong's Review of Medical Physiology*. 24th edn. New York: Lange Medical Publications, 2012

Benumof JL. *Anesthesia for Thoracic Surgery*. 2nd edn. Philadelphia: W.B. Saunders Company, 1995

Bernard GR, Artigas A, Brigham KL, et al. The American-European Consensus Conference on ARDS. Definitions, mechanisms, relevant outcomes, and clinical trial coordination. *Am J Respir Crit Care Med* 1994; **149**(3 Pt 1): 818–24

Blank RS, de Souza DG. Anesthetic management of patients with an anterior mediastinal mass: continuing professional development. *Can J Anaesth* 2011; **58**(9): 853–9

Borley NRA. *Instant Physiology*, 2nd edn. Malden, MA, ed. Oxford: Blackwell Publishing, 2005

Cipolle M, Rhodes M, Tinkoff G. Deadly dozen: dealing with the 12 types of thoracic injuries. *J Emerg MedServices* 2012; **37**(9): 60–5

Davignon K, Kwo J, Bigatello LM. Pathophysiology and management of the flail chest. *Minerva Anestesiolog* 2004; **70**(4): 193–9

Dushianthan A, Grocott MPW, Postle AD, Cusack R. Acute respiratory distress syndrome and acute lung injury. *Postgrad Med J*. 2011; **87**(1031): 612–22

El Oakley RM, Wright JE. Postoperative mediastinitis: Classification and management. *Annals Thorac Surg* 1996; **61**(3): 1030–6

Erdos G, Tzanova I. Perioperative anaesthetic management of mediastinal mass in adults. Eur J Anaesthesiol. 2009; **26**(8): 627–32

Gaissert HA, Burns J. The compromised airway: tumors, strictures, and tracheomalacia. *Surg Clin N Am* 2010; **90**(5): 1065–89

Hlastala MPBAJ. *Physiology of Respiration*, 2nd edn. Oxford: Oxford University Press, 2001

Hurt K, Bilton D. Haemoptysis: diagnosis and treatment. *Acute Med* 2012; **11**(1): 39–45

Jabłoński S, Brocki M, Kordiak J, Misiak P, Terlecki A, Kozakiewicz M. Acute mediastinitis: evaluation of clinical risk factors for death in surgically treated patients. *ANZ J Surg* 2013; **83**(9): 657–63

King PT. The pathophysiology of bronchiectasis. *Int J Chronic Obstr Pulmon Dis* 2009; **4**: 411–9

Kometani T, Okamoto T, Yoshida S, Yoshino I. Acute respiratory distress syndrome after pulmonary resection. *Gen Thorac Cardiovasc Surg* 2013; **61**(9): 504–12

Leigh-Smith S, Harris T. Tension pneumothorax—time for a re-think? *Emerg Med J*. 2005; **22**(1): 8–16

Levitt JE, Gould MK, Ware LB, Matthay MA. Analytic review: the pathogenetic and prognostic value of biologic markers in acute lung injury. *J Intens Care Med* 2009; **24**(3): 151–67

McCulloch P. A simple modle illustrating the balancing forces of lung and chest wall recoil. *Adv Physiol Educ* 2004; **28**(3): 125–7

Merli GJ. Pathophysiology of venous thrombosis and the diagnosis of deep vein thrombosis–pulmonary embolism in the elderly. *Cardiol Clin* 2008; **26**(2): 203–19

Merrill WH, Akhter SA, Wolf RK, Schneeberger EW, Flege JB Jr. Simplified treatment of postoperative mediastinitis. *Ann Thorac Surg* 2004; **78**(2): 608–12

Mossman BT, Shukla A, Heintz NH, Verschraegen CF, Thomas A, Hassan R. New insights into understanding the mechanisms, pathogenesis, and management of malignant mesotheliomas. *Am J Pathol*. 2013; **182**(4): 1065–77

Munis JR. *Just Enough Physiology*. Oxford: Oxford University Press, 2012

Noppen M. Spontaneous pneumothorax: epidemiology, pathophysiology and cause. *Eur Respir Rev* 2010; **19**(117): 217–9

Pocock GR, Christopher D. *Human Physiology: the basis of medicine*, 3rd edn. Oxford: Oxford University Press, 2006

Pramanik B. Hemoptysis with diagnostic dilemma. *Expert Rev Respir Med* 2013; **7**(1): 91–7

Sigalet DL, Montgomery M, Harder J, Wong V, Kravarusic D, Alassiri A. Long term cardiopulmonary effects of closed repair of pectus excavatum. *Pediatr Surg Int* 2007; **23**(5):493–7. Epub 2007/01/26

Soll C, Hahnloser D, Frauenfelder T, Russi EW, Weder W, Kestenholz PB. The postpneumonectomy syndrome: clinical presentation and treatment. European *J Cardio-Thorac Surg* 2009; **35**(2): 319–24

Sukkar MYE-M, El-Munshid H.A, Ardawi MSM. *Concise Human Physiology*, 2nd edn. Oxford: Blackwell Science, 2000

Sylvester JT, Shimoda LA, Aaronson PI, Ward JPT. Hypoxic pulmonary vasoconstriction. *Physiol Rev*. 2012; **92**(1): 367–520

Weibel E. Airways and blood vessels. In: *The Pathway For Oxygen Structure and Function in the Mammalian Respiratory System*. Harvard: Harvard University Press, 1984; 272–301

Weldon E, Williams J. Pleural disease in the emergency department. *Emerg Med Clin N Am* 2012; **30**(2): 475–99, ix–x

West JB. *Respiratory Physiology: the Essentials*, 9th edn. Baltimore: Lippincott Williams & Wilkins, 2012

West JB. *Pulmonary Pathophysiology: the Essentials*, 8th edn. Baltimore: Lippincott Williams & Wilkins, 2013

CHAPTER 5

The inflammatory response to cardiothoracic surgery

William T. McBride and Esther R. McBride

Introduction

This chapter considers the inflammatory response in the context of the overall immune system. The role of the coagulation system in activating the perioperative inflammatory response will be emphasized, In addition, the concept of pro- and anti-inflammatory cytokine balance will also be considered and the effects of imbalance will be described.

The inflammatory response in context

There are classically described two aspects to the immune system (figure 5.1) (1). The innate mechanisms provide protection without specific recognition of antigen and there is no capacity to mount memory to provide an enhanced response on subsequent encounter with antigen. The adaptive or specific response first needs to specifically recognize antigen before mounting a response which includes developing memory such that subsequent exposure to antigen leads to a faster and more enhanced response. In each category there are cellular and humoral elements. For example, the cellular element in the specific response includes B and T lymphocytes, while in the innate response there are neutrophils, natural killer (NK), and mast cells. Lying between the specific and innate

responses are antigen-presenting cells (APCs), which can have specific (antigen recognition) as well as non-specific actions. Chief of these is the dendritic cell (DC) population, which plays a central role in the immune response to infection. This involves antigen recognition in the peripheral tissues, maturation, and migration to lymph nodes where antigen presentation to helper T cells takes place. This leads (in the context of co-stimulation) to antigen-specific responses, as well as in some cases, tolerance.

Controlling these cells are cytokines. These are glycosylated and non-glycosylated polypeptides that are the soluble messengers of the immune system. In addition to their primary direct immunomodulatory effects on T cells and DCs, cytokines may have secondary pro- or anti-inflammatory effects. The mutually opposing biological effects of the pro- and anti-inflammatory mediators has led to the concept of pro- and anti-inflammatory cytokine balance, examples of which are found in the blood, renal tract, and in the lungs.

Cytokines

Pro-inflammatory

Tumour necrosis factor alpha (TNF-α)

Tumour necrosis factor alpha (TNF-α) is a trimer belonging to the tumor necrosis factor/ tumor necrosis factor receptor superfamily

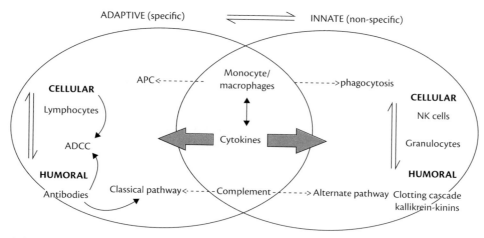

Fig. 5.1 The clotting cascade forms part of the humoral non-specific immune response. NK, natural killer cell; APC, antigen-presenting cell; ADCC, antibody dependent cell mediated cytotoxicity.

Reproduced from McBride WT, Armstrong MA, McBride SJ, 'Immunomodulation: an important concept in modern anaesthesia', Anaesthesia, 51, 5, pp. 465–473, copyright 1996, with permission from The Association of Anaesthetists of Great Britain and Ireland

of proteins. It is produced by vascular endothelial cells and a wide variety of immune cells (2). The main physiological stimulus is bacterial lipopolysaccharide (LPS) in presence of interleukin (IL)1β (2).

When the TNF-α trimer binds to the TNF receptor, aggregation of the receptors occurs prompting their activation through its intracellular cytoplasmic death domain and leading to several pro-inflammatory cellular outcomes including apoptosis and nuclear factor kappa B (NF-κB) activation. Clinical manifestations include pyrexia (hypothalamic effects), acute phase response including C-reactive protein (CRP) (hepatic effects), and generalized inflammation due to endothelial adhesion molecule upregulation. TNF-α counters infection in inflamed tissue by inducing monocytes to become dendritic cells (DCs) promoting adaptive immunity (3).

IL-1α and IL-1β

IL-1α and IL-1β are produced by endothelium, B cells, DC, macrophages, monocytes, and NK cells. They bind to IL-1 receptors and have similar physiological effects to TNF-α. IL1 and TNF-α have a greater pro-inflammatory effect when they act together than each alone. IL-1β in presence of interferon gamma (IFN-γ) stimulates production of TNF-α in human vascular endothelial cells (2). Thus IL-1β is one of the earliest cytokines involved in initiating the pro-inflammatory response, even in the absence of LPS (2). Since IL-1β is generated by perturbations of the coagulation system (see section on Coagulation), it can be appreciated how surgery alone can trigger an IL-1β and TNF-α response which then ignites an overall inflammatory response.

Anti-inflammatory cytokines

IL-10

IL-10 is considered to act as an anti-inflammatory cytokine, suppressing immunological and inflammatory reactions. Its deactivates macrophages, resulting in diminished Type 1 helper T cell (Th1) cytokine production, decreased production of reactive nitrogen or oxygen species and limiting antigen presentation (4). Accordingly, its anti-inflammatory actions involve limiting pro-inflammatory processes, as illustrated by inhibiting production of IL-1β, TNF-α, and IL-8 in LPS stimulated polymorphonuclear (PMN) leukocytes (5). IL-10 amplifies anti-inflammation through stimulating production of the anti-inflammatory cytokines IL-1 receptor antagonist (IL-1ra) and TNF soluble receptors by PMN leukocytes and monocytes (5).

IL-10 is produced in the liver by Kupffer cells. It is also produced extrahepatically by Th lymphocytes and monocytes. IL-10 production correlates with the severity of disease in sepsis and neutralization of IL-10 in mice suffering from septic shock prolongs survival through blocking IL-10 mediated suppression of NK cell function (6).

IL-1 receptor antagonist

IL-1ra is a true receptor agonist binding to, but lacking agonist activity on, the IL-1 receptor. It is produced by monocytes, neutrophils, macrophages, hepatocytes, microglial cells, and fibroblasts. LPS is a potent stimulus for the release of IL-1ra. IL-1ra production is also upregulated by IL-10, IL-4, IFN-γ, and IL-1β (5).

Tumour necrosis factor soluble receptor

TNF receptors are either constitutively expressed (TNFR1) or inducible (TNFR2). When the extracellular domain of these receptors is shed, they are referred to as soluble receptors of TNF (TNFsr type I) (55 kDa receptor) and TNFsr type II (75 kDa receptor). The anti-inflammatory action is mediated by removal of TNF-α receptors from cells, thus reducing TNF-α-mediated pro-inflammatory intracellular signalling as well as by binding free TNF-α. TNFsrs concentration is increased in response to IL-10 (7).

The inflammatory response is only part of the overall immune response and lies within the innate (non-specific) immune response. It is contributed to largely by the humoral component of the complement system (the kallikrein kinin system), aspects of the complement system, and pro-inflammatory cytokines. The cellular component is largely made up of neutrophils whose cargo of degradative enzymes, once disgorged causes local destruction. In non-septic inflammation the inflammatory response arises from contact activation of blood with an endogenous foreign surface such as collagen (in vivo during endothelial damage) or an exogenous non-endothelial surface such as the foreign surface of a cardiopulmonary bypass (CPB) machine and tissue damage leading to activation of the coagulation system.

Localized inflammatory response

An inflammatory response may be localized or systemic. Before considering the systemic, generalized inflammatory response at cardiac surgery, it is necessary to understand the mechanism of a localized normal and appropriate pathophysiological inflammatory response at a site of injury or infection, where the result is protection against infection.

Mechanism of a local inflammatory response

In cardiothoracic surgery, there is an initial breach of the skin, tissues, and vasculature and in the case of cardiac surgery the sternum. This is sufficient to activate the coagulation system, which triggers mechanisms of a localized inflammatory response.

These phenomena are particularly illustrated in an untreated traumatic non-surgical incision where localized inflammation frequently rapidly develops. This is because in areas of local tissue damage or infection, exposure of subendothelial tissue layers activates clotting and complement systems, which in turn trigger an appropriate local pro-inflammatory response; further localized pro-inflammatory mediator production results in the classically described picture of local tissue redness (rubor), pain (dolor), increased temperature (calor) and swelling (tumor) that is attributed to Celsus in the first century BCE.

Local tissue redness (rubor) arises from vasodilation of vascular smooth muscle due to locally released mediators such as bradykinin (secondary to the clotting factor XIIa and kallikrein) as well as histamine from mast cells and the complement product, C5a, together with nitric oxide. This increases circulatory access to the damaged site to allow ingress of leukocytes to deal with infective invaders and causes increased temperature (calor). Furthermore, bradykinin, histamine, and leukotrienes act on endothelial cells to promote capillary leakiness leading to localized swelling (tumor). The increased fluid leak concentrates blood cells in capillaries, slowing the flow and allowing increased adhesion of neutrophils to the endothelial wall. This is further enhanced by local pro-inflammatory cytokines leading to up regulation of endothelial adhesion molecules allowing easier movement of leukocytes through capillaries into inflamed or damaged tissues.

Interaction between clotting and inflammation

The clotting mechanism which is part of the innate response has, likewise, cellular (platelets) and humoral elements (clotting factors).This acts not merely to prevent death by exsanguination but in addition to form a localized clot to provide a temporary barrier preventing entrance of infective organisms. The complex steps within the coagulation system powerfully modulate the overall immune response, of which the inflammatory response is an important part. In turn the inflammatory response can have pro- and anticoagulant effects and at the same time have pro- and anti- effects on the immune response to infection. Thus it is possible for a patient to have marked inflammatory response and still be immunosuppressed with respect to B and T cell function and DC migration and maturation.

Perturbations of the coagulation system at surgery can trigger a localized pro-inflammatory response near to the surgical site and also limit it by concomitant anti-inflammatory effects. Coagulation, anticoagulation, fibrinolysis, and antifibrinolysis are four major elements of the coagulation system and all four are involved in modulating the inflammatory response either by activating or inhibiting it (figure 5.2) (1).

Coagulation

Coagulation is formation of clot and this process tends to be pro-inflammatory. Key players in clot formation are involved in promoting inflammation. For example thrombin and factor Xa enhance production of IL-1. Thrombin induces IL8 production. Factor Xa induces IL-6 and IL-8 production.

Anticoagulation

Anticoagulation is the physiological mechanism that prevents clot formation getting out of control and a small thrombus in a local area of vasculature spreading to compromise vital blood supply. There are three major anticoagulant mechanisms: thrombomodulin–Protein C–Protein S complex (activated Protein C), tissue factor pathway inhibitor (TFPI) and anti-thrombin-III (AT III) are all anti-inflammatory. In humans, recombinant human activated Protein C has antithrombotic as well as anti-inflammatory actions. In rats given LPS, TFPI reduces pulmonary vascular injury by inhibiting leukocyte activation and in baboons, it reduces IL-6 and IL-8. In rats given endotoxin, AT III prevents pulmonary vascular injury by inhibiting leukocyte activation.

Fibrinolysis

Fibrinolysis is proinflammatory and in the context of local injury, fibrinolysis will attract neutrophils into the area as part of the innate immune response. For example, urokinase plasminogen activator (uPA) and its receptor (uPAR) play an important role in fibrinolysis and at the same time promote activation and chemotaxis of neutrophils and lymphocytes (8).

Antifibrinolysis

Antifibrinolysis is anti-inflammatory and the antifibrinolytic drugs, aprotinin and epsilon-aminocaproic acid reduce the IL-8 and IL-6 responses in patients undergoing CPB (9).

Systemic inflammatory response

When local inflammatory processes become systemic and pro-inflammatory mediators that normally act locally, spill into the general circulation then a systemic pro-inflammatory response will develop. Thus local mediators that cause vasodilation, capillary leak, and swelling, will also cause global vasodilation and capillary leak. Untreated, these mediators cause vasoplegia and hypotension. The hypotension further fuels the inflammatory response leading to gut mucosal injury resulting in endotoxin translocation to the circulation while at the same time, renal excretion of pro-inflammatory mediators is compromised (10). A systemic capillary leak leads to pulmonary and generalized tissue oedema. Increased neutrophil adhesion also occurs with neutrophil mediated organ damage.

Typically, the inflammatory response to sepsis and injury is biphasic with an initial systemic inflammatory response syndrome (SIRS) causing multi-organ failure if excessive (figure 5.3). Later, a compensatory anti-inflammatory response arises in parallel to the SIRS that is associated with a decrease in immunity.

Surgery and trauma as triggers of inflammation

Surgery and trauma can trigger both local and systemic inflammatory response in previously healthy non-infected people. During cardiac surgery, it was at first thought that the inflammatory

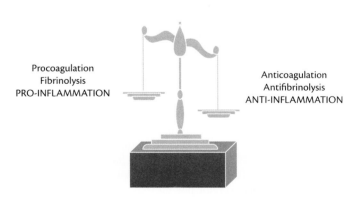

Fig. 5.2 Coagulation and the balance of pro- and anti-inflammation.

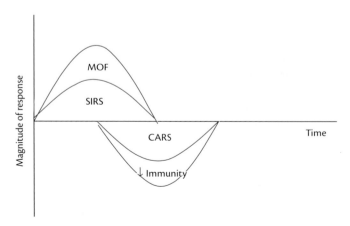

Fig. 5.3 The biphasic response to injury and sepsis.
To begin with there is a systemic inflammatory response syndrome (SIRS) response, which if excessive can lead to multiple organ failure (MOF). Arising in parallel with the SIRS response is the compensatory anti-inflammatory response (CARS).

response arose mainly from the interaction of the patient's blood with the foreign surface of the CPB machine. Evidence for this arose from the observation that patients who undergo minimally invasive coronary artery bypass grafting (CABG) surgery have a significant reduction in some elements of the systemic inflammatory response (leukocyte elastase, platelet beta-thromboglobulin, and complement C3a) compared with patients who undergo conventional CABG surgery with CPB (11). Also in experiments where donor blood passes through an isolated CPB system, there are significant increases in IL-8 and neutrophil adhesion molecule upregulation (12).

However, plasma cytokine pro- and anti-inflammatory response is of almost similar magnitude in patients undergoing off-pump CABG surgery (13). So, the surgical insult and its magnitude are also major contributors to the inflammatory response. Moreover, retransfusion of unwashed mediastinal blood during off-pump CABG surgery significantly accentuates the cytokine inflammatory response (14). This accentuation points to the importance of perturbations of the clotting mechanism triggering the inflammatory response from the outset of surgery and at the same time providing mechanisms to help control that pro-inflammatory response.

Cytokines and the systemic inflammatory response

Shortly after sternotomy in adult patients there is a small and transient increase in plasma pro-inflammatory TNF-α and IL-8. At the end of CPB, there is a further increase in these pro-inflammatory cytokines which normally quickly subsides (12). In isolated CPB experiments, IL-8 is consistently generated in the plasma of the in vitro system (12). Midway through CPB, there is a marked increase in the plasma anti-inflammatory cytokine IL-10 (15). By the next day, this is almost back to baseline normal. Several hours after the IL-10 peak, and possibly stimulated by it, there is a further plasma peak in the anti-inflammatory antagonist to IL-1β, IL1 receptor antagonist (IL-1ra). This response is well reduced 24 hours later. However, to provide ongoing plasma anti-inflammatory protection after 24 hours, there is a more delayed and longer lasting anti-inflammatory response continuing for several days made up of TNF soluble receptor 1 and 2 (TNFsr1 and 2) (12). This pattern is quite similar in paediatric cardiac surgery (15).

Beneficial effects of the perioperative pro-inflammatory response

It has long been known that high cytokine levels following major trauma are associated with higher mortality. However, this does not mean that it is the inflammatory response per se that causes the mortality but merely reflects the magnitude of the surgical insult. In fact, the evidence now points to a controlled pro-inflammatory response having a beneficial effect.

A controlled, time limited and balanced systemic inflammatory response is beneficial to healing and repair in that it heightens the immune system during the time of vulnerability to infection caused by breach of tissues. First, this allows for rapid response to bacterial or viral infection as well as clearance of damaged tissue by macrophages. Second, and of great importance, an early and self-limiting pro-inflammatory response activates human adipose tissue-derived mesenchymal stem cells (ASCs) to stimulate

regeneration of injured tissues (16). The problem arises if the pro-inflammatory response is excessive and unbalanced by the accompanying anti-inflammatory response.

Normal versus abnormal pro- and anti-inflammatory responses

A pro-inflammatory response is abnormal if it becomes excessive or exceeds the capacity of the anti-inflammatory response to contain it and in this situation, there is a risk of organ damage (10). It is also an abnormal response if it becomes sustained, i.e., lasts longer than several days when prolonged TNF-α and IL-6 may be detrimental to healing and repair (17,18).

An anti-inflammatory response is normal if it develops quickly after the commencement of the pro-inflammatory response, thus preventing unwanted pro-inflammatory effects of the inflammatory response. However, an anti-inflammatory response is abnormal if it is excessive or prolonged when there may be an associated immunosuppression and risk of sepsis. For example, IL10 inhibits immune cells required for optimal pathogen protection (19). The IL-10 GCC haplotype has been associated with production of relatively high levels of IL-10, which down-regulate expression of major histocompatibility complex class I and class II molecules potentially contributing to duration of viral infection among immunosuppressed individuals. Also, in septic mice, neutralization of IL-10 confers survival benefit (20).

Factors determining the magnitude of inflammatory responses

Surgical factors

Surgical factors include duration of surgery, and cross-clamp time as well as choice of anaesthetic.

Patient factors

Patient factors include co-morbidities such as renal dysfunction which may alter renal excretion of pro-inflammatory mediators. Impaired cardiac function may compromise organ perfusion, especially splanchnic perfusion predisposing to endotoxin translocation to the circulation and heightening pro-inflammatory responses. Co-existing malignancy at thoracic surgery can alter baseline pro- and anti-inflammatory plasma balance (21). Previous exposure to endotoxin may precondition protective responses conferring protection (22). Also, it is possible that genetic polymorphisms, may help to determine the magnitude of the pro- and anti-inflammatory responses. Polymorphisms that heighten a pro-inflammatory response may in certain contexts confer protection against sepsis while at the same time increase chance of multiple organ dysfunction if the pro-inflammatory response becomes excessive. Conversely, polymorphisms that promote the anti-inflammatory response may well protect against organ failure but increase risk of infection. Hypo- and hyper-secretor genes of TNF-α are good illustrations of this balance.

TNF-α hypo/hyper secretor polymorphisms

Guanine (G) to adenine (A) transitions at the 252 site within the TNF-β- gene (TNF B2/B1 polymorphism respectively) and the –308 site in the TNF-α promoter region have both been associated with greater TNF-α secretion after endotoxin (figure 5.4) (23).

While TNF hyper-secretor polymorphism TNF-308A is linked with greater renal complications, it appears that TNF hyper-secretor

Table 5.1 Influence of genotype on inflammatory response to cardiac surgery

	TNFB2/B2 (42)	TNFB1/B1 or B1/B2	
TNF-α (pg ml⁻¹)	11.3 ± 1.3	7.8 ± 0.7	P=0.013
IL-6 (pg ml⁻¹)	153 ± 27	87 ± 7	P=0.010
Pulm dysfunction	24%	6%	P=0.016

In a study of 95 patients undergoing cardiac surgery, tumour necrosis B2 (TNF) factor gene polymorphism was associated with an enhanced systemic inflammatory response and increased cardiopulmonary morbidity.

Data from Tomasdottir H, Hjartarson H, Ricksten A, Wasslavik C, Bengtsson A, Ricksten SE. Tumor necrosis factor gene polymorphism is associated with enhanced systemic inflammatory response and increased cardiopulmonary morbidity after cardiac surgery. Anesth Analg 2003;97:944–9.

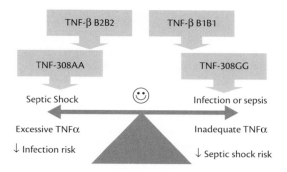

Fig. 5.4 The diagram summarizes which genes promote TNF-α production leading to risk of septic shock but decreasing infection risk. On the other hand the genes which lead to reduced TNF-α responses heighten risk of infection or sepsis but decrease risk of septic shock. The theoretical ideal place is to be is a heterozygote in the middle!.

genotypes may provide protection against infection and sepsis (24,25). So hyper-secretion may predispose to development of an excessive inflammatory response and so to SIRS and renal dysfunction, yet at the same time protect against sepsis. This has led to the suggestion that the best advantage is to carry the polymorphisms for a balanced pro- and anti-inflammatory response (26).

In a study of 95 patients undergoing cardiac surgery, TNF B2 gene polymorphism was associated with an enhanced systemic inflammatory response and increased cardiopulmonary morbidity such as pulmonary dysfunction (27) (table 5.1).

Intermediate TNF production genotypes prolong survival
In a study of 88 critically ill patients with multiple organ dysfunction syndrome, patients predisposed to a balanced cytokine response (e.g. intermediate interleukin-10/TNF-α producers) demonstrated the longest survival times, although overall mortality was unchanged (26). The authors of this study concluded that balanced pro- and anti-inflammatory cytokine genotypes prolonged patient survival time (26).

Endogenous control of inflammation

Reducing pro-inflammation
Mechanisms that reduce the ongoing generation of pro-inflammatory mediators help control inflammation. IL-10 rapidly increases during cardiac surgery, and so reduces the IL-8 response, down-regulates the IL-8 receptor, as well as down-regulating the IL-8 promotor, IL-17 (28). Additionally, it reduces IL-8-induced neutrophil chemotaxis, and C5a-induced monocyte chemotaxis (29).

Increases in the anti-inflammatory cytokines
The phased plasma anti-inflammatory cytokine response compensates for any unwanted systemic effects of pro-inflammatory mediators. Also, the constant presence in plasma of background anti-inflammatory cytokines such as IL-1ra and TNFsr1 and 2 provides protection against any spill over into the circulation of locally produced pro-inflammatory cytokines. This anti-inflammatory protective shield has been elsewhere called 'safe systemic cytokine capacity' (10).

Renal control
The kidneys have the ability to preferentially clear the pro-inflammatory cytokines. However, this protective anti-inflammatory shield can be overwhelmed if plasma clearance of pro-inflammatory mediators becomes compromised. In healthy subjects, the pro-inflammatory cytokine clearance is primarily a renal dependent process (30). In patients with renal failure, compensatory non-renal mechanisms are employed such as higher baseline concentrations of anti-inflammatory mediators (10).

Renal clearance of systemic pro-inflammatory cytokines
The kidneys are important in clearing pro-inflammatory cytokines. Monomeric TNF-α as well as IL-1β and IL-8, which are all pro-inflammatory cytokines, are less than 20 kDa in molecular weight, meaning that they are relatively easily filtered by the glomerulus, which preferentially allows filtration of molecules less than 20 kDa. In contrast, the anti-inflammatory cytokines (IL-10, IL-1ra, and TNFsr) are greater than 20 kDa and thus less readily filtered by the glomerulus. Although the biologically active form of TNFα is a trimer, greater than 20 kDa in molecular weight, the kidney can still contribute to its clearance. This is because the trimer exists in equilibrium with its dimeric and monomeric forms, and removal of the monomer by the glomerulus would ultimately lead to a decrease in the plasma concentration of the biologically active trimer. In light of this, it has been suggested that the kidney helps restore altered plasma pro- and anti-inflammatory cytokine homeostasis during cardiac surgery through preferential filtration and removal of pro-inflammatory cytokines (10,31).

Endogenous kidney protection
Increased plasma IL-10
Increased plasma anti-inflammatory IL-10 was renoprotective in a murine model of cisplatin mediated renal injury and a rat model of renal transplantation where the kidney was subjected to warm ischaemia (34).

Intrarenal anti-inflammatory cytokine response
The kidneys have the ability to develop an endogenous intrarenal anti-inflammatory cytokine response. Since pro-inflammatory cytokines, by virtue of their molecular weights, are preferentially filtered by the glomeruli in comparison with their larger molecular weight anti-inflammatory counterparts, this means that

pro-inflammatory cytokines are found in the glomerular filtrate without the same degree of protection as found in the plasma. It is here that the urinary anti-inflammatory cytokine response may be important (35,36). Even before there are significant increases in plasma IL-1ra and TNFsr, much larger increases in urinary IL-1ra and urinary TNFsr develop and last for at least 24 hours (35,36). The early development of the urinary anti-inflammatory cytokine response, together with its high concentration in relation to the later plasma anti-inflammatory response, strongly suggest that the kidney is able to generate its own anti-inflammatory response so as to allow for the safe disposal of the filtered pro-inflammatory cytokines. Normally IL-1β, TNF-α, and IL-8 are not detectable in the urine (35). This possibly reflects the efficient manner by which the tubular cells absorb and dispose of these filtered cytokines. However, it is likely that the anti-inflammatory cytokine response detectable in the urine is a renal compensatory response to pro-inflammatory cytokine activity more proximally in the nephron. Consequently, it is hardly surprising that the magnitude of the urinary IL-1ra response correlates with the subclinical renal injury detected after cardiac surgery (35).

During cardiac surgery and in a porcine model of infrarenal aortic ischemia, significant increases develop in the urinary concentration of another anti-inflammatory cytokine, transforming growth factor beta-1 (TGFβ-1) (37,38). It is thought that endogenous renal TGFβ-1 promotes tissue regeneration following acute injury. An anti-inflammatory protease inhibitor purified from human urine called ulinastatin is increased in the urine of patients following cardiac surgery, and is thought to protect against sepsis induced renal injury (39).

Conclusion

The inflammatory response is a normal physiological response to surgery promoting defence against infection and wound healing. However, the response should be self-limiting and its effects should be balanced by a compensatory anti-inflammatory response which should also be self-limiting and not excessive.

References

1. McBride WT, Armstrong MA, McBride SJ. Immunomodulation: an important concept in modern anaesthesia. *Anaesthesia* 1996; **51**: 465–73

2. Ranta V, Orpana A, Carpen O, Turpeinen U, Ylikorkala O, Viinikka L. Human vascular endothelial cells produce tumor necrosis factor-alpha in response to proinflammatory cytokine stimulation. *Crit Care Med* 1999; **27**: 2184–7

3. Chomarat P, Dantin C, Bennett L, Banchereau J, Palucka AK. TNF skews monocyte differentiation from macrophages to dendritic cells. *J Immunol* 2003; **171**: 2262–9

4. Beamer GL, Flaherty DK, Assogba BD et al. Interleukin-10 promotes Mycobacterium tuberculosis disease progression in CBA/J mice. *J Immunol* 2008; **181**: 5545–50

5. Cassatella MA, Meda L, Gasperini S, Calzetti F, Bonora S. Interleukin 10 (IL-10) upregulates IL-1 receptor antagonist production from lipopolysaccharide-stimulated human polymorphonuclear leukocytes by delaying mRNA degradation. *J Exp Med* 1994; **179**: 1695–9

6. Hiraki S, Ono S, Kinoshita M, et al. Neutralization of IL-10 restores the downregulation of IL-18 receptor on natural killer cells and interferon-gamma production in septic mice, thus leading to an improved survival. *Shock* 2012; **37**: 177–82

7. Seitz M, Loetscher P, Dewald B, Towbin H, Gallati H, Baggiolini M. Interleukin-10 differentially regulates cytokine inhibitor and chemokine release from blood mononuclear cells and fibroblasts. *Eur J Immunol* 1995; **25**: 1129–32

8. Roelofs JJ, Rowshani AT, van den Berg JG, et al. Expression of urokinase plasminogen activator and its receptor during acute renal allograft rejection. *Kidney Int* 2003; **64**: 1845–53

9. Greilich PE, Brouse CF, Whitten CW, Chi L, Dimaio JM, Jessen ME. Antifibrinolytic therapy during cardiopulmonary bypass reduces proinflammatory cytokine levels: a randomized, double-blind, placebo-controlled study of epsilon-aminocaproic acid and aprotinin. *J Thorac Cardiovasc Surg* 2003; **126**: 1498–1503

10. Baker R, Allen S, Armstrong MA, McBride WT. Editorial. Role of the kidney in perioperative inflammatory responses. *Br J Anaesth* 2002; **88**: 330–4

11. Gu YJ, Mariani MA, van Oeveren W, Grandjean JG, Boonstra PW. Reduction of the inflammatory response in patients undergoing minimally invasive coronary artery bypass grafting. *Ann Thorac Surg* 1998; **65**: 420–4

12. McBride WT, Armstrong MA, Crockard AD, McMurray TJ, Rea JM. Cytokine balance and immunosuppressive changes at cardiac surgery: contrasting response between patients and isolated CPB circuits. *Br J Anaesth* 1995; **75**: 724–33

13. Gormley SM, McBride WT, Armstrong MA, et al. Plasma and urinary cytokine homeostasis and renal function during cardiac surgery without cardiopulmonary bypass. *Cytokine* 2002; **17**: 61–5

14. Allen SJ, McBride WT, McMurray TJ, et al. Cell salvage alters the systemic inflammatory response after off-pump coronary artery bypass grafting surgery. *Ann Thorac Surg* 2007; **83**: 578–85

15. McBride WT, Armstrong MA, Gilliland H, McMurray TJ. The balance of pro and anti-inflammatory cytokines in plasma and bronchoalveolar lavage (BAL) at paediatric cardiac surgery. *Cytokine* 1996; **8**: 724–9

16. Heo SC, Jeon ES, Lee IH, Kim HS, Kim MB, Kim JH. Tumor necrosis factor-alpha-activated human adipose tissue-derived mesenchymal stem cells accelerate cutaneous wound healing through paracrine mechanisms. *J Invest Dermatol* 2011; **131**: 1559–67

17. Badr G, Badr BM, Mahmoud MM, Mohany M, Garraud O. Treatment of diabetic mice with undenatured whey protein accelerates the wound healing process by enhancing the expression of MIP-1 alpha, MIP-2, KC, CX3CL1 and TGF-beta in Wounded Tissue. *BMC Immunol* 2012; **13**: 32

18. Ashcroft GS, Jeong MJ, Ashworth JJ, et al. Tumor necrosis factor-alpha (TNF-alpha) is a therapeutic target for impaired cutaneous wound healing. *Wound Repair Regen* 2012; **20**: 38–49

19. Couper KN, Blount DG, Riley EM. IL-10: the master regulator of immunity to infection. *J Immunol* 2008; **180**: 5771–7

20. Hiraki S, Ono S, Tsujimoto H, et al. Neutralization of interleukin-10 or transforming growth factor-beta decreases the percentages of CD4+ CD25+ Foxp3+ regulatory T cells in septic mice, thereby leading to an improved survival. *Surgery* 2012; **151**: 313–22

21. Atwell DM, Grichnik KP, Newman MF, Reves JG, McBride WT. Balance of proinflammatory and antiinflammatory cytokines at thoracic cancer operation. *Ann Thorac Surg* 1998; **66**: 1145–50

22. Bennett-Guerrero E, Ayuso L, Hamilton-Davies C, et al. Relationship of preoperative antiendotoxin core antibodies and adverse outcomes following cardiac surgery. *JAMA* 1997; **277**: 646–50

23. Waterer GW, Quasney MW, Cantor RM, Wunderink RG. Septic shock and respiratory failure in community-acquired pneumonia have different TNF polymorphism associations. *Am J Respir Crit Care Med* 2001; **163**: 1599–604

24. Jaber BL, Liangos O, Pereira BJ, Balakrishnan VS. Polymorphism of immunomodulatory cytokine genes: implications in acute renal failure. *Blood Purif* 2004; **22**: 101–11

25. Majetschak M, Obertacke U, Schade FU, et al. Tumor necrosis factor gene polymorphisms, leukocyte function, and sepsis susceptibility in blunt trauma patients. *Clin Diagn Lab Immunol* 2002; **9**: 1205–11

26. Reid CL, Perrey C, Pravica V, Hutchinson IV, Campbell IT. Genetic variation in proinflammatory and anti-inflammatory cytokine production in multiple organ dysfunction syndrome. *Crit Care Med* 2002; **30**: 2216–21

27. Tomasdottir H, Hjartarson H, Ricksten A, Wasslavik C, Bengtsson A, Ricksten SE. Tumor necrosis factor gene polymorphism is associated with enhanced systemic inflammatory response and increased cardiopulmonary morbidity after cardiac surgery. *Anesth Analg* 2003; **97**: 944–9

28. Reich K, Garbe C, Blaschke V, et al. Response of psoriasis to interleukin-10 is associated with suppression of cutaneous type 1 inflammation, downregulation of the epidermal interleukin-8/CXCR2 pathway and normalization of keratinocyte maturation. *J Invest Dermatol* 2001; **116**: 319–29

29. Vicioso MA, Garaud JJ, Reglier-Poupet H, Lebeaut A, Gougerot-Pocidalo MA, Chollet-Martin S. Moderate inhibitory effect of interleukin-10 on human neutrophil and monocyte chemotaxis in vitro. *Eur Cytokine Netw* 1998; **9**: 247–53

30. Bocci V, Paulesu L, Pessina GP. The renal catabolic pathways of cytokines. *Contrib Nephrol* 1993; **101**: 55–60

31. Kudo S, Goto H. Intrarenal handling of recombinant human interleukin-1alpha in rats: mechanism for proximal tubular protein reabsorption. *J Interferon Cytokine Res* 1999; **19**: 1161–8

32. Chatterjee PK, Hawksworth GM, McLay JS. Cytokine-stimulated nitric oxide production in the human renal proximal tubule and its modulation by natriuretic peptides: A novel immunomodulatory mechanism? *Exp Nephrol* 1999; **7**: 438–48

33. Gerritsma JS, Hiemstra PS, Gerritsen AF et al. Regulation and production of IL-8 by human proximal tubular epithelial cells in vitro. *Clin Exp Immunol* 1996; **103**: 289–94

34. Deng J, Kohda Y, Chiao H. et al. Interleukin-10 inhibits ischemic and cisplatin-induced acute renal injury. *Kidney Int* 2001; **60**: 2118–28

35. Gormley SM, McBride WT, Armstrong MA et al. Plasma and urinary cytokine homeostasis and renal dysfunction during cardiac surgery. *Anesthesiology* 2000; **93**: 1210–6

36. Gormley SMC, McBride WT, Armstrong MA, et al. Plasma and urinary cytokine homeostasis and renal function during cardiac surgery without cardiopulmonary bypass. *Cytokine* 2002; **17**: 61–5

37. McBride WT, Prasad PS, Armstrong M, et al. Cytokine phenotype, genotype, and renal outcomes at cardiac surgery. *Cytokine* 2013; **61**: 275–84

38. Baker RC, Armstrong MA, Allen SJ, Barros D'Sa AAB, McBride WT. Methylprednisolone reduces urinary transfroming growth factor beta-1 concentration at aortic surgery. *Euro J Anaesthesiol* 2003; **20**: 12–13

39. Park KH, Lee KH, Kim H, Hwang SO. The anti-inflammatory effects of ulinastatin in trauma patients with hemorrhagic shock. *J Korean Med Sci* 2010; **25**: 128–34

CHAPTER 6

Cardiovascular and pulmonary pharmacology

David Smith

Introduction

This chapter covers aspects of cardiovascular and pulmonary pharmacology relevant to anaesthesia for cardiovascular and thoracic surgery in adults and children, including the pharmacology of anaesthetic agents. Drugs are listed alphabetically in each section. Details of basic pharmacokinetics and the more general aspects of cardiovascular pharmacology can be found in suggestions for further reading.

Pharmacokinetic perspectives

Effects of age

Cardiothoracic surgery is successfully undertaken in increasingly elderly patients, so an understanding of specific pharmacokinetic issues in this population is important to effective provision of perioperative care. These patients often have co-morbid disease that may directly affect pharmacokinetics, or they may be taking medicines that modify the pharmacokinetics of drugs given in the perioperative period. Hepatic enzyme activity and creatinine clearance both decrease with age, reducing hepatic and renal drug clearance. The elderly also have a higher ratio of fat to lean body mass that can alter the effective volume of distribution of drugs (see remifentanil). In addition, the minimal alveolar concentration (MAC) of volatile anaesthetic agents decreases with age (1).

Similarly, with improvements in technology and in the understanding of complex cardiovascular physiology, a significant amount of surgery for congenital defects within the thorax is undertaken in neonates and infants. There are several important pharmacokinetic differences between these patients and adults, and larger inter-individual variations in response to drugs.

Drug distribution

Neonates have a relatively high proportion of body water in the first few days after birth, with lower concentrations of plasma proteins and lower protein binding of drugs, leading to an increased concentration of free drug in the plasma. Whilst the total body water normalizes during the first week of life, the lower protein binding capacity and the proportionally larger extra-cellular compartment remain into infancy. In addition, neonatal blood has a lower pH, changing the established ratios between bound and unbound drug fractions.

Drug clearance

The majority of enzyme systems do not function at adult levels for several months after birth, in particular the cytochrome P_{450} family and various cholinesterases. Renal clearance of drugs is also diminished as a result of a lower relative number of nephrons that are also immature; creatinine clearance in the neonate is around 10% of the adult weight-related value. However, metabolism of drugs in the older child and young teenager may exceed adult rates.

Obesity

In common with the general population, a large proportion of both adult and paediatric cardiothoracic surgical patients are significantly overweight. Morbidly obese patients have a higher proportion of body fat than normal, which may alter the usual pattern of drug distribution. In particular, lipid soluble drugs can accumulate to a significant extent in the excess body fat, dramatically increasing recovery times following long procedures.

Drug infusions

A drug given by infusion, with no loading bolus, will take five elimination half-times to reach an approximately steady state plasma concentration (97% of steady state). In practice it may take longer to achieve steady state unless the whole infusion system is purged before the infusion begins, to eliminate the slack, or 'back-lash', in the driving mechanism of the infusion device and the dead space in the intravenous catheter. This is critically important for the low-rate drug infusions used in neonates and infants, when it can take up to 45 minutes before effective drug delivery begins if the system is not purged beforehand.

The elimination rate of many drugs given by infusion is determined by the duration of the infusion. This is termed the 'context-sensitive half-time', the time taken for the plasma concentration to decrease to half the value present at the end of the infusion. The context-sensitive half-time can be significantly longer than the half-time based on a simple single-compartment pharmacokinetic model. This occurs because most drugs are distributed in three (or more) compartments. For short duration infusions the drug concentration in peripheral compartments remains lower than the plasma concentration, so recovery depends upon the standard half-time derived from the single compartment model. However, for infusions that have reached steady state, the concentration in the peripheral compartment is the same as that

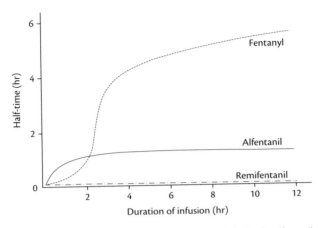

Fig. 6.1 Context-sensitive half-time against duration of infusion for alfentanil, fentanyl, and remifentanil.

Table 6.1 Compounds released from the lung

Adenosine	5-hydroxytryptamine	Plasminogen activator
Heparin	Leukotrienes A4, B4, C4, D4, E4	Prostaglandins I2, E, F
Histamine	Nitric oxide	Surfactant

Table 6.2 Compounds cleared or metabolized by the lung

Adenosine	Chlorpromazine	Metaraminol
Amphetamine	Fentanyl	Methadone
Angiotensin I	5-Hydroxytryptamine	Morphine
Atrial natriuretic peptide	Imipramine	Norephedrine
Bradykinin	Isoprenaline	Prostaglandins E1, E2, F2a
Bupivacaine	Lidocaine	Steroids

in plasma, and there may be a significantly large mass of drug in the peripheral compartment that maintains plasma concentrations by redistribution for a long period after the infusion stops (figure 6.1).

Drugs and the lung

The importance of the lungs in the pharmacokinetics of drugs is often forgotten (2). Several metabolic pathways are present in the endothelial tissues and alveoli (table 6.1), and many drugs are metabolized in the lung, including sympathomimetics, antihistamines, opioids and local anaesthetics (table 6.2).

Cardiopulmonary bypass

The pharmacokinetic profiles of a number of drugs are significantly altered by cardiopulmonary bypass (CPB) and associated procedures. An understanding of the underlying mechanisms is important for maintaining effective therapeutic drug concentrations during CPB.

Heparinization

Anticoagulation with large doses of heparin before CPB causes the release of tissue lipases that hydrolyse plasma triglycerides. The resulting increased concentration of plasma free fatty acids increases competition with drugs for protein binding sites.

Haemodilution

At the start of CPB there is a 40–50% increase in circulating blood volume, due to admixture with the circuit prime, that is associated with a proportional decrease in haematocrit, a reduction in the concentrations of proteins such as albumin and α_1 acid glycoprotein, and a decrease in the total plasma concentration of circulating drugs. Drugs with a small volume of distribution undergo proportionally greater dilution than drugs with a large volume of distribution, because plasma concentrations of drugs with large volumes of distribution tend to be maintained by redistribution of drug from extravascular compartments.

Protein binding

A reduced concentration of plasma proteins causes an increase in the unbound drug fraction, especially for those drugs that are highly protein bound. After CPB, the inflammatory response may cause an increased concentration of α_1 acid glycoprotein, which may increase binding of acidic drugs.

Regional blood distribution

Systemic arterial hypotension occurs during CPB as a result of reduced blood viscosity and possibly changes in systemic vascular resistance. This alters renal and hepatic blood flow, reducing renal drug clearance and hepatic metabolism of drugs. Poorly perfused tissues may become acidotic and trap some pH-sensitive drugs, which are then released back into the circulation when perfusion improves.

Hypothermia

Reduction of core body temperature reduces renal and hepatic blood flow, reduces the rate of enzyme-linked reactions and alters ligand-receptor binding. This results in increased plasma concentrations of drugs given by infusion, unless the administration rate is reduced. Hypothermia reduces cerebral electrical activity and reduces anaesthetic requirements.

Acid–base balance

Hypocarbia and alkalosis increase the potency of lipophilic drugs such as fentanyl, while hypercarbia and acidosis increase the potency of hydrophilic drugs such as morphine.

Isolation of the lungs

The lungs act as a reservoir for basic drugs such as opioids, propofol and thiopental. During CPB, isolation of the pulmonary circulation reduces pulmonary sequestration of drugs given during this time. On resumption of a normal circulation, drugs sequestered before the start of CPB may be liberated into the systemic circulation if the circulating concentration has decreased during CPB, or taken up if the concentration has increased. Some drugs are metabolized in the lungs, and this process may be modified by lung isolation during CPB (see the section on Drugs and the lung).

Drug adsorption

Many anaesthetic drugs bind to the plastics in the CPB circuit, including thiopental, fentanyl (and other opioids in proportion to their lipid solubility), and propofol.

Anaesthetic pharmacology during cardiopulmonary bypass

Anaesthesia may be maintained during CPB by either intravenous or volatile agents, or a combination of the two. If using an intravenous infusion, care must be taken that it is started in time to achieve a stable steady state plasma concentration before CPB commences (see Drug infusions). Spillage of volatile anaesthetic agents destroys polycarbonate plastics (e.g. reservoir shell, pump head cover plates) if the liquid agent comes into contact with them.

Intravenous anaesthesia

Propofol at an infusion rate between 3–5 mg/kg/hr is the principal agent used in adults, although it is also a good choice for paediatric patients. Midazolam may also be used at an infusion rate of 0.07 mg/kg/hr, although this is not really an anaesthetic. There is a decrease in total blood concentration of both drugs with the onset of CPB, but there is a concomitant proportional increase in the free fraction of the drug as a result of both a reduced concentration of plasma proteins and a heparin-induced decrease in protein binding. Metabolism and elimination are also reduced, particularly if the core temperature decreases (3,4). As a result of these changes, the effective plasma concentrations of propofol or midazolam are maintained or even increased during CPB, so infusion rates do not need to be adjusted at the onset of CPB if the delivery rate and the plasma concentration have stabilized.

Volatile anaesthesia

The uptake of volatile anaesthetics during CPB is determined by the blood:gas partition coefficient (increases as temperature decreases), tissue–gas solubility (increases as temperature decreases) and uptake by the oxygenator. There is rapid initial wash-in and wash-out of most volatile agents during CPB, with increasing solubility as perfusate temperature decreases. Haemodilution reduces the blood:gas partition coefficient, so that the effects of mild hypothermia and haemodilution at the onset of CPB cancel each other out for the majority of volatile anaesthetic agents.

Solubility

The uptake ('wash-in') and elimination ('wash-out') of volatile agents during CPB is inversely proportional to blood:gas partition coefficient (see Inhalation agents). The blood:gas partition coefficients for halogenated volatile anaesthetics decrease with crystalloid haemodilution and increase with hypothermia (5,6). Relatively insoluble agents (e.g. isoflurane, partition coefficient 1.4 at 37°C) are more rapidly taken up or eliminated by the oxygenator than more soluble agents (3). The wash-in of isoflurane has an initial rapid phase if there is no isoflurane present in the circulation, with a much slower late phase, and a wash out half-life of around 13 min (7,8). However, Loomis (9) found a washout half-life of 19 ± 5.5 min, and blood concentrations of isoflurane between 0.5 and 1.2% with vaporizer settings between 1.5 and 3.0%.

Oxygenator

Uptake of volatile anaesthetics varies greatly depending on the type of oxygenator that is used, with uptake being virtually non-existent with the newer 'plasma-tight' polymethylpentane (PMP) membranes compared with polypropylene (PPL) (10). When oxygenators with PMP membranes are used it is important to ensure that blood concentrations of volatile anaesthetics are adequate before going on CPB. Increasing oxygenator gas flow increases the uptake of volatile anaesthetics, whilst changes in pump flow rate have no effect on uptake (3).

The exhaust gas concentration of volatile agents is roughly half the setting on the vaporizer dial with PPL membranes (10), though the exhaust concentrations reflect those measured in arterial blood (11). An exhaust isoflurane concentration of 0.3–0.5% produces a bispectral index (BIS) value around 45 during CPB. A 20% lower oxygenator exhaust concentration of isoflurane is required to maintain BIS at 40–50 during mild hypothermic CPB, as opposed to the start of CPB, though the requirement increases back to pre-CPB levels by the end of rewarming (12,13).

Some form of scavenging of oxygenator exhaust gases is advisable if volatile anaesthetics are administered during CPB (14). Even if volatile anaesthetics are not used on CPB, the oxygenator is the main route of escape for volatile agents given before CPB, so there is still an atmospheric pollution risk from volatile agents given beforehand. However, this pollution risk also exists before CPB, as volatile anaesthetics can escape from the open mediastinum (15).

Drugs acting on the airways
Bronchodilators
Adrenaline
When nebulized into the upper airways adrenaline is a potent bronchodilator that is useful in asthmatic crises, treatment of acute stridor, and to reduce the swelling associated with acute upper airway obstruction. However, it can also increase the viscosity of mucus. A solution of 1:1000 (1 mg/mL) can be nebulized neat, or diluted with 0.9% saline, in a dose of 400 µg/kg to a maximum of 5 mg, repeated after 30 min if necessary. The duration of effect is around two hours.

Anticholinergic agents
Acetylcholine is released from muscarinic receptors in the airways under the influence of vagal activity. Inhaled ipratropium blocks this pathway and is poorly absorbed systemically, overcoming the issue of side effects resulting from the lack of selectivity of atropine. Although the duration of action of ipratropium is long, the onset of action is slow and it is not useful in acute bronchospasm.

Beta-2 adrenergic agonists
These agents act directly on β_2 adrenoceptors in airway smooth muscle, and are the first-line treatment for bronchoconstriction. Salbutamol is the classic drug in this group, multiples of 100 µg ('one puff') are usually given by metered dose inhaler. In an emergency, 2–10 separate doses may be given, although nebulized salbutamol 2.5–5 mg is preferred.

Glucocorticoids
Inhaled steroids, such as beclomethasone and fluticasone, increase the number and responsiveness of β_2-adrenoceptors

in the airways, while also reducing the inflammatory response, thereby reducing the hypersecretion of mucus. Systemic glucocorticoids (e.g. prednisolone) may be necessary in acute severe asthma or chronic obstructive pulmonary disease (COPD) that is not responding to conventional treatment. Care must be taken to provide appropriate steroid supplementation in the perioperative period if the prescribed dose of prednisolone is sufficient to induce adrenal suppression (more than 10 mg daily in an adult). Intravenous hydrocortisone is usually used for this, 20 mg being equivalent to 5 mg of oral prednisolone.

Leukotriene antagonists

These drugs act by blocking the effect of cysteinyl leukotrienes at leukotriene receptors, inhibiting smooth muscle constriction and proliferation, and reducing inflammation. Examples are montelukast and zafirlukast, and they are only available as oral preparations.

Mast cell stabilizers

Chromones, such as sodium chromoglycate and sodium nedocromil, inhibit mast cell degranulation thereby reducing the inflammatory response. They are administered by metered dose inhaler, but are of limited use in acute bronchospasm.

Methylxanthines

These drugs act by impairing the breakdown of cyclic AMP through inhibition of phosphodiesterases. Their narrow therapeutic range and poor side effect profile has reduced their use, particularly as first line therapy. Examples are aminophylline and theophylline.

Cough suppressants

Centrally acting agents, such as codeine or dextromethorphan, depress the cough centre in the medulla. Peripherally acting agents, such as local anaesthetics, inhibit the afferent arm of the cough reflex. Probably the most effective treatment is humidification of the airways by simple methods like steam inhalation.

Mucolytics

These drugs (carbocysteine, methyl cysteine hydrochloride, dornase alfa) reduce the viscosity of sputum and make it easier for the patient to clear their airways. Patients with COPD and cystic fibrosis are often prescribed these drugs for regular use.

Anaesthetics and sedatives

Although the aim of general anaesthesia is to produce unconsciousness through central nervous system depression, all anaesthetic agents affect cardiovascular or respiratory function to a greater or lesser extent.

Inhalation agents

Volatile anaesthetic agents in current clinical use in man include desflurane, halothane, isoflurane, and sevoflurane (table 6.3). Xenon, a noble gas extracted by fractional distillation of air, has anaesthetic properties but is currently too expensive for routine clinical use. The relative potencies of the volatile anaesthetics are described by the minimal alveolar concentration (MAC), the partial pressure at steady state that suppresses reflex movement in response to skin incision in 50% of the population. The MAC decreases with age (1), but there is no equivalent of MAC for

Table 6.3 Physical properties of inhaled anaesthetic agents

Agent	Boiling point (°C)	Blood:gas	MAC
Desflurane	23.5	0.42	6.6%
Halothane	50.2	2.40	0.75%
Isoflurane	48.5	1.40	1.17%
Nitrous oxide	−88.0	0.47	105%
Sevoflurane	58.5	0.70	1.8%
Xenon	−108	0.14	71%

describing the effects of inhalation agents delivered by the CPB oxygenator.

The blood:gas partition coefficient is the ratio of mass of agent in the blood phase to the mass of agent in the gaseous phase at equilibrium. Agents with a high blood:gas partition coefficient have a slow onset and offset of action, because they exert a low partial pressure in the blood phase so transfer from the blood into the brain is slow.

At steady state, the alveolar partial pressure of a volatile anaesthetic is in equilibrium with that in the brain, so that the end-tidal concentration reflects the cerebral concentration. However, the different volatile agents approach steady state equilibrium at differing rates over several hours, such that true equilibrium is rarely achieved in clinical practice.

All the halogenated hydrocarbon volatile anaesthetic agents reduce calcium flux into the cardiomyocyte, reducing sarcoplasmic reticular calcium release, with a reduction in myocardial contractility. There is also a decrease in systemic, coronary, and pulmonary vascular resistances, with the newer agents desflurane, isoflurane, and sevoflurane having greater effects than halothane. Volatile agents, except for desflurane, also depress sympathetic activity and impair baroreceptor-mediated reflex tachycardia in response to low systemic arterial pressure.

There is little evidence that the cardiovascular effects of most volatile anaesthetic agents at clinical concentrations adversely affect the diseased heart (table 6.4), although desflurane may worsen myocardial ischaemia as it increases sympathetic activity at concentrations above 0.5 MAC. Halothane may induce ventricular premature beats, particularly in the presence of high circulating concentrations of catecholamines, as a result of ventricular re-entrant circuits; these may progress to ventricular tachycardia or fibrillation (VT or VF) if there is a sudden increase in catecholamine activity.

Desflurane

A halogenated methyl ether, less than 0.02% is metabolized. Its low boiling point makes it difficult to administer by a conventional vaporizer, so it is delivered from a special device that heats it to 39°C at two atmospheres pressure. Although its low blood:gas partition coefficient allows rapid onset and offset of action, it has a pungent odour that limits its usefulness as an induction agent. Desflurane has a relatively high MAC which makes it expensive to use. Its main cardiovascular effect is vasodilation, but at concentrations above 0.5–1 MAC it can produce tachycardia and

Table 6.4 Cardiovascular and respiratory effects of volatile agents

	Desflurane	Isoflurane	Sevoflurane	Xenon
Heart rate	Mild increase	Increase	No effect	Mild decrease
Contractility	Minimal	Mild decrease	Mild decrease	No effect
Systemic resistance	Decrease	Decrease	Mild decrease	No effect
Blood pressure	Decrease	Decrease	Mild decrease	No effect
Respiratory rate	Increase	Increase	Increase	Mild decrease
Tidal volume	Decrease	Decrease	Mild decrease	Mild increase
P_aCO_2	Increase	Increase	Mild increase	No effect

hypertension that may limit its usefulness in patients with cardio-vascular disease (16).

Halothane

A halogenated hydrocarbon, halothane is still occasionally used for inhalation induction as it is sweet-smelling and non-irritant, but it is slow in onset and has largely given way to the newer volatile agents in current practice as a result of its association with hepatic dysfunction. It has significant cardiovascular effects; vagal stimulation decreases heart rate, it sensitizes the heart to catecholamines (leading to arrhythmias), and there is significant depression of myocardial contractility and conduction. Halothane also increases cerebral blood flow more than the other volatile agents, leading to increased intracranial pressure above 0.6 MAC. Any of the newer volatile agents are better choices for cardiothoracic anaesthesia.

Isoflurane

A halogenated methyl ether, only 0.2% is metabolized, the remainder being excreted by the lungs. Although it has a pungent odour that limits its usefulness as an induction agent, isoflurane produces useful bronchodilation. The main cardiovascular side effect of isoflurane is a reduction in systemic vascular resistance, with minimal effect on myocardial contractility. Provided coronary perfusion pressure is maintained, the coronary steal phenomenon reported to be associated with isoflurane is not an issue (17). At concentrations up to 1 MAC cerebral autoregulation is preserved, providing a good balance of decreased cerebral metabolic rate for oxygen ($CMRO_2$) and mildly increased cerebral blood flow.

Sevoflurane

A halogenated isopropyl methyl ether, sevoflurane is metabolized in the liver, about 3.5% being metabolized to release fluoride ions. However, renal fluoride toxicity has not been reported in man. When used with carbon dioxide absorbents, particularly potassium hydroxide, compounds A–E are produced, but these have not been associated with toxicity in clinical use in humans. Sevoflurane is less irritant than the other volatile anaesthetic agents which, in combination with its low blood:gas partition coefficient, makes it a useful induction agent.

Xenon

An inert gas that is present at 8.7 ppm in the atmosphere, xenon is odourless, not metabolized, and has no known hazards or environmental effects; it appears to be the ideal anaesthetic agent apart from its cost (2000 times that of nitrous oxide) (18,19). In contrast to the other anaesthetic gases and vapours, xenon maintains minute ventilation through a combination of reduced respiratory rate and increased tidal volume, and has significant analgesic and neuroprotective properties. Despite its relatively high density and viscosity, it does not significantly increase the work of breathing. Cardiovascular effects are minimal, but xenon produces an unpredictable increase in cerebral blood flow. The high cost of xenon mandates the use of complex delivery equipment, and recycling of the agent from exhaust anaesthetic gas.

Anaesthetic preconditioning

Pharmacological preconditioning with halogenated ether anaesthetic agents may be of clinical benefit in the broad population of patients having cardiac surgery (20,21), although most of the work has been done with sevoflurane and there are a variety of different clinical protocols. Propofol anaesthesia may be better for those patients who have undergone significant preoperative ischaemic stress, as they may already be maximally preconditioned and are likely to benefit more from the antioxidant, free radical scavenging effects of propofol (22).

Intravenous anaesthetic agents

Etomidate

Has the least effect on the cardiovascular system of any of the intravenous anaesthetic agents, but it is associated with suppression of cortisol production from 2-deoxycortisol in the adrenal glands. This limits its usefulness by infusion, although it may not be a significant clinical issue with a single induction dose (23). The induction dose is 0.15–0.3 mg/kg, although children may need 0.4 mg/kg. Etomidate is associated with significant pain on injection.

Ketamine

The only intravenous anaesthetic agent that does not depress cardiovascular function in normal use. Ketamine has central sympathomimetic activity, producing tachycardia and vasoconstriction that increase myocardial oxygen consumption but offset a direct myocardial depressant action. In patients with impaired autonomic function, the unopposed myocardial depression causes a reduction in cardiac output. Ketamine produces bronchodilation, and has been used for the treatment of severe asthma. It is a useful induction agent in haemodynamically compromised patients, at an intravenous dose of 1–2 mg/kg. Ketamine had significant side effects including hallucinations and psychosis, that limit its routine use but these can be reduced by co-administration of a benzodiazepine. Ketamine can also be given intramuscularly at a dose of 5–10 mg/kg, and by infusion to maintain anaesthesia at a rate of 10–45 µg/kg/min. Finally, ketamine is a useful analgesic in intravenous doses of 0.2–0.5 mg/kg.

Propofol

A highly lipid-soluble phenol derivative. The induction dose is 1.5–2.5 mg/kg, reducing to 1–1.5 mg/kg in elderly and compromised patients, given slowly to minimize the cardiovascular side effects. It can be given as an infusion for the maintenance of anaesthesia at a dose rate of 4–12 mg/kg/hr (3–6 mg/kg/hr in elderly patients) aiming for a plasma concentration of 4–8 µg/mL. Propofol has minimal effect on hypoxic pulmonary vasoconstriction, and may be associated with better lung function in the postoperative period in comparison to a volatile anaesthetic (24,25), so may be useful during thoracic surgery. Propofol is also frequently used to provide anaesthesia for cardiac surgery, to avoid having to give a volatile agent by the CPB oxygenator. Like thiopental, it causes direct myocardial depression and systemic vasodilation but with less tachycardia.

Children require a higher induction dose than adults, typically 2.5–3.5 mg/kg. Their central volume of distribution is 50% greater than in adults and clearance is 25% greater, leading to a 50% greater dose requirement for the maintenance of anaesthesia. Pharmacodynamic effects are similar to those seen in adults.

Dosing of propofol should be based on actual body mass rather than 'ideal' body mass in the obese (26); recovery is faster after short-acting inhalation anaesthesia (e.g. desflurane) than propofol anaesthesia in the morbidly obese (27). (See Drug infusions section).

Thiopental

Thiopental is a sulphur analogue of pentobarbitone. Only 12% of an administered dose is active due to protein binding (80%) or ionization in plasma (8%), but onset of action is rapid due to the high lipid solubility. Recovery following a single bolus dose is also rapid, due to rapid redistribution. Thiopental may release histamine and is associated with bronchospasm in patients with asthma. For induction of anaesthesia is used at a dose of 3–7 mg/kg. In status epilepticus, thiopental is useful as an infusion although elimination can become zero order due to saturation of hepatic cytochrome P_{450}. In addition, thiopental has been recommended for cerebral protection during deep hypothermic circulatory arrest, though there is no evidence to support this in man.

Intravenous sedative agents

Benzodiazepines

Benzodiazepines are often used in cardiac anaesthesia, either for co-induction with another agent such as propofol, or to supplement anaesthesia during CPB. Midazolam is also often used in the mistaken belief that memory for an episode of unintended awareness will be impaired (28). All benzodiazepines cause hypotension as a result of myocardial depression and vasodilation, but to a lesser extent than the intravenous anaesthetic agents. They have little effect on heart rate. Midazolam and diazepam decrease tidal volume and increase respiratory rate. They also decrease hypoxic ventilatory drive, an effect only partially reversed by flumazenil (29). Lipophilic benzodiazepines have a markedly increased volume of distribution and reduced clearance in obese patients.

Clonidine

An α-agonist with 200:1 ratio of $α_2$:$α_1$ activity that is used to treat hypertension, acute and chronic pain, and for sedation during mechanical ventilation in intensive care (ICU). Its benefit in ICU may be related more to suppression of both opiate withdrawal and agitation. Clinidine stimulates $α_2$ receptors in the lateral reticular nucleus to suppress sympathetic outflow, and modulates nociceptive pathways and endogenous opioid release in the spinal cord. Effects are limited at higher doses by increasing $α_1$ activity. The terminal half-life of clonidine is 9–18 hours and approximately 50% of the drug is converted to an active metabolite in the liver. Dose rate should be reduced in renal impairment, as the other 50% is excreted unchanged in the urine.

There is a transient increase in blood pressure due to stimulation of peripheral $α_1$ receptors, followed by a sustained decrease in blood pressure, and relative bradycardia. Cardiac output is well maintained; there is an increased P-R interval and slowing of conduction through the AV node.

Clonidine produces sedation and a 50% reduction in the MAC of volatile anaesthetic agents, but does not induce respiratory depression. It acts synergistically with opioids and contributes to a reduction in the surgical stress response. Although platelets carry $α_2$ receptors, clonidine does not induce platelet aggregation; it blocks adrenaline mediated platelet aggregation.

Dexmedetomidine

The active D-stereoisomer of medetomidine, an $α_2$-adrenoceptor agonist with sedative and analgesic properties. Dexmedetomidine has a similar mechanism of action and effects to clonidine, although it has 1600-times the affinity for $α_2$ receptors compared with $α_1$. Dexmedetomidine is gaining popularity as a sedative agent in critical care, as an infusion of 0.2–1.4 μg/kg/hr.

Neuromuscular blocking drugs

Neuromuscular blocking drugs mostly have no direct effect on the lungs, although some may cause significant histamine release (atracurium, mivacurium) that results in bronchoconstriction. However, the muscle relaxation caused by neuromuscular blockade augments the reduction in functional residual capacity resulting from anaesthesia, and failure to reverse these drugs adequately at the end of surgery can significantly impair lung function in the immediate postoperative period. Reversal of neuromuscular blockade with an anticholinesterase such as neostigmine, can significantly increase bronchial tone and airway secretions as a result of muscarininc inhibition of endogenous acetylcholine, an effect that may not be completely countered by the co-administration of anticholinergic agents such as atropine or glycopyrrolate.

Modern non-depolarizing neuromuscular blocking drugs including atracurium, cis-atracurium, mivacurium, pancuronium, rocuronium, and vecuronium, are bis-quaternary benzylisoquinolines or steroidal molecules that have few direct cardiovascular side effects. The most common cardiovascular and pulmonary side effects of these drugs are caused indirectly by histamine release, particularly seen with atracurium but rarely with the steroidal drugs. Pancuronium is mildly vagolytic and has a very low incidence of histamine release which, combined with its long duration of action, makes it a popular choice for cardiac anaesthesia. Atracurium and vecuronium have a limited volume of distribution, though the dose of atracurium should be calculated on total body mass as there is reduced sensitivity to atracurium in the obese.

Suxamethonium (succinylcholine)

Structurally similar to acetylcholine, suxamethonium increases sympathetic nervous system tone, producing a tachycardia and an increase in systemic vascular resistance that increases myocardial oxygen demand. Unopposed direct muscarinic effects can produce a bradycardia in some patients, particularly after a second dose, and in children.

Sugammadex

This γ-cyclodextrin is an inert, doughnut-shaped structure that can encapsulate steroidal neuromuscular blocking drugs, effectively removing them from the plasma and thereby increasing their diffusion gradient away from the neuromuscular junction. It is most effective for reversing the effect of rocuronium, but also works for vecuronium and less well for pancuronium. The advantage of sugammadex is in avoiding the complex side-effect profile of the anticholinesterase/anticholinergic combinations routinely used to reverse neuromuscular blockade, but it is expensive and only works for the reversal of steroidal neuromuscular blocking drugs.

Opioids

These drugs are the mainstay of perioperative pain management for both cardiovascular and thoracic surgery. They all cause respiratory depression and suppress the cough reflex. Opioids, including morphine 0.5–11 mg/kg (30) and fentanyl 100 µg/kg (31) have been used as sole anaesthetic agents for cardiac surgery (Chapter 1), but provide inadequate anaesthesia with an unacceptable incidence of intraoperative awareness (32), primarily because they are not anaesthetics.

Alfentanil

A synthetic phenylpiperidine derivative, alfentanil has a pK_a of 6.5, so 89% of an injected dose is unionized at plasma pH. This allows it to cross lipid membranes more readily than fentanyl, despite its lower lipid solubility, such that alfentanil has a faster onset of action than fentanyl.

Fentanyl

A highly lipid soluble synthetic opioid derived from piperidine that is 60–80 times more potent than morphine in man. First-pass uptake in the lungs temporarily sequesters around 70–80% of an administered dose, but this is released back into the circulation with a half-life of around 6 min. Large amounts of fentanyl are then taken up into body fat to provide a reservoir of drug that maintains a large effective volume of distribution. Fentanyl is around 80% bound to plasma proteins, principally α_1 acid glycoprotein, but changes in plasma protein concentrations have little effect on the unbound fraction of fentanyl as a result of the large volume of distribution. The pK_a of fentanyl is 8.4, so only 9% of the drug is unionized at plasma pH, accounting for its slower onset of action than alfentanil. Historically, fentanyl was used for cardiac surgery in doses of around 100 µg/kg, but this has given way to a balanced technique in which lower doses of fentanyl are employed. Fentanyl is adsorbed onto the plastics of the CPB circuit. When given by infusion, the elimination rate increases as the duration of infusion increases (See Drug infusions).

Morphine

Morphine is a naturally occurring compound derived from the poppy *Papaver somniferum*. It is a µ receptor agonist and is the compound against which all other opioids are compared. Morphine was the principal perioperative opioid used, often in large doses, in the early days of cardiac anaesthesia, but was associated with significantly prolonged recovery times such that overnight mechanical ventilation was required. With the move to early wakening and extubation after cardiac surgery, morphine is now used almost exclusively for premedication and for postoperative analgesia.

Remifentanil

This ultra-short acting opioid is another synthetic phenylpiperidine. Remifentanil is metabolized by non-specific plasma and tissue esterases to provide an elimination half-life of around three minutes, so it has to be given by infusion for procedures of anything more than a few minutes duration. The duration of action is determined by metabolism rather than redistribution, in distinction to the other opioids. There is increased sensitivity to remifentanil in the elderly as they have a reduced muscle mass and much of its metabolism is by muscle esterases. A loading dose of 1.0 µg/kg followed by an infusion of 0.05–1.0 µg/kg/min provides good conditions for cardiothoracic surgery. A constant plasma concentration during CPB may be achieved by reducing the infusion rate by 30% for each 5°C reduction in blood temperature. Although remifentanil provides excellent haemodynamic stability during cardiothoracic surgery, it can be awkward providing effective analgesia when the infusion is stopped. There are a number of solutions, including reducing the infusion rate gradually in the postoperative period, or loading the patient with significant doses of morphine beforehand.

Sufentanil

A synthetic phenylpiperidine derivative that is 5–10 times more potent than fentanyl. It is 93% protein bound at plasma pH. Elimination is by hepatic metabolism, with an elimination half-life around 160 min. Sufentanil provides effective analgesia for major surgery at doses up to 8 µg/kg, and has been used as a sole anaesthetic agent at doses of 10–30 µg/kg. A maintenance infusion may be used at a rate of 0.2–1.5 µg/kg/hr, with the total dose for the procedure not exceeding 30 µg/kg.

Cardiovascular drugs

Anti-arrhythmic drugs

These drugs have historically been classified by the scheme devised by Vaughan Williams (33) (table 6.5), based on the primary mechanism of the anti-arrhythmic effect. However, some anti-arrhythmic drugs do not fall neatly into a single category for example, sotalol demonstrates class I, II, and III activities, and the classification does not include some drugs that are used for their

Table 6.5 The Vaughan Williams classification of anti-arrhythmic drugs.

Class	Action	Example drugs
Ia	Sodium channel blockade: Increased action potential duration	procainamide, disopyramide
Ib	Sodium channel blockade: Decreased action potential duration	lidocaine, mexiletine
Ic	Sodium channel blockade: No effect on cardiac refractory period	flecainide, propafenone
II	β-adrenoceptor blockade	atenolol, esmolol
III	Potassium channel blockade	amiodarone, bretylium, sotalol
IV	Calcium channel blockade	verapamil, diltiazem

Data from Vaughan Williams EM. Classification of antiarrhythmic drugs. In: Symposium on cardiac arrhythmias. Sandoe E, Flensted-Jensen E, Olesen KH, eds. Sodertalje: AB Astra, 1970: 449–72.

anti-arrhythmic properties such as digoxin, adenosine, which some authors include as Class V. All of these drugs depress conduction through the atrioventricular (AV) node and reduce myocardial contractility to a greater or lesser extent. Drugs in classes I and III also prolong the effective refractory period.

Adenosine

Adenosine is a naturally occurring purine nucleoside that is rapidly metabolized, and has a very short duration of action (half-life < 5 s). Adenosine receptors are present on cardiomyocytes (A1) and on vascular endothelial and smooth muscle cells (A2). Stimulation of A1 receptors directly activates potassium channels and indirectly inhibits adenyl cyclase, decreasing heart rate by inhibition of conduction at sinoatrial (SA) and AV nodes and reducing myocardial contractility. Stimulation of A2 receptors enhances adenyl cyclase activity to produce coronary vasodilation.

Adenosine is used for termination of paroxysmal AV nodal re-entry tachycardia, and narrow- or broad-complex tachycardias of supraventricular origin without haemodynamic compromise. It can be used to differentiate between sinus tachycardia, atrial arrhythmias (fibrillation or flutter) and ventricular tachycardia by producing transient bradycardia and AV block, which allows for easier evaluation of the cardiac rhythm. However, adenosine may worsen tachycardias resulting from accessory AV pathways.

Adenosine needs to be given as a rapid intravenous bolus, followed by a saline flush, initially of 3 mg but escalating to 6, 9, or 12 mg if there is no initial response. Awake patients often complain of chest pain and other side effects include flushing, headache, bronchospasm, and hypotension. However, these side effects are transient, due to the short duration of action.

Amiodarone

Amiodarone contains iodine and has a structure similar to the thyroid hormones, which accounts for its ability to interfere with thyroid function. Amiodarone has a large volume of distribution and is extensively bound to tissues and as a result, it has a half-life of 1–2 months. Amiodarone has broad anti-arrhythmic activity, having class I, II, III, and IV actions. However, it is predominantly a class III drug that acts by antagonism of potassium channels. Indications are stabilization of VF or VT during or immediately after cardiac arrest, or in the perioperative period after cardiac surgery. It can also be used for rate control and cardioversion in atrial fibrillation or flutter, especially if cardioversion is undesirable. In addition, amiodarone has been used prophylactically to reduce the incidence of postoperative atrial fibrillation following cardiac surgery.

Amiodarone needs to be given intravenously in the acute setting, as the onset of effect is too slow by oral administration. An initial infusion of 5 mg/kg (300 mg in most adults) over 1 hour is followed by a further 900 mg over 23 hours. Maintenance doses can be given orally, but may need to be continued intravenously in patients on ICU with impaired gut function. A decrementing regimen of 600 mg daily for 1 week, 400 mg for a further week, and 200 mg daily thereafter, usually produces good rhythm control. Treatment can usually be stopped after one week in atrial fibrillation associated with cardiothoracic surgery, but several weeks are required to achieve a stable therapeutic effect for long-term use.

Amiodarone can produce a bradycardia or complete heart block, together with peripheral vasodilation and reduced myocardial contractility. Importantly, it increases the defibrillation threshold, such that more energy needs to be given for successful cardioversion. Long-term treatment is associated with corneal deposits, optic neuritis that may lead to blindness, photosensitivity, pulmonary fibrosis, hepatic dysfunction, and deranged thyroid function (both hypo- and hyper-thyroidism).

Beta-blockers

Only two drugs in this class are really useful for acute control of arrhythmias, esmolol and sotalol, although beta-blockers are recommended as prophylaxis or treatment for perioperative atrial fibrillation.

Esmolol

Esmolol is a relatively cardioselective beta-blocker with a rapid onset and offset of action. Its action is terminated by red blood cell esterases with a half-life of 10 min. It is used for treatment of acute supraventricular tachycardias, and for short-term treatment of perioperative tachycardia and hypertension. Repeat bolus doses of 10 mg can be titrated to effect; an infusion at 50–200 µg/kg/min can be used where a longer duration of action is required.

Sotalol

Sotalol is a non-selective beta-blocker with additional Class III activity that increases the durations of both the cardiac action potential and refractory period. It is indicated for the treatment of both supraventricular and ventricular arrythmias, and for prevention of paroxysmal supraventricular tachycardia. Sotalol is as effective as amiodarone for the treatment of atrial fibrillation that is associated with cardiothoracic surgery. However, it produces a bradycardia and hypotension that limit its use in this setting in patients with poor left ventricular function. Another important side effect of sotalol is an increased risk of torsades de pointes. To avoid these side effects, sotalol must be given slowly in a dose of 1–1.5 mg/kg infused at 10 mg/min.

Digoxin

A glycoside extracted from the foxglove plant *Digitalis lanata*. Digoxin is excreted unchanged by the kidneys with an elimination half-life of around 35 hours, but this is increased significantly in renal failure. Digoxin has a direct inhibitory effect on cardiac Na^+/K^+ ATP-ase to increase the availability of intracellular calcium. This produces a mild, short-lived positive inotropic effect, but the principal therapeutic effect is increased refractory period and reduced conductivity in the AV node and His bundle, which is augmented by the enhancement by digoxin of the release of acetylcholine at cardiac muscarinic receptors. These effects make digoxin a useful drug for acute treatment of atrial fibrillation, though the onset of action is slower than that of amiodarone. Digoxin is given as a loading dose of 1–1.5 mg over 24 hours, usually in divided doses of 0.5 mg over 2 hours each, followed by maintenance doses of 62.5–500 µg/day. It has a narrow therapeutic index and plasma digoxin concentrations should be maintained within 1–2 µg/L, as toxicity develops above a concentration of 2.5 µg/L. Toxic side effects in acute use are primarily cardiac including atrial and ventricular tachycardias, AV block, junctional rhythm, and ventricular extrasytoles (including bigemini). Toxic effects are more likely when the serum potassium concentration is below 4 mmol/L.

Disopyramide

Disopyramide blocks cardiac sodium channels to reduce the rate of rise of phase 0 of the cardiac action potential, increase the threshold potential, and prolong the refractory period. It is used as a secondary agent in atrial and ventricular tachyarrhythmias, though the ventricular rate should first be controlled with a β-blocker or calcium antagonist when used to treat atrial fibrillation. A loading dose of 2 mg/kg (to a maximum of 150 mg) is given over 5–30 min, followed by an infusion at 0.4–1.0 mg/kg/hr to a maximum dose of 300 mg in the first hour and 800 mg daily. Disopyramide has anticholinergic side effects that limit its tolerability in awake patients, and it may produce hypoglycaemia. It can also prolong the QT interval and provoke torsades de pointes.

Flecainide

An amide local anaesthetic that is similar to lidocaine, flecainide inhibits fast sodium currents into the cardiomyocyte and prolongs phase 0 of the action potential. It is metabolized in the liver to active metabolites that are excreted in the urine along with the parent drug. Flecainide is a potent inhibitor of both atrial and ventricular tachyarrhythmias, including those due to aberrant conducting pathways. A loading dose of 2 mg/kg over 10–30 min (to a maximum of 150 mg) is followed by an infusion of 1.5 mg/kg/hr over the first hour. The infusion rate should then be reduced to 100–250 μg/kg/hr for up to 24 hours, with a maximum dose of 600 mg per day, until oral therapy is established.

Lidocaine (lignocaine)

An amide local anaesthetic, lidocaine reduces the rate of rise of phase 0 of the cardiac action potential through sodium channel blockade, producing an increase in the threshold potential, making it useful for sustained ventricular tachyarrhythmias, especially when these are associated with myocardial ischaemia. Lidocaine is metabolized in the liver, with an elimination half-life around 90 min, so an initial adult bolus dose of 1 mg/kg is followed by an infusion at 1–3 mg/min.

Mexiletine

Mexiletine is an analogue of lidocaine with similar properties and usage.

Calcium channel blockers

This heterogeneous group of drugs block the slow inward calcium current associated with L-type calcium channels. The dihydropyridine drugs (e.g. nifedipine) have minimal myocardial effects and are not effective anti-arrhythmics. Diltiazem and verapamil decrease conduction and increase the refractory period in the AV node. They are indicated for the treatment of paroxysmal supraventricular tachycardia and AV nodal re-entry tachycardia, and for rate control in atrial fibrillation or flutter. Both drugs decrease myocardial contractility. Diltiazem is given by intravenous bolus of 0.25 mg/kg and a subsequent bolus of 0.35 mg/kg, but may also be given as an infusion of 5–15 mg/hr for rate control in atrial fibrillation or flutter. Verapamil is given as an intravenous bolus of 2.5–5 mg over 2 min, with a further 5–10 mg every 15–30 min if there is no response, and the maximum dose is 20 mg.

Positive inotropes

Positive inotropic drugs increase the force of myocardial contraction, usually via cyclic GMP as the final common pathway, usually at the cost of increasing myocardial oxygen consumption. They are used to treat circulatory failure due to impaired myocardial performance. Agents that do not depend on cyclic GMP are calcium salts and calcium sensitizers, cardiac glycosides, and thyroid hormones. The cardiac glycosides have no role in the acute treatment of heart failure, as they are of limited effect and narrow therapeutic range. Catecholamine inotropes (table 6.6) increase myocardial oxygen demand, placing continued stress on an organ that is already failing; they are associated with increased hospital mortality in patients with acute heart failure (34).

Catecholamine inotropes

Adrenaline (epinephrine)

Adrenaline has a half-life of 1–2 min due to rapid metabolism by catechol-O-methyl transferase and it acts at both α- and β-adrenoceptors. The β effects predominate at low dose, with an increase in cardiac index as a result of increased myocardial contractility and peripheral vasodilation. At higher doses the α effect predominates and the systemic and pulmonary vascular resistances increase markedly, as does the heart rate. Adrenaline also increases the basal metabolic rate, stimulating both glycogenolysis and gluconeogenesis, and inhibiting insulin secretion, with a resulting increase in plasma glucose concentration.

Dopamine

Dopamine acts on both α- and β-adrenoceptors, but also on both dopamine D_1 and D_2 receptors, and stimulates endogenous release of noradrenaline. The cardiovascular effects are variable and dose dependent. At low doses, around 5 μg/kg/min, the β effects predominate with an increase in myocardial contractility, heart rate, and cardiac index. At doses above 10 μg/kg/min the α effect predominates, with increased systemic and pulmonary vascular resistances. Dopamine causes splanchnic vasodilation by way of an action on D_1 receptors; this is widely believed to increase urine output and preserve renal function, but this has not been confirmed in clinical trials (35,36).

Dobutamine

A synthetic derivative of isoprenaline, dobutamine has predominantly $β_1$-adrenoceptor activity. It increases myocardial

Table 6.6 Cardiovascular actions of catecholamines

Drug	$α_1$	$α_2$	$β_1$	$β_2$	D_1	D_2
Adrenaline	+++	++	+++	++	nil	nil
Dobutamine	+	nil	+++	+	nil	nil
Dopamine	++	+	++	+++	+++	+++
Dopexamine	nil	nil	+	+++	++	++
Isoprenaline	nil	nil	++	++	nil	nil
Noradrenaline	+++	+++	+	nil	nil	nil

Isoprenaline and noradrenaline are poor inotropes, having primarily lusitropic/vasodilator (isoprenaline) and vasoconstrictor (noradrenaline) actions, but they are included here for completeness

contractility and heart rate, with an increase in cardiac index aided by a mild decrease in systemic vascular resistance. As well as its use in critical care, it is used as an alternative to treadmill exercise for cardiac stress testing.

Dopexamine

A synthetic analogue of dopamine, dopexamine has activity at β_2-adrenoceptors and dopamine D_1 receptors; it may also inhibit the re-uptake of noradrenaline. It increases myocardial contractility and reduces systemic vascular resistance aided by a significant reduction in splanchnic vascular tone), such that there is little increase in myocardial oxygen extraction.

Isoprenaline (isoproterenol)

A synthetic catecholamine with activity at both β_1- and β_2-adrenoceptors, isoprenaline is used to treat severe bradycardia, particularly for β-blocker overdose, and for aiding the diagnosis of conduction disorders during electrophysiological studies. A drawback of isoprenaline is that it also decreases the blood pressure due to significant peripheral vasodilation.

Calcium and calcium sensitizers

Apart from their use in the treatment of hypocalcaemia and hyperkalaemia, calcium salts have been recommended for the treatment of low output states after cardiac surgery. However, despite their beneficial effects in vitro, they provide only transient improvement in blood pressure and they do not increase cardiac index in patients after cardiac surgery (37). They are useful in the treatment of calcium channel antagonist overdose, and for the maintenance of ionized calcium concentrations during massive blood transfusion, but care must be taken as they are extremely damaging to tissues if extravasated.

Levosimendan

This calcium sensitizer binds to troponin C in a calcium-dependent fashion to improve myocardial contractility. Systolic function is augmented, without an increase in myocardial oxygen consumption, whilst diastolic function is maintained because the affinity of levosimendan for troponin C decreases as calcium concentrations decrease during diastole. Activation of ATP-dependent potassium channels in vascular smooth muscle produces vasodilation. Levosimendan is increasingly being used for refractory heart failure after cardiac surgery, and as a prophylactic agent in patients at high risk of post-CPB heart failure (38). The inodilator property of levosimendan persists after the infusion is stopped because the active metabolite OR-1896 has along terminal half life (39).

Phosphodiesterase inhibitors

Phosphodiesterases (PDE) catalyse the hydrolysis of phosphodiester bonds, for example in cyclic AMP and cyclic GMP, and are found widely in 12 known isoforms throughout the body (table 6.7). Through the ubiquitous action of PDE, inhibition of their activity may produce therapeutic effects in the cardiovascular system, the lungs, the inflammatory cascade, and on platelet function.

Drugs available for clinical use to improve myocardial performance inhibit either PDE III or PDE IV. Milrinone is a biguanide and enoximone is an imidazoline derivative. Amrinone, another biguanide, is of historic interest only, as it is no longer widely available.

Enoximone

Enoximone has limited pharmaceutical compatibility with other drugs and needs to be given through a dedicated intravenous line. A loading dose of 0.5–1.0 mg/kg is given over 10–30 min, followed by a maintenance infusion of 5–20 µg/kg/min. Enoximone is oxidized to a sulphoxide that has around 10% of the potency but a five-fold increase in elimination half-life. Plasma concentrations of enoximone and its principal metabolite gradually increase with prolonged infusion, potentially leading to excessive accumulation and a significant contribution of the metabolite to overall drug effect.

Table 6.7 Phosphodiesterase isoforms, their main locations and drugs used to inhibit specific isoforms (caffeine, papaverine and theophylline are non-specific inhibitors)

Type	Location	Inhibitor drug
I	Heart, brain, kidney, liver, muscle	Phenothiazines
II	Adrenal cortex, brain, corpora cavernosa, heart, liver, kidney, airway, platelets	
III	Heart, corpora cavernosa, platelets, smooth muscle, liver, kidney, white cells	Milrinone, piroximone
IV	Kidney, lung, heart, muscle, white cells	Enoximone
V	Corpora cavernosa, platelets, muscle, kidney, platelets	Sildenafil, zaprinast, dipyridamole
VI	Retina	
VII	Skeletal muscle, heart, kidney, airways, white cells	Dipyridamole
VIII	A: testis ovary, gut B: thyroid	Dipyridamole
IX	Spleen, small intestine, brain	Zaprinast
X	Brain	Isobutyl methylxanthine
XI	Skeletal muscle, prostate, kidney, liver, pituitary	Zaprinast, dipyridamole

Milrinone

Milrinone has better pharmaceutical compatibility than enoximone. A loading infusion of 50 µg/kg is followed by a maintenance infusion at 0.25–0.75 µg/kg/min. It is excreted virtually unchanged in the urine, although around 10% is metabolized to a glucuronide first. Milrinone has an elimination half-life of around 60 min that increases in proportion to the degree of renal dysfunction, leading to significant accumulation in patients with renal failure.

Although milrinone and enoximone are dissimilar molecules, their haemodynamc effects are remarkably similar. There is approximately a 25–30% increase in cardiac index and a 20% decrease in both central venous and pulmonary artery occlusion pressures, associated with decreases in systemic vascular resistance and blood pressure (40). Vasodilation leads to relative hypovolaemia, and care should be taken with intravascular volume management in patients with impaired ventricular function or who are already hypovolaemic. Simultaneous administration of a vasoconstrictor, such as norepinephrine or vasopressin, will frequently be necessary to maintain an acceptable blood pressure. Pulmonary vasodilation makes these drugs useful in right ventricular failure.

Phosphodiesterase inhibitors are often combined with catecholamine inotropes to produce a synergistic effect on intracellular cAMP, with catecholamines activating adenyl cyclase and phosphodiesterase inhibitors reducing the breakdown of cAMP (41).

Novel inotropes

Istaroxime

Istaroxime has positive lusitropic activity by way of inhibition of sarcolemmal Na/K-ATPase (to increase intracellular calcium concentration), and stimulation of calcium ATPase in sarcoplasmic reticulum to stimulate extrusion of calcium from the cytosol and thereby increase calcium stores for release in the next cardiac cycle. Istaroxime produces a dose-dependent increase in cardiac output, with no effect on blood pressure, heart rate or arrhythmia (42). However, further evaluation is needed before this novel agent is introduced into routine clinical practice.

Omecamtiv mecarbil

Omecantiv activates myosin ATPase to increase the hydrolysis of ATP and increase the force of myocardial contraction, increasing cardiac output and ejection fraction whilst decreasing the heart rate; there is little effect on myocardial oxygen consumption (43).

Vasodilators

Vasodilator drugs can be classified according to their mode of action:

1. Drugs that activate protein kinase (the nitrates and nitric oxide, nesiritide, prostacyclin, PDE inhibitors)

2. Drugs acting through the autonomic nervous system (β adrenergic blocking drugs, isoprenaline, phentolamine, urapidil)

3. Drugs acting by ion channels (calcium antagonists, potassium channel openers, hydralazine)

Many of the drugs in these groups have primary effects other than vasodilation; for example, the PDE inhibitors are primarily inotropes, so this section will consider only those drugs with a primary vasodilator mode of action that are useful in the context of cardiothoracic surgery. Many of these compounds may produce non-selective pulmonary vasodilation that will increase ventilation–perfusion mismatch.

Systemic vasodilators

Enalaprilat

The active form of the pro-drug enalapril, a calcium channel blocker. Enalaprilat is ineffective orally, and is only available in the intravenous formulation.

Fenoldopam

A selective dopamine D_1 receptor antagonist that produces smooth muscle relaxation, particularly in the renal circulation, and inhibits tubular sodium resorption. It is an effective vasodilator in hypertensive emergencies. Fenoldopam may be useful in cardiac patients at high risk of renal dysfunction (44), and has been used as prophylaxis against contrast-induced nephropathy. Onset of action is rapid and maintenance infusion rate is 0.1–0.3 µg/kg/min.

Glyceryl trinitrate

Glyceryl trinitrate (GTN) is an organic nitrate usually given by infusion at 0.5–10 µg/kg/min. At low dose rates, GTN primarily produces venodilation. As a result, venous return decreases so decreasing left ventricular end-diastolic pressure. The resulting decrease in left ventricular wall tension, coupled with coronary vasodilation, may increase cardiac output in patients with heart failure. Increasing dose rates produce systemic hypotension and a reflex tachycardia. Tachyphylaxis, and occasionally methaemoglobinaemia, limit the effectiveness of GTN.

Hydralazine

A potassium channel opener that produces direct arterial vasodilation with little effect on venous capacitance. The diastolic blood pressure is reduced proportionally more than the systolic. Hydralazine provokes a reflex tachycardia, and an increase in myocardial contractility. It has a relatively slow onset and is a long-acting drug. Bolus doses of hydralazine 5–10 mg can be repeated at 10–20 min intervals then followed, if necessary, by an infusion of 50–150 µg/min.

Labetalol

A drug with both non-specific β-adrenoceptor and $α_1$-adrenoceptor blocking activity, labetalol is a useful antihypertensive agent in young patients who are likely to mount a significant tachycardia in response to the majority of other vasodilators. Incremental bolus doses of 5 mg every 2–3 minutes (to a maximum of 200 mg) can be followed by an infusion of 0.5–2.0 mg/min. Side effects are bradycardia and reduced myocardial contractility due to the predominant beta activity (7:1 when given intravenously).

Nicardipine

Nicardipine is short-acting dihydropyridine calcium channel blocker that has an elimination half-life of 40 minutes. It produces arterial vasodilation with minimal venodilation, and no reflex tachycardia. Additionally, it is also a potent coronary vasodilator. An initial bolus dose of 2.5 mg over five minutes can be repeated at 10-minute intervals to a maximum dose of 12.5 mg and can be followed by an infusion of 2–15 mg/hr.

Phentolamine

A competitive α adrenoceptor blocker with an affinity for α_1 adrenoceptors that is three times that for α_2 adrenoceptors. Phentolamine is given intravenously as increments of 0.5–2 mg titrated to effect. A peak effect is seen after 1–2 min, and its duration of action is up to 20 min. Phentolamine is used for the acute treatment of hypertension, and is especially useful in patients with phaeochromocytoma and for acute hypertensive reactions in patients on monoamine oxidase inhibitors.

Phenoxybenzamine

A long-acting non-selective α-adrenoceptor blocker that is slow in onset, the peak effect from an intravenous dose being seen after 1 hour, and the plasma half-life is 24 hours. The effect may persist for several days, as the affinity for α-adrenoceptors is very high and recovery requires synthesis of new receptors.

Sodium nitroprusside

Sodium nitroprusside (SNP) is an organic prodrug that produces arteriolar and venous dilation through the production of NO. It must be reconstituted for infusion in 5% dextrose solution. The light orange-coloured solution that results must be protected from sunlight or cyanide ions will be liberated; the solution then becomes brown or blue and must be discarded. The dose range is up to 6 µg/kg/min, although this should be limited to 4 µg/kg/min for longer-term use and the patient should be monitored for signs of cyanide toxicity (metabolic acidosis and increased mixed venous oxygen saturation due to impaired aerobic metabolism) and methaemoglobinaemia. Acute cyanide toxicity is treated with sodium nitrite (10 mL of a 3% solution given over 5 min) followed by an infusion of 12.5 g sodium thiosulphate in 50 mL 5% dextrose over 10 min. Dicobalt edetate can also be used to chelate the cyanide ions. Methaemoglobinaemia is treated with 1–2 mg/kg of intravenous methylene blue. The half-life of SNP is short, leading to a duration of action of 10 min or less. Elimination is complex as a variety of different pathways are involved, but the basic pathway is the liberation of cyanide in the erythrocyte and its subsequent conversion to thiocynate.

SNP is a potent arterial vasodilator, but venous dilation also occurs and the decrease in blood pressure can be sudden and dramatic, with a reflex tachycardia. The tachycardia is less pronounced in patients with heart failure, and a useful increase in cardiac index accompanies the reduction in afterload. In common with other NO donors, SNP inhibits hypoxic pulmonary vasoconstriction, increasing the shunt fraction.

Urapidil

An α_1-adrenoceptor antagonist and a centrally acting 5-hydroxytryptamine 1A receptor agonist. Unlike some other α_1-adrenoceptor antagonists, urapidil does not elicit reflex tachycardia, which may be related to its weak β_1-adrenoceptor antagonist activity and increased centrally mediated vagal tone. An initial slow bolus dose of 25 mg can be repeated at five-minute intervals to a maximum of 100 mg. A maintenance infusion of 9–30 mg/hr is started once arterial pressure is reduced sufficiently. The elimination half-life of urapidil is between 2.7 and 4.8 hours, but it increases to around 15 hours in patients with liver impairment. Urapidil pharmacokinetics are relatively unaffected by renal impairment.

Nesiritide

A recombinant brain natriuretic peptide that induces arterial and venous dilatation by increasing cyclic-GMP activity. It is not an inotrope, and has no effect on heart rate. Onset is rapid following bolus doses of 0.25–2 µg/kg, and the effect is sustained with infusions of 5–30 ng/kg/min. Acute tolerance does not develop, unlike GTN, and there are also fewer side effects (45–47).

Selective pulmonary vasodilators

Nitric oxide

Nitric oxide (NO) is synthesized endogenously from L-arginine by nitric oxide synthase and this enzyme is found in two isoforms:

1. Constitutive—a calcium/calmodulin dependent form that is stimulated by cGMP. Found in endothelium, neurones, skeletal, and cardiac muscle, and platelets.

2. Inducible—generated in response to inflammation in endothelium, vascular smooth muscle, macrophages, and neutrophils. Non-physiological quantities of NO are produced when it is activated during septic shock that may be cytotoxic and lead to the formation of free radicals.

NO is available for medical use in cylinders containing various low concentrations of NO in nitrogen. In high concentrations of oxygen, it spontaneously converts to NO_2, which is highly toxic. NO is indicated in doses up to 40 ppm for the management of severe adult respiratory distress syndrome, although it probably has little effect on survival, and pulmonary hypertension. NO is corrosive to mild steel, so metal components of delivery equipment should be made of stainless steel. Calibrated delivery systems that synchronize injection to the inspiratory phase of the ventilator are the optimal method for administering inhaled NO, but continuous flow systems can also be used. Whichever form of delivery is used, monitoring of inhaled concentrations of both NO and NO_2 is important for minimizing toxicity.

Inhaled NO has no systemic effect, as it is rapidly inactivated in red blood cells. Endogenous NO is produced in response to shear stresses in small arteries and arterioles to provide a continuous vasodilator tone; it also inhibits platelet aggregation. Overproduction of NO by inducible nitric oxide synthase in septic shock produces hypotension and capillary leak.

The basal pulmonary vasodilator tone is inhibited during hypoxia, leading to pulmonary hypertension and ventilation–perfusion mismatch. Inhaled NO can reverse these effects, and is particularly effective in treating pulmonary hypertension in infants after cardiac surgery.

Excessive administration of NO produces methaemoglobinaemia, particularly in children or those patients with methaemoglobin reductase deficiency, but this is rarely significant. Environmental concentrations should not exceed 25 ppm as an 8-hr time-weighted average, though scavenging should not be required if the theatre or ICU is well ventilated.

SNP and GTN are both 'NO donors' that exert their effects either by release of NO or by metabolism to NO in smooth muscle.

Prostaglandins

Alprostadil (PGE₁), dinoprostone (PGE₂), prostacyclin (epoprostenol, PGI₂), and iloprost (a stable analogue of prostacyclin) are vasodilator prostaglandins. Alprostadil and dinoprostone are used to maintain ductal patency in duct-dependent congenital heart disease. All are potent inhibitors of platelet aggregation, which limits their usefulness as systemic vasodilators. Prostacyclin and iloprost are useful for patients with pulmonary hypertension and they can be nebulized to minimize their systemic effects.

Sildenafil

Sildenafil is competitive inhibitor of PDE V, which is responsible for degradation of cGMP and is found in the arterial smooth muscle of the lungs and penis. Sildenafil acts selectively in both these areas without inducing vasodilation elsewhere.

Vasoconstrictors

These drugs are used to counteract the decrease in systemic vascular resistance following induction of anaesthesia, or in vasoplegic patients on CPB. Care must be taken that the cardiac output is not impaired by excessive doses of vasoconstrictor drugs, particularly when left ventricular function is poor. Renal vascular resistance is also increased, so that renal blood flow and glomerular filtration rate may decrease.

Ephedrine

Ephedrine occurs naturally in some plants, but is synthesized for medical use. It has both direct and indirect α- and β-adrenoceptor activity. It also inhibits monoamine oxidase (caution in patients taking monoamine oxidase inhibitors), so that tachyphylaxis is common as noradrenaline stores are depleted by repeated administration. Bolus doses of 3–6 mg in adults increase cardiac output and heart rate, and increase vascular tone. Ephedrine is also a respiratory stimulant and bronchodilator.

Metaraminol

A synthetic agent that has both direct and indirect activity, primarily on α_1-adrenoceptors. Bolus doses of 0.5–2.0 mg are used to increase the systemic vascular resistance, although the pulmonary vascular resistance is also increased so that right heart failure or an increased right to left intracardiac shunt may occur. Its β-adrenoceptor activity is too weak to counteract the reduction in cardiac output that frequently occurs.

Norepinephrine (noradrenaline)

Norepinephrine is an endogenous catecholamine with primarily α_1- but also significant β-adrenoceptor activity, noradrenaline is synthesized for medical use. The synthetic drug has less β activity than the naturally occurring form. It is given at a rate of 0.05–0.5 μg/kg/min to increase systemic vascular resistance, although the pulmonary vascular resistance also increases. Peripheral vasoconstriction also causes a significant decrease in renal, hepatic, and splanchnic blood flows.

Phenylephrine

A direct acting synthetic α_1 agonist. Bolus doses of 50–100 μg are given to increase systemic vascular resistance, though ten times this may be needed to produce an effect in vasoplegic patients on CPB for example in those patients on ACE inhibitors.

Vasopressin

Presented as a synthetic analogue (arginine vasopressin), vasopressin is given at a rate of 0.02–0.12 units/kg/hr. It is a powerful vasoconstrictor, particularly useful in vasoplegic patients on CPB or in septic shock. It also causes fluid retention through an anti-diuretic effect, and can produce myocardial ischaemia and significant decreases in splanchnic blood flow.

Conclusion

A thorough understanding of the pharmacology of anaesthetic agents and other drugs, particularly cardiovascular drugs, is important to enable cardiothoracic anaesthetists to manage these often complex patients safely and effectively.

Further reading

Peck TE, Hill SA, Williams M. *Pharmacology for Anaesthesia and Intensive Care*, 3rd edn. Cambridge: Cambridge University Press, 2008

Kaski JC (ed.) *Drugs in Cardiology*. Oxford: Oxford University Press, 2010

References

1. Nickalls RWD, Mapleson WW. Age-related iso-MAC charts for isoflurane, sevoflurane and desflurane in man. *Br J Anaesth* 2003; **91**(2): 170–4
2. Boer F. Drug handling by the lungs. *Br J Anaesth* 2003; **91**(1): 50–60
3. Mets B. The pharmacokinetics of anesthetic drugs and adjuvants during cardiopulmonary bypass. *Acta Anaesth Scand* 2000; **44**(3): 261–73
4. Dawson PJ, Bjorksten AR, Blake DW, Goldblatt JC. The effects of cardiopulmonary bypass on total and unbound plasma concentrations of propofol and midazolam. *J Cardiothorac Vasc Anesth* 1997; **11**(5): 556–61
5. Feingold A. Crystalloid hemodilution, hypothermia, and halothane blood solubility during cardiopulmonary bypass. *Anesth Analg* 1977; **56**(5): 622–6
6. Goucke CR, Hackett LP, Barrett PH, Ilett KF. Blood concentrations of enflurane before, during, and after hypothermic cardiopulmonary bypass. *J Cardiothorac Vasc Anesth* 2007; **21**(2): 218–23
7. Zhou J-X, Liu J. Dynamic changes in blood solubility of desflurane, isoflurane, and halothane during cardiac surgery. *J Cardiothorac Vasc Anesth* 2001; **15**(5): 555–9
8. Henderson JM, Nathan HJ, Lalande M, Winkler MH, Dubé M. Washin and washout of isoflurane during cardiopulmonary bypass. *Can J Anaesth* 1988; **35**(6): 587–90
9. Loomis CW, Brunet D, Milne B, Cervenko FW, Johnson GD. Arterial isoflurane concentration and EEG burst suppression during cardiopulmonary bypass. *Clin Pharmacol Ther* 1986; **40**(3): 304–13
10. Wiesenack C, Wiesner G, Keyl C, et al. In vivo uptake and elimination of isoflurane by different membrane oxygenators during cardiopulmonary bypass. *Anesthesiology* 2002; **97**(1): 133–8
11. Lockwood GG, Sapsed-Byrne SM, Adams S. A comparison of anaesthetic tensions in arterial blood and oxygenator exhaust gas during cardiopulmonary bypass. *Anaesthesia* 1999; 54: 434–6
12. Liu EHC, Dhara SS. Monitoring oxygenator expiratory isoflurane concentrations and the Bispectral Index to guide isoflurane requirements during cardiopulmonary bypass. *J Cardiothorac Vasc Anesth* 2005; **19**(4): 485–7
13. Lundell JC, Scuderi PE, Butterworth JF. Less isoflurane is required *after* than *before* cardiopulmonary bypass to maintain a constant Bispectral Index value. *J Cardiothorac Vasc Anesth* 2001; **15**(5): 551–4
14. McNulty SE, Bartkowski R, Schmitz T. Should the gas outlet port on membrane oxygenators be routinely scavenged during cardiopulmonary bypass? *J Cardiothorac Vasc Anesth* 1992; **6**(6): 697–9
15. Mierdl S, Byhahn C, Abdel-Rahman U, Matheis G, Westphal K. Occupational exposure to inhalational anesthetics during cardiac surgery on cardiopulmonary bypass. *Ann Thorac Surg* 2003; **75**(6): 1924–7
16. Ebert TJ, Muzi M. Sympathetic hyperactivity during desflurane anesthesia in healthy volunteers. A comparison with isoflurane. *Anesthesiology* 1993; **79**(3): 444–53
17. Agnew NM, Pennefather SH, Russell GN. Isoflurane and coronary heart disease. *Anaesthesia* 2002; **57**(4): 338–47

18. Dingley J, Ivanova-Stoilova TM, Grundler S, Wall T. Xenon: recent developments. *Anaesthesia* 2000; **54**: 335–46

19. Sanders RD, Franks NP, Maze M. Xenon: no stranger to anaesthesia. *Br J Anaesth* 2003; **91**(5): 709–17

20. Symons JA, Myles PS. Myocardial protection with volatile anaesthetic agents during coronary artery bypass surgery: a meta-analysis. *Br J Anaesth* 2006; **97**(2): 127–36

21. Yu CH, Beattie WS. The effects of volatile anesthetics on cardiac ischemic complications and mortality in CABG: a meta-analysis. *Can J Anaesth* 2006; **53**(9): 906–18

22. Jakobsen C-J, Berg H, Hindsholm KB, Faddy N, Sloth E. The influence of propofol versus sevoflurane anesthesia on outcome in 10,535 cardiac surgical procedures. *J Cardiothorac Vasc Anesth* 2007; **21**(5): 664–71

23. Morel J, Salard M, Castelain C, et al. Haemodynamic consequences of etomidate administration in elective cardiac surgery: a randomized double-blinded study. *Br J Anaesth* 2011; **107**(4): 503–9

24. Spies C, Zuane U, Pauli MH, Boeden G, Martin E. A comparison of enflurane and propofol in thoracic surgery. *Anaesthesist* 1991; **40**(1): 14–8

25. Speicher A, Jessberger J, Braun R, Hollnberger H, Stigler F, Manz R. Postoperative pulmonary function after lung surgery. Total intravenous anesthesia with propofol in comparison to balanced anesthesia with isoflurane. *Anaesthesist* 1995; **44**(4): 265–73

26. Servin F, Farinotti R, Haberer JP, Desmonts JM. Propofol infusion for maintenance of anesthesia in morbidly obese patients receiving nitrous oxide. A clinical and pharmacokinetic study. *Anesthesiology* 1993; **78**(4): 657–65

27. Juvin P, Vadam C, Malek L, Dupont H, Marmuse JP, Desmonts JM. Postoperative recovery after desflurane, propofol, or isoflurane anesthesia among morbidly obese patients: a prospective, randomized study. *Anesth Analg* 2000; **91**(3): 714–9

28. Myles PS. Prevention of awareness during anaesthesia. *Best Pract Res Clin Anaesthesiol* 2007; **21**: 345–55

29. Mora CT, Torjman M, White P. Effects of diazepam and flumazenil on sedation and hypoxic ventilatory response. *Anesth Analg* 1989; **68**(4): 473–8

30. Lowenstein E, Hallowell P, Levine FH, Daggett WM, Austen WG, Laver MB. Cardiovascular responses to large doses of intravenous morphine in man. *N Engl J Med* 1969; **281**(25): 1389–93

31. Stanley TH, Webster LR. Anesthetic requirements and cardiovascular effects of fentanyl-oxygen and fentanyl-diazepam-oxygen anesthesia in man. *Anesth Analg* 1978; **57**(4): 411–6

32. Lowenstein E. Morphine 'anesthesia'—a perspective. *Anesthesiology* 1971; **35**(6): 563–5

33. Vaughan Williams EM. A classification of antiarrythmic actions revisited after a decade of new drugs. *J Clin Pharmacol* 1984; **24**(4): 129–47

34. Mebazaa A, Parissis J, Porcher R, et al. Short-term survival by treatment among patients hospitalized with acute heart failure: the global ALARM-HF registry using propensity scoring methods. *Intensive Care Med* 2011; **37**(2): 290–301

35. Bellomo R, Chapman M, Finfer S, et al. Low-dose dopamine in patients with early renal dysfunction: a placebo-controlled randomised trial. *Lancet* 2000; **356**: 2139–43

36. Marik PE. Low-dose dopamine: a systematic review. *Intensive Care Med* 2002; **28**: 877–83

37. Zaloga GP, Strickland RA, Butterworth JF, Mark LJ, Mills SA, Lake CR. Calcium attenuates epinephrine's beta-adrenergic effects in postoperative heart surgery patients. *Circulation* 1990; **81**(1): 196–200

38. Siirilä-Waris K, Suojaranta-Ylinen R, Harjola V-P. Levosimendan in cardiac surgery. *J Cardiothorac Vasc Anesth* 2005; **19**(3): 345–9

39. Kivikko M, Lehtonen L, Colucci WS. Sustained hemodynamic effects of intravenous levosimendan. *Circulation* 2003; **107**(1): 81–6

40. Feneck RO. Intravenous milrinone following cardiac surgery: I. Effects of bolus infusion followed by variable dose maintenance infusion. *J Cardiothorac Vasc Anesth* 1992; **6**(5): 554–62

41. Royster RL, Butterworth JF, Prielipp RC, et al. Combined inotropic effects of amrinone and epinephrine after cardiopulmonary bypass in humans. *Anesth Analg* 1993; **77**(4): 662–72

42. Ghali JK, Smith WB, Torre-Amione G, et al. A phase 1–2 dose-escalating study evaluating the safety and tolerability of istaroxime and specific effects on electrocardiographic and hemodynamic parameters in patients with chronic heart failure with reduced systolic function. *Am J Cardiol* 2007; **99**(2A): 47A–56A

43. Cleland JG, Teerlink JR, Senior R, et al. The effects of the cardiac myosin activator, omecamtiv mecarbil, on cardiac function in systolic heart failure: a double-blind, placebo-controlled, crossover, dose-ranging phase 2 trial. *Lancet* 2011; **378**(9792): 676–83

44. Cogliati AA, Vellutini R, Nardini A, et al. Fenoldopam infusion for renal protection in high-risk cardiac surgery patients: A randomized clinical study. *J Cardiothorac Vasc Anesth* 2007; **21**(6): 847–50

45. Elkayam U, Akhter MW, Singh H, Khan S, Usman A. Comparison of effects on left ventricular filling pressure of intravenous nesiritide and high-dose nitroglycerin in patients with decompensated heart failure. *Am J Cardiol* 2004; **93**(2): 237–40

46. Publication Committee for the VMAC investigators. Intravenous nesiritide vs nitroglycerin for treatment of decompensated heart failure: a randomized controlled trial. *JAMA* 2002; **287**(12): 1531–40

47. Burger AJ, Horton DP, LeJemtel T, et al. Effect of nesiritide (B-type natriuretic peptide) and dobutamine on ventricular arrhythmias in the treatment of patients with acutely decompensated congestive heart failure: the PRECEDENT study. *Am Heart J* 2002; **144**: 1102–8

CHAPTER 7

Diagnosis and assessment of cardiac disease

Silvana F. Marasco and Martin G. Hiscock

Introduction

The diagnosis of cardiac conditions, as with other body systems, begins with a thorough medical history and examination. In general, adult cardiac patients tend to be older most commonly in their 60s and 70s, and will often downplay symptoms, attributing them to ageing. A high degree of suspicion is needed therefore in any elderly patient presenting with fatigue or decreasing exercise tolerance. More typical symptoms of angina and shortness of breath often go unrecognized by patients who expect heart pain to be painful, and assume shortness of breath is due to lung pathology. In contrast, some patients will present in extremis after no warning symptoms, or more commonly after ignoring symptoms for months. In this chapter, we will review the diagnosis and assessment of heart disease, concentrating on coronary artery disease (CAD) and aortic stenosis, being the two most common surgically correctable cardiac pathologies in adults.

Diagnosis

CAD and aortic stenosis can present with similar symptoms. Aortic stenosis can also present with palpitations and/ or syncope and both of these symptoms tend to develop fairly late in the disease process. Patients presenting with any symptoms suspicious of cardiac disease require a thorough clinical examination. A harsh ejection systolic murmur is diagnostic of aortic stenosis but CAD will often not present diagnostic features to the clinician. A 12-lead electrocardiogram (ECG) should be performed for it can provide a wealth of information to the astute clinician. Electrocardiographic features such as ST changes of ischaemia or infarction, poor R wave progression, arrhythmias, left ventricular hypertrophy, left ventricular strain, all assist in the final diagnosis.

Stress echocardiography

If there is any suspicion of CAD in a patient who is symptomatically stable, stress echocardiography should be the next investigation. Most commonly, an exercise stress test is undertaken with the patient on a treadmill. Bicycle exercise can also be used for those patients who are unable to exercise on the treadmill. Another option is inotropic induced stress, typically with dobutamine, for patients who cannot exercise at all or if there is a suspicion of non-viable myocardium. The main diagnostic feature, induced by stress is segmental wall motion abnormalities (SWMAs). A normal response to exercise is the augmentation of function in all mycardial segments. Ischaemia is identified by SWMAs, most commonly manifesting as poor thickening of muscle rather than motion abnormalities which can be influenced by translation or tethering. Rest and stress images are compared to identify global dysfunction such as left ventricular enlargement or shape change. Inducible SWMAs indicate a significant flow limitation at peak stress and generally correlate with significant coronary lesions. The sensitivity of stress echocardiography is limited, however, in normal ventricles, even with multivessel or single vessel disease.

Coronary angiography

Coronary angiography is the next investigation in an individual with a positive stress test, or with sufficient suspicion of CAD based on symptoms and history. Angiography allows delineation of the coronary anatomy, assessment of CAD and formulation of a management plan of medical management, percutaneous coronary intervention (PCI) or coronary artery bypass graft (CABG) surgery.

One of the most recent advances in coronary angiography is the use of the radial artery for access. This site is becoming increasingly popular for diagnostic and interventional coronary angiography. The main benefit is the ease of cannulation due to its superficial position and its ability to be readily compressed. It also allows patients to immedaitely ambulate after the procedure rather than lying supine for several hours while femoral compression is in place (1–3). However, few other benefits have been convincingly proven, and there could be a slightly increased rate of PCI failure (4). Although there is a lower incidence of local vascular complications (5), a large multicentred randomized controlled trial found no difference in death, myocardial infarction (MI), stroke, or non-CABG related major bleeding.

Preoperative assessment

Preoperative assessment of the cardiac surgical patient encompasses three areas—surgical assessment of suitability for operative intervention, assessment of operative risk, and anaesthetic assessment. Assessment of operative suitability necessitates careful review of the coronary angiogram. Single vessel disease is largely addressed by PCI unless vessel tortuosity or an ostial stenosis makes the risk of the procedure prohibitive. In a patient referred for surgical revascularization, assessment of the 'target' coronary vessels is crucial. Size, distribution, run off, and viability of the

Table 7.1 Indications for revascularization in stable angina or silent ischaemia

	Subset of CAD by anatomy	Class [a]	Level [b]
For prognosis	Left main > 50% [c]	I	A
	Any proximal LAD> 50% [c]	I	A
	2VD or 3VD with impaired LV function [c]	I	B
	Proven large area of ischaemia (> 10% LV)	I	B
	Single remaining patent vessel > 50% stenosis [c]	I	C
	1VD without proximal LAD and without > 10% ischaemia	III	A
For symptoms	Any stenosis >50% with limiting angina or angina equivalent, unresponsive to OMT	I	A
	Dyspnoea/CHF and >10% LV ischaemia/viability supplied by > 50% stenotic artery	IIa	B
	No limiting symptoms with OMT	III	C

[a] Class of recommendation, [b] Level of evidence, [c] With documented ischaemia or FFR < 0.80 for angiographic diameter stenosis 50–90%.

CAD, coronary artery disease; CHF, chronic heart failure; FFR, fractional flow reserve; LAD, left anterior descending; LV, left ventricle; OMT, optimal medical therapy, VD, vessel disease.

Reproduced from Wijns W et al., 'Guidelines on myocardial revascularization', *European Heart Journal*, 2010, **31**, 20, pp. 2501–2555, by permission of the European Society of Cardiology and Oxford University Press

Table 7.2 Indications for coronary artery bypass graft (CABG) surgery vs. percutaneous coronary intervention in stable patients with lesions suitable for both procedures and low predicted surgical mortality

Subset of CAD by anatomy	Favours CABG	Favours PCI
1VD or 2VD- non-proximal LAD	IIb C	I C
1VD or 2 VD	I A	IIa B
3VD simple lesions, full functional revascularization achievable with PCI, SYNTAX score ≤ 22	I A	IIa B
3VD complex lesions, incomplete revascularization achievable with PCI, SYNTAX score* > 22	I A	III A
Left main (isolated or 1VD, ostium/shaft)	I A	IIa B
Left main (isolated or 1VD, distal bifurcation)	I A	IIb B
Left main + 2 VD or 3 VD, SYNTAX score ≤ 32	I A	IIb B
Left main + 2VD or 3VD, SYNTAX score ≥ 33	I A	III B

CABG, coronary artery bypass grafting; CAD, coronary artery disease; LAD, left anterior descending; LV, left ventricle; PCI, percutaneous coronary intervention; VD, vessel disease.

*see text for details.

Reproduced from Wijns W et al., 'Guidelines on myocardial revascularization', *European Heart Journal*, 2010, **31**, 20, pp. 2501–2555, by permission of the European Society of Cardiology and Oxford University Press

territory being supplied are all paramount to the success of the procedure. Vessels with heavy calcification, chronic occlusion and poorly visualized lumen, multiple stenoses, or distal vessel disease may not be technically operable.

European guidelines on myocardial revascularization address the appropriateness of revascularization and the relative merits of CABG and PCI (6). There is strong evidence for revascularization on symptomatic grounds in patients with persistent limiting symptoms despite optimal medical therapy, and on prognostic grounds in patients with significant left main disease, proximal left anterior descending artery disease, and multivessel disease (table 7.1).

The guidelines also support surgical revascularization over PCI, in all anatomical subsets of CAD except for single or double vessel disease not involving the proximal left anterior descending artery (table 7.2). The most recent trial data with 5-year follow-up reinforces this view (7).

Anatomical scoring systems

Clinical risk in coronary revascularization strategies can also be assessed by means of anatomical scoring systems. The most widely used and tested is the SYNTAX score (8), which is a weighted score based on the features of each lesion iincluding bifurcation, thrombus, total occlusion, size of vessel, calcification, and the amount of myocardium distal to each lesion. In the SYNTAX trial (9), the distribution of the SYNTAX scores in both the CABG and PCI arms were superimposed, and followed a normal distribution. Interestingly, in the nested registry trials, the distribution of the SYNTAX scores were no longer superimposed, with the CABG patients exhibiting higher scores than the PCI patients. A higher SYNTAX score has now been shown in multiple studies to be a

good discriminator of poorer outcomes with PCI and is an independent predictor of major adverse cardiac events (SYNTAX score >33) (10,11). In contrast to PCI, the SYNTAX score has little predictive ability in surgical revascularization, probably because vessels are grafted distal to any lesion making the morphology of the lesions irrelevant (12).

The use of the SYNTAX score has since been further refined by the addition of fractional flow reserve measurements to guide coronary intervention by elucidating the actual functional significance of individual coronary lesions in the FAME study (13). This 'functional SYNTAX' score has further improved risk stratification of PCI patients, mainly by reclassifying a significant proportion of the higher risk groups into lower risk categories.

Myocardial viability

Myocardial viability is extremely important for success of coronary revascularization. The first indication of large segments of non-viable muscle come from the patient history. Absence of angina, particularly in those who do not have diabetes, is a concerning feature, as are symptoms of LV failure. Poor R wave progression on ECG should raise suspicion.

Echocardiography

Echocardiography will prove diagnostic in many patients and when assessing the myocardium, wall thickness is visualized in early systole. Normal myocardial thickness is 11–12 mm with thickening of >2 mm in systole indicating viable myocardium. Scar is identified as thinned and echodense tissue. A dobutamine stress echocardiogram is valuable in assessing viability. Dobutamine leads to increased heart rate, blood pressure, and contractility. It also vasodilates causing a coronary steal phenomenon. Viability is indicated by abnormal resting segments, which show improvement with low-dose dobutamine. Biphasic response of hibernating myocardium best predicts recovery of myocardial function after revascularization. Low-dose dobutamine increases coronary flow leading to recruitment of contractile reserve, which improves wall motion of the dysfunctional myocardium. With increased dose of dobutamine there is no further increase in coronary blood flow because of limiting stenoses leading to myocardial ischaemia, and a worsening of wall motion is seen.

Radioisotope scanning

Thallium

A thallium scan is also a useful test to assess myocardial viability (14). Thallium (^{201}Tl) is a potassium analogue and is driven into the cell by the Na^+–K^+ ATPase pump. Thus uptake is directly proportional to regional myocardial blood flow, and defects at rest indicate areas of ischaemia. Following the initial high extraction of ^{201}Tl there is a continuous washout of cellular ^{201}Tl. A normal scan indicates a low risk for cardiac events even in the presence of CAD on angiography. Viability is indicated by redistribution of a resting defect or reversibility of a stress (exercise) defect. Thus in ischaemia demonstrated during exercise, delayed imaging will show improvement with rest. This does not occur with hibernation but reinjection four hours after exercise with more than 50% uptake in the previously low uptake areas indicates hibernating myocardium. A true fixed defect indicates scar from prior MI. Same-day reinjection followed by a scan at three to four hours has reduced the false negative rate of this test from 50% to 10% (15,16). When <50% of maximal uptake is seen at rest, there is little chance of improvement with revascularization.

Technetium

Technetium-99m Sestamibi scanning is an alternative to thallium scanning (17). Technetium 99m pyrophosphate tissue uptake is dependent in part on tissue calcium accumulation. Thus necrotic areas, particularly border zones, which still have an intact blood supply, will take up the radiotracer avidly. It is useful in determining whether or not a patient has had an acute MI in the setting of equivocal ECG and enzyme results. However, it has low sensitivity in subendocardial infarction. A severe fixed defect is usually non-viable whereas a mild defect is frequently viable. Unlike ^{201}Tl significant redistribution in the myocardium does not occur so requiring both stress and resting imaging with this tracer. Increased sestamibi lung activity is a marker of multivessel coronary disease and extensive myocardium at risk which indicate a poor prognosis without coronary revascularization. A normal scan is associated with a low cardiac event rate, even in the presence of CAD on angiography.

Positron emission tomography

Positron emission tomography (PET) for myocardial viability compares metabolism (tracer = ^{18}fluorodeoxyglucose, FDG) to flow (tracer = ^{13}N-ammonia or ^{82}rubidium). ^{11}C-labelled acetate has been used as a marker of oxidative metabolism and thus viability. 90% of segments with FDG:flow mismatch demonstrate improved function after revascularization (18–20). Increased FDG uptake to flow ratio reflects a change to increased anaerobic glycolysis in the ischaemic zone. PET scanning for viability is more sensitive and specific than thallium scanning (21,22). PET has been considered the reference method of viability assessment for some years. However, magnetic resonance imaging (MRI) has more recently been shown to be as sensitive and specific as PET scanning (23), but with some improvement in tissue characterization, because of its better spatial resolution.

Magnetic resonance imaging

MRI has superseded PET scanning as the gold standard for myocardial viability. Gadolinium-based contrast agent is used to detect non-viable myocardium which shows up as hyperenhancement. MRI has high diagnostic accuracy in assessing the transmural extent of myocardial scar. However its sensitivity in detecting viability and predicting recovery of wall motion is not superior to other imaging techniques (24). In a study of 31 patients with ischaemic heart failure, PET and MRI imaging were compared (25). Eleven percent of segments defined as viable by PET showed some degree of MRI hyperenhancement. PET and MRI otherwise correlated well in terms of quantitative assessment of infarct size. MRI has been shown to accurately predict those segments that will not recover functionally after revascularization (26). The most recent study compared single-photon emission computed tomography (SPECT) and cardiac MRI, with coronary angiography as the reference standard, in 752 patients with suspected coronary heart disease (23). This clearly demonstrated that cardiac MRI had high diagnostic accuracy in CAD and was superior to SPECT.

Availability of conduits

Once the cardiac assessment has identified a surgically treatable condition, then the patient assessment with regards to suitability of surgery needs to be undertaken. In patients referred for coronary revascularization, this requires the presence of adequate conduit. Internal mammary arteries are sometimes but not commonly imaged during coronary angiography. Bilateral internal mammary artery conduit can be used in most patients but is associated with increased sternal wound infection rates in diabetics, obese patients, and patients with chronic obstructive airways disease or conditions with chronic cough. A suitable long saphenous vein can usually be found in most patients but may be unavailable in patients with varicose veins, previous varicose vein stripping, or severe peripheral vascular disease (either because of concerns about the wound healing or because the vein has been used for lower limb bypass surgery). Other venous conduit such as short saphenous veins and cephalic veins are associated with poor patency rates and are rarely used any more. Radial arteries are assessed for suitability by palpation and the Allen's test which assesses the presence of a patent palmar arch (27). An abnormal Allen's test is apparent by pallor in the index finger and thumb after releasing pressure on the distal ulnar artery while maintaining pressure on the distal radial artery. Duplex scanning can also be used to assess the patency of the palmar arch and also gives information on caliber and calcification which can make the radial artery unusable.

Aortic stenosis

Contraindications of aortic valve replacement

Surgical assessment of aortic stenosis is more straightforward. Severe aortic stenosis should always be referred for surgical repair unless there is a contraindication. Severe calcification of the aorta commonly known as a porcelain aorta, is a contraindication to surgical aortic valve replacement (AVR). Although there are surgical strategies including aortic endarterectomy or aortic root replacement for dealing with this complication, many centres would now preferentially use a transcatheter aortic valve implanat (TAVI) (Chapter 9) (28–31). Although there are no other 'technical' contraindications to surgical AVR, these patients are often elderly and frail and there may pre-existing patient contraindications to surgery.

Timing of surgery

Isolated aortic valve replacement

Timing of AV surgery in patients with aortic stenosis is important. Rapid progression and sudden death in truly asymptomatic patients is rare. Therefore, surgical intervention is generally not recommended because of the risks of prosthetic valve complications and so the risks of surgery must be weighed against the risks of sudden death in asymptomatic patients (32–34). Patients with symptomatic severe aortic stenosis have a significant increase in cardiac mortality and morbidity, and symptomatically and prognostically improved by AVR (35–38). Many patients who deny symptoms but have a high gradient are not truly asymptomatic because they limit their physical activity. Exercise testing can be used in these patients to elucidate the extent of exercise limitation. Exercise testing in asymptomatic patients with aortic stenosis is controversial, being common in Europe, with very low complication rates (39–41), but is generally considered too risky to undertake in the USA and Australia (42,43). However, useful information can be gained from exercise testing in asymptomatic patients and in demonstrating exercise limitation for which the patient's management will be significantly changed from conservative medical management to surgical intervention.

Combining aortic valve replacement with other heart surgery

Replacement of a stenotic AV while the patient is undergoing other cardiac surgery such as coronary revascularization has a different set of triggers for intervention. In general, even mild to moderate aortic stenosis will progress over about five years in patients with CAD (36,44). Thus most surgeons would consider combining AVR with CABG surgery, if the mean gradient is greater than or equal to 20 mmHg. Interestingly, the smaller bioprosthetic valves will have a similar pressure gradient (often 15–20 mmHg in 19 mm valves). Whereas it increase over time in a diseased native AV, this pressure gradient should not increase in a prosthetic valve. So combining AVR with CABG surgery avoids the risks of resternotomy in a patient with patent grafts to undertake an isolated AVR in a few years' time when the AV stenosis becomes severe and symptomatic.

Aortic stenosis in the presence of low transvalvular flows

Another variant of aortic stenosis which must be accurately identified is low flow/low gradient aortic stenosis. In those patients with underlying cardiac failure and poor ventricular function, an AV with severe calcification and valve area less than 1.0 cm² may only exhibit a low gradient. These patients may be incorrectly diagnosed as having only mild to moderate aortic stenosis and so continue medical treatment, when in fact they have end-stage severe aortic stenosis, for which AV replacement will have prognostic

and symptomatic benefit. It is, however, extremely important to distinguish between a cardiomyopathy secondary to the aortic stenosis versus another underlying myocardial condition, in which case, AV replacement alone is unlikely to improve symptoms or prognosis. The appropriate investigation at this stage is a dobutamine stress echocardiogram (45,46). The inotropic effect of the dobutamine provides augmentation of the stroke volume, increasing flow across the stenotic AV and increasing the gradient. In true severe aortic stenosis, the calculated AV area will not change. In 'pseudo-aortic stenosis', however, where the underlying myocardial dysfunction is not due to the aortic stenosis, the augmented flow across the valve results in only a mild increase in transvalvular gradient with an accompanying mild increase in valve area. It is important to note that failure to increase the transvalvular gradient at all denotes an absence of contractile reserve which increases surgical risk (47,48). Obviously, all of these patients with low flow-low gradient severe aortic stenosis have a higher operative risk. They also have a higher mortality without surgical intervention. However, patients without contractile reserve have a poorer prognosis both with and without surgery (49). Poor contractile reserve has been correlated with extent of myocardial fibrosis preoperatively on MRI (50). Not surprisingly, the degree of myocardial fibrosis is fixed without any improvement or reversal seen on repeat MRI nine months after successful AVR (51). Despite this, there are studies that have shown improvement in symptoms and improvement in left ventricular function in patients with no contractile reserve on preoperative dobutamine echocardiography (48,52). Paradoxical low flow aortic stenosis has also been described whereby the low gradient severe aortic stenosis exists in the setting of preserved left ventricular function (47,53). The mechanism is thought to be related to high afterload but probably also represents a 'subclinical' early myocardial dysfunction.

Predicting outcome after cardiac surgery

History of modelling outcome

In the 1980s, a number of large cohort studies were published, which showed the benefit of coronary artery bypass grafting in patients with CAD. As the number of patients undergoing surgical coronary revascularization rapidly rose, it became clear that results varied amongst hospitals and surgeons. Some of these differences in mortality rates may have been related to the quality of care provided. However, a large part of the differences was due to patient factors such as cardiac function and comorbidities stemming an interest in risk stratification.

The US Society of Thoracic Surgeons (STS) and the European System for Cardiac Operative Risk Evaluation (EuroSCORE) scores are the most common risk stratification indices used today. However, prior to their development, other methods of risk stratification existed and were widely used. The Montreal Heart Model was one of the first published models and was based on 500 patients at a single institution. Significant risk factors were poor ejection fraction (<30%), unstable angina, recent MI, heart failure, age >65 years, emergency surgery, reoperation, and obesity (body mass index > 30) (54). The Parsonnet model was developed later in the 1980s and was based on 3500 patients at multiple sites (55). It stratified patients into risk 'bands' and was widely used throughout the 1990s. An update was also published in the 1990s that eliminated some of the subjective fields and reweighted the remaining variables (56). The Cleveland Clinic clinical severity score was also developed in the 1980's using 5,051 of its patients having primarily CABG surgery (57,58). The same model was also used in an important study exploring the gender differences in outcomes of CABG (59). As had been previously identified (60,61). women had higher unadjusted mortality rates (4.9% v 3.0%) and serious morbidity rates (15.0% v 9.2%). However, they also had a different distribution of risk factors, and when risk-stratified according to preoperative severity score, no statistically significant sex differences in mortality or morbidity remained.

The Northern New England Model was also developed in the late 1980s and identified eight variables that predicted mortality including age, sex, body surface area, comorbidity score, reoperation, ejection fraction, left ventricular end-diastolic pressure, and priority at surgery (62). Although this model has good discrimination and calibration, the observed mortality rates are lower than predicted (63).

Influence of anaesthesia and surgery on outcome

All of the scores mentioned in the previous section allow preoperative evaluation and stratification of risk. However, outcomes are also influenced by surgical and anaesthetic techniques (64,65). Factors such as intraoperative blood loss, surgical or anaesthetic misadventure, length of time on cardiopulmonary bypass and cross clamp time, and adequacy of myocardial preservation, will all influence outcomes. None of these factors will be known preoperatively although some can be loosely predicted. Further risk stratification as the patient arrives in the intensive care unit (ICU) allows such factors to be incorporated into a model that also includes preoperative factors. Perhaps the most widely used and validated score for ICU patients is the APACHE II/III score (Acute Physiology and Chronic Health Evaluation). Although designed for general intensive care patients, it has been evaluated in cardiothoracic surgical patients (66,67).

EuroSCORE

The EuroSCORE was developed during the 1990s, with the aim of devising a simple and pragmatic risk adjustment model based on easily collectable data that could be used for both preoperative risk assessment and post-hoc comparison of surgical performance based on contemporary European data. The original EuroSCORE was developed based on data collection carried out over three months in 1995 on all adult patients who underwent cardiac surgery with cardiopulmonary bypass in 132 centres in 8 countries (68). Complete information on 19 030 patients was collected for analysis. However, centres volunteered to take part, a component of self-selection has already occurred and so the score may not reflect the true risk in less adept centres. However, numerous studies have shown that the EuroSCORE provides reliable risk prediction in cardiac surgery at international, hospital or unit level (69,70). Two versions were eventually developed, a complex logistic version and a simpler additive version, both of which provide reliable results. The logistic EuroSCORE was developed to provide more accuracy in

predicting risk in higher risk patients. The EuroSCORE was revised in 2011, using more up-to-date data.

Limitations of risk models applied to valve surgery

One of the problems with cardiac risk models is that they are designed to predict mortality in CABG patients and do not seem to be as accurate in valve surgery patients, particularly higher risk valve patients. Invariably, these models tend to overestimate the risk in higher risk patients. This has been shown in multiple studies, whereby the logistic EuroSCORE has been shown to overestimate mortality risk in AVR patients by a factor of between 3 to 7 in patients whose observed mortality was 5–10% (71) and by a factor of almost 3 in patients whose observed mortality was less than 20% (72). Similar findings have been reported in other studies (73,74). The reason for this over-prediction is because the model is designed so that CABG is considered the baseline risk, and any added procedure such as a valve repair or replacement is estimated as an additive risk. This over-prediction seems to be amplified with time which is hardly surprising given that the original dataset was collected in 1995.

Thus it has been proposed that the use of the EuroSCORE is inappropriate to risk stratify patients with aortic stenosis, particularly if a decision to withhold surgery based on a prediction of high surgical mortality risk in those patients (73). This has implications as to the rejection of surgery for high-risk AVR patients with the plan to offer them percutaneous valve replacement instead (discussed later).

Society of Throacic Surgeons predicted risk of mortality

In contrast to the EuroSCORE, the current STS Predicted Risk of Mortality (STS- PROM) algorithm for AVR is based on a patient population undergoing isolated AVR from 2002 to 2006 in over 800 centres in the USA. A total of 67 292 patients who were added to the database over that time period were used to develop the algorithm. Predictor variables were identified and model coefficients estimated on a sample of 60% of that population and then the remaining 40% were used as a validation sample to assess model fit, discrimination and calibration. The model now contains 24 covariates for AV mortality and has risk models developed for nine end points (discussed in subsequent sections).

Multiple studies have now shown a greater accuracy with the STS-PROM model compared with the EuroSCORE. A recent study has shown an observed mortality much closer to the expected with an underestimation by a factor of 0.8, rather than an overestimation by a factor of 3 as demonstrated in some of the studies mentioned earlier (75). Another study by the same author found the logistic EuroSCORE to report an expected mortality of 50.9% versus observed mortality of 15.6% in patients in the highest 10% risk percentile for surgical AVR. In contrast the STS-PROM tends to under-predict with an expected versus observed mortality of 13.3% versus 18.8% (70).

EuroSCORE II has just been released on the EuroSCORE. org website and has been designed to address the problem of over-prediction of risk. Some of the input variables have been changed but recent validation studies have so far not demonstrated significant improvements in the prediction of risk in higher-risk cases (76,77).

Risk factors not included in models

One of the problems with both the risk algorithms outlined previously is that there are multiple risk factors known to impact on outcomes which are not included in the models. Factors such as previous chest irradiation, porcelain aorta, liver disease, or general frailty are not taken into account. This is not to say that they have been discounted as being relevant. The reason some factors are not included is because they cannot be accurately quantified and recorded (for example general frailty), or they occur with such limited frequency to be validated as a covariate as for example irradiation of the chest. Because these 'unquantifiable' factors, patients are increasingly being referred for percutaneous valve implants with these types of comorbidities. Unfortunately the EuroSCORE assessment is then being applied and used for justification for not referring these patients on for surgical AVR. A recent meta-analysis of percutaneous valve replacement outcomes concluded that the actual 30-day mortality rates were substantially lower than the expected mortality rates as predicted by EuroSCORE (78). Interestingly, there seems to be a dearth of publications using the STS-PROM to validate percutaneous valve replacement. However, the STS-PROM has been mandated as the entry criteria selection tool for the enrolment of patients in two percutaneous AV replacement trials in the US by the Food and Drug Administration. A minimum STS-PROM score of 8 is included in the entry criteria. The latest iteration of the STS-PROM includes fields specific to transcatheter aortic valve implantation (TAVI). Ideally, however, a specific risk algorithm needs to be developed for TAVI utilizing data collected from patients who have undergone TAVI. Obviously this also needs to be done following adequate training and allowing time for completion of a learning curve in this procedure. Some of the potential risks in TAVI are also different to standard surgical AVR and therefore utilizing a dataset of TAVI patients to determine outcomes and risk prediction of certain complications will be necessary in the future.

Outcomes other than mortality

Prediction of mortality alone is no longer sufficient to truly predict a patient's course through the hospital admission. Other outcomes such as neurological complications, prolonged length of stay, or deep sternal wound infection, have significant impact in terms of morbidity and hospital costs. The latest STS-PROM algorithm includes risk models for eight end points other than mortality. These include predictions of: permanent stroke, defined as a central neurological deficit lasting longer than 72 hours; renal failure defined as a new requirement for dialysis, or a doubling of the preoperative serum creatinine with a peak over 2.0 mg/dL; prolonged ventilation (greater than 24 hours); deep sternal wound infection; reoperation for any reason; prolonged postoperative length of stay (more than 14 days); short postoperative length of stay (less than 6 days); and major morbidity or mortality (a composite end point).

Impediments to risk stratification

One of the problems inherent in any risk modelling is the time required to build the databases to produce an accurate algorithm. This requires either reliance on clinical staff such as hospital medical officers to input data, which is prone to incomplete and inaccurate data entry, or the employment of specific data managers, which adds to the cost of running a hospital department and also relies to a degree on data collection by clinical staff. The use of hospital administrative claims data has been investigated, to enable efficient, accurate risk stratification. Because there is a financial incentive for hospitals to accurately capture this data, it is often complete. However, the use of this data alone does not give sufficient information for risk modelling. The addition of 'present-on-admission' codes and a limited set of numerical laboratory data obtained on admission have been shown to produce an accurate risk stratification model for CABG and other non-cardiac surgery (79). Key clinical findings which are expensive to collect added little to that model in terms of predictive power and resulted in only small reductions in hospital-level bias.

Conclusion

Diagnosis of heart disease can sometimes be made based on symptoms and examination. Most frequently, it will require further technical investigations to establish the type and extent of disease and whether surgical interventions is appropriate. Today, risk scoring is fundamental to cardiac surgery as it allows comparison of outcomes between individual surgeons and institutions and also to provide the patient with information as to the risks of surgery.

References

1. Chase AJ, Fretz EB, Warburton WP, et al. Association of the arterial access site at angioplasty with transfusion and mortality: the M.O.R.T.A.L study (Mortality benefit Of Reduced Transfusion after percutaneous coronary intervention via the Arm or Leg). *Heart* 2008; **94**: 1019–25
2. Montalescot G, Ongen Z, Guindy R, et al. Predictors of outcome in patients undergoing PCI. Results of the RIVIERA study. *Int J Cardiol* 2008; **129**: 379–87
3. Rao SV, Ou FS, Wang TY, et al. Trends in the prevalence and outcomes of radial and femoral approaches to percutaneous coronary intervention: a report from the National Cardiovascular Data Registry. *JACC Cardiovasc Interv* 2008; **1**: 379–86
4. Jolly SS, Amlani S, Hamon M, Yusuf S, Mehta SR. Radial versus femoral access for coronary angiography or intervention and the impact on major bleeding and ischemic events: a systematic review and meta-analysis of randomized trials. *Am Heart J* 2009; **157**: 132–40
5. Jolly SS, Yusuf S, Cairns J, et al. Radial versus femoral access for coronary angiography and intervention in patients with acute coronary syndromes (RIVAL): a randomised, parallel group, multicentre trial. *Lancet* 2011; **377**: 1409–20
6. Wijns W, Kolh P, Danchin N, et al. Guidelines on myocardial revascularization. *Eur Heart J* 2011; **31**: 2501–55
7. Mohr FW, Morice MC, Kappetein AP, et al. Coronary artery bypass graft surgery versus percutaneous coronary intervention in patients with three-vessel disease and left main coronary disease: 5-year follow-up of the randomised, clinical SYNTAX trial. *Lancet* 2013; **381**: 629–38
8. Sianos G, Morel MA, Kappetein AP, et al. The SYNTAX Score: an angiographic tool grading the complexity of coronary artery disease. *EuroIntervention* 2005; **1**: 219–27
9. Serruys PW, Morice MC, Kappetein AP, et al. Percutaneous coronary intervention versus coronary-artery bypass grafting for severe coronary artery disease. *N Engl J Med* 2009; **360**: 961–72
10. Garg S, Stone GW, Kappetein AP, Sabik JF, 3rd, Simonton C, Serruys PW. Clinical and angiographic risk assessment in patients with left main stem lesions. *JACC Cardiovasc Interv* 2010; **3**: 891–901

11. Wykrzykowska JJ, Garg S, Girasis C, et al. Value of the SYNTAX score for risk assessment in the all-comers population of the randomized multicenter LEADERS (Limus Eluted from A Durable versus ERodable Stent coating) trial. *J Am Coll Cardiol* 2010; **56**: 272–7

12. Mohr FW, Rastan AJ, Serruys PW, et al. Complex coronary anatomy in coronary artery bypass graft surgery: impact of complex coronary anatomy in modern bypass surgery? Lessons learned from the SYNTAX trial after two years. *J Thorac Cardiovasc Surg* 2011; **141**: 130–40

13. Tonino PA, Fearon WF, De Bruyne B, et al. Angiographic versus functional severity of coronary artery stenoses in the FAME study fractional flow reserve versus angiography in multivessel evaluation. *J Am Coll Cardiol* 2010; **55**: 2816–21

14. Loong CY, Anagnostopoulos C. Diagnosis of coronary artery disease by radionuclide myocardial perfusion imaging. *Heart* 2004; **90**(Suppl 5): v2–9

15. Gehi AK, Ali S, Na B, Schiller NB, Whooley MA. Inducible ischemia and the risk of recurrent cardiovascular events in outpatients with stable coronary heart disease: the heart and soul study. *Arch Intern Med* 2008; **168**: 1423–8

16. Lauer MS, Lytle B, Pashkow F, Snader CE, Marwick TH. Prediction of death and myocardial infarction by screening with exercise-thallium testing after coronary-artery-bypass grafting. *Lancet* 1998; **351**: 615–22

17. Paeng JC, Lee DS, Cheon GJ, et al. Consideration of perfusion reserve in viability assessment by myocardial Tl-201 rest-redistribution SPECT: a quantitative study with dual-isotope SPECT. *J Nucl Cardiol* 2002; **9**: 68–74

18. Tillisch J, Brunken R, Marshall R, et al. Reversibility of cardiac wall-motion abnormalities predicted by positron tomography. *N Engl J Med* 1986; **314**: 884–8

19. Haas F, Haehnel CJ, Picker W, et al. Preoperative positron emission tomographic viability assessment and perioperative and postoperative risk in patients with advanced ischemic heart disease. *J Am Coll Cardiol* 1997; **30**: 1693–700

20. Di Carli MF, Asgarzadie F, Schelbert HR, et al. Quantitative relation between myocardial viability and improvement in heart failure symptoms after revascularization in patients with ischemic cardiomyopathy. *Circulation* 1995; **92**: 3436–44

21. Beanlands RS, Nichol G, Huszti E, et al. F-18-fluorodeoxyglucose positron emission tomography imaging-assisted management of patients with severe left ventricular dysfunction and suspected coronary disease: a randomized, controlled trial (PARR-2). *J Am Coll Cardiol* 2007; **50**: 2002–12

22. Ghesani M, Depuey EG, Rozanski A. Role of F-18 FDG positron emission tomography (PET) in the assessment of myocardial viability. *Echocardiography* 2005; **22**: 165–77

23. Greenwood JP, Maredia N, Younger JF, et al. Cardiovascular magnetic resonance and single-photon emission computed tomography for diagnosis of coronary heart disease (CE-MARC): a prospective trial. *Lancet* 2012; **379**: 453–60

24. Allman KC, Shaw LJ, Hachamovitch R, Udelson JE. Myocardial viability testing and impact of revascularization on prognosis in patients with coronary artery disease and left ventricular dysfunction: a meta-analysis. *J Am Coll Cardiol* 2002; **39**: 1151–8

25. Klein C, Nekolla SG, Bengel FM, et al. Assessment of myocardial viability with contrast-enhanced magnetic resonance imaging: comparison with positron emission tomography. *Circulation* 2002; **105**: 162–7

26. Kim RJ, Fieno DS, Parrish TB, et al. Relationship of MRI delayed contrast enhancement to irreversible injury, infarct age, and contractile function. *Circulation* 1999; **100**: 1992–2002

27. Brzezinski M, Luisetti T, London MJ. Radial artery cannulation: a comprehensive review of recent anatomic and physiologic investigations. *Anesth Analg* 2009; **109**: 1763–81

28. Zingone B, Gatti G, Spina A, et al. Current role and outcomes of ascending aortic replacement for severe nonaneurysmal aortic atherosclerosis. *Ann Thorac Surg* 2010; **89**: 429–34

29. Svensson LG, Sun J, Cruz HA, Shahian DM. Endarterectomy for calcified porcelain aorta associated with aortic valve stenosis. *Ann Thorac Surg* 1996; **61**: 149–52

30. Rokkas CK, Kouchoukos NT. Surgical management of the severely atherosclerotic ascending aorta during cardiac operations. *Semin Thorac Cardiovasc Surg* 1998; **10**: 240–6

31. King RC, Kanithanon RC, Shockey KS, Spotnitz WD, Tribble CG, Kron IL. Replacing the atherosclerotic ascending aorta is a high-risk procedure. *Ann Thorac Surg* 1998; **66**: 396–401

32. Kelly TA, Rothbart RM, Cooper CM, Kaiser DL, Smucker ML, Gibson RS. Comparison of outcome of asymptomatic to symptomatic patients older than 20 years of age with valvular aortic stenosis. *Am J Cardiol* 1988; **61**: 123–30

33. Pellikka PA, Nishimura RA, Bailey KR, Tajik AJ. The natural history of adults with asymptomatic, hemodynamically significant aortic stenosis. *J Am Coll Cardiol* 1990; **15**: 1012–7

34. Ross J, Jr., Braunwald E. Aortic stenosis. *Circulation* 1968; **38**: 61–7

35. Bonow RO, Carabello BA, Kanu C, et al. ACC/AHA 2006 guidelines for the management of patients with valvular heart disease: a report of the American College of Cardiology/American Heart Association Task Force on Practice Guidelines (writing committee to revise the 1998 Guidelines for the Management of Patients With Valvular Heart Disease): developed in collaboration with the Society of Cardiovascular Anesthesiologists: endorsed by the Society for Cardiovascular Angiography and Interventions and the Society of Thoracic Surgeons. *Circulation* 2006; **114**: e84–231

36. Carabello BA. Indications for valve surgery in asymptomatic patients with aortic and mitral stenosis. *Chest* 1995; **108**: 1678–82

37. Connolly HM, Oh JK, Orszulak TA, et al. Aortic valve replacement for aortic stenosis with severe left ventricular dysfunction. Prognostic indicators. *Circulation* 1997; **95**: 2395–400

38. Connolly HM, Oh JK, Schaff HV, et al. Severe aortic stenosis with low transvalvular gradient and severe left ventricular dysfunction: result of aortic valve replacement in 52 patients. *Circulation* 2000; **101**: 1940–6

39. Clyne CA, Arrighi JA, Maron BJ, Dilsizian V, Bonow RO, Cannon RO, 3rd. Systemic and left ventricular responses to exercise stress in asymptomatic patients with valvular aortic stenosis. *Am J Cardiol* 1991; **68**: 1469–76

40. Linderholm H, Osterman G, Teien D. Detection of coronary artery disease by means of exercise ECG in patients with aortic stenosis. *Acta Med Scand* 1985; **218**: 181–8

41. Otto CM, Pearlman AS, Kraft CD, Miyake-Hull CY, Burwash IG, Gardner CJ. Physiologic changes with maximal exercise in asymptomatic valvular aortic stenosis assessed by Doppler echocardiography. *J Am Coll Cardiol* 1992; **20**: 1160–7

42. Areskog NH. Exercise testing in the evaluation of patients with valvular aortic stenosis. *Clin Physiol* 1984; **4**: 201–8

43. Atwood JE, Kawanishi S, Myers J, Froelicher VF. Exercise testing in patients with aortic stenosis. *Chest* 1988; **93**: 1083–7

44. Kearney LG, Ord M, Buxton BF, et al. Progression of aortic stenosis in elderly patients over long-term follow up. *Int J Cardiol* 2012

45. Monin JL, Monchi M, Gest V, Duval-Moulin AM, Dubois-Rande JL, Gueret P. Aortic stenosis with severe left ventricular dysfunction and low transvalvular pressure gradients: risk stratification by low-dose dobutamine echocardiography. *J Am Coll Cardiol* 2001; **37**: 2101–7

46. Nishimura RA, Grantham JA, Connolly HM, Schaff HV, Higano ST, Holmes DR, Jr. Low-output, low-gradient aortic stenosis in patients with depressed left ventricular systolic function: the clinical utility of the dobutamine challenge in the catheterization laboratory. *Circulation* 2002; **106**: 809–13

47. Jander N, Minners J, Holme I, et al. Outcome of patients with low-gradient 'severe' aortic stenosis and preserved ejection fraction. *Circulation* 2011; **123**: 887–95

48. Quere JP, Monin JL, Levy F, et al. Influence of preoperative left ventricular contractile reserve on postoperative ejection fraction in low-gradient aortic stenosis. *Circulation* 2006; **113**: 1738–44

49. Monin JL, Quere JP, Monchi M, et al. Low-gradient aortic stenosis: operative risk stratification and predictors for long-term outcome: a multicenter study using dobutamine stress hemodynamics. *Circulation* 2003; **108**: 319–24

50. Weidemann F, Herrmann S, Stork S, et al. Impact of myocardial fibrosis in patients with symptomatic severe aortic stenosis. *Circulation* 2009; **120**: 577–84

51. Dweck MR, Joshi S, Murigu T, et al. Midwall fibrosis is an independent predictor of mortality in patients with aortic stenosis. *J Am Coll Cardiol* 2011; **58**: 1271–9

52. Tribouilloy C, Levy F, Rusinaru D, et al. Outcome after aortic valve replacement for low-flow/low-gradient aortic stenosis without contractile reserve on dobutamine stress echocardiography. *J Am Coll Cardiol* 2009; **53**: 1865–73

53. Hachicha Z, Dumesnil JG, Bogaty P, Pibarot P. Paradoxical low-flow, low-gradient severe aortic stenosis despite preserved ejection fraction is associated with higher afterload and reduced survival. *Circulation* 2007; **115**: 2856–64

54. Paiement B, Pelletier C, Dyrda I, et al. A simple classification of the risk in cardiac surgery. *Can Anaesth Soc J* 1983; **30**: 61–8

55. Parsonnet V, Dean D, Bernstein AD. A method of uniform stratification of risk for evaluating the results of surgery in acquired adult heart disease. *Circulation* 1989; **79**: I3–12

56. Parsonnet V, Bernstein AD, Gera M. Clinical usefulness of risk-stratified outcome analysis in cardiac surgery in New Jersey. *Ann Thorac Surg* 1996; **61**: S8–11; discussion S33–4

57. Higgins TL, Estafanous FG, Loop FD, Beck GJ, Blum JM, Paranandi L. Stratification of morbidity and mortality outcome by preoperative risk factors in coronary artery bypass patients. A clinical severity score. *JAMA* 1992; **267**: 2344–8

58. Myles PS, Williams NJ, Powell J. Predicting outcome in anaesthesia: understanding statistical methods. *Anaesth Intensive Care* 1994; **22**: 447–53

59. Koch CG, Higgins TL, Capdeville M, Maryland P, Leventhal M, Starr NJ. The risk of coronary artery surgery in women: a matched comparison using preoperative severity of illness scoring. *J Cardiothorac Vasc Anesth* 1996; **10**: 839–43

60. Eaker ED, Kronmal R, Kennedy JW, Davis K. Comparison of the long-term, postsurgical survival of women and men in the Coronary Artery Surgery Study (CASS). *Am Heart J* 1989; **117**: 71–81

61. Krumholz HM, Douglas PS, Lauer MS, Pasternak RC. Selection of patients for coronary angiography and coronary revascularization early after myocardial infarction: is there evidence for a gender bias? *Ann Intern Med* 1992; **116**: 785–90

62. O'Connor GT, Plume SK, Olmstead EM, et al. A regional prospective study of in-hospital mortality associated with coronary artery bypass grafting. The Northern New England Cardiovascular Disease Study Group. *JAMA* 1991; **266**: 803–9

63. Orr RK, Maini BS, Sottile FD, Dumas EM, O'Mara P. A comparison of four severity-adjusted models to predict mortality after coronary artery bypass graft surgery. *Arch Surg* 1995; **130**: 301–6

64. Slogoff S, Keats AS. Does perioperative myocardial ischemia lead to postoperative myocardial infarction? *Anesthesiology* 1985; **62**: 107–14

65. Merry AF, Ramage MC, Whitlock RM, et al. First-time coronary artery bypass grafting: the anaesthetist as a risk factor. *Br J Anaesth* 1992; **68**: 6–12

66. Becker RB, Zimmerman JE, Knaus WA, et al. The use of APACHE III to evaluate ICU length of stay, resource use, and mortality after coronary artery by-pass surgery. *J Cardiovasc Surg (Torino)* 1995; **36**: 1–11

67. Turner JS, Mudaliar YM, Chang RW, Morgan CJ. Acute physiology and chronic health evaluation (APACHE II) scoring in a cardiothoracic intensive care unit. *Crit Care Med* 1991; **19**: 1266–9

68. Roques F, Nashef SA, Michel P, et al. Risk factors and outcome in European cardiac surgery: analysis of the EuroSCORE multinational database of 19030 patients. *Eur J Cardiothorac Surg* 1999; **15**: 816–22; discussion 22–3

69. Davis KB, Chaitman B, Ryan T, Bittner V, Kennedy JW. Comparison of 15-year survival for men and women after initial medical or surgical treatment for coronary artery disease: a CASS registry study. Coronary Artery Surgery Study. *J Am Coll Cardiol* 1995; **25**: 1000–9

70. Dewey TM, Brown D, Ryan WH, Herbert MA, Prince SL, Mack MJ. Reliability of risk algorithms in predicting early and late operative outcomes in high-risk patients undergoing aortic valve replacement. *J Thorac Cardiovasc Surg* 2008; **135**: 180–7

71. Brown ML, Schaff HV, Sarano ME, et al. Is the European System for Cardiac Operative Risk Evaluation model valid for estimating the operative risk of patients considered for percutaneous aortic valve replacement? *J Thorac Cardiovasc Surg* 2008; **136**: 566–71

72. Leontyev S, Walther T, Borger MA, et al. Aortic valve replacement in octogenarians: utility of risk stratification with EuroSCORE. *Ann Thorac Surg* 2009; **87**: 1440–5

73. Kalavrouziotis D, Li D, Buth KJ, Legare JF. The European System for Cardiac Operative Risk Evaluation (EuroSCORE) is not appropriate for withholding surgery in high-risk patients with aortic stenosis: a retrospective cohort study. *J Cardiothorac Surg* 2009; **4**: 32

74. Wendt D, Osswald BR, Kayser K, et al. Society of Thoracic Surgeons score is superior to the EuroSCORE determining mortality in high risk patients undergoing isolated aortic valve replacement. *Ann Thorac Surg* 2009; **88**: 468–74; discussion 74–5

75. Dewey TM, Herbert MA. Editorial comment: Predicting operative risk: a worthy task—an elusive goal. *Eur J Cardiothorac Surg* 2009; **36**: 797–8

76. Howell NJ, Head SJ, Freemantle N, et al. The new EuroSCORE II does not improve prediction of mortality in high-risk patients undergoing cardiac surgery: a collaborative analysis of two European centres. Eur J Cardiothoracic Surg 2013;44(6):1006–11

77. Barili F, Pacini D, Capo A, et al. Does EuroSCORE II perform better than its original versions? A multicentre validation study. Eur Heart J 2013;34(1):22–9

78. Coeytaux RR, Williams JW, Jr., Gray RN, Wang A. Percutaneous heart valve replacement for aortic stenosis: state of the evidence. *Ann Intern Med* 2010; 153: 314–24

79. Fry DE, Pine M, Jordan HS, et al. Combining administrative and clinical data to stratify surgical risk. *Ann Surg* 2007; **246**: 875–85

CHAPTER 8

Diagnosis and assessment of lung disease

Giorgio Della Rocca and Cecilia Coccia

Introduction

Improvements in surgical technique and perioperative care have reduced the incidences of complications that are associated with thoracic surgery. However, these improvements have also increased the number of patients who are now deemed operable (1). The incidence of postoperative pulmonary complications after lung resection is related not only to lung tissue removed but also related to alterations in chest wall mechanics caused by the thoracotomy itself (table 8.1) (2–4). All spirometric measurements fall precipitously immediately after surgery and do not return to normal until 6–8 weeks postoperatively (5). Importantly, postoperative pulmonary dysfunction appears to be less common after video-assisted thoracoscopic surgery (VATS) procedures than after formal thoracotomy (6,7). The aim of this chapter is to outline the diagnosis and assessment of lung disease in patients presenting for thoracic surgery.

Clinical evaluation

A complete medical history and a good physical examination may identify important patient risk factors. Age, history of smoking, comorbidities (including cardiovascular disease), nutritional status (8), preoperative induction chemotherapy, oxygen therapy, exercise tolerance and intolerance, chest pain, unexplained dyspnoea or cough, should all be noted (9). Presence of decreased breath sounds, wheezes, crackles, or a prolonged expiratory phase on physical examination may establish the extent of the disease and identify any undiagnosed pulmonary pathology. Particular attention should be paid to symptoms related to postural changes such as coughing and dyspnoea that occur in the supine position, because they may indicate intrathoracic compression and shift of the mediastinum and/or airways.

Assessment of lung function

Parameters that are recommended for preoperative evaluation of patients are listed in table 8.2.

Spirometry

Spirometry helps to identify the degree of respiratory disease and allows optimization of medical treatment prior to surgery. It is a reliable method of differentiating between obstructive airways disorders such as chronic obstructive pulmonary disease and asthma and restrictive lung diseases where the size of the lungs is reduced, such as fibrotic lung disease (Chapter 4). Spirometry is the most effective way of determining the severity of chronic obstructive pulmonary disease (COPD). Some parameters have been shown

Table 8.1 Respiratory complications following thoracotomy

1. Loss of integrity of the respiratory muscles (incision), rib resection
2. Chest wall mechanic dysfunction
3. Reduction of functional residual capacity
4. Pain of high intensity
5. Ineffective cough and so sputum retention
6. Reductions in tidal volume and vital capacity
7. Atelectasis
8. Tachypnoea, dyspnoea
9. Gas exchange impairment
10. Pulmonary infections
11. Respiratory failure

Table 8.2 Preoperative assessment of respiratory function for thoracic surgery

All patients
FEV_1
DLCO
Arterial blood gas analysis
Patients with borderline function
Quantitative ventilation/perfusion scan
Quantitative CT scan
Dynamic contrast-enhanced perfusion MRI
Patients with PPO FEV1 and PPO DLCO < 40% predicted
Exercise testing: systemic oxygen consumption ($\dot{V}O_2max$)

FEV_1, forced expiratory volume in 1 second; DLCO, diffusing lung capacity for carbon monoxide or gas transfer factor; CT, computerized tomography; MRI, magnetic resonance imaging; PPO, predicted postoperative.

to have prognostic value in assessing postoperative lung function. Spirometry should be assessed when the patient is clinically stable and receiving the maximal bronchodilator therapy. However, the success of spirometry depends on the full cooperation of the patient.

Forced expiratory volume

Forced expiratory volume in 1 second (FEV_1) provides an indirect measure of pulmonary reserve. Most studies recommend FEV_1 thresholds for safe resections as more than 2 L for pneumonectomy and more than 1.5 L for lobectomy (10,11). However, the use of absolute values have never been generally accepted, because they do not take into consideration gender, height, weight, and age. Importantly, such thresholds do not take into account the functional contribution of the tissue to be excised. Commonly, predicted postoperative (PPO) values of FEV_1, as percentages of normal, are more often used and a PPO FEV_1 of > 80% has been accepted as indicating that the patient is fit to undergo pneumonectomy without any further evaluation (12–14).

Diffusing capacity of the lung for carbon monoxide

Diffusing capacity of the lungs for carbon monoxide or gas transfer factor (DLCO) is a measurement of alveolar oxygen exchange (Chapter 4) (3). DLCO is a surrogate measurement of the oxygen uptake capacity of the lungs and reflects the integrity of the alveolar membrane and pulmonary capillary blood flow. Abnormal DLCO values may represent a defect in gas exchange that may be at the level of the alveolar epithelium, the pulmonary vasculature, or the interstitium (9). Preoperative DLCO is an independent predictor of morbidity and mortality after pulmonary resection (3,5,13,15). When the DLCO is less than 80%, postoperative pulmonary complications are more frequent and when it is less than 60%, mortality is increased (8). A low preoperative DLCO has been associated with an increased incidence of readmission to the hospital and a poorer long-term quality of life (16,17). Some patients may have good spirometric values but a very low DLCO because of diffuse interstitial lung disease and they require more considered assessment before proceeding to surgery. For these reasons, measurement of DLCO is now recommended for all patients being evaluated for lung resection (13,14,18).

Arterial blood gases

Measurement of arterial blood gases (ABGs) is the only objective test that does not depend on patient cooperation. In addition, measurement of ABGs is also the only easily repeatable test of respiratory function that can be used throughout perioperative period. ABGs provide information about the ability of the lung to exchange oxygen and carbon dioxide between the pulmonary vascular bed and the alveoli. Hypoxaemia is caused by parenchymal damage and is a predictor of the requirement for mechanical ventilation after surgery.

Hypercapnia is an estimate of the severity of COPD and is a marker of poor ventilatory function. An arterial oxygen tension (PaO_2) of less than 60 mmHg (8 kPa) or an arterial carbon dioxide tension ($PaCO_2$) of greater than 45 mmHg (6 kPa) have been used as cut-off thresholds for pulmonary resection (1). Although cancer resections have now been successfully undertaken or even combined with volume reduction in patients who do not meet these criteria, they remain useful as warning indicators of increased risk (8,13). An arterial oxyhaemoglobin saturation with oxygen (SaO_2)

of less than 90% and $PaCO_2$ greater than 45 mmHg are associated with poor ventilatory function, but have not been shown to be independent risk factors for postoperative death or increased rates of complications (19–22). Patients who have a SaO_2 less than 90% or $PaCO_2$ greater than 45 mmHg (6 kPa) should have additional evaluation prior to proceeding to lung resection (8).

Assessment of regional lung function

As an estimate of the amount of functioning tissue that will be lost with resection of the lung, the concept of PPO values was recently introduced. The percentage of PPO (%PPO) for FEV_1 and DLCO are now routinely used for establishing risk assessment thresholds instead of absolute values.

Anatomic calculations

Anatomic calculations are a simple method of assessing regional lung function that are reliable predictors of postoperative lung function (23). Anatomic calculations are based on the number of segments of the lungs to be resected that is the PPO value is a fraction of remaining segments or subsegments from the total of 19 (table 8.3). The simplest formula to calculate PPO FEV_1 is:

$$PPO\ FEV_1 = preoperative\ FEV_1 \times \left[1 - \frac{\text{unobstructed elements to be removed}}{19} \right]$$

The PPO FEV_1 can be converted into %PPO FEV_1 using standard equations. In addition, the PPO and %PPO DLCO can be determined using the same formula. Anatomic calculations usually overestimate the extent of functional loss, because destroyed or collapsed lung parenchyma might be resected with little loss of function (23). The %PPO FEV_1 calculated after lobectomy is strongly correlated with the actual postoperative FEV_1 (24,25). The anatomic method can also be applied to segmentectomies (26).

Table 8.3 Lung lobar segments

Right lung	Left lung
A) Upper right lobe	**A) Upper left lobe**
1) Apical	1–2) Apicoposterior
2) Posterior	3) Anterior
3) Anterior	4) Sperior lingula
B) Middle right lobe	5) Inferior lingula
4) Lateral	**B) Lower right lobe**
5) Medial	6) Apical
B) Lower right lobe	7) Anterobasal
6) Apical	8) Laterobasal
7) Anterobasal	9) Posterobasal
8) Mediobasal	
9) Laterobasal	
10) Posterobasal	

Quantitative computerized tomography scanning

Quantitative computerized tomography (CT) scanning is a simple, commonly available method of assessing regional lung function. The total functional lung volume (TFLV) is identified by semiautomated analyses. The part of the lung to be resected is calculated as the regional functional lung volume (RFLV) (2). This method has been reported to be simpler and more accurate in the prediction of postoperative FEV_1 in patients undergoing pulmonary resection (27,28).

Radionucleotide ventilation/perfusion scanning

The usefulness of radionucleotide perfusion scanning was established in the 1970s by a study showing that functional loss 3 months after pneumonectomy could be accurately predicted by perfusion scanning using intravenous technetium-99 macroaggregates (29). Patients are scanned in four projections and images obtained by a γ-camera using single-photon emission computed tomography (SPECT). The technetium particles are trapped in the capillary bed of the lungs and emit γ-rays proportional to regional pulmonary perfusion. Quantification of regional perfusion is performed by a system-integrated program. The perfusion scintigraphy is the most used method to predict postoperative lung function in lung cancer patients undergoing pneumonectomy. The estimation of the %PPO FEV_1 in patients who undergo pneumonectomy can be calculated by obtaining preoperative FEV_1 and the quantitative ventilation perfusion scan to obtain the fraction of the total lung perfusion present in the lung to be resected, using the following formula (13).

$$PPO\ FEV_1 = FEV_1 - pre \times (1 - \text{fraction of total perfusion resected lung})$$

The PPO FEV_1 can then be converted into the %PPO FEV_1 using standard equations. The PPO and %PPO DLCO following pneumonectomy can be determined using the same formula. For pneumonectomy there is a strong correlation between the postoperative FEV_1 expressed as percentage predicted and calculated from the quantitative lung perfusion scans, and the actual values (30,31). Traditionally, a PPO FEV_1 of 0.8 L based on perfusion scintigraphy, was the minimal accepted FEV_1 for patients undergoing resection (32). However, 0.8 L as a single value cannot be used to discriminate between patients of different age, size, sex, and levels of cardiovascular fitness. Scintigraphy is not widely employed in assessing patients for lobectomy, because of the difficulty in interpreting the contribution of individual lobes to overall ventilation or perfusion. Either ventilation or perfusion scintigraphy can be used to predict postoperative lung function but there is no additional benefit in performing both (24,25,30,33). Importantly, scintigraphy results may underestimate actual postoperative values (33,34).

Dynamic contrast-enhanced perfusion magnetic resonance imaging

The most recently established method is contrast-enhanced perfusion magnetic resonance imaging (MRI) to calculate the regional pulmonary blood volume. This technique requires some expertise as well as appropriate software, but has been shown to reliably predict postoperative values (27,35). Regional pulmonary blood volume is calculated from the signal intensity-time course curve. Perfusion MRI is superior to SPECT, in predicting postoperative FEV (35).

Approach to assessment of regional lung function

Tumors that obstruct the airway may create a ventilation/perfusion (V/Q) mismatch. If a portion of a segment or lobe is partially or completely atelectatic, surgical resection may not have the predicted negative impact on postoperative function (8). A right-sided pneumonectomy in a patient with 60% perfusion to the lung may be more prone to postoperative complications than in a patient with only 15% perfusion. In this setting a quantitative V/Q study should always requested to calculate the impact on the postoperative predicted performance (8).

Alterations to the standard calculations should also be considered in the management of patients with severe emphysema. Patients with predominantly upper lobe emphysema and a lesion within the same lobe may tolerate surgery better than predicted because of lung volume reduction (8,13).

Although less accurate than other techniques, calculating PPO-lung function based on anatomic values is the simplest way of predicting postoperative function. More sophisticated methods should be reserved for borderline patients (2,23). Only the number of segments that are patent on imaging or bronchoscopy, to be resected should be subtracted from the total number of functional segments. In patients who require additional evaluation then availability, cost, and local expertise usually determine the choice of method (2).

Assessment of cardiopulmonary reserve

Cardiopulmonary exercise testing

Cardiopulmonary exercise testing (CPET) assesses cardiopulmonary reserve. CPET measures the electrocardiograph, heart rate, minute ventilation, and systemic oxygen uptake in response to exercise (8,12). Testing should be performed in a controlled environment. Measured values are dependent on pulmonary function, cardiovascular function, and oxygen use by peripheral tissues, thus assessing the overall fitness of a patient (2). However, CPET requires expertise that is not universally available. The most widely used exercise tests are maximal or symptom-limited incremental exercise tests on a treadmill or bicycle. CPET allows for formal evaluation of the cardiopulmonary reserve that may be needed to survive the stress of surgery; it is particularly useful in high-risk patients (8,36).

The most important measurement in CPET is the level of work achieved, measured as maximum systemic oxygen uptake ($\dot{V}O_2$max). $\dot{V}O_2$max may measured directly or indirectly or may be calculated. $\dot{V}O_2$ in the lungs is representative of $\dot{V}O_2$ at the cellular level. With an increase in the cellular respiration from exercise, there is a predictable increase in $\dot{V}O_2$, which is related to age, sex, weight, and type of work performed. $\dot{V}O_2$ increases with exercise until it plateaus and a further increase in work does not result in any further rise and this is the $\dot{V}O_2$max (37). Increasingly, CPET is being used because it provides the best index of functional capacity and $\dot{V}O_2$max, as well as estimating both cardiac and pulmonary reserves that are not available from other modalities (9).

Systematic review and meta-analysis has found that lower levels of $\dot{V}O_2$max are associated with increased incidences of complications after lung resection (38). Until recently, a $\dot{V}O_2$max of greater than 20 mL/kg/min, or greater than 75% of predicted, was considered sufficient to undergo pneumonectomy, whereas a $\dot{V}O_2$max of less than 10 mL/kg/min or less than 40% of predicted would preclude any resection (39). Most recently, the $\dot{V}O_2$max value precluding any resection was lowered to 35% of predicted (13). A cutoff of 15 mL/kg/min is considered to be sufficient for lobectomy (2,14,21,40,41). The inability to measure $\dot{V}O_2$max in patients who are unable to reach peak exertion because of limiting comorbidities is an important limitation. However, calculation of an oxygen uptake efficiency slope has been suggested to allow for better prediction of surgical outcomes in patients with limited exercise capacity (8,36).

Low-technology tests

Lack of access to CEPT equipment and expertise often necessitates the use of simpler forms of testing.

Walking test

In the walking test, patients are asked to walk as far as they can, and good performance has been reported to predict survival in those with COPD and pulmonary hypertension (42,43). However, its value in predicting outcome after pulmonary resection are equivocal (44–46), and the interpretation of the results are not standardized (8).

Shuttle walking test

The shuttle walking test requires that patients walk back and forth between two markers set 10 m apart. Walking speed is set by an audio signal that is increased every minute. The test is completed when the patient is too short of breath to maintain the required speed. Unlike the walking test, the shuttle walking test is more reproducible. In addition, it better correlates with $\dot{V}O_2$max and walking more than 400 m is associated to a $\dot{V}O_2$ of more than 15 mL/kg/min (14,47–49). Some studies indicate that it is poorly correlated with pulmonary complication at lower range but the shuttle walking test is useful to stratify low-risk groups (49,50).

Stair climbing tests

Stair climbing has been established as a reliable screening test of pulmonary function and a predictor of cardiopulmonary morbidity after lung resection (51,52). Under the supervision of a health care professional, patients are asked to walk up at their own pace, as many flights of stairs as possible and only to stop for reasons of exhaustion, limiting dyspnoea, leg fatigue, or chest pain. During the test, heart rate, pulse oximetry, time, and height climbed are measured, and then ergometric variables are calculated. The advantages of stair climbing are ready availability, low cost, and the familiarity of patients with this kind of exercise. Being able to climb less than 12 m has been associated with 2–13-fold higher rates of complication and mortality compared to a patient that is able to climb more than 22 m (13,52). The height reached correlates with $\dot{V}O_2$max and patients who can climb 22 m or more can proceed directly to surgery because they generated high values of $\dot{V}O_2$max (53). In contrast, patients who are unable to perform stair climbing because of comorbidities, have an increased mortality (52).

Exercise induced pulse oximetry desaturation

The role of exercise induced pulse oximetry desaturation in the stratification has yet to be defined but it is a good marker of postoperative complications (54,55). Desaturation of more than 4% during exercise has been associated with a worse outcome (56).

Assessment for lung resection

Algorithm for the assessment of the lung function

Preoperative pulmonary function tests are useful to identify patients who are at risk of developing postoperative complications but they cannot predicted by them alone. Evidence-based guidelines have been published by many of the thoracic societies (12–14). A stepwise approach to preoperative pulmonary evaluation is described in figure 8.1 (2).

Whilst FEV$_1$ and DLCO predict morbidity of patients undergoing thoracotomy, they do not in those undergoing VATS (8,57). In patients with severe emphysema, a PPO FEV$_1$ of 40% underestimates the actual postoperative function because it does not account the effect reducing lung volume (1,13). In patients undergoing chemotherapy, the diffusing capacity of the lungs is usually decreased and a 21% or more decrease in DLCO and PPO DLCO% have been found to be associated with pulmonary complications (58).

Risks related to surgery

Surgical centre and surgeon experience can play a role in mortality and morbidity (59). The effects of pulmonary resection on respiratory function depends on the function and volume of the excised lung parenchyma. Removal of nonfunctional lung tissue such as a bullae, may improve or at least, result in no deterioration in lung function. In addition, excising a tumour may allow the remaining lung to re-expand. However, in most patients, thoracic surgery results in some functional impairment (60).

Lobectomy results in less impairment than pneumonectomy. After lobectomy, the remaining lobes rapidly expand to fill the vacant space. However, this adaptation may take up to three months. The degree of functional impairment depends on the number of segments that are excised. For example, lobectomy of the middle lobe which is constituted of two segments, has less functional impact than lobectomy of the right inferior lobe which has five segments. If the parenchyma of the remaining lung is normal, ABGs remain in the normal range both at rest and during exertion. Respiratory function has been found to be proportional to the amount of functioning lung parenchyma that is preserved (62). Increasingly, less extensive resections such as sleeve-lobectomies or segmentectomies, are used for patients with limited pulmonary reserve.

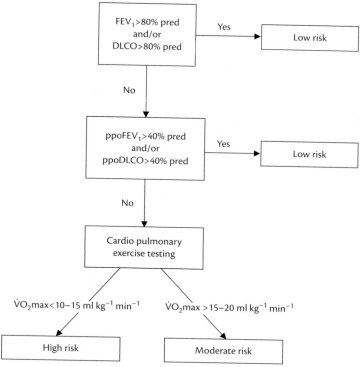

Fig. 8.1 Algorithm for preoperative pulmonary evaluation.
Where: FEV_1, forced expiratory volume in 1 second; DLCO, Diffusing lung capacity for carbon monoxide or gas transfer factor; PPO, predicted postoperative; pred, predicted; $\dot{V}O_2max$, maximum systemic oxygen uptake.

Pulmonary function is also less impaired after VATS than after thoracotomy (7). VATS lobectomy leads to only a 15% loss in vital capacity and FEV_1, whereas, thoracotomy leads to losses of 23% and 29%, respectively (62). Postoperative levels of PaO_2, $SaO2$, peak flow rates, FEV_1, and forced vital capacity, are all better in patients who undergo VATS compared to thoracotomy (6).

Patient-related risk

Although much of the assessment of patient is to estimate perioperative risk, it is also important to consider the long-term implications of lung resection on pulmonary function and exercise tolerance (8). Postoperatively, FEV_1 is lower than PPO FEV_1 then worsens for the first three months before improving by the sixth month (64). Patients, especially those with little reserve, should be evaluated considering this expected fluctuation in pulmonary physiology. When assessing potential long-term disability, it is crucial to assess comorbidity to provide patients with realistic expectations. Age greater than 70 years, obesity, heart disease, and renal impairment will all reduce the likelihood of a favorable outcome.

Chronic obstructive pulmonary disease

Patients with COPD should be optimised before surgery with pharmacological treatment for about 5 to 10 days to reduce pulmonary hyperinflation, airway obstruction and to minimise postoperative complications (65,66). Additionally, these patients should undergo a preoperative program of chest physiotherapy to educate them to cough properly and inhale deeply to reduce the incidence of pulmonary complications (67). Smoking cessation for 8 weeks prior to surgery is also recommended, even

for patients not afflicted with COPD, to decrease in sputum production, improve ciliary action, macrophage activity, and small airway function. Even 12 to 24 hours prior to surgery, smoking cessation is useful because carboxyhemoglobin has a half-life of 6 hours (68–70).

Asthma

Patients with asthma should continue their therapy to ensure that they are asymptomatic and have a peak expiratory flow of more than 80% of predicted or that is their personal best value. Bronchial hyperactivity may cause bronchospasm during tracheal intubation. Inhaled β_2 agonists and systemic corticosteroids will reduce the risk of bronchospasm if given for 5 days prior to surgery (71).

Obstructive sleep apnoea

Patients with obstructive sleep apnoea should be evaluated on the basis of the presence of the following symptoms and signs: persistent snoring every night for at least 6 months, respiratory pauses during sleep as recounted by a partner, waking up with the sensation of suffocation, daytime sleepiness, arterial hypertension, and dysmorphic craniofacial and oro-pharyngeal anomalies.

Comorbidities

Each comorbidity increase the perioperative morbidity and the mortality in a manner that is hard to predict. The presence of more preoperative pathologies makes more difficult quantify how symptomatic the patients will be after pulmonary resections (72). Figure 8.2 describes a rational approach of how the different preoperative diseases can be evaluated to quantify the operative risk.

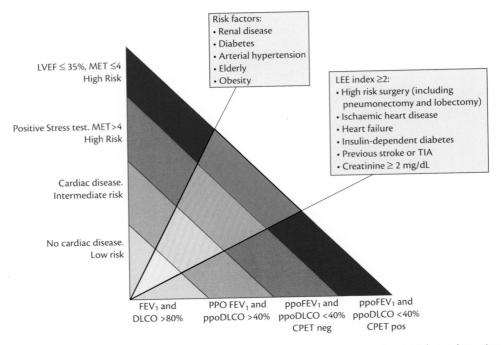

Fig. 8.2 Risk of lung resections based on preoperative cardiopulmonary evaluation, type of surgery, and on other clinical risk factors (grey triangle). VEF, left ventricular ejection fraction; MET, metabolic equivalent of task; FEV$_1$, forced expiratory volume in one second; PPO, predicted postoperative value; CPET, cardiopulmonary exercise test; TIA, transient ischaemic attack.

Conclusion

No single test should exclude a patient from thoracic surgery (8). Once reports are available on comorbidity disease, cardiovascular risk, pulmonary function, and exercise tolerance, they should be considered by a multidisciplinary team who will provide counseling regarding the risks, benefits, and alternatives to surgical treatments for lung cancer (8). Each patient should be informed of and accept the risks of surgery as well as the impact that it will have their lifestyle (14). Anesthesiologists are not gate-keepers and generally, they will meet the patients at the very end of their assessment for thoracic surgery when they should participate in the discussion of the risks and benefits of surgery (1). In the preoperative assessment, the anesthesiologists should identify the risks, optimize functional reserves and manage perioperative procedures to improve the outcome from thoracic surgery (1).

References

1. Slinger PD, Johnston MR. Preoperative assessment: an anesthesiologist's perspective. *Thorac Surg Clin* 2005; **15**(1): 11–25
2. von Groote-Bidlingmaier F, Koegelenberg CFN, Bolliger CT. Functional evaluation after lung resection. *Clin Chest Med* 2011; **32**: 773–82
3. Ferguson MK, Lehman AG, Bolliger CT, Brunelli A. The role of diffusing capacity and exercise tests. *Thorac Surg Clin* 2008; **18**(1): 9–17.
4. Busch E, Verazin G, Antkowiak JG, Driscoll D, Takita H. Pulmonary complications in patients undergoing thoracotomy for lung carcinoma. *Chest* 1994; **105**(3): 760–6
5. Bastin R, Moraine JJ, Bardocsky G, Kahn RJ, Mélot C. Incentive spirometry performance. A reliable indicator of pulmonary function in the early postoperative period after lobectomy? *Chest* 1997; **111**: 559–63
6. Nakata M, Saeki H, Yokoyama N, Kurita A, Takiyama W, Takashima S. Pulmonary function after lobectomy: video-assisted thoracic surgery versus thoracotomy. *Ann Thorac Surg* 2000; **70**: 938–41
7. Nomori H, Ohtsuka T, Horio H, Naruke T, Suemasu K. Difference in the impairment of vital capacity and 6-minute walking after a lobectomy performed by thoracoscopic surgery, and anterior limited thoracotomy, an anteroaxillary thoracotomy, and a posterolateral thoracotomy. *Surg Today* 2003; **33**: 7–12
8. David EA, Marshall MB. Physiologic evaluation of lung resection candidates. *Thorac Surg Clin* 2012; **22**: 47–54
9. Banki F. Pulmonary assessment for general thoracic surgery. *Surg Clin N Am* 2010; **90**: 969–84
10. Peters RM, Clausen JL, Tisi GM. Extending resectability for carcinoma of the lung in patients with impaired pulmonary function. *Ann Thorac Surg* 1978; **26**(3): 250–60
11. Boushy SF, Billig DM, North LB, Helgason AH. Clinical course related to preoperative and postoperative pulmonary function in patients with bronchogenic carcinoma. *Chest* 1971; **59**(4): 383–91
12. Colice GL, Shafazand S, Griffin JP, Keenan R, Bolliger CT. Physiologic evaluation of the patient with lung cancer being considered for resectional surgery. ACCP Evidenced-based clinical practice guidelines (2nd Edition). **Chest** 2007; **132**: 161S–177S
13. Brunelli A, Charloux A, Bolliger CT, et al. The European Respiratory Society and European Society of Thoracic Surgeons clinical guidelines for evaluating fitness for radical treatment (surgery and chemoradiotherapy) in patients with lung cancer. *Eur J Cardiothor Surg* 2009; **36**: 181–4
14. Lim E, Baldwin D, Beckles M, et al. Guidelines on the radical management of patients with lung cancer. *Thorax* 2010; **65**(Suppl 3): iii1–27
15. Santini M, Fiorello A, Vicidominici G, Di Crescenzo VG, Laperuta P. The role of diffusion capacity in predicting complication after lung resection for cancer. *Thorac Cardiovasc Surg* 2007; 55: 391–4
16. Ferguson MK, Little L, Rizzo L, et al. Diffusing capacity predicts morbidity and mortality after pulmonary resection. *J Thorac Cardiovasc Surg* 1988; **96**(6): 894–900

17. Bousamara N, Presberg KW, Chammas JH. Early and late morbidity in patients undergoing pulmonary resection with low diffusion capacity. *Ann Thorac Surg* 1996; **62**: 968–74

18. Ferguson MK, Vigneswaran WT. Diffusing capacity predicts morbidity after lung resection in patients without obstructive lung disease. *Ann Thorac Surg* 2008; **85**(4): 1158–64

19. Chetta A, Tzani P, Marangio E, Carbognani P, Bobbio A, Olivieri D. Respiratory effects of surgery and pulmonary function testing in the preoperative evaluation. *Acta Biomed* 2006; **7**(2): 69–74

20. Turner SE, Eastwood PR, Cecins NM, Hillman DR, Jenkins SC. Physiologic responses to incremental and self-paced exercise in COPD: a comparison of three tests. *Chest* 2004; **126**(3): 766–73

21. Morice RC, Peters EJ, Ryan MB, Putnam JB, Ali MK, Roth JA. Exercise testing in the evaluation of patients at high risk for complications from lung resection. *Chest* 1992;**101**(2): 356–61

22. Harpole DH, Liptay MJ, DeCamp MM Jr, Mentzer SJ, Swanson SJ, Sugarbaker DJ. Prospective analysis of pneumonectomy: risk factors for major morbidity and cardiac dysrhythmias. *Ann Thorac Surg* 1996; **61**(3): 977–82

23. Koegelenberg CF, Bolliger CT. Assessing regional lung function. *Thorac Surg Clin* 2008; **18**(1): 19–29

24. Bolliger CT, Guckel C, Engel H, et al. Prediction of functional reserves after lung resection: comparison between quantitative computed tomography, scintigraphy, and anatomy. *Respiration* 2002; **69**(6): 482–9

25. Zeiher BG, Gross TJ, Kern JA, Lanza LA, Peterson MW. Predicting postoperative pulmonary function in patients undergoing lung resection. *Chest* 1995; **108**(1): 68–72

26. Takizawa T, Haga M, Yagi N, et al. Pulmonary function after segmentectomy for small peripheral carcinoma of the lung. *J Thorac Cardiovasc Surg* 1999; **118**: 536–41

27. Ohno Y, Koyama H, Nogami M, et al. Postoperative lung function in lung cancer patients: comparative analysis of predictive capability of MRI, CT, and SPECT. *AJR Am J Roentgenol* 2007; **189**(2): 400–8.

28. Wu MT, Pan HB, Chiang AA, et al. Prediction of post-operative lung function in patients with lung cancer: comparison of quantitative CT with perfusion scintigraphy. *AJR Am J Roentgenol* 2002; **178**(3): 667–72

29. Olsen GN, Block AJ, Tobias JA. Prediction of postpneumonectomy pulmonary function using quantitative macroaggregate lung scanning. *Chest* 1974; **66**(1): 13–6

30. Corris PA, Ellis DA, Hawkins T, Gibson GJ. Use of radionuclide scanning in the preoperative estimation of pulmonary function after pneumonectomy. *Thorax* 1987; **42**:285–91

31. Boysen PG, Harris JO, Block AJ, Olsen GN. Prospective evaluation for pneumonectomy using perfusion scanning: follow-up beyond one year. *Chest* 1981; **80**: 163–6

32. Olsen GN, Block AJ, Swenson EW, Castle JR, Wynne JW. Pulmonary function evaluation of the lung resection candidate: a prospective study. *Am Rev Respir Dis* 1975; **111**: 379–87

33. Win T, Tasker AD, Groves AM, et al. Ventilation-perfusion scintigraphy to predict postoperative pulmonary function in lung cancer patients undergoing pneumonectomy. *AJR Am J Roentgenol* 2006; **187**(5): 1260–5

34. Williams AJ, Cayton RM, Harding LK, Mostafa AB, Matthews HR. Quantitative lung scintigrams and lung function in the selection of patients for pneumonectomy. *Br J Dis Chest* 1984; **78**: 105–12

35. Ohno Y, Hatabu H, Higashino T, et al. Dynamic perfusion MRI versus perfusion scintigraphy: prediction of postoperative lung function in patients with lung cancer. *AJR Am J Roentgenol* 2004; **182**(1): 73–8

36. Kasikcioglu E, Toker A, Tanju S, et al. Oxygen uptake kinetics during cardiopulmonary exercise testing and postoperative complications in patients with lung cancer. *Lung Cancer* 2009; **66**(1): 85–8

37. Datta D, Lahiri B. Preoperative evaluation of patients undergoing lung resection surgery. *Chest* 2003; **123**, 2096–103

38. Benzo R, Kelley GA, Recchi L, Hofman A, Sciurba F. Complications of lung resection and exercise capacity: a meta-analysis. *Respir Med* 2007; **101**: 1790–7

39. Bolliger CT, Jordan P, Soler M, et al. Exercise capacity as a predictor of postoperative complications in lung resection candidates. *Am J Respir Crit Care Med* 1995; **151**(5): 1472–80

40. Smith TP, Kinasewitz GT, Tucker WY, Spillers WP, George RB. Exercise capacity as a predictor of post-thoracotomy morbidity. *Am Rev Respir Dis* 1984; **129**(5): 730–4

41. Wang JS, Abboud RT, Evans KG, Finley RJ, Graham BL. Role of CO diffusing capacity during exercise in the preoperative evaluation for lung resection. *Am J Respir Crit Care Med* 2000; **162**(4 Pt 1): 1435–44

42. Cote CG, Pinto-Plata V, Kasprzyk K, Dordelly LJ, Celli BR. The 6-min walk distance, peak oxygen uptake, and mortality in COPD. *Chest* 2007; **132**: 1778–85

43. Oudiz RJ, Barst RJ, Hansen JE, et al. Cardiopulmonary exercise testing and six-minute walk correlations in pulmonary arterial hypertension. *Am J Cardiol* 2006; **97**: 123–6

44. Holden DA, Rice TW, Stelmach K, Meeker DP. Exercise testing, 6-min walk, and stair climb in the evaluation of patients at high risk for pulmonary resection. *Chest* 1992; **102**: 1774–9

45. Markos J, Mullan BP, Hillman DR, et al. Preoperative assessment as a predictor of mortality and morbidity after lung resection. *Am Rev Respir Dis* 1989; **139**; 902–10

46. Pierce RJ, Copland JM, Sharpe K, Barter CE. Preoperative risk evaluation for lung cancer resection: predicted postoperative product as a predictor of surgical mortality. *Am J Respir Crit Care Med* 1994; **150**(4): 947–55

47. Singh SJ, Morgan MD, Hardman AE, Rowe C, Bardsley PA. Comparison of oxygen uptake during a conventional treadmill test and the shuttle walking test in chronic airflow limitation. *Eur Respir J* 1994; 7(11): 2016–20

48. Swinburn CR, Wakefield JM, Jones PW. Performance, ventilation, and oxygen consumption in three different types of exercise test in patients with chronic obstructive lung disease. *Thorax* 1985; **40**(8): 581–6

49. Swinburn CR, Wakefield JM, Jones PW. Performance, ventilation, and oxygen consumption in three different types of exercise test in patients with chronic obstructive lung disease. *Thorax* 1985; **40**(8): 581–6

50. Win T, Jackson A, Groves AM et al. Relationship of shuttle walk test and lung cancer surgical outcome. *Eur J Cardiothorac Surg* 2004; **26**(6): 1216–9

51. Bolton JW, Weiman DS, Haynes JL, Hornung CA, Olsen GN, Almond CH. Stair climbing as an indicator of pulmonary function. *Chest* 1987; **92**(5): 783–8

52. Brunelli A, Al Refai M, Monteverde M, Borri A, Salati M, Fianchini A. Stair climbing test predicts cardiopulmonary complications after lung resection. *Chest* 2002; **121**(4): 1106–10

52. Brunelli A, Refai M, Xiumé F, et al. Performance at symptom-limited stair-climbing test is associated with increased cardiopulmonary complications, mortality, and costs after major lung resection. *Ann Thorac Surg*, 2008; **86**(1): 240–7

53. Brunelli A, Xiume F, Refai M, et al. Peak oxygen consumption measured during the stair-climbing test in lung resection candidates. *Respiration* 2010; **80**(3): 207–11

54. Ninan M, Sommers KE, Landreneau RJ, et al. Standardized exercise oximetry predicts postpneumonectomy outcome. *Ann Thorac Surg* 1997; **64**(2): 328–32

55. Rao V, Todd TR, Kuus A, Buth KJ, Pearson FG. Exercise oximetry versus spirometry in the assessment of risk prior to lung resection. *Ann Thorac Surg* 1995; **60**(3): 603–8

56. Brunelli A, Refai M, Xiumé F, Salati M, et al. Oxygen desaturation during maximal stair-climbing test and postoperative complications after major lung resections. *Eur J Cardiothorac Surg* 2008; **33**(1): 77–82

57. Berry MF, Villamizar-Ortiz NR, Tong BC, et al. Pulmonary function tests do not predict pulmonary complications after thoracoscopic lobectomy. *Ann Thorac Surg* 2010; **89**(4): 1044–51

58. Takeda S, Funakoshi Y, Kadota Y, et al. Fall in diffusing capacity associated with induction therapy for lung cancer: a predictor of postoperative complication? *Ann Thorac Surg* 2006; **82**(1): 232–6

59. Schipper PH, Diggs BS, Ungerleider RM, Welke KF. The influence of surgeon specialty on outcomes in general thoracic surgery: a national sample 1996 to 2005. *Ann Thorac Surg* 2009; **88**(5): 1566–72

60. Tzani P, Chetta A, Olivieri D. Patient assessment and prevention of pulmonary side-effects in surgery. *Curr Opin Anesth* 2011; **24**: 2–7

61. Olsen GN. Pre and postoperative evaluation and management of the thoracic surgical patient. In: Fishman AP, ed. *Pulmonary Diseases and Disorders*, 2nd ed. New York: Mc-Graw-Hill, 1988; 2413–32

62. Brusasco V, Ratto GB, Crimi P, Sacco A, Motta G. Lung function after upper sleeve lobectomy for bronchogenic carcinoma. *Scand J Thor Cardiovasc Surg* 1988; **22**: 73–78

63. Kaseda S, Aoki T, Hangai N, Shimizu K. Better pulmonary function and prognosis with video-assisted thoracic surgery than with thoracotomy. *Ann Thorac Surg* 2000; **70**: 1644–6

64. Nezu K, Kushibe K, Tojo T, Takahama M, Kitamura S. Recovery and limitation of exercise capacity after lung resection for lung cancer. *Chest* 1998; **113**(6): 1511–6

65. Alberg AJ, Ford JG, Samet JM. Epidemiology of lung cancer: ACCP evidence-based clinical practice guidelines (2nd edition). *Chest* 2007; **132**(Suppl 3): 29S–55S

66. Papi A, Casoni G, Caramori G, et al. COPD increases the risk of squamous histological subtype in smokers who develop non-small cell lung carcinoma. *Thorax* 2004; **59**: 679–81

67. Van Tilburg PM, Stam H, Hoogsteden HC, van Klaveren RJ. Pre-operative pulmonary evaluation of lung cancer patients: a review of the literature. *Eur Respir J* 2009; **33**(5): 1206–15

68. Nakagawa M, Tanaka H, Tsukuma H, et al. Relationship between the duration of the preoperative smoke-free period and the incidence of postoperative pulmonary complications after pulmonary surgery. *Chest* 2001; **120**(3): 705–10

69. Barrera R, Shi W, Amar D, et al. Smoking and timing of cessation: impact on pulmonary complications after thoracotomy. *Chest* 2005; **127**(6): 1977–83

70. Mason DP, Subramanian S, Nowicki ER, et al. Impact of smoking cessation before resection of lung cancer: a Society of Thoracic Surgeons General Thoracic Surgery Database study. *Ann Thorac Surg* 2009; **88**(2): 362–70

71. Bapoje SR, Whitaker JF, Schulz T, et al. Preoperative evaluation of the patients with pulmonary disease. *Chest* 2007; **4**: 53–61

72. Bolliger CT, Jordan P, Soler M, et al. Pulmonary function and exercise capacity after lung resection. *Eur Respir J* 1996; **9**(3): 415–21

CHAPTER 9

Structural cardiac intervention

Mario Carminati and Angelo Micheletti

Introduction

Structural heart disease includes a wide spectrum of non-coronary heart diseases ranging from septal defects to acquired valvular diseases. This heterogeneous group of diseases includes congenital defects, surgical sequelae, and acquired diseases that were previously treated exclusively surgically and where catheter-based interventions have become a feasible and effective option over the last decade.

Recent and continuous technological progresses have led to the development of new devices and procedures that greatly improve the chance to effectively treat structural heart diseases both in children and adult patients and, following initial encouraging results, such new techniques are still receiving fast and wide implementation. Therefore structural heart disease interventions are emerging as a new branch of percutaneous treatments in the field of interventional cardiology.

This new branch is characterized by some typical aspects, as follows:

1. Selection of the patients is crucial in order to increase the success of interventions and reduce the complications.

2. Proper selection requires a multidisciplinary approach that involves cardiac imaging specialists, clinical cardiologists, interventional cardiologists, interventional paediatricians, cardiac surgeons, and anaesthesiologists.

3. The role of imaging is becoming more and more essential to support such interventions as every procedure, from the initial planning and intraoperative monitoring, to the assessment of the acute result and follow up, requires a careful mostly noninvasive evaluation.

4. The necessity of continuous training and knowledge of the variety of materials and devices available to treat the different diseases.

5. The current cardiac catheterization laboratory should be equipped and adapted to hold multimodality imaging capabilities in order to perform hybrid procedures.

Therefore, the aim of this chapter is to go through the different types of structural diseases along with the different interventional procedures developed to address them as a first-line treatment option.

Septal defects

Atrial septal defect

Surgical treatment of the main patterns of atrial septal defect (ASD) is described in Chapter 21. The presence of haemodynamically significant left-to-right (L-R) shunt that is a ratio of pulmonary blood flow to systemic blood flow of >1.5:1.0 and/or right heart volume overload without significant pulmonary hypertension (PH) are indications for ASD closure. PH alone does not preclude closure but diagnostic cardiac catheterization is mandatory to calculate pulmonary vascular resistance and to assess pulmonary circulation vasoreactivity.

Haemodynamic evaluation with an ASD balloon occlusion test is also necessary in selected cases of ASD associated with RV and/or LV dysfunction, in order to determine whether patients would benefit from closure. The European Soceity of Cardiology (ESC) guidelines for ASD closure (1) are presented in table 9.1. Defect closure results in symptomatic improvement, regression of both right chamber size and PH. Benefits from closure are not age dependent (2), although the best outcome is seen in young patients with less functional impairment (3,4). If closure is performed in adolescence or childhood, life expectancy returns to normal (3,4).

Transcatheter closure of ASD has been practised for over 30 years and is now established as the standard technique for definitive treatment of ostium secundum (OS) ASDs. Many devices are currently on the market and most use the dual-disc system for closure. Percutaneous closure is unfeasible for the other variants of ASD such as the sinus venosus or ostium primum types and OS ASD associated with partial anomalous pulmonary venous drainage. To be eligible for transcatheter implantation of an occluding device, a secundum ASD must meet certain criteria, concerning size, margins and proximity to other structures. Before closure, a full diagnostic study using two-dimensional transoesophageal echocardiography (2DTOE) is needed to determine the size of the ASD, the presence of margins, and the absence of other associated defects. The three-dimensional (3D) TOE is useful to determine the anteroposterior and superoinferior diameters of the defect and to determine if there is more than one defect in the septum (5).

TOE is also pivotal in guiding percutaneous closure. Coupled with fluoroscopy, TOE provides detailed and reliable, real-time information to the operator, enabling visualization of devices

Table 9.1 Indications for ASD closure

Class Ib	Patients with significant shunt (signs of RV volume overload) and pulmonary vascular resistance (PVR) < 5 Wood units (WU) should undergo ASD closure regardless of symptoms.
Class Ic	Device closure is the method of choice for secundum ASD closure when applicable.
Class IIa	All ASDs regardless of size in patients with suspicion of paradoxical embolism (exclusion of other causes) should be considered for intervention.
Class IIb	Patients with PVR ≤5 WU but <2/3 systemic vascular resistance (SVR) or pulmonary artery pressure (PAP) <2/3 systemic pressure (baseline or when challenged with vasodilators, preferably nitric oxide, pulmonary to systemic flow ratio Qp:Qs or after targeted pulmonary arterial hypertension therapy and evidence of net L-R shunt with Qp:Qs > 1.5) may be considered for intervention.
Class III	ASD closure must be avoided in patients with Eisenmenger pathophysiology.

Reproduced from Baumgartner H et al., 'Task Force on the Management of Grown-Up Congenital Heart Disease of the European Society of Cardiology (ESC); Association of European Paediatric Cardiology (AEPC). ESC Guidelines for the management of grown-up congenital heart disease (new version 2010)', *European Heart Journal*, 2010, **31**, **23**, pp. 2915–2957, by permission of the European Society of Cardiology and Oxford University Press

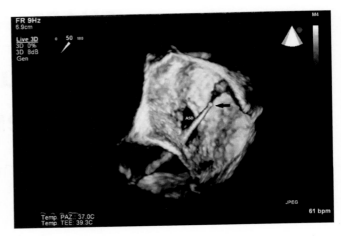

Fig. 9.2 RT3DTOE view of the atrial septum from the left atrial side. A catheter (arrow) is seen crossing the ASD. (See also figure in colour plates section)

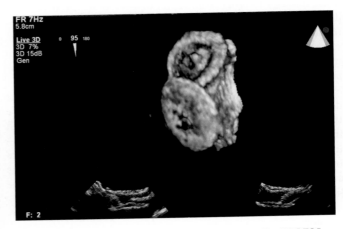

Fig. 9.3 Two devices have been implanted in two separate ASDs: RT3DTOE confirms their correct placement, with partial overlapping. (See also figure in colour plates section)

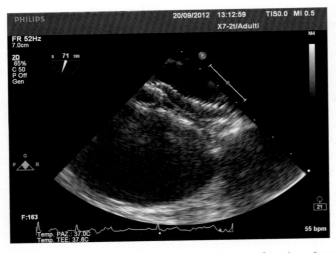

Fig. 9.1 2D TOE view of the atrial septum after implantation of Amplatzer Septal Occluder device.

during deployment and release and immediate evaluation of the results (figure 9.1).

Real-time 3D TOE (RT3DTOE) is a recent innovation in echocardiographic imaging, based on miniaturized matrix-array transducers, that allows three-dimensional imaging in real time without the need for multiple-beat acquisition and is particularly useful for guidance of percutaneous procedures (6). RT3DTOE enables accurate localization of guidewires and catheters when crossing the defects, and monitoring of device deployment and release (figure 9.2). In cases where multiple devices are used, RT3DTOE provides information on their arrangement and relationship with surrounding structures (figure 9.3).

Intracardiac echocardiography (ICE) is a useful, albeit expensive, technique for guidance of percutaneous procedures. ICE overcomes the need for tracheal intubation and general anesthesia but is only feasible in adults and older children because of the considerable size of the probe and only provides monoplane bidimensional imaging.

Percutaneous closure has a success rate up to 98%, which is comparable to that of surgical closure but with a lower complication rate at less than 0.5%. Periprocedural complications may include:

◆ Air or clot embolization in handling the catheters and flushing.

◆ Cardiac perforation by the guide wire or delivery sheath.

◆ Device embolization or dislocation.

◆ Thrombus development on the occluder device or guide wire. However, starting antiplatelet therapy the day before implantation and providing a sufficient anticoagulation with heparin (ACT >250 s) during the procedure will minimize the risk.

◆ Arrhythmias such as supraventricular extrasystoles or atrial fibrillation are mostly transient. Atrioventricular block after large device implantation usually resolves after device removal.

- Acute pulmonary oedema may occur in presence of LV dysfunction as ASD closure reducing L-to-R shunt increases LV preload and cardiac output at the expense of left atrial hypertension which may result in pulmonary oedema.

- Infection and/or endocarditis; the risk is minimized by periprocedural antibiotic therapy.

- Erosion and cardiac perforation is the most feared, late, possible complication occurring in less than 0.05% of cases and is mostly due to oversized devices.

Antiplatelet therapy should be continued for 6 months after implantation; it could vary from a minimum of 100 mg aspirin daily to a combination of aspirin and clopidogrel (75 mg daily). Antibiotic prophylaxis for infective endocarditis (IE) is strongly recommended for the same period.

Patent foramen ovale

The fossa ovalis is the remnant of patent foramen ovale (PFO) after anatomical closure which usually occurs within first year of life (7). The lack of closure results in PFO whose characteristics can vary in terms of anatomy, size and degree of shunting. It occurs in about one quarter of the general population and has been associated with various diseases such as cryptogenic ischaemic events, both cerebral and peripheral, due to paradoxical embolism, orthostatic desaturation observed in orthodeoxia-platypnoea syndrome, decompression illness observed in divers, and migraine. Paradoxical embolism occurs when a thrombus passes from venous to arterial circulation through the PFO. Although in several cases a thrombus was detected by echocardiography in the PFO (8,9), usually, in patients with cryptogenic stroke and PFO, no thrombus can be seen at the level of PFO. Therefore paradoxical embolism remains a presumptive diagnosis and should be considered in the following cases: (a) an arterial source of the thromboembolism is not found; (b) potential R-to-L shunting through the PFO is seen on echocardiography; and (c) thrombus in the venous circulation is detected. However, the clinical guidelines in neurology and cardiology are still not able to offer a consensus opinion and controversial studies have failed to clarify the issue of the benefits of percutaneous closure versus medical therapy (10). This controversy can be partially explained by the heterogeneity of factors that are involved in cryptogenic stroke: patient's clinical features, prothrombotic states, venous return problems, which may increase the risk of venous thrombosis, and finally PFO characteristics that increase the possibility of right-to-left shunting; among these characteristics, atrial septal aneurysm (ASA) plays a major role. ASA is defined as a redundant and hypermobile portion of interatrial septum with more than 10 mm excursion from the centre line during cardiac cycle; it may facilitate the passage of thrombotic material from RA to LA, increasing the size of the PFO by shifting to the left, especially in any conditions in which RA pressure exceeds LA pressure, like the Valsalva manoeuver.

Several instrumental techniques are available for the accurate assessment of PFO. Transthoracic echocardiography (TTE) (second harmonic mode) is used to evaluate cardiac structure, interatrial septum motility, and potential causes of cardiac embolism (11,12). It is also recommended that TOE should be performed in almost all the patients suspected of having a PFO (figure 9.4) (13). TOE, done with a bubble test, can be useful in diagnosing a clinically relevant intracardiac shunt at rest and after a Valsalva

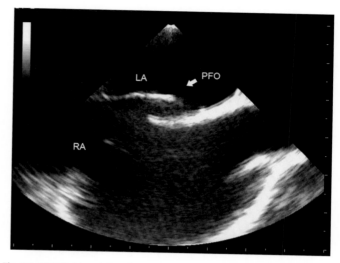

Fig. 9.4 2DTOE: bicaval view showing thick septum secundum, thin oval fossa membrane.

manoeuvre. The intra-atrial shunt is defined as the presence of contrast in the left atrium within the first three to five cardiac cycles after contrast has entered the right atrium. Shunt quantification is mild or moderate when there are fewer than 20 bubbles and severe when there are 20 or more bubbles. When bubbles are detected in the left atrium after three to five cardiac cycles, an arteriovenous pulmonary shunt is suspected.

Indication for closure

Current guidelines recommend PFO closure for:

- Patients who experience an ischaemic event recurrence while receiving optimal medical treatment or who cannot tolerate medical treatment (14,15).

- Platypnoea orthodeoxia syndrome.

- Professional divers with PFO and divers after a decompression illness who are not discontinuing diving.

Transcatheter closure is currently the first choice procedure for definitive treatment of PFO.

Many devices are approved and most have the double umbrella design with deployment of LA disc, alignment of LA disc at the left side of atrial septum, and the deployment of the RA disc.

Procedure should be guided by fluoroscopy and TOE in order to properly visualize all the steps of implantation and in this regard, RT3DTOE can be very helpful (figure 9.5).

ICE is an effective but expensive alternative, which is inserted through a second venous access.

Procedural complications are the same as for ASD device closure apart from risk of pulmonary oedema which is not encountered in such a procedure. Overall the rate of procedural complications is estimated to be less than 1%.

Antiplatelet therapy should be continued for 6 months after implantation: it could vary from a minimum of 100 mg aspirin daily to a combination of aspirin and clopidogrel (75 mg daily) although optimal therapy has not been defined yet. Antibiotic prophylaxis is strongly recommended for the same period.

Close follow up should assess any residual shunt in terms of anatomical characteristics and quantification. The presence of a

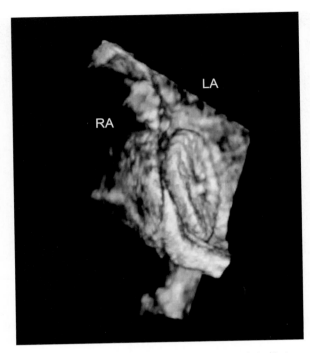

Fig. 9.5 RT3DTOE: right and left disk of Amplatzer® PFO Occluder device, embracing the interatrial septum. (See also figure in colour plates section)

residual shunt increases the risk of ischaemic event recurrence 3.4 times higher. Residual shunt device closure could be considered for moderate to severe shunt, which are likely to persist after the first 1–2 years of follow up.

Ventricular septal defect

Ventricular septal defect (VSD) can be either congenital or acquired. Congenital VSD is the most common congenital heart disease (CHD) accounting for almost 20% of all malformations (16). The different patterns of VSD are reviewed in Chapter 21. Acquired VSD is rare in adults without congenital heart disease and can be seen in different conditions, as follows:

♦ After myocardial infarction (MI), VSD may complicate a small proportion of patients at an incidence of about 0.2%. Being in a necrotic tissue, it is like a tear rather than a discrete hole and there can be multiple defects. VSD usually occurs within the first week of the initial MI and is associated with very high morbidity and mortality (17).

♦ As a result of trauma.

♦ Associated with a history of endocarditis.

♦ After previous cardiac surgery as a residual VSD. It is reported in 1% to 6% of cases who have undergone VSD patch closure and is quite often due to patch dehiscence (18).

For both congenital and acquired VSDs, the magnitude and direction of the shunt are determined by the size of the defect, LV/RV systolic and diastolic function, the presence of right ventricular outflow tract obstruction and PVR. Several clinical problems may occur. A large L-to-R shunt causes LV volume overload presenting with heart failure and, particularly in infancy and childhood with failure to thrive and repeated respiratory infections. Large VSD with large L-R shunt is associated with PH and, if untreated, ends up in severe pulmonary vascular disease as in Eisenmenger syndrome.

In case of outlet VSD, less commonly perimembranous, there is a risk for prolapse of the right coronary or non coronary cusp of the aortic valve, resulting in progressing aortic regurgitation (AR).

Considering residual VSD, subaortic discrete obstruction and/or double-chambered RV may develop, the latter being the result of a high velocity VSD jet lesion on RV endothelium. Finally arrhythmias can occur although less frequently than in other forms of CHD.

Indications for closure

Indications for closure are symptoms of heart failure and/or signs of left heart volume overload. In children, the presence of haemodynamically significant left-to-right shunt, as in large VSD, usually requires surgical closure in the first months of life in order to prevent overt cardiac failure, PH worsening into pulmonary vascular disease, aortic regurgitation and arrhythmias. Moderate-sized VSD should also be closed if symptomatic and/or LV volume overload. Even small VSDs should be closed if associated with an episode of infective endocarditis or with aortic valve cusp prolapse causing progressive aortic valve regurgitation.

In VSD evaluation, TTE is mandatory to assess all the characteristics in terms of position, size, number, association with other congenital defects or aortic valve dysfunction, direction of the shunting, relationship with tricuspid valve and its chordal apparatus, the presence of aneurysmal tissue, and the distance between the VSD and aortic valve.

Three dimensional (3D) TTE has acquired an important role in evaluating VSD size and shape. It displays an en face view of the VSD from both ventricles which allows to identification of the specific features and to differentiate the anatomy of the various defects providing useful information with which to plan the correct therapeutic strategy, especially in oval and linear VSD shaped, apical and postinfarction defects (19,20). Recently preprocedural assessment of postinfarction defects by cardiac magnetic resonance (CMR) imaging has been suggested, potentially providing detailed anatomic imaging of size, location, and tissue margins (21). In some selected cases a diagnostic cardiac catheterization is needed to calculate pulmonary vascular resistance and to assess pulmonary circulation vasoreactivity. ESC guidelines for VSD closure are summarized in table 9.2 (1).

Percutaneous VSD closure

(a) Congenital VSD. Although surgical closure remains the treatment of choice with low operative mortality and good long-term results, it is still associated with morbidity, the need for sternotomy, and cardiopulmonary bypass. Therefore, it is unsurprising that much effort have been put over the years to develop less invasive techniques. Transcatheter closure has become a valid and alternative procedure (22) to be considered in cases who have increased risk factors for surgery, had previous multiple cardiac operations or VSDs that are poorly accessible for surgical closure. Indeed inlet, malalignment type VSDs, VSDs associated with straddling or overriding atrioventricular valves, or aortic valve prolapse and regurgitation, doubly committed VSDs classically cannot be treated using a transcatheter approach. However, successful transthoracic device closure of doubly committed VSDs under TOE guidance has recently been described (23).

Table 9.2 Indications for VSD closure

Class I	Patients with symptoms that can be attributed to L–R shunting through the VSD and who do not have severe pulmonary vascular disease should undergo surgical VSD closure.
Class I	Asymptomatic patients with evidence of LV volume overload attributable to the VSD should undergo surgical VSD closure.
Class IIa	Patients with a history of IE should be considered for surgical VSD closure.
Class IIa	Patients with VSD-associated prolapse of an aortic valve cusp causing progressive AR shoul be considered for surgery
	Patients with VSD and PAH should be considered for surgery when there is still net L-R shunt (Qp:Qs >1.5) present and PAP or PVR are <2/3 systemic values (baseline or when challenged with vasodilators, preferably nitric oxide, or after targeted pulmonary PAH therapy).
Class III	Closure must be avoided in Eisenmenger VSD and when exercise-induced desaturation is present.
	If the VSD is small, not subarterial, does not lead to LV volume overload or PH, and if there is no history of IE, surgery should be avoided.

Reproduced from Baumgartner H et al., 'Task Force on the Management of Grown-Up Congenital Heart Disease of the European Society of Cardiology (ESC); Association of European Paediatric Cardiology (AEPC). ESC Guidelines for the management of grown-up congenital heart disease (new version 2010)', *European Heart Journal*, 2010, **31**, **23**, pp. 2915–2957, by permission of the European Society of Cardiology and Oxford University Press.

Currently, percutaneous closure of congenital muscular and perimembranous VSD is routinely performed under general anaesthesia with fluoroscopy and 2DTOE guidance (24,25). In most cases 2DTOE provides accurate information about VSD position, morphology and size and its relationship with adjacent cardiac structures mainly aortic valve and tricuspid valve apparatus (figure 9.6). Then 2DTOE allows real-time continuous imaging during device release confirming the right position and ruling out significant residual shunt and interference with tricuspid, mitral, and aortic valve function (Figure 9.7). Recently, 3DTOE has been applied to enhance periprocedural evaluation of VSDs with good results in term of additional information about shape and dimensions.

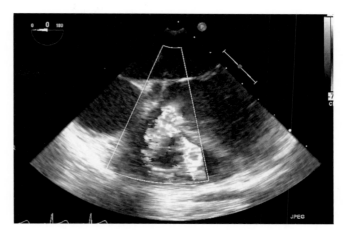

Fig. 9.6 2D Color TOE. Perimembranous VSD. (See also figure in colour plates section)

Furthermore, 3DTOE often yields accurate guidance for positioning of the delivery system and deployment of the occluder device.

Routinely, right and left heart catheterizations are performed, antibiotic prophylaxis is administered, and heparinization (100 IU/kg) is given to achieve an activated clotting time more than 200 s.

For muscular VSD (mVSD), the device available is the Amplatzer Muscular Ventricular Septal Defect Occluder, which is a self-expandable device made of nitinol wires, consisting of two discs having a diameter 8 mm larger than a central connecting waist, 7 mm long. Ideally it is only suitable for patients weighing more than 5 kg because of the issue of the devices size for vascular access. However, in some selected cases, the device can be implanted in infants weighing <5 kg, using a hybrid approach. Overall complication rate for mVSD closure is reported about 5% (26,27); major complications include embolization of the device, rhythm disturbances, cardiac perforation, and stroke.

For perimembranous VSD (pmVSD), the presence of a 2 mm or more rim of tissue between the aortic valve and the defect is considered a prerequisite for device closure. The device available is the Amplatzer Membranous Ventricular Septal Occluder, which is

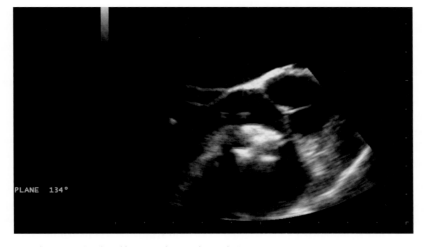

Fig. 9.7 2D TOE long axis view: perimembranous VSD closed by muscular Amplatzer device.

characterized by two discs of unequal size. In fact the aortic rim of the asymmetric left ventricular disc exceeds the dimensions of the connecting waist by only 0.5 mm in order to avoid impingement on the aortic valve whereas the apical portion is 5.5 mm larger than the waist; the right ventricular disc is symmetrical. It is suitable for patients weighing more than 8–10 kg again because of the issue of vascular access.

(b) Acquired VSD. A percutaneous approach is feasible for:

- post MI VSDs: percutaneous closure during acute phase of MI has high morbidity and mortality, up to 70%, with low rate of successful closure (28). In the chronic phase, 2–4 weeks after MI, morbidity and mortality are low with high rate of complete closure; therefore the transcatheter approach can be considered the first choice treatment. The devices currently available are the Amplatzer muscular device and the more recent Amplatzer post-infarct muscular ventricular septal defect device. Procedure is performed under general anaesthesia, TOE monitoring and fluoroscopy.

- Post surgical, residual VSDs: transcatheter closure has become first choice treatment considering the high rate of success and low rate of complications compared with further open heart surgery (29, 30). TOE guidance is required in addition to fluoroscopy and angiography all throughout the procedure.

Fistulas

Patent ductus arteriosus

If the ductus arteriosus does not spontaneously close, there is a patent ductus arteriosus (PDA). PDA accounts for 5 to 10% of all CHD in children, more frequent in females than in males. In adults it is usually an isolated finding. From anatomical point of view PDAs can vary considerably in their shape, size and attachment to the aorta; usually the narrowest part of the PDA is the pulmonary arterial end. The most common type is a funnel-shaped ductus with a localized narrowing at the pulmonary artery junction.

PDA results in L-R shunt with potential left heart volume overload and pulmonary artery (PA) pressure overload. Clinical and haemodynamic features depend on size, length and age at presentation; especially the size should be correlated to the age and weight of the patient. A small PDA is usually not associated with either symptoms or signs of volume/pressure overload. A moderate to large PDA may present predominantly with left heart failure due to volume overload or right heart failure due to PA and RV pressure overload. Large PDAs, if not closed in time, generally develop into Eisenmenger syndrome. Quite rare complications, regardless of the size, are endoarteritis and aneurysm formation, with left main coronary compression.

TTE evaluation gives accurate information about ductal anatomy and physiology and is practically feasible in almost all infants, children and in many adults. In selected adult cases computerized tomography (CT) angiography with 3D reconstruction can provide a complete assessment.

Indication for closure

PDA should be closed in patients with signs of LV volume overload even if asymptomatic (class I) and in patients with pulmonary artery hypertension (PAH) but pulmonary artery pressure (PAP) less than two thirds of systemic pressure or pulmonary

vascular resistance (PVR) less than two thirds of systemic vascular resistance (SVR) (class I). Closure should be considered in small PDA with continuous murmur and normal LV and PAP (class IIa) whereas should be avoided in 'silent' duct, very small with no murmur, and in PDA Eisenmenger (class III) (1).

Percutaneous PDA closure

Percutaneous closure of a PDA can be performed in those cases who meet criteria for body weight and ductal size and it's feasible and safe in children weighing more than 5 kg with PDA diameter of 2.5–3 mm. In smaller-weight babies this option is still under debate, whereas larger PDAs are currently best managed with surgery. In adults, percutaneous closure is the first choice treatment, even if cardiac surgery is indicated for other concomitant cardiac lesions, because calcification of the ductus increases surgical complications. Usually the procedure is carried out under general anaesthesia in infants and children and with local anaesthesia in adolescents and adults. Heparin (100 UI/kg) is administered thereby reducing the risk related to arterial puncture, especially in small babies. Antibiotic prophylaxis is indicated as well.

The PDA anatomical characteristics guide the choice of proper occlusion device because different types are worldwide currently available. Small ducts can be closed using coils such as Cook detachable coil, whereas large PDAs can be addressed, according to the anatomy, using different devices as an Amplatzer Duct Occluder Device (ADO) I or its modification ADO II (31) or a mVSD Amplatzer Occluder or an ASD Amplatzer Occluder (32).

Periprocedural complications may include:

◆ Air or clot embolization in handling the catheters and flushing.

◆ Device embolization or dislocation. Embolization can occur more often after coil release; according to the size, coil can embolize into the pulmonary arteries or the aorta and subsequently into all the arterial tree including intracranial arteries. Wherever it embolizes, coil can be retrieved using specific catheters. In case of dislocation or malposition, device can cause left pulmonary artery stenosis or aortic stenosis associated, quite often, with residual shunting.

◆ Haemolysis. It is a rare but serious complication usually after coil PDA occlusion, related to a residual flow at the end of the procedure. If it happens, it is difficult to eliminate as long as the residual shunt is closed using other coils.

◆ Infection and/or endocarditis; the risk is minimized by periprocedural antibiotic therapy.

Antibiotic prophylaxis for IE is recommended for 6 months after the procedure.

Coronary fistulae

Coronary fistulae are abnormal connections between any coronary artery or its branches and any of the cardiac chambers or coronary sinus. They may be:

◆ Congenital. The feeding vessel is most commonly the right coronary followed by the anterior interventricular artery and the circumflex artery. The entry point is usually the right ventricle followed by the right atrium, coronary sinus, left ventricle, and pulmonary artery.

♦ Acquired. After thoracic surgery or after right heart biopsies in transplant patients or as a consequence of an aneurysmal artery erosion. They are usually smaller than congenital fistulae and the entry point is usually the right ventricle.

Many fistulae are asymptomatic and discovered due to the presence of pathological murmur. In addition, they may close spontaneously. Coronary fistula-related symptoms generally depends on ischaemia in the territory supplied by the feeding artery due to a steal phenomenon and high output cardiac failure: exertional shortness of breath, angina, atrial or ventricular arrhythmias (33). Infective endocarditis and rupture, though quite rare, have been reported as well. A proper visualization of fistulae may be difficult by echochardiogram due to the dilatation and tortuosity of the feeding coronary; therefore CMR imaging or CT angiography can be valuable diagnostic tools although coronary angiography remains the gold standard technique.

Indications for closure

Treatment of asymptomatic fistulae remains controversial. If a conservative strategy is adopted then follow up angiography may be reasonable because some fistulae increase in size with time. Symptomatic fistulae or those that have progressively increased in size or are associated with a high shunt volume causing left or right heart volume overload should be closed. If technically feasible, percutaneous closure should be considered as the first approach. Depending on the size, it can be performed with coils or vascular plugs with the aim of releasing the appropriate device as distally into the fistula as possible in order to avoid proximal ischaemia related to inadvertent occlusion of the feeding vessel or one of its branches.

Pulmonary arteriovenous fistulae

Pulmonary arteriovenous fistulae are direct connections between the pulmonary artery and pulmonary vein leading to right–left shunting. They are a typical manifestation of an autosomal dominant disease known as hereditary haemorrhagic teleangiectasia (HHT) (34). These fistulae can be simple, with a single feeding artery, or complex, with multiple arteries; they can be single, limited to one lobe or segment or, more often, multiple involving more than one lobe or segment. Symptoms and signs include transient ischaemic attack, paradoxical embolism, haemoptysis, haemothorax, hypoxaemia, right heart failure, and pulmonary hypertension. The best screening test is contrast echocardiography which has a sensitivity of >90%; this can be complemented by CT scan.

Indication for closure

Closure is recommended even for asymptomatic fistulae fed by an artery more than 3 mm diameter in order to prevent embolic events. In case of multiple fistulae, it is advised to treat them in a staged fashion to minimize the risk of pulmonary infection as a consequence of pulmonary infarction. Contraindications to treatment are active pulmonary infection and/or greater than moderate pulmonary hypertension.

Percutaneous closure

Percutaneous embolization is the first-choice approach, when technically feasible, considering the significant morbidity and mortality related to surgical therapy. Closure can be achieved using coil or vascular plug with very high technical success rate. Potential complications unique to this procedure include pleuritic chest pain or pleural effusion (10–35%) and pulmonary infarction with subsequent infection. After successful occlusion, recanalization can occur in up to 17%; therefore, contrast echo and/or CT follow-up along with antibiotic prophylaxis should be recommended in all the cases.

Vascular obstructions

Aortic coarctation

Coarctation of the aorta is considered as part of a generalized arteriopathy and not just a circumscript narrowing of the aorta. It occurs as a discrete stenosis most commonly seen in periductal region (35,36) or as a long, hypoplastic segment. It accounts for 5–8% of all CHD and may occur in isolation or in association with other anomalies: bicuspid aortic valve (up to 80%) subvalvular, valvular or supravalvular aortic stenosis, mitral valve stenosis (as seen in Shone complex: subaortic stenosis and supra-valve mitral ring), hypoplastic left heart syndrome, aberrant subclavian artery. Coarctation of the aorta can be associated with Turner, Williams–Beuren, or congenital rubella syndromes, neurofibromatosis, Takayasu aortitis, or trauma.

Signs and symptoms depend on the severity of the coarctation; when severe, closure of the arterial duct after birth will result in critical aortic obstruction, LV dilatation and dysfunction, and low cardiac output state with metabolic acidosis. Untreated, death ensues quickly. In less severe forms the anomaly may become evident during childhood when a murmur may be heard and femoral pulses found to be of reduced volume where as in adulthood the most common sign is systemic hypertension (35,36). Symptoms may include headache, nosebleeds, dizziness, shortness of breath, abdominal angina, claudication, leg cramps, exertional leg fatigue, and cold feet. Some life-threatening conditions may complicate the natural course of coarctation of the aorta: left heart failure, intracranial haemorrhage (from berry aneurysm of circle of Willis), aortic rupture/dissection, infective endocarditis, premature coronary and cerebral artery disease.

Indications for intervention

The standard management of native coarctation in infants and young children is surgical repair. In adolescent and adult patients a significant coarctation is regarded as being present when there is a systolic blood pressure gradient between the upper and lower limb of at least 20 mmHg or less than 20 mmHg in the presence of systemic hypertension (37). Indications for intervention in adults (class IC) for significant aortic coarctation include also pathological blood pressure response during exercise or prominent LV hypertrophy (1). Key features, prior to any treatment, are the aortic arch morphology and the branching pattern of the head and neck vessels. Therefore CMR and CT imaging are the preferred non-invasive techniques to evaluate the entire aorta in adults while cardiac catheterization is still the gold standard at many centres, before and after treatment; a peak-to-peak gradient more than 20 mmHg is indicative of a significant coarctation in the absence of well developed collaterals.

Percutaneous treatment

Currently, balloon angioplasty is mainly indicated in re-coarctation in infants and young children providing excellent acute relief of obstruction but being associated with high rate of coarctation recurrence and important concerns regarding aneurysm formation and dissection (37,38). For older children, adolescents and adults with native or recurring or residual coarctation of the aorta, angioplasty with covered or non-covered stent implantation, has become first choice treatment if anatomy is appropriate (figure 9.8). The use of covered stents has significantly reduced the incidence of dissection and aneurysm formation at the site of treated coarctation; furthermore, stents can be re-dilated later in life in case of re-coarctation or residual stenosis. Biologically absorbable stents are still in development. Procedure is generally performed under general anaesthesia, which reduces sympathetic drive so may result in a falsely low gradient across a coarctation.

Acute complications may include stent migration which is, the most important one occurring in 5% of cases, cerebrovascular accident, seen more frequently in older patients and femoral artery injury resulting in leg ischaemia or retroperitoneal bleeding. Regarding late complications, the incidence of aortic dissection or aneurysm formation following stenting is reported at approximately 10% of cases, most commonly at the site of the narrowest segment of coarctation of the aorta. The vast majority of aneurysms are small and can be managed conservatively. Successful stenting is usually effective in lowering systemic blood pressure but during follow-up at least a third of patients remain hypertensive demonstrating that coarctation of the aorta is not purely an isolated mechanical obstruction but a complex aortic vasculopathy involving arterial stiffness and elasticity, endothelial function, and the renin–angiotensin system. Hypertension is the most important long-term complication, being a key determinant of late morbidity and mortality (39). The most relevant predictor of problematic hypertension late after repair is the age of the patient at the time of treatment; the lowest incidence is seen in those repaired under 1 year of age. All coarctation patients require regular follow-up, including accurate evaluation of aorta imaging to document the post-interventional anatomy and complications.

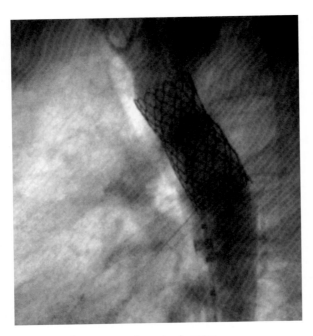

Fig. 9.8 Angiography post covered stent implantation.

Stenosis of pulmonary arteries

Stenosis of pulmonary arteries is caused by narrowing of the main pulmonary trunk, pulmonary arterial bifurcation or pulmonary branches. It can be classified as:

◆ Congenital, usually in cono-truncal heart defects such as tetralogy of Fallot or pulmonary atresia or in the context of certain syndromes as Williams–Beuren, Noonan, congenital rubella, or Alagille.

◆ Acquired, in patients already operated, at the site of pulmonary artery banding or systemic to pulmonary shunt anastomosis or after arterial switch operation; in patients with vasculitis, particularly in Takayasu arteritis, or following irradiation or extrinsic compression by tumors.

The stenosis may vary in position (proximal or peripheral), in severity, in extent (discrete or diffuse—hypoplastic), and number (single or multiple).

A single diseased branch may not give symptoms whereas multiple stenosis usually lead to RV overload and dysfunction and consequently reduced exercise capacity and/or dyspnoea. Peripheral stenosis may progress in severity (1).

Indication for intervention

A stenosis at any level should be treated, regardless of symptoms, when echo Doppler maximal gradient is >64 mmHg (max velocity > 4 m/s), provided that RV function is normal (class I of recommendation). Peripheral pulmonary stenosis, regardless of symptoms, should be considered for treatment if >50% diameter narrowing and RV systolic pressure >50 mmHg and/or lung perfusion abnormalities are present (class IIa of recommendation) (1). Because echocardiography has its own limitations in assessing pulmonary stenosis expecially if peripheral, CMR and CT imaging frequently provide additional important information. Cardiac catheterization may be required to confirm the extent, severity and level of obstruction.

Percutaneous treatment

In case of young patients the treatment of choice is simple or cutting balloon angioplasty; restenosis occurs in less than 12% (40). In adult patients, angioplasty with stent implantation is currently the key treatment technique (figure 9.9).

Valvular diseases

Pulmonary valve stenosis

Pulmonary valve (PV) stenosis is a quite common CHD, occurring in about 5 out of every 10 000 livebirths and accounts for 80–90% of all right ventricular outflow tract (RVOT) obstructions. It can be an isolated lesion or associated with other CHD, up to 50%. Its inheritance rate ranges from 1.7 to 3.6%. PV is the characteristic cardiac finding in Noonan syndrome and in several rarer conditions such as Leopard syndrome and neurofibromatosis type 1.

Considering the anatomy, three different forms of pulmonary stenosis may be encountered:

◆ Dome shaped valve, the most common, characterized by a narrow central opening but a preserve mobile valve base, fused commissures and normal arterial walls.

◆ Dysplastic valve occurs in 15–20% of cases and is characterized by poorly mobile cusps and myxomatous thickening. It is characteristic of Noonan syndrome.

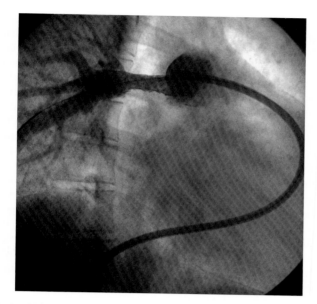

Fig. 9.9 Right PA angiography post implantation of 39 XL Andramed stent.

◆ Bottle-shaped valve with thickened pulmonary trunk forming an hourglass narrowing at the level of the sinutubular junction.

In all forms, dilatation of pulmonary trunk and left pulmonary artery usually occurs. Elevated RV pressure results in RV hypertrophy mainly in the infundibular region. In case of severe obstruction, there may be a small RV cavity with reduced compliance and increased end diastolic pressure leading to so-called restrictive physiology; in the concomitant presence of an ASD, right to left shunting will occur with a resultant reduction in pulmonary blood flow and cyanosis. If RV pressure is suprasystemic, myocardial ischaemia may ensue, leading to myocardial fibrosis and eventually congestive cardiac failure.

The neonate with critical pulmonary stenosis typically presents in congestive heart failure or with deep cyanosis due to right–left shunt at the atrial level; having a duct-dependent pulmonary circulation, as soon as the arterial duct closes, clinical conditions get worse and worse. Beyond the neonatal periods, most cases of pulmonary stenosis remain asymptomatic as the RV and right atrium compensate to maintain resting cardiac output. With advancing age, reduced exercise tolerance, and fatigue are the most common symptoms. In adults, a stenotic pulmonary valve may calcify late in life.

Indication for intervention and percutaneous valvuloplasty
Echocardiography is essential to assess the nature and severity of the valvular stenosis: a peak Doppler systolic gradient less than 40 mmHg is considered as a mild obstruction, 40 to 70 mmHg moderate and greater than 70 mmHg severe. On cardiac catheterization, a RV to PA peak to peak systolic pressure gradient less than 30 mmHg is considered mild; between 30 and 50 mmHg associated with RV systolic pressure approaching the systemic pressure, is considered moderate; greater than 50 mmHg with RV systolic exceeding the systemic arterial pressure, is considered severe. Neonates presenting with critical pulmonary stenosis should be commenced on prostaglandin infusion as soon as possible to maintain ductal patency until percutaneous valvuloplasty is provided; PDA is useful both for catheter positioning

and preservation of pulmonary blood flow during balloon occlusion of outflow tract. Successful dilatation rate is about 95%; in the few cases where cyanosis persists, stabilization on prostaglandin is slow or the therapy is not tolerated, ductal stenting, or a systemic-to-pulmonary shunt should be considered.

Asymptomatic infants should be treated electively around the age of 9 to 12 months in case of severe pulmonary stenosis. Older children and adults with at least moderate stenosis judged by cardiac catheterization should undergo percutaneous valvuloplasty, irrespective of symptoms and age (1). Procedure is conventionally performed under general anaesthesia using a transfemoral approach. Ideal balloon diameter for effective dilatation is 110–120% of the annular diameter measured by echocardiography. A final resting gradient of less than 30 mmHg across the pulmonary valve should be achieved at any patient age; dysplastic valves are associated with higher residual gradients and less consistent outcomes. In neonates and infants catheterization is technically more challenging and complications are more frequent. Major complications include RVOT rupture with cardiac tamponade and injury to the tricuspid valve, leaving significant regurgitation. Dynamic infundibular obstruction with resulting hypotension and hypoxia is a particular risk mainly for infants with critical stenosis. Although the majority of patients will only have trivial or mild pulmonary regurgitation following valvuloplasty, moderate to severe insufficiency can occur and in these cases, percutaneous pulmonary valve implantation should be considered (41). Minor complications include vascular access injury, transient arrhythmias, and infection. Over 85% of patients treated with valvuloplasty are free from reintervention up to 9 years later.

Right ventricular outflow tract dysfunction
RVOT and/or pulmonary trunk dysfunction is a growing clinical problem in older children and adults after repair of CHD, either manifesting as an obstructive lesion or as pulmonary regurgitation. Thus far, surgical pulmonary valve (PV) replacement using valved conduits or biological valves has been an effective and safe procedure with low morbidity and mortality. However, considering the limited lifespan of such conduits and valves, the majority of patients have to undergo several open-heart procedures during their life times; therefore management strategies have been always based on intervening as late as possible to reduce the number of surgeries but before RV dysfunction has become irreversible. Unfortunately the right timing for PV replacement is still controversial. Over the last decade percutaneous pulmonary valve implantation (PPVI) has become a feasible, safe and effective non-surgical technique that enables treatment of both conduit stenosis and regurgitation. Currently, two devices are available:

◆ the Melody valve (Medtronic, MN), which is composed of a segment of bovine jugular vein with a central valve. It comes in three different sizes according to the outer balloon diameters: 18, 20, and 22 mm (figure 9.10).

◆ The Edward Sapien valve (Edwards Lifesciences LLC, Irvine, CA), which consists of three bovine pericardial leaflets hand-sewn to a stainless steel stent. It is available in 23 and 26 mm diameter sizes. The most significant limitation is the suitability of this procedure as only patients with a RV to PA conduit can be considered good candidates because conduit allows for safe

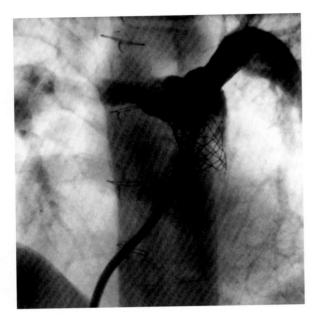

Fig. 9.10 AP view: pulmonary artery angiography after 22mm Melody Valve and LPA CP stent implantation.

anchoring of the device. Therefore there remains a large number of CHD operated patients are unsuitable for PPVI: patients presenting with significant pulmonary regurgitation secondary to previous surgery such as following tetralogy of Fallot transannular patch repair, whose outflow tracts are markedly dilated and very distensible.

Patient selection prior to PPVI is crucial and should fulfil both clinical and morphological criteria. Clinical indications in the context of RV pressure overload and pulmonary stenosis are based on RV systolic pressure: >65% of systemic pressure in symptomatic patients or >75% of systemic pressure in asymptomatic patients (1,42). Clinical indications in the context of RV volume overload and pulmonary regurgitation are based on a combined assessment of RV end-diastolic volume and systolic function (from CMR imaging), cardiopulmonary exercise testing and the presence of ventricular arrhythmia. Morphological criteria depends on two factors: size and shape of implantation site and coronary artery anatomy to rule out any compression due to the expansion of the RVOT. On CMR 3D whole heart images, the anatomical relationship of the coronary arteries and the proposed implantation size can be judged.

Major procedural complications include homograft rupture with haemodynamic compromise, device dislodgement, hypercarbia, and elevation of LV filling pressure requiring mechanical ventilation, coronary compression, ventricular arrhythmias, obstruction of origin of right pulmonary artery, perforation of PA causing bleeding, bronchial bleeding due to guide wire injury, and entrapment of delivery system in the tricuspid valve apparatus causing significant regurgitation.

Median follow-up data show good freedom from re-operation and re-catheterization, being >70% at five years after PPVI.

Aortic valve stenosis

The gold standard of treatment in aortic valve stenosis is surgery. However, patients at high-risk for conventional surgery may benefit from alternative procedures. Medical therapy and/or balloon angioplasty have limited benefit, with a mortality rate after 2 years which is approximately 70% (43). In recent years, transcatheter aortic valve implantation (TAVI) has been widely used in high-risk patients with a stenotic aortic valve. This procedure is based on a transcatheter implantation of a bioprosthetic aortic valve, either through peripheral arteries (femoral and subclavian arteries), or directly through the apex of the left ventricle using a mini-thoracotomy (transapical TAVI). In inoperable patients, TAVI is superior to medical theraphy and/or balloon angioplasty, with a mortality rate at 1 year of 31% vs. 50% (44) and at 2 years of 43% vs. 68% (43).

There is a group of medium-to-high risk patients who could be candidates for both TAVI and conventional surgery. In this patient population, TAVI is not superior to conventional surgery in terms of procedural or medium-term mortality (45,46); the incidences of residual aortic valve regurgitation, peripheral vascular damages and stroke, are higher in patients receiving a TAVI (45); major bleeding and blood transfusion are more likely to complicate conventional surgery (46).

At present, the role of TAVI in inoperable patients appears well established, while a debate exists as to its application in high-risk patients who could, however, receive conventional surgery. As a result, the rate of patients referred to TAVI greatly varies in different countries and institutions. The recently released guidelines of the American Heart Association, the American Society of Echocardiography, the European Association of Cardiothoracic Surgery, the Society of Cardiovascular Anesthesiologists, and other scientific associations offer a comprehensive view on this issue, including the inclusion and exclusion criteria for a TAVI procedure (47). The prerequisites are the presence of a calcific aortic valve stenosis with echocardiographic criteria of severity; symptoms clearly related to the aortic valve disease and the presence of a high-risk profile for conventional aortic valve replacement surgery.

Mitral valve regurgitation

Conventional surgery that is mitral valve repair or replacement, is the standard of care for mitral valve regurgitation. However, high-risk patients for conventional surgery may be treated with a transcatheter approach and edge-to-edge repair. The MitraClip® (Abbott Vascular, Abbott Park, IL) is a device for percutaneous mitral valve repair by clipping the edges of the anterior and posterior mitral valve leaflets. It is delivered via the femoral vein, through a trans-septal approach to the mitral valve. Patients eligible for this treatment are elderly, at high-risk for conventional surgery and with functional mitral valve regurgitation. A careful preoperative assessment of the mitral valve and the mechanism leading to regurgitation is mandatory and based on 2D- and 3DTOE. The study of mitral valve function aims to confirm that the anatomical pattern and size of the two leaflets is adequate to allow the procedure. A recent meta-analysis (48) found that the immediate procedural success ranges from 72% to 100%, with a reported 30-days mortality of 0% to 7.8%. One-year survival rate was 75–90%.

Anaesthetic considerations

From the point of view of the anaesthetist, the anaesthetic management of structural heart interventions may cover the whole scenario of sedation, general anaesthesia, and regional anaesthesia. The choice of the technique depends on the age of the patient, the haemodynamic conditions and of course the nature of the procedure.

In paediatric patients, simple procedures may be performed under sedation. Ketamine may be used intramuscularly at a dose of 3 to 7 mg/kg, or intravenously at a dose of 1 mg/kg bolus followed by additional smaller doses or continuous infusion. Other alternatives include midazolam and low-dose opioids.

For the majority of the interventional procedures, general anesthesia is required. The preparation of the patient and the techniques of anaesthesia are described in Chapter 21. The choice of a short- (propofol) or long- (midazolam) acting hypnotic agent depends on the expected postoperative care: some patients may be directly sent to the ward, while others require an overnight stay in an Intensive Care Unit. Monitoring includes standard electrocardiography, end-tidal CO_2, and invasive arterial blood pressure unless undertaking very simple procedures. Reliable vascular access is mandatory, since all the interventional procedures carry the risk for haemorragic shock due to vessel lesions.

A specific issue is represented by the choice of the anaesthesia for TAVI and MitraClip® procedures.

Transapical TAVI is usually performed under general anaesthesia and mechanical ventilation. Conversely, different options are available for transarterial TAVI. Data from the Italian Registry Observant reported about 75% of the procedures performed under local anaesthesia, with or without conscious sedation (46). There are advantages and disadvantages of both general and local anaesthesia. General anaesthesia allows the peri-procedural monitoring of cardiac function with the TOE, and provides the substrate for an eventual surgical closure of the femoral access (49,50); local anaesthesia may safer for patients with severe chronic obstructive pulmonary disease, and allow a faster recovery (51). In general, institutions at the beginning of their experience with TAVI prefer general anaesthesia, whereas most experienced operators often shift to local anaesthesia.

In contrast to TAVI, the backbone of peri-procedural imaging for MitraClip® inplantation is TOE. For this reason, the great majority of these procedures are carried on under general anaesthesia, to allow for prolonged TOE examination. However, there are reports of cases done under local anaesthesia and sedation with low-doses of midazolam (2 mg) and propofol (20–60 mg for the whole procedure) (52,53).

References

1. Baumgartner H, Bonhoeffer P, De Groot NM, et al. Task Force on the Management of Grown-Up Congenital Heart Disease of the European Society of Cardiology (ESC); Association of European Paediatric Cardiology (AEPC). ESC Guidelines for the management of grown-up congenital heart disease (new version 2010). *Eur Heart J* 2010; **31**: 2915–57

2. Humenberger M, Rosenhek R, Gabriel H, et al. Benefit from atrial septal defect closure in adults: impact of age. *Eur Heart J* 2011; **32**: 553–60

3. Murphy JG, Gersh BJ, McGoon MD, et al. Long-term outcome after surgical repair of isolated atrial septal defect. Follow-up at 27 to 32 years. *N Engl J Med* 1990; **323**: 1645–50

4. Roos-Hesselink JW, Meijboom FJ, Spitaels SE, et al. Excellent survival and low incidence of arrhythmias, stroke and heart failure long-term after surgical ASD closure at young age. A prospective follow-up study of 21–33 years. *Eur Heart J* 2003; **24**: 190–7

5. Lodato JA, Cao QL, Weinert L, et al. Feasibility of real-time three-dimensional transoesophageal echocardiography for guidance of percutaneous atrial septal defect closure. *Eur J Echocardiogr* 2009; **10**: 543–8

6. Taniguchi M, Akagi T, Watanabe N, et al. Application of real-time three-dimensional transesophageal echocardiography using a matrix array probe for transcatheter closure of atrial septal defect. *J Am Soc Echocardiogr* 2009; **22**: 1114–20

7. Anderson RH, Brown NA, Webb S. Development and structure of the atrial septum. *Heart* 2002; **88**: 104–10

8. Kearney LG, Srivastava PM. Thrombus entrapped in a patent foramen ovale: a potential source of pulmonary and systemic embolism. *Heart and Lung Circ* 2010; **19**: 58–60

9. Mascarenhas V, Kalyanasundaram A, Nassef LA, Lico S, Qureshi A. Simultaneous massive pulmonary embolism and impending paradoxical embolism through a patent foramen ovale. *JACC* 2009; **53**: 1338

10. Furlan AJ, Reisman M, Massaro J, et al. Closure or medical therapy for cryptogenic stroke with patent foramen ovale. *N Eng J Med* 2012; **366**: 991–9

11. Weytjens C, Cosyns B, Schoors D, et al. Second harmonic transthoracic echocardiography: the new reference screening method for the detection of patent foramen ovale. *Eur J Echocardiogr* 2004; **5**: 449–52

12. Maffè S, Dellavesa P, Zenone F, et al. Transthoracic second harmonic two- and three-dimensional echocardiography for detection of patent foramen ovale. *Eur J Echocardiogr* 2010; **11**: 57–63

13. Van Camp G, Franken P, Melis P, Cosyns B, Schoors D, Vanoverschelde JL. Comparison of transthoracic echocardiography with second harmonic imaging with transesophageal echocardiography in the detection of right to left shunts. *Am J Cardiol* 2000; **86**: 1284–7

14. European Stroke Organisation (ESO) Executive Committee; ESO Writing Committee. Guidelines for management of ischaemic stroke and transient ischaemic attack 2008. *Cerebrovasc Dis* 2008; **25**: 457–507

15. Furie KL, Kasner SE, Adams RJ, et al. Guidelines for the prevention of stroke in patients with stroke or transient ischaemic attack: a guideline for healthcare professionals from the American Heart Association/ American Stroke Association. *Stroke* 2011; **42**: 227–76

16. Rudolph AM. Ventricular septal defect. In: Rudolph AM, ed. *Congenital Diseases of the Heart: Clinical-Physiological Considerations*, 2nd ed. Armonk NY: Futura Publishing Company, 2001; 197–244

17. Crenshaw BS, Granger CB, Birnbaum Y, for the GUSTO-I Trial Investigators. Risk factors, angiographic patterns and outcomes in patients with ventricular septal defect complicating acute myocardial infarction. *Circulation* 2000; **101**: 27–32

18. Roos-Hesselink JW, Meijboom FJ, Spitaels SE, et al. Outcome of patients after surgical closure of ventricular septal defect at a young age: longitudinal follow-up of 22–34 years. *Eur Heart J* 2004; **25**: 1057–62

19. Nygren A, Sunnegard J, Berggren H. Preoperative evaluation and surgery in isolated ventricular septal defects: a 21 years perspective. *Heart* 2005; **83**: 198–204

20. Mercer-Rosa L, Seliem MA, Fedec A, Rome J, Rychik J, Gaynoret JW. Illustration of the additional value of real-time 3-dimensional echocardiography to conventional transthoracic and transesophageal 2-dimensional echocardiography in imaging muscular ventricular septal defects: Does this have any impact on individual patient treatment? *J Am Soc Echocardiogr* 2006; **19**: 1511–9

21. Artis NJ, Thomson J, Plein S, Greenwood JP. Percutaneous closure of postinfarction ventricular septal defect: cardiac magnetic esonance-guided case selection and postprocedure evaluation. *Can J Cardiol* 2011; **27**: 869.e3–5

22. Lock JE, Block PC, McKay RG, Baim DS, Keane JF. Transcatheter closure of ventricular septal defects. *Circulation* 1988; **78**: 361–8

23. Chen Q, Chen LW, Wang QM, Cao H, Zhang GC, Chen DZ. Intraoperative device closure of doubly committed subarterial ventricular septal defects: initial experience. *Ann Thorac Surg* 2010; **90**: 869–74.

24. Janorkar S, Goh T, Wilkinson J. Transcatheter closure of ventricular septal defects using the Rashkind device: initial experience. *Catheter Cardiovasc Interv* 1999; **46**: 43–8

25. Kalra GS, Verma PK, Dhall A, Singh S, Arora R. Transcatheter device closure of ventricular septal defects: immediate results and intermediate follow-up. *Am Heart J* 1999; **138**: 339–44

26. Carminati M, Butera G, Chessa M, et al. Transcatheter closure of congenital ventricular septal defects: results of the European Registry. *Eur Heart J* 2007; **28**: 2361–8

27. Chessa M, Carminati M, Cao QL, et al. Transcatheter closure of congenital and acquired muscular ventricular septal defects using the Amplatzer device. *J Invasive Cardiol* 2002; **14**: 322–7

28. Thiele H, Kaulfersch C, Daenhert I,et al. Immediate primary transcatheter closure of postinfarction ventricular septal defects. *Eur Heart J* 2009; **30**: 81–8

29. Dua JS, Carminati M, Lucente M, Transcatheter closure of post-surgical residual ventricular septal defects: early and mid-term results. *Catheter Cardiovasc Interv* 2010; **75**: 246–55

30. Pedra CA, Pontes SC Jr, Pedra SR, et al. Percutaneous closure of post-operative and post-traumatic ventricular septal defects. *J Invasive Cardiol* 2007; **19**: 491–5

31. Jaspal D, Chessa M, Piazza L, et al. Initial experience with the new Amplatzer Duct Occluder II. *J Invasive Cardiol* 2009; **21**: 401–5

32. Pedra CA, Sanches SA, Fontes VF. Percutaneous occlusion of the patent ductus arteriosus with the Amplatzer device for atrial septal defect. *J Invasive Cardiol* 2003; **15**: 413–17

33. Qureshi SA. Coronary arterial fistulas. *Orphanet J Rare Dis* 2006; **1**: 51

34. Faughnam ME, Granton JT, Young LH. The pulmonary vascular complications of hereditary haemorrhagic teleangiectasia. *Eur Respir J* 2009; **33**: 1186–94

35. Oechslin EN. Does a stent cure hypertension? *Heart* 2008; **94**: 828–9

36. Matsui H, Adachi I, Uemura H, Gardiner H, Ho SY. Anatomy of coarctation, hypoplastic and interrupted aortic arch: relevance to interventional/surgical treatment. *Expert Rev Cardiovasc Ther* 2007; **5**: 871–80

37. Forbes Tj, Garekar S, Amin Z, et al. Congenital cardiovascular interventional study consortium (CCISC). Procedural results and acute complications in stenting native and recurrent coarctation of the aorta in patients over 4 years of age: a multi-institutional study. *Catheter Cardiovasc Interv* 2007; **70**: 276–85

38. Rao PS. Coarctation of the aorta. *Curr Cardiol Rep* 2005; **7**: 425–34

39. Forbes TJ, Moore P, Pedra CA, et al. Intermediate follow-up following intravascular stenting for treatment of coarctation of the aorta. *Catheter Cardiovasc Interv* 2007; **70**: 569–77

40. Mori Y, Nakanishi T, Niki T, et al. Growth of stenotic lesions after balloon angioplasty for pulmonary artery stenosis after arterial switch operation. *Am J Cardiol* 2003; **91**: 693–8

41. Lurz P, Coats L, Khambadkone S, et al. Percutaneous pulmonary valve implantation: impact of evolving technology and learning curve on clinical outcome. *Circulation* 2008; **117**: 1964–72

42. Nordmeyer J, Khambadkone S, Coats L, et al. Risk stratification, systematic classification, and anticipatory management strategies for stent fracture after percutaneous pulmonary valve implantation. *Circulation* 2007; **115**: 1392–7

43. Makkar RR, Fontana GP, Jilaihawi H, et al. Transcatheter aortic-valve replacement for inoperable severe aortic stenosis. *N Engl J Med* 2012; **366**: 1696–704

44. Leon MB, Smith CR, Mack M, et al. Transcatheter aortic-valve implantation for aortic stenosis in patients who cannot undergo surgery. *N Engl J Med* 2010; **363**: 1597–607

45. Kodali SK, Williams MR, Smith CR, et al. Two-year outcomes after transcatheter or surgical aortic-valve replacement. *N Engl J Med* 2012; **366**: 1686–95

46. D'Errigo P, Barbanti M, Ranucci M, et al. Transcatheter aortic valve implantation versus surgical aortic valve replacement for severe aortic stenosis: Results from an intermediate risk propensity-matched population of the Italian OBSERVANT study. *Int J Cardiol* 2013 **167**: 1945–52

47. Holmes Dr Jr, Mack MJ, Kaul S, et al. 2012 ACCF/AATS/SCAI/STS expert consensus document on transcatheter aortic valve replacement. *JACC* 2012; **59**: 1200–54.

48. Munkholm-Larsen S, Wan B, Tian DH, et al. A systematic review on the safety and efficacy of percutaneous edge-to-edge mitral valve repair with the MitraClip system for high surgical risk candidates. *Heart* 2014; **100**: 473–8.

49. Ree RM, Bowering JB, Schwarz SK. Case series: anesthesia for retrograde percutaneous aortic valve replacement-experience with the first 40 patients. *Can J Anaesth* 2008; **55**: 761–8

50. Billings FT 4th, Kodali SK, Shanewise JS. Transcatheter aortic valve implantation: anesthetic considerations. *Anesth Analg* 2009; **108**: 1453–62

51. Behan M, Haworth P, Hutchinson N, et al. Percutaneous aortic valve implants under sedation. *Catheter Cardiovasc Interv* 2008; **72**: 1012–5

52. Teufel T, Steinberg DH, Wunderlich N, et al. Percutaneous mitral valve repair with the MitraClip® system under deep sedation and local anaesthesia. *EuroIntervention* 2012; **8**: 587–90

53. Ussia GP, Barbanti M, Tamburino C. Feasibility of percutaneous transcatheter mitral valve repair with the MitraClip system using conscious sedation. *Catheter Cardiovasc Interv* 2010; **75**: 1137–40

CHAPTER 10

Blood gases, clinical chemistry, and acid–base

David Story and Philip J. Peyton

Introduction

Patient monitoring in cardiac and thoracic surgery presents particular difficulties. Major shifts in fluid balance and manipulations of body temperature are often part of the surgical procedure, and complicate the interpretation of blood gas analysis and metabolic management particularly in more extensive surgery (1). Further, one-lung ventilation changes pulmonary physiology and interferes with the measurement and interpretation of indices of gas exchange and oxygenation (2). For these reasons, the aim of this chapter is to review the interpretation of blood gas, clinical chemistry, and acid–base measurements in patients undergoing cardiothoracic anaesthesia and critical care.

Point-of-care measurements

Hospital central laboratories allow clinicians to measure a wide variety of blood constituents, including plasma chemistry, cellular components, and clotting. In critical care areas, including operating rooms (ORs), central laboratories usually have the disadvantages of transport distance and processing times (often hours), which may undermine their use in clinical decisions in perioperative care of cardiothoracic patients (3). Point-of-care testing refers to testing close to the patient, even at the bedside. Some devices are literally hand held, but have important limitations. In this section, point-of-care testing will refer to laboratory bench mounted machines within critical care areas: ORs, post-anaesthesia care unit (PACU), or intensive care unit (ICU). Point-of-care testing largely eliminates transport times and provides information in clinically useful timeframes, often minutes (3).

Point-of-care testing of blood samples falls into several broad groups with some overlap (3). The first is coagulation with the activated clotting time and thromboelastography (TEG), which are discussed elsewhere (Chapter 16). The second group of tests comprises the three classic blood gas variables: partial pressures of oxygen, carbon dioxide, and pH. Clinical chemistry (table 10.1) overlaps with acid–base chemistry (4–6) and is provided by specific electrodes added to blood gas machines (7,8): this often includes sodium, potassium, chloride, lactate, calcium, and glucose. A further component is haemoglobin measurement and co-oximetry (9). An important point is that all clinical blood tests discussed are performed at 37°C (10). Therefore if a patient's temperature varies from 37°C (usually hypothermic in the OR and early postoperative

period (11) some variables, particularly gas partial pressures and derived variables, will differ between the measured and actual values. The alpha-stat and pH-stat approaches to acid–base regulation (Chapter 11) attempt to deal with these temperature-related differences.

Carbon dioxide

Control of carbon dioxide is central to control of perioperative acid–base status. Blood gas machines directly measure the partial pressure of carbon dioxide using a Severinghaus electrode (10). Carbon dioxide is widely measured in mmHg or the SI unit kPa (conversion: 1 mmHg = 0.13 kPa). Changes in the arterial partial pressure of carbon dioxide are associated with respiratory acidosis and alkalosis. These changes can aggravate or attenuate any co-existing metabolic acid–base changes.

The relationship between the alveolar P_ACO_2 (or arterial partial) pressure of carbon dioxide and alveolar ventilation V_A is described by the universal alveolar equation for an excreted gas (12,13):

$$P_ACO_2 = P_ICO_2 + K \times \frac{VCO_2}{V_A} \qquad \text{(Equation 10.1)}$$

Table 10.1 Bedside guide to changes in acid–base variables in primary disorders

Primary disorder	pH	PaCO$_2$ mmHg	Bicarbonate, mmol/L	Base-excess, mmol/L
Acute respiratory acidosis	<7.35	>45	(pCO$_2$–40)/10 + 24*	0*
Acute respiratory alkalosis	>7.45	<35	24 –(40– pCO$_2$)/5*	0*
Metabolic acidosis	<7.35	40 + SBE*	<22	<– 3
Metabolic alkalosis	>7.45	40 + SBE/2*	>26	> 3
Chronic respiratory acidosis	<7.40	>45	(pCO$_2$ – 40)/3 + 24*	(pCO$_2$ – 40)/2*
Chronic respiratory alkalosis	>7.40	<35	24 – (40 – pCO$_2$)/2*	(pCO$_2$–40)/2*

*Expected compensation in primary disorder, modified from (4) and (15). Where PaCO$_2$, arterial carbon dioxide tenson, mmHg: millimetres of mercury, SBE standard base excess

Where P_ICO_2 is the partial pressure of inspired carbon dioxide, K is a constant, and VCO_2 is the production of carbon dioxide (usually mL) per minute. In the absence of rebreathing or supplemental CO_2 the P_ICO_2 is assumed to be zero and Equation 10.1 is simplified to its more familiar form (Equation 10.2):

$$P_ACO_2 = K \times \frac{VCO_2}{V_A} \qquad \text{(Equation 10.2)}$$

An increase in the measured arterial partial pressure of carbon dioxide is most often due to decreased alveolar minute ventilation secondary to decreased total minute ventilation and/or increased dead physiological dead space: a greater proportion of lung segments have high ventilation/perfusion units (dead space). Conversely, decreased partial pressure of carbon dioxide is associated with increased alveolar ventilation.

The partial pressure of end-tidal carbon dioxide is measured using different (usually infra-red) technology. Arterial to end-tidal gradients for carbon dioxide are often due to a combination of ventilation/perfusion mismatch and difference between the measuring temperatures in the blood gas machine (37°C) and the expired gas analyser which is often closer to body temperature.

Oxygen

Control of oxygen is important in cardiac anaesthesia and is a central focus of thoracic anaesthesia. The partial pressure of oxygen in blood is measured using a Clark electrode (10). Like carbon dioxide, oxygen is widely measured in mmHg or the SI unit kPa. There are cascading decreases in the partial pressure of oxygen between the atmosphere and arterial or venous blood. Interpretation of the arterial or venous partial pressure of oxygen involves several factors.

The universal alveolar gas equation for an absorbed gas (12,13) links the alveolar partial pressure of oxygen with the inspired partial pressure of oxygen, alveolar ventilation, and oxygen consumption.

$$P_AO_2 = P_IO_2 - K \times \frac{VO_2}{V_A} \qquad \text{(Equation 10.3)}$$

From Equation 10.3, alveolar hypoxia, and arterial hypoxaemia, can be associated with decreased inspired oxygen as a result of decreased barometric pressure and/or decreased fraction of inspired oxygen, decreased alveolar ventilation, or increased oxygen consumption.

Other respiratory causes of hypoxaemia include lung units with low ventilation perfusion ratios or true shunt (no ventilation); or diffusion limitation (12). Quantifying these abnormalities in gas exchange requires determining the difference between a measure of alveolar partial pressure of oxygen and the arterial partial pressure. Clinically, it is not possible to determine alveolar ventilation and so the arterial partial pressure of carbon dioxide is used as an indirect or inverse measure. For clinical utility the alveolar gas equation (Equation 10.4) combines the universal gas equations for carbon dioxide (Equation 10.2) and oxygen (Equation 10.3).

$$P_AO_2 = P_IO_2 - \frac{P_ACO_2}{RR} \qquad \text{(Equation 10.4)}$$

Where RR is the respiratory exchange ratio: $\frac{VCO_2}{VO_2}$.

The alveolar gas equation allows us to estimate the partial pressure of oxygen in an ideal lung unit (ventilation/perfusion ratio of 1) for the given inspired oxygen, ventilation and oxygen consumption. This ideal partial pressure is required to estimate impaired gas exchange using the alveolar to arterial oxygen gradient; other aids are the ratio of arterial partial pressure of oxygen to the inspired fraction of oxygen (PaO_2/FiO_2 ratio), and the shunt equation (14). The alveolar arterial oxygen gradient is usually less than 15 mmHg in healthy younger people and less than 37.5 mmHg in healthy older people (15). Increasing alveolar–arterial oxygen gradient is associated with impaired gas exchange particularly ventilation / perfusion mismatch and diffusion limitation (15).

The PaO_2/FiO_2 ratio (14,15) is widely used in critical care medicine. For a healthy person with an arterial partial pressure of oxygen of 85 mmHg breathing room air (0.21 fraction) the PaO_2/FiO_2 ratio is about 400. A PaO_2/FiO_2 ratio of less than 300 represents impaired gas exchange and less than 200 severely impaired gas exchange. The PaO_2/FiO_2 ratio will be further decreased with hypoventilation as indicated by hypercapnia. Like all monitoring modalities, the alveolar gas equation and the PaO_2/FiO_2 ratio have limitations particularly with higher inspired oxygen fractions (FiO_2) (14) and altered barometric pressure (15).

Oximetry

Many blood gas machines report the haemoglobin concentration and oxygen saturation from co-oximetry (9). These devices have technology related to pulse oximetry where absorption of light of known wavelengths is associated with haemoglobin species. In co-oximetry at least four wavelengths of light are used to detect the four principal haemoglobin species: oxyhaemoglobin, reduced (deoxy) haemoglobin, methaemoglobin, and carboxyhaemoglobin. The total haemoglobin concentration is the sum of these four species. The haemoglobin saturation measured using the amount of oxyhaemoglobin divided by the sum of all four haemoglobin species is the fractional haemoglobin (Equation 10.5) (HbO_2) (9).

$$HbO_2 = \text{oxyhaemoglobin/(oxyhaemoglobin + reduced}$$
$$\text{haemoglobin + methaemoglobin + carboxyhaemoglobin)}$$
$$\text{(Equation 10.5)}$$

The haemoglobin saturation is usually reported, however, as the functional haemoglobin saturation (9) (SO_2, Equation 10.5), omitting the methaemoglobin and carboxyhaemoglobin contents (Equation 10.6):

$$SO_2 = \text{oxyhaemoglobin/(oxyhaemoglobin +}$$
$$\text{reduced haemoglobin)} \qquad \text{(Equation 10.6)}$$

The functional haemoglobin saturation more closely reflects the saturation measured by pulse oximeters, which use two wavelengths to estimate the oxyhaemoglobin and reduced haemoglobin

(9). While arterial oxygen measurements are most frequently measured during thoracic and cardiac surgery, there is growing use of central venous and mixed venous oxygen saturations.

Hydrogen ion concentration

The third component of routine blood gas analysis is pH, which is a mathematical transformation of the hydrogen ion (H$^+$) concentration (Equation 10.7) (10):

$$pH = \log_{10}\left(\frac{1}{H^+}\right) \qquad \text{(Equation 10.7)}$$

Hydrogen ion concentration is the central mechanism for (patho) physiologic effects of acid–base changes. pH is measured with a glass electrode (10). The reference range for pH (which has no units) is 7.35 to 7.45. The corresponding hydrogen ion reference range is 35 to 45 nmol/L. In many instances clinically important acidosis is a pH less than 7.25; however, in patients at risk of pulmonary hypertension, a clinically important effect may occur at a higher or more alkaline levels of pH.

Bicarbonate and base-excess

Two derived acid–base variables are bicarbonate and base-excess (box 10.1) (6,10). Blood gas machines calculate bicarbonate from the measured pH and partial pressure of carbon dioxide using the Henderson–Hasselbalch equation (10). Bicarbonate can be used to qualitatively (6,15,16) assess whether acid–base changes are primary respiratory or mixed disorders or mixed disorders (table 10.1). The bicarbonate approach does not, however, quantify the changes. An important point is that the reference value for

---

Box 10.1 A brief history of base-excess

One problem with using bicarbonate as a measure of metabolic acid-base status is that the plasma bicarbonate concentration is partly dependent on the partial pressure of carbon dioxide. Base-excess was developed by Sigaard-Anderson from Denmark, who studied blood equilibrated with an atmosphere of 40 mmHg carbon dioxide to eliminate respiratory acid-base effects. He defined base-excess as the amount of strong acid (HCl) in mmol/L required to return an alkaline blood sample to pH 7.40 at 37°C, pCO$_2$ 40 mmHg (6,10). In an acidaemic sample this would be the amount of strong base (NaOH) required to return the blood to pH 7.40. Opponents of base-excess from the United States pointed out, and continue to do so, that the pH buffering of blood in vitro differed from blood in-vivo because in vivo blood is in continuity with the extracellular fluid which has less pH buffering capacity. Sigaard-Andersen produced a modified, more physiologic, variable he called the standard base-excess also known as the plasma or extracellular fluid (ECF) base-excess. The mirror image to base-excess is the base-deficit. Despite the greater physiological utility of the standard base-excess, many clinicians, particularly nephrologists in the United States, prefer to use 'rules of thumb' to determine if a disorder is a primary disorder with compensation or a mixed respiratory and metabolic disorder (27). Table 10.1 demonstrates how base-excess simplifies this process.

---

bicarbonate is assumed to be exactly 24 mmol/L when determining expected compensatory changes for primary acid–base disorders.

Base-excess is a more useful quantitative measure of metabolic acid–base status (box 10.1). Blood gas machines calculate standard base-excess from the measured pH and calculated bicarbonate using the Van Slyke equation (9). For reasons that are unclear, some blood gas machines report both the standard base-excess (SBE) and the original, but less reliable, actual base-excess (ABE). The standard base-excess is preferred clinically (10). The reference range for standard base-excess is –3 to 3 mmol/L. As a patient develops a greater metabolic acidosis the base-excess becomes more negative and the base-deficit which is the mirror image, becomes more positive. A clinically important acidosis may be a base-excess of –5 mmol/L or less (17).

Sodium

Sodium is the major cation (positive ion) in the plasma and extracellular fluid (4,6). It is the most important single factor governing extracellular water distribution and osmotic pressure (7). Hyponatraemia and hypernatraemia and the rapidity of their correction are associated with adverse events and mortality (5,18). Further, sodium concentration is an important part of several physiologically important calculated variables (table 10.2) including osmolality, water deficit, anion-gap, strong ion difference, and strong-ion-gap. The strong ion difference is a central component of the Stewart approach to acid–base disorders (box 10.2). Assessment of plasma sodium concentration is central to individualized fluid therapy (5).

While central laboratories assays use indirect electrodes, blood gas machines use ion-specific electrodes (7,8). Ion-specific electrodes are less sensitive to changes in plasma solids including albumin than the central laboratory assays. While the relatively rare psuedohyponatraemia that is associated with increased plasma solids (7,8), is often mentioned, a far more frequent but rarely mentioned phenomenon is apparent increases in measured plasma sodium concentration associated with decreased plasma albumin with many central laboratory assays (8). In contrast to high turn over central laboratory assays, the ion-specific electrodes used in point-of-care machines are less sensitive to changes in albumin and are the preferred method to determine sodium for patients with varying plasma albumin concentrations, common in cardiothoracic surgery (8).

Potassium

While potassium is the principal intracellular cation, deviations in the plasma that is extracellular, concentration do, however, often indicate important disturbances in body potassium homeostasis and are associated with important arrhythmias (7,9,19). This is particularly so after cardiopulmonary bypass. In blood gas machines, plasma potassium is measured using an ion-specific electrode (7,8). Patients presenting for cardiothoracic surgery often have renal impairment, both acute and chronic ranging in severity from mild increases in plasma creatinine, and decreased glomerular filtration rate, to requiring renal replacement therapy. Patients with renal impairment are at increased risk of hyperkalaemia, which can be exacerbated by respiratory acidosis secondary to relative hypoventilation (Equation 10.1 and Equation 10.2) and hyperchloraemic acidosis from fluid therapy (5). While the plasma concentration of potassium is small compared to sodium, the contribution of potassium to derived variables such

Table 10.2 Derived measures using sodium

Osmolality, mosmol/L = 2Na$^+$ + glucose + urea
Altered total Body water = 140 × Ideal body water / measured sodium
Altered − Ideal = water deficit
Anion-gap, mmol/L = Na$^+$ + K$^+$ − Cl$^-$ − HCO$_3^-$
Albumin corrected anion gap = anion gap − (42-measured albumin)/4
Measured strong-ion-difference, meq/L = Na+K+2Ca+2 Mg-Cl-Lactate
Strong-ion-gap= Measured strong ion difference − bicarbonate − albumin/4−phosphate/3

Box 10.2 Stewart approach to acid–base

The major difference between Stewart's quantative approach to acid-base disorders and the widely used bicarbonate centred approach is the suggested mechanism for metabolic (non-respiratory) changes (4,6,15,16). In Stewart's approach, instead of bicarbonate being the primary mechanism for metabolic changes, bicarbonate is a dependent marker of, not the mechanism for, changes in hydrogen ion concentration and therefore pH. Stewart's mechanism for changes in pH is changes in the strong-ion-difference (concentrations of completely dissociated ions), and the concentration of weak (partly dissociated) acids. The most important strong cations in plasma are sodium ions and to a lesser extent potassium, calcium and magnesium ions. The important, measured, strong anions in plasma are chloride and lactate (21). As the difference in the sum of strong cations minus the strong anions: the strong ions difference (table 10.2) decreases there is greater acidosis (lower pH) associated with decreased bicarbonate. The converse is true with increased strong-ion-difference with greater alkalosis.

The other mechanism controlling the metabolic acid–base status is the total weak acids. In plasma the important weak acids are albumin, and to a lesser extent, phosphate (16). As the concentration of total weak acids increases acidosis increases, however, decreased weak acids, particularly albumin, with associated alkalosis is more common in critically ill patients. In Stewart's approach the role and interpretation of the partial pressure of carbon dioxide is similar to the bicarbonate centred approach. Stewart's approach can be integrated with base-excess by examining the base-excess effects of strong ions (particularly sodium and chloride), weak acids (particularly albumin) and other ions 16 17). Using the albumin corrected anion gap is now accepted by many of those using bicarbonate centred approaches. Stewart's approach is often misrepresented in the literature, particularly nephrology literature (27), as being in competition with the bicarbonate and base-excess approaches to metabolic acid–base disorders. While Stewart's approach challenges the central mechanistic role of bicarbonate it does not eliminate bicarbonate as a marker of acid–base changes. The use of bicarbonate rules-of-thumb is largely qualitative while Stewart's is a detailed quantitative approach. Stewart's approach can be used to enhance the use of base-excess, a quantitative measure of acid–base change (16,17).

as the anion gap and measured strong ion difference can vary by several meq/L, supporting inclusion of potassium in these calculations for patients undergoing cardiothoracic surgery.

Chloride

Quantitatively chloride is the dominant anion in plasma and the extracellular fluid. The importance of measuring chloride for understanding clinical chemistry has often been underestimated (20). In blood gas machines, plasma chloride is measured using an ion-specific electrode (8,9). Hyperchloraemic metabolic acidosis secondary to fluid therapy is a frequent event both in operating rooms and ICUs. From a (qualitative) bicarbonate point of view hyperchloremic acidosis is a narrow anion gap metabolic acidosis (15). From a Stewart point of view (box 10.2), if all other variables were the same, the decrease in base-excess and bicarbonate is quantitatively inversely related in a one to one ratio to increases in chloride: a 1 mmol/L increase in chloride is associated with a 1 mmol/L decrease in bicarbonate and base-excess (16). The overall acid–base status or severity of acidaemia, will also depend on the cation concentration: hyperchloraemic metabolic acidosis is a relative phenomenon (21). Patients with hyponatraemia can have significant hyperchloraemic metabolic acidosis with chloride concentrations in the reference range but a decreased strong-ion-difference. While clinical evidence is still emerging, sodium chloride fluid therapy, and resulting hyperchloraemia has been associated with organ dysfunction, notably renal dysfunction (16).

Lactate

Lactate is both a metabolic product and substrate (15). Increased lactate is associated with increased lactate production and/ or decreased lactate clearance (15). Increased lactate, often with acidaemia, is associated with increased complications and mortality in the perioperative period (15,22). In hospitalized patients the upper limit of the reference range for blood lactate is about 1.5 mmol/L. While the rate of lactate change is important, an absolute blood concentration of greater than 4 mmol/L is likely to be clinically important (22). Lactate is an anion that is completely dissociated in plasma and extracellular fluid and is therefore a strong anion. In the past, lactic acidosis has been inferred from metabolic acidosis with widened anion gap (table 10.2) (22). Because blood gas machines can now routinely measure lactate, the role of calculating the anion gap in patients with metabolic acidosis has changed (22). In the past, a widened anion gap was used to determine if other anions, including lactate, were associated with acidosis. The anion gap only plays this role if lactate analysis is not immediately available or as a measure of other unmeasured anions once lactate is accounted for (15,22). A more detailed version is the strong-ion-gap (table 10.2) (23). Like chloride a 1 mmol/L increase in lactate is associated with a 1 mmol/L decrease in bicarbonate and base-excess, if other factors particularly the sodium concentration remain, constant (21). In critical care patients, the anion gap should be routinely corrected for changes that usually are the result of decreases in plasma albumin (4). Albumin, however, is not measured in standard point-of-care machines.

Calcium

Calcium is a cation with important roles in physiological function including coagulation, cardiac rhythm, inotropy, and vascular tone (15,24). While often incorrectly called ionized calcium, free calcium, as opposed to bound calcium, is the biologically important component of plasma calcium (15,24). In the perioperative period, hypocalcaemia is most often associated with the transfused blood products due to binding with citrate. Following massive transfusion mortality has been associated with the severity of hypocalcaemia (24).

Glucose

Glucose is the central metabolic substrate. Hyperglycaemia is common among patients during and after cardiothoracic surgery, some of whom will have undiagnosed diabetes mellitus. Frequents measurement of blood glucose is a cornerstone for managing perioperative patients with known diabetes mellitus (25). While there has been enthusiasm for tight control of perioperative glucose, recent studies in patients in ICU and undergoing cardiac surgery have found that tight glucose control is associated with increased mortality and morbidity (26). Currently, moderate control appears the preferred approach; that is, blood glucose 5 to 10 mmol/L, avoiding both hyperglycaemia with risks including infections and hypoglycaemia with risks including neuronal injury (25–27).

Conclusion

Measurement of arterial blood gases, acid–base balance and clinical chemistry is fundamental to the care of patients undergoing cardiothoracic anaesthesia and critical care. Not only does it allow diagnosis of the complications of cardiothoracic surgery but it allows assessment of effectiveness of their treatment.

References

1. Harrington DK, Ranasinghe AM, Shah A, Oelofse T, Bonser RS. Recommendations for haemodynamic and neurological monitoring in repair of acute type a aortic dissection. *Anesthesiol Res Pract* 2011; **2011**: 949034
2. Bruells CS, Rossaint R. Physiology of gas exchange during anaesthesia. *Eur J Anaesthesiol* 2011; **28**(8): 570–9
3. Rhee AJ, Kahn RA. Laboratory point-of-care monitoring in the operating room. *Curr Opin Anaesthesiol* 2010; **23**(6): 741–8
4. Kellum JA. Disorders of acid–base balance. *Crit Care Med* 2007; **35**(11): 2630–6
5. Kaplan LJ, Kellum JA. Fluids, pH, ions and electrolytes. *Curr Opin Crit Care* 2010; **16**(4): 323–31
6. Story DA. Bench-to-bedside review: A brief history of clinical acid-base. *Critical Care* 2004; 8: 253–8
7. Hood JS, Scott MG. Physiology and disorders of water, electrolyte, and acid-base metabolism. In: Burtis CA, Ashwood ER, Bruns DE, eds. *Tietz Textbook of Clinical Chemistry and Molecular Diagnostics*, 5th ed. Philadelphia: Elsevier, 2012; 1609–35
8. Story DA, Morimatsu H, Egi M, Bellomo R. The effect of albumin concentration on plasma sodium and chloride measurements in critically ill patients. *Anesth Analg* 2007; **104**(4): 893–7
9. Scott MG, LeGrys VA, Hood JL. Electrolytes and blood gases. In: Burtis CA, Ashwood ER, Bruns DE, eds. *Tietz Textbook of Clinical Chemistry and Molecular Diagnostics*, 5th ed. Philadelphia: Elsevier, 2012; 807–35
10. Severinghaus J, Astrup P, Murray J. Blood gas analysis and critical care medicine. *Am J Resp Crit Care Med* 1998; **157**: S114–S22
11. Karalapillai D, Story DA, Calzavacca P, Licari E, Liu YL, Hart GK. Inadvertent hypothermia and mortality in postoperative intensive care patients: retrospective audit of 5050 patients. *Anaesthesia* 2009; **64**(9): 968–72
12. Eskaros S, Papadakos P, Lachman B. Respiratory Monitoring. In: Miller R, ed. *Miller's Anaesthesia*, 7th ed. Philadelphia: Churchill Livingstone, 2010; 1411–41
13. Story DA. Alveolar oxygen partial pressure, alveolar carbon dioxide partial pressure, and the alveolar gas equation. *Anesthesiology* 1996; **84**(4): 1011
14. Kathirgamanathan A, McCahon RA, Hardman JG. Indices of pulmonary oxygenation in pathological lung states: an investigation using high-fidelity, computational modelling. *Br J Anaesth* 2009; **103**(2): 291–7
15. Bersten AD, Soni N, editors. *Oh's Intensive Care Manual*, 6th ed. Philadelphia: Butterworth Heinemann, 2009.
16. Kellum JA, Elbers PWG, editors. *Stewart's Textbook of Acid–Base*. Amsterdam: AcidBase.Org, 2009
17. Story DA, Morimatsu H, Bellomo R. Strong ions, weak acids and base excess: a simplified Fencl-Stewart approach to clinical acid-base disorders. *Br J Anaesth* 2004; **92**(1): 54–60
18. Stelfox HT, Ahmed SB, Zygun D, Khandwala F, Laupland K. Characterization of intensive care unit acquired hyponatremia and hypernatremia following cardiac surgery. *Can J Anaesth* 2010; **57**(7): 650–8
19. Sedlacek M, Schoolwerth AC, Remillard BD. Electrolyte disturbances in the intensive care unit. *Semin Dial* 2006; **19**(6): 496–501
20. Yunos NM, Bellomo R, Story D, Kellum J. Bench-to-bedside review: Chloride in critical illness. *Crit Care* 2011; **14**(4): 226
21. Story DA, Morimatsu H, Bellomo R. Hyperchloremic acidosis in the critically ill: one of the strong-ion acidoses? *Anesth Analg* 2006; **103**(1): 144–8
22. Jansen TC, van Bommel J, Bakker J. Blood lactate monitoring in critically ill patients: a systematic health technology assessment. *Crit Care Med* 2009; **37**(10): 2827–39
23. Story DA. Filling the (strong ion) gap. *Crit Care Med* 2008; **36**(3): 998–9
24. Ho KM, Leonard AD. Concentration-dependent effect of hypocalcaemia on mortality of patients with critical bleeding requiring massive transfusion: a cohort study. *Anaesth Intensive Care* 2011; **39**(1): 46–54
25. Killen J, Tonks K, Greenfield J, Story DA. New insulin analogues and perioperative care of patients with type 1 diabetes. *Anaesth Intensive Care* 2010; **38**(2): 244–9
26. Egi M, Finfer S, Bellomo R. Glycemic control in the ICU. *Chest* 2011; **140**(1): 212–20
27. Adrogue HJ, Gennari FJ, Galla JH, Madias NE. Assessing acid–base disorders. *Kidney Int* 2009; **76**(12): 1239–47.

CHAPTER 11

Cardiopulmonary bypass

Marco Ranucci

Introduction

Cardiopulmonary bypass (CPB) is used in the great majority of operations on the heart. Whenever the procedure requires opening of the cardiac chambers, CPB is mandatory to replace the heart's pump function. For isolated coronary artery bypass graft (CABG) surgery, it is technically possible to perform the procedure without CPB that is off-pump. Off-pump coronary artery bypass (OPCAB) regained popularity in the mid-1990s, and is still routinely or occasionally performed in some institutions (Chapter 20). However, the rate of OPCAB reached a plateau in the early decade of the new millennium, settled at about 20% of the total coronary operations in the USA (1).

During heart surgery, CPB is used to replace the functions of the heart and lungs by diverting blood from the patient's venous system towards a pump then an artificial lung so bypassing the heart and lungs. This is undertaken with or without arresting the heart and by returning the blood into the arterial system after being oxygenated and depleted of excess carbon dioxide (CO_2).

Cardiopulmonary bypass circuit

A standard CPB circuit includes venous cannulae, left-heart venting cannula, a venous blood reservoir, a pump, an oxygenator, an arterial line filter, and an arterial cannula. A system of tubings connects the various items of the CPB circuit. Thermal management is obtained by a heat-exchanging system incorporated in the oxygenator or by an external one.

Venous cannulas and venous cannulation

Depending on the type of the surgical operation, one or two venous cannulae may be used. Venous cannulation aims to divert all the blood from the systemic venous circulation into the CPB circuit. This may be achieved by simply placing a single, two-staged, venous cannula through the right atrium inside the inferior vena cava: the blood from the inferior vena cava is drained through the venous cannula tip, and the blood from the superior vena cava reaches the right atrium and is drained by an additional set of holes (figure 11.1). This cannulation is commonly used in CABG surgery and for surgery of the aortic valve and/or ascending aorta. Due to the presence of a large cannula inside the right atrium, this cannulation does not allow opening the right atrium and makes it technically difficult to open the left atrium. Therefore, operations requiring a direct access to the right or left atrium, such as atrial septal defect closure and mitral valve or tricuspid valve surgery, require two venous cannulae. These

cannulae are placed and snared inside the inferior and superior vena cava so preventing systemic venous blood entering the cardiac chambers (figure 11.2).

Both cannulation techniques require first opening of the chest and direct access to the heart. An alternative approach to venous cannulation may be achieved indirectly, through the femoral or the right internal jugular veins, which does not require direct access to the heart. The cannulae may be placed percutaneously or by surgical cut-down and direct exposure of the femoral vein. Indirect venous cannulation, together with a femoral artery cannulation, is used to establish CPB before opening the chest; this is a safety procedure to unload the heart so as to limit the risk of damage to the heart and major vessels during sternotomy in redo surgery or whenever the chest conditions are hostile, such as presence of previously implanted artificial vessel grafts or previously implanted and patent coronary artery grafts. Additionally, indirect venous cannulation using the jugular, femoral, or both veins, is used for a mini-thoracotomy approach for atrial septal defect, aortic valve, and mitral valve surgery.

Left heart venting

Despite a total drainage of the systemic venous blood, the left heart chamber is not totally drained because de-oxygenated blood from the arterial bronchial blood flow drains into the left atrium. Although the bronchial blood flow is only 1% to 2% of the cardiac output, it is enough to progressively load the left heart chambers. Therefore, adequate measures must be taken to

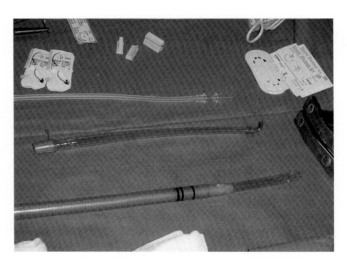

Fig. 11.1 Single-stage venous cannula and ascending aorta cannula.

drain this blood flow back into the CPB circuit. This procedure is known as venting of the left heart chambers and specific cannulae are included in the CPB circuit to fulfill this requirement. Left heart venting may be obtained by diverting blood from the ascending aorta, usually using the cardioplegia delivery cannula, either in a passive, gravitational fashion, or actively using a dedicated roller pump. This approach is mainly used for CABG operations. Direct venting of the left atrium may be also undertaken with a direct cannulation of left atrium. Additional methods include cannulation and active suction from the pulmonary veins or the pulmonary artery.

Venous blood reservoir

The venous blood reservoir, also known as *cardiotomy reservoir*, may be either constituted of a hard shell container (figure 11.3) or a collapsible bag (figure 11.4). When a collapsible bag is used, the blood is always passively drained siphoned from the heart chambers using gravity. If a hard-shell reservoir is used then the blood may be drained passively or actively, by applying a negative pressure to the reservoir which is called vacuum-assisted drainage. Vacuum-assisted drainage better empties the cardiac chambers, and reduces the size of venous cannulae and tubing required.

Pumps

The pump included in the CPB circuit actively pumps the blood from the venous reservoir into the oxygenator. Pumps used for CPB have roller or centrifugal mechanisms.

Roller pumps (figure 11.5) use an occlusive mechanism that comes into direct contact with a specific part of the CPB tubing. When the pump rotates, the tubing is squeezed against a back-plate, propelling blood forward. The amount of blood being pumped in each rotation depends on the tubing size (internal diameter) and on the diameter of the pump head. The blood flow is regulated by the pump speed in revolutions per minute. Based on simple calculations, the total pump flow is estimated and shown in a display. The precision of this calculation depends on the quality of the 'occlusion' of the pump head. Insufficient occlusion leads

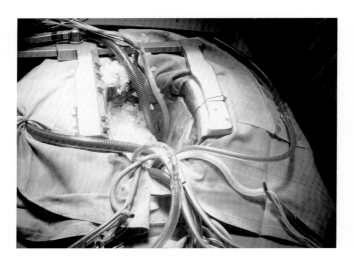

Fig. 11.2 Bicaval venous cannulation and ascending aorta cannulation.

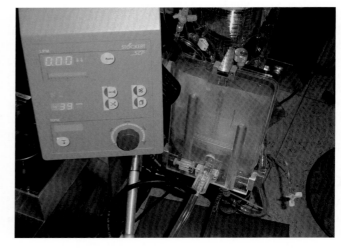

Fig. 11.4 Collapsible soft-bag venous reservoir.

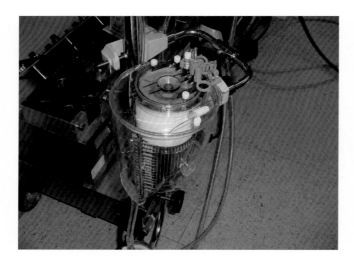

Fig. 11.3 Hard-shell venous cardiotomy reservoir.

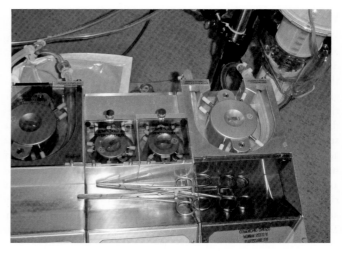

Fig. 11.5 Roller pump.

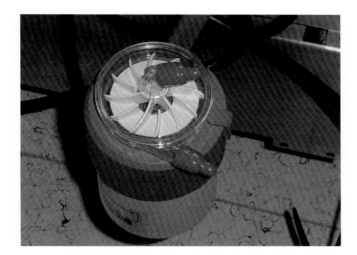

Fig. 11.6 Centrifugal pump.

Table 11.1 Differences between roller and centrifugal pumps

Roller Pump	Centrifugal Pump
Occlusive	Non-occlusive
Pump flow (relatively) constant	Pump flow dependent on pre- and afterload
Pump flow calculated	Pump flow directly measured
Spallation of the tubing	No spallation
Haemolysis dependent on degree of tubing occlusion	Minimal haemolysis
May cause massive air embolism	Small air bubbles are not pumped
Platelet damage	Less platelet consumption in long pump runs
Lower safety profile	Higher safety profile
Lower cost	More expensive

to an overestimation of the actual pump flow, whereas excessive occlusion damages blood cells and dangerously mechanical stresses the tubing.

Centrifugal pumps (figure 11.6) generate blood flow by imparting kinetic energy to the blood. Some pumps are based on a nested cones constrained vortex, while others use vertical vane impellors. In both cases, blood enters the upper part of the pump, and is propelled out through a lateral escape port. Centrifugal pumps are very different from the roller pumps in practice, and the main differences are summarized in table 11.1. Basically, the pump speed (rpm) is only one of the determinants of pump flow, and no mathematical calculation can be applied to assess the actual pump flow. For this reason, a direct measurement of blood flow is required, using a flow transducer placed on the arterial line. Centrifugal pumps are not occlusive at all, and crucially, the arterial line must be clamped whenever they are stopped, to prevent back flow and so drainage of blood into the reservoir from the aorta. The kinetic energy that is imparted to the blood is variable, and depends on the venous blood pressure at the inlet and

on the arterial line resistances. At a stable pump speed, the pump flow is directly proportional with the inlet pressure (preload) and inversely proportional with the arterial resistances (afterload); therefore resembling the natural functioning of the left ventricle.

Being non-occlusive, centrifugal pumps are safer in event of accidental cross-clamping of the arterial line as zero flow will occur, which is in contrast to the roller pumps that will exert increasing pressure on the circuit causing rupture of the arterial line. Another safety benefit is that centrifugal pumps will not pump forward small amounts of air that have accidentally entered the circuit, because small air bubbles receive less kinetic energy than blood. However, when large amounts of air enter the circuit, gaseous embolism may still occur. Finally, especially when the duration of CPB is prolonged, centrifugal pumps cause less damage to red blood cells and consumption of platelets (2,3).

In North America, centrifugal pumps are used for the great majority of CPB procedures whereas their routine use is less established in Europe and other continents. The explanation for this disparity is that, despite centrifugal pumps having a better safety profile, studies have not found a significant difference in patient outcome when they have been compared roller pumps (4,5).

Oxygenators

The oxygenator is an artificial lung that oxygenates and removes CO_2 from the systemic venous blood. The first routinely used oxygenators achieved the gas transfer by direct contact between blood and gas (mainly oxygen). Bubble oxygenators were still in use until the early 1990s, and were based on bubbling oxygen (O_2) directly into the venous blood. Nowadays, the oxygenators currently used for routine CPB are membrane oxygenators (figure 11.7). These oxygenators have a semipermeable membrane that separates blood and gas, and the gas transfer is either by transmembrane diffusion or micropores. The membrane can be flat, or formed into hollow fibres. In the latter, blood flows outside and gas inside, the fibres. The gas mixture is a combination of air and O_2, at variable flow rates. Nitrous oxide is avoided, due to the risk of gas bubble size increase and volatile anaesthetic agents may be administered according to the instructions of the oxygenator's manufacturer.

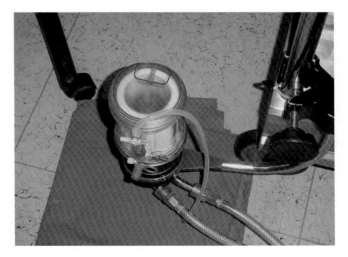

Fig. 11.7 Hollow-fibre oxygenator.

The oxygenator follows the same gas transfer rules of the native lung but with some important differences. As in the native lung, the gas transfer depends on the membrane permeability—the equivalent of the alveolo-capillary membrane—which, in turn, depends on the diameter of the micropores or the thickness of the membrane. O_2 and CO_2 transfer across the membrane follows their pressure gradients. As in the native lung, the ratio of ventilation to perfusion (Va/Qc) is important determinant of the efficacy of the gas transfer. O_2 transfer is the most critical process. Whilst the new-generation oxygenators are safe with respect to O_2 transfer even when CPB is prolonged, O_2 transfer suffers from a time-related impairment, due to the adsorption of proteins and platelets on to the surface of the hollow-fibres. A progressive plasma-leak may further deteriorate the efficiency of hollow-fibre oxygenators. If O_2 transfer becomes insufficient then the perfusionist may may compensate by increasing the O_2 content of the gas mixture of the sweep gas to the oxygenator.

Due to its high solubility, CO_2 removal is much more efficient in the oxygenators compared to the lungs. For this reason, the Va/Qc during CPB must be controlled far below the normal value of 0.8. Usually, a gas flow around 25% to 30% of the pump flow is enough to maintain the arterial CO_2 tension ($PaCO_2$) within the normal range. The $PaCO_2$ can be adjusted at the desired value by increasing or decreasing the gas flow rate through the oxygenator.

Arterial line filters

The routine use of arterial line filters is recommended by all the existing CPB guidelines. Arterial line filters represent a safety measure to prevent gaseous embolism as well as particulate embolism by microaggregates, fat, or plasticizers from the CPB circuit. They are structured as a filtering net with 20–40 μm pore size.

Leukocyte-depleting filters appear to reduce the inflammatory response to CPB (6). However, leukodepleting filters may activate neutrophils (7,8), and the recently released Society of Thoracic Surgeons—Society of Cardiovascular Anesthesiologists Blood Conservation Guidelines do not recommend their use during CPB (9).

Arterial cannulas and arterial cannulation

In routine CPB, the arterial cannula closes the loop of the CPB circuit by returning the oxygenated blood into the systemic circulation, and is usually placed at the level of the ascending aorta (figure 11.8). However, different sites of arterial cannulation may be used, and theoretically, every large artery may be used for this purpose. As discussed in the section on cannulation of the femoral artery, it may be used for safety reasons. Femoral artery cannulation reverses the systemic circulation and rarely, hypoperfusion of the brain is possible. Other cannulation sites include the right subclavian artery, which is particularly useful for surgery of acute ascending aortic dissection (Chapter 22).

Heat-exchanging system

Control of the patient's body temperature is achieved using a heat-exchanging system. As well as different degrees of hypothermia induced during CPB, this system provides a control over the inevitable fall in body temperature due to the contact of blood with a large foreign surface. All oxygenators include a heat-exchanger, which is composed of folded layers of aluminium separating blood from non-sterile water that flows counter-currently within the heat-exchanger. An external console regulates the temperature of

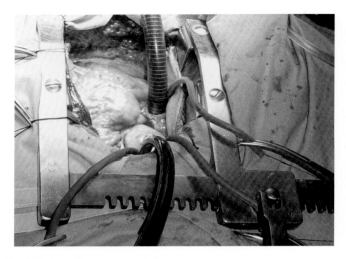

Fig. 11.8 Ascending aorta cannulation.

the water and allows the patient to be cooled or rewarmed. The patient's temperature should be monitored with adequate sensors, which may be placed on the skin, in the oesophagus, rectum or bladder, or on the tympanic membrane.

Monitoring the quality of cardiopulmonary bypass and the adequacy of pump flow

Standard controls during cardiopulmonary bypass

CPB is a dynamic procedure inducing many pathophysiological changes in the patient's homeostasis. A strict control of the effects of CPB and monitoring of the adequacy of the pump flow rate are mandatory. Table 11.2 includes the parameters that should be measured during CPB which should be done at a frequency dependent on local protocols but at least, at the onset of CPB and then every 30 minutes.

Some of these parameters including haematocrit, $PaCO_2$, PaO_2, mixed venous haemoglobin oxygen saturation, sodium and potassium concentrations, may be measured continuously with sensors placed on the arterial and venous line of the CPB circuit. Additional parameters such as near-infrared spectroscopy and thromboelastography may be also included depending on the operation and institutional practice.

Setting the pump flow rate and confirming adequacy of flow

Traditionally, the 'normal' pump flow (L/min) is established based on the body surface area (m²) and expressed as L/min/m². Under normothermic conditions, the pump flow should be settled at around 2.8–3.0 L/min/m². Under hypothermic conditions, this value may decrease in a linear fashion with temperature, and during the widely used, moderate hypothermia (32°C) CPB, the pump flow rate is usually about 2.4–2.6 L/min/m². This standardized concept of the 'normal' pump flow has been recently questioned by a number of observations. Low values (<22–24%) of haematocrit/haemoglobin during CPB have been associated with adverse outcomes in a number of retrospective studies (see Haemodilution)

Table 11.2 Parameters to be measured and documented during CPB

Biochemical Haematologic	Haemodynamic	Respiratory	Metabolic
Na^+ concentration	Pump flow	Gas flow	HCO_3^-
K^+ concentration	Mean arterial pressure	FiO_2	Base excess
Ionized Ca^{2+} concentration	Central venous or pulmonary artery pressure	PaO_2	SvO_2
Haematocrit or haemoglobin concentration		SaO_2	Lactate concentration
Activated clotting time or heparin/protamine assays	Urine output	$PaCO_2$	Temperature (blood and core)
			Glucose

(10–14). Severe haemodilution during CPB decreases the arterial O_2 content, and as a consequence, the systemic O_2 delivery (DO_2) is decreased unless the pump flow rate is increased, and this decrease in the DO_2 may in turn result in an inadequate O_2 supply to the peripheral organs. This condition is similar to that experienced by patients under cardiogenic or distributive shock, where the DO_2 is inadequate to sustain the systemic oxygen uptake oxygen ($\dot{V}O_2$). Whenever the DO_2 falls below a 'critical' value, the $\dot{V}O_2$ decreases, and to sustain the O_2 needs the anaerobic energy production is triggered, with a resulting metabolic acidosis and lactate formation (figure 11.9).

Some studies have identified that an inadequate DO_2 during CPB is the main determinant of the adverse outcomes including acute kidney injury that is observed after severe haemodilution during CPB (15–17). The critical value of the DO_2 during moderate hypothermia CPB is around 260–270 mL/min/m² (15–17). Below this value, lactate production progressively increases (18), and the likelihood of experiencing an acute kidney injury also increases (17). These observations result in a new concept as to

how the adequacy of the pump flow rate should be determined; this is based not only on the body surface area and the temperature, but also takes into account the arterial O_2 content in order to maintain the DO_2 above the critical value of 260 mL/min/m². The nomogram in figure 11.10 links the haematocrit with the pump flow rate needed to maintain the DO_2 above the critical value.

Anticoagulation during cardiopulmonary bypass

Anticoagulation during CPB is achieved using intravenous unfractionated heparin (UFH) (Chapter 16), at a variable loading dose of between 300–400 IU, before cannulation of the major vessels. This is then supplemented by additional boluses during CPB if required. To exert its anticoagulant properties, heparin needs the cofactor antithrombin (AT). AT is a natural anticoagulant, which inactivates the small doses of thrombin formed under normal circumstances. Heparin causes AT to inactivate not only thrombin, but also FIXa, FXa, FXIa, and FXIIa, 2000 times faster than normal. As discussed in Chapter 17, monitoring of anticoagulation during CPB is traditionally based on the activated clotting time (ACT), with a target ACT value settled at 450–480 seconds. This target ACT is more conventional than a well-established cut-off value, actually being based on an experiment carried on nine monkeys in 1978 (19). ACT has several important limitations including a lack of correlation with heparin concentration (20), it is poorly reproducible and changes depending on the activator that is used for example celite or kaolin, and the device used (21). More sensitive tools are the heparin-monitoring systems, which provide an in-vitro assessment of the heparin responsiveness by measuring the ACT in presence of different heparin concentrations (figure 11.11) (22). These devices can provide a useful information for determining the correct dose of protamine to inactivate heparin after weaning from CPB (22,23).

About 20% of the patients undergoing cardiac surgery have a poor response to heparin and referred to as 'heparin resistant' (9). Many factors contribute to a poor sensitivity to heparin are listed in table 11.3 (24–26).

When heparin resistance is encountered, the correct approach is diagnosis. Some patients who have thrombocytosis or increased

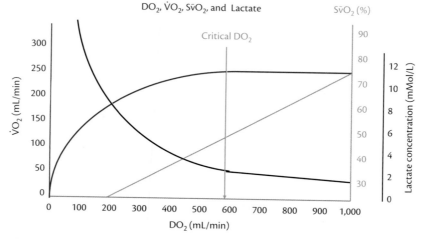

Fig. 11.9 The relationship between oxygen delivery (DO_2), oxygen uptake ($\dot{V}O_2$), mixed venous oxygen saturation ($S\bar{v}O_2$), and lactate formation.

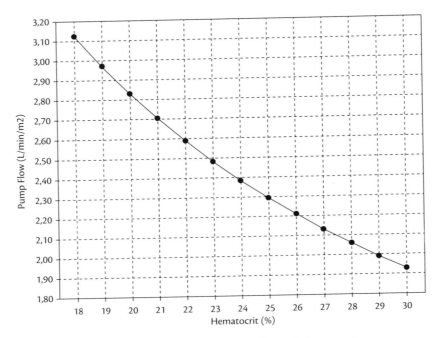

Fig. 11.10 A nomogram to maintain the DO_2 above the critical level by adjusting the pump flow to the haematocrit.

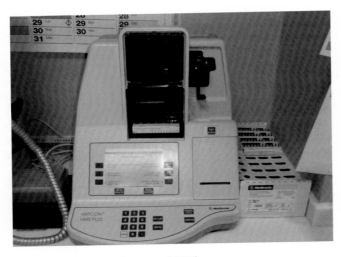

Fig. 11.11 Heparin monitoring system (HMS®).

Table 11.3 Main causes for a reduced heparin sensitivity ('heparin resistance')

Reduced heparin availability	Reduced antithrombin availability	Increased thrombin generation
Low amounts of active heparin in the drug preparation	Congenital antithrombin deficiency (rare)	Advanced age
	Acquired antithrombin deficiency due to chronic heparin administration, infections, liver disease	Diabetes mellitus
Incorrect heparin administration		Open heart procedures
Thrombocytosis		Prolonged Cardiopulmonary bypass
Heparin sequestration by Endothelium	Leukocytes Proteins	Congenital thrombophilic pattern

thrombin generation, may simply require additional heparin whilst others who AT values less than 80% before going on CPB, require AT concentrate and yet others need both the interventions. AT concentrate is recommended over the use of fresh frozen plasma to correct AT-dependent heparin resistance (9,27–29). Low levels of AT at the end of the operation or in the first 48 hours after the operation are associated with adverse outcomes (30,31), and the use of purified AT appears a reasonable option to prevent this outcome (9), although class I evidence is still lacking.

After successfully weaning from CPB, heparin is reversed using protamine sulphate, at a dose that remains controversial. Recently, it has been recognized that the conventional dose ratio of 1.3:1 protamine to heparin leads to excessive administration of protamine, and the current trend is to use a lower dose ratio, based on an initial 1:1 protamine to heparin. The use of heparin monitoring systems may allow to accurate estimation of the dose of protamine required to reverse heparin (22,32,33). Other near-patient tests that may be useful in diagnosing residual heparin effect after protamine administration include thromboelastography and thromboelastometry. A difference in the reaction time or coagulation time between blood samples with or without heparinase is suggestive for the need of additional protamine supplementation (figure 11.12).

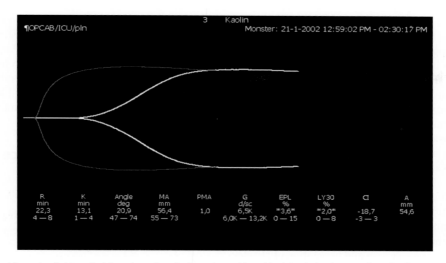

Fig. 11.12 Thromboelastographic tracing (with and without heparinase) of a patient with residual circulating heparin. (See also figure in colour plates section)

Blood activation

Material-dependent blood activation

Whenever blood comes in contact with foreign surfaces, a material-dependent blood activation through the contact phase is triggered. CPB, with its extensive contact surface area between blood and plasticizers, is a classical model of contact-phase activation.

Contact phase activation leads to the formation of a layer of proteins and cells on the foreign surface, as a result of a complex interaction between plasma proteins, coagulation factors, platelets, fibroblasts, and other blood cells, including leukocytes and red cells.

Fibrinogen is the main determinant of the initial protein layer on the foreign surface. This fibrinogen adhesion is mainly due to the interaction between the hydrophobic foreign surface and specific hydrophilic adhesion sites of fibrinogen. Other plasma proteins such as albumin and γ-globulins, are included in this initial protein layer. Once fibrinogen becomes bound, platelets will adhere to it, through the GPIIb-IIIa receptor. Therefore, in a time-dependent fashion, a final layer of proteins, platelets, and other blood cells will be formed.

The coagulation cascade is triggered by contact with foreign surfaces through the formerly defined intrinsic pathway (Chapter 16). The blood zymogen factor XII (also known as Hageman factor) is activated by contact into its active enzymatic form FXIIa. This activation is the result of the interaction between negatively charged surfaces and specific, positively charged lysine groups. FXII activation will in turn activate the pre-kallikrein, the high-molecular-weight kininogen, and FXI. This process leads to an auto-activation and amplification, leading to increased production of FXIIa (34).

As a result of the intrinsic pathway activation, and through the contribution of FIX and FX, prothrombin (FII) is activated to thrombin (FIIa). In the past, because of thrombin generation during CPB and the consequent need for thrombin antagonization with heparin, the contact phase was believed to be responsible for the majority of the thrombin formed during CPB. Recently, it has been established that simple material-dependent activation causes a relatively small amount of thrombin generation (35–37),

and most of the thrombin is generated by the extrinsic pathway, as a result of a material-independent blood activation.

Material-independent blood activation

During CPB, thrombin generation is greatly enhanced. The main pathway leading to thrombin generation starts with tissue factor (TF) release. Soluble TF is released from the surgical wound and its concentration increases during heart surgery (36). Cell-bound TF is expressed by the epicardium, myocardium, adventitia, and bone, and all these structures are injured during heart surgery (36,38). Thrombin generation triggered by TF release follows the extrinsic coagulation pathway. The current view is that, once TF is released from the damaged endothelial surface, it generates small amounts of thrombin (initiation). Thrombin activates platelets (amplification) and on the platelet surface a further, larger thrombin generation occurs (propagation). This large amount of thrombin triggers the conversion of fibrinogen to fibrin finally promoting stable clot formation (39).

TF released from the injured tissues is largely found in the pericardial shed blood. Once this blood is aspirated back into the CPB circuit and subsequently, enters into the systemic circulation, it triggers thrombin generation. Separation of shed blood from the systemic circulation greatly reduces thrombin generation (see Shed-blood management and Mini-CPB).

Biocompatibility of the cardiopulmonary bypass materials

The CPB circuit is composed by a number of different biomaterials: including polyvinyl chloride (tubings), silicone (roller pump tubings), polycarbonate (solid parts, hard shells), polypropylene (hollow fibres of the oxygenator), polyester (filtering nets), polyurethanes (potting and defoaming sponges), and aluminium (heat exchanger). All these foreign surfaces are recognized as 'non-self' by the human organism, and once the blood comes in contact with them, the various biochemical and cellular cascades described earlier are activated.

In order to improve the biocompatibility of the materials used for the CPB circuit, different additional surface treatments or coatings were introduced and applied in clinical practice during the last two decades of the twentieth century. The basic purpose of all these treatments is the attempt to mimic a natural endothelial surface, therefore reducing the reaction to 'non-self' materials.

The first generation of biocompatible treatments was based on surface bonding of heparin molecules. The natural endothelium actually contains heparin-like molecules, called glycosaminoglycans (GAGs), which contribute to the anticoagulant properties of the endothelium. In these heparin-bonded materials, heparin is either ionically or covalently bonded. Ionic-bonded heparin treatments are presently almost abandoned, whereas covalently bonded heparin surfaces are still used.

Heparin-bonded CPB circuits have been widely studied in in-vitro models, animal experiments, and humans for cardiac surgery. The majority of studies demonstrate that heparin-bonded surfaces decrease the inflammatory reaction to CPB, blunting complement activation and the release of cytokines, so inducing less activation of the haemostatic system and prevention of platelet adhesion and activation as well as a preservation of platelet count (40–44). These findings generated the hypothesis that the routine use of these materials might result in an improved postoperative outcome, by reducing a number of complications such as bleeding, atrial fibrillation, kidney failure, and lung dysfunction, which may be directly or indirectly linked to the activation of the inflammatory and coagulation systems.

However, a large multi-centre randomized controlled trial (RCT) of low-risk patients failed to demonstrate any difference in terms of postoperative outcome when treated with an ionic-bonded heparin circuit and oxygenator compared to a conventional circuit (45), which has tempered enthusiasm towards these materials. Subsequently, a second RCT could only demonstrate minor beneficial effects in a population of high-risk patients (46).

After these preliminary clinical experiences, new biocompatible treatments were released by a number of manufacturers of CPB circuits and oxygenators. The new-generation coatings include poly-2-methoxyethylacrylate; phosphorylcholine; siloxane/caprolactone; polyethylene oxide chains, and sulphate/sulphonate groups.

Recently, two meta-analyses addressed the clinical role of biocompatible surfaces for routine CPB in cardiac surgery. In 2007, Mangoush and coworkers (47) evaluated 46 RCTs of heparin-bonded circuits compared to conventional circuits. When pooled together, the results were in favour of heparin-bonded circuits with respect to the incidence of blood transfusions and re-sternotomy, with a shorter duration of mechanical ventilation and hospital length of stay. Subsequently, a second meta-analysis (48), inclusive of non-heparin bonded biocompatible materials, confirmed a lower incidence of transfusion of concentrate red cells and atrial fibrillation in patients treated with biocompatible surfaces, with a shorter duration of intensive care unit and hospital length of stay. However, when only high-quality studies were included, only the incidence of atrial fibrillation and the intensive care unit length of stay remained significantly in favour of the biocompatible surface-treated group.

Biocompatible surfaces certainly represent an improvement in the quality of CPB circuits, and are nowadays included in a great number of commercially available CPB equipment. However, if used as the sole method for limiting blood activation during CPB their effect is limited. The main reason is that they have a direct impact only on the material-dependent blood activation, leaving intact the material-independent pathways. Indeed, thrombin generation is mainly dependent on retransfusion of blood shed into the chest. The use of open circuits with large shed blood retransfusion could obscure the improvements in biocompatibility of extra-corporeal circuits (49,50), and the overall effects of the material independent blood activation including blood–air interface, cardiotomy suction and haemolysis, may blunt the effect of biocompatible surfaces (51).

Special issues in the practice of cardiopulmonary bypass

Haemodilution

Haemodilution during CPB is inevitable, due to the fluids used to prime the circuit and for cardioplegia. Until the mid-1990s, haemodilution during CPB was not of general concern, and opinion was that haematocrit values in the range of 18–20% were acceptable, and even favourable, in terms of peripheral capillary perfusion.

Haemodilution determines a number of physical, haemodynamic, and metabolic effects. According to the Hagen-Poiseuille equation, flow (Q) is generated in presence of a pressure gradient (ΔP) and limited by flow resistance (R):

$$Q = \Delta P / R$$

Resistance is, in turn, dependent on the radius (r) of the conduit (a vessel or the CPB circuit), the length (l) of the conduit, and the viscosity (η) of the fluid:

$$R = 8\eta l / \pi r^4$$

And therefore the flow is:

$$Q = \Delta P(\pi r^4 / 8\eta l)$$

This means that the resistance decreases linearly with decreased viscosity, and for a given flow, pressure decreases linearly with decreased viscosity. Haematocrit is the main determinant of blood viscosity (figure 11.13). The relative viscosity of blood is greatly increased for haematocrit values above 50%; however, haemodilution

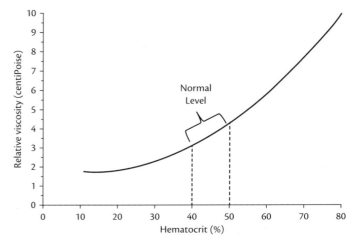

Fig. 11.13 Relationship between haematocrit and relative blood viscosity.

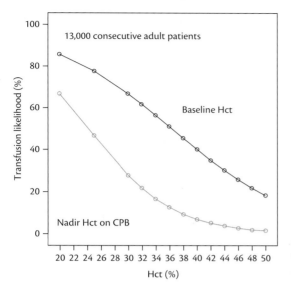

Fig. 11.14 Effects of anaemia and haemodilution on the transfusion risk. CPB, cardiopulmonary bypass

Table 11.4 Beneficial effects of haemodilution control during cardiopulmonary bypass

- Preservation of peripheral vascular resistance
- Preservation of functional capillary density
- Maintenance of adequate perfusion pressure
- Maintenance of blood flow to critical organs (kidney, brain)
- Preservation of the oxygen delivery
- Preservation of coagulation factors concentrations (fibrinogen and FXIII)
- Decreased blood transfusion incidence

section, propriety systems are available to guarantee this approach in an integrated system.

Perfusion pressure

During CPB, because the flow generated by the roller or the centrifugal pump is continuous, there is no pulse pressure, and the mean arterial pressure (MAP), together with the peripheral resistances is the determinant of flow to the various organs. As discussed in the Haemodilution section, perfusion pressure is strongly dependent on pump flow rate and on blood viscosity, which is determined by haemodilution and blood temperature. Because of the decrease in blood viscosity with haemodilution as a result of the mixing of the crystalloid prime, the onset of CPB is often accompanied by systemic arterial hypotension. Cytokine release may also contribute to the hypotension at the start of CPB.

The ideal MAP during CPB has never been established, but the lower limit is generally agreed to be 50–60 mmHg (56). This value has been recognized as the lowest acceptable level to maintain cerebral blood flow autoregulation (57). However, the level may be lower during anaesthesia and hypothermia. Potential benefits of perfusion at a relatively low MAP include less shed blood in the surgical field, with less need for aspiration of shed blood, less heart perfusion from collateral vessels, less trauma to the blood cells and a lower embolic load to the brain.

Maintenance of a higher perfusion pressure of 70–80 mmHg may be justified by a number of pathophysiological considerations. First, as previously discussed, the need for a high pump flow rate to counteract the deleterious effects of haemodilution so as to maintain an adequate DO_2 inevitably leads to a higher perfusion pressure. In addition, for a number of high-risk patients who are older and have chronic hypertension or peripheral vascular disease, the perfusion pressure may require to be higher. Carotid artery disease may also require that the perfusion pressure is maintained higher to maintian cerebral perfusion.

Perfusion of the kidney is also very dependent on perfusion pressure with a decrease in renal blood flow when the MAP is lower than 70 mmHg in a normal kidney, and lower than 100 mmHg in presence of a renal vascular disease. In a retrospective series, Fisher and coworkers observed that patients who developed postoperative acute kidney injury had longer periods of low perfusion pressure defined as less than 60 mmHg, during CPB than patients with preserved postoperative renal function (58).

Currently, there is only one RCT comparing a low- (50–60 mmHg) to a high-perfusion pressure (target 80–100 mmHg) (59). The results favoured the high-perfusion pressure for a combined

leading to a haematocrit decrease from 40% to 20% causes a decrease in relative blood viscosity of about 30%. For a given pump flow, this means a decrease in the perfusion pressure of about 30%. In haemodynamic terms, *haemodilution leads to hypotension.*

Blood viscosity is even one of the major determinants of peripheral capillary perfusion. Studies conducted with a Hamster window chamber model can be used investigate microcirculation under different conditions of blood viscosity. The functional capillary density (FCD) is an expression of the microcirculation viability; FCD is directly associated with survival in haemorrhagic shock (52). Maintenance of blood viscosity is essential to preserve FCD (53) and improves survival in haemorrhagic shock (54). Under CPB conditions, the second major factor determining blood viscosity is temperature: relative viscosity linearly increases with decreasing temperature. Therefore, in order to maintain an acceptable blood viscosity, a correct coupling of haemodilution and temperature is warranted, with higher values of haemodilution allowed for lower levels of blood temperature.

Haemodilution leads to a decrease in coagulation factor activity, and fibrinogen and factor XIII concentrations may be particularly affected (55), leading to postoperative bleeding. Additionally, the level of haemodilution during CPB is a strong predictor for the number of units of concentrated red cells transfused. In a series of 13 000 consecutive adult patients, we observed that the nadir values of haematocrit during CPB below 30% was more predictive for concentrated red cell transfusions than the baseline haematocrit (figure 11.14). Finally, as discussed previously, low haematocrit values during CPB may trigger an inadequate DO_2, which in turn is a determinant of adverse outcomes. There is presently little doubt that levels of haematocrit should be preserved during CPB (table 11.4).

Various technical measures are available to achieve this goal including: minimization of priming volume with adequate oxygenators and circuits, vacuum-assisted venous drainage, retro-prime, ultrafiltration. As will be discussed in the mini-CPB

index of adverse cardiac and neurological outcomes, but the study was underpowered to provide conclusive evidence. A high-perfusion pressure management may more appropriate for patients with peripheral vascular disease and impairment of blood flow to brain, kidney, and gut mucosa. However, this strategy may increase the embolic load to the brain if achieved by using higher pump flow rates.

Loss of pulsatillity has been identified by some the cause of poor organ perfusion and in particular, the kidney (60). However, a large RCT (61) failed to demonstrate any advantage of pulsatile over continuous flow during CPB in terms of postoperative morbidity, mortality, and renal function. Nowadays, there are still some investigations in the field of pulsatile CPB flow, but for routine CPB practice continuous flow is the standard of care.

Management of shed blood

As discussed in the earlier section on Blood Activation, one of the main determinants of blood activation, and in particular, thrombin generation, is the re-infusion of shed blood into the systemic circulation during CPB. Shed blood contains both micro- and macro-particles including lipids, bone fragments, and wax, that are aspirated into the CPB circuit. For this reason, separation of shed blood from the CPB circulation has been recommended by a number of workers (62–66). Shed blood can be separated from the systemic CPB flow by collecting it into a dedicated reservoir. This shed-blood reservoir could be physically separated from the venous reservoir such as a collapsible bag in closed circuits, or included in a single hard-shell reservoir with separate chambers for systemic venous blood and shed blood. Shed blood can be processed in a cell-saver before re-transfusion into the systemic circulation, therefore significantly reducing the amount of circulating enzymes of thrombin generation (36,63,64). Clinical studies have demonstrated that thrombin generation is significantly blunted during CPB without cardiotomy suction (65) or with a separate cardiotomy reservoir and cell-saver use (66). Despite being based on sound theoretical concepts, elimination of the cardiotomy reservoir and shed-blood processing produced equivocal results in the published clinical trials. Although the majority of the studies have confirmed that shed blood is responsible for increased thrombin generation, neutrophil count, platelet activation, and release of cytokines (65,67–69), there is a limited evidence of a clinically relevant benefit of closed CPB circuits with shed-blood separation (70). Extensive blood processing with mechanical cell salvage systems may cause a consumption coagulopathy, and one RCT observed a higher blood transfusion rate in patients treated with washed shed blood and lipid filtration (71).

Ultrafiltration

Ultrafiltration during and after CPB (modified ultrafiltration) is intended to physically remove excess of fluids and biochemically remove inflammatory mediators. Excessive haemodilution during and after CPB may be treated by removing fluid by ultrafiltration. Conventional ultrafiltration is run during CPB with a haemofilter inserted into the CPB circuit. Modified ultrafiltration is initiated after completion of the operation, with the CPB cannulas still in place and before protamine reversal of heparin. Blood is actively aspirated from the arterial line, fluid is removed with a haemofilter, and blood is returned into the venous line.

Many randomized controlled studies investigated the efficacy of ultrafiltration in decreasing blood loss and transfusions. A meta-analysis (72) demonstrated that patients treated with ultrafiltration had significantly less blood loss, but only when modified ultrafiltration was used. Blood transfusion was also significantly reduced in patients who underwent ultrafiltration (0.73 units per patient), but again this effect was significant only when modified ultrafiltration was applied. Additional benefits of ultrafiltration include the reduction of circulating inflammatory mediators (73,74), improved cardiovascular performance (73,75), and better neurological outcome (76). However, these effects appear to be clinically relevant mainly when modified ultrafiltration is applied in paediatric patients (77).

Hypothermia versus normothermia

Hypothermia during CPB was widely used until the early 1990s, with the purpose of decreasing the metabolic organ demand, increasing tolerance to ischaemia, and protecting brain in case of accidental pump failure. Subsequently, the majority of the institutions shifted to moderate hypothermia or normothermia in routine adult cardiac operations, confining deep hypothermia to some paediatric cases and adult cases undergoing highly complex surgery.

Currently, the data is inconclusive regarding outcome from warm (>33°C) compared to cold (25–30°C) CPB. A meta-analysis of RCTs that used neurological injury as the outcome found no significant differences between cold and warm strategies of thermal management in coronary artery surgery (78).

Blood viscosity is inversely related to body temperature, and the resulting increase in viscosity at lower temperatures may allow maintenance of a higher perfusion pressure despite severe haemodilution. Conversely, hypothermia may affect the activity of the coagulation factors and platelet function. However, this effect is transient and reversed once normal body temperature is re-established. To date, trials have not shown any differences in transfusion rates in between cold and warm approaches to thermal management during CPB (79,80) even if a trend in favour of normothermia has been identified by some workers (81,82).

At present, there is no evidence that one form of thermal management is superior to another. Neurological dysfunction is probably more related to the approach to thermal management rather than to actual temperature used. Specifically, the rate of rewarming from hypothermia should be gradual rate and active warming of the patient should be avoided when the blood temperature is more 37°C when using normothermia. Further details on temperature and pH management are provided in Chapter 14.

Mini-systems for cardiopulmonary bypass

In the earlier section on Special Issues, we have addressed a number of technical issues which may improve the quality of the perfusion and the patients' outcome. These are the containment of haemodilution, use of biocompatible CPB circuits, and the use of closed circuits that separate the shed blood then process it before re-retransfusion and use of centrifugal pumps.

Taken individually, these measures have demonstrated only limited beneficial effect or none at all. As previously discussed, the causes of adverse outcomes from CPB are multifactorial involving material-dependent reaction, material-independent reaction, biochemical and cellular activation of coagulation and inflammation pathways, and specific organ reactions to an inadequate DO_2. Given the multifactorial causes, it is unlikely that a single intervention will result in a significant improvement in outcome. Therefore, combining a number of strategies may be required. This approach is known as minimally invasive CPB or mini-CPB and has been recently applied clinically and its effect on outcome tested.

A mini-CPB circuit is composed of a centrifugal pump, closed circuit with biocompatible treatment, low priming volume, and separation of shed-blood. In the majority of the system manufactured and commercially available there is no collapsible venous reservoir, and the venous line is directly connected to the inlet port of the centrifugal pump. This allows a negative pressure on the venous return, with a lower size of the venous line and cannulas. A collapsible venous reservoir may be included in the system to accept additional 'reserve' blood or fluids. Left heart venting is achieved by direct connection of the venting line to the venous line, therefore creating an active suction on the left heart chambers.

The direct connection of both the systemic venous return line and the venting line to the inlet of the centrifugal pump, without an interposed cardiotomy reservoir, leads to some technical and safety issues. In mini-CPB systems, the patient is the 'cardiotomy reservoir'. The fluid loading of the patient and CPB circuit represents a continuum that the perfusionist has only limited ability to influence using the CPB circuit. However, the anaesthetist can modify the system by infusing IV fluids, vasodilation, or vasoconstriction. Indeed, the management of a mini-CPB circuit requires close team-work between the cardiac surgeon, anesthesiologist, and perfusionist.

Because there is active suctioning of the systemic venous blood and left heart venting directly into CPB circuit, air may enter the system. In conventional CPB, air entering the venous line or by left-heart venting line is not problematic as it is separated from the blood once it arrives into the venous reservoir(s). In absence of a venous reservoir, air can be pumped through the oxygenator into the arterial line and finally reach the patient. To prevent this catastrophic event occurring, all the commercially available mini-CPB systems have one or more safety devices such as bubble detectors, filters and automatic clamps, which detect and purge air from the circuit. These devices add complexity to the CPB system that has been postulated result in mini-CPB being less safe than conventional systems (83).

Mini-CPB systems have been widely investigated for their impact on outcome. However, the majority of the RCTs were underpowered to detect clinically important differences (83–86). Some studies have found mini-CPB associated with a lower rate of blood transfusion (87–90), better renal function (87,88,91), better neurologic outcome (88,91) and a lower incidence of low cardiac output syndrome postoperatively (88).

One large propensity-adjusted study found that in CABG surgery, the outcome from mini-CPB systems was similar to that of off-pump CABG surgery (92). In a recent systematic review and meta-analysis (93), mini-CPB systems confirmed a significantly lower need for transfusions (odds ratio 0.4, 95% confidence interval 0.26–0.63, $p < 0.001$).

Therefore, the available evidence indicates that mini-CPB reduces blood transfusion in cardiac surgery, and possibly improve some other outcomes. However, the complexity of mini-CPB

Table 11.5 Main incidents reported during CPB

Type of incident	Rate	Reports
Air bubbles entering the circuit	1/491	Jenkins et al. 1997[95]
	1/385	Groenenberg et al. 2010[94]
Visible clots in the circuit or coagulation problems	1/4864	Charriere et al. 2007[96]
	1/317	Groenenberg et al. 2010[94]
	1/771	Mejak et al. 2000[97]
Heater-cooler failure or cooling/rewarming problems	1/314	Jenkins et al. 1997[95]
	1/1305	Groenenberg et al. 2010[94]
Protamine reactions or allergic reaction to drugs	1/783	Mejak et al. 2000[97]
	1/1702	Charriere et al. 2007[96]
	1/317	Groenenberg et al. 2010[94]
Aortic or arterial lesion at the cannulation site	1/1792	Charriere et al. 2007[96]
	1/839	Groenenberg et al. 2010[94]

requires a steep learning curve to master the technique, and this along with increased cost, have limited the use of the technique in clinical practice and confined it to experienced institutions.

Emergencies during cardiopulmonary bypass

CPB completely replaces the function of heart and lungs during cardiac surgery. Therefore, even if rare, equipment failure is potentially life-threatening. The Dutch Perfusion Incident Survey found that equipment failure occurred at an incidence of 1 in 16 episodes of CPB, with an associated incidence of adverse outcomes occurring 1 in 1236 (94). However, 41% of the incidents was the failure to reach and maintain an ACT of more than 400 seconds which is not a true incident. Anaphylactic reactions to fluids, blood products, or medications represented 51% of the incidents, visible clots in the CPB circuit represented 32% of the incidents. A summary of the main incidents reported during CPB is provided in table 11.5.

CPB incidents leading to serious injury or death are rare, in the range of 0.03% to 0.8%, according to published surveys (94–97). Adequate safety devices including automatic clamps, arterial line filters, manometers, and gas line filters should always be included in the CPB circuit to prevent adverse event resulting from any incidents. Some of the incidents are related to simple hardware failure, and before use the correct functioning of the CPB circuit should be confirmed using a check-list

Emergencies due to failure of the mains electrical power supply or rupture of the circuit or oxygenator represent catastrophic events. Although rare, these incidents should be prepared for using simulation training for hand cranking and replacement of the circuit and oxygenator.

Conclusion

CPB management remains a key aspect in the present scenario of cardiac surgery. The great technological improvements achieved in the last decades contributed to limit, but not to eliminate the potential adverse effects linked to the exposure of blood to the foreign surfaces. Further developments are warranted for achieving a truly 'biocompatible' CPB circuit.

References

1. Kerendi F, Morris CD, Puskas JD. Off-pump coronary bypass surgery for high-risk patients: only in expert centers? *Curr Opin Cardiol* 2008; **23**: 573–8

2. Wheeldon DR, Bethune DW, Gill RD. Vortex pumping for routine cardiac surgery: a comparative study. *Perfusion* 1990; **5**: 135–43

3. Linneweber J, Chow TW, Kawamura M, Moake JL, Nosè Y. In vitro comparison of blood pump induced platelet microaggregates between a centrifugal and roller pump during cardiopulmonary bypass. *Int J Artif Organs* 2002; **25**: 549–55

4. Andersen KS, Nygreen EL, Grong K, Leirvaag B, Holmsen H. Comparison of the centrifugal and roller pump in elective coronary artery bypass surgery—a prospective, randomized study with special emphasis upon platelet activation. *Scand Cardiovasc J* 2003; **37**: 356–62

5. Keyser A, Hilker MK, Diez C, Philipp A, Foltan M, Schmid C. Prospective randomized clinical study of arterial pumps used for routine on pump coronary bypass grafting. *Artif Organs* 2011; **35**: 534–42

6. Farsak B, Gunaydin S, Yildiz U, Sari T, Zorlutuna Y. Clinical evaluation of leukocyte filtration as an alternative anti-inflammatory strategy to aprotinin in high-risk patients undergoing coronary revascularization. *Surg Today* 2012; **42**: 334–41

7. Warren O, Wallace S, Massey R, et al. Does systemic leukocyte filtration affect perioperative hemorrhage in cardiac surgery? A systematic review and meta-analysis. *ASAIO J* 2007; **53**: 514–21

8. Bakhtiary F, Moritz A, Kleine P, et al. Leukocyte depletion during cardiac surgery with extracorporeal circulation in high-risk patients. *Inflamm Res* 2008; **57**: 577–85

9. Ferraris VA, Brown JR, Despotis GJ, et al. 2011 Update to The Society of Thoracic Surgeons and the Society of Cardiovascular Anesthesiologists Blood Conservation Clinical Practice Guidelines. *Ann Thorac Surg* 2011; **91**: 944–82

10. Ranucci M, Pavesi M, Mazza E, et al. Risk factors for renal dysfunction after coronary surgery: the role of cardiopulmonary bypass technique. *Perfusion* 1994; **9**: 319–26

11. Fang WC, Helm RE, Krieger KH, et al. Impact of minimum hematocrit during cardiopulmonary bypass on mortality in patients undergoing coronary artery surgery. *Circulation* 1997; **96** (suppl II): 194–9

12. Habib RH, Zacharias A, Schwann TA, Riordan CJ, Durham SJ, Shah A. Adverse effects of low hematocrit during cardiopulmonary bypass in the adult: should current practice be changed? *J Thorac Cardiovasc Surg* 2003; **125**: 1438–50

13. Swaminathan M, Phillips-Bute BG, Conlon PJ, Smith PK, Newman MF, Stafford-Smith M. The association of lowest hematocrit during cardiopulmonary bypass with acute renal injury after coronary artery bypass surgery. *Ann Thorac Surg* 2003; **76**: 784–92

14. Ranucci M, Biagioli B, Scolletta S, et al. Lowest hematocrit on cardiopulmonary bypass impairs the outcome in coronary surgery: An Italian Multicenter Study from the National Cardioanesthesia Database. *Tex Heart Inst J* 2006; **33**: 300–5

15. Ranucci M, Isgrò G, Romitti F, Mele S, Biagioli B, Giomarelli P. Anaerobic metabolism during cardiopulmonary bypass: predictive value of carbon dioxide derived parameters. *Ann Thorac Surg* 2006; **81**: 2189–95

16. Ranucci M, Romitti F, Isgrò G, et al. Oxygen delivery during cardiopulmonary bypass and acute renal failure after coronary operations. *Ann Thorac Surg* 2005; **80**: 2213–20

17. de Somer F, Mulholland JW, Bryan MR, Aloisio T, Van Nooten GJ, Ranucci M. O2 delivery and CO2 production during cardiopulmonary bypass as determinants of acute kidney injury: time for a goal-directed perfusion management? *Crit Care* 2011; **15**: R192

18. Ranucci M, De Toffol B, Isgrò G, Romitti F, Conti D, Vicentini M. Hyperlactatemia during cardiopulmonary bypass: determinants and impact on postoperative outcome. *Crit Care* 2006; **10**: R167

19. Young JA, Kisker CT, Doty DB. Adequate anticoagulation during cardiopulmonary bypass determined by activated clotting time and the appearance of fibrin monomer. *Ann Thorac Surg* 1978; **26**: 231–40

20. Despotis GJ, Summerfield MD, Joist JH, et al. Comparison of activated coagulation time and whole blood heparin measurements with laboratory plasma anti Xa-heparin concentration in patients having cardiac operations. *J Thorac Cardiovasc Surg* 1994; **108**: 1076–82

21. Bosch YP, Ganushchak YM, de Jong DS. Comparison of ACT point-of-care measurements: repeatability and agreement. *Perfusion* 2006; **21**: 27–31.

22. Despotis GJ, Joist JH, Hogue CW, Jr. et al. More effective suppression of hemostatic system activation in patients undergoing cardiac surgery by heparin dosing based on heparin blood concentrations rather than ACT. *Thromb Haemost* 1996; **76**: 902–8

23. Ranucci M, Aronson S, Dietrich W, et al. Patient blood management during cardiac surgery: do we have enough evidence for clinical practice? *J Thorac Cardiovasc Surg* 2011; **142**: 249. e1–32

24. Ranucci M, Isgrò G, Cazzaniga A, Soro G, Menicanti L, Frigiola A. Predictors for heparin resistance in patients undergoing coronary artery bypass grafting. *erfusion* 1999; **14**: 437–42

25. Ranucci M, Isgrò G, Cazzaniga A, et al. Different patterns of heparin resistance: therapeutic implications. *Perfusion* 2002; **17**: 199–204

26. Dietrich W, Spannagl M, Schramm W, Vogt W, Barankay A, Richter JA. The influence of preoperative anticoagulation on heparin response during cardiopulmonary bypass. *J Thorac Cardiovasc Surg* 1991; **102**: 505–14

27. Spiess B. Treating heparin resistance with antithrombin or fresh frozen plasma. *Ann Thorac Surg* 2008; **85**: 2153–60

28. Williams MR, D'Ambra AB, Beck JR, et al. A randomized trial of antithrombin concentrate for treatment of heparin resistance. *Ann Thorac Surg* 2000; **70**: 873–7

29. Avidan MS, Levy JH, Scholz J, et al. A phase III, double-blind, placebo-controlled, multicenter study on the efficacy of recombinant human antithrombin in heparin-resistant patients scheduled to undergo cardiac surgery necessitating cardiopulmonary bypass. *Anesthesiology* 2005; **102**: 276–84

30. Ranucci M, Frigiola A, Menicanti L, Ditta A, Boncilli A, Brozzi S. Postoperative antithrombin levels and outcome in cardiac operations. *Crit Care Med* 2005; **33**: 355–60

31. Garvin S, Muehlschlegel JD, Tjörvi E, et al. Postoperative activity, but not preoperative activity, of antithrombin is associated with major adverse cardiac events after coronary artery bypass graft surgery. *Anesth Analg* 2010; **111**: 862–9

32. Jobes DR, Aitken GL, Shaffer GW. Increased accuracy and precision of heparin and protamine dosing reduces blood loss and transfusion in patients undergoing primary cardiac operations. *J Thorac Cardiovasc Surg* 1995; **110**: 36–45

33. Ohata T, Sawa Y, Ohtake S, et al. Clinical role of blood heparin level monitoring during open heart surgery. *Jpn J Thorac Cardiovasc Surg* 1999; **47**: 600–6

34. Vogler EA, Siedlecki CA. Contact activation of blood plasma coagulation: A contribution from the Hematology at Biomaterial Interfaces Research Group The Pennsylvania State University. *Biomaterials* 2009; **30**: 1857–69

35. Boisclair SJ, Lane DA, Philippou H. Mechanisms of thrombin generation during surgery and cardiopulmonary bypass. *Blood* 1993; **82**: 3350–7

36. Edmunds LH, Colman RW. Thrombin during cardiopulmonary bypass. *Ann Thorac Surg* 2006; **82**: 2315–22

37. Gikakis N, Khan MMH, Hiramatsu Y, et al. Effect of factor Xa inhibitors on thrombin formation and complement and neutrophil activation during in-vitro extracorporeal circulation. *Circulation* 1996; **94** (Suppl II): 341–6

38. Drake TA, Morrissey JH, Edgington TS. Selective cellular expression of tissue factor in human tissues. *Am J Path* 1989; **134**: 1087–96

39. Hoffman M, Munroe DM. A cell-based model of hemostasis. *Thromb Haemost* 2001; **85**: 958–65

40. Fosse E, Thelin S, Svennevig JL, et al. Duraflo II coating of cardiopulmonary bypass circuits reduces complement activation, but does

not affect the release of granulocyte enzymes: A European multicentre study. *Eur J Cardiothorac Surg* 1997; **11**: 320–7

41. Gu YJ, van Oeveren W, Akkerman C, Boonstra PW, Huyzen RJ, Wildevuur CR. Heparin-coated circuits reduce the inflammatory response to cardiopulmonary bypass. *Ann Thorac Surg* 1993; **55**: 917–22

42. Moen O, Hogasen K, Fosse E, et al. Attenuation of changes in leukocyte surface markers and complement activation with heparin-coated cardiopulmonary bypass. *Ann Thorac Surg* 1997; **63**: 105–11

43. Spiess BD, Vocelka C, Cochran RP, Soltow L, Chandler WL. Heparin-coated bypass circuits (carmeda) suppress the release of tissue plasminogen activator during normothermic coronary artery bypass graft surgery. *J Cardiothorac Vasc Anesth* 1998; **12**: 299–304

44. te Velthuis H, Baufreton C, Jansen PG, et al. Heparin coating of extracorporeal circuits inhibits contact activation during cardiac operations. *J Thorac Cardiovasc Surg* 1997; **114**: 117–22

45. Wildevuur CR, Jansen PG, Bezemer PD, et al. Clinical evaluation of Duraflo II heparin treated extracorporeal circulation circuits (2nd version). The European Working Group on heparin coated extracorporeal circulation circuits. *Eur J Cardiothorac Surg* 1997; **11**: 616–23

46. Ranucci M, Mazzucco A, Pessotto R, et al. Heparin-coated circuits for high-risk patients: a multicenter, prospective, randomized trial. *Ann Thorac Surg* 1999; **67**: 994–1000

47. Mangoush O, Purkayastha S, Haj-Yahia S, et al. Heparin-bonded circuits versus nonheparin-bonded circuits: an evaluation of their effect on clinical outcomes. *Eur J Cardiothorac Surg* 2007; **31**: 1058–69

48. Ranucci M, Balduini A, Ditta A, Boncilli A, Brozzi S. A systematic review of biocompatible cardiopulmonary bypass circuits and clinical outcome. *Ann Thorac Surg* 2009; **87**: 1311–9

49. de Haan J, Boonstra PW, Tabuchi N, van Oeveren W, Ebels T. Retransfusion of thoracic wound blood during heart surgery obscures biocompatibility of the extracorporeal circuit. *J Thorac Cardiovasc Surg* 1996; **111**: 272–5

50. de Haan J, Schönberger J, Haan J, van Oeveren W, Eijgelaar A. Tissue-type plasminogen activator and fibrin monomers synergistically cause platelet dysfunction during retransfusion of shed blood after cardiopulmonary bypass. *J Thorac Cardiovasc Surg* 1993; **106**: 1017–23

51. McCarthy PM, Yared JP, Foster RC, Ogella DA, Borsh JA, Cosgrove DM,3rd. A prospective randomized trial of Duraflo II heparin-coated circuits in cardiac reoperations. *Ann Thorac Surg* 1999; **67**: 1268–73

52. Kerger H, Saltzman DJ, Menger MD, Messmer K, Intaglietta M. Systemic and subcutaneous microvascular Po2 dissociation during 4-h hemorrhagic shock in conscious hamsters. *Am J Physiol* 1996; **270**: H827–36

53. Cabrales P, Tsai AG, Intaglietta M. Increased plasma viscosity prolongs microhemodynamic conditions during small volume resuscitation from hemorrhagic shock. *Resuscitation* 2008; **77**: 379–86

54. Cabrales P, Tsai AG, Intaglietta M. Hyperosmotic-hyperoncotic vs. hyperosmotic-hyperviscous small volume resuscitation in hemorrhagic shock. *Shock* 2004; **22**: 431–7

55. Ternström L, Radulovic V, Karlsson M. Plasma activity of individual coagulation factors, hemodilution and blood loss after cardiac surgery: a prospective observational study. *Thromb Res* 2010; **126**: e128–33

56. Murphy GS, Hessel GA II, Groom RC. Optimal perfusion during cardiopulmonary bypass: an evidence-based approach. *Anesth Analg* 2009; **108**: 1394–417

57. Lassen NA. Cerebral blood flow and oxygen consumption in man. *Physiol Rev* 1959; **39**: 183–238

58. Fisher UM, Weissenberger WK, Warters RD, Geissler HJ, Allen SJ, Mehlhorn U. Impact of cardiopulmonary bypass management on postcardiac surgery renal function. *Perfusion* 2002; **17**: 401–6

59. Gold JP, Charlson ME, Williams-Russo P, et al. Improvement of outcomes after coronary artery bypass. A randomized trial comparing intraoperative high versus low mean arterial pressure. *J Thorac Cardiovasc Surg* 1995; **110**: 1302–11

60. Kim HK, Son HS, Fang YH, Park SY, Hwang CM, Sun K. The effects of pulsatile flow upon renal tissue perfusion during cardiopulmonary bypass: a comparative study of pulsatile and nonpulsatile flow. *ASAIO J* 2005; **51**: 30–6

61. Abramov D, Tamariz M, Serrick CI, et al. The influence of cardiopulmonary bypass flow characteristics on the clinical outcome of 1820 coronary bypass patients. *Can J Cardiol* 2003; **19**: 237–43

62. Ranucci M, Pazzaglia A, Isgrò G, et al. Closed, phosphorylcholine-coated circuit and reduction of systemic heparinization for cardiopulmonary bypass: the intraoperative ECMO concept. *Int J Artif Organs* 2002; **25**: 875–81

63. De Somer F, Van Belleghem Y, Caes F, et al. Tissue factor as the main activator of the coagulation system during cardiopulmonary bypass. *J Thorac Cardiovasc Surg* 2002; **123**: 951–8

64. Albes JM, Stohr IM, Kaluza M, et al. Physiological coagulation can be maintained in extracorporeal circulation by means of shed blood separation and coating. *J Thorac Cardiovasc Surg* 2003; **126**: 1504–12

65. Aldea GS, Soltow LO, Chandler WL, et al. Limitation of thrombin generation, platelet activation and inflammation by elimination of cardiotomy suction in patients undergoing coronary artery bypass grafting treated with heparin-bonded circuits. *J Thorac Cardiovasc Surg* 2002; **123**: 742–55

66. Koster A, Yeter R, Buz S, et al. Assessment of hemostatic activation during cardiopulmonary bypass for coronary artery bypass grafting with bivalirudin: results of a pilot study. *J Thorac Cardiovasc Surg* 2005; **129**: 1391–4

67. Jensen E, Andreasson S, Bengtsson A. Influence of two different perfusion systems on inflammatory response in pediatric heart surgery. *Ann Thorac Surg* 2003; **75**: 919–25

68. Lindholm L, Westerberg M, Bengtsson A, Ekroth R, Jensen E, Jeppsson A. A closed perfusion system with heparin coating and centrifugal pump improves cardiopulmonary bypass biocompatibility in elderly patients. *Ann Thorac Surg* 2004; **78**: 2131–8

69. Schonberger JP, Everts PA, Hoffmann JJ. Systemic blood activation with open and closed venous reservoirs. *Ann Thorac Surg* 1995; **59**: 1549–55

70. Jewell AE, Akowuah EF, Suvarna SK, Braidley P, Hopkinson D, Cooper G. A prospective randomized comparison of cardiotomy suction and cell saver for recycling shed blood during cardiac surgery. *Eur J Cardiothorac Surg* 2033; **23**: 633–6

71. Rubens FD, Boodhwani M, Mesana T, Wozny D, Wells G, Nathan HJ. The cardiotomy trial: a randomized, double-blind study to assess the effect of processing of shed blood during cardiopulmonary bypass on transfusion and neurocognitive function. *Circulation* 2007; **116** (11 Suppl): I89–97

72. Boodhwani M, Williams K, Babaev A, Gill G, Saleem N, Rubens FD. Ultrafiltration reduces blood transfusions following cardiac surgery: a meta-analysis. *Eur J Cardiothorac Surg* 2006; **30**: 892–7

73. Bogă M, Islamoğlu, Badak I, et al. The effects of modified hemofiltration on inflammatory mediators and cardiac performance in coronary artery bypass grafting. *Perfusion* 2000; **15**: 143–50

74. Tassani P, Richter JA, Eising GP, et al. Influence of combined zero-balanced and modified ultrafiltration on the systemic inflammatory response during coronary artery bypass grafting. *J Cardiothorac Vasc Anesth* 1999; **13**: 285–91

75. Blanchard N, Toque Y, Trojette F, Quintard JM, Benammar A, Montravers P. Hemodynamic and echocardiographic effects of hemofiltration performed during cardiopulmonary bypass. *J Cardiothorac Vasc Anesth* 2000; **14**: 393–8

76. Luciani GB, Menon T, Vecchi B, Auriemma S, Mazzucco A. Modified ultrafiltration reduces morbidity after adult cardiac operations: a prospective, randomized clinical trial. *Circulation* 2001; **104** (12 Suppl 1): I253–I259

77. Groom RC, Froebe S, Martin J, et al. Update on pediatric perfusion practice in North America: 2005 survey. *J Extra Corpor Technol* 2005; **37**: 343–50

78. Rees K, Beranek-Stanley M, Burke M, Ebrahim S. Hypothermia to reduce neurologic damage following coronary artery bypass surgery. *Cochrane Database Syst Rev* 2006; **1**: CD002138

79. Nathan HJ, Parlea L, Dupuis JY, et al. Safety of deliberate intraoperative and postoperative hypothermia for patients undergoing coronary artery surgery: a randomized trial. *J Thorac Cardiovasc Surg* 2004; **127**: 1270–5

80. Stensrud PE, Nuttall GA, de Castro MA, et al. A prospective, randomized study of cardiopulmonary bypass temperature and blood transfusion. *Ann Thorac Surg* 1999; **67**: 711–5

81. Christenson JT, Maurice J, Simonet F, Velebit V, Schmuziger M. Normothermic versus hypothermic perfusion during primary coronary artery bypass grafting. *Cardiovasc Surg* 1995; **3**: 519–24

82. Birdi I, Regragui I, Izzat MB, Bryan AJ, Angelini GD. Influence of normothermic systemic perfusion during coronary artery bypass operations: a randomized prospective study. *J Thorac Cardiovasc Surg* 1997; **114**: 475–81

83. Nollert G, Schwabenland I, Maktav D, et al. Miniaturized cardiopulmonary bypass in coronary artery bypass surgery: marginal impact on inflammation and coagulation but loss of safety margins. *Ann Thorac Surg* 2005; **80**: 2326–32

84. Abdel-Rahman U, Ozaslan F, Risteski PS, et al. Initial experience with a minimized extracorporeal bypass system: is there a clinical benefit? *Ann Thorac Surg* 2005; **80**: 238–44

85. Kamiya H, Kofidis T, Haverich A, Klima U. Preliminary experience with the mini-extracorporeal circulation system (Medtronic resting heart system). *Interact CardioVasc Thorac Surg* 2006; **5**: 680–2

86. Beghi C, Nicolini F, Agostinelli A, et al. Mini-cardiopulmonary bypass system: results of a prospective randomized study. *Ann Thorac Surg* 2006; **81**: 1396–1400

87. Huybregts RAJM, Morariu AM, Rakhorst G, et al. Attenuated renal and intestinal injury after use of a mini-cardiopulmonary bypass system. *Ann Thorac Surg* 2007; **83**: 1760–7

88. Remadi JP, Rakotoarivelo Z, Marticho P, Benamar A. Prospective randomized study comparing coronary artery bypass grafting with the new mini-extracorporeal circulation Jostra System or with a standard cardiopulmonary bypass. *Am Heart J* 2006; **151**: 198.e1–198.e7

89. Perthel M, El-Ayoubi L, Bendisch A, et al. Clinical advantages of using mini-bypass systems in terms of blood product use, postoperative bleeding and air entrainment: an in vivo clinical perspective. *Eur J Cardiothor Surg* 2007; **31**: 1070–5

90. Castiglioni A, Verzini A, Pappalardo F, et al. Minimally invasive closed circuit versus standard extracorporeal circulation for aortic valve replacement. *Ann Thorac Surg* 2007; **83**: 586–91

91. Remadi JP, Rakotoarivello Z, Marticho P, et al. Aortic valve replacement with the minimal extracorporeal circulation (Jostra MECC System) versus standard cardiopulmonary bypass: a randomized prospective trial. *J Thorac Cardiovasc Surg* 2004; **128**: 436–41

92. Mazzei V, Nasso G, Salamone G, et al. Prospective randomized comparison of coronary bypass grafting with minimal extracorporeal circulation system (MECC) versus off-pump coronary surgery. *Circulation* 2007; **116**: 1761–7

93. Ranucci M, Castelvecchio S. Management of mini-cardiopulmonary bypass devices: is it worth the energy? *Curr Opin Anaesthesiol* 2009; **22**: 78–83

94. Groenenberg I, Weerwind PW, Everts PA, Maessen JG. Dutch perfusion incident survey. *Perfusion* 2010; **25**: 329–36

95. Jenkins OF, Morris R, Simpson JM. Australasian perfusion incident survey. *Perfusion* 1997; **12**: 279–88

96. Charrière J, Pélissié J, Verd C, et al. Survey: retrospective survey of monitoring/safety devices and incidents of cardiopulmonary bypass for cardiac surgery in France. *J Extracorpor Technol* 2007; **39**: 142–57

97. Mejak BL, Stammers A, Rauch E, Vang S, Viessman T. A retrospective study on perfusion incidents and safety devices. *Perfusion* 2000; **15**: 51–61

CHAPTER 12

Extracorporeal membrane oxygenation

Thomas Langer, Eleonora Carlesso, and Luciano Gattinoni

Definition

Extracorporeal membrane oxygenation (ECMO) is the general term used to define a technique that allows gas exchange to be performed outside of the body in order to support the failing heart and/or lungs. Despite being the most commonly used term, 'ECMO' is not entirely correct. Indeed, extracorporeal membrane lungs do add oxygen (O_2) and remove carbon dioxide (CO_2) from the blood so the term extracorporeal gas exchange (ECGE) would therefore be more appropriate. However, for the sake of simplicity, we will use the term ECMO in this chapter.

Introduction

ECMO allows to partial to total support of the functions of the heart and/or lungs to be temporarily performed. It is however very important to note that ECMO itself does not cure the underlying pulmonary and/or cardiovascular disorder. The use of ECMO only allows one to 'buy time' so as to investigate, diagnose and treat the pathology that caused organ failure.

Two major categories of ECMO exist that are veno-arterial (figure 12.1) and venovenous (figure 12.2). In the case of veno-arterial configuration, blood is drained from a vein, pumped through the membrane lung, and delivered in the arterial tree through a cannulated artery (usually the femoral artery). This type of setting, having the artificial lung in parallel with the native lung, has the great advantage of also providing cardiac support. Very importantly, in this configuration of veno-arterial ECMO with femoral arterial access, the oxygenated blood is pumped retrogradely through the aorta and, depending on the interactions between heart and ECMO pump, retrograde aortic flow may be insufficient to reach the proximal circulation (coronary arteries and cerebral perfusion) (1).

In the venovenous configuration blood is drained from a vein, pumped through the membrane lung and delivered back into the patient's venous system. The artificial lung is in series with the native lung so oxygenated blood is delivered to the pulmonary artery but no cardiovascular support is provided. This chapter will focus on the use of venovenous ECMO for the treatment of respiratory failure.

Historical aspects on the use of ECMO for respiratory support

Pioneering use of ECMO and the NIH trial

The first successful use of ECMO in a patient with post-traumatic respiratory failure was described by Hill and colleagues in 1972 using the Bramson membrane lung (2). A few years later Bartlett and co-workers reported the successful use of ECMO in neonates with respiratory distress (3). These promising results led to the design of a large multicenter randomized trial performed in the United States and sponsored by the National Institutes of Health (NIH). Interestingly, this was the first randomized controlled trial ever performed in the field of intensive care medicine. The aim was to compare the outcome of patients with adult respiratory distress syndrome (ARDS) treated with veno-arterial ECMO in addition to mechanical ventilation versus patients treated with conventional mechanical ventilation alone (4). The trial was stopped after the randomization of 90 patients, as the mortality was around 90% in both treatment groups. Importantly, however, the only difference in mechanical ventilation settings between the two groups was a lower inspired oxygen concentration (FiO_2) in the ECMO arm (oxygen toxicity being a serious concern at that time). In addition, mechanical ventilation was applied using high tidal volume and airway pressures in both groups, because their deleterious effects had not yet been fully recognized. Moreover, ECMO was applied in veno-arterial mode, which likely led to marked increases in ventilation–perfusion ratios of the native lungs, as standard mechanical ventilation was applied to poorly perfused lungs. Furthermore, the risks and complications (mainly bleeding) associated with the use of the cumbersome extracorporeal circuits of that time need to be kept in mind. Indeed, the reported daily transfusion rate of patients treated with ECMO was close to 5 litres of blood. For these reasons the disappointing and discouraging results of the NIH study led to the abandonment of the ECMO technique worldwide.

The concept of CO_2 removal and lung rest

Kolobow and Gattinoni, however, kept looking to 'lung rest' as the ideal milieu to allow lung healing. This was achieved by removing the metabolically produced CO_2 extracorporeally through the use of membrane lungs and by keeping the natural lungs ventilated

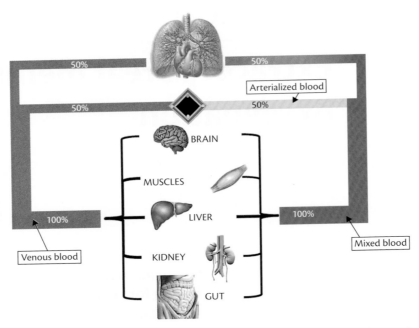

Fig. 12.1 Schematic representation of a veno-arterial ECMO circuit. For simplicity the case of a patient with complete pulmonary shunt is represented, i.e. a patient where the native lungs do not contribute to gas exchange.
Venous blood is drained through a cannula placed in the venous system and pumped through the membrane lung. In figure, 50% of cardiac output is pumped through the artificial lung. Blood exiting from the membrane lung (in this case 50% of cardiac output) is completely oxygenated and cleared of CO_2. Thereafter it is delivered back to the arterial system, in this case through a cannula placed in the femoral artery. Here arterialized blood mixes with venous blood arriving from the failing lungs, and mixed blood perfuses the organs and tissues with retrograde flow. As can be noted, the retrograde flow does not assure an adequate oxygenation of the coronary arteries and of the brain. Moreover, the native lungs can be substantially underperfused, depending on the amount of blood shunted through the membrane lung. Blue represents venous blood, light gray represents arterialized blood exiting the artificial lung, while dark gray represents mixed blood, i.e. a mixture of venous blood arriving from the native lungs and arterialized blood arriving from the artificial lung. Percentages represent percentages of circulating blood volume (for more details see the text). (See also figure in colour plates section)

at low pressures and frequencies (5) or even completely motion-less (6). Uncontrolled studies performed at the University of Milan (7,8) strongly suggested that this type of respiratory support strategy might be associated with an improved outcome in patients who could not be treated safely by means of conventional mechanical ventilation.

The promising results reported in these uncontrolled observations caught the interest of American critical care physicians and a new randomized controlled trial was performed. Notably, this trial was performed after a training consisting in the treatment of seven healthy sheep and two patients with ARDS (one who survived and one who died) with low-flow extracorporeal CO_2 removal (9). The authors reported that a total of 193 hours of support with extracorporeal CO_2 removal were performed on humans in order to learn the technique, meaning that the complex pathophysiology of extracorporeal gas exchange and the complex interactions between artificial and native diseased lung were 'learned' in approximately 8 days. The lack of experience of the investigators could therefore be one of the factors that contributed to the results of the randomized controlled trial performed in Salt Lake City, Utah, by Morris and colleagues (9) that found no difference between the two treatment arms.

Technical improvements, "CESAR" trial and the H1N1 flu pandemic

The impressive technical improvements made in the last decade have greatly increased safety and efficacy of new generation

ECMO systems. Indeed, the introduction of polymethylpentene membranes (10) has significantly improved gas exchange performance and reduced the occurrence of plasma leakage, thus allowing the use of membrane lungs for longer periods. Moreover, the implementation of centrifugal pumps has led, compared to roller blood pumps, to a significant reduction in haemolysis (11,12). Finally, the engineering of biocompatible non-thrombogenic components that are currently employed to coat fibres and circuitry have significantly reduced the need for profound systemic anticoagulation, thus limiting the occurrence of bleeding complications in patients treated with ECMO.

In 2009 a British randomized control trial on the efficacy and economic assessment of ECMO versus conventional mechanical ventilation, the so called 'CESAR trial' was published (13). In this study the treatment arm was performed in a single, high-volume centre, capable of treating patients with ECMO, while control patients were treated either in the hospital of origin or in the nearest participating hospital to the study that was considered an 'expert centre'. Therefore, patients were randomized to be transferred to a high-volume ECMO centre or to peripheral expert centres. The primary outcomes were survival and severe disability at 6 months from randomization; both were significantly better in patients allocated to treatment by ECMO (75% of patients actually received respiratory support with ECMO). Despite criticisms of the randomization design and a lack of data relative to the treatment of control patients, this pragmatic study showed a survival benefit for patients treated in

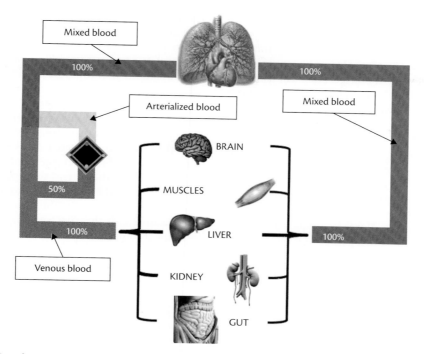

Fig. 12.2 Schematic representation of a venovenous ECMO circuit. For simplicity the case of a patient with complete pulmonary shunt is represented, i.e. a patient where the native lungs do not contribute to gas exchange.
Venous blood is drained through a cannula placed in the venous system and pumped through the membrane lung. In the figure, 50% of cardiac output is pumped through the artificial lung. Blood exiting from the membrane lung (in this case 50% of cardiac output) is completely oxygenated and cleared from CO_2. Thereafter it is delivered back into the venous system (see Cannulation section for additional details). Here, arterialized blood mixes with venous blood and is pumped by the heart through the native, failing lungs. As can be noted, blood with high oxygen saturation passes through the lungs and is thereafter pumped by the heart in order to perfuse organs and tissues. An important difference compared to the veno-arterial approach is that 100% circulating volume reaches the native lungs (see figure 12.1 for comparison). Blue represents venous blood, light gray represents arterialized blood exiting the artificial lung, while dark gray represents mixed blood, i.e. a mixture of venous blood arriving from the native lungs and arterialized blood arriving from the artificial lung. Percentages represent percentages of circulating blood volume (for more details see the text). (See also figure in colour plates section)

a high-volume centre in which respiratory support with ECMO is available.

However, the greatest single reason for the resurgence of interest in ECMO was the H1N1 flu pandemic of 2009, which caused, in infected patients, an acute pneumonia characterized by extremely severe hypoxaemia. In Australia and New Zealand ECMO was basically used as a rescue therapy in severely hypoxaemic patients who could not be managed safely with conventional mechanical ventilation alone. The outstanding results reported in *JAMA* (14) encouraged western countries to prepare themselves for the upcoming H1N1 pandemic. This was made possible also thanks to a joint political effort that made expensive ECMO resources available to several centres throughout Europe. The success rates in this category of patients were excellent and reached approximately 70% of survival. In the UK, a study comparing patients with H1N1-related ARDS treated with ECMO with well-matched patients with ARDS who were not treated with ECMO (not referred to an ECMO centre), clearly demonstrated the impressive advantage of this technique compared to conventional mechanical ventilation (15). In Italy, as in other countries, a network was established at a national level leading to a survival rate of about 70% (16). We might therefore conclude that the H1N1 flu pandemic has provided a very powerful drive, far beyond whatever randomized trial, for the use of ECMO in patients with severe ARDS.

At the time of writing the Extracorporeal Membrane Oxygenation for Severe adult respiratory distress syndrome (EOLIA) randomized control trial on the use of ECMO as an adjunct to mechanical ventilation in patients with ARDS is ongoing in France. The results of the trial should be available soon and will hopefully provide further insight into the usefulness of ECMO for the treatment of patients with ARDS.

Physiology of extracorporeal gas exchange

During veno-venous ECMO a portion of venous blood (up to 60–70% of cardiac output) is shunted through the artificial, membrane lung. Gas exchange takes place at the interface between blood and membrane fibres (similarly to the alveolar–capillary membrane in natural lungs) and can be divided in oxygenation (addition of oxygen to venous blood) and CO_2 removal (elimination of CO_2 from venous blood).

Oxygenation

Oxygenation is mainly determined by the extracorporeal flow rate, or, more correctly, by the ratio between extracorporeal flow rate and patient's cardiac output. The higher that this ratio is then the higher the impact on systemic oxygen values. Another way to increase oxygen delivery through the membrane lung is to increase haemoglobin levels (17). With venovenous ECMO, blood with an unphysiologically high haemoglobin oxygen saturation is delivered to the pulmonary circulation. An increase of pulmonary shunt fraction is observed due to a partial loss of hypoxic vasoconstriction (18). Nevertheless, sufficient oxygenation can usually be assured with veno-venous ECMO, through the increased oxygen content of shunted blood, provided high blood flow rates are used.

Carbon dioxide removal

In contrast to oxygenation, the main determinant of extracorporeal CO_2 removal is not extracorporeal blood flow, but the sweep gas flow that is the volume of gas per minute ventilating the membrane lung. Only the dissolved part of CO_2, which constitutes a small fraction of total CO_2 blood content, can be removed through the extracorporeal artificial lung. Novel techniques designed to enhance the ability to remove also that part of CO_2 that is chemically bond to water—i.e. bicarbonate ions—by the means of local acidification of blood are currently under investigation (19).

Technical aspects

Cannulation approaches

Venovenous ECMO is classically performed with dual-site cannulation. In this setting two large veins are cannulated percutaneously or surgically and vascular cannulae are inserted and connected to the extracorporeal circuit. Usual approaches include femorojugular cannulation (i.e. drainage from a femoral vein and reinfusion from the internal jugular vein (figure 12.3)) and femorofemoral cannulation (i.e. drainage from a femoral vein and reinfusion through a cannula placed in the contralateral femoral vein (figure 12.4)). A third option is single site cannulation with the use of bicaval dual lumen catheters (20). These catheters allow to perform venovenous ECMO using a single venous access, usually through the right internal jugular vein. Blood is drained from the superior and inferior vena cava through two dedicated ports and is pumped through a respiratory membrane. Oxygenated and CO_2-cleared blood is then returned to the patient through a separate lumen with its port situated in the right atrium and oriented toward the tricuspid valve (figure 12.5). The major advantage of bicaval dual lumen catheters is that they avoid femoral access, thus enabling the patient to perform passive and active physical therapy (21). Positioning of these catheters is however challenging and their correct placement is crucial in order to minimize recirculation (22) and avoid potentially severe complications including ventricular rupture (23). Techniques reported for the placement of these catheters include image-guidance (24), pressure-guidance (25), and the use of transesophageal or transthoracic echocardiography (26,27).

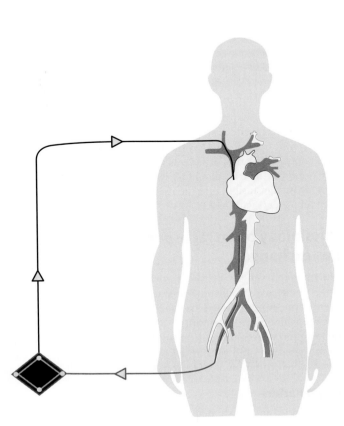

Fig. 12.3 Schematic representation of dual-site venovenous ECMO using femorojugular vascular access. Blood is drained from a vascular cannula placed in the inferior vena cava through a femoral vein and reinfused through a cannula placed in the right internal jugular vein.

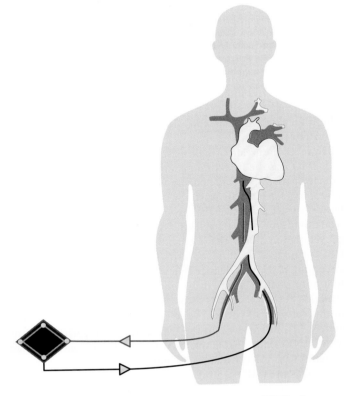

Fig. 12.4 Schematic representation of dual-site venovenous ECMO using femorofemoral vascular access. Blood is drained from a cannula placed in the inferior vena cava through the right femoral vein and reinfused through a second cannula placed through the controlateral femoral vein. The drainage cannula is usually positioned in the inferior vena cava above the renal veins, while the reinfusion cannula is positioned more cranial, close to the right atrium in order to minimize recirculation.

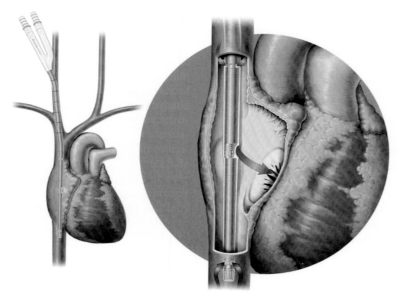

Fig. 12.5 Schematic representation of a single site venovenous ECMO using a bicaval dual-lumen catheter. Bicaval dual-lumen catheters are usually placed through the right internal jugular vein and advanced into the inferior vena cava. Venous blood is drained from the superior and inferior venae cavae and pumped through the artificial lung. The oxygenated and carbon dioxide-cleared blood is thereafter returned to the patient through a dedicated lumen with its port in the right atrium directed toward the tricuspid valve.
Reproduced by kind permission of Maquet Cardiopulmonary AG.

Complications during venovenous ECMO

The most common complication during venovenous ECMO is bleeding, which occurs in approximately 30% of patients and is likely due to the need for continuous heparin infusion and to a certain degree of platelet and endothelial dysfunction which is typical of critical ill patients (28). Other possible but rare complications include infection at the site of cannula insertion, systemic thromboembolism due to thrombus formation within the arterial site of the membrane, entrance of air in the extracorporeal circuit, and haemolysis.

Priming solutions for extracorporeal circuits

At the moment of initiation of extracorporeal circulation the patient is connected to the ECMO system. Prior to patient connection, the system is filled with a priming solution. Current generation ECMO systems have small priming volumes of around 600 mL and therefore do not require the routine use of blood products and are usually primed with crystalloid solutions. Despite the small priming volume, a moderate acute haemodilution occurs at extracorporeal circulation initiation as 600 mL of crystalloid solution is almost instantly added to the patient's blood. Given the effects on acid-base balance of acute haemodilution (29) and the possible role of chloride-rich crystalloid solutions in worsening renal function (30), normal saline should be avoided and a more balanced solution should be preferred in order to minimize acid base derangements (31,32).

Pharmacokinetic changes during ECMO

Appropriate drug therapy that is adequate plasma and tissue drug levels is fundamental in critically ill patients. Its achievement is, however, complicated by the fact that pharmacokinetics are typically altered in critically ill patients, mainly due to changes in drug *distribution* (increased distribution volume

and reduced albumin levels), *metabolism* (changes in hepatic clearance), and *elimination* (reduction in renal clearance) (33). In patients supported with ECMO, drug sequestration into the ECMO circuit needs to be taken into account, especially for lipophilic molecules, that can increase the volume of distribution and decrease drug clearance and thus lead to therapeutic failure (34).

Mechanical ventilation during ECMO

The optimal approach to mechanical ventilation in patients receiving respiratory support has yet to be fully defined, although the ECMO system has been developed to provide lung rest that is to apply mechanical ventilation as gently as possible. In our opinion, if the patients are on mechanical ventilation, it is very important to adopt a strategy which allows to minimize unphysiologically high transpulmonary pressures (*stress*) and volumes (*strain*), thus limiting the occurrence of ventilator-induced lung injury (35). However, it is also important to keep the lung open to some extent, in order to avoid diffuse alveolar collapse with the resulting increase in pulmonary vascular resistance which can lead to acute failure of the right ventricle requiring conversion to veno-arterial ECMO.

Present and future directions: ECMO as an alternative to mechanical ventilation

Several centres are starting to use ECMO as an alternative to invasive mechanical ventilation in awake spontaneously breathing patients. This type of approach to respiratory failure is well established in patients awaiting lung transplantation (36,37) and is increasingly considered as the gold standard (38). Moreover, some reports have been published on the use of ECMO as an alternative to mechanical ventilation in patients with acute exacerbation of chronic obstructive pulmonary disease (39,40). Respiratory support with ECMO in combination with spontaneous breathing has also been described also in a series of patients with ARDS (41,42) and has been extensively studied in an ovine model of oleic acid-induced experimental ARDS (43).

Conclusion

The use of ECMO is increasing worldwide due to the drive arising from recently published trials and the excellent results obtained during the H1N1 flu pandemic. The impressive progress in ECMO technology has substantially improved safety and cost-effectiveness of this technique. ECMO is a valuable technique to support gas exchange in any type of respiratory failure as an adjunct to, or even as an alternative to mechanical ventilation. The potential complications associated to the technique, mainly bleeding, need however to be kept in mind.

References

1. Mayo Clinic. Femoral Cannulation and Veno-Arterial ECMO, 2013. http://www.youtube.com/watch?v=NGGA-8zXVGE (accessed 9 July 2014)
2. Hill JD, O'Brien TG, Murray JJ, et al. Prolonged extracorporeal oxygenation for acute post-traumatic respiratory failure shock-lung syndrome. Use of the Bramson membrane lung. N Engl J Med 1972; 286: 629–34
3. Bartlett RH, Gazzaniga AB, Jefferies MR, Huxtable RF, Haiduc NJ, Fong SW. Extracorporeal membrane oxygenation ECMO. cardiopulmonary support in infancy. Trans Am Soc Artif Intern Organs 1976; 22: 80–93
4. Zapol WM, Snider MT, Hill JD, et al. Extracorporeal membrane oxygenation in severe acute respiratory failure. A randomized prospective study. JAMA 1979; 242: 2193–6
5. Gattinoni L, Kolobow T, Tomlinson T, et al. Low-frequency positive pressure ventilation with extracorporeal carbon dioxide removal LFPPV-ECCO2R.: an experimental study. Anesth Analg 1978; 57: 470–7
6. Gattinoni L, Pesenti A, Kolobow T, Damia G. A new look at therapy of the adult respiratory distress syndrome: motionless lungs. Int Anesthesiol Clin 1983; 21: 97–117
7. Gattinoni L, Agostoni A, Pesenti A, et al. Treatment of acute respiratory failure with low-frequency positive-pressure ventilation and extracorporeal removal of CO2. Lancet 1980; 2: 292–4
8. Gattinoni L, Pesenti A, Mascheroni D, et al. Low-frequency positive-pressure ventilation with extracorporeal CO2 removal in severe acute respiratory failure. JAMA 1986; 256: 881–6
9. Morris AH, Wallace CJ, Menlove RL, et al. Randomized clinical trial of pressure-controlled inverse ratio ventilation and extracorporeal CO2 removal for adult respiratory distress syndrome. Am J Respir Crit Care Med 1994; 149: 295–305
10. Toomasian JM, Schreiner RJ, Meyer DE, et al. A polymethylpentene fiber gas exchanger for long-term extracorporeal life support. ASAIO J 2005; 51: 390–7
11. Barrett CS, Jaggers JJ, Cook EF, et al. Pediatric ECMO outcomes: comparison of centrifugal versus roller blood pumps using propensity score matching. ASAIO J 2013; 59: 145–51
12. Yamagishi T, Kunimoto F, Isa Y, Hinohara H, Morishita Y. Clinical results of extracorporeal membrane oxygenation ECMO. support for acute respiratory failure: a comparison of a centrifugal pump ECMO with a roller pump ECMO. Surg Today 2004; 34: 209–13
13. Peek GJ, Mugford M, Tiruvoipati R, et al. Efficacy and economic assessment of conventional ventilatory support versus extracorporeal membrane oxygenation for severe adult respiratory failure CESAR: a multicentre randomised controlled trial. Lancet 2009; 374: 1351–63
14. Davies A, Jones D, Bailey M, et al. Extracorporeal membrane oxygenation for 2009 influenza A H1N1. acute respiratory distress syndrome. JAMA 2009; 302: 1888–95.
15. Noah MA, Peek GJ, Finney SJ, et al. Referral to an extracorporeal membrane oxygenation center and mortality among patients with severe 2009 influenza AH1N1.. JAMA 2011; 306: 1659–68
16. Patroniti N, Zangrillo A, Pappalardo F, et al. The Italian ECMO network experience during the 2009 influenza A H1N1. pandemic: preparation for severe respiratory emergency outbreaks. Intensive Care Med 2011; 37: 1447–57
17. Schmidt M, Tachon G, Devilliers C, et al. Blood oxygenation and decarboxylation determinants during venovenous ECMO for respiratory failure in adults. Intensive Care Med 2013; 39: 838–46
18. Lamy M, Eberhart RC, Fallat RJ, Dietrich HP, Ratliff J, Hill JD. Effects of extracorporeal membrane oxygenation ECMO. on pulmonary hemodynamics, gas exchange and prognose. Trans Am Soc Artif Intern Organs 1975; 21: 188–98
19. Zanella A, Patroniti N, Isgrò S, et al. Blood acidification enhances carbon dioxide removal of membrane lung: an experimental study. Intensive Care Med 2009; 35: 1484–7
20. Javidfar J, Brodie D, Wang D, et al. Use of bicaval dual-lumen catheter for adult venovenous extracorporeal membrane oxygenation. Ann Thorac Surg 2011; 91: 1763–8
21. Turner DA, Cheifetz IM, Rehder KJ, et al. Active rehabilitation and physical therapy during extracorporeal membrane oxygenation while awaiting lung transplantation: a practical approach. Crit Care Med 2011; 39: 2593–8
22. van Heijst AF, van der Staak FH, de Haan AF, et al. Recirculation in double lumen catheter veno-venous extracorporeal membrane oxygenation measured by an ultrasound dilution technique. ASAIO J 2001; 47: 372–6
23. Hirose H, Yamane K, Marhefka G, Cavarocchi N. Right ventricular rupture and tamponade caused by malposition of the Avalon cannula for venovenous extracorporeal membrane oxygenation. J Cardiothorac Surg 2012; 7: 36
24. de Bucourt M, Teichgraber UK. Image guided placement of extracorporeal life support through bi-caval dual lumen venovenous membrane oxygenation in an interventional radiology setting—initial experience. J Vasc Access 2012; 13: 221–5
25. Langer T, Vecchi V, Belenkiy SM, Cancio LC, Gattinoni L, Batchinsky AI. Pressure-guided positioning of bicaval dual-lumen catheters for venovenous extracorporeal gas exchange. Intensive Care Med 2013; 39: 151–4
26. Dolch ME, Frey L, Buerkle MA, Weig T, Wassilowsky D, Irlbeck M. Transesophageal echocardiography-guided technique for extracorporeal membrane oxygenation dual-lumen catheter placement. ASAIO J 2011; 57: 341–3
27. Tabak B, Elliott CL, Mahnke CB, Tanaka LY, Ogino MT. Transthoracic echocardiography visualization of bicaval dual lumen catheters for veno-venous extracorporeal membrane oxygenation. J Clin Ultrasound 2012; 40: 183–6
28. Rice TW, Wheeler AP. Coagulopathy in critically ill patients: part 1: platelet disorders. Chest 2009; 136: 1622–30
29. Scheingraber S, Rehm M, Sehmisch C, Finsterer U. Rapid saline infusion produces hyperchloremic acidosis in patients undergoing gynecologic surgery. Anesthesiology 1999; 90: 1265–70
30. Yunos NM, Bellomo R, Hegarty C, Story D, Ho L, Bailey M. Association between a chloride-liberal vs chloride-restrictive intravenous fluid administration strategy and kidney injury in critically ill adults. JAMA 2012; 308: 1566–72
31. Carlesso E, Maiocchi G, Tallarini F, et al. The rule regulating pH changes during crystalloid infusion. Intensive Care Med 2011; 37: 461–8
32. Langer T, Carlesso E, Protti A, et al. In vivo conditioning of acid–base equilibrium by crystalloid solutions: an experimental study on pigs. Intensive Care Med 2012; 38: 686–93

33. Smith BS, Yogaratnam D, Levasseur-Franklin KE, Forni A, Fong J. Introduction to drug pharmacokinetics in the critically ill patient. *Chest* 2012; **141**: 1327–36

34. Shekar K, Roberts JA, McDonald CI, et al. Sequestration of drugs in the circuit may lead to therapeutic failure during extracorporeal membrane oxygenation. *Crit Care* 2012; **16**: R194

35. Gattinoni L, Protti A, Caironi P, Carlesso E. Ventilator-induced lung injury: the anatomical and physiological framework. *Crit Care Med* 2010; **38**: S539–48

36. Crotti S, Iotti GA, Lissoni A, et al. Organ allocation waiting time during extracorporeal bridge to lung transplantation affects outcomes. *Chest* 2013; **144**: 1018–25

37. Fuehner T, Kuehn C, Hadem J, et al. Extracorporeal membrane oxygenation in awake patients as bridge to lung transplantation. *Am J Respir Crit Care Med* 2012; **185**: 763–8

38. Del Sorbo L, Ranieri VM, Keshavjee S. Extracorporeal membrane oxygenation as 'bridge' to lung transplantation: what remains in order to make it standard of care? *Am J Respir Crit Care Med* 2012; **185**: 699–701

39. Abrams DC, Brenner K, Burkart KM, et al. Pilot study of extracorporeal carbon dioxide removal to facilitate extubation and ambulation in exacerbations of chronic obstructive pulmonary disease. *Ann Am Thorac Soc* 2013; **10**: 307–14

40. Crotti S, Lissoni A, Tubiolo D, et al. Artificial lung as an alternative to mechanical ventilation in COPD exacerbation. *Eur Respir J* 2012; **39**: 212–5

41. Hoeper MM, Wiesner O, Hadem J, et al. Extracorporeal membrane oxygenation instead of invasive mechanical ventilation in patients with acute respiratory distress syndrome. *Intensive Care Med* 2013;**39**: 2056–7.

42. Wiesner O, Hadem J, Sommer W, Kühn C, Welte T, Hoeper MM. Extracorporeal membrane oxygenation in a nonintubated patient with acute respiratory distress syndrome. *Eur Respir J* 2012; **40**: 1296–8

43. Langer T, Vecchi V, Belenkiy SM, et al. Extracorporeal gas exchange and spontaneous breathing for the treatment of ARDS: an alternative to mechanical ventilation? *Crit Care Med* 2013; **42**: e211–20

CHAPTER 13

Mechanical support of the circulation

Vladimir Saplacan, Mario Gaudino, and Massimo Massetti

Introduction

The number of patients suffering from advanced heart failure is ever growing (1). Myocardial ischaemia is the most frequent aetiology and, despite medical advancements, almost one third of patients following myocardial infarction will develop heart failure over the following 10 years as a result of ventricular remodelling (2). Whilst heart transplantation can be used to treat advanced heart failure (Chapter 23), this treatment remains limited due to the low number of donors (1). Historically, mechanical circulatory support (MCS) was regarded as only a life-saving treatment. However, it is now frequently used electively or in relative urgency rather than in just vital emergencies to ensure patients a good quality of life (3). Ninety-five percent of all the MCS are ventricular assist devices (VAD) (4). For these reasons, the aim of this chapter is to review the use of MCS to treat heart failure and its complications.

Indications

The decision to implant a MCS is multifactorial and depends on aetiology of heart failure and the long-term strategy. The choice of devices depends on several factors, including patient status, potential for weaning, and duration of the intended assistance (5,6). Broadly, VADs can be used as a bridge to recovery or heart transplantation or as a destination therapy.

Bridge to recovery

Initially limited to only a few days, the duration of MCS has increased with new technology so allowing support of stunned myocardium for much longer intervals of up to several weeks (6–9). Survival in this group of patients is strongly dependent on the aetiology of heart failure (6,9).

Bridge to transplantation

In the absence of immediate availability of a donor, MCS can support patients with chronic heart failure awaiting transplantation so allowing them to mobilize and return home with a reasonable quality of life (6,10). A patient's chance of heart transplantation when supported with a VAD support is 70–80% (6). In the 2008 report of the International Society of Heart Lung Transplantation (ISHLT), 33% of patients who were transplanted had mechanical assistance and 22% had a left ventricular assist device (LVAD) (11). Bridging to heart transplantation with MCS does not adversely influence long-term survival compared to a non-assisted population (11). Decompensated patients who became unstable with multiple organ failure (MOF) or pulmonary arterial hypertension (PAH) do not benefit from immediate transplantation. However, with a long-term VAD, MOF, and PAH may be reversible over several months (12,13).

Destination therapy

Their success in bridging patients to heart transplantation has led to use of VADs as an alternative to transplantation. The Randomized Evaluation of Mechanical Assistance for the Treatment of Congestive Heart Failure (REMATCH) trial demonstrated that patients with end-stage heart failure who are ineligible for transplantation, have a superior survival rate (52% vs. 25% at 1 year and 23% vs. 8% at 2 years) and a better quality of life using VAD compared to medical treatment (14). The Interagency Registry for Mechanically Assisted Circulatory Support (INTERMACS) report has confirmed the prognostic benefits with a 55% 1 year survival in patients having a LVAD as a destination therapy (15).

Patient selection

The most important factor that determines a favourable outcome following implantation, is the patient selection for MCS (16). The New York Heart Association classification is unsuitable for choosing the therapy for patients with advanced heart failure and the INTERMACS profile with seven clinical and prognostic levels, should instead be used (Table 13.1) (17).

In general, VAD implantation can be considered for patients who are severely symptoms despite optimal drug therapy:

- Left ventricular ejection fraction (LVEF) <25%
- Peak exercise systemic oxygen consumption < 12 mL/kg min,
- Frequent hospitalizations during the previous year for heart failure
- Dependency intravenous positive inotropic treatment
- Progressive MOF
- Right ventricle dysfunction (18).

Table 13.1 Intermacs level of limitation at time of implant

INTERMACS level	Time frame for intervention
Level 1. Critical cardiogenic shock	**Within hours**
Patients with life-threatening hypotension despite rapidly escalating inotropic support, critical organ hypoperfusion, often confirmed by worsening acidosis and/or lactate levels.	
Level 2. Progressive decline	**Within few days**
Patient with declining function despite intravenous inotropic support. Worsening renal function, nutritional depletion, inability to restore volume balance.	
Level 3. Stable but inotrope-dependent	**Weeks or months**
Patient with stable blood pressure, organ function, nutrition, and symptoms on continuous intravenous positive inotropic support or on temporary circulatory support device or both.	
Inability to wean from positive inotropes or support.	
Level 4. Symptoms at rest	**Weeks or months**
Stable patient but with daily symptoms of congestion at rest or during activity of daily living, under high doses of diuretics.	
May fluctuate from level 4 to level 5.	
Level 5. No exercise tolerance	**Variable**
Comfortable at rest and with daily living activities but unable to tolerate a greater work-load. Predominantly living within the house. May have underlying refractory elevated volume status, and renal dysfunction.	
Level 6. Poor exercise tolerance	**Variable**
Patient without evidence of fluid overload, comfortable at rest and with activities of daily living and minor activities outside the home. Fatigues after the first few minutes of any meaningful activity (e.g. walking).	
Level 7. Advanced NYHA III class	**Usually not indicated for circulatory support**
Patients without current or recent episodes of unstable fluid balance, living comfortably with meaningful activity limited to mild physical exertion.	

NYHA: New York Heart Association

Adapted from *The Journal of Heart and Lung Transplantation*, **28**, 6, Stevenson LW et al., 'INTERMACS profiles of advanced heart failure: the current picture', pp. 535–541, Copyright 2009, with permission from the International Society for Heart and Lung Transplantation and Elsevier

Considerations prior to implantation of ventricular assist devices

Haemodynamic criteria

The frequently used implantation criteria are those defining cardiogenic shock including systolic arterial pressure <80 mmHg or mean arterial pressure < 65 mmHg, oliguria <0.5 mL/kg/hr, pulmonary capillary wedge pressure (PCWP) >18 mmHg, central venous pressure (CVP) >15 mmHg and cardiac index < 2.0 L/min/m^2 under maximal drug therapy (18,19). Stroke volume measurement (<25 mL) is an alternative if a low cardiac index is compensated by tachycardia (1). Indeed, an extremely rigorous and dogmatic use of these haemodynamic criteria may unduly delay implantation and be responsible for increased morbidity and mortality. Moreover, there are patients who are well adapted to a low chronic output but do not have severe symptoms. Conversely, there are patients who still have a well preserved cardiac output but who are developing MOF (1,16). The survival of patients implanted with an LVAD who are in an almost irreversible critical state

(INTERMACS level 1) at one year is lower than that of more stable patients (INTERMACS 3) (73% vs. 82%) (15).

Renal function

Renal failure before implantation is a very important prognostic factor for mechanical assistance (1,20). Serum creatinine >2.5 mg/dl (221 mmol/L), blood urea nitrogen (BUN) > 40 mg/dl (14.3 mmol/L), glomerular filtration rate <0.5 mL/kg/min or chronic dialysis are associated with a worse outcome (1,21). To ensure patients with a potential to recover are not excluded, the duration of cardiogenic shock and basic renal function must be assessed (16).

Right ventricular function

Between 13–44% of patients develop right ventricular (RV) failure following implantation of an LVAD which significantly contributes to mortality and morbidity (21,22). RV failure associated with LVAD can be anticipated knowing that 20–30% of the patients have a degree of RV failure at the time of LVAD implantation

(1,21). For these reasons, the function of the RV must be assessed echocardiographically to determine the size of the RV and its function including tricuspid annular plane systolic excursion, pulmonary artery pressure (21). Several variables have been identified as preimplantation risk factors for developing RV failure, including RV dilation, as defined by an end diastolic volume >200 mL and end-systolic volume >177 mL, CVP >15 mmHg, transpulmonary gradient >15 mmHg and pulmonary vascular resistance >4 Wood units, major tricuspid insufficiency and altered RV geometry (relation between the short and long axes), ventricular arrhythmia, increased ratio of RV/LV end-diastolic diameter ratio >0.72 and a bilirubin >2.5 mg/dL with ascites and pleural effusions (16,21,22). Preoperatively, management with diuretics, positive inotropes, pulmonary vasodilators and possibly intra-aortic balloon pump (IABP) and ultrafiltration should assist the patient in attaining a CVP less than15 mmHg (21).

Heart valve function

Although it is often difficult because of LV failure, assessment of aortic regurgitation is essential before implanting an LVAD. Aortic valve regurgitation, even if only moderate, may adversely influence LVAD function increasing trans-aortic valve gradient and worsening regurgitation requiring closure of the aortic orifice or bioprosthetic replacement of the valve (16,21).

Significant mitral stenosis should be corrected so as not to alter LVAD loading (23). Mitral insufficiency does not impair LVAD function but should be corrected in the prospect of weaning mechanical support. If severe, tricuspid insufficiency should be corrected to protect the RV and so as not interfere with the loading of the LVAD (21). Structural defects, such as foramen ovale, should be closed so as to avoid a right-to-left shunt and post-LVAD hypoxia (16).

Pulmonary function

Pulmonary dysfunction requiring mechanical ventilation is a negative prognostic factor (1). Functional respiratory parameters that are usually acceptable prior to LVAD implantation are forced expiratory volume at 1 second >50% of predicted, forced vital capacity >50% of predicted, and diffusing capacity of the lung for CO of 50% of predicted (16). LVAD reduces RV afterload but fixed PAH can induce RV failure (21). Despite this risk, LVAD implantation may reduce PAH and allow cardiac transplantation with long-term results comparable to those to patients transplanted who are free from PAH (24).

Hepatic function

Hepatic dysfunction is associated with unfavourable outcome (1). Coagulation disorders secondary to hepatic dysfunction may result in polytransfusion with RV failure and polyimmunization risk (1,21). Hepatic fibrosis or cirrhosis are contraindications (16). Preoperative supplementation with vitamin K is beneficial for malnourished patients (21).

Nutrition

Early parenteral nutrition prior to VAD implantation reduces infection and improves prognosis (1). Malnourishment with a body mass index <22 kg/m² and an albumin level <1.5 g/dL significantly increase the perioperative risk. Despite a higher incidence of infective complications obesity is not a contraindication to LVAD (21).

Table 13.2 Classification of assist devices

Characteristic	Classification
Propulsion	Volume displacement, centrifugal pump, or axial pump
Flow character	Pulsatile or continuous
Placement site	Intra- or extra-corporeal
Energy source	Electrical, pneumatic and magnetic
Assistance duration	Short- or long-term
Assisted ventricle	Left, right, biventricular, or total artificial heart

Devices

There a number of assist devices that are in perpetual evolution and improvement. The characteristics of the devices are classified in table 13.2. As the number of different devices are too numerous, only the most commonly used devices will be briefly presented in the following subsections.

Short-term devices

Short-term assist devices are usually implanted in emergencies. The main purpose is to ensure the patient's survival and to allow time for consideration of subsequent possible treatment strategies. The ideal system must allow an easy emergency implantation and produce adequate systemic perfusion with the minimum of adverse effects (25,26).

Intra-aortic balloon pump

Although not technically a VAD, intra-aotic balloon pumps (IABPs) are widely used in first instance for mechanical assistance of the circulation. A double-lumen balloon catheter placed within the descending thoracic aorta provides aortic counterpulsation by balloon inflation during diastole (figure 13.1) so increasing aortic diastolic pressure and consequently, improving coronary perfusion. In addition, balloon deflation during systole reduces LV parietal pressure so reducing myocardial oxygen consumption, and after-load leading to a moderate increase of cardiac output (26,27). IABP insertion, preferably under fluoroscopic monitoring, is performed percutaneously using the Seldinger technique or inserted directly into an artery, as may be required in the presence of hypotension, obesity, or arteriopathy. Balloon inflation and deflation is usually triggered using an electrocardiograph signal. When the signal is scrambled by the electrocautery then the intra-aortic blood flow or the systemic arterial pressure wave can be used (28).

Several factors may influence the performance of IABPs including their position that should ideally be located immediately distal to the left subclavian artery, the inflation volume (30–40 mL for an adult), the inflation/deflation timing and several patient-related factors such as heart rate and rhythm, mean arterial pressure, aortic valve competence and aortic wall compliance (27). The main contraindications to the use of IABPs are aortic insufficiency as it increases regurgitation and worsens LV dysfunction, sepsis, aortic dissection, and severe peripheral arterial disease (3).

With regard to the activation timing, the pressure increase resulting from balloon inflation is superimposed on the dicrotic notch of the aortic pressure curve which is the aortic valve closure.

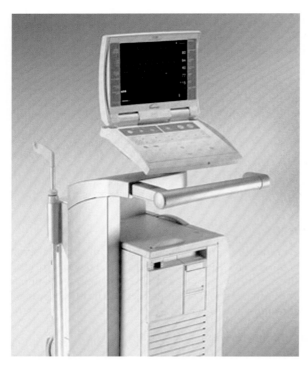

Fig. 13.1 IABP console.
Reproduced from Maquet Cardiovascular—Cardiac Assist with permission

Early inflation and late deflation will adversely affect ventricular ejection, so increasing myocardial oxygen consumption, whilst late inflation and early deflation reduce its positive effect on coronary perfusion (27).

Weaning from IABP is performed in presence of a stable hemodynamic profile under minimal inotropic support, by gradually reducing (over 6–12 hours) either the ratio between IABP inflation and the native heart beats, or the volume inflation of the balloon (6). When the use of IABP is prolonged then heparin anticoagulation is generally used. In the postoperative period, heparin is started 4–6 hr post surgery to minimize the risk of bleeding (3).

Lower limb ischaemia is the most important complication of IABPs, occurring in between 9–25% of patients, whilst haematoma at the femoral puncture site and pseudoaneurysm are less frequent complications (27). Dissection of the aorta by guide wire or catheter may occur, as may renal and mesenteric artery embolization. Thrombocytopenia, from mechanical trauma to the platelets, occurs in up to 50% of patients. Balloon rupture occurs rarely in 1–2% of patients. It is identified by the presence of blood in the gas drive line and requires balloon removal (27,29). However, recently published research questions the efficacy of IABP in the treatment of post-myocardial infarction cardiogenic shock (30).

Impella

The Impella (Abiomed Inc, Danvers, MA) is a battery-powered endovascular axial pump placed within the LV through the aortic valve (31). Two models are available, providing either partial (Impella 2.5) or complete haemodynamic support (Impella 5.0) and they are licensed for use for up to 7 days in the USA and 10 days in Europe (26).

Compared with IABP that increases cardiac output by about 0.5 L/min, the Impella provides a larger increase in cardiac output

and more unloading of the left heart so it is a better solution for a patient with unstable hemodynamic condition (26,31,32). Pump flow depends upon the LV preload (dependent on RV function and pulmonary vascular resistance) and LV afterload (a high systemic vacular resistance will reduce flow) (25). The Impella can be used to drain the LV in patients under extracorporeal life support (ECLS) or to assist a failing RV following heart transplantation with the Impella implanted into the pulmonary artery (25).

The main contraindications to the use of an Impella are aortic insufficiency, aortic stenosis (because of the difficulty accessing the LV and the risk of embolism), hypertrophic heart disease, LV thrombus, myxomatous mitral valve (as a billowing valve blocks the inflow orifice), interventricular septal defect, arterial atherosclerosis, and severe RV failure. The 2.5 L model is preferred, as it may be rapidly implanted percutaneouly without vascular exposure, and has a low incidence of complications including haemorrhage 6%, vascular complications 4% and haemolysis <1% (26,33).

Abiomed BVS 5000

Abiomed BVS 5000 (Abiomed Cardiovascular, Inc, Danvers, MA) is a paracorporeal pulsatile pump for mono- or bi-ventricular support. Each pump contains an atrial and ventricular polyurethane chamber within a polycarbonate tube and polyurethane valves to ensure unidirectional blood flow. Inflow cannulae, fixed onto the atria, ensure filling of the atrial chamber by gravity. Filling depends upon blood volume and pump positioning with respect to the patient and usually, the atrial chamber is set 25 cm below the right atrium. The console pressurizes the ventricular chamber to provide ejection. Outflow cannulae are implanted into the ascending aorta or pulmonary artery. The pump functions asynchronously with the native heart rate and automatically adjusts itself to pre- and after-load with minimal input. When used for BiVAD, serial functioning of the pumps requires adjustment according to individual native ventricular output. This device is mainly used for post-cardiotomy cardiogenic shock for up to 15 days. Heparin anticoagulation is required to maintain an activated clotting time (ACT) between 150 to 200 seconds (27–29).

Centrifugal pumps

Centrifugal pumps are the first choice in refractory cardiac arrests and severe cardiogenic shock. They are commonly referred to as ECLS or extra-corporeal membrane oxygenation (ECMO) (figure 13.2). These devices consist of a centrifugal pump (which is less destructive to blood elements than roller pumps when used for long-term support), frequently an oxygenator, and cannulae to connect the device to the patient. The pump is often implanted in a veno-arterial femoral configuration for BiVAD but can also be used in a central configuration when the chest is open as a right or left VAD. Heparin anticoagulation is required during their use.

Indications for implantation are cardiogenic shock of different aetiologies including post-cardiotomy, following myocardial infarction, drug intoxication, myocarditis, hypothermia, and refractory cardiac arrest. Depending on the aetiology, the average survival is 20–30% (9). Contraindications include brain death, multiorgan failure, and major disorders of coagulation (34).

Serious complications are usually related to the peripheral vessels that were used for implantation or to bleeding from the peripheral

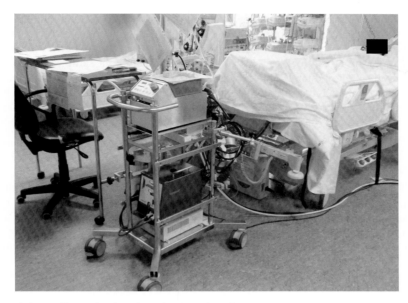

Fig. 13.2 ECMO and IABP assistance being used in a patient in an intensive care unit setting.

and central cannulation sites. Vascular complications, including haemorrhage, dissection, and acute ischaemia, may require emergency surgical treatment. Bleeding requires surgical revision, especially from central cannulation. Should bleeding persists despite surgery, correction of the haemostasis is required with transfusion of packed red cells, fresh-frozen plasma, fibrinogen, and platelets. Rarely, anticoagulation discontinuation over a few hours, while maintaining the pump at high speed, is required to stop bleeding and, exceptionally, the use of recombinant factor VII (60–90 µg/kg), with the potential risk of circuit thrombosis (35).

Insufficient flow rates may be due to inadequate preload, requiring optimization of fluid balance and checking the positioning of the cannulae, pump malfunction, and excessive afterload. Other complications include fibrin deposits within the oxygenator, requiring checking of the anticoagulation or even circuit exchange, gas embolism, and pulmonary oedema caused by an increased end diastolic LV pressure. In the latter, intraventricular stasis must be immediately treated by increasing cardiac performance with positive inotropes and IABP or by directly draining the left heart chambers by means of a surgical or percutaneous technique (35). LV apical surgical drainage allows the switch to a left-left support after right ventricular function recovery and can allow support lasting several weeks.

Long-term devices

Pulsatile devices were the first generation of long-term assist devices. Implantable systems have proven their efficacy but they have drawbacks including their large size, requirement for the percutaneous supply of power through a large pneumatic line and their noisiness (36). The second-generation assist devices are small in size, have continuous flow pumps without a pump chamber or valves and have a satisfactory mechanical performance (37,38). These characteristics have led to their use as a destination therapy. The third-generation devices benefit from magnetic or hydrodynamic levitation, improved durability, blood washing to reduce the risk of thrombosis, and interaction with the patient's

haemodynamics (such as flow modification during variations of pre- and after-load) (38).

First-generation: pulsatile pumps (pneumatic or electric)

Paracorporeal

The THORATEC PVAD (Thoratec Laboratories Corp, Pleasanton, CA) is a paracorporeal pneumatic pulsatile device with polycarbonate external pumps used for mono- or bi-ventricular support. The left inflow cannula is placed in either the left atrium or ventricular apex and the outflow one is inserted into the ascending aorta. For the RVAD, the inflow cannula is placed into the right atrium and the outflow one within the pulmonary artery. Cannulae penetrate the upper abdominal skin and the artificial ventricles rest on the patient's abdomen. Extracorporeal position allows use for BSA (body surface area) between 0.73–2.5 m² (5).

The flow is independent from native heart function and the pump has several functioning modes: fixed-rate mode (independent from native heart frequency); synchronous mode (ejection triggered by R wave); and fill-to-empty mode (flow regulated by pump filling). For BiVAD configuration, the RVAD flow is slightly inferior to the LVAD one to avoid pulmonary congestion.

Its main use is as bridge to transplantation. Optimal timing for heart transplantation depends on multi-organ recovery (3–5 weeks on average) and side effects (such as intrathoracic adhesions due to long-term use, which may complicate transplantation in patients with altered platelet function associated with anticoagulation therapy) (25).

Patients in critical condition (INTERMACS Class 1) benefit most from a biventricular implantation with a bridge-to-heart transplantation success rate of 71.3% and a post-heart transplantation survival of almost 90% at 1 year (39).

Intracorporeal LVAD

Implantable pulsatile LVADs are left support devices using an electric or pneumatic pusher-plate displacement pump. They are power-supplied via a percutaneous cable and ensure outflows of 10 L/min allowing the patient to be discharged home. They are implanted either intraperitoneally or in a preperitoneal pocket in the left upper abdomen. Due to pumps sizes, small-size patients are excluded (the minimal body area required for Thoratec Heart Mate XVE is 1.5 m^2) (5). The inflow cannula is fixed to the LV apex and the outflow one is connected to the ascending aorta. They are used as bridge to heart transplantation and as destination therapy. In the ISHLT 2005 report, among 655 patients, survival with pulsatile supports was 83% and 50% at 1 month and one year respectively when utilized as bridge to heart transplantation (40).

◆ HeartMate XVE LVAD (Thoratec Laboratories Corp, Pleasanton, CA): This device had a first pneumatic version and then an electrical one. The pump internal surfaces in contact with blood are coated with titanium microspheres to stimulate a neointima formation and reduce thrombogenicity (thrombo-embolic risk below 5% despite the absence of an anticoagulant therapy). Long-term anticoagulation is not necessary and only platelets inhibitors are prescribed (41).

◆ Novacor LVAD (World Heart, Inc, Oakland, CA): This is a reliable device but with a high rate of thrombotic complications despite anticoagulation. Used as a bridge to transplantation, results of more than 2000 implantations worldwide over the last 20 years are comparable with those of paracorporeal devices (25).

Total artificial heart

One of the most used total artifical hears (TAHs) is the Cardiowest TAH (CardioWest Technologies, Inc, Tucson, AZ). This provides pneumatic biventricular support, with an intrathoracic implantation in an orthotopic position and powered by an external console. Its dimensions limit its use to large chests (BSA >1.7 m^2 and sternum–column distance >10 cm) (42).

Its implantation requires native heart explantation under CPB, while keeping the atrial cuffs to allow suturing artificial ventricles. Outflow prostheses are anastomosed onto the ascending aorta and pulmonary artery. Anticoagulation therapy together with platelet inhibitor is necessary aiming for an international normalized ratio (INR) of 2 (28).

In a large study on over 700 TAHs implanted as a bridge to transplantation, 79% of patients have been transplanted with an 85.9% survival at 1 year (42).

Second-generation: rotary axial flow pumps

These small size devices connected via a transcutaneous cable to the external console propel the blood through a high-speed rotor (8000–12 000 rpm) providing a 6–8 L/min flow. Blood component destruction is caused by high-speed rotation together with turbulence induced by contact bearings. This increases thrombus formation and risk of embolic events. Whilst pump function is less sensitive to pre- or after-load variations, hypovolaemia can cause left ventricle suction with subsequent arrhythmias. Pump dysfunction may induce a backflow equivalent to acute aortic insufficiency due to the absence of valves within the device (38).

Jarvik 2000 (Jarvik Heart, Inc, New York, NY)

This miniaturized pump is implanted into the LV through median sternotomy or left thoracotomy (thus allowing the implantation of the outflow cannula onto the ascending or descending thoracic aorta), with or without CPB. The energy driveline is either tunnelled through the abdomen wall or fixed with a titanium pedestal screwed into the skull (retro-auricular, reducing the infectious risk due to the vascularity of the scalp and pedestal immobility) (43). The operating mode includes a pump intermittent low speed option, allowing for left ventricular ejection and aortic valve washing.

Micromed de Bakey (MicroMed Cardiovascular, Inc, Houston, TX) and HeartMate II (Thoratec Laboratories Corp, Pleasanton, CA)

These pumps are implanted through median sternotomy within a preperitoneal pocket connected to the LV apex and ascending aorta. Results are satisfactory, with nearly 80% of patients transplanted, weaned off, or living under support at 18 months post-implantation. Survival post-transplantation at 1 year is similar to the general population (86%). Patients supported by these LVADs had a survival rate at 12 and 18 months of 73% and 72%, greater than survival under pulsatile VADs (36).

Third-generation: the levitation principle

These are continuous flow centrifugal pumps (apart from the axial pump Incor (Berlin Heart GmbH, Berlin Germany)), with a suspended impeller rotating in the blood flow. The contact-free rotation reduces wear and heat production (potentially increase of durability), diminishes blood components destruction, and ensures a better washing of the impeller, thus reducing thrombotic risk inside the pump. Centrifugal pump flow is more dependent on pressure variations of pre- and post-load than axial pump flow, reducing the risk of ventricular suction during hypovolaemia or arrhythmia incidents and restraining the increase of post-capillary pulmonary pressures during exercise (38).

The most diffused models are HVAD Heartware (HeartWare Corp), VentrAssist (Ventracor Ltd), DuraHeart (Terumo Corp). These pumps are implanted into the left ventricle apex and the outflow prosthesis is fixed onto the ascending aorta. Despite their small size, delivered flows are high (up to 10 L/min). Its use for biventricular failure has been reported (double implantation), with a survival of 82% at 30 days (38,44).

Postoperative complications

Suboptimal functioning of the LVAD

Beside the rare instance of pump malfunction, suboptimal flow can be related to a variety of factors including aortic regurgitation and an intracardiac shunt.

Undiagnosed aortic regurgitation

The reduction of preoperative aortic transvalvular gradient, due to LV dysfunction with a low systemic arterial pressure and high EDLVP, may mask the diagnosis of aortic regurgitation that will worsen after implantation of a LVAD. Clinically, it results in a systemic peripheral hypoperfusion associated with a high LVAD outflow (3).

Undiagnosed intracardiac shunt

Septal defects that are undiagnosed and untreated, will result in a right-to-left shunt with ongoing hypoxia after starting the LVAD (3).

Other causes

RV failure, kinking of the prosthesis, thrombosis of the LVAD's valves, intermittent aspiration of the free ventricular wall or septum into the inflow cannula because of malpositioning or hypovolaemia, and arrhythmias, can all cause suboptimal functions of LVADs.

Bleeding

Bleeding in the early postoperative period may be surgical in origin: for example, extensive dissection and suboptimal technique, or from haematological causes, including a post-CPB coagulopathy, liver dysfunction due to low cardiac output, preoperative undernutrition and anti-vitamin K treatment, haemodilution because of bleeding and intravascular filling, and hypothermia. Almost 50% of patients have bleeding and the blood loss is usually significant. Frazier and colleagues reported 635 mL over 12 hr for an axial pump and 2405 mL/12 hr for a pulsatile LVAD (45). Heparin is usually stopped during day 1 and restarted when bleeding reduces to 30 mL/hr over 3 hr (6). In the intensive care unit, once the patient has rewarmed and platelets and coagulation factors have been transfused, reoperation for haemostasis is eventually considered if haemorrhage continues. Platelets and red blood cells should be administered after leukocyte filtration to avoid hyperimmunization of patients awaiting transplantation (3). During the late postoperative period, a low pump flow associated with a low output despite adequate intravascular filling, and high intracardiac pressures suggest cardiac tamponade. In 15 to 50% of cases, patients with second- and third-generation continuous flow devices often present with gastrointestinal bleeding caused by the loss of pulsatility and associated with an acquired von Willebrand disease (46).

Infection

The REMATCH trial found that sepsis was the leading cause of death in patients with long-term LVAD, with an incidence of 30–40% (14). The most common infection are with *Staphylococcus*, *Pseudomonas*, *Enterococcus* and *Candida* (5). Infection is less frequent with continuous compared with pulsatile flow pumps (11.8% vs. 28.3%) (15). Using aggressive antibiotic therapy, most patients will reach transplantation, but pump infection (endocarditis) requires either the device to explanted and exchanged or heart transplantation, and both at a high risk (3). Despite their high incidence, infections when well treated, do not seem to have an adverse impact on pre- and post-transplantation mortality and post-transplantation infection rate is not significantly increased (5,46).

Thromboembolism

A third of the patients with LVAD will suffer an embolic event (5). Of the neurological adverse events reported in the REMATCH trial, 47% were transient. Increased afterload and reduced preload can lead to stasis in the ascending aorta, fusion of aortic valve leaflets and thrombosis of the ascending aorta (5,48). Anticoagulation is required for all devices except the Thoratec HeartMate XVE, which has a very low rate of thromboembolic events at 2–4% per patient year (41).

Haemolysis

Haemolysis is a complication associated most frequently with axial flow pumps, the Heart Mate II having a hemolysis reported incidence of 3% (37). This is because the impeller rotates at high-speed in axial pumps and negative pressure is generated in the inflow cannula. Other causes of haemolysis include kinking of the prostheses (which can be avoided with proper position of the pump and reinforcement of outflow tracts), and incorrect positioning of the left intraventricular inflow cannula with intermittent obstruction by the septum or the free wall. Haemolysis, as evidenced by increases in the blood concentration of lactic dehydrogenase and plasma free haemoglobin concentration, is often transient and can be decreased by reducing pump rotation speed or by correcting any technical problems (21).

Dysrhythmias

Although supraventricular arrhythmias are usually well tolerated by patients with a VAD, atrial fibrillation should be treated because of the risk of thrombosis and potential impairment of VAD filling. In the case of refractory ventricular fibrillation under LVAD, pump filling can be maintained temporarily if pulmonary resistances are low as may occur in paediatric surgery during the Fontan cavo-pulmonary shunt (16). However, if the pulmonary pressure is high during the early post-implantation period, a RVAD is often necessary (49).

Right heart failure

In the immediate postoperative period, alterations of ventricular interdependence as a result of deviation of the interventricular septum to the left, and increased RV preload caused by a high LVAD flow should be limited by reducing the LVAD output (6). Pulmonary vasoconstriction from a post-CPB inflammatory response is an additional risk factor for RV failure (3). Once the RV failure occurs, inadequate filling of the LVAD results in a low systemic output. Despite phosphodiesterase inhibitors, beta-2 agonists and pulmonary dilators such as nitric oxide, about 10% of patients will require right-sided mechanical assist (49).

Device failure

In the REMATCH trial, device failure is the second most common cause of death in patients with long-term LVAD occurring in 13% in the first year and 63% by the end of the second year (14). Failure may be caused by a variety of the device components and generally, it is a minor defect. Major dysfunctions are rare but disastrous and may necessitate emergency reoperation and replacement of the pump (3).

Immunologic effects and allosensitization

Alteration of the T-cell function, hyper-reactivity of the B-cell and a high frequency of circulating antiphospholipid and anti-human leukocyte antigen (HLA) antibodies are observed during LVAD. The progressive reduction in cellular immunity increases the risk of infection and the allosensitization to HLAs may prolong the duration of pretransplant waiting times and generate acute rejection. An immunosuppressor treatment such as immunoglobulin therapy in association with cyclophosphamide administration, reduces the risk of rejection (5,50–52).

Conclusion

Continuous advancements and refinements of technology have made mechanical assistance devices a highly valuable resource for the management of patients both with acute and chronic congestive heart failure. The recent development of spoke and hub systems and ECMO networks have enabled this therapy to be delivered even in tertiary care centres so further expanding its possibilities and indications for the use of ECMO. Future developments are likely to further improve VADs safety and effectiveness, so that an increasing proportion of patients suffering from cardiac failure will benefit from the technology of circulatory assistance (50).

References

1. Miller LW. Patient selection for the use of ventricular assist devices as bridge to transplantation. *Ann Thorac Surg* 2003; **75**: S66–71
2. Lietz K, Miller LW. Left ventricular assist devices: evolving devices and indications for use in ischemic heart disease. *Curr Opin Cardiol* 2004; **19**: 613–8
3. Sun BC, Harter R, Gravlee GP. Devices for cardiac support and replacement. In: Hensley FA, Martin DE, Gravlee GP, eds. *A Practical Approach to Cardiac Anesthesia*. Philapedlphia PA: Lippincott Williams & Wilkins, 2008; 587–603
4. Frazier OH, Delgado RM. Mechanical circulatory support for advanced heart failure: where does it stand in 2003? *Circulation* 2003; **108**: 3064–8
5. Aggarwal S, Cheema F, Oz MC, Naka Y. Long term mechanical circulatory support. In Cohn LH, ed. *Cardiac surgery in the adult*. New York NY: McGraw Hill Companies, 2008; 1609–29
6. Dempster K, Tsui S. Mechanical circulatory support. In: Ghosh S, Falter F, Cook DJ, eds. *Cardiopulmonary Bypass*. Cambridge UK: Cambridge University Press, 2009; 106–24
7. Simon MA, Kormos RL, Murali S, et al. Myocardial recovery using ventricular assist devices: prevalence, clinical characteristics and outcomes. *Circulation* 2005; **112**: I-32–I-36
8. Christian TF, Gitter MJ, Miller TD, Gibbons RJ. Prospective identification of myocardial stunning using technetium-99m sestamibi-based measurements of infarct size. *J Am Coll Cardiol* 1997; **30**: 1633–40
9. Massetti M, Tasle M, Le Page O, et al. Back from irreversibility: extracorporeal life support for prolonged cardiac arrest. *Ann Thorac Surg* 2005; **79**: 178–84
10. Allen JG, Weiss ES, Schaffer JM, et al. Quality of life and functional status in patients surviving 12 months after left ventricular assist device implantation. *J Heart Lung Transplant* 2010; **29**: 278–85
11. Taylor DO, Edwards LB, Aurora P, et al. Registry of the International Society for Heart and Lung Transplantation: Twenty-fifth Official Adult Heart Transplant Report—2008. *J Heart Lung Transplant* 2008; **27**: 943–56
12. Salzberg SP, Lachat ML, Harbou vK, Zund G, Turina MI. Normalization of high pulmonary vascular resistance with LVAD supporting heart transplantation candidates. *Eur J Cardiothorac Surg* 2005; **27**: 222–5
13. Mikus E, Stepanenko A, Krabatsch T, et al. Reversibility of fixed pulmonary hypertension in left ventricular assist device support recipients. *Eur J Cardiothorac Surg* 2011; **40**: 971–7
14. Rose EA, Gelijns AC, Moskowitz AJ, et al. Long term use of a left ventricular assist device for end stage heart failure. *N Engl J Med* 2001; **345**: 1435–43
15. Kirklin JK, Naftel DC, Kormos RL, et al. Second INTERMACS annual report: More than 1,000 primary left ventricular assist device implants. *J Heart Lung Transplant* 2010; **29**: 1–10
16. Aaronson KD, Patel H, Pagani FD. Patient selection for left ventricular assist device therapy. *Ann Thorac Surg* 2003; **75**: S29–35
17. Stevenson LW, Pagani FD, Young JB. INTERMACS profiles of advanced heart failure: the current picture. *J Heart Lung Transplant* 2009; **28**: 535–41
18. McMurray JJ, Adamopoulos S, Anker SD, et al. ESC Guidelines for the diagnosis and treatment of acute and chronic heart failure 2012. *Eur Heart J* 2012; **14**: 803–69
19. Reynolds HR, Hochman JS. Cardiogenic shock: current concepts and improving outcomes. *Circulation* 2008; **117**: 686–97
20. Vanzetto G, Akret C, Bach V, et al. Assistance circulatoire extracorporelle percutanée dans les défaillances hémodynamiques aigues graves: experience monocentrique chez 100 patients consecutifs. *Can J Cardiol* 2009; **25**: e179–86
21. Slaughter MS, Pagani FD, Rogers JG, et al. Clinical management of continuous-flow left ventricular assist devices in advanced heart failure. *J Heart Lung Transplant* 2010; **29**: S1–39
22. Kukucka M, Stepanenko A, Potapov E, et al. Right-to-left ventricular end-diastolic diameter ratio and prediction of right ventricular failure with continuous-flow left ventricular assist devices. *J Heart Lung Transplant* 2011; **30**: 64–9
23. Oz MC, Rose EA, Levin HR. Selection criteria for placement of left ventricular assist devices. *Am Heart J* 1995; **129**: 173–7
24. Zimpfer D, Zrunek P, Sandner S, et al. Post-transplant survival after lowering fixed pulmonary hypertension using left ventricular assist devices. *Eur J Cardiothorac Surg* 2007; **31**: 698–702
25. Loisance D. Mechanical circulatory support: a clinical reality. *Asian Cardiovasc Thorac Ann* 2008; **16**: 419–31
26. Naidu SS. Novel percutaneous cardiac assist devices: the science of and indications for hemodynamic support. *Circulation* 2011; **123**: 533–43
27. McGee EC, McCarthy PM, Moazami N. Temporary mechanical circulatory support. In: Cohn LH ed. *Cardiac Surgery in the Adult*. New York NY: McGraw Hill Companies, 2008; 507–33
28. DiNardo JA, Zvara DA. Mechanical circulatory support. In: DiNardo JA, Zvara DA, eds. *Anesthesia for Cardiac Surgery*. Hoboken NJ: Blackwell Publishing, 2008; 375–408
29. Bojar RM. *Manual of Perioperative Care in Adult Cardiac Surgery*. Hoboken NJ: Blackwell Publishing, 2005; 339–466
30. Thiele H, Zeymer U, Neumann FJ, et al. IABP-SHOCK II Trial Investigators. Intraaortic balloon support for myocardial infarction with cardiogenic shock. *N Engl J Med* 2012; **367**: 1287–96
31. Reesink KD, Dekker AL, Van Ommen V, et al. Miniature intracardiac assist device provides more effective cardiac unloading and circulatory support during severe left heart failure than intraaortic balloon pumping. *Chest* 2004; **126**: 896–902
32. Seyfarth M, Sibbing D, Bauer I, et al. A Randomized clinical trial to evaluate the safety and efficacy of a percutaneous left ventricular assist device versus intra-aortic balloon pumping for treatment of cardiogenic shock caused by myocardial infarction. *J Am Coll Cardiol* 2008; **52**: 1584–8
33. Catena E, Milazzo F, Merli M, et al. Echocardiographic evaluation of patients receiving a new left ventricular assist device: the Impella_ recover 100. *Eur J Echocardiogr* 2004; **5**: 430–7
34. Beckmann A, Benk C, Beyersdorf F, et al. A Position article for the use of extracorporeal life support in adult patients. *Eur J Cardiothorac Surg* 2011; **40**: 676–81
35. Ruggieri VG, Guinet P, Abouliatim I, Felix C, Flecher E. Les complications de l'ECMO et leur prise en charge. In: Flecher E, Seguin P, Verhoye JP, eds. *ECLS et ECMO Guide pratique*. Berlin: Springer, 2010; 49–64
36. Pagani FD, Miller LW, Russell SD, et al. Extended mechanical circulatory support with a continuous-flow rotary left ventricular assist device. *J Am Coll Cardiol* 2009; **54**: 312–21
37. Miller LW, Pagani FD, Russell SD, et al. Use of a continuous-flow device in patients awaiting heart transplantation. *N Engl J Med* 2007; **357**: 885–96
38. Pagani F. Continuous-flow rotary left ventricular assist devices with '3rd generation' design. *Semin Thorac Cardiovasc Surg* 2008; **20**: 255–63
39. Moriguchi J, Davis S, Jocson R, et al. Successful use of a pneumatic biventricular assist device as a bridge to transplantation in cardiogenic shock. *J Heart Lung Transplant* 2011; **30**: 1143–7
40. Deng MC, Edwards LB, Hertz MI, et al. Mechanical circulatory support device database of the International Society for Heart and Lung Transplantation: Third Annual Report—2005. *J Heart Lung Transplant* 2005; **24**: 1182–7

41. Slater JP, Rose EA, Levin HR, et al. Low thromboembolic risk without anticoagulation using advanced-design left ventricular assist device.*Ann Thorac Surg* 1996; **62**: 1321–8

42. Morris RJ. Total artificial heart—Concepts and clinical use. *Semin Thorac Cardiovasc Surg* 2008, **20**: 247–54

43. Majert-Hohlweg B, Gutwald R, Siegenthaler MP, Schmelzeisen R. Implantation of the Jarvik 2000 left ventricular assist device: role of the maxillo facial surgeon. *Eur J Cardiothorac Surg* 2005; **28**: 337–9

44. Krabatsch T, Potapov E, Stepanenko A, et al. Biventricular circulatory support with two miniaturized implantable assist devices.*Circulation* 2011; **124**[suppl 1]: S179–86

45. Frazier OH, Gregoric ID, Cohn WE. Initial experience with non-thoracic, extraperitoneal, off-pump insertion of the Jarvik 2000 heart in patients with previous median sternotomy. *J Heart Lung Transplant* 2006; **25**: 499–503

46. Aggarwal A, Pant R, Kumar S, et al. Incidence and management of gastrointestinal bleeding with continuous flow assist devices. *Ann Thorac Surg* 2012; **93**: 1534–40

47. Sinha P, Chen JM, Flannery M, Scully BN, Oz MC, Edwards NM. Infections during left ventricular assist device support do not affect posttransplant outcomes. *Circulation* 2000; **102**[suppl III]: III-194–III-199

48. Rose AG, Park SJ, Bank AJ, Miller LW. Partial aortic valve fusion induced by left ventricular assist device. *Ann Thorac Surg* 2000; **70**: 1270–4

49. Vural KM. Ventricular assist device applications. *Anadolu Kardiyol Derg* 2008; **8** [suppl 2]: 117–30

50. Frazier OH. Prologue: ventricular assist devices and total artificial hearts. A historical perspective. *Cardiol Clin* 2003; **21**: 1–13

51. Schuster M, Kocher A, John R, Hoffman M, et al. B-cell activation and allosensitization after left ventricular assist device implantation is due to T-cell activation and CD40 ligand expression. *Human immunology* 2002; **63**: 211–20

52. Itescu S, Ankersmit JH, Kocher AA, Schuster MD. Immunobiology of left ventricular assist devices. *Prog Cardiovasc Dis* 2000; **43**: 67–80

CHAPTER 14

Hypothermia and circulatory arrest

Jeremy M. Bennett, Andrew Shaw, and Chad Wagner

Introduction

Induced, or therapeutic, hypothermia has been used for cardiac surgical patients undergoing cardiopulmonary bypass (CPB) since the 1960s. Early work was undertaken in the 1940s with animal models, though it was not until the 1950s when Bigelow and his group were able to demonstrate feasibility of hypothermia and cardiac surgery with dog experiments (1). Until recently, patients undergoing CPB received therapeutic hypothermia at temperatures approaching 28°C. Despite the use of hypothermia at these temperatures with good outcomes, continued concerns related to perceived increases in ventricular dysrhythmias, prolonged sedation and emergence from CPB, and coagulopathic bleeding, prompted interest in mild hypothermia or normothermia for most cardiac surgery. Additionally, concerns related to worsened neurological outcomes with warmer temperatures have not been shown, and 'mild' hypothermia at temperatures of 32–36°C have neuroprotective effects for patients post-cardiac arrest (2). Consequently, more patients are undergoing cardiac surgical procedures with CPB utilizing mild hypothermia or normothermic temperatures. For procedures where complete arrest of the circulation is required, deep or profound hypothermia remains the mainstay of therapy to reduce the ischaemic consequence to organs and neurological function.

In this chapter we will discuss the underlying physiology and mechanistic effects of hypothermia on organ protection during cardiac surgery and CPB. Further discussion on organ changes along with temperature monitoring will be addressed. The benefits and risks of hypothermia will be discussed along with indications for its use. The definitions of body temperature that are used in this chapter are presented in table 14.1.

Physiology of hypothermia

First described by Bigelow and colleagues in 1950 using animal models (1), the protective effects of hypothermia on organ function have allowed increasingly complex cardiac, aortic, neurological, and other surgical procedures to be undertaken without resultant harm to the patient. Hypothermia, along with a cardioplegic solution, reduces the metabolic requirements of the myocardium and allows periods of reduced or complete absence of blood flow to be utilized for cardiac surgical procedures. Additionally hypothermia

Table 14.1 Definitions of body temperature

Term	Temperature (°C)
Hyperthermia	> 37
Normothermia	35–37
Mild hypothermia	32–35
Moderate hypothermia	25–31
Deep hypothermia	18–24
Profound hypothermia	< 18

results in proportional decreases in metabolic requirements of the brain, spinal cord, renal, hepatic, and splanchnic tissues resulting in total body decreased oxygen requirement and prolonging time until ischaemic injury occurs.

Traditional teaching of hypothermic organ protection revolves around the decrease in metabolic oxygen consumption of tissues by approximately 7 to 8% per centigrade decrease in body temperature (3). At 32°C the metabolic rate is decreased by 45% and further declines to one-half the normal requirement at 28°C. A decrease in metabolic rate reduces the amount of oxygen required to maintain cellular function and therefore aerobic metabolism can continue for brief periods of compromised blood flow and oxygen supply without resulting in devastating injury. Additionally, waste by-products and anaerobic metabolism are decreased in proportion to the decreased metabolic rate. While hypothermia is known to be protective, the exact degree and mechanism to which tissue injury is reduced continues to be investigated. Mild hypothermia has been previously demonstrated to result in improved outcomes when combined with high-dose inhalational anaesthetic agents (isoflurane) or even barbiturate-induced coma (4), suggesting that additional factors, beyond the traditional teaching of a reduction in metabolic rate, are responsible for the protective effect of hypothermia.

Additional protective mediators are believed to be due to stabilization of neuronal and cellular membranes, a reduction in free oxygen radicals (5), and a reduction in excitatory amino acids such as glutamate, leukotrienes, protein kinase C, and a reduced calcium influx all of which may trigger cellular apoptosis (6). As a mediator of glutamate excitotoxicity, nitric oxide may increase neuronal cellular damage during periods of ischaemia and the synthesis of nitric oxide has been shown to be reduced during hypothermia and may play a supplementary protective role (7).

Deep hypothermic circulatory arrest

Profound or, as it is more often referred, deep hypothermic circulatory arrest (DHCA), undertaken at body temperatures of less than 18°C is a well-known and beneficial modality used for congenital heart surgery, aortic arch reconstruction, pulmonary endarterectomy, and additional procedures. Beyond the significant reduction in whole-body oxygen and metabolic requirements, the cessation of blood flow created by circulatory arrest provides for optimal operating conditions allowing the surgeon to work in a near 'bloodless' field. Circulatory arrest otherwise leads to tissue hypoxia, which affects all aerobic functions, particularly the production of adenosine triphosphate (ATP), which leads to failure of energy-dependent cell functions (8). Failure of the ATPase pump ensues, leading to intracellular accumulation of sodium and chloride ions. This leads to depolarization, resulting in an inflow of calcium ions with the end result being hydrolysis of mitochondrial and plasma membranes. Excessive depolarization leads to a build up of excitatory amino acids glutamate and aspartate.

During ischaemia there is insufficient ATP production for glutamate and glial reabsorption. Anaerobic metabolism leads to the production of lactate, causing a decrease in intracellular pH and further stimulating release of glutamate and aspartate. Left unabated, cellular calcium homeostasis cannot be achieved leading to progressive cellular dysfunction and apoptosis (8).

Hypothermia and continued antegrade cerebral perfusion are the most effective measures to maintain aerobic glycolysis in the presence of reduced flow. Circulatory arrest helps to reduce anaerobic glycolysis and accompanying acidosis by eliminating continued glucose supply (9). Besides hypothermia there are several pharmacological neuroprotective agents listed in table 14.2 that have been, and are still, utilized to attenuate the cellular ischemic response. Anaesthetic management for organ protection will be discussed later in this chapter.

Organ function during hypothermia

Cardiac function

Hypothermia affects cardiac, renal, respiratory, coagulation, and other organ system functions. The cardiovascular system undergoes several changes: bradycardia and a reduction in cardiac output and, due to alterations of myocardial calcium kinetic impairment of isovolumetric relaxation and the early phase of ventricular relaxation develops resulting in impaired diastolic function (10). Along with a slowing of the heart rate a concomitant increase in ventricular irritability occur, even at normal pH and electrolyte composition. As the body continues to cool the heart rate further declines until at temperatures between 25 and 30°C the increasing ventricular irritability gives way to sustained ventricular fibrillation that is often refractory to electrical cardioversion or medical treatment. This fibrillatory state and subsequent

Table 14.2 Potential neuroprotective agents

Drug	Neuroprotective effect
Steroids	Decrease proinflammatory response
Barbiturates	Decrease CMRO$_2$, CBF, free fatty acids, free radicals, and cerebral oedema. Protective in focal ischaemia
Mannitol	Reducing cerebral oedema, scavenging free radicals, protecting the kidneys by lowering renal vascular resistance, preserving tubular integrity and reducing endothelial oedema
Furosemide	Blocking renal reabsorption of sodium and increasing renal blood flow
Insulin	Controlling hyperglycaemia, preventing intracellular acidosis
Calcium channel blockers	Blockade of voltage-sensitive and NMDA-activated neuronal calcium channels, decreasing calcium influx into cytoplasm
Lidocaine	Selective blockade of sodium channels in neuronal membranes, reducing CMRO$_2$
Dexmedetomidine	Inhibition of ischaemia-induced norepinephrine release, protective in both focal and global ischaemia
Remacemide	Glutamate antagonist
Acadesine	Mitigates the effects of reperfusion injury
Beta-adrenergic blockers	Decreasing inflammatory response

Adapted from *Journal of Cardiothoracic and Vascular Anaesthesia*, 24, 4, Svyatets M et al., 'Perioperative management of deep hypothermic circulatory arrest', pp. 644–655, Copyright 2010, with permission from Elsevier.

CMRO$_2$: cerebral metabolic rate for oxygen; CBF: cerebral blood flow; NMDA: *N*-methyl-d-aspartate.

cardiac decompensation was such a significant complication during early experimental studies of hypothermia that this fuelled further interest in extracorporeal circulation technology (11). At first, an increase in catecholamines drives an increase in contractility. However, as temperature continues to decline, a negative inotropic state develops. This negative contractility does not appear to be related to the decrease in heart rate as was demonstrated by Lewis and colleagues (12) when the heart rate was maintained at a set rate by external pacing. An inverse relationship developed with an increased heart rate with worsening contractility in hypothermic patients at less than 33°C. Changes in the electrocardiograph (ECG) that seen with mild hypothermia include an increased PR interval, widening of the QRS complex, and the appearance of the Osborne J wave. Systemic vascular resistance increases along with central venous pressure, which ultimately maintains mean arterial pressure despite worsening cardiac function.

Systemic carbon dioxide production

As the metabolic rate decreases with hypothermia, the production of waste by-products is decreased. The amount of carbon dioxide produced by the body is decreased and minute volume of the mechanical ventilator or sweep gas rate to the oxygenator on the CPB machine, require adjustment to maintain PaCO$_2$ within the physiological range.

Coagulation

As body temperature decreases, the haematologic system is adversely affected, often with impairment of coagulation and increased bleeding necessitating transfusion of blood products. Platelet function is often the most dramatically affected with increased bleeding times. A decrement in platelet count is frequently seen, due to sequestration in the liver and possibly the spleen, which partially improves with rewarming (13). Further platelet impairment beyond that expected due to platelet interaction with the extracorporeal tubing, roller pumps, or protamine-induced alteration to platelet aggregation has been seen, suggesting that hypothermia alone has adverse effects on platelet function (14). Enzymatic function in the coagulation cascade is also affected with mild prolongation of the prothrombin time and activated partial thromboplastic time (15). A recent meta-analysis demonstrated an increase in surgical blood loss and transfusion requirement in surgical patients with even mild hypothermia (34–36ºC), suggesting that these effects are clinically important (16).

Renal function

Alteration in renal function and electrolyte composition are frequently areas of concern in patients undergoing induced hypothermia. Impairments of glomerular filtration rate (GFR), renal blood flow, and vascular resistance, with an increased urinary output frequently occur as hypothermia develops. In early studies a decrease in urinary output was seen and was attributed to decreased GFR, renal blood flow, and increased afferent renal arteriole resistance (17) with subsequent concern for worsened renal outcomes. However, more recent studies of patients undergoing mild hypothermia following cardiac arrest compared to normothermic controls have not demonstrated a worsened renal function despite mild increases in serum creatinine (18). Additional studies undertaken in a neurosurgical intensive care patient population undergoing induced hypothermia demonstrated mild renal dysfunction with an increased diuresis and significant electrolyte disturbances as temperature reduction was undertaken (19). An increased free-water diuresis often occurs during hypothermia, which may be due to impaired antidiuretic hormone activity, further promoting electrolyte alterations resulting in cardiac arrhythmias. Hyponatraemia, hypokalaemia, hypomagnesaemia, and hypophosphataemia are all frequently encountered along with a mild reduction in serum calcium concentration during hypothermia. These changes are due to renal alterations of GFR and blood flow in addition to intracellular movement with cooling. Management of these changes should be performed judiciously as extracellular shift occurs during rewarming and may lead to elevated plasma levels that could be harmful.

Blood gas management

Blood gas management is additionally affected by hypothermia with increased solubility of oxygen and carbon dioxide. Though oxygen has greater affinity for haemoglobin at colder temperatures, the extent of reduced oxygen requirement results in a net improvement in aerobic function.

As the blood temperature decreases carbon dioxide becomes more soluble with a subsequent reduction in $PaCO_2$ and development of respiratory alkalosis. Acid–base management of patients undergoing hypothermia often revolves around alpha-stat or pH-stat management. Alpha-stat management seeks to maintain electrochemical neutrality with *temperature uncorrected* blood gas values—that is the blood sample is measured at 37ºC and interpreted uncorrected for body temperature. Autoregulated cerebral blood flow is maintained while limiting the degree of cerebral vasodilation and potential embolic burden.

Originally a pH-stat approach to acid–base management was used during hypothermic CPB. Carbon dioxide is added to the sweep gas to the oxygenator management to maintain the pH near 7.4 when the arterial blood gas is measured at 37ºC and then interpreted corrected to body temperature. This *temperature-corrected* strategy results in cerebral vasodilation and luxuriant cerebral blood flow, which may increase the risk of embolic burden to the brain. However, pH-stat management has been shown to improve cortical oxygenation in an animal model of newborn pigs (20) and has been shown to improve outcomes when combined with alpha-stat management in congenital heart surgery (21).

In a recent systematic review, Abdul and colleagues (8) reviewed 16 studies of patients undergoing DHCA. Seven papers demonstrated improved neurologic outcomes with alpha-stat acid–base management; another four indicated improved outcomes with pH-stat management, while the remainder were inconclusive. Of the four indicating improvement with pH-stat management, three were performed in paediatric populations while all seven studies indicating superiority of alpha-stat management were performed in adult patients. They thus concluded that alpha-stat management should be the preferred blood gas management strategy in adults while pH-stat management should be preferred in the paediatric surgical population. This issue remains controversial, however, and current institutional preferences may not follow these general rules.

Temperature monitoring

With induced hypothermia, the site of temperature monitoring is important. Surrogates for core body temperature include bladder, rectal, and pulmonary artery catheter thermistors, while brain temperature is more closely approximated by nasopharyngeal, tympanic membrane, and invasive jugular bulb thermistors (22). Jugular bulb temperatures are often considered the gold standard due to the proximity to the carotid arteries as well as the aortic cannula through which warming or cooling of the patient is performed. During the induction of hypothermia and subsequent rewarming it is important to identify which body location is guiding therapy as significant variation between sites is frequently seen. During active rewarming, nasopharyngeal temperature measurements have been shown to lag behind those made in the jugular venous bulb with the potential to underestimate the brain temperatures and so cerebral hyperthermia may develop. Rewarming to hyperthermic temperatures that is more than 37ºC, may result in increased neurological impairment and/or stroke risk. In a study assessing rewarming strategy, aggressive rewarming resulted in worse neurocognitive outcomes when compared to slower rates of rewarming (23). This was attributed to brain temperatures that were in excess of those measured at the core and nasopharyngeal sites, suggesting that hyperthermia contributed to the neurologic outcomes. Additionally, hyperthermia may aggravate any neurological injury that has occurred due to micro- or macro-embolization (9). During rewarming the brain temperature should not be allowed to exceed 37°C with some preferring to maintain brain surrogate temperatures at 36°C to reduce the risk of hyperthermia. Core temperatures often lag behind surrogates of cerebral monitoring during active rewarming. The difference between the core and brain temperature site should not exceed 10°C to reduce gaseous formation and hyperthermic neurologic injury. A core temperature of 34–35°C is often considered reasonable for adequate rewarming and the initiation of separation from CPB.

Hypothermia for coronary artery bypass grafting and valve surgery

Cardiac surgery can be a lifesaving procedure but end organ damage from ischaemia related to CPB is problematic, especially with regards to neurological damage and cognitive impairment. Although the incidence of major adverse events like stroke may be low 0.5–2% in CPB patients (24) and 3–12% in aortic arch surgery with DHCA, the postoperative implications of cognitive dysfunction are great. More subtle neuropsychological impairment after CPB has been reported in 15–80% of adult patients, and 100% in the elderly (25). The cause of neurologic injury is not fully delineated or uniform but may be related to acute cerebrovascular accident, microemboli, hypoperfusion (watershed infarctions), and depressive illness associated with coronary artery disease. Specific interventions used to reduce the risk of neurological damage include: degree of hypothermia and warming during CPB, mechanical interventions to reduce micro-emboli in the CPB machine, controlling acid–base balance and glucose management (26).

The utilization of hypothermia in cardiac surgery varies across centres and around the world. One Canadian study (27) surveyed cardiac centres in 2011 and found that 97% routinely cool patients for CPB; with 66% cooling to 34°C and 34% cooling to 32°C. Centres also vary in how they measure temperature with core body temperature being measured via tympanic membrane, nasophraynx, oesophagus, bladder, rectum, pulmonary artery catheter, and jugular venous bulb. It is a common assumption that CPB outflow temperature is the best indication of jugular venous blood temperature. In general a bladder temperature of 34°C is considered adequate rewarming, the critical issue is not to induce hyperthermia.

The clinical impact of postoperative hypothermia in cardiac surgery is debatable. Hypothermia is known to be associated with coagulopathy, increased incidence of wound infection and prolonged hospital stay (29–31). Insler and colleagues (32), in a large retrospective review, found that patients with a body temperature in the intensive care unit (ICU) of less than 36°C had prolonged intubation, longer durations of stay in ICU and hospital, increased red blood cell transfusion and increased mortality. In contrast, Nathan and colleagues (27) did a prospective randomized controlled trial (RCT) that extended hypothermia into the postoperative period, and found no differences in bleeding, cardiac outcomes, or durations of hospital or ICU stay. In addtion, animal studies have clearly demonstrated a large protective effect of mild hypothermia in the setting of ischaemia followed by reperfusion (33,34).

The difficulty in interpreting the many studies is that the level of hypothermia (i.e. mild, moderate or deep), is not always defined consistently and the rewarming protocols are not described (35). Moderate hypothermia may provide more organ protection with

specific evidence to support its use as found in one clinical (36) and multiple animal studies (37–39). There are as yet limited data from RCTs to declare an evidence-based optimal temperature. Where temperature is measured is extremely important, especially during rewarming where bladder and rectal temperature monitoring can underestimate temperature in high blood flow organs such as the kidney and brain (40). Jugular venous bulb measurement is the gold standard for temperature measurement of the brain. But this technique is invasive and not without risk, Avoidance of hyperthermia is arguably more important than any debate of normothermia vs. hypothermia outside of the necessity for DHCA (28). As stated previously, impairments in memory, attention, and psychomotor function can be observed in 30–80% of patients (41). This decline may be recoverable but has also been linked with late cognitive decline.

While mild to moderate hypothermiawas adopted early for cardiac surgery because of empiric evidence from animal research, some workers began looking at the safety of normothermic CPB. The Warm Heart Study (42) was a RCT that compared normothermic and hypothermic CPB for coronary artery bypass grafting (CABG) surgery. There was no significant difference in outcomes between the two groups and the authors concluded normothermic cardiac surgery was safe and highlight the potential benefits of normothermia with respect to myocardial preservation without detrimental neurological outcomes. In contrast, another prospective trial evaluated normothermia versus hypothermia in patients undergoing CABG surgery and found that hypothermic CPB attenuated early neurological decline, and this difference remained significant at thee months following surgery.

A Cochrane review (26) of RCTs that compared normothermic and hypothermic CPB in patients undergoing CABG surgery was reported in 2011, including 17 trials but only four of which reported neurological outcomes. They found a trend towards a reduction in the incidence of non-fatal stroke in the hypothermic group but also a trend for increased non-stroke related perioperative deaths. When pooling all adverse outcomes including stroke, perioperative death, myocardial infarction, low-output syndrome and intra-aortic balloon pump use, there was no significant difference in outcome between hypothermia or normothermia.

Outside of CPB for CABG surgery, there is limited evidence to guide temperature management in standard mitral or aortic valve surgery. In one small trial of 60 patients undergoing aortic valve replacement with hypothermia or normothermia on CPB found no difference between the two groups for neurological or cardiac outcomes (44). Aside from neuroprotection, a key issue is myocardial preservation, for which there is limited data in CABG surgery. However, there is probable value in minimally invasive mitral valve surgery (45). This surgical technique requires femoral arterial and venous cannulation and there is no cross clamp of the ascending aorta and therefore, no cardioplegia. Myocardial preservation is achieved by cooling to 28°C and then inducing ventricular fibrillation. In this situation moderate hypothermia is mandatory for myocardial preservation, despite the lack of clinical trials evaluating such a benefit.

Deep hypothermic circulatory arrest

Deep hypothermic CPB with periods of DHCA is commonly used for surgical repair and replacement of the aortic arch and sometimes, for descending thoracic and thoracoabdominal aortic surgery, as well as for more complex aortic aneurysms (46–47). The reason for its use is it allows the surgeon to visualize the inside of the arch during the period of circulatory arrest with the benefit of bloodless exposure and allows more time for reconstruction of the aortic arch. Importantly, deep hypothermia decreases brain metabolism and oxygen requirements thus permitting a longer period of interrupted perfusion to the brain (48). However, disadvantages of DHCA include prolonged duration of CPB, coagulopathy and alteration in organ function: including to kidney, brain, intestinal mucosa, alveolar epithelium, liver, and pancreas.

Based on data from eight centres in the USA and Europe, the risk of neurological injury after aortic arch surgery ranges from 3–12%, renal dysfunction 5–14%, pulmonary insufficiency 5–39%, left ventricular failure and low cardiac output syndrome 7–34% (25). Risk factors for global ischaemia include increased duration of circulatory arrest and CPB, diabetes and hypertension. In DHCA, transient neurologic injury occurs in 5.9–28% of patients, and irreversible injury 1.8–13.6% of patients. Focal deficits are believed to be secondary to embolic phenomena.

Alternatives to DHCA for aortic arch surgery are normothermic CPB or mild to moderate hypothermia, and both of these techniques require uninterrupted brain perfusion. The safety and effectiveness of arch repair done under lesser degrees of hypothermia is based on small case series and non-randomized comparative studies.

For descending or thoracoabdominal repairs hypothermia allows excellent exposure and prevents blood loss that can occur with left heart bypass, relying on modalities such as the 'clamp and sew' technique. Some centres use DHCA for catastrophic aortic rupture. This involves emergent aortic cannulation (if possible, otherwise axillary, innominate or femoral artery cannulation is preferred) and using the pump sucker from the CPB machine to return aortic blood loss to the venous system of the circuit. This is rescue therapy, and one centre (46) advocates its use only if the bleeding is controlled and the entire body is being sufficiently perfused and cooled.

While providing for optimal operating conditions, the disadvantages of DHCA limit its overall utility to a few operations. The increased coagulopathy, cardiac dysfunction, neurological impairment, oedema formation, and increased operating times are continuing concerns and must be aggressively managed. Attempts to minimize the degree of hypothermia, relying on mild to moderate hypothermia, have been actively studied and promoted.

Antegrade and retrograde cerebral perfusion

Selective perfusion of the brain during deep hypothermia can be done with retrograde or antegrade cerebral perfusion (ACP). ACP has a number of advantages and drawbacks (table 14.3). ACP can be hemispheric, with right axillary subclavian or innominate artery cannulation, or bihemispheric with added cannulation of the left common carotid artery. ACP is thought to be superior to retrograde cerebral perfusion (RCP) for cerebral protection because it achieves near physiological perfusion with homogeneous distribution of blood that may extend the safe time of circulatory arrest (49). ACP of the brain may yield improved neurologic benefit over retrograde perfusion, possibly due to more homogenous blood flow, reduced interruption of cerebral blood flow, and improved cellular uptake of oxygen (50). With ACP during

Table 14.3 Advantages and disadvantages of antegrade cerebral perfusion

Advantages	Disadvantages
Better ability to match the demands of brain metabolism	Risk of arterial wall dissection
Ability to flush brain metabolites	Malperfusion
Better control of brain temperature	Embolism of atheromatous aortic arch vessel plaques

DHCA, flow occurs at 10–20 mL/kg/min, aiming for a mean arterial pressure measured at the right radial artery of 40–70 mmHg (49,51).

Recently, the implementation of the trifurcated graft for ACP (figure 14.1) allows a significant reduction in the duration of circulatory arrest time, bihemispheric selective cerebral perfusion and avoidance of anastomosis near atheroma (48). The authors of this paper advocate the routine use of right axillary cannulation, as it is effective in reducing permanent neurologic injury and increases the ease of selective cerebral perfusion, as demonstrated in figure 14.2.

RCP is achieved by cannulating the superior vena cava with flows maintained between 300–500 mL/min with corresponding mean pressures of 25–35 mmHg. RCP allows for deep and homogeneous cooling of the brain, flushes arterial debris, which may reduce risk of embolism and delays the onset of acidosis. RCP is more effective in the absence of atherosclerotic disease, but in general the partial perfusion provided by RCP is insufficient to maintain cerebral metabolism.

Strategies vary by institution, some advocating that DHCA alone may be sufficient for limited aortic arch replacement with a short circulatory arrest time (30–40 minutes). More extensive repairs will require DHCA and ACP, and in cases with high embolic risk DHCA plus RCP is recommended.

Anaesthetic management of deep hypothermic circulatory arrest

Anaesthesia during DHCA begins with the standard patient monitoring for any type of cardiac surgery, and institution-dependent monitoring such as a pulmonary artery (PA) catheter. Arterial catheter placement is usually via the right radial artery as the left may become occluded during surgery. In addition, a left radial or femoral arterial line is necessary if subclavian or axillary cannulation is anticipated as right radial pressures will not reflect whole body perfusion pressure.

Transoesophageal echocardiography is standard of care in most cardiac procedures, especially in aortic work for assessment of cannula placement, myocardial function and filling. Temperature measurement can be tympanic, nasopharynx, oesophagus, bladder, and rectum, PA catheter, or jugular venous bulb. CPB outflow temperature is the best indicator of jugular venous blood temperature. As stated previously, jugular venous blood temperature is the gold standard of the different measurements. Other monitoring may include electroencephalograph (EEG), somatosensory evoked potential (SSEP) and near infrared spectroscopy (NIRS). NIRS deserves special mention in that a recent survey found that

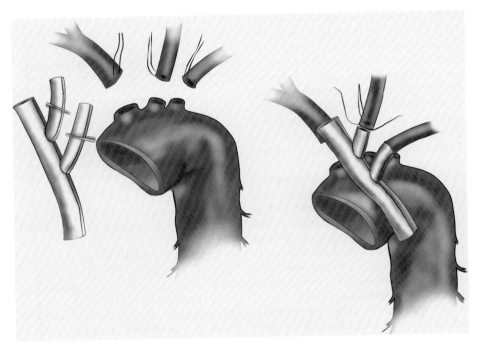

Fig. 14.1 Anastomosis of the three limbs of the trifurcated graft to the head vessels.

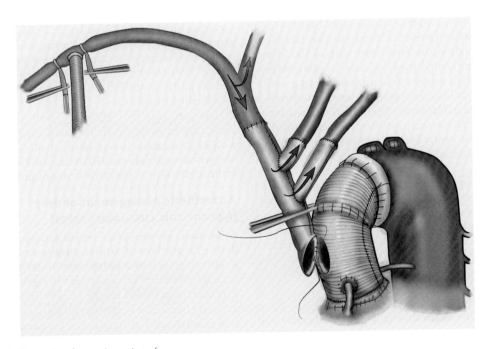

Fig. 14.2 Anastomosis of trifurcated graft to main aortic graft.

the majority of high volume aortic centers are using cerebral NIRS routinely (52). Use of NIRS monitoring can help guide the duration of circulatory arrest as well as cerebral perfusion techniques. In a study evaluating NIRS monitoring and postoperative outcomes Orihashi and colleagues (53) demonstrated that a 22% reduction from baseline in cerebral oxygen saturation (baseline 70% and decrease <55%) was associated with worsened postoperative neurologic outcomes, especially when the time of decrement

extended beyond 5 minutes. A drop in cerebral oxygen saturation to less than 55% is indicative of neurological compromise and has been associated with adverse clinical outcomes including neurological dysfunction (54). A disadvantage of NIRS is that blood flow in the external carotid artery may yield inaccurate cerebral saturation values and that NIRS cannot differentiate between embolus and malperfusion. A proposed possible algorithm for management of low cerebral oximetry readings is detailed in Chapter 32.

The EEG is useful to ensure that cerebral electrical quiescence is achieved prior to undertaking circulatory arrest. However, electrical silence of the EEG can be affected by neurologic insult prior to true neurologic 'silence' and should not be considered an absolute measure. The overall duration of DHCA can be extended by further decrease in temperature, but overall time of arrest without brain perfusion is estimated to be 29 minutes at 15°C, up to 40 minutes at 10°C (55). This timeframe can be increased with RCP or selective ACP, though the best neuroprotective modality remains a short circulatory arrest time. DHCA can also be used for thoracic aorta surgery and thoracoabdominal aortic aneurysm surgery (Chapter 22). Hypothermia increases the maximum cross-clamp time without spinal cord ischaemia from 20 minutes to 50 minutes at 32°C. Using DHCA, several studies of patients with extensive thoracoabominal resections show a lesser overall incidence of acute renal failure, need for dialysis and liver damage in the hypothermia group (46,47,58,59).

Circulatory arrest is initiated when the core body temperature is less than 18°C and ideally with electrical silence for at least three minutes using either EEG or bispectral index monitoring. Most anaesthetists pack the head in ice, and some data support the use of barbiturates or etomidate to aid EEG suppression. Cooling should be slow, for at least 30 minutes, as rapid cooling may create an imbalance between oxygen delivery. High dose steroids have been shown to improve neurologic outcomes thought to be due to the decrease in proinflammatory cytokines (56). However, the possibility of high-dose steroids leading to an increased risk of sepsis in combination with the clinically deleterious effect of hyperglycaemia on outcomes has tempered its use. Some centres administer mannitol, or furosemide before the initiation of DHCA. The combination of mannitol and/or furosemide has been shown to possibly preserve renal function in ischaemic conditions (57).

As discussed in the section on blood gas management, in adults undergoing hypothermic surgery the alpha-stat technique maintains physiologic coupling between cerebral blood flow and metabolism; cerebral oedema from over perfusion may therefore be less likely. Rewarming should be undertaken slowly, aiming for a bladder temperature of 34°C and/ or esophageal temperature of 36°C. The clinical benefits of mild hypothermia in the immediate post-pump period far outweigh the bleeding risk.

Conclusion

Hypothermia has been used for over 50 years in cardiac surgery. Its proven benefits in extending the safe time for aortic arch and descending aorta surgery is evident. Data to date do not support a need for hypothermia in on-pump CABG surgery, and a current large trial is nearing completion assessing hypothermia versus normothermia in valve replacement surgery (see clinicaltrials.gov NCT01338961).

References

1. Bigelow WG, Lindsay WK, Greenwood WF. Hypothermia; its possible role in cardiac surgery: an investigation of factors governing survival in dogs at low body temperatures. *Ann Surg* 1950; **132**: 849–66
2. Mild therapeutic hypothermia to improve the neurologic outcome after cardiac arrest. *N Engl J Med* 2002; **346**: 549–56
3. Michenfelder JD, Milde JH. The relationship among canine brain temperature, metabolism, and function during hypothermia. *Anesthesiology* 1991; **75**: 130–6
4. Todd MM, Warner DS. A comfortable hypothesis reevaluated. Cerebral metabolic depression and brain protection during ischaemia. *Anesthesiology* 1992; **76**: 161–4
5. Globus MY, Busto R, Lin B, et al. Detection of free radical activity during transient global ischaemia and recirculation: effects of intrais-chemic brain temperature modulation. *J Neurochem* 1995; **65**: 1250–6
6. Bickler PE, Buck LT, Hansen BM. Effects of isoflurane and hypothermia on glutamate receptor-mediated calcium influx in brain slices. *Anesthesiology* 1994; **81**: 1461–9
7. Kader A, Frazzini VI, Baker CJ, et al. Effect of mild hypothermia on nitric oxide synthesis during focal cerebral ischaemia. *Neurosurgery* 1994; **35**: 272–7; discussion 7
8. Abdul Aziz KA, Meduoye A. Is pH-stat or alpha-stat the best technique to follow in patients undergoing deep hypothermic circulatory arrest? *Interact Cardiovasc Thorac Surg* 2010; **10**: 271–82
9. Ginsberg MD, Busto R. Combating hyperthermia in acute stroke: a significant clinical concern. *Stroke* 1998; **29**: 529–34
10. Lauri T, Leskinen M, Timisjarvi J, et al. Cardiac function in hypothermia. *Arctic Med Res* 1991; **50**(Suppl 6): 63–6
11. Spencer FC, Bahnson HT. The present role of hypothermia in cardiac surgery. *Circulation* 1962; **26**: 292–300
12. Lewis ME, Al-Khalidi AH, Townend JN, et al. The effects of hypothermia on human left ventricular contractile function during cardiac surgery. *J Am Coll Cardiol* 2002; **39**: 102–8
13. Pina-Cabral JM, Ribeiro-da-Silva A, Almeida-Dias A. Platelet sequestration during hypothermia in dogs treated with sulphinpyrazone and ticlopidine—reversibility accelerated after intra-abdominal rewarming. *Thromb Haemost* 1985; **54**: 838–41
14. Ortmann E, Klein AA, Sharples LD, et al. Point-of-care assessment of hypothermia and protamine-induced platelet dysfunction with multiple electrode aggregometry (Multiplate(R)) in patients undergoing cardiopulmonary bypass. *Anesthes Analg* 2013; **116**: 533–40
15. Staab DB, Sorensen VJ, Fath JJ, et al. Coagulation defects resulting from ambient temperature-induced hypothermia. *J Trauma* 1994; **36**: 634–8
16. Rajagopalan S, Mascha E, Na J, et al. The effects of mild perioperative hypothermia on blood loss and transfusion requirement. *Anesthesiology* 2008; **108**: 71–7
17. Morales P, Carbery W, Morello A, et al. Alterations in renal function during hypothermia in man. *Ann Surg* 1957; **145**: 488–99
18. Zeiner A, Sunder-Plassmann G, Sterz F, et al. The effect of mild therapeutic hypothermia on renal function after cardiopulmonary resuscitation in men. *Resuscitation* 2004; **60**: 253–61
19. Polderman KH, Peeroedeman SM, Girbes AR. Hypophosphatemia and hypomagnesemia induced by cooling in patients with severe head injury. *J Neurosurg* 2001; **94**: 697–705
20. Pirzadeh A, Schears G, Pastuszko P, et al. Effect of deep hypothermic circulatory arrest followed by low-flow CPBon brain metabolism in newborn piglets: comparison of pH-stat and alpha-stat management. *Pediatr Crit Care Med* 2011; **12**: e79–86
21. Duebener LF, Hagino I, Sakamoto T, et al. Effects of pH management during deep hypothermic bypass on cerebral microcirculation: Alpha-stat versus pH-stat. *Circulation* 2002; **106**: I-103–I-8
22. Bissonnette B, Sessler DI, LaFlamme P. Intraoperative temperature monitoring sites in infants and children and the effect of inspired gas warming on esophageal temperature. *Anesth Analg* 1989; **69**: 192–6
23. Grigore AM, Grocott HP, Mathew JP, et al. The rewarming rate and increased peak temperature alter neurocognitive outcome after cardiac surgery. *Anesth Analg* 2002; **94**: 4–10, table of contents
24. Gilman S. Neurological compliccations of open heart surgery. *Ann Neurol*1990; **28**: 475–6
25. Svyatets M, Tolani K, Zhang M, et al. Perioperative management of deep hypothermic circulatory arrest. *J Cardiothorac Vasc Anesth* 2010; **24**: 644–55
26. Rees K, Beranek S, Burke M, et al. Hypothermia to reduce neurological damage following coronary artery bypass surgery. *Cochrane Database Syst Rev* 2001: 1–51
27. Nathan HJ, Lavallee G. The management of temperature during hypothermic cardiopulmonary bypass: Canadian survey. *Cana J Anaesthesia* 1995; **42**: 669–71

28. Grocott HP, Mackensen GB, Grigore AM. Postoperative hyperthermia is associated with cognitive dysfunction after coronary artery bypass surgery. *Stroke* 2002; **33**: 537–41

29. Bush HL, Hydo LJ, Fisher E, et al. Hypothermia during abdominal aortic aneurysm repair: the high price of avoidable morbidity. *J Vasc Surg* 1995; **21**: 392–400

30. Schmeid H, Kurz A, Sessler DI, et al. Mild hypothermia increases blood loss and transfusion requirements during total hip arthroplasty. *Lancet* 1996; **347**: 289–92

31. Kurz A, Sessler DI, Lenhardt R. Perioperative normothermia to reduce the incidence of surgical wound infection and shorten hospitalization. *N Engl J Med* 1996; **334**: 289–92

32. Insler S, O'Connor ML, Nelson D, et al. Association between post-operative hypothermia and adverse outcome after coronary artery bypass surgery. *Ann Thorac Surg* 2000; **70**: 175–81

33. Xue D, Huang ZG, Smith KE, et al. Immediate or delayed mild hypothermia prevents focal cerebral infarction. *Brain Res* 1992; **587**: 66–72

34. Busto R, Globus MY, Dietrich WD, et al. Effect of mild hypothermia on ischaemia induced release of neurotransmitters and free fatty acids in the rat brain. *Stroke* 1989; **20**: 904–10

35. Roman P, Grigore AM. Pro; Hypothermic CPBshould be used routinely. *J Cardiothorac Vasc Anesth* 2012; **26**: 945–48

36. Martin TD, Craver JM, Gott JP, et al. Prospective randomized trial of retrograde warm blood cardioplegia: myocardial benefit and neurologic threat. *Ann Thorac Surg* 1994; **57**: 298–302

37. Qing M, Vazqueai-Jimenez JF, Klosterhalflen B, et al. Influence of temperature during CPBon leukocyte activation, cytokine balance and post-operative organ damage. *Shock* 2001; **15**: 372–77

38. Liu AY, Bian H, Huang LE, et al. Transient cold shock induces the heat shock response upon recovery at 37 degrees C in human cells. *J Biol Chem* 1994; **269**: 14678–775

39. Qing M, Vazqueai-Jimenez JF, Schumacher K, et al. Moderate hypothermia during CPBincreases intramyocardial synthesis of heat shock protein 72. *J Thorac Cardiovasc Surg* 2002; **124**: 724–31

40. Belway D, Tee R, Nathan HJ, et al. Temperature management and monitoring practices during adult cardiac surgery under cardiopulmonary bypass: results of a canadian national survey. *Perfusion* 2011; **26**: 395–400

41. Selnes OA, Goldsborough MA, Borowicz LM, et al. Neurobehavioral Sequelae of cardiopulmonary bypass. *Lancet* 1999; **353**: 1601–9

42. Warm Heart Investigators. Randomised trial of normothermic versus hypothermic coronary bypass surgery. *Lancet* 1994; **343**:559–63

43. Loop FD, Higgins TL, Panda R, et al. Myocardiac protection during cardiac operations. Decreased mortality and lower cost with blood cardioplegia and coronary sinus perfusion. *J Thorac Cardiovasc Surg* 1992; **103**: 1104–11

44. Fakin R, Zimpfer D, Sodeck GH, et al. Influence of temperature management on neurocognitive function in biological aortic valve replacement: A prospective randomized trial. *J Cardiovasc Surg* 2011; **53**: 107–12

45. Umakanthan R, Leacche M, Petracek MR, et al. Safety of minimally invasive mitral surgery without aortic cross clamp. *Ann Thorac Surg* 2008; **85**: 1544–9

46. Fehrenbacher J, Siderys H, Terry C, et al. Early and late results of descending thoracic and thoracoabdominal aortic aneurysm open repair with deep hypothermia and circulatory arrest. *J Thorac Cardiovasc Surg* 2010; **140**: S154–60

47. Griepp RB, Luozzo G. Hypothermia for aortic surgery. *J Thorac Cardiovasc Surg* 2013; **145**: S56–8

48. Luozzo G, Griepp RB. Cerebral protection for aortic arch surgery: deep hypothermia. *Semin Thorac Cardiovasc Surg* 2012; **24**: 127–30

49. Bachet J, Guilmet D, Goudot B, et al. Antegrade cerebral perfusion with cold blood: a 13 year experience. *Ann Thorac Surg* 1999; **67**: 1874–78

50. Misfeld M, Leontyev S, Borger MA, et al. What is the best strategy for brain protection in patients undergoing aortic arch surgery? A single center experience of 636 patients. *Ann Thorac Surg* 2012; **93**: 1502–8

51. Di Eusanio M, Schepens MA, Morshuis WJ, et al. Brain protection using antegrade selective cerebral perfusion: a multicenter study. *Ann Thorac Surg* 2003; **76**: 1181–8

52. Murkin JM. NIRS: A standard of care for CPB vs. and evolving standard for selective cerebral perfusion. *J Extracorp Technol* 2009; **41**: P11–4

53. Orihashi K, Sueda T, Okada K, et al. Near-infrared spectroscopy for monitoring cerebral ischaemia during selective cerebral perfusion. *Eur J Cardio-Thorac Surg* 2004; **26**: 907–11

54. Leyvi G, Bello R, Wasnick JD, et al. Assessment of cerebral oxygen balance during deep hypothermic circulatory arrest by continuous jugular bulb venous saturation and near-infrared spectroscopy. *J Cardiothorac Vasc Anesth* 2006; **20**: 826–33

55. McCullough JN, Zhang N, Reich DL, et al. Cerebral metabolic suppression during hypothermic circulatory arrest in humans. *Ann Thorac Surg* 1999; **67**: 1895–9

56. Shum-Tim D, Tchervenkov CI, Jamal AM, et al. Systemic steroid pretreatment improves cerebral protection after circulatory arrest. *Ann Thorac Surg* 2001; **72**: 1465–71

57. Hanley MJ, Davidson K. Prior mannitol and furosemide infusion in a model of ischemic acute renal failure. *Am J Physiol* 1981; **241**: F556–64

58. Kulik A, Castner CF, Kouchoukos NT. Outcomes after thoracoabdominal aortic aneurysm repair with hypothermic circulatory arrest. *J Thorac Cardiovasc Surg* 2011; **141**: 953–60

59. Weiss AJ, Lin HM, Bischoff MS, et al. A propensity score-matched comparsion of deep versus mild hypothermia during thoracoabdominal surgery. *J Thorac Cardiovasc Surg* 2012; **143**: 186–93

CHAPTER 15

Myocardial protection during cardiac surgery

Michael G. Irwin and
Gordon Tin Chun Wong

Introduction

Despite major advances in cardiac surgery, such surgery is still inevitably accompanied by significant physiological insult. Over past several decades, despite significant improvements in perioperative myocardial protection, there has been an ever ageing population and increasing prevalence of chronic diseases such as diabetes mellitus (DM). These factors along with the popularity of percutaneous coronary intervention (PCI), have led to patients now presenting for CABG often being more elderly, with more co-morbidities and have more complex lesions accompanied by poor target vessels that lengthens surgical time and are, thus, more susceptible to injury. This chapter will briefly review the history of myocardial protection, provide an updated overview of current cardioprotective strategies and discuss some of the novel approaches to reducing myocardial damage from ischaemia–reperfusion (I-R) injury.

History of myocardial preservation

Perhaps the idea of protecting the heart perioperatively began with Bigelow who proposed that hypothermia would allow the surgeon to operate on an unperfused heart (1) Lewis and Taufic successfully closed an atrial septal defect with the aid of deep systemic hypothermia and brief circulatory arrest (2). The following year, Gibbon and colleagues performed the first successful operation to close a large secundum atrial septal defect using cardiopulmonary bypass (CPB). However, it soon became obvious that irreversible damage occurred to the heart as well as the brain after prolonged periods of global ischaemia.

Melrose and associates were among the first to use potassium citrate to provide cardiac arrest on demand. However, the high concentration of potassium citrate induced focal myocardial necrosis and its use was abandoned in the United States; however, potassium-based cardioplegia continued to be used in Europe, particularly in Germany. Bretschneider and others experimented with different chemical additives and developed a solution which was then widely used in many centres (3). Later on, a lower potassium concentration was used to reversibly arrest the heart without inducing the focal myocardial necrosis (4). In England, different formulations of cardioplegic solutions were assessed using an isolated rat heart (5), eventually leading to the development of the St Thomas' Hospital cardioplegic solution (6). Blood as the delivery solution for the cardioplegic mixture was the next big development (7). The rationale being that blood has a better buffering and oxygen-carrying capacity. Non-cardioplegic techniques also were available and were used then and even now by some centres and mainly focussed on various permutations of fibrillation of the heart, aortic clamping, and hypothermia. These have been used with success in selected centres and patient groups but are essentially mostly suited to procedures restricted to the heart surface.

The quest to improve myocardial preservation then took a rather unusual turn when Murry and colleagues observed that intermittent ischaemia intentionally applied to the myocardium actually improved its ability to withstand subsequent ischaemia of greater magnitude (8). This adaptive phenomenon was termed ischaemic preconditioning and its existence probably accounts for the apparent efficacy of intermittent cross-clamping with fibrillation. Though the cumbersome nature of its application rendered it unattractive for routine practice, it inspired many researchers to examine the underlying molecular mechanisms. It became apparent that certain ligand receptor interactions can activate similar pathways and replicate the preconditioning response. Interestingly, many of these preconditioning pharmacomimetics include drugs that are already in perioperative use such as volatile anaesthetics and opioids. It was later observed that mechanical ischaemia at the time of reperfusion could also produce protection (postconditioning) and this, also, could be induced by the same drugs (pharmacological postconditioning). Przyklenk and others observed that an ischaemic stimulus applied to the circumflex coronary artery protected the territory supplied by the left anterior descending coronary artery and, from this observation, spawned the concept of remote preconditioning, which can circumvent many of the limitations of direct ischaemic preconditioning (9). As details of mechanisms of cardioprotection continue to accumulate in the laboratory, translation to the clinical setting has been disappointing. Part of the reason is that diseased and senescent myocardium does not behave like the normal myocardium of animals in the laboratory. In addition, patients with coronary artery disease may already be preconditioned such that preconditioning drugs confer little additional benefit.

Myocardial protection

Minimizing ischaemia–reperfusion injury

Conceptually, myocardial protection requires a combination of delaying the trespass of the ischaemic threshold by lowering metabolic demand and then secondarily mitigating the adverse consequences of reperfusion as the blood supply is restored. Reperfusion results in inflammation and oxidative damage through the induction of oxidative stress rather than restoration of normal function. Damage in the cardiomyocyte occurs from a confluence of effects from diverse biological pathways, which include disruptions in ion homeostasis, dissipation in mitochondrial membrane potential, and generation of free radicals. Restored blood flow carries white blood cells, which release inflammatory factors and free radicals in response to tissue damage. Reintroduction of oxygen into cells damages cellular proteins, DNA, and the plasma membrane. This damage may exacerbate the problem by releasing more free radicals. These reactive species may also act indirectly in redox signalling to turn on apoptosis. Leukocytes and platelet aggregation may also cause ischaemia by binding to the endothelium of small capillaries and obstructing them. There are also alterations in nitric oxide metabolism that affect vascular reactivity with endothelial dysfunction. Manifestations of cardiac injury include reversible injurious states such as myocardial stunning, as well as irreversible damage in the form of apoptosis and necrosis.

As mortality rates are now reasonably low in cardiac surgery, many hundreds to thousands of patients are required in clinical trials to demonstrate any significant differences in mortality or major morbidities. Consequently, many of the clinical studies evaluating efficacy of cardioprotective interventions may be powered to detect differences only in surrogate outcomes such as biochemical markers of cardiac damage. However, a recent meta-analysis of over 18 000 patients concluded that elevation of creatine kinase-MB (CKMB) or troponin in the first 24 hours was independently associated with increased intermediate to long-term mortality risk in patients undergoing CABG surgery (10). Therefore, interpretation of data from studies may well translate into novel therapy.

Cardioplegia-based cardioprotection

Minimizing myocardial oxygen requirement (MvO_2) is pivotal in myocardial preservation as this favourably adjusts the supply demand balance to delay the onset of ischaemia. Emptying of the heart with the establishment CPB significantly reduces the external work performed by the heart and, thereby, reducing MvO_2. Cardioplegia decreases the membrane resting potential of cardiac cells and arrests the heart in diastole which further reduces the metabolic demands of the heart. A key component of the technique relies on the solution having a high potassium concentration that establishes a more positive resting membrane thus creating a 'depolarized' arrest. Hypothermia is the other key component, as it 'indiscriminately' reduces the metabolic rate of tissues, irrespective of whether the heart is beating or fibrillating.

Apart from reducing oxygen demand, cardioplegic solutions by virtue of selective delivery into the coronary circulation, may also reduce injury by modifying metabolic substrate supply and utilization (11). Oxygen, glucose, and amino acid delivery are improved. The acidity of the immediate environment as well as the rate of metabolism can be manipulated with the use of buffers and temperature control, respectively. Composition of the cardioplegia is also designed to mitigate calcium overload by the use of chelating agents and oedema by use of a hyperosmolar solution delivered with a moderate infusion pressure.

Temperature

Initially, hypothermic cardioplegic solutions were delivered in line with the notion of lowering the myocardial temperature. However, this technique results in myocardial hypothermia and delays in recovery of myocardial metabolism and function (12). Further, hypothermia only contributes fractionally more in reducing MvO_2 but it increases plasma viscosity, increases sludging and activates cold agglutinins (13). It also shifts the oxygen haemoglobin dissociation curve to the left, thus impairing oxygen delivery. For these reasons, some practitioners have turned to warm cardioplegia. There may be slight differences in terminology, but in general, cold cardioplegia ranges between 4 and 15°C, tepid or lukewarm cardioplegia is 28–30°C and warm cardioplegia 32–37°C. Fan and colleagues performed a meta-analysis of 41 trials, including 5789 patients between the years 1992 and 2005, addressing the question of warm versus cold cardioplegia (14). They failed to find any statistical difference in the incidences of clinical events but warm cardioplegia was associated with improved postoperative cardiac index and reduced postoperative CKMB and cardiac troponin concentrations.

Blood versus crystalloid solutions

Crystalloid based cardioplegia solutions are inexpensive, simple to prepare and thus widely available but its administration is accompanied by the infusion of large amounts of fluids to the patient. Compared to the crystalloid counterpart, blood cardioplegia is more similar to blood in terms of osmotic pressure and composition and should provide higher oxygen delivery, greater buffering and, possibly, free radical scavenging ability. These theoretical advantages are outweighed by increased cost and complexity and may not translate to clear clinical benefits across all groups. Results from a meta-analysis of 34 trials that pooled data from over 900 patients, showed a modest reduction in the incidence of low cardiac output syndrome, a reduction of CKMB release after 24 hours (seven trials, 821 patients), but similar incidences of myocardial infarction (MI) (23 trials, 4316 patients) and death (17 trials, 4022 patients) (15). The investigators made several cautionary remarks regarding the generalizability of their findings, in that the included trials were small and spanned over 25 years and many co-interventions made the analysis difficult.

Antegrade versus retrograde delivery

The full potential of cardioplegia can only be realized if it can be uniformly distributed to the at-risk myocardium. Like the aforementioned variables, there is no 'one size fits all' approach to cardioplegia delivery. The solution may be administered continuously or intermittently in an antegrade fashion that is through the aortic root, coronary ostia or even bypass conduits once the distal anastomosis has been completed. Although it is simple and mimics normal coronary blood flow, its delivery is limited in the presence significant aortic insufficiency, either as a primary or acquired pathology as a result of heart manipulation as in mitral valve surgery. Its distribution in hearts with advanced coronary atherosclerosis or in areas that have poor collateral circulation may also be questionable.

Some of the limitations of the antegrade approach may be circumvented by delivering the solution in a retrograde fashion through the coronary venous system via cannulation of the coronary sinus. This approach, however, is limited by anatomical variability in the venous system that can result in underperfusion of the septum and right ventricle. To improve the efficiency of induction of cardiac arrest, an initial infusion via the antegrade approach may still be required. Infusion pressure using the retrograde approach should be carefully monitored to limit perivascular haemorrhage and oedema. To take advantage of both routes, combined retrograde with continuous or intermittent antegrade delivery are also used. However, retrospective analysis of over 7000 patients comparing retrograde with a combination approach showed no substantial advantage of the combination approach in CABG with or without concurrent valve replacement (16).

Non-cardioplegia based techniques

Fibrillation

Intermittent fibrillation with aortic cross clamp, together with hypothermia, was a major technique for myocardial protection from the very early days of cardiac surgery. Interestingly, the protection afforded by this method rested on the principle of ischaemic preconditioning, although this technique was not actually scientifically 'discovered' until 1986 (8). It was also simple in execution and avoided the hazards associated with cardioplegia delivery. The surgeon can perform the distal anastomosis on a quiet field during fibrillation then the proximal anastomosis may be completed with a beating heart. In single centre analyses this technique is safe (17,18), and there is a suggestion that diastolic dysfunction following separation from CPB is less using the fibrillation technique (19).

Conditioning of the myocardium

Conditioning confers different forms of cardioprotection and can reduce not just infarct size but arrhythmia and contractile dysfunction. Although different factors and their receptors can initiate the process, it is the activation of kinase signalling pathways and, ultimately, mitochondrial manipulation that produce the protection. These cardioprotective signalling pathways include extracellular-regulated kinase (ERK)1/2, phosphatidylinositol 3 kinase (PI3K)/Akt, protein kinase C and protein kinase G. They lead to the inactivation of mitochondrial glycogen synthase kinase-3β (GSK-3β) and this inhibits the opening of the mitochondrial permeability transition pore (MPTP), which plays a crucial role in myocardial necrosis (20). Reactive oxygen species (ROS) production in mitochondria, where the mitochondrial ATP-dependent potassium channels play an essential role, is also involved in the cardioprotective mechanism (figure 15.1).

Classification and modes of conditioning

The types of conditioning are listed in table 15.1. Preconditioning refers to application of the protective stimulus prior to infarction. Although subsequent reperfusion can salvage myocardium after sustained ischaemia, the reperfusion itself paradoxically induces 'reperfusion injury' which decreases the benefits. The protective stimulus, however, can also be applied at the onset of reperfusion, thereby attenuating reperfusion injury and this is known as postconditioning. When the conditioning stimulus is applied

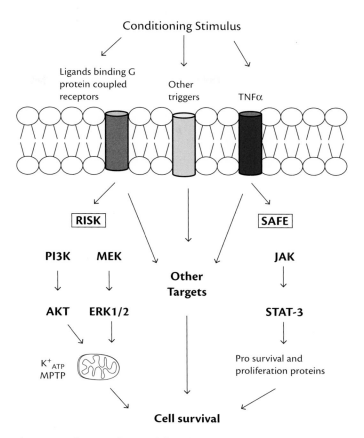

Fig. 15.1 Mechanisms of myocardial conditioning.
Some of the signalling mechanisms of myocardial conditioning. One pathway involves activating a group of protein kinases that is collectively called the reperfusion injury salvage kinases (RISK). These include PI3K (phosphatidylinositol 3 kinase), Akt (protein kinase B), MEK (mitogen-activated protein kinase) and (ERK)1/2 extracellular regulated kinase (ERK)1/2. This pathway maybe triggered by factors such as adenosine or opioids activating G protein coupled receptors. These then act on, among other targets, the mitocohondrial permeability transition pores and potassium ATP channels. Another pathway termed survivor activating factor enhancement (SAFE) is initiated by tumour necrosis factor alpha (TNFα) and involves JAK (Janus kinase) and STAT-3 (signal transducer and activator of transcription-3).
Reprinted from Journal of Molecular and Cellular Cardiology, 47, 1, Lecour S, 'Activation of the protective Survivor Activating Factor Enhancement (SAFE) pathway against reperfusion injury: Does it go beyond the RISK pathway?', pp. 32–40, Copyright 2009, with permission from Elsevier.

directly to the target organ it is referred to as 'local conditioning'. Interestingly, though, it has been discovered that conditioning of one organ or tissue (e.g. skeletal muscle) can actually protect another distal organ (e.g. the heart) and this is known as 'remote conditioning'. Furthermore, the remote ischaemic conditioning procedure can be applied before and during sustained ischaemia and at the onset of reperfusion.

Ischaemic preconditioning

Although exciting in concept, the application of intermittent myocardial ischaemia subjects the patient to the risks of arrhythmia, embolic events, and damage to vascular endothelium as well as prolonging surgical time. There is, however, evidence that ischaemic preconditioning may provide additional myocardial protection over cardioplegia alone. A meta-analysis of 22 trials

Table 15.1 Types of myocardial conditioning and their characteristics

Mode of stimulus	Ischaemia	Cycles of brief intermittent non lethal ischaemia
	Pharmacological	Use of drugs or agents to mimic endogenous triggers
		May be receptor or non receptor mediated
	Others	Hypoxia, trauma
Site of application	Local	Stimulus applied to the circulation supplying the organ of interest
	Remote	Stimulus applied to a circulation distal to the organ of interest
Timing of stimulus	Preconditioning	Stimulus applied before lethal ischaemia reperfusion injury
	Perconditioning	Stimulus applied during lethal ischaemia reperfusion injury
	Postconditioning	Stimulus applied at the time of reperfusion
Protective window	Acute	Powerful but short duration
	Chronic	Less intense but with a longer duration

using predominately aortic cross-clamping to apply the ischaemic stimulus revealed a small reduction in ventricular arrhythmias, inotrope requirement and intensive care unit (ICU) stay in the treated groups. These benefits were evident even when the analyses were restricted to those who received cardioplegia, but not when restricted to those who received intermittent cross-clamp fibrillation (22).

Ischaemic postconditioning

Attenuation of reperfusion injury from postconditioning is via the prevention of rapid changes in intracellular pH and generation of ROS. Within a few minutes of myocardial ischaemia, the interstitial and intracellular pH values rapidly decrease due to the accumulation of protons. These are then washed out upon reperfusion, and acidosis is corrected through the sarcolemmal Na^+/H^+ exchanger, which results in a massive Na^+ influx. Intracellular Na^+ accumulation stimulates the passive, inverted action of the sarcolemmal Na^+/Ca^{2+} exchanger causes intracellular Ca^{2+} overload, which results in myocardial cell death or contractile dysfunction. Therefore, the rapid normalization of intracellular pH enhances myocardial damage in the early stage of reperfusion and a gradual correction of low intracellular pH by acidic reperfusion is preferable as it should be cardioprotective through inhibition of the opening of the mitochondrial permeability transition pore (MPTP), preventing the activation of Ca^{2+}-dependent protease and reducing the gap junction communication involved in spreading cell death. The cardioprotective effects of ischaemic postconditioning are associated with the maintenance of low intracellular pH during reperfusion and are comparable to the effects of acidic reperfusion. The same autacoids that precondition the myocardium (e.g. opioids, adenosine, bradykinin) also activate the PI3K/Akt and ERK1/2 kinase signalling pathway, known as the reperfusion

injury risk kinases (RISK) pathway. The RISK pathway inactivates GSK-3β, which inhibits MPTP opening at reperfusion. The 'survivor activating factor enhancement (SAFE)' pathway which results from activation of the JAK-STAT pathway by cytokines, has also been implicated in ischaemic postconditioning, but it is less well understood. An evaluation in a small trial in adult valve surgery showed reduced peak CKMB release but equal troponin-I and less use of inotropes (23).

Volatile anaesthetic agents and cardioprotection

It was discovered that certain volatile anaesthetic agents mimic some of the biological effects of ischaemic preconditioning, employing similar signal transduction pathways. Adenosine type 1 (A_1) receptors, protein kinase C (PKC), inhibitory guanine nucleotide binding (Gi) proteins, ROS, and mitochondrial and sarcolemmal K_{ATP} channels have been implicated. There also appears to be important roles for prosurvival kinases such as PI3K/Akt40 and the transcription factor hypoxia-inducible factor-1 (HIF-1). Volatile anaesthetics also produce coronary vasodilation by activating K_{ATP} channels or by affecting intracellular Ca^{2+} homeostasis in vascular smooth muscle. Sevoflurane can increase collateral blood flow to ischaemic myocardium and improve the functional recovery of coronary vascular reactivity and nitric oxide release in isolated hearts after global ischaemia. They may also attenuate apoptosis after ischaemia/reperfusion and shift the myocardium into an 'anti-apoptotic' state by modulation of proteins of the BCL-2 family. Consequently, the use of volatile agents, particularly sevoflurane, as a primary anaesthetic agent has undergone a resurgence in popularity despite previous concerns over their negative inotropic effects.

Symons and Myles (24) undertook a meta-analysis of 27 clinical trials and, although there are data supporting a cardioprotective effect for volatile anaesthetics administered during coronary surgery, the optimal dosing and timing for administration have not been determined. It seems that for maximal protection administration of volatile agents is required throughout the entire duration of surgery.

Propofol and cardioprotection

As discussed in a previous section, ROS have been implicated in ischaemia–reperfusion injury (IRI). Propofol appears to be a powerful antioxidant with effects similar to alpha-tocopherol. It protects against cardiac IRI mainly via enhancement of endogenous antioxidant capacity in the myocardium (25), and this is totally different from isoflurane preconditioning. Propofol reduced ROS-induced lipid peroxidation and attenuated IRI in isolated rat hearts, in a dose-dependent manner and can prevent hydrogen peroxide-mediated exacerbation of tumour necrosis factor (TNF)-α cellular toxicity (26), which might be a mechanism whereby it attenuates hydrogen peroxide-induced cardiac dysfunction. More recently it has also been shown that propofol postconditioning confers protection against myocardial as well as cerebral IRI, probably by maintaining the activity of the prosurvival PI3K/Akt pathway, which is important considering that both organs are at risk during CPB. In addition, experimentally, propofol has been shown to be cardioprotective when used at a relatively high dose solely during ischaemia or when applied in a clinically relevant model of normothermic blood cardioplegic arrest and CPB. High-dose propofol during CPB attenuates postoperative myocardial cellular damage compared with isoflurane or low-dose propofol during CABG, whereas the cardioprotective effects of isoflurane did not differ from that of a low-dose propofol regimen. Similarly, more recent clinical trial results show that the use of isoflurane-opioid anaesthesia in comparison with propofol–opioid anaesthesia does not afford additional benefit in terms of postoperative troponin-I release as well as 1-year cardiac morbidity and mortality.

Opioids and cardioprotection

Investigators realized early in the study of cardiac conditioning that opioid receptor activation is involved with cardiac protection, in particular the delta and kappa receptor subtypes. Intravenous morphine could mimic the effects of ischaemic preconditioning, albeit using a high dose (27,28). The requirement for activation of delta and kappa receptors by morphine may explain the relatively high doses necessary to trigger cardioprotection. High morphine doses would cause prolonged respiratory depression and sedation and would be impractical for large scale clinical use. However, even a single dose of 40 mg morphine can improve myocardial performance after CPB (29). The introduction of remifentanil with its favourable pharmacokinetic profile enabled clinical trials of opioid cardioprotection to be conducted. A meta-analysis of remifentanil use in cardiac surgery of 1473 patients showed that its use is associated with a reduction in cardiac troponin release, time of mechanical ventilation, and length of hospital stay (30).

Combining protective strategies

Different agents seem to possess confer some cardioprotection but may differ in their properties. This was shown clinically in a review of outcomes of over 10 000 patients undergoing cardiac procedures where sevoflurane was more beneficial than propofol to patients without severe preoperative ischaemic heart disease or those undergoing non-CABG cardiac surgery (31). In contrast, propofol appeared better for those with ischaemic heart disease or undergoing acute or urgent surgery, with cardiovascular instability. Whether synergism occurs when various modes of myocardial conditioning are combined is controversial. The addition of remote ischaemic preconditioning to standardized isoflurane anaesthesia did not confer any benefit in a recent CABG study, both being a form of preconditioning (32). Interestingly synergism with preconditioning may occur when protection is initiated by different means (26,33).

Myocardial conditioning for special circumstances

Diabetic myocardium

The consequences of I-R injury are greater for the myocardium of diabetic patients with higher mortality following MI (34). There is a greater risk of low cardiac output syndrome (35) and prolonged ICU stay. Coincidently experimental models of diabetic ischaemia reperfusion injury show that the diabetic heart is more resistant to the effect of myocardial conditioning, whether this is mechanical (36) or pharmacological (37). There is also disruption of cardioprotective signalling pathways in the diabetic myocardium (38). Oxidative stress in tissues of diabetic patients may be pivotal in the pathogenesis of the many complications of this disease (39).

Interestingly, the administration of N-acetylcysteine, an oxygen radical scavenger, can restore the preconditioning effect of isoflurane during hyperglycaemia (40). Although the bulk of the literature favours volatile anaesthetics in the realm of myocardial conditioning, a group of researchers have investigated the antioxidant, rather than conditioning properties of propofol in providing cardioprotection in diabetes (41). A small study has shown some benefits of large doses of propofol in reducing markers of myocardial damage following CPB (25). Therefore, there may be a specific role for propofol in this group of patients.

Scenescent myocardium

Advanced age is an independent factor for significant cardiac dysfunction following cardiac surgery. Increased sensitivity to the harmful effects of I-R may be related to alterations in calcium homeostasis (42) in addition to a number of other intracellular changes. Evidence from clinical data suggests that senescent myocardium is more resistant to the preconditioning effects of intermittent ischaemia. Experimental studies point to a beneficial role for exercise and caloric restriction in restoring the sensitivity of the aged myocardium to cardiac conditioning (43).

Conclusion

As the patient population becomes increasing older and surgical procedures more complex, better myocardial preservation techniques are needed more than ever. Advances in basic science are frequently providing potential therapies for testing in the clinical setting. Cardioplegia perhaps still represents the cornerstone of myocardial protection. Conditioning of the myocardium may add incremental benefits to ameliorate the adverse biochemical consequences of I-R injury. However, the optimal choice or combination and the mode of delivery of these agents remain to be elucidated. In particular, more work is required to utilize this technique in aged or diseased myocardium which may require adjunctive treatments to restore their sensitivity to cardioprotection. One should not overlook measures, such as introducing perioperative medications that may benefit patients, such as HMG coarctation of the aorta reductase inhibitors (statins). The benefits of even the best intraoperative myocardial protection may pale into insignificance if it is not accompanied by optimal patient preparation, meticulous surgical technique and vigilance in post-operative care. As such anaesthesiologists maybe called to expand their sphere of influence beyond the operating room to optimise cardioprotection.

Further reading

Cordell AR. Milestones in the development of cardioplegia. *Ann Thorac Surg* 1995; **60**: 793–6

Hausenloy DJ, Boston-Griffiths E, Yellon DM. Cardioprotection during cardiac surgery. *Cardiovasc Res* 2012; **94**: 253–65

Przyklenk K. Efficacy of cardioprotective 'conditioning' strategies in aging and diabetic cohorts: the co-morbidity conundrum. *Drugs & Aging* 2011; **28**: 331–343.

Boengler K, Schulz R, Heusch G: Loss of cardioprotection with ageing. *Cardiovasc Res* 2009; **83**: 247–61

Davignon J. Beneficial cardiovascular pleiotropic effects of statins. *Circulation* 2004; **109**(23 suppl 1),III-39–III-43

Collard CD, Body SC, Shernan SK, Wang S, Mangano DT. Preoperative statin therapy is associated with reduced cardiac mortality after coronary artery bypass graft surgery. *J Thorac Cardiovasc Surg* 2006; **132**(2): 392–400

References

1. Bigelow WG, Lindsay WK, Greenwood WF. Hypothermia; its possible role in cardiac surgery: an investigation of factors governing survival in dogs at low body temperatures. *Ann Surg* 1950; **132**: 849–66

2. Lewis FJ, Taufic M. Closure of atrial septal defects with the aid of hypothermia; experimental accomplishments and the report of one successful case. *Surgery* 1953; **33**: 52–9

3. Bretschneider HJ. Uberlebenszeit und Weider-Belbungxzeit des Herzens bei normo und Hypothermic. *Verh Dtsch Ges Kreisl-Forsh* 1964; **30**: 11–34

4. Gay WA, Jr., Ebert PA. Functional, metabolic, and morphologic effects of potassium-induced cardioplegia. *Surgery* 1973; **74**: 284–90

5. Hearse DJ, Stewart DA, Braimbridge MV. Cellular protection during myocardial ischemia: the development and characterization of a procedure for the induction of reversible ischemic arrest. *Circulation* 1976; **54**: 193–202

6. Cordell AR. Milestones in the development of cardioplegia. *Ann Thorac Surg* 1995; **60**: 793–6

7. Follette DM, Mulder DG, Maloney JV, Buckberg GD. Advantages of blood cardioplegia over continuous coronary perfusion or intermittent ischemia. Experimental and clinical study. *J Thorac Cardiovasc Surg* 1978; **76**: 604–19

8. Murry CE, Jennings RB, Reimer KA. Preconditioning with ischemia: a delay of lethal cell injury in ischemic myocardium. *Circulation* 1986; **74**: 1124–36

9. Przyklenk K, Bauer B, Ovize M, Kloner R, Whittaker P. Regional ischemic 'preconditioning' protects remote virgin myocardium from subsequent sustained coronary occlusion. *Circulation* 1993; **87**: 893–9

10. Domanski MJ, Mahaffey K, Hasselblad V, et al. Association of myocardial enzyme elevation and survival following coronary artery bypass graft surgery. *JAMA* 2011; **305**: 585–91

11. Vinten-Johansen J, Thourani VH. Myocardial protection: an overview. *J Extra-corp Technol* 2000; **32**: 38–48

12. Fremes SE, Weisel RD, Mickle DA, et al. Myocardial metabolism and ventricular function following cold potassium cardioplegia. *J Thorac Cardiovas Surg* 1985; **89**: 531–46

13. Mauney MC, Kron IL. The physiologic basis of warm cardioplegia. *Ann Thorac Surg* 1995; **60**: 819–23

14. Fan Y, Zhang A-M, Xiao Y-B, Weng Y-G, Hetzer R. Warm versus cold cardioplegia for heart surgery: a meta-analysis. *Eur J Cardiothorac Surg* 2010; **37**: 912–9

15. Guru V, Omura J, Alghamdi AA, Weisel R, Fremes SE. Is blood superior to crystalloid cardioplegia? A meta-analysis of randomized clinical trials. *Circulation* 2006; **114**: I331–8

16. Arom KV, Emery RW, Petersen RJ, Bero JW. Evaluation of 7,000+ patients with two different routes of cardioplegia. *Ann Thorac Surg* 1997; **63**: 1619–24

17. Raco L, Mills E, Millner RJW. Isolated myocardial revascularization with intermittent aortic cross-clamping: experience with 800 cases. *Ann Thorac Surg* 2002; **73**: 1436–9

18. Boethig D, Minami K, Lueth JU, El-Banayosy A, Breymann T, Koerfer R. Intermittent aortic cross-clamping for isolated CABG can save lives and money: experience with 15307 patients. *Thorac Cardiovasc Surgeon* 2004; **52**: 147–51

19. Casthely PA, Shah C, Mekhjian H, et al. Left ventricular diastolic function after coronary artery bypass grafting: a correlative study with three different myocardial protection techniques. *J Thorac Cardiovasc Surg* 1997; **114**: 254–60

20. Granfeldt A, Lefer DJ, Vinten-Johansen J. Protective ischaemia in patients: preconditioning and postconditioning. *Cardiovasc Res* 2009; **83**: 234–46

21. Lecour S. Activation of the protective survivor activating factor enhancement (SAFE) pathway against reperfusion injury: Does it go beyond the RISK pathway? *Journal of Molecular and Cellular Cardiology* 2009; **47**: 32–40

22. Walsh SR, Tang TY, Kullar P, Jenkins DP, Dutka DP, Gaunt ME. Ischaemic preconditioning during cardiac surgery: systematic review and meta-analysis of perioperative outcomes in randomised clinical trials. *Euro J Cardiothorac Surg* 2008; **34**: 985–94

23. Luo W, Li B, Chen R, Huang R, Lin G. Effect of ischemic postconditioning in adult valve replacement. *Eur J Cardiothorac Surg* 2008; **33**: 203–8

24. Symons JA, Myles PS. Myocardial protection with volatile anaesthetic agents during coronary artery bypass surgery: a meta-analysis. *Br J Anaesth* 2006; **97**: 127–36

25. Xia Z, Huang Z, Ansley DM. Large-dose propofol during cardiopulmonary bypass decreases biochemical markers of myocardial injury in coronary surgery patients: a comparison with isoflurane. *Anesth Analg* 2006; **103**: 527–32

26. Huang Z, Zhong X, Irwin MG, et al. Synergy of isoflurane preconditioning and propofol postconditioning reduces myocardial reperfusion injury in patients. *Clin Sci* 2011; **121**: 57–69

27. Schultz JE, Rose E, Yao Z, Gross GJ. Evidence for involvement of opioid receptors in ischemic preconditioning in rat hearts. *Am J Physiol Heart Circ Physiol* 1995; **268**: H2157–61

28. Schultz JE, Hsu AK, Gross GJ. Morphine mimics the cardioprotective effect of ischemic preconditioning via a glibenclamide-sensitive mechanism in the rat heart. *Circ Res* 1996; **78**: 1100–4

29. Murphy GS, Szokol JW, Marymont JH, et al. Opioids and cardioprotection: the impact of morphine and fentanyl on recovery of ventricular function after cardiopulmonary bypass. *J Cardiothorac Vasc Anesth* 2006; **20**: 493–502

30. Greco M, Landoni G, Biondi-Zoccai G, et al. Remifentanil in cardiac surgery: a meta-analysis of randomized controlled trials. *J Cardiothorac Vasc Anesth* 2012; **26**: 110–6

31. Jakobsen CJ, Berg H, Hindsholm KB, Faddy N, Sloth E. The influence of propofol versus sevoflurane anesthesia on outcome in 10,535 cardiac surgical procedures. *J Cardiothorac Vasc Anesth* 2007; **21**: 664–71

32. Lucchinetti E, Bestmann L, Feng J, et al. Remote ischemic preconditioning applied during isoflurane inhalation provides no benefit to the myocardium of patients undergoing on-pump coronary artery bypass graft surgery: lack of synergy or evidence of antagonism in cardioprotection? *Anesthesiol* 2012; **116**: 296–310

33. Li T, Wu W, You Z, et al. Alternative use of isoflurane and propofol confers superior cardioprotection than using one of them alone in a dog model of cardiopulmonary bypass. *Euro J Pharmacol* 2012; **677**: 138–46

34. Norhammar A, Lindbäck J, Rydén L, Wallentin L, Stenestrand U. Improved but still high short- and long-term mortality rates after myocardial infarction in patients with diabetes mellitus: a time-trend report from the Swedish Register of Information and Knowledge about Swedish Heart Intensive Care Admission. *Heart* 2007; **93**: 1577–83

35. Rao V, Ivanov J, Weisel RD, Ikonomidis JS, Christakis GT, David TE. Predictors of low cardiac output syndrome after coronary artery bypass. *J Thorac Cardiovasc Surg* 1996; **112**: 38–51

36. Kersten JR, Toller WG, Gross ER, Pagel PS, Warltier DC. Diabetes abolishes ischemic preconditioning: role of glucose, insulin, and osmolality. *Am J Physiol Heart Circ Physiol* 2000; **278**: H1218–H24

37. Kim HS, Cho JE, Hwang KC, Shim YH, Lee JH, Kwak YL. Diabetes mellitus mitigates cardioprotective effects of remifentanil preconditioning in ischemia-reperfused rat heart in association with anti-apoptotic pathways of survival. *Eur J Pharmacol* 2010; **628**: 132–9

38. Wang B, Raedschelders K, Shravah J, et al. Differences in myocardial PTEN expression and Akt signalling in type 2 diabetic and nondiabetic patients undergoing coronary bypass surgery. *Clin Endocrinol* 2011; **74**: 705–13

39. Giacco F, Brownlee M. Oxidative stress and diabetic complications. *Circ Res* 2010; **107**: 1058–70

40. Kehl F, Krolikowski JG, Weihrauch D, Pagel PS, Warltier DC, Kersten JR. N-Acetylcysteine Restores Isoflurane-induced Preconditioning against myocardial infarction during hyperglycemia. *Anesthesiol* 2003; **98**: 1384–90

41. Ansley DM, Raedschelders K, Chen DDY, Choi PT. Rationale, design and baseline characteristics of the PRO-TECT II study: PROpofol CardioproTECTion for Type II diabetics: A randomized, controlled trial of high-dose propofol versus isoflurane preconditioning in patients undergoing on-pump coronary artery bypass graft surgery. *Contemp Clin Trials* 2009; **30**: 380–5

42. O'Brien JD, Ferguson JH, Howlett SE. Effects of ischemia and reperfusion on isolated ventricular myocytes from young adult and aged Fischer 344 rat hearts. *Am J Physiol Heart Circ Physiol* 2008; **294**: H2174–H83

43. Shim YH. Cardioprotection and ageing. *Korean J Anesthesiol* 2010; **58**: 223–30

CHAPTER 16

Antithrombotic and antiplatelet therapy

David Royston

Introduction

Anticoagulant drugs such as the coumarins and direct thrombin inhibitors are required to prevent and treat thrombotic complication. The anticoagulant heparin is fundamental to the conduct of cardiopulmonary bypass (CPB). Starting with aspirin, antithrombotic drugs been been used to treat coronary artery disease and it complications. More recently, drugs that specifically target platelet surface receptors are being used. A knowledge of all these drugs are essential to cardiac anaesthesia so this chapter will review these drugs.

Thrombosis

Arterial and venous thromboses are a major cause of morbidity and mortality. Arterial thrombosis is the most common cause of myocardial infarction (MI), ischemic stroke, and limb gangrene. Arterial thrombi, which typically form under high shear conditions, consist of platelet aggregates held together by small amounts of fibrin. Because of the predominance of platelets, strategies to inhibit arterial thrombogenesis focus mainly on drugs that inhibit platelet function, but include anticoagulants for prevention of cardioembolic events in patients with atrial fibrillation or mechanical heart valves.

Deep vein thrombosis (DVT) may lead to pulmonary embolism (PE) and to the post-phlebitic syndrome. Venous thrombi, which form under low shear conditions, are composed mainly of fibrin and trapped red cells, and contain relatively few platelets. With the predominance of fibrin in venous thrombi, anticoagulants are the agents of choice for the prevention and treatment of DVT and venous thromboembolism (VTE). VTE is the leading cause of preventable in-hospital mortality with up to 300,000 deaths annually in the USA (1) and a similar number within France, Germany, Spain, Italy, Sweden, and the UK (2). The incidence of VTE is about 20% higher in men than in women and increases with age in both sexes.

Overview of normal platelet function and haemostasis

When there is tissue or endothelial injury, the initial response to provide primary haemostasis is formation of a platelet plug. The platelet has multiple receptors on its surface, which when stimulated, produce a shape change. The glycoprotein Ib (GpIb) receptor is expressed at all times and binds to von Willebrand factor (vWF) that is exposed on the vessel if there is endothelial injury. Amplification pathways to enhance the generation of the primary haemostatic plug involve receptors for adensosine diphospahate (ADP), thrombin and thromboxane A2. These amplification pathways have been the focus of attention of the most recent attempts to inhibit platelet function. With platelet shape change there is expression of the glycoprotein IIb/ IIIa (GpIIb/ IIIa) receptor. This binds fibrinogen molecules to provide bridging between adjacent platelets.

Overview of generation of thrombin and fibrin for haemostasis

The aim of the coagulation phase of haemostasis is the generation of fibrin from the fibrinogen holding the primary plug together in order to bind and stabilize the weak platelet haemostatic plug. This process requires proteolysis of the fibrinogen by thrombin. Thrombin has a highly specific action on fibrinogen to cleave the molecule at only two sites. Thrombin achieves this with clusters of charged and polar amino acid residues distributed unevenly on its surface. The active site of the molecule is surrounded by a number of negatively charged amino acid residues and away from this are positively charged exosites to allow the very specific alignment and cleavage of fibrinogen. The anionic sites are used by various anticoagulants to aid in inhibition of thrombin (figure 16.1).

The coagulation system relies primarily on a group of soluble factors that circulate in the plasma. These factors are synthesized in the liver and expressed into the circulation. Most coagulation factors are identified by Roman numerals, the active form denoted by the lower case 'a'. They circulate in an inactive, zymogen form and become active after proteolytic cleavage. The exception to this is Factor VII, which can circulate as an active protease. Apart from Factor XIII, which is a transglutaminase, all the active factors are serine proteases related to the digestive enzyme trypsin. Other factors in the coagulation process, such as tissue factor, Factor V, factor VIII, and high molecular weight kininogen (HK) act as co-factors.

Blood coagulation is intended to be localized to the area where the original platelet plug was formed by first restricting the chain of reactions to a surface, such as platelet phospholipids and second, through a series of inhibitors intended to constrain the reaction to the site of injury. Historically, the blood coagulation system is divided into two initiating pathways: the tissue factor

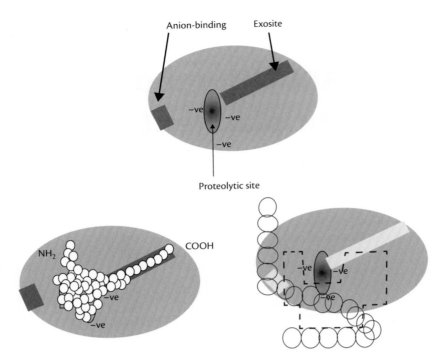

Fig. 16.1 Upper section shows a schematic diagram of thrombin molecule. The active proteolytic site is surrounded by a ring of negative charge. A section of the fibrinogen molecule interacts with the negatively charged ring around the active site as well as the active site itself. Also shown are two anionic binding sites. The positively charged exosite shown on the right hand side also interacts with the fibrinogen molecule. This is likely important in both orienting the fibrinogen molecule correctly within the active site and maintaining a strong bond between the enzyme and its substrate.

In the lower panel the use of the anionic sites to bind and augment orientation of anticoagulant proteins is shown. In the lower right schematic the polypeptide of native hirudin is shown attached to the active site together with the tail of the molecle aligned in one exosite. The other exosite binds to glycosaminoglycans (heparan and chondroitin) and also to heparin. This is shown for an 18 saccharide sequence of heparin (open circles) attached to antithrombin through the pentasaccharide sequence and orienting this molecule through attachment to an exosite to ensure maximal effect of the antithrombin

(extrinsic) pathway and the contact factor (intrinsic) pathway that meet at a final common pathway whereby Factor Xa converts prothrombin to thrombin. One molecule of Factor Xa generates about 50 thrombin molecules explaining the recent burst of interest in orally active inhibitors of Factor Xa.

Agents acting by indirect interference with thrombin generation

Heparins

These are available in two forms. Unfractionated heparin, which is a naturally occurring substance, and low-molecular-weight heparins (LMWHs) that are chemical modifications of unfractionated heparin. The pharmacology of both these groups of compounds has been extensively reviewed elsewhere (3–7).

Unfractionated heparin

Unfractionated heparin (UFH) is a naturally occurring negatively charged sulphated polysaccharide glycosaminoglycan. Heparin is mostly located in lungs, intestine and liver in mammals, and is now derived from porcine gut. The number and sequence of the saccharides is variable, producing a heterogeneous collection of polysaccharides. Molecular weights range from 3000 to 30 000 Da, with a mean of 15 000 Da representing 40 to 50 saccharides in length. There is no apparent difference between any of the

available forms of unfractionated heparin (UFH) with respect to their pharmacology or anticoagulant profile (4).

Mechanism of action of unfractionated heparin

Heparin has a direct anti-inflammatory action in humans and has a wide spectrum of activity with enzymes, hormones, biogenic amines, and plasma proteins. Heparin alone has no anticoagulant activity but requires a plasma cofactor originally designated as antithrombin III (AT III), now simply called antithrombin (AT). AT has an intrinsic low level of anticoagulant activity, mediated by a strongly electropositive arginine centre that binds to the serine centre of proteases of the coagulation cascade. The binding of heparin to AT is highly specific via a pentasaccharide sequence found in about one third of molecules. The binding of heparin and the subsequent anticoagulant activity depends on the saccharine chain length.

The binding of the AT molecule to thrombin is suicidal in the thrombin–antithrombin (T-AT) complex but the heparin molecule is able to reversibly disengage from this complex unchanged. The inhibition of thrombin activation also prevents the amplification feedback by thrombin on factors V and VIII. In contrast, the inhibition of factors IXa, Xa, and XIIa requires only that the heparin should bind AT to form the heparin-AT complex (4). This explains why LMWHs and the synthetic pentasaccharide fondaparinux, can act as inhibitors of Factor Xa but not necessarily thrombin.

At high blood levels (>4 IU/mL), heparin is capable of binding heparin co-factor II, potentiating its inactivation of bound activated thrombin (8). This action does not require the specific pentasaccharide but does require heparins of greater than 7200 Da or 24 saccharide units in length. Heparin also stimulates the release of tissue factor pathway inhibitor (TFPI), which binds and neutralizes the tissue factor-VIIa complex, reducing prothrombinase production via the extrinsic pathway. Plasma concentrations of TFPI rise 2–6-fold following injection with unfractionated and LMWHs.

Metabolism/elimination

Elimination is non-linear and occurs by two separate processes. The rapid saturable phase of heparin clearance is due to cellular degradation. In particular, macrophages internalize the heparin, then depolymerize and desulphate it. This process explains the poor bioavailability after low-dose subcutaneous injection, as the slow rate of absorption barely exceeds the capacity of the cellular degradation. Significant plasma levels can only be achieved following a loading dose.

There is great variability in the plasma concentration of heparin in relation to the dose administered. After intravenous injection more than 50% of heparin circulates bound to plasma proteins including platelet factor 4, histidine-rich glycoprotein, vitronectin, fibronectin, and von Willebrand factor. The first three of these also neutralize heparin's activity and reduce its bioavailability. Raised levels of these proteins may account for the heparin resistance sometimes seen in malignancy and inflammatory disorders (3). Plasma levels also decline rapidly due to redistribution and uptake by endothelial cells and macrophages.

The slower phase of heparin elimination is due to renal excretion. As the dose of heparin is increased, the elimination half-life increases and the anticoagulant response is exaggerated. At a dose of 25 units/kg the half-life is about 30 minutes, rising to about 150 minutes with a bolus dose of 400 units/kg. Surprisingly, no consistent report of the effects of renal or hepatic dysfunction on the pharmacokinetics of heparin have been described (3,4).

Therapeutic effects

Heparin is given to slow the process of thrombin generation and activity and therefore 'anticoagulate' the patient. The therapeutic target dose will depend on the indication. As there is a marked variation in response between individuals to the effect of a fixed dose of unfractionated heparin, regular monitoring of anticoagulation must be routinely performed typically using a coagulation test initiated by contact activation. The plasma version of this is the activated partial thromboplastin time (APTT). The therapeutic range most commonly quoted is an APTT between 1.5 and 2.5 times the control value. The whole blood version of the APTT used when higher doses are administered is the automated or activated clotting time (ACT). This is the standard of care used in cardiac surgical practice and typically the ACT is maintained above about 400–480 seconds. The benefit and limitations of these tests is discussed in Chapter 17.

Clinical use of heparin

For thromboembolic prophylaxis, UFH is administered either as 'low-dose' (5000 U subcutaneously 8 or 12 hourly) or 'adjusted-dose' heparin (3500 U 8 or 12 hourly which is then adjusted to maintain the APTT to about 3–5 seconds above control level. Overviews of clinical trials have shown low dose subcutaneous UFH produces an over 50% reduction in the incidence of

venous thrombosis, and fatal and non-fatal pulmonary embolism (9) without an increase in major or fatal haemorrhage. However LMWH have been shown to be safer and more effective, with significant reductions in recurrence of thrombosis and major haemorrhage (10).

For treatment of established thromboembolic disease higher concentrations are needed to prevent thrombus propagation. Recommended regimens for the treatment of DVT with UFH include an intravenous loading dose of 5000 to 10 000 U, then a continuous infusion of 1300 U per hour, adjusted to maintain the APTT 1.5 to 2.5 times control. The most common reason for failure of treatment is inadequate anticoagulation, particularly within the first 24 hours—a problem which is overcome by the loading dose (11).

Adverse effects of heparin

Until 2008, the standard test of heparin potency was different between the USA Pharmacopeia (USP) standard and that of the World Health Organization's (WHO) International Standard or International Unit (IU). In 2008, the USP adopted new manufacturing controls for heparin. This was due to a number of cases of severe hypotension, sometimes leading to death, being reported between 2005 and 2007. The source for the heparin was a manufacturer in China and In March 2008 the FDA identified 'oversulfated chondroitin sulfate' (OSCS) as a contaminant in this heparin. The OSCS contaminant is manmade and mimics the activity of unfractionated heparins activity in the USP tests of potency of the time.

In-vitro and in-vivo studies (12) showed that OSCS directly activated the kinin–kallikrein pathway in human plasma with subsequent generation of bradykinin. In addition, OSCS induced generation of C3a and C5a, potent anaphylatoxins derived from complement proteins. Adopting the WHO IU standards allows early detection of a contaminant.

The new agent now has about a 10% reduction in 'anticoagulant' potency compared to the previous USP standard. The current WHO standard has a potency of 122 IU/mg heparin. The reduced potency should have no clinical effect as dosing regimen are tailored to individual patient needs. The US Food and Drug Administration therefore did not change the approved labeling for heparin nor the recommended ranges of doses.

Haemorrhage

Although hemorrhage is rare in patients on prophylactic doses of either UFH or LMWHs, it is a frequent complication of higher dose heparin therapy. Many factors increase the risk of hemorrhage including the length of treatment, presence of cardiac, hepatic or renal dysfunction, aspirin or other non-steroidal anti-inflammatory drug (NSAID) therapy and recent surgery, trauma, or invasive procedures. The incidence of major bleeding is around 5% with an estimated daily frequency of fatal, major and all types of haemorrhage in patients receiving therapeutic anticoagulation as 0.05%, 0.8%, and 2.0% respectively. This is approximately twice the level expected in the absence of anticoagulation (13).

Thrombocytopenia

Heparin-induced thrombocytopenia (HIT) is a complication with an incidence of 1.0–1.5% of patients receiving intravenous heparin. Affected patients usually are receiving high doses, though

Table 16.1 The 4 T's scoring system for suggesting a patient has Type II Heparin induced thrombocytopenia

4 T's	2 points	1 point	0 point
Thrombocytopenia	Platelet count fall >50% or lowest platelet count >20x10^9/L	Platelet count fall 30–50% or lowest platelet count 10–19 x10^9/L	Platelet count fall <30% or Lowest platelet count <10 x10^9/L
Timing of platelet count fall	Clear onset between days 5–10 or platelet fall ≤1 day (prior heparin exposure within 30 days)	Consistent with days 5–10 fall, but not clear (e.g. missing platelet counts); onset after day 10 or fall ≤1 day (prior heparin exposure 30–100 days ago)	Platelet count fall <4 days without recent exposure
Thrombosis or other sequelae	New thrombosis (confirmed); skin necrosis; acute systemic reaction postintravenous unfractionated heparin (UFH) bolus	Progressive or recurrent thrombosis; Non-necrotizing (erythematous) skin lesions; Suspected thrombosis (not proven)	None
O**T**her causes for thrombocytopenia	None apparent	Possible	Definite

With a total score of 6–8 the probability is high (>80%), Intermediate with a score of 4–5 and low (<5%) with a score of 0–3.

Reproduced from Lo GK et al., 'Evaluation of pretest clinical score (4 T's) for the diagnosis of heparin-induced thrombocytopenia in two clinical settings', *Journal of Thrombosis and Haemostasis*, **4**, 4, pp.759–765, Copyright 2006, with permission from International Society on Thrombosis and Haemostasis and John Wiley and Sons

rare cases have been attributed to flushing lines with heparin. Two distinct clinical syndromes have been described (14). Type I involves a mild thrombocytopenia with a platelet count that rarely falls below 100×10^9/L, which occurs during the first few days of treatment and usually recovers rapidly even if heparin is continued. The underlying mechanism involves the action of heparin as a mild direct platelet aggregator and no specific treatment is required.

Type II HIT is characterized by a delayed onset of a severe, progressive thrombocytopenia with platelet counts below 100×10^9/L, and often below 50×10^9/L. Heparin has to be stopped completely for platelet count to recover, typically over a seven day period. The mechanism of HIT Type II is immunological. Heparin binds platelet factor 4 to form a molecule that stimulates the production of an immunoglobulin G (IgG) antibody. This antibody binds heparin-platelet factor 4 to produce an immune complex, all three parts of which are capable of binding to platelets. These complexes have two separate effects. First, they coat platelets and increase their removal from the circulation by the reticuloendothelial system. Second, they cause activation of platelets and the coagulation cascade (14).

A clinical score system (4 T's) has been suggested to help with raising clinical suspicion (table 16.1). This system has been validated in clinical practice (15). The most serious complication associated with Type II HIT is new thromboembolic events, due to platelet-rich thrombi. Arterial and venous thrombosis may occur. In patients receiving therapeutic doses of porcine heparin, 0.4% exhibited manifestations of thrombosis, most commonly lower limb thrombosis, and thrombotic cerebrovascular accident.

Low-molecular-weight heparin
Structure/activity
LMWHs are produced from UFH by depolymerization. It is this depolymerization that produces marked differences in the properties of LMWHs and leads to their clinical advantages over UFHs (5,6). LMWHs have mean molecular weights of 4000 to 6500 Da, although

the range is 2000 to 10 000 Da. The production methods used and source material of the UFH lead to significant variations between the different commercial preparations are shown in table 16.2.

The LMWHs also differ in the distribution of their fragment molecular weights, their potency (anti-Xa, antithrombin and anticoagulant activities) and, consequently, in their biodynamic patterns, recommended dose regimen, and efficacy/safety ratio (7), as shown in table 16.3. The anticoagulant properties of LMWHs are not identical (16). The proportion of LMWH containing the pentasaccharide responsible for binding AT is less than in the parent UFH (5,6). The reduced amount of this pentasaccharide results in less in-vitro inhibition of thrombin via AT. However the LMWH-AT complex is able to inhibit Xa. Although the LMWHs have a weak anti-IIa action, their high bioavailability and long half-life mean that the anti-Xa action is four times greater than for UFH.

LMWHs do not bind to endothelial cells or macrophages, and so are not subject to the degradation that UFH suffers. Only about 10% of LMWH is protein bound and they are resistant to inactivation by platelet factor 4. LMWHs thus have nearly complete bioavailability. They exhibit linear pharmacokinetics with proportionality between anti-Xa (and anti-IIa in some cases) plasma concentration and dose. Urinary excretion of anti-Xa activity for enoxaparin, dalteparin, and nadroparin, all given at doses for prevention of venous thrombosis, is between 3 and 10% of the injected dose. However, these drugs differ in the extent of their non-renal clearance, resulting in different apparent elimination half-life values. Although the clearance of LMWH is dependent on renal excretion this is not clinically apparent until clearance values <15 mL/min are achieved. When given at doses recommended for prevention of venous thromboembolism the LMWHs do not significantly cross the placenta.

Studies of LMWHs given as prophylaxis show they are associated with wound haematomas but not an increased incidence of haemorrhage. In contrast a significant reduction in major haemorrhage is seen when LMWHs are used to treat established thrombosis (6,11).

Table 16.2 Generic and trade names and method of production of low molecular weight heparins. Also included is the average molecular mass, together with percentage of molecules with molecular weights between 2000 and 6000 Da, showing differences in molecular size distribution by compound.

Preparation	Trade name(s)	Method of production	Weight average molecular mass	% between 2000–6000 Da
Nardroparin	Fraxiparine Selaparin	Nitrous acid depolymerization and fractionation	4200	85
Enoxaparin	Clexane Lovenox	Benzylation followed by alkaline depolymerisation	3900	75
Dalteparin	Fragmin	Nitrous acid depolymerization and gel filtration	5700	80
Tinzaparin	Logiparin Innohep	Depolymerisation with heparinase	6000	64
Certoparin	Alphaparin Sandoparin	Depolymerisation with isoamylnitrate	5100	63
Ardeparin	Normiflo	Peroxidative cleavage	6000	
Reviparin	Clivarine	Nitrous acid depolymerization and chromatographic separation	4000	

Table 16.3 Potency (as anti Xa activity and Anti Xa to IIa activity), plasma half-life and bioavailability of the commercially available low molecular weight heparins compared to unfractionated heparin

Preparation	Anti Xa activity (Unit/ mg)	Anti Xa to IIa Ratio	Half-life (min)	Bioavailability (%)
Unfractionated Heparin		1	30–150	10–20
Nadroparin	95	3.6:1	132–162	89
Enoxaparin	105	3.8:1	129–180	91
Dalteparin	130	2.7:1	119–139	87
Tinzaparin	83	1.9:1	111	90
Certoparin	88	2.0:1	240	90
Ardeparin	100	1.9:1	200	90
Reviparin	130	3.6:1	180	90

Therapeutic effects of lmwh

Because of the differences among LMWHs, the clinical profile cannot be extrapolated to another one or generalized to the whole LMWH family. These differences lead to a major problem with providing a potency reference standard. This has a profound impact on licensing generic versions.

Adverse effects of lmwh

The principle adverse effect of LMWH is haemorrhage. Unlike UFH, there is no absolute antidote such as protamine. LMWHs have a high incidence of cross-reaction with the heparin-dependent antibody found in HIT. If no cross-reaction occurs using platelet aggregometry, anticoagulation can be safely undertaken with a LMWH.

Pentasaccharides

Structure activity and mechanism of action

Fondaparinux is a synthetic preparation of the pentasaccharide sequence found in heparin. This allows manufacture to a high degree of purity and uniformity. The antithrombotic activity of fondaparinux is the result of antithrombin (AT)-mediated selective inhibition of Factor Xa which is about 300 times the innate neutralization of Factor Xa by AT. Fondaparinux does not interact with AT to inactivate thrombin and has no known effect on platelet function.

In healthy individuals with normal kidney function, about 80% of a single subcutaneous dose is eliminated in urine as unchanged drug in 72 hours. The elimination half-life is 17 to 21 hours. Fondaparinux is administered by subcutaneous injection and has 100% bioavailability. In healthy adults fondaparinux is more than 90% bound to AT. It does not bind significantly to other plasma proteins including platelet factor 4 or red blood cells. The anti-Xa activity of the drug increases with increasing drug concentration, reaching maximum values in approximately two hours. In 2002 fondaparinux was licensed for VTE prevention in orthopaedic surgery patients, where it appears to be more effective than LMWH for VTE prophylaxis (17).

Special populations

Fondaparinux clearance is decreased about 25% in patients older than 75 years and by about 30% in patients weighing less than 50 kg. Fondaparinux elimination is prolonged in patients with renal impairment being approximately 50% lower in patients with severe renal impairment (< 30 mL/min) compared to patients with normal renal function.

Emerging developments

Idraparinux is a second-generation pentasaccharide with sulphate group substitution on the pentasaccharide leading to a half-life of about 80 hours. A study comparing idraparinux with a vitamin K antagonist to prevent stroke in patients with atrial fibrillation was stopped early due to excess bleeding in the idraparinux arm. The molecule has been modified further to add a biotin moiety. This idrabiotaparinux is rapidly (<10 min) removed from the circulation following intravenous injection of avidin, an egg derived protein with low antigenicity. Idrabiotaparinux is in clinical trials and should be available in the next 2–3 years

Oral vitamin K antagonists

Since being licensed for human use in the early 1950s this class of drug has been, until recently, the only orally available anticoagulant. This is despite multiple problems including a narrow therapeutic index, slow onset and offset times, multiple food and drug interactions, together with genetic variations in metabolism. A recently published review outlines the pharmacology and guidelines for use and management of these drugs (18). Certain aspects will be briefly reviewed for warfarin as the example drug.

Warfarin inhibits the vitamin K-dependent synthesis of biologically active forms of clotting factors II, VII, IX, and X, as well as the regulatory factors, protein C and protein S. The process is shown diagrammatically in figure 16.2. The precursors of these factors require carboxylation of their glutamic acid residues to allow the

coagulation factors to bind to phospholipid surfaces such as that of the activated platelet. The carboxylation reaction will proceed only if the carboxylase enzyme is able to convert a reduced form of vitamin K (vitamin K hydroquinone) to vitamin K epoxide. The vitamin K epoxide is in turn recycled back to vitamin K and vitamin K hydroquinone by another enzyme, the vitamin K epoxide reductase (VKOR).Warfarin inhibits epoxide reductase (specifically the VKORC1 subunit), thereby diminishing available vitamin K and vitamin K hydroquinone in the tissues. When this occurs, the coagulation factors are no longer carboxylated and are thus biologically inactive.

Warfarin is the archetypical drug affected by multiple interactions. This is because of interference with the metabolic pathways by not only other drugs but also genetic polymorphisms. Warfarin consists of a racemic mixture of two active enantiomers—R- and S- forms. S-warfarin has five times the potency of the R-isomer. The enantiomers of warfarin are differentially metabolized by human cytochrome P450 (CYP). R-warfarin is metabolized primarily by CYP1A2 and CYP3A4. S-warfarin is metabolized primarily by CYP2C9 (figure 16.1). The efficacy of warfarin is affected mainly when metabolism of S-warfarin is altered. A few selected examples of various drugs and non-proprietary agents interactions with warfarin is shown in table 16.4. It is therefore not surprising that there is little correlation among dose, serum concentration, and therapeutic effect, necessitating individualized dosing guided by monitoring the prothrombin time or international normalized ratio (INR). Warfarin is used in a number of chronic thrombotic and thromboembolic-prone conditions. These, together with the recommended INR range for effective prophylaxis, are shown in table 16.5.

When warfarin is newly started, it may temporarily promote clot formation. This is because the level of protein C and protein S are also dependent on vitamin K activity. Warfarin causes decline in protein C levels (half-life 14 hours) and therefore, reduced degradation of factor Va and factor VIIIa. The haemostasis system becomes temporarily biased towards thrombus formation. If thrombosis occurs it typically presents as skin necrosis and gangrene of limbs. Co-administration of heparin with warfarin therapy for four to five days is required, until the full effect of warfarin has been achieved.

The risk of severe bleeding is small (a median annual rate of 0.9 to 2.7% has been reported) and any benefit needs to outweigh this risk when warfarin is considered as a therapeutic measure. Risk of bleeding is augmented if the INR is out of range (due to overdose or drug interactions), when combined with antiplatelet drugs such as clopidogrel, aspirin, or other NSAIDs, and in elderly patients. Warfarin will pass through the placental barrier and may cause fetal bleeding, in addition coumarins are teratogens.

Reversal of warfarin effect can be achieved in many ways depending on the urgency of the situation. Stopping the drug will return the INR to <1.5 in about 3–5 days. 2 mg of oral vitamin K will return INR to normal within 24 hours and the same dose intravenously within about 4–6 hours. Note that intravenous vitamin K contains Cremophor EL, a potent cause of anaphylactoid and anaphylactic reactions. More recently prothrombin complex has been licensed for rapid reversal of effect (less than 1 hour). The dose is 30 factor IXa equivalent units/kg. This replaces the prior treatment with 15 mL/kg of fresh frozen plasma.

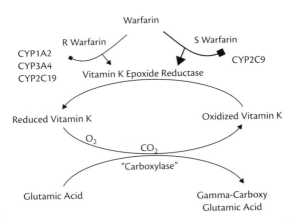

Fig. 16.2 Schematic diagram showing mechanism of action of the vitamin K antagonist warfarin. The glutamic acid residues of certain coagulation factors require addition of as carboxy moiety to achieve full activity. The carboxylation reaction will proceed only if the carboxylase enzyme is able to convert a reduced form of vitamin K to vitamin K epoxide at the same time. The vitamin K epoxide is in turn recycled back to reduced vitamin K by vitamin K epoxide reductase (VKOR). Warfarin inhibits epoxide reductase thereby slowing this reaction sequence. Also shown are the metabolic pathways of the two enantiomers of warfarin. Clinically and functionally the S enantiomer is most important and is metabolized by the CYP2C9 cytochrome system.

Table 16.4 Compounds recognized to interact with warfarin therapy to increase or decrease potency, as shown by effects on prothrombin time/INR. Also shown are the proposed mechanisms for this action.

Drugs that change plasma concentration of Warfarin	Additive anticoagulant effect with no change in plasma concentration	Unknown mechanisms
Prolonged prothrombin time/increase bleeding risk		
Inhibit S isomer clearance 　Metronidazole 　Sulphinpyrazone 　Trimethaprim 　Disulphiram	Inhibit vitamin K cycle 　Acetaminophen (paracetamol) 　Antibiotics inhibiting gut vitamin K	Ketoconazole/fluconazole Tamoxifen Phenytoin Erythromycin
Inhibit R isomer clearance 　Cimetidine 　Omeprazole 　Ciprofloxacin 　Metronidazole	Inhibit coagulation and/or platelet function 　Heparin 　Aspirin/clopidogrel	
Inhibit both S & R isomer clearance 　Amiodarone		
Reduced prothrombin time/ decrease bleeding risk		
Reduced absorption 　Cholestyramine	Altered diet especially vitamin K-rich foods such as liver, spinach, broccoli, and Brussel sprouts	Penicillins
Increased metabolism 　Barbiturates 　Rifampicin 　Griseofulvin 　Carbamazepine 　St Johns Wort		

Table 16.5 Recommended international normalised ratio (INR) targets for various thromboprophylactic and treatment plans with vitamin K antagonists such as warfarin

Indication	INR
Treatment of venous thrombosis 6 weeks for calf vein and 3–6 months for proximal deep vein thrombosis	2.0–3.0
Treatment of pulmonary embolism for at least 6 months	2.0–3.0
Prevention of systemic embolism	2.0–3.0
Tissue heart valves	2.0–3.0
To prevent systemic embolism after acute myocardial infarction	2.0–3.0
To prevent recurrent myocardial infarction	2.5–3.5
Valvular heart disease	2.0–3.0
Atrial fibrillation. Over age 75 consider lower range (1.5–2.5) due to increased risk of intracranial bleed	2.0–3.0
Bileaflet mechanical valve in aortic position	2.0–3.0
Mechanical prosthetic valves with cage	2.5–3.5
Systemic recurrent emboli	2.5–3.5

Agents acting by direct inhibition of thrombin or activated factor X

Intravenous direct thrombin inhibitors

The basic pharmacology of these compounds has been recently reviewed elsewhere (19,20). Historically the agents developed are analogues of hirudin that bind to the proteolytic site of thrombin and an anionic exosite (bivalent inhibitor) (shown for hirudin in figure 16.1) or the proteolytic site only (monovalent). The hirudin-like molecules are made by recombinant technology. Lepirudin and desirudin mimic natural hirudin but with amino acid and sulphate substitutions; bivalirudin has a unique structure with a dodecapeptide attached to the active binding site moiety by four glycine residues and is shown in figure 16.3. Argatroban is also a synthetic derivative of arginine. All of these compounds inhibit both free and bound thrombin and none are affected by platelet factor 4.

Clinical pharmacology

These medications are indicated for the treatment and prevention of thrombosis in patients with HIT. Bivalirudin is also licensed for use during percutaneous coronary interventions/angioplasty procedures. Table 16.6 outlines the basic pharmacokinetic profile

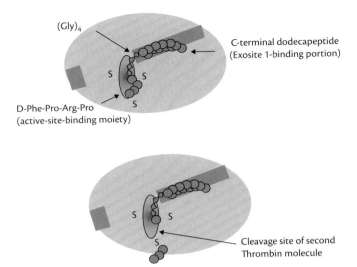

(Gly)₄

C-terminal dodecapeptide
(Exosite 1-binding portion)

D-Phe-Pro-Arg-Pro
(active-site-binding moiety)

Cleavage site of second
Thrombin molecule

Fig. 16.3 Schematic to show, in the upper panel the binding of bivalirudin to the thrombin molecule. Binding of the dodecapeptide is at the anion binding site used by fibrinogen and the 4 amino acid residue D-Phe-Pro-Arg-Pro to the active proteolytic site. Lower panel shows effect of a second thrombin molecule to cleave the Pro-Arg bond of the active site of thrombin binding moiety to stop the direct antithrombin action.

of each drug. The main points are that the recombinant hirudins are highly affected by renal function whereas agatroban is entirely metabolized in the liver requiring the dose to be lowered and slowing reversal of anticoagulant effects. There is no antidote to any of these agents so the antithrombin effect cannot be reversed pharmacologically.

Bivalirudin has renal excretion but also a unique metabolic elimination process. A second thrombin molecule can cleave the

Pro-Arg bond of the active site binding moiety to metabolize biva-lirudin (figure 16.3). This obviously improves safety in patients with impaired renal function. However if used during CPB, the blood flow in the system cannot be allowed to stop otherwise thrombin and clot will form in the stagnant blood.

The anticoagulant effect of thrombin inhibitors is monitored by the aPTT or ACT (table 16.6) with the coagulation time increasing in a dose-dependent manner. Argatroban also inhibits the prothrombin time in a dose-dependent manner. This has implications when transferring patients to long-term anticoagulation with vitamin K antagonists. The individual effects of argatroban and a vitamin K antagonist on the INR can be calculated using a nomogram available in the prescribing information. The major adverse effect is haemorrhage, which may be life threatening. In addition, the recombinant hirudins are also associated with allergic/anaphylactic reactions that limit their use whereas allergy to bivalirudin or argatroban is rare.

Oral direct thrombin inhibitors

The only oral direct thrombin inhibitor currently available is dabigatran, which is an orally active competitive direct thrombin inhibitor administered as the prodrug dabigatran etexilate mesylate. The active drug is able to inhibit both free and clot-bound thrombin and thrombin induced platelet activation. It has low protein binding and is not metabolized by cytochrome P450, but dabigatran is predominantly excreted unchanged in the urine.

The formulation of the capsules is highly acidic and was associated with an increased incidence of gastritis in the RE-LY (Randomized Evaluation of Long-term Anticoagulant Therapy) study (21). Of more importance, the bioavailability of the drug after oral administration is about 6–7%. This is increased to about 75% if the capsule is chewed prior to swallowing and the patient should be warned to swallow the capsule whole.

Table 16.6 Basic pharmacokinetics, monitoring method and excretion of the four available intravenous direct thrombin inhibitors. Also shown are the conditions for reductions in dose in patients with renal or hepatic failure.

Drug	Administration	Half-life	Dosing schedule	Monitoring	Renal Excretion	Dose reductions
Desirudin	Intravenous and Subcutaneous	2–3 hours after intravenous injection	15mg b.d.	APTT of 1.5 times control. Stop drug if > 2 times control	40–50%	3 fold reduction with creatinine clearance 30–49mL/min. 9 fold reduction with creatinine clearance < 30 mL/min
Lepirudin	Intravenous	1.3 hours in health men 2 hours in both health females & over 70 year. 2 days with creatinine clearance < 15 mL/min	Load of 0.4 mg/kg followed by continuous infusion of 0.15mg/kg/hour	APTT 1.5–2.5 times control	45–50%	Creatinine clearance < 60ml/min or plasma creatinine > 1.5mg/dL (124µmol/L)
Bivalirudin	Intravenous	25 minutes. Coagulation tests within normal limits after 2 hours	0.75mg/kg bolus then 1.75mg/kg/hr		25–50%	Creatinine Clearance <30ml/min infusion rate to 1mg/kg/min
Agatroban	Intravenous	Coagulation tests are within normal limits 4 hours after discontinuing infusion	2µg/kg/min increasing to 10µg/kg/min based on raising APTT2–3 fold	APTT, ACT	None	Hepatic failure/impairment

APTT, activated partial thromboplastin time; ACT, activated clotting time

Dabigatran has a predictable pharmacokinetic/pharmacodynamic profile, allowing for a fixed-dose regimen. Peak plasma concentrations of dabigatran are reached approximately two hours after oral administration. Because the drug is predominantly excreted by the kidneys, the recommendation is that the dose of the drug should be reduced from 150 mg twice daily to 75 mg twice daily if the estimated creatinine clearance is 30–50 mL/min.

Dabagatran is licensed to prevent VTE after knee and hip replacement in Europe and as a means of reducing stroke risk in patients with chronic atrial fibrillation in other markets.

The RE-LY study (21) was a multi-centre trial comparing two blinded doses of dabigatran (110 mg twice daily and 150 mg twice daily) with open-label warfarin (dosed to target INR of 2 to 3) in patients with non-valvular, persistent, paroxysmal, or permanent atrial fibrillation A total of 18 113 patients were randomized and followed for a median of 2 years.

The conclusions from this study were that dabigatran given at a dose of 110 mg was associated with rates of stroke and systemic embolism that were similar to those associated with warfarin as well as lower rates of major hemorrhage (2.71% versus 3.36%; $p = 0.003$). Dabigatran administered at a dose of 150 mg, as compared with warfarin, was associated with lower rates of stroke and systemic embolism but similar rates of major hemorrhage at 3.11% ($p = 0.31$ compared to warfarin). Despite this finding, the US Food and Drug Administration chose to license only the 150 mg twice-daily regimen and not the 110 mg dose.

As with other agents the major risk is for bleeding which may be life threatening. At the time of writing there are reports from post-marketing surveillance of 260 deaths directly due to bleeding in dabigatran-treated patients. This may lead to changes in regulatory approval.

There is no specific antidote to dabigatran and if surgery or an intervention is planned then it is recommended to discontinue the drug for 2–5 days depending on renal function. The manufacturers recommend longer times should also be considered for patients undergoing major surgery, spinal puncture, or placement of an epidural catheter. The prescribing information suggests that due to the low protein binding then it may be possible to remove about 60% of dabigatran in 2–3 hours by dialysis, but this has not been reported in clinical practice.

Oral inhibitors of activated factor X

This group of drugs bind to and inhibit factor Xa directly without a requirement for antithrombin. Antithrombotic activity is specific for factor Xa with no effect on other components of the coagulation cascade. As a class of antithrombotic agents, the major advantage of direct factor Xa inhibitors lies in their small size and ability to inactivate circulating and bound factor Xa. The rapid onset and offset of action also means that there is no need to monitor the anticoagulant effect. The inhibitors of activated factor X developed to date generally bind in an L-shaped conformation, where one group of the ligand occupies the anionic S1 pocket and another group of the ligand occupies the aromatic S4. Examples of two molecules (rivaroxaban and apixaban) are shown in figure 16.4.

Apixaban, betrixaban, edoxaban, and rivaroxaban are the most advanced in their period of clinical development. Both apixaban and rivaroxaban have licensed indications in Europe and in the latter case in the USA. Edoxaban was licensed in Japan only for thromboprophylaxis after major orthopaedic surgery in April 2011. The pharmacokinetic profiles for these four anti-Xa antagonists are shown in table 16.7. Only betrixaban is unaffected by renal function. All of the agents have protein binding of about 90% meaning they will be difficult to remove by dialysis. Studies have shown that all the agents will induce a prolongation of coagulation times by 2–3 hours following ingestion. There are no clinical trials to show a specific antagonist to this effect. However, a recent study in blood of volunteers who took rivaroxaban or dabagatran showed that administration of prothrombin complex reversed the rivaroxaban but not the dabigatran effect (22).

There are a large number of phase II/III studies of oral factor Xa inhibitors currently underway. Of specific interest are patients with an acute coronary syndrome (ACS) receiving dual

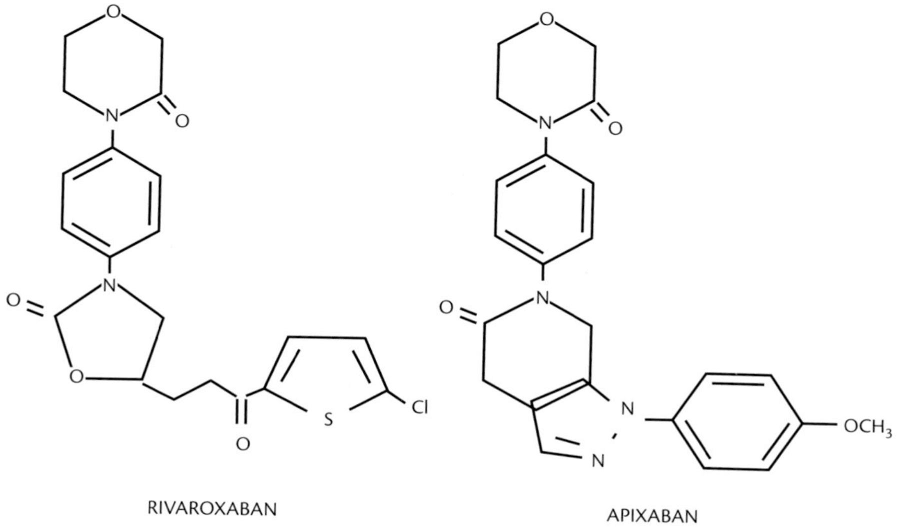

Fig. 16.4 Chemical structures for the activated factor X antagonists rivaroxaban and apixaban to show the L shaped structure of this class of compound. This molecular configuration allows binding of the upper part of the molecule to the anionic S1 pocket and the foot of the molecule to the aromatic S4 pocket.

Table 16.7 Data for basic pharmacology of the four orally active Factor Xa inhibitors rivaroxaban, apixaban, edoxaban and betrixaban

Drug	Prodrug	Bioavailability	Half-life	Dosing schedule	Metabolism	Renal Excretion	Dose reduction criteria
Rivaroxaban	No	90%	9 hours. 12–16 hours over 75 years of age	Once or twice daily	CYP34A	35%	Age over 75 years. Caution if creatinine clearance <49mL/min
Apixaban	No	50–80%	12 hours	Once or twice daily	CYP3A4	25%	NR
Edoxaban	No	45%	9–11hours	Once daily		35%	NR
Betrixaban	No	45–50%	20 hours	Once daily		5%	NR

NR, no reduction

antiplatelet medication as they are most likely to present for a cardiac intervention.

The results of the studies published thus far have been confusing. The APPRAISE study of apixaban in ACS was terminated early because of increased fatal intracranial bleeding (23). However, in the ATLAS ACS2-TIMI 51 study (24) with rivaroxaban there was a benefit with the lower but not the higher dose and an increase in non-fatal intracranial haemorrhage. It may be that this class of compound will mainly be of benefit to replace vitamin K antagonists, but it may have safety issues when taken with antiplatelet therapy. The safety of these agents, when it is necessary to perform urgent surgery or following trauma, has not been determined. Only rivaroxaban currently has specific instructions for use with reduced renal function and advanced age included in the product specification. This information also states that epidural haematomas have been reported during rivaroxaban administration. It is certain that the other agents will also have limitations agreed with regulatory authorities as appropriate.

Antiplatelet agents

As acute arterial occlusion leading to myocardial infarction or stroke is a leading cause of death world wide it is not surprising that considerable effort has been placed into developing drugs that will affect platelet function and reduce these cardiovascular events. In the earlier days acetyl salicylic acid (ASA) was the mainstay of therapy. With increasing knowledge of the mechanism(s) of action of platelet activation more recent therapies have concentrated on specific receptor inhibition.

The platelet can be activated in a number of different ways. The early targets for pharmacological intervention were suppression of cyclo-oxygenase with ASA and phosphodiesterase with dipyridamole. More recently, the major focus of pharmacological interventions has been to inhibit receptors at the platelet surface. In particular, there has been a considerable interest in inhibition of purinergic receptors and those binding fibrinogen (the IIb/IIIa receptor). Agents that inhibit binding of vWF to the GpIb receptor are in early clinical development. Inhibitors of the protease-activated receptor 1 (thrombin receptor) on the platelet surface have reached phase II/III studies but have shown increased bleeding so development is currently suspended. The targets and agents in clinical use or development are shown in figure 16.5.

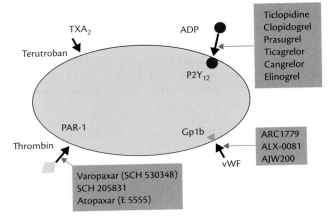

Fig. 16.5 Schematic figure showing platelet receptors currently targets of novel drug research. Also shown are the various drugs that have been administered in humans. The thromboxane A_2 (TXA_2) receptor inhibitor terutroban is being studied in stroke prevention. Inhibitors of the protease activated receptor type 1 (PAR-1) receptor activated by thrombin (Varopaxar and Atopaxar) have been studied in patients with acute coronary syndrome and have development on hold due to the observation of increased bleeding in this setting. The inhibitors of the binding of von Willebrand factor (vWF) to the glycoprotein Ib receptor on the platelet are in early development. For the antagonists of the action of ADP at the $P2Y_{12}$ receptor ticlopidine is of historic interest only and elinogrel (a competetive reversible inhibitor with a 12 hour half-life) is in phase 3 studies in humans.

Acetyl salicylic acid

Aspirin is the registered trade name of the ASA first produced by the Bayer Company, and thus ASA will be used. Prostaglandin H-synthase 1 and 2 (also known as cyclo-oxygenase (COX) 1 and 2) catalyse the conversion of arachidonic acid to prostaglandin H_2 (PGH_2). Human platelets and vascular endothelial cells process PGH_2 to produce primarily thromboxane A_2 (TXA_2) and PGI_2, respectively (25). TXA_2 induces platelet aggregation and vasoconstriction, whereas PGI_2 inhibits platelet aggregation and induces vasodilatation. Platelet thromboxane A_2 synthesis is reduced by about 98% following ASA administration. Whereas TXA_2 is largely a COX-1-derived product, COX-2-mediated PGI_2 production is insensitive to ASA inhibition at conventional antiplatelet doses.

ASA is rapidly absorbed in the stomach and upper intestine. Peak plasma levels occur 30 to 40 min after ASA ingestion, and inhibition of platelet function is evident by one hour. The oral bioavailability of regular ASA tablets is approximately 40 to 50% over a wide range of doses (26). The plasma concentration of ASA decays with a half-life of 15 to 20 min. Despite this rapid clearance of ASA from the circulation, the platelet-inhibitory effect lasts for the life span of the platelet because ASA irreversibly inactivates platelet COX-1 (27). ASA also acetylates the enzyme in megakaryocytes. The mean life span of human platelets is approximately 5 to 10 days (28). Therefore, about 10 to 12% of circulating platelets are replaced every 24 h. Normal primary haemostasis requires about 20–30% of normal platelet numbers/function. This suggests that cessation of ASA ingestion for 48 hours will result in a return to a normal haemostatic activity.

Numerous studies have shown a risk reduction of about 15–20% for myocardial ischaemia, stroke with doses starting at about 60 mg daily (29,30). However, some patients are resistant to these doses of ASA and may be more prone to recurrent cardiovascular events (31). The antiplatelet effect of ASA at low doses, the lack of dose–response relationship in clinical studies evaluating its antithrombotic effects, and its side effects, in particular bleeding, has been shown to be dose dependent in patients with stroke and acute coronary syndrome (32,33). These factors all support the use of as low a dose of ASA in the prophylaxis and treatment of thromboembolic disorders (table 16.8).

Dipyridamole

Dipyridamole has vasodilator and antiplatelet properties. The mechanism of action of dipyridamole is to increase intracellular cyclic AMP and thus inhibit the platelet shape change. Dipyridomole is eliminated primarily by biliary excretion as a glucuronide conjugate and is subject to enterohepatic recirculation. Dipyridamole is highly bound to plasma proteins. Following an oral dose of dipyridamole tablets, the average time to peak concentration is about 75 minutes. The decline in plasma concentration fits a two-compartment model. The alpha half-life (the initial decline following peak concentration) is approximately 40

Table 16.8 The lowest effective daily dose of acetyl salicylic acid to reduce the risk of thrombotic events by condition

Disorder	Lowest effective daily dose (mg)
Transient ischaemic attack or ischaemic stroke*	50
Men at high cardiovascular risk	50
Hypertension	75
Stable angina	75
Unstable angina*	75
Severe carotid artery stenosis*	75
Polycythaemia vera	100
Acute myocardial infarction	160
Acute ischaemic stroke*	160

In those conditions marked with an asterisk higher doses have been studied but did not show added benefit.

minutes and the beta half-life is approximately 10 hours which is consistent with the twice-daily oral dose regimen. The absorption of dypyridamole from conventional formulations is quite variable and may result in low systemic bioavailability of the drug. A newer formulation with greater bioavailabilty and a fixed combination of modified-release dipyridamole and low-dose aspirin has been studied and licensed to reduce recurrent stroke incidence (34).

Specific platelet receptor inhibitors
Purinergic receptors

There are three known subtypes of ADP receptors on platelets: P2X$_1$, P2Y$_1$, and P2Y$_{12}$ (figure 16.6). ADP binds to the P2Y$_1$ receptor to initiate the platelet aggregation process and to the P2Y$_{12}$ receptor, which amplifies and completes the platelet aggregation process. Sustained ADP-induced platelet aggregation requires co-activation of P2Y$_1$ and P2Y$_{12}$ receptors. Without

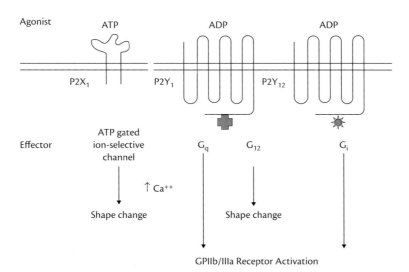

Fig. 16.6 Schematic figure of the three parts of the purinergic receptor on platelets, together with their mechanism of platelet activation. The two seven-transmembrane receptors act through G protein mechanisms. The P2Y$_1$ receptor initiates the platelet aggregation process and the P2Y$_{12}$ receptor amplifies and completes the aggregation process. Continued stimulation of this receptor is needed to prevent platelet disaggregation.

continued $P2Y_{12}$ activation, aggregated platelets disaggregate. Due to this the $P2Y_{12}$ receptor and its inhibition have been the focus of recent clinical drug development.

Thienopyridines

Thienopyridines selectively inhibit ADP-induced platelet aggregation with no direct effects on arachidonic acid metabolism. All of the thienopyridines are prodrugs. Of major clinical interest is that clopidogrel is metabolized into 2-oxo-clopidogrel through a cytochrome P450-dependent pathway. The most important of these clinically is the 2C19 variant. This intermediate metabolite is then hydrolysed and generates a highly labile thiol active metabolite. The active metabolite of clopidogrel belongs to a family of eight stereoisomers, only one of which is biologically activity. Prasugrel is not detected in plasma following oral administration. It is rapidly hydrolysed by esterase in the intestine to a thiolactone, which is then converted to the active metabolite by a single step, primarily by CYP3A4 and CYP2B6, and to a lesser extent by CYP2C9 and CYP2C19. The active metabolite of prasugrel is metabolized to two inactive highly protein bound compounds by S-methylation or conjugation with cysteine. Clopidogrel is also metabolised by esterases to produce an inactive carboxylic acid derivative thought to represent over 80% of circulating metabolites.

The active metabolites of both clopidogrel and prasugrel couple through a irreversible covalent disulfide bridge to the $P2Y_{12}$ receptor, rendering the receptor unresponsive to its agonist for the remainder of their lifespan (about 7 to 10 days). Return of global platelet function requires the generation of a new platelet pool.

Following oral administration, about 80% of the dose of prasugrel and about 50% of clopidogrel is absorbed and these figures are not affected by food ingestion. Peak plasma concentrations of the active metabolite occur approximately 30 minutes after dosing. Repeat daily doses do not lead to accumulation of the active metabolite, which has an elimination half-life of about 7 hours in both cases. Both drugs are highly protein bound (>95%). Approximately 70% of the prasugrel dose is excreted in the urine and 30% in the faeces as inactive metabolites. The corresponding figures for clopidogrel are about 50% by each route.

With both drugs the recommendation is to give a loading dose followed by a once daily maintenance dose. For clopidogrel the recommendation is a 300 mg load and 75 mg per day and for prasugrel 60 mg and 10 mg, respectively. With prasugrel platelet inhibition reaches about 50% one hour after a loading dose of 60 mg. Steady state inhibition of about 70% occurs after 3–5 days with a maintenance dose of 10 mg per day. Platelet aggregation returns to baseline values over 5–9 days reflecting production of a new platelet population. With clopidogrel at a dose of 75 mg once daily platelet inhibition reaches a steady state of 40–60% inhibition after 3–7 days of therapy. Platelet aggregation and bleeding time return to baseline values in about 5 days after stopping therapy.

Therapeutic Effects of Thienopyridines
Both clopidogrel and prasugrel are indicated for use in patients with acute coronary syndromes including patients with unstable angina or non-ST-elevation myocardial infarction (NSTEMI) and patients with ST-elevation myocardial infarction (STEMI) when managed with primary or delayed percutaneous coronary intervention (PCI). The principal adverse outcome related to the use of thienopyridines is bleeding. In the TRITON TIMI 38 study (35) comparing prasugrel with clopidogrel, the classification of

bleeding was according to the original TIMI definitions of major (clinically overt bleeding associated with a fall in hemoglobin ≥5 g/dL, or intracranial hemorrhage) and TIMI minor (overt bleeding associated with a fall in hemoglobin of ≥3 g/dL but <5 g/dL). At the doses used major bleeding occurred more commonly in the prasugrel arm and for this drug bleeding was also more common in patients with a body weight less than 60kg and those over the age of 75 years. In the study population 213 of 6741 patient allocate to prasugrel and 224 of 6716 allocated to clopidogrel required surgical revascularisation with coronary artery bypass grafting (CABG). Major bleeding was reported in 11.3% of prasugrel compared to 3.6% in clopidogrel-treated patients with significantly increased rates of fatal bleeding, need for reoperation and requirement for red cell transfusion of ≥5 units in the prasugrel patients (36).

Patient having surgery within three days of stopping the study medication had rates of major/minor bleeding of 26.7% for prasugrel and 5% for clopidogrel. This fell to 11.3% and 3.4% respectively for patients having surgery 4–7 days after stopping study medication. Currently, the prescribing information suggests clopidogrel is stopped for 5 days prior to surgery and prasugrel for 7 days. In addition the information for prasugrel states that this drug should not be started in patients likely to undergo surgical revascularization. There is also a warning about administration to patients older than 75 years of age and those with a body weight of less than 60kg due to the increased incidence of intracranial bleeding.

The clopidogrel prescribing information now contains a warning about a group of patients, identified as poor metabolizers of clopidogrel based on their CYP 2C19 state, who are at greater risk of ischaemic events despite taking clopidogrel (37). Drugs that modify the CYP450 2C19 and 3A4 isoenzymes may alter the effectiveness of clopidogrel but not prasugrel therapy (38,39). An example of the former is the proton pump inhibitor omeprazole. Ingestion of omeprazole with clopidogrel showed platelet ADP response was reduced by about 20% by day 5. In experimental studies when clopidogrel and atorvastatin, a CYP3A4 substrate, are present at equimolar concentrations in vitro, clopidogrel metabolism is inhibited by >90%. It has also been shown that atorvastatin, in a dose dependant manner reduced platelet activation (40). It may seem surprising that despite these known interactions, there is no evidence that this is clinically relevant as shown by a lack of a statistically discernable effect on cardiovascular outcomes (30).

Adenosine polyphosphate analogues

Ticagrelor

Ticagrelor, formerly known as AZD6140, is the first of a new class of antiplatelet agents, the cyclo-pentyl-triazolo-pyrimidines. Similar to the thienopyridines, ticagrelor is an oral $P2Y_{12}$ receptor antagonist. Ticagrelor has a binding site different from ADP making it a reversible allosteric antagonist. Unlike the thienopyridines, ticagrelor is not a prodrug, and therefore does not require metabolic activation in order to inhibit platelets. Since ticagrelor does not require metabolic activation, it avoids the variability seen with the CYP450 system. However the parent drug is metabolized, principally by the CYP3A group of cytochrome to about 10 metabolites. The major metabolite, AR-C124910X, is formed by O-de-ethylation of the parent. Exposure to AR-C124910XX represents about 30% of peak and 40% of overall exposure to ticagrelor.

This metabolite is as active as ticagrelor in inhibiting ADP induced platelet aggregation. Both the parent and major metabolite are nearly 100% protein bound. Ticagrelor is about 36% bioavailable after oral administration and is rapidly absorbed with a maximum plasma concentration at 1.5 h. based on analysis of radiolabeled drug. Levels of unchanged ticagrelor and AR-C124910XX were <0.05% in the urine, indicating that renal clearance of ticagrelor and AR-C124910XX is of minor importance.

Inhibition of platelet activity (IPA) using ADP stimulated platelet aggregation showed 88% platelet inhibition with ticagrelor. Ticagrelor inhibited platelets to a greater extent than did a 600 mg loading dose of clopidogrel at 2 hours (mean IPA, ~90% versus ~40%, respectively). In this study (41), other measures of platelet function showed more rapid and robust inhibitory activity (typically three- to fivefold greater effectiveness) for ticagrelor compared to clopidogrel.

The two drugs were also studied in a head to head comparison in the PLATO (PLATelet inhibition and patient Outcomes) study (42). This was a trial in more than 18,000 patients hospitalized for an ACS, with or without ST-segment elevation. Ticagrelor was given in a loading dose of 180 mg, followed by a dose of 90 mg twice daily. Patients in the clopidogrel group received a 300 mg loading dose followed by 75 mg daily. In patients undergoing CABG surgery, it was recommended that the study drug be withheld for five days in the clopidogrel group and for 24 to 72 hours in the ticagrelor group. All patients received aspirin. In patients who went on to have CABG surgery, there was an early (at one month) difference in cardiovascular death, which continued out to one year follow up (7.9% with clopidogrel v 4.1% ticagrelor $p = 0.009$). This striking benefit was unrelated to any excess bleeding in either group (43).

In the PLATO study the groups did not differ significantly in the rates of CABG-related TIMI major bleeding trial (11.6% and 11.2%, respectively; $p = 0.43$), despite the fact that ticagrelor was only withheld for 24 to 72 hours prior to surgery while clopidogrel was withheld for five days. It is somewhat strange that the prescribing information for ticagrelor states that the drug should be withheld for five days prior to surgery.

Ticagrelor has adenosine as a potential breakdown product and drug administration is associated with effects that could be related to this. In particular patients receiving ticagrelor had significantly more episodes of dyspnoea (10% to 20%) and ventricular pauses lasting more than 3 seconds (6%). Contraindications for ticagrelor are active pathological bleeding and a history of intracranial bleeding.

Plasma concentrations of ticagrelor are slightly increased (12–23%) in elderly patients, women, patients of Asian ethnicity, and patients with mild hepatic impairment. The pharmacodynamics of ticagrelor and not materially affected in patients with severe renal impairment. Ticagrelor has to be taken twice daily which is a disadvantage in respect of compliance as the effects of missing doses of ticagrelor will increase the risk for stent thrombosis.

Cangrelor

Cangrelor is a $P2Y_{12}$ purinoreceptor antagonist discovered by manipulation of ATP. It is given by intravenous injection and has been shown to have a short half-life of about 2.6 minutes. Steady-state inhibition levels of ADP-induced platelet aggregation were achieved within 30 minutes of infusion of cangrelor titrated up to 4 µg/kg/min. These effects were stable until the end of the study at 72 hours. Return of baseline platelet aggregation was reestablished in 70% of volunteers within one hour of infusion termination.

Cangrelor acts directly at the $P2Y_{12}$ receptor without need for conversion in the liver to an active metabolite. Plasma concentrations of cangrelor are unaffected by severe renal or hepatic impairment. Cangrelor was being studied in two large-scale Phase III studies. The Cangrelor versus standard tHerapy to Achieve optimal Management of Platelet inhibitION (CHAMPION) before (CHAMPION PCI) or after (CHAMPION PLATFORM) PCI trials were both ended early following a decision by the interim analysis review committee (IARC) that the study would not demonstrate the 'persuasive' clinical efficacy needed for regulatory approval. The standard therapy comparator was a loading dose of clopidogrel of 600 mg. Subsequently, a small study has used cangrelor as a bridge to revascularization surgery after discontinuing clopidogrel.

Table 16.9 compares and contrasts the basic pharmacology and safety data for the available purinergic receptor antagonists.

Glycoprotein (GP) IIb/IIIa antagonists

Two types of GP IIb/IIIa receptor antagonists are available: non-competitive (a monoclonal antibody) and competitive (a peptide and a peptidomimetic). Abciximab, is a chimeric compound modified from an original murine monoclonal antibody to reduce its immunogenicity. The ability of abciximab to bind to the vitronectin receptor and the leukocyte receptor (MAC-1) may also contribute to the anti-inflammatory properties of this drug. The drug is taken up by the reticular endothelial system where it is degraded by proteolysis.

Eptifibatide is a cyclic heptapeptide containing six amino acids and one mercaptopropionyl (des-amino cysteinyl) residue. Tirofiban is a non-peptide but peptidomimetic. Both agents mimic the arginine-glycine-aspartate (RGD) sequences on fibrinogen. They contain either the RGD sequence itself or a similar sequence. The therapeutic efficacy of these drugs depends on maintaining plasma levels high enough to compete with fibrinogen for GP IIb/IIIa. Neither agent is significantly metabolized, and both are renally excreted. Neither tirofiban nor eptifibatide react with the vitronectin or MAC-1 receptor.

Comparator data for the three available agents are shown in table 16.10. All three drugs are administered as a bolus followed by a continuous intravenous infusion. Following intravenous bolus administration of abciximab, free plasma concentrations decrease very rapidly but high receptor affinity results in a long biological half-life of 12–24 hours Platelet function generally recovers over the course of 48 hours, although abciximab remains in the circulation for 15 days or more in a platelet-bound state. GP IIb/IIIa receptor occupancy by abciximab exceeds 30% at 8 days and 10% at 15 days. Abciximab can redistribute from the originally bound platelet to newly produced platelets.

Tirofiban is cleared from the plasma largely by renal excretion, with about 65% of an administered dose appearing in urine as unchanged tirofiban. Tirofiban is not highly protein bound to plasma proteins and the unbound fraction in human plasma is 35%.

The pharmacokinetics of eptifibatide are linear and dose related for bolus doses ranging from 90 to 250 µg/kg and infusion

Table 16.9 Data to compare and contrast the basic pharmacology and certain safety aspects of the available purinergic receptor antagonists

Drug	Clopidogrel	Prasugrel	Cangrelor	Ticagrelor
Chemical structure	Thienopiridine		ADP analogue	Cyclopentyl-trazolo-pyrridine (ADP analogue)
Prodrug	Yes		No	
Administration	Oral	Oral	Intravenous	Oral
Time to peak effect	Dose dependant	2 hour	30 min	2 hour
Platelet inhibition with ADP stimulus 2 hours following loading dose	40–50%	70–90%	90–100%	80–90%
Half-life	6 hours	8 hours	1.5 to 3 min	6–12 hours
Time to steady state platelet inhibition	4–5 days	2–4 days	30 min	2–3 days
Reversible	No		Yes	
Time to recovery of platelet aggregation	5 days	7 days	60–90 min	24–48 hours
Safety with prior CVA	Yes	No	NA	Yes
Non-CABG bleeding		Increased risk		Increased risk
CABG bleeding		Increased risk		Reduced risk

CABG, coronary artery bypass graft; CVA, cerebrovascular accident; ADP, adenosine diphosphate.

The risk of CABG and non-CABG related bleeding is in comparison to standard dose clopidogrel therapy.

Table 16.10 Basic pharmacology data for the one noncompetitive (monoclonal antibody) and the two competitive inhibitors of the glycoprotein IIb/IIIa receptor

Compound	Chemistry	Plasma half life	Biological half life	Clearance mechanism
Abciximab	Monoclonal antibody	10 minutes	12–24 hours	Reticulo-endothelium
Tirofiban	Peptidomimetic	2 hours	4–8 hours	Renal
Eptifibatide	Polypeptide	2.5 hours	4–6 hours	Renal

rates from 0.5 to 3.0 µg/kg/min. Administration of a single 180 µg/kg bolus combined with an infusion produces an early peak level, followed by a small decline prior to attaining steady state (within 4–6 hours). The extent of eptifibatide binding to human plasma protein is about 25%. Renal clearance accounts for approximately 50% of total body clearance, with the majority of the drug excreted in the urine as eptifibatide or deaminated eptifibatide. No major metabolites have been detected in human plasma.

The benefit of GP IIb/IIIa inhibitors is mainly limited to patients with unstable angina or NSTEMI. The most notable conditions where benefit is shown are in troponin-positive patients, whether or not they undergo revascularization. Abciximab is the only GP IIb/IIIa inhibitor observed to provide a significant survival advantage in diabetic patients undergoing PCI with angioplasty or stent placement. Abciximab also has the greatest weight of data supporting safety of use in patients with severe renal insufficiency. The current ACC/AHA guidelines recommend a platelet GP IIb/IIIa antagonist in patients with moderate- to high-risk ACS in whom catheterization and PCI are planned (Class I, Level A).

As with all anticoagulant and antiplatelet agents bleeding is always a risk. The main concern is when these agents are given with heparin. With abciximab the incidence of bleeding decreases to only about 2% when used with low-dose heparin (70 U/kg) and further studies have reported major bleeding rates that are at least as low, if not lower, than that due to heparin alone. With tirofiban the addition of heparin does not significantly alter inhibition of platelet aggregation, but does increase the average bleeding time, as well as the number of patients with bleeding times prolonged to more than 30 minutes. This has obvious implications in patients having a period of extracorporeal circulation.

Thrombocytopenia occurs with all GP IIb/IIIa receptor antagonists, with an incidence of ranging from 1.1% to 5.6% in clinical studies. An immune mechanism is believed to be responsible. It has been suggested that the binding of the antagonist to GP IIb/IIIa receptors leads to the exposure of binding sites to pre-existing or induced antibodies. An alternate mechanism is direct activation of platelets by GP IIb/IIIa antagonists. Thrombocytopenia induced by these mechanisms occurs within the first 24 hours of administration. All patients receiving parenteral GP IIb/IIIa antagonists should be monitored within 24 hours of initiation of therapy for development of thrombocytopenia and the drug discontinued if this occurs.

Treatment with GpIIb/IIIa receptor antagonists is contraindicated in patients with:

- Known hypersensitivity to any component of the product, and in the case of abciximab, any murine protein.

- A history of bleeding diathesis, or evidence of active abnormal bleeding within the previous 30 days.

- Severe hypertension (systolic blood pressure >200 mmHg or diastolic blood pressure >110 mmHg) not adequately controlled on antihypertensive therapy.

- Major surgery or history of major trauma within the preceding 4–6 weeks.

- History of stroke within 30 days or any history of haemorrhagic stroke for tirofiban and eptifibatide. This duration is increased to 2 years prior to the use of abciximab.

- Current or planned administration of another parenteral GP IIb/IIIa inhibitor.

- A history of intracranial haemorrhage, intracranial neoplasm, arteriovenous malformation or aneurysm.

- A history of thrombocytopenia following prior exposure to a GpIIb/IIIa receptor inhibitor.

For abciximab additional criteria contraindicating its use are:

- Administration of oral anticoagulants within 7 days unless prothrombin time ≤1.2 times control.

- Use of intravenous dextran before percutaneous coronary intervention, or intent to use it during intervention.

- Presumed or documented history of vasculitis.

Tirofiban is also contraindicated with a history, symptoms, or findings suggestive of aortic dissection or pericarditis. As both tirofiban and eptifibatide are principally cleared by the kidney, both should have the dose of the maintenance infusion reduced to half with an estimated creatinine clearance less than 50 mL/min. Both are also contraindicated in patients receiving chronic renal dialysis.

Administration of abciximab may result in the formation of human anti-chimeric antibodies (HACA) that could potentially cause allergic or hypersensitivity reactions (including anaphylaxis), thrombocytopenia, or diminished benefit upon re-administration.

Conclusion

Many patients presenting for cardiothoracic surgery and in particular CABG surgery, will be receiving antithrombotic agents and some a coumarin anticoagulant. All patients undergoing heart surgery with CPB will require treatment with the anticoagulant heparin. A good understanding of the pharmacology of these agents provides a sound basis for the conduct of cardiac anaesthesia.

References

1. Tapson VF. Acute pulmonary embolism. *N Engl J Med* 2008; **358**(10): 1037–52
2. Cohen AT, Agnelli G, Anderson FA, et al. Venous thromboembolism (VTE) in Europe. The number of VTE events and associated morbidity and mortality. *Thromb Haemost* 2007; **98**(4): 756–64
3. Hirsh J. Heparin [see comments]. *N Engl J Med* 1991; **324**(22): 1565–74
4. Hirsh J, Dalen JE, Deykin D, Poller L. Heparin: mechanism of action, pharmacokinetics, dosing considerations, monitoring, efficacy, and safety. *Chest* 1992; **102**(4 Suppl): 337s–351s
5. Hirsh J, Levine MN. Low molecular weight heparin. *Blood* 1992; **79**(1): 1–17
6. Hirsh J, Levine MN. Low molecular weight heparin: laboratory properties and clinical evaluation. A review. *Eur J Surg Suppl* 1994; **571**: 9–22
7. Frydman A. Low-molecular-weight heparins: an overview of their pharmacodynamics, pharmacokinetics and metabolism in humans. *Haemostasis* 1996; **26**(Suppl 2): 24–38
8. Tollefsen DM, Majerus DW, Blank MK. Heparin cofactor II. Purification and properties of a heparin-dependent inhibitor of thrombin in human plasma. *J Biol Chem* 1982; **257**(5): 2162–9
9. Gallus AS. Anticoagulants in the prevention of venous thromboembolism. *Baillières Clin Haematol* 1990; **3**(3): 651–84
10. Green D, Hirsh J, Heit J, Prins M, Davidson B, Lensing AW. Low molecular weight heparin: a critical analysis of clinical trials. *Pharmacol Rev* 1994; **46**(1): 89–109
11. Litin SC, Gastineau DA. Current concepts in anticoagulant therapy. *Mayo Clin Proc* 1995; **70**(3): 266–72
12. Kishimoto TK, Viswanathan K, Ganguly T, et al. Contaminated heparin associated with adverse clinical events and activation of the contact system. *N Engl J Med* 2008; **358**(23): 2457–67
13. Landefeld CS, Beyth RJ. Anticoagulant-related bleeding: clinical epidemiology, prediction, and prevention [see comments]. *Am J Med* 1993; **95**(3): 315–28 Issn: 0002–9343
14. Linkins LA, Warkentin TE. The approach to heparin-induced thrombocytopenia. *Semin Respir Crit Care Med* 2008; **29**(1): 66–74
15. Lo GK, Juhl D, Warkentin TE, Sigouin CS, Eichler P, Greinacher A. Evaluation of pretest clinical score (4 T's) for the diagnosis of heparin-induced thrombocytopenia in two clinical settings. *J Thromb Haemost* 2006; **4**(4): 759–65
16. Fareed J, Walenga JM, Hoppensteadt D, Huan X, Racanelli A. Comparative study on the in vitro and in vivo activities of seven low-molecular-weight heparins [published erratum appears in *Haemostasis* 1988; **18**(4–6): following 389]. *Haemostasis* 1988; **18**(Suppl 3): 3–15
17. Turpie AG, Bauer KA, Eriksson BI, Lassen MR. Superiority of fondaparinux over enoxaparin in preventing venous thromboembolism in major orthopedic surgery using different efficacy end points. *Chest* 2004; **126**(2): 501–8
18. Ansell J, Hirsh J, Hylek E, Jacobson A, Crowther M, Palareti G. Pharmacology and management of the vitamin K antagonists: American College of Chest Physicians Evidence-Based Clinical Practice Guidelines (8th Edition). *Chest* 2008; **133**(6 Suppl): 160S–198S
19. Di Nisio M, Middeldorp S, Buller HR. Direct thrombin inhibitors. *N Engl J Med* 2005; **353**(10): 1028–40
20. Lee CJ, Ansell JE. Direct thrombin inhibitors. *Br J Clin Pharmacol* 2011; **72**(4): 581–92
21. Connolly SJ, Ezekowitz MD, Yusuf S, et al. Dabigatran versus warfarin in patients with atrial fibrillation. *N Engl J Med* 2009; **361**(12): 1139–51
22. Eerenberg ES, Kamphuisen PW, Sijpkens MK, Meijers JC, Buller HR, Levi M. Reversal of rivaroxaban and dabigatran by prothrombin complex concentrate: a randomized, placebo-controlled, crossover study in healthy subjects. *Circulation* 2011; **124**(14): 1573–9
23. Alexander JH, Lopes RD, James S, et al. Apixaban with antiplatelet therapy after acute coronary syndrome. *N Engl J Med* 2011; **365**(8): 699–708
24. Mega JL, Braunwald E, Wiviott SD, et al. Rivaroxaban in patients with a recent acute coronary syndrome. *N Engl J Med* 2012; **366**(1): 9–19
25. Majerus PW. Arachidonate metabolism in vascular disorders. *J Clin Invest* 1983; **72**(5): 1521–5
26. Pedersen AK, FitzGerald GA. Dose-related kinetics of aspirin. Presystemic acetylation of platelet cyclooxygenase. *N Engl J Med* 1984; **311**(19): 1206–11
27. Roth GJ, Stanford N, Majerus PW. Acetylation of prostaglandin synthase by aspirin. *Proc Natl Acad Sci U S A* 1975; **72**(8): 3073–6
28. Najean Y, Ardaillou N, Dresch C. Platelet lifespan. *Annu Rev Med* 1969; **20**: 47–62

29. Collaborative meta-analysis of randomised trials of antiplatelet therapy for prevention of death, myocardial infarction, and stroke in high risk patients. *Br Med J* 2002; **324**(7329): 71–86

30. Patrono C, Baigent C, Hirsh J, Roth G. Antiplatelet drugs: American College of Chest Physicians Evidence-Based Clinical Practice Guidelines (8th Edition). *Chest* 2008; **133**(6 Suppl): 199S–233S.

31. Hankey GJ, Eikelboom JW. Aspirin resistance. *Lancet* 2006; **367**(9510): 606–17

32. Slattery J, Warlow CP, Shorrock CJ, Langman MJ. Risks of gastrointestinal bleeding during secondary prevention of vascular events with aspirin—analysis of gastrointestinal bleeding during the UK-TIA trial. *Gut* 1995; **37**(4): 509–11

33. Peters RJ, Mehta SR, Fox KA, et al. Effects of aspirin dose when used alone or in combination with clopidogrel in patients with acute coronary syndromes: observations from the Clopidogrel in Unstable angina to prevent Recurrent Events (CURE) study. *Circulation* 2003; **108**(14): 1682–7

34. Halkes PH, van Gijn J, Kappelle LJ, Koudstaal PJ, Algra A. Aspirin plus dipyridamole versus aspirin alone after cerebral ischaemia of arterial origin (ESPRIT): randomised controlled trial. *Lancet* 2006; **367**(9523): 1665–73

35. Wiviott SD, Braunwald E, McCabe CH, et al. Prasugrel versus clopidogrel in patients with acute coronary syndromes. *N Engl J Med* 2007; **357**(20): 2001–15

36. Montalescot G, Wiviott SD, Braunwald E, et al. Prasugrel compared with clopidogrel in patients undergoing percutaneous coronary intervention for ST-elevation myocardial infarction (TRITON-TIMI 38): double-blind, randomised controlled trial. *Lancet* 2009; **373**(9665): 723–31

37. Shuldiner AR, O'Connell JR, Bliden KP, et al. Association of cytochrome P450 2C19 genotype with the antiplatelet effect and clinical efficacy of clopidogrel therapy. *JAMA* 2009; **302**(8): 849–57

38. Mega JL, Close SL, Wiviott SD, et al. Cytochrome p-450 polymorphisms and response to clopidogrel. *N Engl J Med* 2009; **360**(4): 354–62

39. Mega JL, Close SL, Wiviott SD, et al. Cytochrome P450 genetic polymorphisms and the response to prasugrel: relationship to pharmacokinetic, pharmacodynamic, and clinical outcomes. *Circulation* 2009; **119**(19): 2553–60

40. Lau WC, Waskell LA, Watkins PB, et al. Atorvastatin reduces the ability of clopidogrel to inhibit platelet aggregation: a new drug-drug interaction. *Circulation* 2003; **107**(1): 32–7

41. Gurbel PA, Bliden KP, Butler K, et al. Randomized double-blind assessment of the ONSET and OFFSET of the antiplatelet effects of ticagrelor versus clopidogrel in patients with stable coronary artery disease: the ONSET/OFFSET study. *Circulation* 2009; **120**(25): 2577–85

42. Wallentin L, Becker RC, Budaj A, et al. Ticagrelor versus clopidogrel in patients with acute coronary syndromes. *N Engl J Med* 2009; **361**(11): 1045–57

43. Held C, Asenblad N, Bassand JP, et al. Ticagrelor versus clopidogrel in patients with acute coronary syndromes undergoing coronary artery bypass surgery: results from the PLATO (Platelet Inhibition and Patient Outcomes) trial. *J Am Coll Cardiol* 2011; **57**(6): 672–84

CHAPTER 17

Haemostasis management

David Royston

Introduction

The haemostatic system involves a complex interaction between the vascular, platelet, coagulation, and fibrinolytic systems to prevent blood loss and localize thrombus to the site of injury. Bleeding can arise from abnormalities in any one, or a combination, of these components. The early rational for improving haemostatic control was to prevent exposure to blood and blood products in order to reduce the risk of viral transmission particularly for hepatitis C and human immunodeficiency virus (HIV). Current concerns of the strong association between increased volumes of blood transfusions and adverse outcome (see Chapter 18) has now become the significant driver.

The first part of this chapter discusses the use of laboratory based and point-of-care (POC) devices to guide therapy and improve haemostasis. The second part of the chapter is devoted to pharmaceutical agents to reduce bleeding after major surgery and especially cardiac surgery.

Techniques based on measurement of haemostasis variables

Laboratory test of coagulation

The tests used in the haematology setting are unlike those in clinical chemistry with regard to a calibration normal value. In haematology laboratory practice the 'normal' range is derived from disease-free subjects and defined as results falling within two standard deviations above and below the mean for this population. Therefore 5% of healthy subjects will have a result outside the normal range

The first-line laboratory clotting tests are the activated partial thromboplastin time (APTT) and the prothrombin time (PT). The APTT is used to determine the integrity of the intrinsic pathway and the prothrombin time the extrinsic system and both tests are affected by inhibition of the final pathway. All of the components of the coagulation cascade are intrinsically in the plasma whereas an external stimulus (tissue thromboplastin) is required for clot in the extrinsic system. The division of the coagulation cascade into intrinsic, extrinsic and common pathways has little validity but is a useful concept for interpreting laboratory clotting tests. An additional test that can be part of a coagulation screen is a measure of the concentration of fibrinogen in the plasma. All these tests are conducted in citrated plasma that has subsequently been re-calcified.

Activated partial thromboplastin time

The APTT is abnormal with deficiencies of factors VIII, IX, and XI, and inhibitors of the intrinsic and common pathway factors (including lupus anticoagulant and therapeutic anticoagulation with heparin). Marked variations in the reagents (1) and clot detection methods (2) lead to differences in the sensitivity of each test to the effect of heparin. Historically, kaolin was used as the activator (explaining a prior name for the test of the kaolin cephalin clotting time (KCCT)), but is now rarely used in automatic analysers as its opacity makes the optical detection of fibrin clot difficult.

Prothrombin time and international normalized ratio

The PT and its derived value of international normalized ratio (INR) are measures of the extrinsic pathway of coagulation (factors I, II, V, VII, and X). They are used to determine the clotting tendency of blood, in the measure of vitamin K antagonists such as warfarin, liver damage, and vitamin K status. For an accurate measurement, the proportion of blood to citrate needs to be fixed at one part anticoagulant to nine parts whole blood; if too much or too little blood is added to the collection tube this will impact the result. Following recalcification of the plasma, tissue factor is added and the time the sample takes to clot is measured. Most automatic analysers use an optical technique as with the APTT, but some use a mechanical measurement that eliminates interferences from lipaemic and icteric samples.

The result (in seconds) for a prothrombin time will vary according to the type of analytical system employed and variations between different batches of manufacturer's tissue factor used to perform the test. To overcome this potential problem each manufacturer assigns an International Sensitivity Index (ISI) for tissue factor in their kit. The ISI value indicates how a particular batch of tissue factor compares to an international reference tissue factor. The ISI is usually between 1.0 and 2.0. The INR is the ratio of a patient's prothrombin time to a control sample, raised to the power of the ISI value for the analytical system used.

$$INR = (\text{Test time/Control time})^{ISI}$$

This effectively standardizes the results when assessing the dose of vitamin K antagonists. However, the results for INR and APTT do not predict bleeding prior to surgery or invasive interventions (3,4) nor do they correlate with postoperative drains blood loss after cardiac surgery (5). Laboratory tests of coagulation have however been shown of benefit in certain transfusion algorithms (6).

Activated clotting time

The activated clotting time (ACT) was described by Hattersley in 1966, when it was used as a means of speeding up blood coagulation in patients with advanced hepatic failure. Three types of

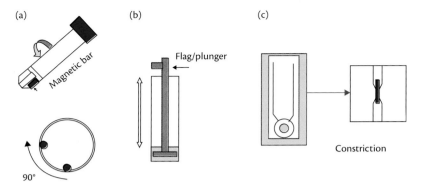

Fig. 17.1 Mechanisms of three commercial devices to measure activated clotting time.
(a) A schematic of the system used in the Hemocron® response system, in which 2 mL of whole blood is added to the test tube containing either celite or kaolin as activator. In this system both are presented as powders so the tube needs to be gently agitated to provide appropriate mixing. The tube is rotated and the position of the magnetic bar is monitored; when the blood clots the bar moves with the rotating tube. The system stops to give the activated clotting time when the magnet travels for 90 degrees. (b) An illustration of the Medtronic® system cuvette. Whole blood (0.4 mL) is injected into the cuvette, which contains a suspension of kaolin together with 0.05 M calcium chloride. The plunger is forced downwards, braking off a daisy wheel shaped lower end and the plunger is lifted and allowed to fall under gravity. The rate at which the plunger falls through the blood is monitored and as the blood clots the viscosity in the cuvette rises and the rate of falling slows. There is optical detection of flag motion, which stops the clock when it is greater than 10% slower than the initial measure. The clot mass does not need to be as stable as with the Hemochron system so fibrin formation alone will result in the test halting. (c) The reaction cuvette is the Hemochron® junior signature, now called the signature Elite. This cuvette must be prewarmed in the measuring test chamber. A drop of whole blood is placed into the cuvette reservoir and the system takes 15 μL of this sample to mix with the activating reagents. In this system they are silica, kaolin, phospholipids, and buffers. The blood is pumped back and forth through a constriction. As the blood clots its motion changes and this is measured using light emitting diodes. The clot endpoint is when this motion falls below a prespecified rate.
Reproduced with kind permission from Medtronic and Hemochron.

commercial system are currently available that not only use different blood sample sizes and activators but more importantly, different principles of detection (figure 17.1). The Hemochron® tube system uses a glass tube containing a magnet. The time for clot formation is taken as the time to carry this magnet through a 90° angle. The Medronic® system uses a plastic cuvette and detects the rate of descent of a flag attached to a daisy wheel system as it passes through the activated sample. There are also cartridge systems that require very small whole blood samples. For example, Hemochron have a device called the Elite, which relies on the detection of cessation of flow through a constriction. Abbott laboratories offer an ACT test in their I-STAT range of cartridges. This test uses a synthetic substrate that is cleaved by thrombin. The product of this thrombin-substrate reaction is an electro active compound that is detected amperometrically.

Results for the ACT systems correlate but do not give the same duration for blood clotting due to differences in the activators and detection systems (7). Additionally, the ACT does not accurately reflect the heparin content of the blood of the patient in clinical practice. The ACT was found to be unrelated to heparin activity, as measured by a chromogenic factor Xa assay (8). In addition an ACT based system failed to predict the heparin bolus dose necessary to achieve a target ACT (9). This may be due to the effect on the ACT of hypothermia, haemodilution, factor concentrations, and platelet numbers and functions, especially those affected by certain drugs such as aprotinin, GpIIb/IIIa inhibitors, or epoprostenol.

Given these problems it is therefore somewhat surprising that studies have shown that getting improved control of heparinization and its antagonism using ACT-based systems will contribute to improved postoperative haemostasis and reduced transfusion requirements (10,11). Unfortunately from a clinician's perspective the studies produced two conflicting strategies. The Medtronic

based system (11) showed improved haemostasis with an increased dose of heparin to achieve a target ACT and no change in protamine dosing whereas the Hemochron-based system (10) suggested no change in heparin dose but reducing the dose of protamine.

Monitoring coagulation using viscoelastic point-of-care devices

The value of laboratory-based tests has been questioned in the acute perioperative setting, due to a lack of information on platelet function and the interaction between clotting factors, platelets, and red cells, as the tests are determined in plasma rather than whole blood. There are also delays from blood sampling to obtaining results leading to a lag time before intervention.

There are currently thee commercially available devices to assess whole blood coagulation by assessing the viscoelastic properties of whole blood: thrombelastography (TEG®) (figure 17.2), rotation thrombelastometry (ROTEM®) (figures 17.3 and 19.5), and Sonoclot® signature analysis (figure 17.4). In the classic TEG® the blood is placed in a cup into which a pin is placed. The cup oscillates by a few degrees and this motion is transmitted along a torsion wire as the blood coagulates. The ROTEM® system is almost identical in principle, apart from the fact that the cup is fixed and the pin rotates. In the Sonoclot® system an oscillating plastic probe is introduced into the blood and changes in oscillating frequency are transduced into the 'signature'. These devices and their use and limitations have been the subject of a recent review (12).

Viscoelastic coagulation tests have been used successfully to guide therapies and have been incorporated in a variety of algorithms aimed at reducing haemostatic product transfusion requirements in the patient having cardiac surgery. Including POC tests in a multimodal transfusion guideline was assessed as a Class 1 recommendation, with an evidence level graded as A in the Society of Thoracic Surgeons and Society of

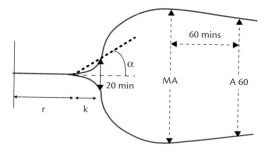

Fig. 17.2 Thromboelastogram.

Variables derived from thrombelastogram (TEG®) trace

Time to initial fibrin formation is reaction time (r-time) time between r time and trace becoming 20 mm wide is related to kinetics of clot formation (k-time). This is also related to the alpha angle derived from a line between trace being 2 and 20 mm wide. Maximum amplitude (MA) is greatest width for trace. Clot retraction or lysis was originally defined as ratio of MA at 60 minutes following MA to the MA itself. Certain algorithm have shortened this to 30 minutes.

TEG ® Hemostasis Analyzer Tracing image is used by permission of Haemonetics Corporation. TEG® and Thrombelastograph® are registered trademarks of Haemonetics Corporation in the US, other countries or both.

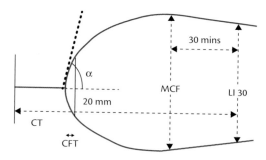

Fig. 17.3 Rotational thrombmoelastometry.

Variables derived from rotational thrombelastometry (ROTEM®). Time to the trace getting to 2 mm wide is coagulation time (CT). The time between this point and the trace getting to 20 mm wide is the clot formation time (CFT). For this device the alpha angle is derived from a tangent to the curve drawn from the 2 mm wide trace point. MCF represents maximum clot firmness as the equivalent of the TEG® MA. The lysis index at 30 minutes (LI 30) is derived from the ratio of the measured clot firmness at 30 minutes beyond the CT compared to the MCF expressed as a percentage.

Reproduced with kind permission from ROTEM.

Cardiothoracic Anesthesiologists practice guidelines (13). There are two major problems for the clinician. First, there have been no head-to-head comparisons of the various devices and/or the published algorithm to suggest which, if any has a better clinical role in modifying haemostatic function. Second, because of the differences in the method of measurement and the results obtained (table 17.1), the values of variables derived for a TEG®-derived algorithm cannot be directly utilized when measurements are made with the ROTEM®, and vica versa. Finally, the inclusion of a preoperative POC test does not improve the prediction of postoperative bleeding above that of standard laboratory tests (14).

Monitoring platelet function

Although it is well known a defect in platelet function associated with a period of cardiopulmonary bypass (CPB), the explosive driver to develop POC methods to assess platelet reactivity is in monitoring the effects of platelet active medications given early after vascular stent placement. This has lead to certain reference values of

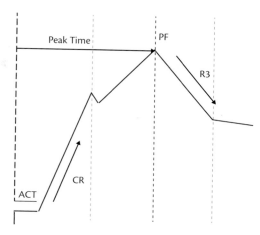

Fig. 17.4 Sonoclot.

Variables derived from Sonoclot® signature. Time to change in slope of viscosity is the activated clotting time (ACT) and the maximum slope of the initial viscosity change with time, reflecting initial fibrin polymerization and clot formation, is the clot rate (CR). The platelet function (PF) is a complex index derived from the timing and quality of clot retraction (shown as R3). PF is reported as being between 0 (no retraction) to 5, representing strong platelet function (clot retraction occurs earlier and is strong with a sharp peak in the signature after fibrin formation).

Reproduced with kind permission from Sienco.

results that reflect the chance of not of having some major adverse cardiovascular event major adverse cardiovascular event (15).

A variety of these systems, which use different methods of determining platelet reactivity have been described and some of these are shown in table 17.2. One of the fundamental problems about using these methods is that results trend in the same direction but correlate extremely poorly. For example, in a subgroup analysis from one large randomized study the correlation between platelet inhibition to adenosine diphosphate (ADP) measured by light transmission aggregometry was poorly correlated with the signal from the VerifyNow® P2Y$_{12}$ test ($r^2 = 0.16$) (16). Similarly, in a small unblinded single centre study the correlation (r^2) between platelet inhibition measured by flow cytometry to assess vasodilator-associated phosphorylation (VASP) and the VerifyNow® P2Y$_{12}$ test was 0.08 (17).

There are limited non-blinded single centre studies to show these systems may be of some value in assessing the risk of increased bleeding (18) or optimum timing of surgery (19) after ingestion of clopidogrel. Currently these systems are increasingly being used in the interventional cardiology and intensive care settings to monitor efficacy of interventions to inhibit platelet function. Nonetheless, it is certain that over the lifetime of this book these devices will be investigated as means of assessing the value of drug withdrawal or platelet transfusions at the time of planned interventions.

Techniques based on pharmacological interventions

Desmopressin

Desmopressin (1-desamino-8-d-arginine vasopressin [DDAVP]) is an analogue of the naturally occurring arginine vasopressin: one of its trade names being DDAVP. After parenteral injection (subcutaneous, intramuscular or intravenous) the plasma concentrations of Factor VIII and von Willebrand factor rise in a dose-dependant

Table 17.1 Data from four variables derived from thrombelastography (TEG®) and thrombelastometry (ROTEM®) used commonly in algorithms intended to guide transfusion therapy Data are normal ranges for each device derived from manufacturer literature when coagulation is activated by intrinsic coagulation system activator i.e. kaolin for TEG® and in-TEM cartridge (partial thromboplastin phospholipids) for ROTEM®

	TEG®	ROTEM®
Time to 2 mm amplitude	R time / 3–8 minutes	CT (clotting time) / 2–4 minutes
Period from 2 to 20 mm amplitude	k time / 1–3 minutes	CFT (clot formation time) / 40–100 seconds
Alpha angle	Slope from 2–20mm amplitude / 55–78°	Slope of tangent at 2 mm amplitude / 71–82°
Maximum strength	MA (maximum amplitude) / 51–69 mm	MCF (maximum clot firmness) / 52–72 mm

Data are normal ranges for each device derived from manufacturer literature when coagulation is activated by intrinsic coagulation system activator i.e. kaolin for TEG® and in-TEM cartridge (partial thromboplastin phospholipids) for ROTEM®.

Table 17.2 Outline of various commercially available devices for measurement of platelet function showing great variability in principles of measurement and detection end-points

Device	Measurement principle	Comments
Light transmission aggregation	Transmission of light following agonist stimulation in platelet-rich plasma	Regarded as the gold standard but very time and technician dependent so certainly not a point-of-care test
Whole blood aggregometry For example ChronoLog Aggregometer (Havertown, PA, USA)	Electrical impedance between two electrodes immersed in whole blood after agonist stimulation Platelet inhibition is calculated as (1 − residual impedance/baseline impedance) × 100.	Has tended to seen as a laboratory based test system rather than point-of-care.
VerifyNow® (Accumetrics, San Diego, CA, USA)	Turbidimetric optical detection of platelet aggregation in citrated whole blood.	Test cartridges available to assess inhibition of platelets by aspirin (arachidonic acid stimulus), $P2Y_{12}$ inhibitors (ADP and thrombin receptor activation peptide, TRAP) and GpIIb/IIIa receptor antagonists (TRAP)
Platelet function analyser 100 PFA-100® (Dade Behring, Deerfield, IL, USA)	Assesses platelet aggregation in citrated whole blood under high shear stress. 'Closure time' is the time necessary to occlude a microscopic aperture in a membrane coated with collagen and either ADP or adrenaline/epinephrine	Has shown good correlation with laboratory tests in von Willebrand factor deficiency. However the device cannot easily produce a value for platelet inhibition in the presence of $P2Y_{12}$ inhibitors.
Plateletworks® (Helena Laboratories, Beaumont, TX, USA)	Two-step method using a cell counter to measure total platelet count in whole blood anticoagulated with EDTA before and after exposed to an agonist. The difference in the platelet count between samples provides a direct measurement of platelet aggregation and is reported as percent aggregation.	
Platelet Mapping (Haemonetics, Braintree, MA, USA)	Modified thrombelastography®. Measurement of maximal clot strength (maximum amplitude of the trace) are performed with heparin to eliminate thrombin activity: Stimuli for inducing activation are: (1) Kaolin for maximal haemostatic activity; (2) Reptilase and Factor XIII to isolate the fibrin contribution to the clot strength. The contribution of the ADP or ThromboxaneA2 (TxA2) receptors to the clot formation is provided by the addition of ADP or arachidonic acid.	Requires 4 cuvette simultaneously for a single assay. None automated system so very susceptible to user technique.
Multiplate® (Roche, Basel, Switzerland)	Extension of whole blood aggregometry in a 5-channel machine. The increase in impedance is monitored every 0.5 seconds and is transformed to arbitrary aggregation units (AU) and plotted against time. The most important parameter is the area under the aggregation curve (AUC). AUC is recorded as Units or U Two other parameters are displayed Aggregation (in AU) is the maximum height of the curve during the measurement period and the velocity (in AU/min) is the maximum slope of the curve.	Each test cuvette contains 2 sets of impedance electrodes and values must agree by over 98% for the result to be displayed. Agonist available include ristocetin (GPIb), arachidonic acid (aspirin) ADP ($P2Y_{12}$ inhibitors) collagen (GpVI receptor) and TRAP (GpIIb/IIIa inhibitors)

Light transmission aggregation is a laboratory-based test and all others can be used as point-of-care tests in operating rooms, intensive care or interventional cardiology settings.

manner and peak about 30–60 minutes after administration. The rise is transient implying release of these factors from storage sites. This also explains the marked tachyphylaxis after repeat dosing. Desmopressin has no effect on platelet count or aggregation, but enhances platelet adhesion to the vessel wall. The parenteral form of DDAVP is presented in ampoules containing 4 μg/mL and the recommended dose is 0.3 μg/kg. This should be given intravenously over about 20 minutes as DDAVP also causes the release of prostacyclin and stimulates extra renal vasopressin V_2 receptors to cause marked hypotension in about 40% of patients.

Considerable interest in this compound in cardiac surgery was stirred by a report in 1986 suggesting a positive benefit for this agent in patients having high-risk surgeries (20). Continuing experience unfortunately failed to show any overall benefit in those patients having uncomplicated elective procedures (21). However, desmopressin may have significant benefits in patients with acquired platelet dysfunction. This has been shown in heart surgery for patients taking aspirin mono therapy (22,23). The group in St Louis have also shown that DDAVP was of significant benefit in a patient population with platelet dysfunction, as defined by a point-of care-platelet function analyser following a period of CPB (24).

Drugs acting by platelet inhibition

The concept of inhibition of platelets during the period of CPB to allow normal function at the end of this period has been termed the platelet paradox. In the same year as desmopressin was shown to have a benefit in cardiac surgical practice a proof of concept study of the use of prostacyclin (now termed epoprostenol) was also published from North America (25). While there was a significant reduction in postoperative chest drain loss and a reduction in transfusion volume, the effect was achieved only at the expense

of needing continuous high-dose norepinephrine infusion to counteract the vasodilator properties of the epoprostenol.

Drugs acting on the fibrinolytic system

Mechanisms of action

These compounds fall into two classes. The lysine analogue antifibrinolytics (tranexamic acid and epsilon-aminocaproic acid [EACA]) and the serine protease inhibitor aprotinin, which acts to inhibit free but not, bound plasmin. As illustrated in figure 17.5, there is a considerable difference between the mechanism of action of these two groups of agents in relation to their ability to affect haemostasis and clot lysis.

Of particular relevance is their role in the inhibition of fibrinolysis. Once a fibrin surface has formed, fibrinolysis is activated with the generation of plasmin. Plasmin can escape from its fibrin-binding site fairly easily, and therefore a mechanism exists to neutralize the enzyme. The body's naturally occurring inhibitor is α_2-antiplasmin or α_2-plasmin inhibitor (α_2-PI). Alpha$_2$-PI will react and neutralize free plasmin with a time constant of approximately 0.01 second. This is the fastest enzyme/ inhibitor reaction found thus far in nature and attests to the need for not having free plasmin in the circulation as it is a digestive enzyme and will degrade a number of intravascular proteins including the clotting factors. In contrast to this extraordinary rapid inhibition of free plasmin, if this enzyme is generated in its normal position on the fibrin strand via the action of tissue plasminogen activator (t-PA) then α_2-PI will only slightly inhibit this process. This natural inhibitor therefore has little if any action on bound plasmin; indeed the time constant for this reaction is greater than five minutes. It is therefore apparent that α_2-PI is a powerful inhibitor of free plasmin (associated with 'pathologic' fibrinolysis) but does

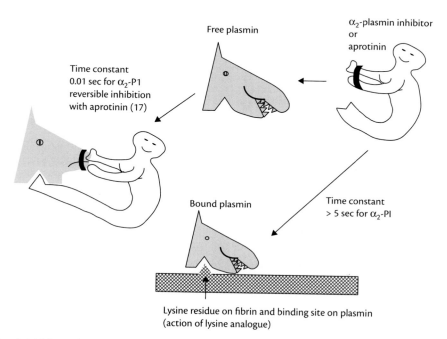

Fig. 17.5 Binding of alpha-2 plasmin inhibitor and aprotonin to plasmin.
The differences in action of the naturally occuring serine protease inhibitor α_2-plasmin inhibitor and aprotinin to bind free plasmin. Alpha$_2$ plasmin inhibitor binding is suicidal and non-reversible. In contrast, lysine analogues, such as tranexamic acid and epsilon aminocaproic acid, occupy lysine binding sites to prevent binding of plasmin to active lysine residue site on the fibrin molecule.

not act as an anti-fibrinolytic agent for 'appropriate' or 'physiological' fibrinolysis (figure 17.6 top right panel) (26). Alpha$_2$-plasmin inhibitor does however have an interesting effect on the haemostatic process. Administration of t-PA produces an increase in both the amount and duration of bleeding from cut wounds. The administration of α_2-PI inhibits this process and returns the duration and quantity of skin bleeding towards normal values (figure 17.6 top left panel) (26). This site-specificity of α_2-PI ensures that haemostasis will be maintained, and physiological or appropriate clot lysis will not be prevented.

Aprotinin and the serine protease inhibitors act in the same way as the naturally occurring inhibitor to rapidly inactivate free plasmin but have little effect on bound plasmin following t-PA administration. Separate studies have shown that lysis of clot, induced by t-PA, is not significantly inhibited in the presence of high doses of aprotinin (figure 17.6 middle right panel) (27). Nonetheless, and as found with α_2-PI, the haemostatic defect induced by t-PA, prolonged and increased bleeding from cutaneous wounds, is inhibited in the presence of high doses of aprotinin (figure 17.6 middle left panel) (28,29). Aprotinin's effect on functional fibrinolysis, shown as the lytic activity of plasma on human fibrin layers containing plasminogen has also been demonstrated in patients before, during and at the conclusion of CPB (30). The increased lytic activity observed at the end of CPB was not inhibited by the presence of aprotinin. These data support the concept that in physiologic terms aprotinin is not an antifibrinolytic agent but will improve the haemostatic defect associated with excess fibrinolytic activity.

The mode of action of the lysine analogue antifibrinolytics is in complete contrast to the actions of the plasmin inhibitors. The lysine analogues are designed to prevent excessive plasmin formation by mimicking lysine, fitting into plasminogen's lysine-binding site and thus preventing the binding of plasminogen to fibrin.

It is thus not surprising that results from similar animal studies as those described earlier, but using lysine analogue antifibrinolytics, contrast with those achieved with plasmin inhibitors (α_2-PI or aprotinin). The lysine analogues had no effect on the t-PA associated bleeding (figure 17.6 lower left panel) (29). As anticipated, and unlike the natural enzyme inhibitors, the lysine analogues act primarily to inhibit t-PA induced fibrinolysis (figure 17.6 lower right panel) (27).

Efficacy of pharmacological interventions

The observations just described may go some way to explaining apparent reported differences in the efficacy of these agents to reduce bleeding and transfusion burden in a variety of surgeries.

Cardiac surgery

Overall in cardiac surgical practice there is evidence for a reduction in red cell transfusion with all three agents (31) (table 17.3). Studies in those patients receiving aspirin prior to surgery show a consistent effect with aprotinin and no effect in the one study investigating tranexamic acid (32). There are no studies of the effects of EACA with aspirin and no data for the effects of tranexamic acid in patients receiving thienopyridines up to the time of surgery. Aprotinin has been shown to have significant benefits to reduce transfusions in this group of patients operated with (33,34) or without (35) CPB. However, these studies are either small or retrospective.

There is also some discussion as to benefits of these drugs with increasing patient risk. The data in table 17.3 show the proportion of patients receiving at least one red blood cell transfusion in patients having adult cardiac surgery and orthopedic surgery from the most recent Cochrane database review (31). This database includes the published data from the Blood Conservation Using Antifibrinolytics in a Randomized Trial (BART) (36) study, which was designed to investigate patients at a higher risk of massive bleeding/transfusion. Even with these potentially higher transfusion risk patients included the rates of transfusion in the control groups for the lysine analogues are much lower than in the aprotinin group. This leads to the suggestion that aprotinin has been studied mainly in those patients at a higher risk of bleeding and transfusion.

A separate argument is that the patients enrolled in the BART study were only low- or moderate-risk patients. This suggestion comes from a recent retrospective analysis from one centre in Canada. This retrospective analysis also suggested a lower incidence of massive haemorrhage, associated with a significant reduction in mortality in very high-risk patients given aprotinin compared to tranexamic acid treated patients (37). The universal applicability of this data is unclear as the risk score used was a bespoke system derived and used in that particular centre. Nonetheless a reduced mortality with aprotinin compared to tranexamic acid has also been shown, again in a retrospective analysis from a large European centre (38).

Orthopaedic and hepatic transplantation surgery

Data for proportions of patient receiving transfusions associated with a variety of orthopaedic surgeries also shows that aprotinin and tranexamic acid are effective but EACA has no effect. Again this may reflect the complexity of the surgery. As shown in table 17.3, the control subject transfusion rates vary greatly with drugs studied and are opposite to the observations for cardiac surgery.

Finally, the differences in apparent efficacy may be related to the dose of drug being used. Currently there is no unified, evidenced-based approach to dosing of the lysine analogues. The only publication to specifically address this issue showed a plateau in effect to reduce bleeding with a total dose of tranexamic acid of 3 g (39). With aprotinin, there is strong data to support a significant dose response to reduce transfusion burden with cardiac, hepatic and orthopaedic surgeries (40).

Safety issues

Lysine analogues

EACA for intravenous infusion is not available in the majority of world markets. This was in part due to a number of reports in the late 1970s and early 1980s of effects on muscle, ranging from myalgia to frank rhabdomyolysis, renal failure, and death. While these reports usually involved chronic administration, the acute effect of a rapid infusion is hypotension and, typically, bradycardia, although other arrhythmias are also associated with its use.

For tranexamic acid the main focus of safety has been the nervous system. Multiple studies, again in the late 1970s and early 1980s reported on the use of tranexamic acid to prevent rebleeding in patients with acute subarachnoid haemorrhage. The effectiveness of this intervention was unfortunately offset by the finding that mortality and stroke were increased because of an increased incidence of vasospasm of the cerebral arteries leading to increased

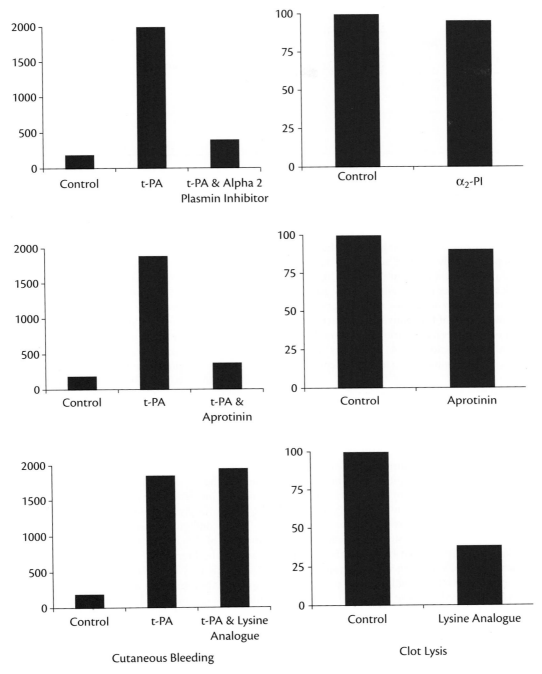

Fig. 17.6 Cutaneous bleeding, clot lysis and tissue plasminogen activator.
Histograms showing effects of tissue type plasminogen activator (t-PA) on cutaneous bleeding time (left panels) and lysis of preformed clot (right panels). Also shown is effect of addition of the serine protease inhibitor alpha$_2$ plasmin inhibitor (α_2-PI) (top panels) or aprotinin (middle panels) on these effects. Lower panels show the effects of lysine analogues on these two experimental systems. Data in top panels from Weitz JI, Leslie B, Hirsh J, Klement P. Alpha 2-antiplasmin supplementation inhibits tissue plasminogen activator-induced fibrinogenolysis and bleeding with little effect on thrombolysis. J Clin Invest 1993, 91(4),1343–50. Data for clot lysis in the middle and lower panels from Fears R, Greenwood J, Hearn J, Howard B, S, Morrow G, Standring R. Inhibition of the fibrinolytic and fibrinogenolytic activity of plasminogen activators in vitro by the antidotes ε-aminocaproic acid,tranexamic acid and aprotinin. Fibrinolysis 1992, 6, 79–86. Data for the middle and lower panels for cutaneous bleeding from de-Bono DP, Pringle S, Underwood I. Differential effects of aprotinin and tranexamic acid on cerebral bleeding and cutaneous bleeding time during rt-PA infusion. Thromb Res 1991, 61(2), 159–63. Histograms show serine protease inhibitors significantly affect cutaneous bleeding but have little effect on clot lysis. Lysine analogues are powerful antifibrinolytics against clot lysis but have no effect on t-PA induced cutaneous bleeding.

Table 17.3 Data for the proportion of patients receiving a red-cell transfusion with cardiac or orthopaedic surgery

Surgery type	Aprotinin		Tranexamic acid		Epsilon-aminocaproic acid	
	Treatment	Control	Treatment	Control	Treatment	Control
Cardiac	2431 / 5329	2728 / 4168	459 / 1578	617 / 1428	97 / 338	130 / 311
	45.6%	65.4%	29%	43.2%	28.7%	41.8%
Orthopaedic	131 / 655	177 / 491	193 / 722	329 / 659	105 / 150	108 / 154
	20%	36%	27%	50%	70%	70%

Data is summed from randomized controlled trials collated in Cochrane database: Henry DA, Carless PA, Moxey AJ, et al. Anti-fibrinolytic use for minimising perioperative allogeneic blood transfusion. Cochrane Database Syst Rev 2011(3),CD001886. Data show effect of administration of aprotinin, tranexamic acid and epsilon-aminocaproic acid (EACA). Table shows all interventions show benefit with cardiac surgery but differ in proportion of patients given blood in control groups implying more studies in higher risk patients with aprotinin compared to tranexamic acid or EACA. With orthopaedic surgery there was no benefit for administration of EACA but from a much higher baseline transfusion rate than either tranexamic acid or aprotinin.

mortality from cerebral ischaemia (41). More recently, the focus of attention has been on perioperative seizure activity. A number of reports have appeared in the recent literature showing highly significant increased risk of post-operative seizure activity especially in those patients having surgery where a cardiac chamber was opened (42,43). The mechanism of this potential has been known for many years as lysine analogues have marked structural homology with gamma aminobutyric acid (GABA) and act as competitive inhibitors in the central nervous system leading to convulsive activity (44).

Although the most effective dose to reduce transfusions without side effects is undetermined the timing of administration may have an impact. The original **C**orticosteroid **R**andomisation **A**fter **S**ignificant **H**ead injury (CRASH) study was followed by a second study, CRASH-2 (45) investigating the use of tranexamic acid in patients with trauma and evidence of bleeding, based on heart rate and systolic blood pressure, or were thought likely to be bleeding by the emergency physician. The results of that study showed a significant reduction in mortality in patients receiving the treatment. However, the mechanism of this was unclear, as there was no effect of tranexamic acid on transfusions. A subsequent post hoc analysis of the data (46) showed that this mortality benefit was only seen if tranexamic acid was given within 3 hours of the trauma. If given after three hours the mortality in the tranexamic acid treated patients was increased by about 50%. (Risk ratio 1.44 95% CI 1.12–1.84 p = 0.004.) The mechanism of this observation is currently opaque.

Aprotinin

The Bayer Company voluntarily suspended the marketing of aprotinin in November 2007. The reason for this was the publication in the *New England Journal of Medicine* of three observational studies (47–49) questioning the safety of this medication, and most importantly, some preliminary data from a randomized study suggesting an increased mortality in aprotinin-treated patients. The data from the three observational studies had been reviewed by the Food and Drug Administration (FDA) in the United States of America (USA) in September of 2007 and found not to provide sufficient evidence to show a negative benefit/risk ratio for aprotinin in the licensed indications.

The reasons for this are complex and based on the methods of analysis of the data that were prospectively collected but retrospectively analysed. To perform this analysis, the authors of the studies used a statistical method called propensity analysis that allows the data to be analysed as if it were from a randomized trial. To do this the groups of data take into account all of the other variables that may contribute to the outcome. These are termed confounders and have to be equally matched between groups before any conclusion as to if the significance of the outcome being associated with the treatment can be made. The Mangano propensity score included a number of 'risk factors' for adverse outcome, such as duration of education that the FDA advisors felt were inappropriate so they reanalysed the data using more conventional risk factors to develop their propensity score and found no significant association between aprotinin use and adverse outcome apart from need for new dialysis.

A subsequent analysis of the McSPI dataset showed that this was mainly due to a very high incidence of new dialysis in patients operated in German centres (50). The data from that country showed the incidence of new dialysis/haemofiltration was higher than the incidence of a predefined significant increase in plasma creatinine implying this intervention was for non-renal reasons.

The second study discussed by the FDA advisors came from analysis of a very large database used to administer and cost contain the Premier Hospitals group in the USA (48). As such it contains very little data of clinical relevance and this may, in part explain significant anomalies in the conclusions reached. In addition to an increased mortality signal in the aprotinin-treated patients the analysis showed a highly significant reduction in mortality associated with having hypertension, currently smoking, having had a recent myocardial infarction, stroke and being older. The FDA panel concluded that the database was unsuitable for addressing the relative safety of aprotinin in cardiac surgery.

The final retrospective review (49) was deemed not to be appropriate for inclusion in a benefit/ risk analysis as there was a major difficulty in matching the various confounders between the patient groups. The supplementary data associated with the article showed a 'matched pair' analysis that showed no mortality signal at 30 days or 1 year. However even this analysis failed to match the groups for age, red cell transfusion and year of surgery.

The FDA committee did, however, note that aprotinin therapy was associated with a small, transient but statistically significant risk of a creatinine rise of more than 44 μmol on the days after surgery. Typically, this rise occurred in about 8% of treated patients and lasted for 9 days. The mechanism is exactly the same as found with aminoglycosides and contrast media and is due to the proximal tubule reuptake mechanism being overloaded by the aprotinin being recycled from the glomerular filtrate.

The other more concerning safety issue is anaphylactic reactions after a second exposure. This is most likely in the six months following the first exposure and has been reported as presenting as a minor rash up to a lethal reaction. The recommendation was that aprotinin is not used within six months of the first exposure.

The BART study was published in May of 2008 (36) and had the benefit of being a blinded, randomized controlled trial. The conclusion reached by the authors was that aprotinin was no more effective than tranexamic acid at preventing the primary end-point of massive bleeding and was associated with an increased mortality. However, the Bayer Company, who held the marketing authorization for aprotinin, were sent raw, albeit somewhat redacted data from the study and questioned the conclusions in the published paper. This led the regulatory authority in Canada (Health Canada) to call together an expert panel, which met in December 2008. They concluded (51) there were a number of limitations to the BART analysis. The main two identified were:

♦ The exclusion of 137 patients from the analysis after randomization. This cohort included a number of dead patients, none of whom received aprotinin. When these patient data were included in the analysis the mortality signal became non-significant. The panel concluded that there while there were numerically more deaths in the aprotinin-treated patients but this could have occurred by chance.

♦ More worrisome was an unusually large number of reclassifications of outcomes from the originally reported data, with a large (approximately 75%) change rate in primary outcome (massive postoperative bleeding). Reclassifications were in opposite directions for aprotinin versus tranexamic acid and aminocaproic acid, favouring the latter, and these changes increased with the duration of the study. The panel concluded that this aspect was not satisfactorily explained

In a subsequent statement (52), Health Canada explained the reason for allowing the licence to be regranted, but also highlighted that the way heparin was used for anticoagulation during in the BART study was inconsistent. There was also a lack of appropriate monitoring of patients' anticoagulation with the ACT as the reagent could be influenced by aprotinin.

Subsequently, the European Medicines Agency has also revisited the aprotinin data and also concluded that the BART data, as published was not to be included in the benefit/risk analysis and they have also recommended the license is restored for aprotinin use in Europe.

Conclusion

POC testing of coagulation to accurately diagnose and direct treatment of coagulapathy combined with the use of pharmaceutical agents to minimize bleeding has greatly transformed the care of patients undergoing heart surgery so as to minimize blood loss and transfusion.

References

1. Shapiro GA, Huntzinger SW, Wilson JE, 3rd. Variation among commercial activated partial thromboplastin time reagents in response to heparin. *Am J Clin Pathol* 1977; **67**(5): 477–80

2. D'Angelo A, Seveso MP, D'Angelo SV, Gilardoni F, Dettori AG, Bonini P. Effect of clot-detection methods and reagents on activated partial thromboplastin time (APTT). Implications in heparin monitoring by APTT. *Am J Clin Pathol* 1990; **94**(3): 297–306

3. Segal JB, Dzik WH. Paucity of studies to support that abnormal coagulation test results predict bleeding in the setting of invasive procedures: an evidence-based review. *Transfusion* 2005; **45**(9): 1413–25

4. Chee YL, Crawford JC, Watson HG, Greaves M. Guidelines on the assessment of bleeding risk prior to surgery or invasive procedures. British Committee for Standards in Haematology. *Br J Haematol* 2008; **140**(5): 496–504

5. Gravlee GP, Arora S, Lavender SW, et al. Predictive value of blood clotting tests in cardiac surgical patients. *Ann Thorac Surg* 1994; **58**(1): 216–21

6. Nuttall GA, Oliver WC, Santrach PJ, et al. Efficacy of a simple intraoperative transfusion algorithm for nonerythrocyte component utilization after cardiopulmonary bypass. *Anesthesiology* 2001; **94**(5): 773–81

7. Bosch YP, Ganushchak YM, de Jong DS. Comparison of ACT point-of-care measurements: repeatability and agreement. *Perfusion* 2006; **21**(1): 27–31

8. Despotis GJ, Summerfield AL, Joist JH, et al. Comparison of activated coagulation time and whole blood heparin measurements with laboratory plasma anti-Xa heparin concentration in patients having cardiac operations. *J Thorac Cardiovasc Surg* 1994; **108**(6): 1076–82

9. Garvin S, FitzGerald DC, Despotis G, Shekar P, Body SC. Heparin concentration-based anticoagulation for cardiac surgery fails to reliably predict heparin bolus dose requirements. *Anesth Analg* 2010; **111**(4): 849–55

10. Jobes DR, Aitken GL, Shaffer GW. Increased accuracy and precision of heparin and protamine dosing reduces blood loss and transfusion in patients undergoing primary cardiac operations. *J Thorac Cardiovasc Surg* 1995; **110**(1): 36–45

11. Despotis GJ, Joist JH, Hogue CW, Jr., et al. The impact of heparin concentration and activated clotting time monitoring on blood conservation. A prospective, randomized evaluation in patients undergoing cardiac operation. *J Thorac Cardiovasc Surg* 1995; **110**(1): 46–54

12. Ganter MT, Hofer CK. Coagulation monitoring: current techniques and clinical use of viscoelastic point-of-care coagulation devices. *Anesth Analg* 2008; **106**(5): 1366–75

13. Ferraris VA, Ferraris SP, Saha SP, et al. Perioperative blood transfusion and blood conservation in cardiac surgery: the Society of Thoracic Surgeons and The Society of Cardiovascular Anesthesiologists clinical practice guideline. *Ann Thorac Surg* 2007; **83**(5 Suppl): S27–86

14. Lee GC, Kicza AM, Liu KY, Nyman CB, Kaufman RM, Body SC. Does Rotational Thromboelastometry (ROTEM) Improve Prediction of Bleeding After Cardiac Surgery? *Anesth Analg* 2012; **115**(3): 499–506

15. Price MJ, Endemann S, Gollapudi RR, et al. Prognostic significance of post-clopidogrel platelet reactivity assessed by a point-of-care assay on thrombotic events after drug-eluting stent implantation. *Eur Heart J* 2008; **29**(8): 992–1000

16. Storey RF, Angiolillo DJ, Patil SB, et al. Inhibitory effects of ticagrelor compared with clopidogrel on platelet function in patients with acute coronary syndromes: the PLATO (PLATelet inhibition and patient Outcomes) PLATELET substudy. *J Am Coll Cardiol* 2010; **56**(18): 1456–62

17. Alstrom U, Granath F, Oldgren J, Stahle E, Tyden H, Siegbahn A. Platelet inhibition assessed with VerifyNow, flow cytometry and PlateletMapping in patients undergoing heart surgery. *Thromb Res* 2009; **124**(5): 572–7

18. Dalen M, van der Linden J, Lindvall G, Ivert T. Correlation between point-of-care platelet function testing and bleeding after coronary artery surgery. *Scand Cardiovasc J* 2012; **46**(1): 32–8

19. Mahla E, Suarez TA, Bliden KP, et al. Platelet function measurement-based strategy to reduce bleeding and waiting time in clopidogrel-treated patients undergoing coronary artery bypass graft surgery: the timing based on platelet function strategy to reduce

clopidogrel-associated bleeding related to CABG (TARGET-CABG) study. *Circ Cardiovasc Interv* 2012; **5**(2): 261–9

20. Salzman E, Weinstein M, Weintraub R, et al. Treatment with desmopressin acetate to reduce blood loss after cardiac surgery. *N Engl J Med* 1986; **314**: 1402–10

21. Carless PA, Henry DA, Moxey AJ, et al. Desmopressin for minimising perioperative allogeneic blood transfusion. *Cochrane Database Syst Rev* 2004(1): CD001884

22. Dilthey G, Dietrich W, Spannagl M, Richter JA. Influence of desmopressin acetate on homologous blood requirements in cardiac surgical patients pretreated with aspirin. *J Cardiothorac Vasc Anesth* 1993; **7**(4): 425–30

23. Sheridan DP, Card RT, Pinilla JC, et al. Use of desmopressin acetate to reduce blood transfusion requirements during cardiac surgery in patients with acetylsalicylic-acid-induced platelet dysfunction. *Can J Surg* 1994; **37**(1): 33–6

24. Despotis GJ, Levine V, Saleem R, Spitznagel E, Joist JH. Use of point-of-care test in identification of patients who can benefit from desmopressin during cardiac surgery: a randomised controlled trial. *Lancet* 1999; **354**(9173): 106–10

25. Fish KJ, Sarnquist FH, van Steennis C, et al. A prospective, randomized study of the effects of prostacyclin on platelets and blood loss during coronary bypass operations. *J Thorac Cardiovasc Surg* 1986; **91**(3): 436–42

26. Weitz JI, Leslie B, Hirsh J, Klement P. Alpha 2-antiplasmin supplementation inhibits tissue plasminogen activator-induced fibrinogenolysis and bleeding with little effect on thrombolysis. *J Clin Invest* 1993; **91**(4): 1343–50

27. Fears R, Greenwood H, Hearn J, Howard B, Humphreys S, Morrow G, Standring R. Inhibition of the fibrinolytic and fibrinogenolytic activity of plasminogen activators in vitro by the antidotes ε-aminocaproic acid,tranexamic acid and aprotinin. *Fibrinolysis* 1992; 6: 79–86

28. Garabedian HD, Gold HK, Leinbach RC, et al. Bleeding time prolongation and bleeding during infusion of recombinant tissue-type plasminogen activator in dogs: potentiation by aspirin and reversal with aprotinin. *J Am Coll Cardiol* 1991; **17**(5): 1213–22

29. de-Bono DP, Pringle S, Underwood I. Differential effects of aprotinin and tranexamic acid on cerebral bleeding and cutaneous bleeding time during rt-PA infusion. *Thromb Res* 1991; **61**(2): 159–63

30. Dietrich W, Spannagl M, Jochum M, et al. Influence of high-dose aprotinin treatment on blood loss and coagulation patterns in patients undergoing myocardial revascularization. *Anesthesiology* 1990; **73**(6): 1119–26

31. Henry DA, Carless PA, Moxey AJ, et al. Anti-fibrinolytic use for minimising perioperative allogeneic blood transfusion. *Cochrane Database Syst Rev* 2011(3): CD001886

32. McIlroy DR, Myles PS, Phillips LE, Smith JA. Antifibrinolytics in cardiac surgical patients receiving aspirin: a systematic review and meta-analysis. *Br J Anaesth* 2009; **102**(2): 168–78

33. Lindvall G, Sartipy U, van der Linden J. Aprotinin reduces bleeding and blood product use in patients treated with clopidogrel before coronary artery bypass grafting. *Ann Thorac Surg* 2005; **80**(3): 922–7

34. van der Linden J, Lindvall G, Sartipy U. Aprotinin decreases postoperative bleeding and number of transfusions in patients on clopidogrel undergoing coronary artery bypass graft surgery: a double-blind, placebo-controlled, randomized clinical trial. *Circulation* 2005; **112**(9 Suppl): I276–80

35. Bittner HB, Lehmann S, Rastan A, Mohr FW. Impact of clopidogrel on bleeding complications and survival in off-pump coronary artery bypass grafting. *Interact Cardiovasc Thorac Surg* 2012; **14**(3): 273–7

36. Fergusson DA, Hebert PC, Mazer CD, et al. A comparison of aprotinin and lysine analogues in high-risk cardiac surgery. *N Engl J Med* 2008; **358**(22): 2319–31

37. Karkouti K, Wijeysundera DN, Yau TM, McCluskey SA, Tait G, Beattie WS. The risk-benefit profile of aprotinin versus tranexamic acid in cardiac surgery. *Anesth Analg* 2010; **110**(1): 21–9

38. Sander M, Spies CD, Martiny V, Rosenthal C, Wernecke KD, von Heymann C. Mortality associated with administration of high-dose tranexamic acid and aprotinin in primary open-heart procedures: a retrospective analysis. *Crit Care* 2010; **14**(4): R148

39. Horrow JC, Van Riper DF, Strong MD, Grunewald KE, Parmet JL. The dose-response relationship of tranexamic acid. *Anesthesiology* 1995; 82(2): 383–92

40. Kovesi T, Royston D. Pharmacological approaches to reducing allogeneic blood exposure. *Vox Sang* 2003; 84(1): 2–10

41. Vermeulen M, Lindsay KW, Murray GD, et al. Antifibrinolytic treatment in subarachnoid hemorrhage. *N Engl J Med* 1984; **311**(7):432–7

42. Martin K, Wiesner G, Breuer T, Lange R, Tassani P. The risks of aprotinin and tranexamic acid in cardiac surgery: a one-year follow-up of 1188 consecutive patients. *Anesth Analg* 2008; **107**(6): 1783–90

43. Murkin JM, Falter F, Granton J, Young B, Burt C, Chu M. High-dose tranexamic Acid is associated with nonischemic clinical seizures in cardiac surgical patients. *Anesth Analg* 2010; **110**(2): 350–3

44. Furtmuller R, Schlag MG, Berger M, et al. Tranexamic acid, a widely used antifibrinolytic agent, causes convulsions by a gamma-aminobutyric acid(A) receptor antagonistic effect. *J Pharmacol Exp Ther* 2002; **301**(1): 168–73

45. Shakur H, Roberts I, Bautista R, et al. Effects of tranexamic acid on death, vascular occlusive events, and blood transfusion in trauma patients with significant haemorrhage (CRASH-2): a randomised, placebo-controlled trial. *Lancet* 2010; **376**(9734): 23–32

46. Roberts I, Shakur H, Afolabi A, et al. The importance of early treatment with tranexamic acid in bleeding trauma patients: an exploratory analysis of the CRASH-2 randomised controlled trial. *Lancet* 2011; **377**(9771):1096–101, 1101 e1–2

47. Mangano DT, Tudor IC, Dietzel C. The risk associated with aprotinin in cardiac surgery. *N Engl J Med* 2006; **354**(4): 353–65

48. Schneeweiss S, Seeger JD, Landon J, Walker AM. Aprotinin during coronary-artery bypass grafting and risk of death. *N Engl J Med* 2008; **358**(8): 771–83

49. Shaw AD, Stafford-Smith M, White WD, et al. The effect of aprotinin on outcome after coronary-artery bypass grafting. *N Engl J Med* 2008; **358**(8): 784–93

50. Ott E, Mazer CD, Tudor IC, et al. Coronary artery bypass graft surgery—care globalization: the impact of national care on fatal and nonfatal outcome. *J Thorac Cardiovasc Surg* 2007; **133**(5): 1242–51

51. Health Canada. Final Report–Expert advisory panel on Trasylol (aprotinin). http://www.hc-sc.gc.ca/dhp-mps/medeff/advise-consult/eapgce_trasylol/final_rep-rap-eng.php. Accessed 21 May 2014

52. Health Canada. Health Canada endorsed important safety information on Trasylol. http://www.healthycanadians.gc.ca/recall-alert-rappel-avis/hc-sc/2011/14107a-eng.php. Accessed 22 August 2014.

CHAPTER 18

Blood management

Gavin J. Murphy, Nishith N. Patel, and Nicola Curry

Introduction

Blood management is a term that encompasses the transfusion of blood components or use of therapeutic adjuncts aimed at preventing or treating coagulopathic haemorrhage and acute anaemia. Optimal blood management is central to achieving good clinical outcomes in cardiac surgery because these procedures are characterized by:

1. A high red blood cell (RBC) requirement; cardiac surgery utilizes a significant proportion of all RBC, ranging from 5–7% in the UK (1) to 25% in the USA (2).

2. A high prevalence of coagulopathy and severe bleeding that often necessitates administration of non-RBC components (15–25%) or emergency resternotomy (5–10%).

3. Highly monitored environments, which facilitate the use of therapeutic treatment adjuncts that reduce bleeding and transfusion and can improve outcome.

This chapter will consider the evidence for effective blood management in cardiac surgery. A schematic of the multifaceted components of good blood management is described in table 18.1.

Red blood cell transfusion

Bleeding and acute anaemia

Bleeding is a feature of all invasive surgical procedures and in cardiac surgery can often be severe necessitating large volume RBC transfusion in addition to non-RBC components for the treatment of coagulopathy. Emergency resternotomy is performed in some cases to establish whether diathesis control may be best achieved surgically, and this is a useful indicator of the frequency of severe haemorrhage, which in the UK ranges from 2–7% between units (figure 18.1). RBC transfusion rates are much higher than published resternotomy rates, ranging from 45–95% (3), which suggests, albeit indirectly, that a significant proportions of RBC transfusions are administered not for bleeding but for the reversal of anaemia, although these two indications are not mutually exclusive. Perioperative anaemia, defined arbitrarily as a haemoglobin concentration less than 12 g/dL is common, affecting over 75% of patients. It occurs as a consequence of low preoperative red cell mass (a product of the patients haemoglobin concentration, body weight, age, and sex), haemodilution during surgery, including the use of crystalloid prime, perioperative blood loss, and impaired haematopoiesis as a consequence of chronic disease

Table 18.1 Schematic showing components of effective blood management in cardiac surgery

	Diagnosis	Prevention	Treatment
Preoperative	Detailed preoperative assessment Transfusion risk scores	Cessation of antiplatelet agents/anticoagulants Preoperative autologous donation	Treatment of preoperative anaemia and coagulopathy rhEPO
Intraoperative	Point of care tests for early diagnosis and directed treatment of coagulopathy: TEG, ROTEM, PFA	Good surgical technique: Zero tolerance for re-sternotomy or bleeding Cardiopulmonary bypass: low prime volume, retrograde priming, MECB, closed vs. open circuits, circuit coating Optimization of physiological anaemia tolerance: NIRS based algorithms Pharmacological strategies: tranexamic acid, aprotinin, platelet anaesthesia, desmopressin Mechanical cell salvage and autotransfusion Normovolaemic haemodilution and autotransfusion	Platelets, FFP, cryoprecipitate, PCC, fibrinogen concentrate, rFVII
Postoperative	Ponit of care tests: Thromboelastography Platelet aggregometry	Restrictive transfusion thresholds Postoperative cell salvage Appropriate use of blood volume replacement solutions	Resternotomy algorithms

rhEPO: recombinant human erythropoietin; TEG: thromboelastography; ROTEM: rotational thromboelastometry; PFA: platelet function analyser; FFP: fresh frozen plasma; PCC: prothrombin complex concentrate; rFVII: recombinant activated Factor VII; CPB: cardiopulmonary bypass; NIRS: near infrared spectroscopy.

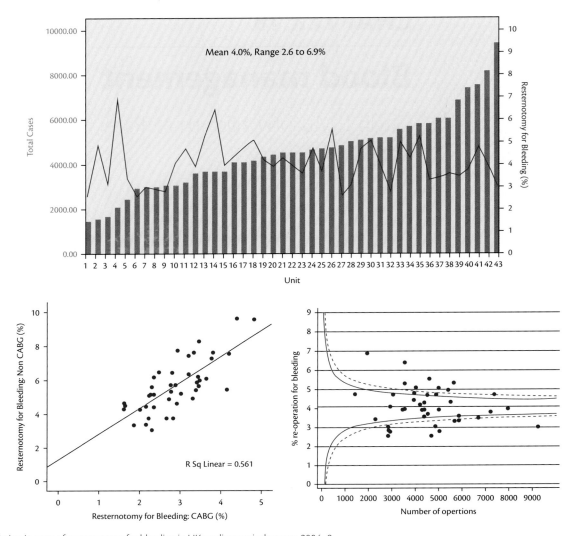

Fig. 18.1 Variation in rates of resternotomy for bleeding in UK cardiac surgical centres 2004–9.
(A) Reopening rates show wide variation between UK centres. This variation is unlikely to be accounted for simply by differences in (B) Caseload or (C) Volume of cases.
n = 189 338.
Unpublished data provided courtesy Ben Bridgewater, Society for Cardiothoracic Surgery in Great Britain and Ireland Database Committee.

e.g. renal disease, or, as a result of a perioperative inflammatory state e.g. the systemic inflammatory response (SIRS) or sepsis. Anaemia increases the risk of bleeding, low cardiac output, acute kidney injury and death in cardiac surgery (4,5). Postoperatively, anaemia slows recovery and mobilization, although these effects are not sustained beyond 6 weeks (6).

When is transfusion of red blood cells indicated?

Whereas RBC transfusion for severe haemorrhage, particularly in patients with incipient hypovolaemic shock, is clearly life-saving, the indications for RBC transfusion in the setting of severe anaemia in cardiac surgery are unclear. Observational studies suggest that reversal of anaemia with RBC transfusion results in an increased risk of major morbidity and mortality beyond that attributable to anaemia alone (figure 18.2). The adverse effects attributable to transfusion are consistent across studies, patient populations and geographical location and show a dose response, with much

higher rates of morbidity associated with larger volume transfusions (5–11). Transfusion-related morbidity has been attributed to the storage lesion, whereby the accumulation of harmful and pro-inflammatory substances in the storage supernatant as well as deterioration in erythrocyte structure and function, are thought to result in post-transfusion inflammation and organ injury in recipients (figure 18.3). Observational data supports such a hypothesis. Koch and colleagues, in a study of 6001 patients at the Cleveland Clinic, demonstrated that transfusion of older blood, stored for more than 14 days, was associated with an increase in pulmonary, renal, and cardiac complications compared to transfusion of blood stored less than 14 days (12).

The results of observational studies must be interpreted with caution however as they are subject to numerous biases. These include residual confounding from unmeasured variables, treatment and regression biases that arise due to more liberal administration of RBC to sicker patients, and publication bias, and it is impossible to establish a causal relationship between transfusion

(a)

Observational Studies

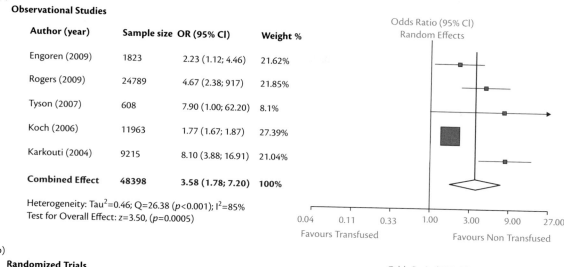

Author (year)	Sample size	OR (95% CI)	Weight %
Engoren (2009)	1823	2.23 (1.12; 4.46)	21.62%
Rogers (2009)	24789	4.67 (2.38; 917)	21.85%
Tyson (2007)	608	7.90 (1.00; 62.20)	8.1%
Koch (2006)	11963	1.77 (1.67; 1.87)	27.39%
Karkouti (2004)	9215	8.10 (3.88; 16.91)	21.04%
Combined Effect	**48398**	**3.58 (1.78; 7.20)**	**100%**

Heterogeneity: Tau^2=0.46; Q=26.38 (*p*<0.001); I^2=85%
Test for Overall Effect: z=3.50, (*p*=0.0005)

(b)

Randomized Trials

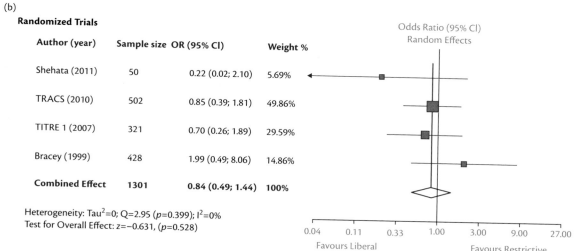

Author (year)	Sample size	OR (95% CI)	Weight %
Shehata (2011)	50	0.22 (0.02; 2.10)	5.69%
TRACS (2010)	502	0.85 (0.39; 1.81)	49.86%
TITRE 1 (2007)	321	0.70 (0.26; 1.89)	29.59%
Bracey (1999)	428	1.99 (0.49; 8.06)	14.86%
Combined Effect	**1301**	**0.84 (0.49; 1.44)**	**100%**

Heterogeneity: Tau^2=0; Q=2.95 (*p*=0.399); I^2=0%
Test for Overall Effect: z=−0.631, (*p*=0.528)

Fig. 18.2 Relationship between RBC transfusion and outcome.
(A) Observational data, adjusted for differences in baseline characteristics demonstrates a consistent association between transfusion and harm (mortality). (B) Randomized trials of restrictive versus liberal transfusion thresholds show no effect of more liberal transfusion on outcome. TRACS, Transfusion Requirements in Cardiac Surgery; TITRE, Transfusion Indication Threshold Reduction. Data from references 7–11, 13, 14, 16.

and adverse outcome from these types of study. Randomized controlled trials (RCTs) that compare restrictive versus liberal transfusion thresholds overcome many of these biases and in contrast do not show an increase in adverse effects attributable to RBC (figure 18.2). These RCTs also have significant limitations, however. They suffer from selection bias in that they exclude high-risk patients who are more likely to receive large-volume blood transfusions and suffer adverse outcomes. They have also tended to be small, single-centre studies that were poorly reported and uniformly demonstrated lack of blinding and allocation concealment, raising the possibility of detection and performance bias (13–16). Performance bias acts to lower the transfusion rate in the liberal arm and increase that in the restrictive arm, reducing the difference in transfusion between the groups. The difference in mean transfusion volume between treatment groups in these RCTs is often less than two units of blood which observational data suggests as having only very modest effects on clinical outcomes.

Recently, a large single-centre RCT, the Transfusion Requirements in Cardiac Surgery (TRACS) trial (16), which compared a liberal haemoglobin transfusion threshold of 10 g/dL versus a restrictive threshold of 8 g/dL in 512 cardiac surgical patients, detected no difference in outcome between groups. This study was limited in that it randomized all eligible patients, including those without severe anaemia, to the intervention arms, resulting in only 78% of patients in the liberal arm receiving a transfusion. In addition, the study was underpowered to detect a difference in outcomes with a high non-inferiority margin of 8%. The age of the blood transfused in this study was on average 3 days old, which also limits the relevance of the study to other countries where storage duration may be as long as 35 days in the UK and 42 days in the USA.

Because of these design limitations, existing RCTs are unable to demonstrate that RBC transfusion causes adverse outcomes. They are valuable, however, as they provide the best available evidence that restrictive transfusion practice in patients with acute anaemia

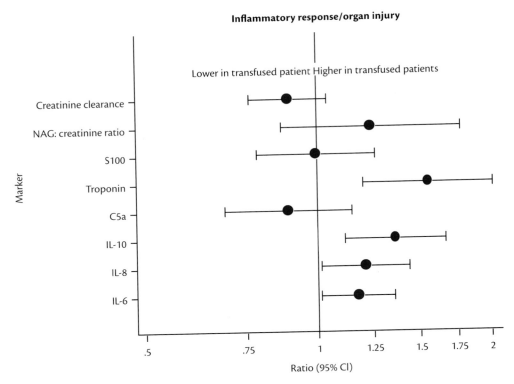

Fig. 18.3 Inflammatory and biochemical response to transfusion of red blood cells. Meta-analysis of individual patient data from six previous randomized trials at the Bristol Heart Institute, n = 230. Odds ratios represent differences between transfused and non-transfused patients for individual biochemical markers of inflammation and organ injury measured over 48 hours postoperatively. Estimates derived from Mixed Models with adjustment for baseline differences, study, and intervention (unpublished data). NAG, N-acetyl-β-d-glucosaminidase, C5a, complement component 5a.

is safe using transfusion thresholds of about 8 g/dL. Importantly, they also indicate that the use of more liberal transfusion thresholds has no clinical benefit. A limitation is that 8 g/dL does not denote the point at which the benefits of transfusion outweigh the risks for individual patients over time, as the critical haematocrit is likely to be highly time and patient specific. Real time measures of regional tissue oxygenation are thought to hold out the greatest hope for a patient specific indicator of the point at which anaemia severity results in incipient hypoxia, and where transfusion is necessary. Suggested modalities have included near infrared tissue oxygenation monitoring and measurement of sublingual microcirculatory oxygen tension; however, there is no high quality evidence to recommend their use currently.

Coagulopathy

Coagulopathy is poorly defined; it may refer to bleeding as a consequence of severe impairment of blood coagulation in the setting of endocarditis or prolonged cardiopulmonary bypass (CPB), or alternatively to a prolonged clotting time as determined by a laboratory test. The lack of a clear definition complicates epidemiological analyses and the development of accurate diagnostic tests and treatments. It remains a significant clinical problem, however, and depending on the definition, and or case-mix affects up to 15–25% (recipients of non-RBC component (17,18)) or 5–15% (emergency resternotomy (19–24)) of cardiac surgery patients. Severe bleeding is associated with adverse outcome and an increase in resource use (figure 18.4), which in turn, reflects the severity of the underlying

illness, complexity of surgery, and/ or the consequences of significant haemorrhage and shock. Adverse effects of coagulopathic bleeding may also be attributable in part, however, to large-volume RBC transfusions or the administration of pro-haemostatic therapies such as platelets and fresh frozen plasma (FFP) transfusion or recombinant activated factor VII. These risks, although offset by the risks of ongoing bleeding in coagulopathic patients may be clinically significant in those without coagulopathy, or when administered to those who are not actively bleeding.

Aetiology

The nature of coagulopathy is heterogeneous and reflects, in the most part, the underlying aetiology:

Antiplatelet drugs

Antiplatelet drugs are ubiquitous in cardiovascular disease because of the survival advantage they confer in stable coronary artery disease (aspirin), as well as in unstable disease/acute coronary syndromes and post percutaneous intervention (ADP receptor antagonists; clopidogrel, prasurgel, GPIIb IIIa inhibitors; tirofiban, abicimixub) (Chapter 16). In elective surgery these drugs can be stopped preoperatively to reduce the risk of residual platelet inhibition and coagulopathic haemorrhage. Early cessation of aspirin has been associated with an increase in preoperative ischaemic events, with only a modest reduction in the risk of bleeding and transfusion, and is not recommended (25). Taking both clopidogrel and aspirin until surgery has been shown to significantly increase the risk of both major bleeding

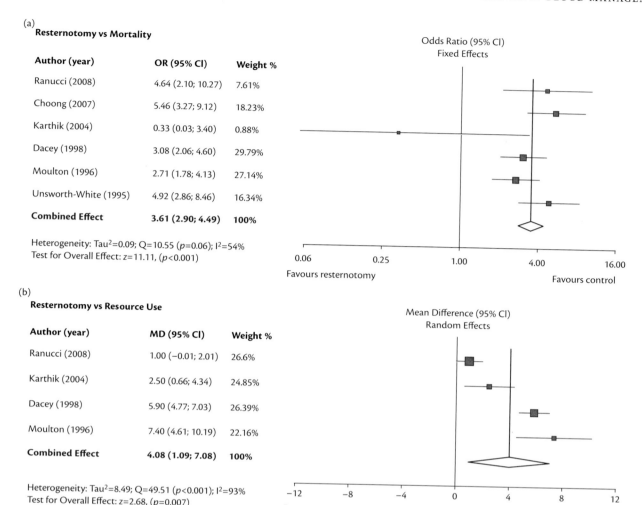

Fig. 18.4 The effect of severe haemorrhage on mortality and resources use.
The association between severe haemorrhage defined as emergency resternotomy following cardiac surgery and (a) mortality, (b) resource use. Data from references 19–24.

and emergency resternotomy (26). Published guidelines indicate that this risk may be reduced by stopping clopidogrel at least three days prior to surgery (27); however, this arbitrary threshold does not reflect the wide inter-patient variability in the degree of platelet inhibition with clopidogrel. Some centres do not routinely stop clopidogrel, without apparent detriment. Alternatively, preoperative assessment of residual platelet inhibition in patients previously receiving clopidogrel as a guide to the timing of surgery has been shown to reduce bleeding in small single-centre studies (28). Prasugel, a new adenosine diphophate (ADP) receptor antagonist, which has more consistent pharmacokinetics and greater efficacy than clopidogrel anecdotally, has been associated with significant haemorrhage.

Platelet inhibition

Platelet inhibition may be evident in patients preoperatively. This may occur as a result of chronic illness (renal or liver disease), or acutely, as is the case in patient presenting with shock or sepsis. Platelets are also activated by the CPB circuit. This results in the release of platelet granules, the formation of microaggregates,

and the expression of pro-inflammatory ligands on the platelet surface (29). Post-CPB, however, platelet responsiveness is blunted via poorly understood mechanisms, resulting in an overall reduction in the capacity of platelets to form aggregates and fibrin thrombi.

Clotting factor depletion

The CPB circuit causes activation of the extrinsic clotting cascade. Typically circuit thrombosis is prevented by the administration of heparin (Chapters 11 and 17). However, heparin acts at the level of anti-thrombin 3, preventing the cleavage of fibrinogen to fibrin. The upstream clotting cascades are therefore continuously activated during CPB. Prolonged CPB subsequently results in clotting factor depletion and diminished clot formation following heparin reversal with protamine (30). Hypothermia and acidosis also inhibit these cascades and can contribute to coagulopathy. Thrombin, which is activated during surgery, also has a range of pro- and anticoagulant effects, including the promotion of fibrinolysis and concomitant platelet activation and inhibition.

Fibrinolysis

As well as activating platelets and coagulation cascades the CPB circuit also results in activation of plasminogen, causing fibrinolysis. Fibrinolysis is increased following prolonged procedures, aspiration of large volumes of unwashed blood from the operative field, and in some situations such as ongoing sepsis, or in the presence of shock.

Diagnosis of coagulopathy

Effective treatment of coagulopathy particularly in a bleeding patient requires accurate and timely diagnosis. The nature of coagulopathy is heterogeneous and is influenced by the aetiology, as described previously, and also by the blood management strategy adopted (e.g. the use of antifibrinolytics and non RBC blood components). Specific defects in the clotting pathway are commonly not detected by standard clotting tests that, with average turn-around-times of plasma-based assays as long as 65 minutes, are also often considered impractical in the setting of ongoing blood loss. Near-patient testing is increasingly advocated in this setting and is discussed in more detail in Chapter 17. The most widely used near patient testing devices include the Thromboelastogram® (TEG) or ROTEM®. These are whole blood viscoelastic tests that evaluate the effects of coagulation factors, platelets, and red cells on overall clotting potential. Both work along similar principles, whereby progressive clot formation in the presence of an activator is measured as impedance to a rotating pin within the clot. The resultant trace can then be used to infer information as to the activity of separate components of the clotting pathway, including the clotting cascade, platelet function, and lysis (figure 18.5 a). These platforms are user friendly and widely used and TEG based treatment algorithms, as initially described by Shore-Lesserson and colleagues in 1999 (figure 18.5 b), have been used in clinical studies to standardize the management of coagulopathic bleeding (31). However, in practice, these tests have limited sensitivity and specificity and a recent systematic review has highlighted the lack of evidence of clinical benefit associated with their use (32). Near patient assessment of platelet aggregometry and alternative laboratory assays such as thrombin generation testing have been shown to accurately predict bleeding and target therapy in small single centre studies. Wider validation of these techniques is awaited.

Treatment of coagulopathy

Without accurate diagnostic tests to identify specific defects in the clotting pathway that are associated with adverse clinical outcomes the management of coagulopathy is often empiric. The clinical efficacy, safety and cost effectiveness of this approach is unclear.

Platelet transfusion

Cardiac surgery utilizes over 17% of all platelet transfusions in the UK (1). Indications for, and effective doses of. platelets are

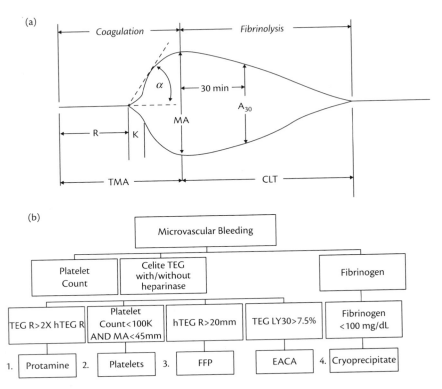

Fig. 18.5 Point of care testing in coagulopathy.
(a) Representative schematic of thromboelastogram (TEG®) output. R refers to the time from the start of measurement until initiation of clotting and may reflect either activity of the intrinsic or extrinsic pathway depending on the activator. The angle α and k time reflect the time from clot initiation to a pre-defined clot thickness. MA refers to maximal clot thickness, all of which are measures of fibrin polymerization. These are indices of platelet activity and fibrin concentrations The LY30 is the ratio of clot thickness at 30 minutes post MA relative to the MA and is a measure of fibrinolysis. (b) Thromboelastogram based treatment algorithm.
Reproduced from Shore-Lesserson L, Manspeizer HE, DePerio M, Francis S, Vela-Cantos F, Ergin MA, 'Thromboelastography-guided transfusion algorithm reduces transfusions in complex cardiac surgery', Anesthesia Analgesia, 88, 2, pp. 312–319, copyright 1999, with permission from International Anesthesia Research Society.

unclear. There are no RCT data outside the haemato-oncology setting that can be used to guide practice, although observational studies report lower mortality rates in trauma patients receiving high-dose platelet transfusion for major blood loss. Some observational studies have demonstrated strong independent associations between platelet administration and adverse events, particularly stroke (17). However, some do not (18) and, it is likely that the risk benefit ratio is highly context specific; i.e. more liberal use may be appropriate in high risk operations where aprotinin has not been given, whereas administration in a patient without significant platelet dysfunction is likely to carry an increased risk.

Fresh frozen plasma and prothrombin complex concentrate

Twelve percent of all FFP in the UK is administered to cardiac surgery patients (1). A meta-analysis of RCTs has demonstrated no clinical benefit from prophylactic FFP administration (33). There is no RCT evidence to guide FFP transfusion in the setting of post-CPB bleeding and its use is generally empirical. FFP from female donors is associated with transfusion-associated lung injury, dyspnoea, and circulatory overload (TRALI, TAD, and TACO), via mechanisms that are poorly understood (34). Prothrombin complex concentrate (PCC) is increasingly being considered as a substitute for FFP in cardiac surgery. PCC is plasma derived and contains standardized, high concentrations of either three or four vitamin K-dependent factors: typically, factors II, VII, IX, and X. PCCs are currently indicated for the treatment of serious or life-threatening bleeding related to vitamin K antagonist therapy. PCC are pathogen inactivated, produce more predictable increases in factor concentrations, have smaller volumes relative to FFP transfusion, and may have greater clinical efficacy (35).

Fibrinogen replacement

Traditionally, fibrinogen is replaced during major blood loss or as part of the management for DIC once the Clauss fibrinogen value falls below 1 g/L. Cryoprecipitate is the first line treatment in the UK for acquired hypofibrinogenaemia, and a standard adult dose (two pools) raises the plasma fibrinogen level by 1 g/L.

There are no clinical data to confirm effectiveness of cryoprecipitate in active bleeding and there is increasing interest in the use of fibrinogen concentrates. These are currently not licensed in the UK but have obvious advantages in light of their reduced infection risk and standardized fibrinogen concentration. Phase II RCTs (36,37) have reported positive outcomes following administration of fibrinogen concentrate, but further evaluation of the safety of these interventions is needed.

Therapeutic treatment adjuncts to reduce transfusion

The safety and efficacy of therapeutic adjuncts to reduce transfusion exposure and prevent coagulopathic bleeding have been evaluated in a series of quantitative meta-analyses (figure 18.6 and figure 18.7).

Cardiopulmonary bypass circuit modification

Haemodilutional anaemia can be avoided by the use of low volume prime or displacement techniques that use the patients' own blood to prime the CPB circuit. Other modifications, such as heparin coating or closed circuits, are designed to reduce postoperative platelet inhibition, either as a result of high heparin doses or intraoperative platelet activation at the air–blood interface, respectively. Mini-CPB circuits combine these advantages with the absence of a venous reservoir and a smaller surface area for blood activation (Chapter 11). A recent systematic review (38) has demonstrated that mini-CPB circuits significantly reduce transfusion and bleeding volumes, and may have modest clinical benefits including a reduction in arrhythmias and neurocognitive decline (figure 18.6 and figure 18.7).

Transfusion of autologous red blood cells

Preoperative autologous donation (PAD) involves the patient donating one or more units of their own blood preoperatively, often in conjunction with the administration of erythropoietin.

Intervention	Author	Sample size	RR (95% CI)	Risk Ratio (95% CI)
Acute Normovolaemic Haemodilution	Davies	1423	0.77 (0.57; 1.04)	
Mechanical cell salvage	Carless	2518	0.77 (0.69; 0.86)	
MECC	Harling	920	0.35 (0.23; 0.53)	
EPO and iron	Alghamdi	361	0.36 (0.16; 0.81)	
Tranexamic acid versus placebo	Henry	3006	0.68 (0.57; 0.81)	
Aprotinin versus placebo	Henry	9497	0.68 (0.63; 0.73)	
Aprotinin versus tranexamic acid/EACA	Henry	5192	0.86 (0.77; 0.97)	
Desmopressin	Carless	1196	0.95 (0.84; 1.07)	

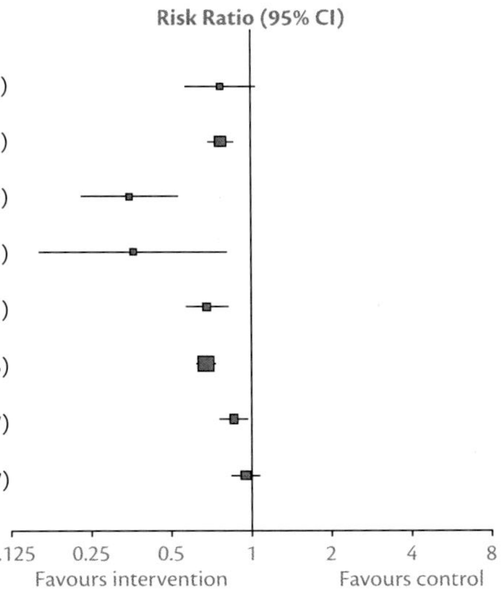

0.125   0.25   0.5   1   2   4   8
Favours intervention   Favours control

Fig. 18.6 Therapeutic adjuncts to reduce blood loss and transfusion.
Forest plot summarizing the effects of commonly used therapeutic adjuncts aimed at reducing bleeding and transfusion on allogeneic red cell exposure in cardiac surgery patients. Data derived from recently published meta-analyses as indicated (38–46). MECC, minimal extracorporeal circulation cardiac surgery; EPO, erythropoietin; EACA, epsilon-amino caproic acid

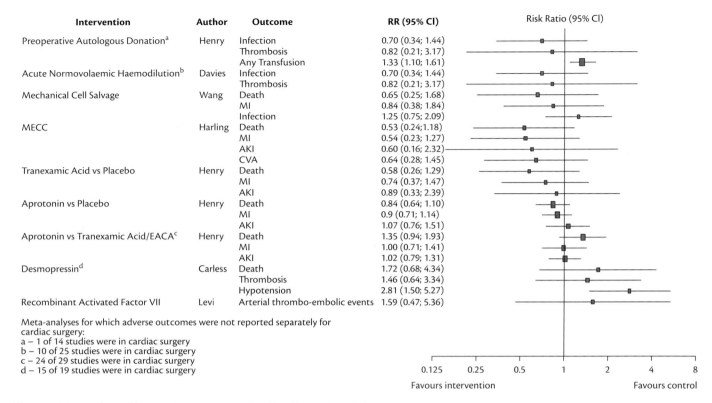

Intervention	Author	Outcome	RR (95% CI)	Risk Ratio (95% CI)
Preoperative Autologous Donation[a]	Henry	Infection	0.70 (0.34; 1.44)	
		Thrombosis	0.82 (0.21; 3.17)	
		Any Transfusion	1.33 (1.10; 1.61)	
Acute Normovolaemic Haemodilution[b]	Davies	Infection	0.70 (0.34; 1.44)	
		Thrombosis	0.82 (0.21; 3.17)	
Mechanical Cell Salvage	Wang	Death	0.65 (0.25; 1.68)	
		MI	0.84 (0.38; 1.84)	
		Infection	1.25 (0.75; 2.09)	
MECC	Harling	Death	0.53 (0.24; 1.18)	
		MI	0.54 (0.23; 1.27)	
		AKI	0.60 (0.16; 2.32)	
		CVA	0.64 (0.28; 1.45)	
Tranexamic Acid vs Placebo	Henry	Death	0.58 (0.26; 1.29)	
		MI	0.74 (0.37; 1.47)	
		AKI	0.89 (0.33; 2.39)	
Aprotonin vs Placebo	Henry	Death	0.84 (0.64; 1.10)	
		MI	0.9 (0.71; 1.14)	
		AKI	1.07 (0.76; 1.51)	
Aprotonin vs Tranexamic Acid/EACA[c]	Henry	Death	1.35 (0.94; 1.93)	
		MI	1.00 (0.71; 1.41)	
		AKI	1.02 (0.79; 1.31)	
Desmopressin[d]	Carless	Death	1.72 (0.68; 4.34)	
		Thrombosis	1.46 (0.64; 3.34)	
		Hypotension	2.81 (1.50; 5.27)	
Recombinant Activated Factor VII	Levi	Arterial thrombo-embolic events	1.59 (0.47; 5.36)	

Meta-analyses for which adverse outcomes were not reported separately for
cardiac surgery:
a – 1 of 14 studies were in cardiac surgery
b – 10 of 25 studies were in cardiac surgery
c – 24 of 29 studies were in cardiac surgery
d – 15 of 19 studies were in cardiac surgery

Fig. 18.7 Adverse effects of therapeutic outcomes to reduce blood loss and transfusion.

Forest plot summarizing the effects of commonly used therapeutic adjuncts aimed at reducing bleeding and transfusion on important clinical outcomes in cardiac surgery. Data derived from published meta-analyses as indicated (38–46). MI, myocardial infarction; MECC, minimal extracorporeal circulation cardiac surgery; AKI, acute kidney injury

This blood is held within the blood bank where it is administered as required during the perioperative period, as an alternative to allogenic RBC. PAD is effective at reducing exposure to allogenic blood (figure 18.6). However, overall exposure to transfused RBC (both autologous and allogenic) is increased, and PAD is not associated with improved clinical outcomes (figure 18.7). PAD may be advantageous where infectious particle transmission risk from allogenic blood is high; however, given its otherwise limited benefits, and relatively high infrastructure costs its adoption has not been widespread.

Acute normovolaemic haemodilution

Acute normovolaemic haemodilution (ANH) involves removing blood from a patient, usually during induction of anaesthesia, replacing it with crystalloid or colloid to maintain circulating volume, and storing the blood for reinfusion during surgery as a response to blood loss, or at the end of surgery. Significant haemodilution reduces the red cell mass lost during surgery, and replacement of losses with autologous blood has better homeostatic properties than colloid or crystalloid. ANH may also improve haemostasis by preventing consumption or loss of clotting factors during prolonged CPB and ANH has been shown to reduce bleeding rates. ANH has not been shown to result in specific clinical benefits to patients beyond reducing transfusion exposure, however (figure 18.6 and figure 18.7). The disadvantages of ANH relate principally to the safety of low haematocrits during surgery, which may increase the risk of neurological, myocardial, and renal injury.

Mechanical cell salvage

Blood lost as a result of acute haemorrhage during surgery can be salvaged using commercially available devices that wash the blood removing plasma proteins, cell fragments and other contaminants of the surgical field, allowing re-infusion of washed autologous cells. This technique significantly reduces RBC exposure (figure 18.6), and improves clinical outcomes including the risk of perioperative infection (figure 18.7). Published guidelines do not recommend the autotransfusion of unwashed salvaged red cells (risk of excessive bleeding) or postoperative shed mediastinal fluid (risk of infection) (27).

Pharmacological interventions

Recombinant human erythropoietin (EPO) is commonly administered along with iron supplementation to reverse chronic anaemia preoperatively in cardiac surgical patients where it has been shown to reduce transfusion exposure without apparent adverse effects (figure 18.6 and figure 18.7). However, the studies included in this meta-analysis (42) were generally of poor quality and underpowered to detect important clinical outcomes. Large RCTs in non-cardiac surgery patients identify an increase in thrombo-embolic events with EPO attributable to rapid increases in viscosity as well as a direct effect on platelet aggregation (47), and, despite published guidelines recommending the use of EPO in cardiac surgery patients preoperatively (27), safe and effective dosing regimens remain to be defined.

Antifibrinolytics

The lysine analogues tranexamic acid and epsilon-amino caproic acid (EACA) act by irreversibly binding to the active site of plasminogen thereby inhibiting clot lysis. Tranexamic acid and EACA reduce transfusion exposure in cardiac surgery but have not been shown to improve clinical outcomes (figure 18.6 and figure 18.7). There is little consensus as to the most effective dose of these agents. High doses have been anecdotally associated with perioperative seizures, although no RCTs to date have identified significant safety concerns with their use. The serine protease inhibitor aprotinin, which acts as an antifibrinolytic as well as having a range of other anti-inflammatory and anti-apoptotic actions, has greater efficacy at reducing transfusion exposure relative to tranexamic acid or EACA (figure 18.6). However, data from RCTs suggests that this is also associated with an increased risk of adverse outcomes including mortality (figure 18.7). For more detailed discussion of anti-fibrinolytics see Chapter 17.

Desmopressin

Desmopressin is a synthetic analogue of arginine vasopressin that induces the release of the contents of endothelial cell-associated Weibel–Palade bodies. The resulting increase in factor VIII and von Willebrand factor concentrations as well as evidence of increased platelet aggregation in response to desmopressin has led to use as a haemostatic agent in cardiac surgery however a Cochrane review has failed to demonstrate any significant reduction in transfusion exposure, or improvement in clinical outcomes (figure 18.6 and figure 18.7).

Factor VII

Recombinant activated factor VII (rFVII) is a potent pharmacological prohaemostatic agent licensed for use in patients with haemophilia. This has led to the off-label use of rFVII for the treatment of severe coagulopathic bleeding in cardiac surgery as an adjunct to conventional non RBC blood components. In a multicentre Phase II RCT rFVII reduced resternotomy for bleeding in patients refractory to conventional components (FFP, platelets); however, this was associated with a non-statistically significant (68%) increase in major thrombotic complications (48), an effect size remarkably similar to that of a systematic review of rFVII in cardiac and non cardiac patients (46).

Transfusion risk scores and integrated blood management

Optimal blood management requires the integration of multiple interventions. The precise combination of these is highly patient specific. Each additional intervention will have an incrementally smaller benefit than would be derived by its use in isolation (incremental cost effectiveness) and potentially the addition of multiple interventions may substantially increase the risk of adverse outcome without significant additional benefit. The most effective combination of interventions is dictated by the relative risk of coagulopathy

and/or anaemia and those patients at greater risk of larger volume blood loss or transfusion will benefit from more intensive blood management. Risk prediction scores for transfusion (49) or massive transfusion (50) have been described; however, these have proven to have limited prognostic accuracy beyond the centre in which they were developed. This is because they do not adjust for institutional or individual blood management preferences such as thresholds for the administration of RBC and non-RBC components or the use of aprotinin versus tranexamic acid. Risk scores for other outcomes are widely used in cardiac surgery, and it is reasonable to suggest that an accurate risk score that can reflect these preferences should have widespread utility in blood management.

Conclusion

Blood management is an important contributor to achieving good patient outcomes in cardiac surgery. Blood management decisions are a central feature of every cardiac surgical procedure undertaken. Existing evidence suggests that restrictive transfusion thresholds are safe in cardiac surgery. More importantly, there is no evidence of benefit and a significant likelihood of harm from more liberal administration of RBC. Coagulopathy has a multifactorial aetiology and is common in these patients, where it is associated with adverse outcome. This condition is poorly defined; however, existing tests lack diagnostic accuracy, and treatment is largely empirical and highly variable. This is an important area for research. There are multiple therapeutic adjuncts that have been shown to prevent severe anaemia, coagulopathy, and transfusion; however, few of these, with the exception of cell salvage, have been shown to improve clinical outcomes. Furthermore, pharmacological strategies such as rhEPO, aprotinin, and rFVII may reduce bleeding and transfusion but worsen clinical outcome. Risk scores that identify those at greatest risk of transfusion or massive transfusion may be used to identify those patients who will benefit most from multiple interventions, or integrated blood management; however, accurate risk scores that have been widely validated have yet to be described.

References

1. Wells AW, Llewelyn CA, Casbard A, et al. The EASTR Study: indications for transfusion and estimates of transfusion recipient numbers in hospitals supplied by the National Blood Service. *Transfus Med* 2009; **19**: 315–28
2. US Department of Health and Human Services. *The 2007 Nationwide Blood Collection and Utilization Survey Report.* Washington, DC: Dept of Health and Human Services, 2007
3. Bennett-Guerrero E, Zhao Y, O'Brien SM, et al. Variation in use of blood transfusion in coronary artery bypass graft surgery. *JAMA* 2010; **304**(14): 1568–75
4. Karkouti K, Wijeysundera DN, Beattie WS. Risk associated with preoperative anemia in cardiac surgery: a multicenter cohort study. *Circulation* 2008; **117**: 478–84
5. Habib RH, Zacharias A, Schwann TA, et al. Role of hemodilutional anemia and transfusion during cardiopulmonary bypass in renal injury after coronary revascularization: implications on operative outcome. *Crit Care Med* 2008; **33**: 1749–56
6. Ranucci M, La Rovere MT, Castelvecchio S, et al. Postoperative anemia and exercise tolerance after cardiac operations in patients without transfusion: what hemoglobin level is acceptable? *Ann Thorac Surg* 2011; **92**: 25–31

7. Koch CG, Li L, Duncan AI, Mihaljevic T, et al. Morbidity and mortality risk associated with red blood cell and blood-component transfusion in isolated coronary artery bypass grafting. *Crit Care Med* 2006; **34**: 1608–16

8. Engoren M, Habib RH, Hadaway J, et al. The effect on long-term survival of erythrocyte transfusion given for cardiac valve operations. *Ann Thorac Surg* 2009; **88**: 95–100

9. Rogers MA, Blumberg N, Saint S, Langa KM, Nallamothu BK. Hospital variation in transfusion and infection after cardiac surgery: a cohort study. *BMC Med* 2009; **7**: 37

10. Tyson GH 3rd, Rodriguez E, Elci OC, et al. Cardiac procedures in patients with a body mass index exceeding 45: outcomes and long-term results. *Ann Thorac Surg* 2007; **84**: 3–9

11. Karkouti K, Wijeysundera DN, Yau TM, et al. (2004) The independent association of massive blood loss with mortality in cardiac surgery. *Transfusion* **44**: 1453–62

12. Koch CG, Li L, Sessler DI, et al. Duration of red-cell storage and complications after cardiac surgery. *N Engl J Med* 2008; **358**: 1229–39

13. Shehata N, Burns LA, Nathan H, et al. A randomized controlled pilot study of adherence to transfusion strategies in cardiac surgery. *Transfusion* 2012; **52**: 91–9

14. Bracey AW, Radovancevic R, Riggs SA, et al. Lowering the hemoglobin threshold for transfusion in coronary artery bypass procedures: effect on patient outcome. *Transfusion* 1999; **39**: 1070–7

15. Murphy GJ, Rizvi SIA, Battaglia F, et al. A pilot randomized controlled trial of the effect of transfusion-threshold reduction on transfusion rates and morbidity after cardiac surgery. *Transfusion Alternatives in Transfusion Medicine* 2007; **9**(Suppl 1): 41–2

16. Hajjar LA, Vincent JL, Galas FR, et al. Transfusion requirements after cardiac surgery: the TRACS randomized controlled trial. *JAMA* 2010; **304**: 1559–67

17. Speiss BD, Royston D, Levy JH et al. Platelet transfusions during coronary artery bypass graft surgery are associated with serious adverse outcomes. *Transfusion* 2004; **44**: 1143–8

18. Karkouti K, Wijeysundera DN, Beattie WS. Platelet transfusions as a risk factor in cardiac surgery. *Transfusion* 2007; **47**: 1739–40

19. Unsworth-White MJ, Herriot A, Valencia O, et al. Resternotomy for bleeding after cardiac operation: a marker for increased morbidity and mortality. *Ann Thorac Surg* 1995; 59: 664–7

20. Moulton MJ, Creswell LL, Mackey ME, Cox JL, Rosenbloom M. Reexploration for bleeding is a risk factor for adverse outcomes after cardiac operations. *J Thorac Cardiovasc Surg* 1996; **111**: 1037–46

21. Dacey LJ, Munoz JJ, Baribeau YR, et al. Reexploration for hemorrhage following coronary artery bypass grafting: incidence and risk factors. Northern New England Cardiovascular Disease Study Group. *Arch Surg* 1998; **133**: 442–7

22. Karthik S, Grayson AD, McCarron EE, Pullan DM, Desmond MJ. Reexploration for bleeding after coronary artery bypass surgery: risk factors, outcomes, and the effect of time delay. *Ann Thorac Surg* 2004; 78: 527–34

23. Choong CK, Gerrard C, Goldsmith KA, Dunningham H, Vuylsteke A. Delayed re-exploration for bleeding after coronary artery bypass surgery results in adverse outcomes. *Eur J Cardiothorac Surg* 2007; **31**: 834–8

24. Ranucci M, Bozzetti G, Ditta A, Cotza M, Carboni G, Ballotta A. Surgical reexploration after cardiac operations: why a worse outcome? *Ann Thorac Surg* 2008; **86**: 1557–62

25. Ferraris VA, Ferraris SP, Moliterno DJ, et al; Society of Thoracic Surgeons. The Society of Thoracic Surgeons practice guideline series: aspirin and other antiplatelet agents during operative coronary revascularization (executive summary). *Ann Thorac Surg* 2005; **79**: 1454–61

26. Nijjer SS, Watson G, Athanasiou T, Malik IS. Safety of clopidogrel being continued until the time of coronary artery bypass grafting in patients with acute coronary syndrome: a meta-analysis of 34 studies. *Eur Heart J* 2011; **32**: 2970–88

27. Ferraris VA, Brown JR, Despotis GJ, et al. 2011 update to the society of thoracic surgeons and the society of cardiovascular anesthesiologists blood conservation clinical practice guidelines. *Ann Thorac Surg* 2011; 91: 944–82

28. Ranucci M, Baryshnikova E, Soro G, Ballotta A, De Benedetti D, Conti D. Surgical and Clinical Outcome Research (SCORE) Group. Multiple electrode whole-blood aggregometry and bleeding in cardiac surgery patients receiving thienopyridines. *Ann Thorac Surg* 2011; **91**: 123–9

29. Weerasinghe A, Taylor KM. The platelet in cardiopulmonary bypass. *Ann Thorac Surg* 1998; **66**: 2145–52

30. Despotis GJ, Avidan MS, Hogue CW Jr. Mechanisms and attenuation of hemostatic activation during extracorporeal circulation. *Ann Thorac Surg* 2001; **72**: S1821–31

31. Shore-Lesserson L, Manspeizer HE, DePerio M, Francis S, Vela-Cantos F, Ergin MA. Thromboelastography-guided transfusion algorithm reduces transfusions in complex cardiac surgery. *Anesth Analg* 1999; **88**: 312–9

32. Afshari A, Wikkelsø A, Brok J, Møller AM, Wetterslev J. Thrombelastography (TEG) or thromboelastometry (ROTEM) to monitor haemotherapy versus usual care in patients with massive transfusion. *Cochrane Database Syst Rev* 2011; **3**: CD007871

33. Casbard AC, Williamson LM, Murphy MF, Reges K, Johnson T. The role of prophylactic fresh frozen plasma in decreasing blood loss and correcting coagulopathy in cardiac surgery. A systematic review. *Anaesthesia* 2004; 59: 550–8

34. Vlaar AP, Hofstra JJ, Determann RM, et al. The incidence, risk factors, and outcome of transfusion-related acute lung injury in a cohort of cardiac surgery patients: a prospective nested case-control study. *Blood* 2011; **117**: 4218–25

35. Demeyere R, Gillardin S, Arnout J, Strengers PF. Comparison of fresh frozen plasma and prothrombin complex concentrate for the reversal of oral anticoagulants in patients undergoing cardiopulmonary bypass surgery: a randomized study. *Vox Sang* 2010; **99**: 251–60

36. Rahe-Meyer N, Pichlmaier M, Haverich A, et al. Bleeding management with fibrinogen concentrate targeting a high-normal plasma fibrinogen level: a pilot study. *Br J Anaesth* 2009; **102**: 785–92

37. Karlsson M, Ternström L, Hyllner M,et al. Prophylactic fibrinogen infusion reduces bleeding after coronary artery bypass surgery. A prospective randomised pilot study. *Thromb Haemost* 2009; **102**: 137–44

38. Harling L, Warren OJ, Martin A, et al. Do miniaturized extracorporeal circuits confer significant clinical benefit without compromising safety? A meta-analysis of randomized controlled trials. *ASAIO J* 2011; **57**: 141–51

39. Henry DA, Carless PA, Moxey AJ, et al. Pre-operative autologous donation for minimising perioperative allogeneic blood transfusion. *Cochrane Database Syst Rev* 2002; **2**: CD003602

40. Davies L, Brown TJ, Haynes S, Payne K, Elliott RA, McCollum C. Cost-effectiveness of cell salvage and alternative methods of minimising perioperative allogeneic blood transfusion: a systematic review and economic model. *Health Technol Assess* 2006; **10**(iii–iv,ix–x), 1–210

41. Carless PA, Henry DA, Moxey AJ, O'Connell D, Brown T, Fergusson DA. Cell salvage for minimising perioperative allogeneic blood transfusion. *Cochrane Database Syst Rev* 2010; **4**: CD001888

42. Alghamdi AA, Albanna MJ, Guru V, Brister SJ. Does the use of erythropoietin reduce the risk of exposure to allogeneic blood transfusion in cardiac surgery? A systematic review and meta-analysis. *J Card Surg* 2006; **21**: 320–6

43. Segal JB, Blasco-Colmenares E, Norris EJ, Guallar E. Preoperative acute normovolemic hemodilution: a meta-analysis. *Transfusion* 2004; **44**: 632–44

44. Henry DA, Carless PA, Moxey AJ, et al. Anti-fibrinolytic use for minimising perioperative allogeneic blood transfusion. *Cochrane Database Syst Rev* 2011; **3**: CD001886

45. Carless PA, Henry DA, Moxey AJ, et al. Desmopressin for minimising perioperative allogeneic blood transfusion. *Cochrane Database Syst Rev* 2004; **1**: CD001884

46. Levi M, Levy JH, Andersen HF, Truloff D. Safety of recombinant activated factor VII in randomized clinical trials. *N Engl J Med* 2010; **363**: 1791–800

47. Corwin HL, Gettinger A, Fabian TC, et al. EPO Critical Care Trials Group. Efficacy and safety of epoetin alfa in critically ill patients. *N Engl J Med* 2007; **357**: 965–76

48. Gill R, Herbertson M, Vuylsteke A, et al. Safety and efficacy of recombinant activated factor VII: a randomized placebo-controlled trial in the setting of bleeding after cardiac surgery. *Circulation* 2009; **120**: 21–7

49. Ranucci M, Castelvecchio S, Frigiola A, Scolletta S, Giomarelli P, Biagioli B. Predicting transfusions in cardiac surgery: the easier, the better: the Transfusion Risk and Clinical Knowledge score. *Vox Sang* 2009; **96**: 324–32

50. Karkouti K, Wijeysundera DN, Beattie WS, et al. Reducing Bleeding in Cardiac Surgery (RBC) Research Group. Variability and predictability of large-volume red blood cell transfusion in cardiac surgery: a multicenter study. *Transfusion* 2007; **47**: 2081–8

CHAPTER 19

Anaesthesia for adult cardiac surgery

R. Peter Alston

Introduction

Cardiac anaesthesia requires the ability to safely provide anaesthesia to patients with advanced cardiovascular disease undergoing major surgical trespass as well as during cardiopulmonary bypass (CPB). To do so, a cardiac anaesthetist needs to have an intimate understanding of the physiology, pathophysiology, and pharmacology of the cardiovascular, pulmonary, and coagulation systems as well as the skills to operate a variety of different technical devices such as pacing boxes and intra-aortic balloon pump (IABP). Therefore cardiac anaesthesia requires the synthesis of all the knowledge from many of the other chapters in this textbook. As most of the heart surgery around the world is undertaken in adults using CPB, to treat acquired heart disease such as coronary artery disease (CAD) and heart valve disease, the aim of this chapter is to address anaesthesia for this group of patients. Anaesthesia for CABG surgery without CPB and minimally invasive cardiac surgery is discussed in Chapter 20.

With a few important exceptions such as emergencies, most cardiac anaesthesiologists apply a standardized anaesthetic technique to all but a few of their patients. Historically, as there is little underlying evidence base for our practice of cardiac anaesthesia, this standardized technique has historically varied from institution to institution and from anaesthetist to anaesthetist. Perpetuating this tradition, this chapter will describe the author's practice of cardiac anaesthesia, which is based on over 30 years of clinical experience. However, it will identify areas where an evidence base exists to guide the practice of cardiac anaesthesia.

Preoperative assessment and preparation

Preoperative assessment of patients underpins safe cardiac anaesthesia. Traditionally, this was often done following admission to hospital a day or more before surgery, which allowed adequate time for assessment and the provision of information to the patient by the anaesthetist who was to administer the anaesthesia. Increasingly, because of financial pressures, patients undergoing heart surgery are day of surgery admissions (DOSAs). Therefore, DOSA requires establishment of outpatient clinics to ensure, not only robust anaesthetic assessment, but also provision of information to patients, and obtaining consent for specific procedures. Ideally, these clinics should be staffed by cardiac anaesthesiologists as they can both assess and advise the patient about their

procedure. However, lesser but effective models would be for routine screening by trained nurses, physician's assistants, nurse anaesthetists, or general anaesthesiologists. If this model is used then it needs to identify high risk patients who are then assessed and advised by experienced cardiac anaesthesiologists.

High-risk patients can usually be identified by mortality prediction score such as the EuroSCORE (Chapter 7). Nonetheless, they may also have some condition that increases the risk of anaesthesia or surgery that is not covered by such scores. In addition, whilst patients may have been adequately assessed by the cardiologist and surgeon, occasionally there may be aspects of their health that have been overlooked, which have an important bearing on risk. When such patients are identified then the cardiac anaesthetists should discuss them with the surgeon and a joint assessment of the risks and benefits of surgery should be made before then discussing the issues with the patient. In addition, sometimes the surgeon will have be referred a patient by a cardiologist that he believes to be high risk and wishes input from an anaesthetist before scheduling the patient for surgery. Again, such patients require assessment by a trained cardiac anaesthetist.

Microbiological screening and eradication

Surgical site infections (SSIs) of the sternal wound, most especially caused by methicillin-resistant *Staphylococcus aureus* (MRSA), are a serious complication of cardiac surgery that are both life threatening and lead to prolonged durations of stay in the critical care areas and hospital. For this reason, patients scheduled for heart surgery should undergo routine microbiological screening for MRSA. If the surgery is elective then patients with positive results require their surgery to be postponed until eradication treatment with antibiotics and antiseptics can be completed. If the surgery is urgent and the patient is MRSA positive, then appropriate antibiotic prophylaxis should be given during surgery.

Prophylactic mouth washing with chlorhexidine gluconate 0.12%, has also been recommended based on one small randomized controlled trial (RCT) that found that one oral rinse preoperatively and twice daily rinses postoperatively in the critical care area reduces both nosocomial infection and mortality (1,2).

Anaemia

Patients who are anaemic, who are scheduled for elective cardiac surgery should be investigate and treated before surgery.

Anaesthetic assessment

As for any patient who is to undergo general anaesthesia, patients scheduled for cardiac surgery should have standard anaesthetic assessment covering airway, previous general anaesthetics, drug history, and past medical history (box 19.1). More than this standard assessment, a thorough review of the cardiac symptoms and investigation is required. Except for major chest trauma, patients scheduled for cardiac surgery have generally had extensive investigations of their heart pathology by angiography, cardiac catheterization, echocardiography, or magnetic resonance imaging (MRI), and all that may be required is to review the reports. However, reviewing the imaging may add useful insight to guide anaesthetic management. In addition, it should be established that are no contraindications to the use of transoesophageal echocardiography (TOE).

Patient's medications

One very important and controversial aspect of preoperative preparation is what medicines are continued or discontinued before surgery. Many drugs that patients are receiving for treatment of their cardiovascular and other disease can influence

Box 19.1 Preoperative assessment

- Confirm consent provided for surgery
- Medical history
- Drug history/allergies
- Presenting history
- Contraindication to insertion of a TOE probe
- Physical examination centred on cardiovascular system
- View chest X-ray
- Coronary angiogram: read report/view images
- Echocardiography: read report/view images
- MRI imaging: read report/view images
- Blood tests
  - Full blood count
  - Coagulation screen
  - Electrolytes
  - Urea and creatinine
  - Blood sugar
  - Liver function tests
- MRSA screening
- Pulmonary function tests
- Carotid doppler report
- Permanent pacemaker—set to fixed rate
- AICD inactivated

TOE, transoesophageal echocardiography; MRI: magnetic resonance imaging; MRSA: methicillin resistant staphylococcus aureus and AICD: automatic implantable cardioverter/defibrillator.

Table 19.1 Possible effects of continuing or discontinuing patient drugs before cardiac surgery

Drug	Continued	Discontinued
Beta-adrenergic blockers Bradycardia	Myocardial ischaemia/increased mortality	
Diuretics	Patient falls after sedative premedication	Fluid overload
ACE inhibitors/renin antagonists	Excessive intra- and postoperative vasodilation	Left ventricular failure/hypertension
Calcium channel blockers	Bradycardia/hypotension	Hypertension
StatinsLower mortality	Increase mortality	
Antiplatelet agents	Increased bleeding	Coronary thrombosis/myocardial infarction
Oral hypoglycaemic agents	Hypoglycaemia	Hyperglycaemia
Insulin	Hypoglycaemia	Hyperglycaemia
Warfarin	Increased bleeding	Intra-cardiac thrombosis
IV nitrates	Hypotension	Myocardial ischaemia
IV heparin	Increased blood loss	Myocardial ischaemia

important intraoperative events. Often, the anaesthetist plays little part in the decision as to whether the patient's drugs are continued or discontinued in the individual patient, as any decision may have already made by the surgeon days or weeks before the surgery. However, it is important that the anaesthetist is aware of the implications of these decisions so that he may influence the surgeon's or institutional protocols. Table 19.1 lays out some of the possible effects of continuing or discontinuing patient drugs.

Statins

With regard to statins, systematic review and meta-analysis indicates that their continuation preoperatively is associated with a 24% reduction in mortality (OR 0.76 [95%CI 0.64, 0.90]) (3). However, the level of evidence is weak as 10 of the 13 included studies were observational, introducing selection bias.

Beta-adrenergic blockers

A review by an international consensus group has recommended beta-adrenergic blockers should not be discontinued in patients who are receiving chronic treatment because it increases mortality (4). However, based a single observational study, the grade of evidence for this recommendation is very low (5).

Warfarin

Patients who are anticoagulated with warfarin or similar drugs should have them discontinued several days before elective surgery. If the prothrombin time international normalized ratio (INR) is still elevated on admission to hospital and surgery is elective, then a small dose of vitamin K (1–2 mg) should be administered and the INR rechecked after a few hours (Chapter 17). If the surgery is urgent then sufficient prothrombin complex concentrate should be given to normalize the coagulation.

Premedication

Traditionally, patients undergoing cardiac anaesthesia were heavily premedicated with opioids and large doses of benzodiazepines, resulting in prolonged sedation following surgery. When patients were electively mechanically ventilated, this was an advantage. Today, such prolonged sedation is a drawback as it impedes recovery especially in the ever-ageing population presenting for surgery. Currently, the author uses small doses of temazepam 10–20 mg PO and if anxiolysis is inadequate on arrival in the anaesthetic/operating room then supplements this intravenously with small doses of an opioid such as fentanyl or a benzodiazepine such as midazolam. In emergency surgery where there is severe cardiovascular compromise such as tamponade, it is prudent to avoid any form of premedication until the patient is in the operating room and monitored.

Alpha-2 adrenergic blockers

The alpha-2 adrenergic blockers clonidine and dexmedetomidine have also been used for premedication either alone or in combination with a benzodiazepine. Indeed, a systematic review and meta-analysis found that their perioperative use reduced myocardial ischaemia (6). However, this lower incidence of ischaemia does not translate into fewer myocardial infarctions or a lower mortality. The lack of affect on patient outcome, along with the side effects of hypotension and bradycardia, may explain why these drugs have not become widely adopted.

Oxygen

In the past, oxygen was commonly administered to patients following premedication, probably to compensate for the respiratory depressant resulting from heavy premedication and prevent hypoxia. Given the lighter premedication that is generally used now along with the availability to pulse oximeters, there is no benefit in routinely administered oxygen unless there is measurable hypoxia, for example as a result of pulmonary oedema.

Preparation for induction of anaesthesia

Pre-arrival preparation

Before the arrival of the patient in the anaesthesia or operating room, most especially in emergencies, the operating room and staff should be present and prepared (box 19.2). All the anaesthetic drugs should be drawn-up in syringes, as well as heparin, an antibiotic, and any cardiovascular drugs that might be required. Cardiovascular drugs usually include syringes of atropine, a pure alpha-adrenergic vasoconstrictor such a meteraminol (0.5 mg/mL), and a dilute solution of a positive inotrope such as epinephrine (adrenaline) 1:10 000. These allow immediate treatment of bradycardia or hypotension to prevent cardiovascular collapse. An infusion of a positive inotrope such as epinephrine (adrenaline) should also be immediately available. In addition, the CPB circuit should be set-up and primed and a surgeon and perfusionist immediately available.

Anaesthetic versus operating room

Following premedication, the patient will arrive in the anaesthetic or operating room depending on your institutional practice. Anaesthetic rooms have a number of benefits, and most

---

> **Box 19.2** Pre-patient arrival check list
>
> - Blood cross-matched and red blood cells available
> - Anaesthetic work stations checked
> - Monitoring equipment switched on and functioning
> - Near-patient testing equipment on and functioning, e.g. blood gas analyser, ACT
> - Sufficient infusion pumps and syringe drivers present
> - Pacing box present and functioning
> - Defibrillator/cardioverter present and functioning
> - Anaesthetic assistants present
> - Operating room staff present and room prepared
> - Heparin, antibiotic, and anaesthetic and cardiovascular drugs prepared and drawn-up
> - Cardiopulmonary bypass circuit set-up and primed
> - Surgeon and perfusionist immediately available

especially, they allow the patient to be set-up and anaesthesia induced in a quiet, controlled environment while the surgical trays are laid out in separate operating room. However, building an anaesthetic room increases capital outlay. Moreover, an important clinical drawback is that the anaesthetized patient then has to be transferred to the operating room. In routine cases transferring a patient to the operating room takes but a few minutes. However, if there is cardiovascular collapse following induction of anaesthesia, rapid institution of CPB may be lifesaving and these few minutes may be precious. So any patient who is assessed to be at risk of cardiovascular collapse, for example ongoing myocardial ischaemia, acute severe valve regurgitation, or tamponade, should always be anaesthetized in the operating room with the surgeon and operating room team scrubbed and prepared for surgery. Wherever the patient is to be anaesthetized, monitoring should be applied (box 19.3), and a preoperative safety check should be performed by all the operating room staff (Chapter 42).

Pacemakers and automatic implantable cardioverter/defibrillators

If the patient has a permanent pacemaker that has not already programmed to a non-sensing mode set at a suitable high rate such as 80 beats per minute, then this may be done before induction of anaesthesia and certainly before the start of surgery as diathermy may inhibit discharge of the pacemaker. On return to the intensive care unit (ICU), the pacemaker should be converted back to a sensing mode to prevent ventricular arrhythmias resulting from pacing on the t-wave. Automatic implantable cardioverter defibrillators (AICD) should also be inhibited before surgery as diathermy may be mistaken by the device for a ventricular arrhythmia and unrequired defibrillation will result.

Neuroaxial and regional techniques

Some anaesthesiologists combine general anaesthesia with a neuroaxial technique such as intrathecal opioids or epidural

Box 19.3 Monitoring

- ◆ Before induction of anaesthesia
  - ECG
  - Pulse oximetry
  - A large bore peripheral IV access (two if large blood loss is anticipated.
  - Arterial line (usually radial artery)
  - Baseline arterial blood gas/blood glucose
  - Near-patient testing of coagulation
  - Cerebral oximetry (if used)
  - Processed EEG (if used)
  - Depth of anaesthesia (if used)
  - Minimally invasive cardiac output monitoring (if used)
- ◆ After induction of anaesthesia
  - Multiple lumen central venous cannulation (before induction if patient unstable)
  - Sheath ± pulmonary artery balloon catheter (if used)
  - TOE probe (if used)

ECG, electrocardiogram; EEG: electroencephalogram,
TOE: transoesophageal echocardiogram.

anaesthesia, or regional techniques such as a paravertebral block. As the thoracic epidural anaesthesia (TEA) is the most controversial of these techniques, it requires further consideration.

There are a number of physiological mechanisms whereby TEA should improve outcome from cardiac surgery and especially CABG surgery. However, a meta-analysis by Svircevic and colleagues found that although TEA combined with general anaesthesia was associated with lower incidences of respiratory complications (relative risk [RR] 0.53 [95% CI 0.40, 0.69]) and supraventricular arrhythmias (RR 0.68 [95% CI 0.50, 093]), it was not associated with significant reductions in mortality (RR 0.81 [95%CI 0.40,1.64]) or myocardial infarction (RR 0.80 [95% CI 0.52,1.24]) (7). Whilst it may be that the sample size of the meta-analysis was too small, the current evidence does not support the view that TEA is associated with myocardial outcome benefits or reduction in mortality.

Risk is the other side of the coin from efficacy and the known unknown is the unquantified risk of epidural haematoma that is associated with using TEA for cardiac anaesthesia. Antiplatelet medications, administration of large doses of heparin for CPB, and the development of coagulopathies might all suggest an increased risk of developing epidural haematoma. Meta-analyses such as Svircivic and colleagues have too small a population size to inform us of the incidence of epidural haematoma (7). So currently, the evidence suggests there are some short-term outcome benefits to be gained by the use of TEA but they come at an unquantified risk of epidural haematoma. Therefore, the risks and benefits of TEA should be assessed on an individual patient basis. If TEA is used then there should be a safe monitoring system to detect epidural haematoma postoperatively and access to MRI for diagnosis.

Intravenous access

At least one large bore IV access (14 g) is essential for administration of intravascular volume replacement as major haemorrhage is an ever present risk of any intrathoracic surgery. A second IV cannula may be prudent in situations when major haemorrhage anticipated for example trauma and aortic dissections. Where peripheral venous access is poor then the use of a large bore central venous cannula is invaluable.

Arterial monitoring line

Although it has no evidence base that it influences outcome, invasive haemodynamic monitoring is one of the hallmarks of cardiac anaesthesia. Before induction of anaesthesia, monitoring should be established in a relaxed environment while providing verbal distraction and reassurance to the patient. Direct measurement of systemic arterial pressure (SAP) is by far the single most useful clinical monitor, as it allows beat-to-beat assessment of the SAP during dynamic phases of the cardiac anaesthesia and surgery. As induction of anaesthesia is one of the most important of such phases, direct measurement of SAP should routinely be established before doing so (figure 19.1). Traditionally, a radial artery was cannulated but the increasing the use of the left radial artery as a conduit for CABG and the right for coronary angiography often forces the use of a brachial or femoral artery. Arterial blood sampling at the time of cannulation for blood gas analysis should be undertaken as it provides a baseline levels for arterial oxygen and carbon dioxide tensions that may valuable in managing weaning patients from mechanical ventilation postoperatively.

Central venous cannulation

Although of minimal value as a monitor of cardiac function, central venous access by way of the internal jugular or subclavian veins, is also essential should inotropic or vasoconstrictor drugs be required. Presently, the author's preference is to routinely use a single, five-lumen catheter as it allows bolusing of drugs centrally, central venous pressure measurement and administration of multiple IV drug infusions including total intravenous anaesthesia (TIVA) (figure 19.2). Many anaesthetists also insert a large-bore pulmonary artery balloon catheter (PABC) sheath catheter in case floating one is required. However, PABC infrequently used now if TOE is available, as this provides far more information about the cardiovascular system so there is currently less indication for the routine insertion of sheaths.

Many anaesthesiologists would place central venous lines following induction of anaesthesia as it is simpler and avoids the patient experiencing any discomfort during insertion. However, if cardiovascular collapse is anticipated then central lines should be placed under local anaesthesia before induction of anaesthesia.

Pharmacological prophylaxis

Alongside anaesthetic consideration, the anaesthetist needs to consider the administration of number of pharmacological agents to minimize the incidence of serious postoperative adverse events associated with cardiac surgery.

Antibiotic prophylaxis

SSI may seem a distant problem when inducing anaesthesia in a patient with cardiovascular disease and so of low priority.

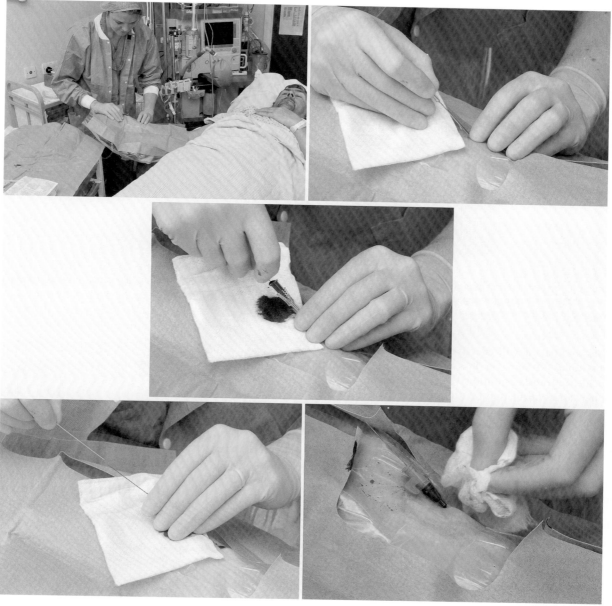

Fig. 19.1 Insertion of radial artery line.
Insertion of an arterial monitoring line into the radial artery to measure systemic arterial pressure, before induction of anaesthesia. Top left: aseptic preparation: Top right: puncture of radial artery with thin walled needle; Middle: insertion of guide wire: Bottom left insertion of cannula over guide wire; Bottom right: arterial cannula in-situ in the radial artery with guide wire still in place.
Photograph supplied by the Department of Medical Illustration, Royal Infirmary of Edinburgh.

However, mediastinal sepsis has at worst has a high mortality and at best, markedly prolongs patients' ICU and hospital stay. Administration of prophylactic antibiotics, although the evidence-base is weak, reduces the incidence of this serious complication of sternotomy (8). So, timely administration of a prophylactic antibiotic should remain high in anaesthesiologists' priorities even in the face of cardiovascular instability (8). The decision as to which antibiotic should be administered and when, what alternatives should be used if there is penicillin allergy and in the presence of MRSA colonization or unknown MRSA status, should be made into an institutional protocol based on the advice

of a microbiologist in conjunction with the surgeons. Further doses of the antibiotic should be given if surgery is prolonged more than 4 hours (8).

Arrhythmia prophylaxis

After cardiac surgery, many patients will develop supraventricular arrhythmias, which may cause cardiovascular compromise, and a few will have ventricular arrhythmias, which can be life-threatening. There is a large body of evidence that indicates that pharmacological prophylaxis including magnesium, amiodarone, beta-adrenergic blockers, some of the calcium channel

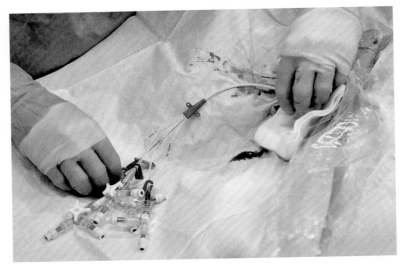

Fig. 19.2 Central venous cannulation.
Insertion of a five-lumen central venous cannula into the right internal jugular vein using a Seldinger technique under asepsis. The insertion of an additional wide bore cannula may be indicated if the use of a pulmonary artery balloon catheter or massive blood loss, is anticipated.
Photograph supplied by the Department of Medical Illustration, Royal Infirmary of Edinburgh.

antagonists, and pacing will effectively reduce the incidence of these arrhythmias (9). However, it is unclear whether this reduction in incidence translates into better clinical outcome (9). For example, new atrial fibrillation that develops after heart surgery will spontaneously resolve within about 6 weeks in most patients. However, in the short term, it can cause profound cardiovascular compromise, most especially in patients who are dependent on the atrial contribution to left ventricular filling to maintain an adequate stroke volume. For this reason, although they have not been recommended for routine use, prophylaxis may be considered for individual patients (9).

Reducing blood loss and transfusion

As there is an overwhelming evidence base that drugs including aprotinin, tranexamic acid, and aminocaproic acid, are efficacious in reducing both blood loss and transfusion as well as sternal re-openings for massive blood loss (Chapters 17 and 18), one such agent should be used. Far more controversial is whether one drug is associated with more adverse events than another (Chapter 17). Intraoperative, mechanical cell salvage during heart surgery will reduce the need for red blood cell transfusion (figure 19.3).

Steroids

Pharmacological immunomodulation of patients undergoing CPB has been proposed as a means of preventing adverse events. Indeed, a recent, large, multicentre RCT was unable to find any significant difference in a composite measure of serious adverse events (SAEs) between patients who received dexamethasone 1 mg/kg or placebo undergoing cardiac surgery with CPB (10). However, dexamethasone was associated with reductions in postoperative infections as well as the durations of mechanical ventilation and ICU and hospital stays. So dexamethasone may be associated with short-term benefits in terms of postoperative management, but it does not prevent SAEs.

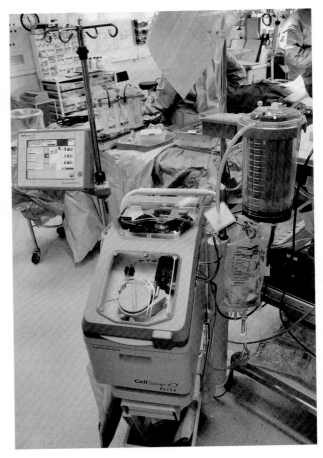

Fig. 19.3 Mechanical cell salvage device.
Mechanical cell salvage minimizes the need for red cell transfusion intraoperatively during routine heart surgery and can been invaluable when massive haemorrhage occurs.
Photograph supplied by the Department of Medical Illustration, Royal Infirmary of Edinburgh.

Induction of anaesthesia

Intravenous induction agents

Following preoxygenation, the author favours a small to moderate dose of fentanyl (250 μg) followed by etomidate (~0.2 mg/kg) then using rocuronium 1 mg/kg, as it results in little hypotension and rapid neuromusclar blockade, facilitating early tracheal intubation. Even with just a single dose, etomidate is associated with measurable adrenal suppression for the first 24 hours after cardiac surgery (11). However, there is no evidence that this physiological derangement translates into adverse patient outcomes. Propofol or thiopentone combined with an opioid can be used just as well if hypotension is corrected with vasoconstrictors and ketamine is favoured by some for induction in patients who are cardiovascularly compromised.

Whatever, agents are used for induction of anaesthesia, if hypotension and/or bradycardia ensue then they should be rapidly corrected by IV administration of a vasconstrictor and/or anticholinergic such as atropine or glycopyrolate. This is most especially so in patients with unstable angina or severe aortic stenosis when cardiovascular collapse may result in cardiac arrest. Positive inotropic agents such as adrenaline or ephedrine are infrequently required to control the cardiovascular system and they are usually not used as first-line treatments because of their adverse effect on myocardial oxygen supply/demand balance in patients with CAD. However, in a small number of circumstances (such as tamponade), it may be prudent to start an IV infusion of a positive inotrope before induction of anaesthesia as no matter what technique is used, cardiovascular collapse may occur on induction. In patients deemed to be 'high risk', consideration should be given to insertion of an intra-aortic balloon pump (IABP) before induction of anaesthesia in patients who are deemed to be 'high risk' as systematic review and meta-analysis indicates that its use is associated with a much lower in-hospital mortality and a much lower incidence of low cardiac output in the postoperative period (12).

Neuromuscular blockade

Pancuronium often in large doses, has long been favoured as the neuromuscular blockade (NMB) for cardiac anaesthesia because its vagolytic action reduces the risk of bradycardia developing during induction of anaesthesia. However, pancuronium's prolonged duration of action when used for cardiac anaesthesia does not facilitate enhanced recovery (13). Infusions of short-acting NMBs may be used, but are generally not required as an intubating dose then supplemental boluses of rocuronium or atracurium may be used successfully.

Cardiac anaesthesia has had poor history of awareness and a further advantage of using a short- rather than a long-acting NMB is that spontaneous movement alerts the anaesthetist to light levels of anaesthesia in the patient. This is most especially so when other clinical signs of depth of anaesthesia are masked during CPB. However, if this approach is taken then the anaesthetist needs to be alert for movement as it requires rapid administration of additional NMB and increasing the depth of anaesthesia to prevent patient harm as result of movement. Alternatively, if NMB is desired throughout surgery then a depth of anaesthesia monitor might be used to identify lightening of anaesthesia.

Following induction of anaesthesia

After IV induction of anaesthesia and obtaining NMB, the trachea should be intubated. A temperature probe should be inserted into the nasopharynx to measure core body temperature. Whilst central venous cannulation is taking place, a urinary catheter should inserted to monitor urine output during and after surgery. Core body temperature may alternatively be measured using a urinary catheter that incorporates a temperature probe. Finally, a TOE probe should be inserted, if indicated, and there are no contraindications. Before surgery, the patient should then be positioned taking care to protect the patient from pressure injuries. After ensuring that the patient is being adequately mechanically ventilated, all monitoring is functional, and anaesthetized then if required, TOE examination should be performed while the patient is being surgically prepped.

If cardiovascular collapse occurs following induction that is not correctable by vasoconstrictors, anticholinergics, and positive inotropes, then the surgeon should surgically prepare the patient, open the sternum and institute CPB with alacrity. Should collapse reach the stage where there is little or no cardiac output, cardiac massage should be instituted. However, it will greatly complicates the institution of CPB and increases the likelihood of an adverse outcome.

Maintenance of anaesthesia

Total intravenous anaesthesia

Maintenance of anaesthesia for cardiac surgery was traditionally a balanced technique including an inhalational agent, opioid, and NMB; but from the late 1960s high-dose opioid anaesthesia was the popular technique. In the last two decades, it has reverted to a balanced technique most commonly using TIVA although techniques using inhalational agents are still favoured by some anaesthesiologists. TIVA has practical advantages as it is easily be administered and controlled by the anaesthetist throughout surgery, and especially during CPB.

Inhalational-based techniques

To administer an inhalational technique throughout surgery requires the mounting of an anaesthetic vaporizer on the CPB machine in the sweep gas supply to the oxygenator along with standard delivery of inhalational agents before and after CPB from an anaesthesia work station. Delivering inhalational agents during CPB presents a number of logistic problems: although supervised by the anaesthetist, administration is under the direct control of the perfusionist; variable transfer of inhalational agent across different oxygenators; the requirement for scavenging gases from the oxygenator exhaust: and requirement to switch-on the anaesthetic vaporizer on the anaesthesia work station when resuming mechanical ventilation before weaning from CPB (14). However, overcoming the practical drawbacks of administering an inhalational anaesthetic agent may have important outcome benefits. Compared to TIVA, systematic review and meta-analysis has associated sevoflurane- and desflurane-based techniques with a lower incidence of myocardial infarction (OR 0.51 [95%CI 0.32–0.84]) and mortality (OR = 0.31 [(95% CI 0.12–0.80]) (15). On this basis, an international consensus group has recommended their use (16).

Sternotomy

Sternotomy is another important surgical event for the anaesthetist as sawing can infrequently transect the right ventricle, right atrium, or aorta and all of which can cause precipitous haemorrhage and hamper establishment of CPB. This a more likely occurrence in re-do sternotomy when the heart may be adhered to the posterior of the sternum. Using alternate cannulation sites such as femoro-femoro allows safe establishment of CPB and decompresses the heart, making cardiac trauma less likely. Traditionally, the surgeon will ask for IPPV to be discontinued during sternotomy so if the pleura is transection then the lung will safely collapse out of the surgical field. However, evidence of the efficacy of this manoeuvre is lacking and it is not required during re-sternotomy because of adhesions.

Anticoagulation for cardiopulmonary bypass

Heparin

The surgeon will request heparin to be administered usually before transecting the distal end of the mammary artery, during CABG surgery and before cannulating the aorta in other forms of heart surgery. Heparin is commonly administered in a dose of 300 IU/kg by slow IV injection. Completion of the administration should be announced so that surgeon and perfusionist know that the patient is anticoagulated so that it is both safe to cannulate and aspirate shed blood from the cardiotomy back into the CPB circuit. The announcement should also trigger blood sampling to measure the activated clotting time (ACT) (Chapter 17). Most especially in emergencies, it is important that measurement of the ACT is not overlooked as failure to do so can delay the safe institution of CPB. There is institutional variation in actual threshold of ACT deemed sufficiently anticoagulated to initiate CPB but usually it is in the range 400–500 s.

Heparin resistance

Much less commonly than in the past when patients with unstable angina were maintained on IV infusions of heparin, some patients will have resistance to heparin because of antithrombin III deficiency. Often additional doses of heparin will take the ACT above the required threshold but sometimes supplying antithrombin III as concentrate or fresh frozen plasma will be required (17) (Chapter 11).

Alternatives to heparin

Also far less common than in the past, because patients with unstable angina are maintained preoperatively on antiplatelet agent rather than heparin, are the number of patients who have heparin-induced thrombocytopenia (HIT) (Chapter 16). There are a variety of different approaches that can be taken to anticoagulation that are beyond the scope of this chapter and readers wishing to know more are referred elsewhere (18).

Cardiopulmonary bypass

Before the surgeon cannulates the aorta, the anaesthetist should ensure that the systemic arterial blood pressure is well controlled using anaesthetic agents, vasodilators and/or head-up positioning, to prevent disruption of the aorta during cannulation. Once the surgeon has cannulated the aorta and venous system and the ACT has reached the required threshold, the surgeon will ask the perfusionist to go on CPB. The perfusionist will release the clamp on the venous line to drain blood and gradually increase the arterial pump flow rate until it reaches the predicted flow rate required ('full flow'). Once full flow is achieved and there is no cardiac output then mechanical ventilation may be discontinued, pulse oximetry should be removed to prevent pressure injury and the monitoring alarms switched-off. If an inhalational technique is being used then the anaesthetist should ensure that the vaporizer is mounted in the sweep gas supply to the oxygenator, it is adequately filled with the anaesthetic agent and it is switched-on at the required level. Although it relationship to blood concentrations is unclear, monitoring oxygenator exhaust levels of inhalational agent using an agent monitor allows detection of supply failure should the vaporizer empty undetected.

Once full pump flow on CPB is established, the surgeon will cross-clamp the aorta and administer cardioplegia to arrest the heart in diastole (Chapter 15). After this point, there is little that the anaesthetist is required to do until the aortic cross-clamp is removed. However, the anaesthetist should remain immediately available as although extremely rare, potentially catastrophic pump accidents or oxygenator failures occur requiring emergency reinstatement of the spontaneous circulation.

Lung management during cardiopulmonary bypass

During CPB, continuous positive airway pressure and vital capacity manoeuvres have been advocated for lung protection. However, a recent meta-analysis indicates that whilst at best, they improve oxygenation in the short-term, these manoeuvres have no long-term outcome benefits (19).

Carbon dioxide insufflation

All open heart surgery will result in entry of air into cavities of the heart and pulmonary blood vessels. Despite extensive manoeuvres by the surgeon to expel air, some may remain when the circulation is restored and that may then embolize. To minimize any harm resulting from such emboli, carbon dioxide is insufflated into the cardiotomy area to denitrogenate the operative field. Thus, any emboli generated would be more rapidly absorbed because of the greater solubility of carbon dioxide compared to nitrogen, so limiting any organ damage. Carbon dioxide insufflation is also used surgically to clear the surgical field of blood.

Glycaemic control

Hyperglycaemia is common during cardiac surgery, because many patients presenting for surgery have diabetes mellitus. Even in patients who do not have diabetes mellitus, the high level of stress associated with cardiac surgery and CPB also promotes hyperglycaemia as does the use of catacholamines. Control of hyperglycaemia requires administration of IV insulin, and frequently in large doses, as patients are often insulin resistant during and after CPB.

Whilst the importance of controlling hyperglycaemia during and after surgery is well accepted, the degree of that control is more controversial. There is some weak evidence from systematic review and meta-analysis that tight compared to 'normal' control is associated with a reduced incidence of early mortality (death in the intensive care unit [ICU] (OR 0.52 [95% CI 0.30, 0.91]); of post-surgical atrial fibrillation (odds ratio (OR 0.76 [95%CI 0.58, 0.99]); the use of epicardial pacing (OR 0.28 [95%CI 0.15, 0.54]); the durations of mechanical ventilation (mean difference (MD) –3.69 [95% CI –3.85, –3.54]) and stay in the ICU (MD –0.57 [95%CI –0.60, –0.55]) days (20). However, tight glycaemic control can result in hypoglycaemia, which has its own intrinsic effect on mortality and morbidity. Yet, this is poorly quantified in this setting so the balance of benefit to risk of this approach over 'normal' control, remains unclear.

Weaning from cardiopulmonary bypass

Weaning from CPB is a crucial stage and so it is essential that the anaesthetist is well prepared for this event. Failure to wean successfully from CPB may not only prolong the surgery but may adversely affect patient outcome. To be adequately prepared, there are many routine tasks and checks that should be undertaken before weaning are listed in box 19.4.

Box 19.4 Pre-weaning from cardiopulmonary bypass checklist

- Anaesthetic assistant present in the operating room or immediately available
- Blood tests
  - Acid–base balance normal—correct metabolic acidosis
  - Potassium concentration > 4.5 < 6.5 mmol/L
  - Haemoglobin concentration > 60 g/L
  - Blood sugar < 10 mmol/ L
  - Calcium concentration > 1.2 mmol/ L
- Monitoring
  - Monitoring in correct mode
  - Alarms re-established
  - Transducers zeroed
  - Arterial pressure trace accurate (aorto-radial discrepancy)
- Rewarmed to 37ºC
- Heart rhythm
  - Pacing box immediately available (even if not required for weaning)
  - Establish sinus rhythm or ventricular or ideally, dual chamber synchronized pacing
    - Cardioversion
    - Anti-arrhythmic drug
    - Epicardial pacing effective
  - Heart rate 60–100 beats per minute
- Cardiovascular function
  - Visual assessment of heart function
  - TOE examination to ensure air eliminated from heart
  - Vasoconstrictor and anticholinergic drawn-up and immediately available
  - Intravascular fluids connected
  - Positive inotropes and infusion devices immediately available/connected/ running
- Coagulation
  - Protamine dose calculated, drawn-up, labelled and placed in separate area from other drugs
  - Activated clotting time > 450 s
  - Blood products ordered (if severe coagulopathy/high volume blood loss anticipated)

(Continued)

Box 19.4 (Continued)

- • Transfusion device in the operating room (if high volume blood loss anticipated)
    - • Near patient test of coagulation if coagulopathy anticipated, e.g. viscoelastic testing
- ◆ Ventilation
    - • Pleural spaces checked for pneumothorax if closed and if opened, suctioned for occult blood loss by the surgeon
    - • Gas supply on 100% oxygen
    - • Breathing circuit is reconnected (if disconnected during CPB)
    - • Lungs fully re-expanded manually (in cooperation with surgeon)
    - • Suction trachea if secretions noted on re-expansion
    - • Mechanical ventilation re-established (confirmation should be sought by surgeon or perfusionist)
- ◆ Anaesthesia
    - • Volatile anaesthetic agent switched-on if inhalational technique being used or
    - • Adequate amounts of drugs available for TIVA

TOE, transoesophageal echocardiography; CPB, cardiopulmonary bypass; TIVA, total intravenous anaesthesia.

Cardiac rate and rhythm

With modern cardioplegia techniques, the heart often resumes contraction in sinus rhythm. Sometimes, a ventricular arrhythmia will occur and defibrillation or cardioversion will usually convert the conduction to sinus rhythm but administration of anti-arrhythmic drugs may be required as well. Sometimes, supraventricular tachycardia will occur and will require synchronized cardioversion to re-establish sinus rhythm. Much more commonly, bradycardias (frequently nodal rhythms), occur and require epicardial pacing to generate an adequate heart rate and synchronized contraction of atria and ventricles, to generate an adequate cardiac output (figure 19.4). Arbitrarily, a rate of 80 beats/min is commonly used, although higher rate should be used if cardiac function is poor.

Lung re-inflation

If one or both pleura have been opened then one or both lungs will have collapsed and they will require to be manually re-expanded by compression of the reservoir bag before weaning. This re-expansion should be done in cooperation with the surgeon most especially when the internal mammary artery has been used. The surgeon should protect the mammary artery during manual inflation as it possible to avulse the graft. In addition, the surgeon may have better vision of the pleural space than the anaesthesiologists so can see whether the lungs are fully expanded. Once the lungs have been fully expanded then mechanical ventilation should be recommenced.

Assessment of cardiac function

Before weaning from CPB, the anaesthetist should make a visual and TOE assessment of cardiac function. Whilst the right ventricle filling and systolic function can be easily assessed by direct vision, the left ventricle is usual hidden from the anaesthesiologist's line of sight and TOE is required to image its function and filling. Whilst it is not be possible to fully assess the

heart's systolic function until it has been volume loaded, one can get a good impression as to whether positive inotropes will be required to support the circulation after weaning. If heart function seems poor then a positive inotropic infusion should be prepared and connected to the patient, if not already running.

Positive inotropic agents

There are a large variety of positive inotropic agents that are used to wean patients off CPB and the evidence base to advocate one inotrope over another is lacking (Chapter 6). However, one systematic review and meta-analysis indicates that levosimendan may be associated with about a 50% reduction in mortality (21). However, levosimendan is not available in many countries and the author most commonly uses epinephine (adrenaline) and/or norepinephrine (noradrenaline).

Communication

Weaning from CPB is a crucial stage of surgery that demands a high level of communication and interaction (Chapter 41). The anaesthetist, surgeon, and perfusionist each have important roles but they must function tightly together as a team to successfully wean patients from CPB. The surgeon should establish that the anaesthetist and perfusionist are aware that he is going start weaning and aspirate the pleural spaces to make sure that there has no occult blood loss. Clear instructions, acknowledgements, confirmations, and communications of any difficulties need to be provided by all three. For example, it should be orally established by the surgeon or perfusionist, and confirmed by the anaesthetist, that the patient is being mechanically ventilated before weaning.

If the surgeon is content that the heart is functioning well, he will instruct the perfusionist to 'come down and come off. Whilst watching the arterial and central venous pressures, the perfusionist will gradually reduce siphonage of venous blood into the reservoir and decrease the pump flow rate until it is zero. As the venous

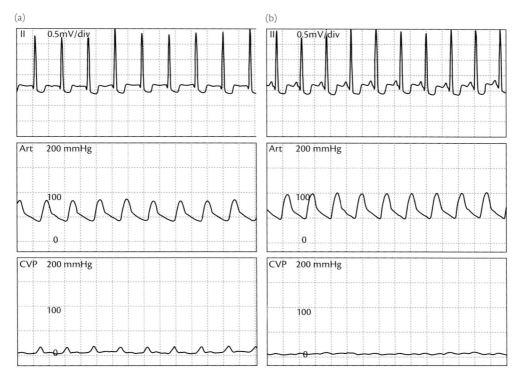

Fig. 19.4 Effect of conversion of nodal to sinus rhythm on systemic arterial pressure.
(a) (left). A screen shot of monitoring showing nodal tachycardia on the electrocardiograph trace with systemic arterial hypotension as measured by the arterial line (Art) and cannon waves on central venous pressure (CVP) tracing. Cannon waves result from atrial systole when tricuspid valve is closed. (b) (right). A screen shot of monitoring showing the beneficial effect of conversion to sinus tachycardia with an increase systemic arterial pressure and loss of cannon waves on CVP.

return to the heart increases, and because of the Frank–Starling mechanism, the cardiac output will increase and the flat arterial trace will resume a pulsatile form. Successful weaning will result in an adequate SAP and a low central venous pressure (CVP). Fine adjustment of the SAP may require administration of aliquots of blood, usually 100 mL, from the pump. If the anaesthetist asks the perfusionist to give blood from the pump, it should be checked with the surgeon that it is safe to do so. For example, the surgeon may have clamped the aortic line or gas might have accumulated in the arterial line. An adequate SAP is difficult to define absolutely but is one that the anaesthetist and surgeon feel mutually comfortable with. Too high a SAP might cause disruption of the aorta during de-cannulation and excessive bleeding whilst too low might result precipitate a vicious spiral of cardiovascular collapse. Once off pump, the surgeon will quickly remove the venous line as if left in situ, it may impair venous return to the heart.

Successful weaning

If most cases, weaning is successful and if the patient is cardiovascularly stable, the surgeon will ask for the protamine, decannulate heart and aorta, secure haemostasis, and then close the sternum and skin. This is usually uneventful, although if the vascular system is under-filled by the anaesthetist then hypotension may occur when the sternum is closed. Sometimes this may also occur if the surgeon decides to close the pericardium because the patient is young and to facilitate future re-sternotomy to replace an aortic prosthetic valve when it fails. Hypotension as a result of hypovolaemia can

usually be prevented by adequate re-infusion of pump blood, cell salvaged blood, or other forms of volume replacement.

Rarely, cardiovascular collapse may occur late after an initial successful weaning, as a result of coronary gas embolism in open heart surgery or graft failure in patients undergoing CABG surgery. Systemic hypotension that is unresponsive to vasoconstrictors, bradycardia unresponsive to atropine and ST changes are hallmarks of such events. Air will preferentially embolize down the right coronary artery because its ostia is at the highest point of the aorta. Elevating the blood pressure with vasoconstrictors, plus or minus a positive inotrope, usually dissipates the gas and recovery of the myocardial ischaemia. Unheralded ventricular tachyarrhythmias can also occur late after a successful wean and are also indicative graft failure. Prompt cardioversion and administration of anti-arrhythmic drugs are required.

Unsuccessful weaning

Systemic hypotension despite intravascular volume loading from the pump, following weaning from CPB is an ominous sign especially if associated with elevated CVP or pulmonary capillary wedge pressure and is unresponsive to boluses of vasoconstrictors. The causes for failure to wean from CPB that are listed in box 19.5.

Diagnosis

Prompt diagnosis of the cause or causes of the cardiovascular dysfunction is most important for accurate applying treatment to avoid the need re-institute CPB. Visually, it is possible to assess the function and filling of the right ventricle and the surgeon can assess pulmonary artery pressure by palpation. If there is a PABC

Box 19.5 Potential causes of failure to wean from cardiopulmonary bypass

- Left and right ventricular dysfunction
  - Systolic ventricular dysfunction
  - Myocardial ischaemia
    - Preoperative myocardial infarction
    - Kinking or spasm of coronary artery bypass graft
    - Coronary embolism—air, atheromatous plaque, thrombus
    - Obstruction of coronary ostia, e.g. malposition of aortic valve prothesis
    - Incomplete coronary artery revascularization
    - Myocardial stunning—inadequate cardioplegia, prolonged duration of aortic cross-clamping
    - Hypoxia—pulmonary oedema, failure to restart mechanical ventilation
- Diastolic ventricular dysfunction
  - Myocardial ischaemia—as for Systolic ventricular dysfunction
  - Pre-existing left ventricular hypertrophy—aortic stenosis, systemic hypertension,
  - Pre-existing right ventricular hypertrophy—pulmonary hypertension secondary to mitral valve or pulmonary disease
  - Pressure overload—systemic or pulmonary vasoconstriction
  - Volume overload—excessive transfusion of blood from CPB circuit or intravascular fluids by anaesthetist
  - Tamponade—closure of pericardium or sternum, hyperinflated lungs, PEEP
- Hypovolaemia
  - Inadequate transfusion of blood from CPB circuit
  - Occult blood loss
  - Vasodilation
  - Preoperative administration of vasodilating drugs—ACE inhibitors
  - Prolonged duration of CPB
  - Sepsis—bacterial endocarditis
- Arrhythmias
  - Atrial fibrillation
  - Heart block
  - Nodal rhythm
- Valve dysfunction
  - Malfunction of prosthetic valve—stuck leaflet
  - Exacerbation of native valve dysfunction—mitral regurgitation
- Dynamic left ventricular outflow tract obstruction
  - Following mitral valve repair
  - Following aortic valve replacement
  - Left ventricular hypertrophy
  - Hypertrophic cardiomyopathy
- High rate of blood loss—inadequate surgical haemostasis
- Hypoxia -
  - Pulmonary oedema
  - Atrial septal defect—patent foramen ovale
  - Venous admixture—low cardiac output

in situ then it is possible to get some estimation of cardiac output, left ventricular function, or peripheral vascular resistance. In this situation, TOE comes into its own as both right and left ventricular filling and function can be assessed as well as the functioning of native and implanted valves.

Recommencing cardiopulmonary bypass

Institution of positive inotropes and/or insertion of an IABP may stabilize the patient, but sometimes cardiovascular collapse continues and a decision should be made to go back on CPB. If protamine has not been given, and as long as the venous line has not been drained, then the surgeon can usually rapidly achieve this by simply reinserting the venous line. Once CPB has been recommenced, the work of the heart will be greatly diminished using a full or partial flow rate so allowing it to recover. If CABG surgery has been undertaken then the surgeon should confirm that graft flow is satisfactory and none of the grafts are kinked. If graft flow is inadequate then the surgeon may need to undertake additional CABG. Rarely, valve replacement or repair has been undertaken then consideration of malfunction of the prosthetic valve or repair. If the surgeon considers this is a serious possibility, or there are TOE findings to this effect, then aortic cross-clamping, cardioplegia, and reopening of the heart may be required to correct the fault.

Hypovolaemia

Hypovolaemia can be diagnosed empirically using the Frank–Starling's Law, by a rising SAP with little increase in CVP, in response to transfusion of aliquots of blood from the pump. No change or a decrease in systemic arterial pressure and an increasing CVP are ominous and suggest marked dysfunction left, right or both ventricles. Hypovolaemia as a result of uncontrolled haemorrhage will usually require re-establishment of CPB and securing of surgical haemostasis.

Heart rate and rhythm

As cardiac output is the product of stroke volume and heart rate, then increasing the heart rate by epicardial pacing will be valuable. The atrial contribution to ventricular filling may be important especially in the setting of a poorly functioning, poorly compliant LV; such LV hypertrophy is associated with aortic stenosis. In this circumstance, synchronized dual-chamber rather than only ventricular pacing, will be beneficial. In the presence of arrhythmias, cardioverting them to sinus rhythm or suppressing them pharmaceutically, to allow effective pacing may also be valuable.

Vasodilation

Vasodilation is common, probably because of the frequent preoperative use of angiotensin-converting enzyme inhibitors and angiotensin blockers in today's patient, and can easily be overlooked as a cause of hypotension. Prolonged CPB commonly also results in vasodilation. Sepsis arising during heart surgery from active endocarditis can also cause profound catecholamine resistant, vasodilation that requires treatment with vasopressin. A high cardiac output as measured by PABC associated with a low SAP, can point to the diagnosis and demonstration of a high aortic-radial SAP gradient will confirm the diagnosis. Again, TOE can also aid diagnosis of vasodilation.

Left ventricular systolic dysfunction

If LV systolic dysfunction is believed to be the cause the haemodynamic instability then institution of positive inotropic support

may all that be required. IABP along with inotropic support, will be necessary for more severe LV systolic function. However, insertion of an IABP can take time and it may be best to elect to go back on CPB to rest the heart while this is done. Sometimes, time resting on CPB is all that is required for the heart to overcome myocardial stunning. This is often the case when the LV is hypertrophied, when myocardial preservation may have been less than optimal. If myocardial ischaemia is diagnosed by ST changes on the ECG or new segmental wall motion abnormality (SWMA) on TOE, and especially if the surgeon feels that revascularization was incomplete, then prompt insertion of an IABP to support coronary blood flow will be required. However, resumption of CPB may be required to allow additional CABGs to be placed by the surgeon.

Right ventricular dysfunction

Despite being able to see its anterior wall, RV dysfunction is often a more difficult diagnosis than LV dysfunction and once made, it is far more challenging to manage. In severe RV dysfunction, PABC measurements or TOE imaging of the left ventricular function may misleadingly indicate hypovolaemia as the diagnosis because of low left heart pressures or small LV end systolic area. In this circumstance, under-filling of the LV represents a failure of forward flow from the RV and not absolute hypovolaemia. Further transfusion will only exacerbate the volume overload of right heart and may cause tricuspid regurgitation, so an accurate diagnosis of RV dysfunction is essential. RV dysfunction may occur in isolation, for example when unvented gas embolizes down the right coronary artery. However, RV dysfunction also occurs secondary to or in combination with LV dysfunction. Indeed, sometimes the extent of LV dysfunction is only unveiled when the RV function is improved.

An elevated CVP in the face of systemic hypotension will impair right coronary perfusion, exacerbating RV dysfunction. Therefore, besides inotropic support, treating RV dysfunction requires reducing CVP and RV after-load whilst maintaining an adequate mean SAP. Starting at 10 ppm, inhaled nitric oxide is probably the most reliable and fastest way to produce pulmonary vasodilation to RV afterload whilst a vasoconstricting inotrope such a norepinephrine (noradrenaline) can be used to maintain an adequate mean SAP. Alternatively, inhaled prostacyclin or IV sildenafil may be used to off-load the RV. IABP is also invaluable in this situation as it also helps maintain an adequate mean SAP and so, right coronary perfusion. Protamine should be administered extremely cautiously when RV dysfunction is severe, as any increase in pulmonary vascular resistance may precipitate cardiovascular collapse.

Dynamic left ventricular outflow tract obstruction

Dynamic left ventricular outflow tract (LVOT) obstruction is a rare but important cause of failure to wean from CPB that is associated with mitral valve repair, aortic valve replacement, and hypertrophic cardiomyopathy. However, it can occur in patients with severe LV hypertrophy in presence of hypovolaemia, vasodilation, and beta-adrenergic agonists. Systolic anterior motion (SAM) of the anterior mitral leaflet into the LVOT during systole will both cause mitral regurgitation and obstruct flow precipitating marked haemodynamic compromise. The diagnosis of dynamic LVOT by SAM is important as the haemodynamic compromise is exacerbated by the standard treatments for failure to wean from

CPB that is increasing doses of positive beta-adrenergic agonists. Moreover, treatment is counterintuitive to standard approaches to cardiovascular dysfunction as beta-adrenergic agonists should be discontinued if they are being and intravascular volume loading and increasing after-load with vasoconstrictors are required.

Protamine administration

Once the surgeon and anaesthetist agree that stable cardiovascular function has been achieved, the surgeon will ask for protamine to be administered to antagonize the remaining heparin. A standard dose of protamine is 1 mg per 100 units of heparin that has been administered. However, judging the amount of active heparin at the end of CPB is difficult and the dose required varies greatly. Again, it is important for the anaesthetist to communicate on starting administration so that perfusionist knows to stop the cardiodotomy suction. This is to prevent contaminating the residual blood in the CPB circuit with protamine and so clotting it and precluding re-establishment of CPB. Finishing the injection of protamine or after an agreed proportion, should also be communicated so that the surgeon knows that the aortic line can safely be removed before it clots.

Confirming complete heparin reversal

No matter which dosing regime is used, it is important to confirm that the ACT has returned to baseline and if not, then the administration of additional protamine is required. However, there may be residual heparin activity even in the presence of a normalized ACT. Undertaking additional near-patient visco-elastic testing of coagulation may identify residual heparin activity as well as other coagulopathies (figure 19.5) (Chapters 17 and 18)

Reactions to protamine

Protamine administration can precipitate a spectrum of reactions, from mild systemic hypotension due to simple histamine release, to full blown anaphylactic reaction (with urticaria, bronchospasm, systemic hypotension, pulmonary hypertension, and right heart failure) (22). The former is commonly the result of excessive speed of administration and can usually be quickly resolved by administering a vasoconstrictor. The latter usually results in cardiovascular collapse that often makes necessary re-administration of a full dose of heparin so that CPB may be quickly recommenced. Sometimes, administration of epinephrine, H1 and H2 antihistamine drugs and a corticosteroid alone with salvage the situation. As an anaphylactoid reaction is an ever-present risk associated with its administration, additional heparin should always be immediately available in case a severe protamine reaction occurs or drawn-up if difficulty is anticipated (e.g. redo heart surgery).

Hypoxia

Hypoxia on weaning from CPB is uncommon, but important to detect, as it can precipitate cardiovascular collapse as it causes myocardial dysfunction. Inadequate re-expansion of the lungs is a simple cause that can be rapidly corrected by alveolar recruitment manoeuvres. Pulmonary oedema is another more serious cause as it is much more difficult to manage. This may arise if there has been severe LV failure before CPB. Lung recruitment, then applying

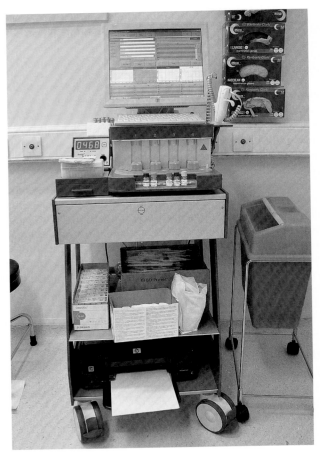

Fig. 19.5 Near patient coagulation testing.
Devices for measuring activated clotting (ACT) (on the left) and viscoelastic assessment of coagulation (on the right). ACT is used to monitoring anticoagulation on cardiopulmonary bypass (CPB) when it is usually maintained >450 s using IV heparin. ACT is also used to assess whether sufficient protamine has been administered to antagonize all heparin activity after weaning from CPB. The viscoelastic device is used to diagnose the presence and character of any coagulopathy following protamine administration.
Photographs supplied by the Department of Medical Illustration, Royal Infirmary of Edinburgh.

positive end-expiratory pressure may be sufficient to obtain adequate oxygenation, but nitric oxide might be required to obtain adequate oxygenation if this is insufficient. Shunting through a septal defect should also be considered and a TOE examination performed to eliminate or confirm this diagnosis.

Securing haemostasis

After successfully weaning from CPB, the surgeon has to decannulate and, importantly, secure haemostasis. However, it is also important to diagnose and treat any coagulopathy that has developed. Traditionally, the failure of blood to clot in the cardiotomy was used by surgeons to clinically diagnose coagulopathy. Laboratory tests of coagulation were also slow to be reported so patients were commonly, empirically, and often unnecessarily, given fresh frozen plasma and platelet concentrate. However, near-patient testing (Chapters 17 and 18), have tempered this and allowed more accurate diagnosis and more targeted treatment.

Chest closure

Once haemostasis has been secured, sternal closure is next important surgical event for the anaesthetist, as it may precipitate hypotension and infrequently, cardiovascular collapse. Hypotension is commonly the result of under-filling following CPB and is simply resolved with intravascular volume transfusion. However, it is important to differentiate under-filling from cardiac dilatation, which is a far more malign cause of hypotension, most especially when associated with poor ventricular systolic function. In this case, sternal closure can cause tamponade and initial treatment is increased support with positive inotropes rather than volume transfusion. Ensuring complete NMB is useful as increased diaphragmatic tone can contribute to the tamponade. If hypotension is not quickly resolved then the surgeon should reopen the sternum until cardiovascular stability can be restored with increased doses of positive inotropes and IABP before attempting to close the sternum again. Rarely, leaving the chest open with a sterile dressing, for a day or two until there is sufficient recovery of cardiac function, is the safest course of action.

Transfer to critical care

Another important event when the patient is vulnerable, is transfer of the patient to critical care (figure 19.6). Moving a patient who is cardiovascularly unstable from the operating table to their bed can be associated with cardiovascular collapse so the anaesthetist needs to remain vigilant of the SAP at this time, as the other members of the operating room team will be preoccupied with their own tasks.

Transferring patient from the operating room to the ICU or recovery areas is also a vulnerable period when there may little immediate technical or human support (figure 19.7). Direct measurement of SAP and ECG are the minimum required for monitoring. Pulse oximetry is also valuable to detect hypoxia. Sedation needs to be continued during transfer as patient emergence from anaesthesia may also cause cardiovascular instability. Mechanical ventilation will also be required and commonly, hand ventilation using a Mapleson C circuit is used and it should be confirmed that there is an adequate reserve of oxygen present in the cylinder before leaving the operating room. If positive inotropes and or vasconstrictors are being administered then they need to be continued and syringe drivers and pump need to have adequate battery reserves to cover transfer. Also, drugs for resuscitation should be taken with the patient in case of emergencies.

On arrival in the critical care area, monitoring needs to be transferred and the patient established on the mechanical ventilator (figure 19.8). IV infusions and drug infusion pumps should be transferred and connected to the mains electrical supply. Once the physical transfer is complete and the patient condition is stable, a full verbal and written handover to medical and nursing staff should be undertaken before the anaesthetist leaves the patient (Chapter 26).

Sternal reopening

Sternal reopening is infrequently required after heart surgery because of ongoing blood loss or tamponade. Patients with excessive blood loss without tamponade can usually be safely transferred back to an operating room for re-exploration is an aseptic environment. However, tamponade major haemorrhage can present as cardiovascular collapse and resuscitation may require emergency sternal reopening in the ICU. Commonly, the patient's trachea has not been extubated so all that is required is to provide anaesthesia and neuromuscular blockade and TIVA is a good approach, especially if surgery is conducted in the ICU. Patients with tamponade, and whose trachea has been extubated, are challenging as any approach to induction of anaesthesia is likely to precipitate cardiovascular collapse that can only be treated by

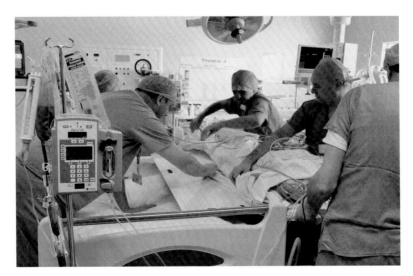

Fig. 19.6 Transferring a patient from the operating table to their bed.
Transferring the patient from the operating table to their bed following heart surgery is a vulnerable period and so merits a high degree of vigilance by the anaesthetist as other operating team members will be distracted by their own tasks. Movement can precipitate hypotension as a result of fluid shifts and most especially in the patient who is cardiovascularly unstable. The anaesthetist should take the lead role directing patient care from this time.
Photograph supplied by the Department of Medical Illustration, Royal Infirmary of Edinburgh.

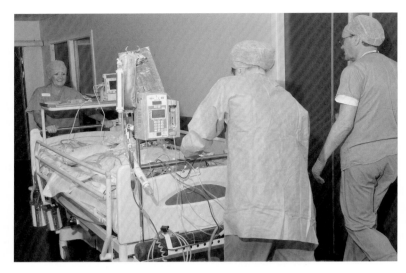

Fig. 19.7 Transfer to the critical care area.
Transferring the patient from the operating room to the critical area is a vulnerable period as there is little technical or human support immediately available. Arterial pressure and ECG is the minimum monitoring during transfer.
Photograph supplied by the Department of Medical Illustration, Royal Infirmary of Edinburgh.

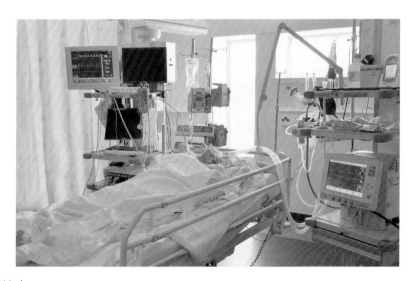

Fig. 19.8 Patient established in critical care.
Patient established fully monitored, on a mechanical ventilator with inotropic infusion in critical care. Having safely established the patient then the anaesthetist must provide a full hand over of relevant information and operative events should be given to the nurse and doctor in charge of the patient and provide all required written instructions (Chapter 26).
Photograph supplied by the Department of Medical Illustration, Royal Infirmary of Edinburgh.

sternal reopening. Wherever the patient is operated on, additional antibiotic prophylaxis should be administered.

Conclusion

Cardiac anaesthesia is a complex procedure that requires a deep understanding of cardiovascular physiology, pathophysiology and pharmacology along with a sound understanding of the delivery of anaesthesia to patients with cardiac disease and during CPB as well as the ability to use TOE. However, successful mastery of these cognitive and practical skills by anaesthesiologists allows

the safe delivery of anaesthesia to tens of thousands of patients around the world every year.

References

1. DeRiso AJ, 2nd, Ladowski JS, Dillon TA, Justice JW, Peterson AC. Chlorhexidine gluconate 0.12% oral rinse reduces the incidence of total nosocomial respiratory infection and nonprophylactic systemic antibiotic use in patients undergoing heart surgery. *Chest* 1996; **109**(6): 1556–61
2. Landoni G, Rodseth RN, Santini F, et al. Randomized evidence for reduction of perioperative mortality. *J Cardiothorac Vasc Anesth* 2012; **26**(5): 764–72

3. Takagi H, Umemoto T. A meta-analysis of controlled studies of pre-operative statin therapy for prevention of postoperative mortality in cardiac surgery. *J Thorac Cardiovasc Surg* 2009; **138**(3): 790–1

4. Landoni G, Augoustides JG, Guarracino F, et al. Mortality reduction in cardiac anesthesia and intensive care: results of the first International Consensus Conference. *Acta Anaesthesiol Scand* 2011; **55**(3): 259–66

5. Ferguson TB, Jr., Coombs LP, Peterson ED. Preoperative beta-blocker use and mortality and morbidity following CABG surgery in North America. *JAMA* 2002; **287**(17): 2221–7

6. Wijeysundera DN, Naik JS, Beattie WS. Alpha-2 adrenergic agonists to prevent perioperative cardiovascular complications: a meta-analysis. *Am J Med* 2003; **114**(9): 742–52

7. Svircevic V, van Dijk D, Nierich AP, et al. Meta-analysis of thoracic epidural anesthesia versus general anesthesia for cardiac surgery. *Anesthesiology* 2011; **114**(2): 271–82

8. Scottish Intecollegiate Guidelines Network. *Antibiotic prophylaxis in surgery (104)*. Edinburgh: SIGN, 2008

9. Cobbe S, Rankin A, Alston RP, et al. Cardiac arrhythmias in coronary heart disease: a national guideline. Edinburgh: SIGN, 2007

10. Dieleman JM, Nierich AP, Rosseel PM, et al. Intraoperative high-dose dexamethasone for cardiac surgery: a randomized controlled trial. *JAMA* 2012; **308**(17): 1761–7

11. Morel J, Salard M, Castelain C, et al. Haemodynamic consequences of etomidate administration in elective cardiac surgery: a randomized double-blinded study. *Br J Anaesth* 2011; **107**(4): 503–9

12. Thomas T, Mohamad B, Arvind R, et al. Preoperative intra aortic balloon pumps in patients undergoing coronary artery bypass grafting. *Cochrane Database Syst Rev* 2011; **19**(1): CD004472 doi: 10.1002/14651858.CD004472.pub3

13. Thomas R, Smith D, Strike P. Prospective randomised double-blind comparative study of rocuronium and pancuronium in adult patients scheduled for elective 'fast-track' cardiac surgery involving hypothermic cardiopulmonary bypass. *Anaesthesia* 2003; **58**(3): 265–71

14. Wiesenack C, Wiesner G, Keyl C, et al. In vivo uptake and elimination of isoflurane by different membrane oxygenators during cardiopulmonary bypass. *Anesthesiology* 2002; **97**(1): 133–8

15. Landoni G, Biondi-Zoccai GG, Zangrillo A, et al. Desflurane and sevoflurane in cardiac surgery: a meta-analysis of randomized clinical trials. *J Cardiothorac Vasc Anesth* 2007; **21**(4): 502–11

16. Landoni G, Augoustides JG, Guarracino F, et al. Mortality reduction in cardiac anesthesia and intensive care: results of the first International Consensus Conference. *Acta Anaesthesiol Scand* 2011; **55**(3): 259–66

17. Avidan MS, Levy JH, van Aken H, et al. Recombinant human antithrombin III restores heparin responsiveness and decreases activation of coagulation in heparin-resistant patients during cardiopulmonary bypass. *J Thorac Cardiovasc Surg* 2005; **130**(1): 107–13

18. Warkentin TE, Greinacher A (eds). *Heparin Induced Thrombocytopenia*, third edn. New York, NY: Marcel Dekker, 2004

19. Schreiber J-U, Lancé MD, de Korte M, et al. The effect of different lung-protective strategies in patients during cardiopulmonary bypass: a meta-analysis and semiquantitative review of randomized trials. *J Cardiothorac Vasc Anesth* 2012; **26**(3): 448–54

20. Haga KK, McClymont KL, Clarke S, et al. The effect of tight glycaemic control, during and after cardiac surgery, on patient mortality and morbidity: A systematic review and meta-analysis. *J Cardiothorac Surg* 2011; **6**: 3–10

21. Landoni G, Biondi-Zoccai G, Greco M, et al. Effects of levosimendan on mortality and hospitalization. A meta-analysis of randomized controlled studies. *Crit Care Med* 2012; **40**(2): 634–46

22. Weiler JM, Gellhaus MA, Carter JG, et al. A prospective study of the risk of an immediate adverse reaction to protamine sulfate during cardiopulmonary bypass surgery. *J Allerg Clin Immunol* 1990; **85**(4): 713–9

CHAPTER 20

Anaesthesia for off-pump coronary artery bypass grafting

Yatin Mehta and Madhur Malik

Introduction

Off-pump coronary artery bypass grafting (OPCABG) is a 'reinvented procedure'. Before cardiopulmonary bypass (CPB) was introduced in 1953, coronary artery bypass grafting (CABG) surgery was done off-pump—that is without a CPB machine on a beating heart. With the availability of CPB, on-pump or conventional (cCABG) became the practice of the time (1). However, OPCAB resurfaced like a phoenix, in the 1980s, especially in isolated series and in centres with limited resources (2). The recent introduction of sophisticated stabilizing devices and exposure techniques, along with an understanding of the anaesthetic management during grafting, has led to widespread use of this technique and has resulted in graft patency rates that are equivalent to cCABG (3,4). Currently, the authors' institution does about 3000 patients for OPCAB procedures per annum. For these reasons and based on the authors experience, this chapter will review the anaesthetic management of off-pump CABG surgery.

Advantages of off- over on-pump coronary artery bypass grafting surgery

Patients undergoing CABG surgery usually have many comorbidities that complicate the deleterious effects of CPB and its management: these include hypothermia, coagulopathy, inflammatory response, interstitial oedema, neurological dysfunction, myocardial dysfunction, renal dysfunction, embolism risk, and others. Of these, the most important as far as patient outcome is end-organ injury, and particularly, neurological, myocardial, and renal dysfunction. OPCAB seems to have fewer deleterious effects on myocardial and renal function (5,6). However, the incidence of neurological dysfunction, and stroke in particular, has not been found to be reduced in patients undergoing OPCAB (7). The explanation for this lack of difference in outcome may be that a good neurological outcome depends on accurate assessment of atheroma in the ascending aorta combined with limiting and accurately applying the aortic cross-clamp.

Reduced postoperative rise in markers of systemic inflammatory response syndrome (SIRS) such as C3a, C5a, tumour necrosis factor (TNF)-α, interleukin (IL)-6, and IL-8 has been reported in patients undergoing OPCAB (8). The effects of CPB on SIRS depend on the balance between pro- and anti-inflammatory mediators. The proinflammatory mediators have an effect on long-term outcome of the patient (9). Therefore the high-risk patients—that is those with comorbidities and left ventricular dysfunction—are expected to benefit the most from OPCAB (2).

The same is evident in the early postoperative course of patients undergoing OPCAB compared with those undergoing CABG surgery in terms of durations of mechanical ventilation, intensive care unit (ICU), and hospital lengths of stay. In addition, the earlier postoperative recovery translates into a decrease in short-term costs. The graft patency rates have also been found to be comparable at one month although the debate on better long-term graft patency with cCABG continues and needs further investigation. Reston and colleagues (10) reviewed 53 studies, of which 10 were randomized control trials (RCTs), five were prospective controlled trials, and 38 were retrospective controlled studies. The total review involved 46 621 patients. With regards to short-term outcomes, they found significantly lower incidences of myocardial infarction (MI), stroke, re-operation for bleeding, renal failure, atrial fibrillation, and wound infection in the OPCAB group. As far as mid-term outcomes, the recurrence of angina was no different (odds ratio [OR] 1.28, 95% CI: 0.79 to 2.05; $p = 0.31$), but the risk of repeat intervention by percutaneous or open strategy (OR 3.63, 95% CI: 1.91 to 6.78; $p < 0.001$) or death was lower in the cCABG group (OR 0.49, 95% CI: 0.29 to 0.82; $p = 0.008$).

Several large RCTs comparing OPCAB with cCABG have recently been published (11–13). The Veterans Affairs Randomized On/Off Bypass (ROOBY) trial enrolled 2203 patients and found that 30-day adverse composite outcome and short-term morbidities were similar between the two groups (11). Follow-up angiograms in 1371 patients who underwent 4093 grafts revealed that the overall rate of graft patency was lower in the off- compared to the on-pump group (83% vs. 88%, $p < 0.01$). A 1-year follow-up study found that the composite adverse outcome that consisted of all-cause death, non-fatal MI, and repeat revascularization was 47% higher with OPCAB (15% versus 10%; $p < 0.001$) (12). The CORONARY trial was conducted in 79 centres in 19 countries, and randomly assigned

4752 patients to OPCAB or cCABG (13). There was no significant difference in the rate of the primary composite outcome
(both around 10%), but OPCAB significantly reduced the rates
of blood-product transfusion (51% vs. 63%; relative risk [RR]
0.80; 95% CI: 0.75 to 0.85; $p < 0.001$), reoperation for bleeding
(1.4% vs. 2.4%; RR 0.61; 95% CI: 0.40 to 0.93; $p = 0.02$), acute kidney injury (28% vs. 32%; RR 0.87; 95% CI: 0.80 to 0.96; $p = 0.01$),
and respiratory complications (5.9% vs. 7.5%; RR 0.79; 95%
CI: 0.63 to 0.98; $p = 0.03$). As with ROOBY, OPCAB increased
the rate of early repeat revascularizations (0.7% vs. 0.2%; hazard ratio, 4.0; 95% CI, 1.34 to 12; $p = 0.01$). These major clinical
trials indicate some benefits of OPCAB, with the quality of the
coronary grafting being a primary determinant of long-term
outcome. It is thus likely that surgical and anaesthetic expertise
with OPCAB are key factors, for which traditional RCT may
overlook (14).

The surgeon's challenges

The indications for OPCAB have been increasing and includes
most patients who would be suitable for cCABG surgery except
those with intracavitary thrombus, malignant arrhythmias,
deep intramyocardial bridging vessels, and CABG surgery combined with valve surgery or left ventricular (LV) aneurysm repair
(15). The patients expected to benefit the most from OPCAB are
patients with poor LV function, renal, or liver dysfunction, and
those with a calcified and/or atheromatous aorta in whom neurological outcome might be better as aortic cannulation and
clamping is avoided (2). This wide range of indications requires
a detailed understanding of the coronary anatomy, the degree
of stenosis, the likelihood of haemodynamic derangement during grafting, requirement of inotropes and intra-aortic balloon
counterpulsation (IABC) by both the anaesthetist as well as the
surgeon.

The surgeon has to first decide the sequence of anastomosis of
coronary arteries based on the coronary angiogram. The more
stenotic vessel is anastomosed first because of the presence of
good collateral circulation from the less stenosed vessel (16).
The collaterals will maintain supply to the area of more stenosed
vessel initially during anastomosis and will supply the area of
less stenosed vessel after anastomosis because of pressure head
differential.

Exposure of the vessels requires heart tilting manoeuvres by
the surgeon, which typically cause haemodynamic derangement.
The various techniques of exposure can be roughly classified into
heart 'rocking' (figure 20.1) and enucleation (figure 20.2).

The area of anastomosis is stabilized by use of stabilizer
devices. Earlier heavy metallic stabilizer devices were available, which worked on the principle of compression and stabilization, but led to significant haemodynamic derangement.
With the availability of suction-based stabilization devices
(figure 20.3)—octopus (Medtronic Octopus® System), urchin,
starfish (Starfish™ Heart Positioner), and the Octopus® 3 Tissue
Stabilizer (Medtronic, Inc, Minneapolis, MN), the myocardial compression and the haemodynamic compromise are less.
Anastomosis of coronaries on the posterior aspect of the heart
requires lifting of the heart, which is aided by the use of the
starfish suction-based stabilizer, which in turn decreases RV
outflow tract obstruction.

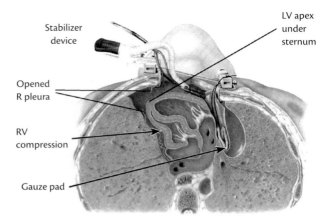

Fig. 20.1 Heart 'rocking'.
Heart rocking consists of displacing the heart with gauze swabs and rocking it
with suction stabilizer devices. This usually results in the right ventricle (RV) being
compressed under the right hemisternum, which is managed in the Trendelenburg
position, preload augmentation and opening the right pleura.

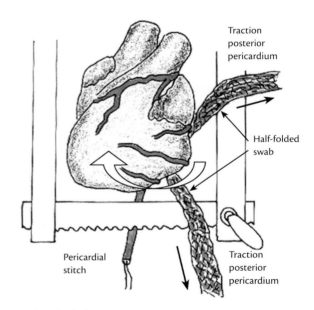

Fig. 20.2 'Enucleation'.
Enucleation consists of enucleating the heart by aspiration by a suction device or
by pulling the pericardium with single or multiple stitches placed in the oblique
sinus.

The anaesthesiologist's challenges

The anaesthetist plays a pivotal role to play in the success of
OPCAB. He or she has to understand the coronary anatomy, the
sequence of anastomosis, the mechanisms behind the haemodynamic derangements during coronary anastomosis and the
manoeuvres required to manage the haemodynamic derangement.

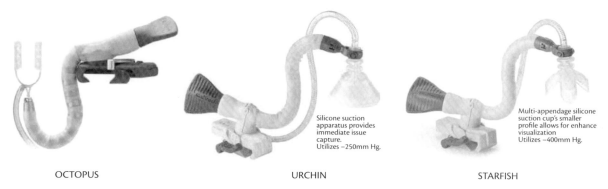

OCTOPUS   URCHIN   STARFISH

Silicone suction apparatus provides immediate issue capture. Utilizes −250mm Hg.

Multi-appendage silicone suction cup's smaller profile allows for enhance visualization Utilizes −400mm Hg.

Fig. 20.3 Suction-based stabilization devices for off-pump surgery. Reproduced with kind permission from Medtronic.

Close communication between the surgeon and the anaesthetist is of paramount importance (Chapter 42).

Mechanisms of haemodynamic derangement and their management

Anastomosing to the left anterior descending and artery and its branches

The left anterior descending (LAD) artery lies on the anterior aspect of heart in the interventricular groove and supplies the anterior wall of the LV and contributes significantly to contractility and stroke volume (SV). Positioning the heart for better exposure of the LAD and its branches (diagonal) may require just a slight traction on pericardial stitches with or without placement of a pericardial swab, and this positioning does not cause significant haemodynamic derangement. However, placement of stabilizer device on the actively contracting anterior wall does decrease the SV and so the cardiac output (CO). Haemodynamic compromise occurs more with anterior and lateral wall compression than with posterior and inferior wall compression (17).

Anastomosing the left circumflex artery and its branches

The left circumflex (LCx) artery runs in the left atrioventricular groove and turns back to reach the crux of the heart. The obtuse marginal arteries (1–4 in number) arise from LCx artery and supply the lateral and posterior aspect of the LV. Exposure of the LCx artery and its branches requires verticalization of the heart which is achieved by pericardial traction and aided by cup-shaped suction devices placed at the apex of heart. However, verticalization of the heart causes haemodynamic derangement by two mechanisms. First, the atria are below the ventricles and thus require higher filling pressure to fill their corresponding ventricle (17,18). Diastolic dysfunction has been reported during verticalization, which again requires higher filling pressures. Second, verticalization may distort the mitral and the tricuspid annuli increasing the severity of valvular regurgitation especially in patients with pre-existing lesions (19). Management of this haemodynamic derangement requires the Trendelenburg position, volume loading to increase filling pressure, and use of inotropes and vasoconstrictors to maintain perfusion pressures. The increase in CO is achieved better with leg elevation as compared to the Trendelenburg position (20,21).

Verticalization of heart is often associated with a marked decrease in amplitude of the electrocardiograph (ECG) due to change in axis of the heart, and transoesophageal echocardiography (TOE) imaging is often lost due to pericardial swabs. Thus, the anaesthetist loses two important monitors during verticalization. Invasive intra-arterial pressure, pulmonary artery pressure, and plethysmography, along with continuous CO and $ScVO_2$, serve as monitors of CO and peripheral perfusion during this period.

Anastomosing the right coronary artery and its branches

The right coronary artery (RCA) runs in the right atrioventricular groove and turns back to supply the right ventricle (RV) and inferior wall of the LV. Positioning the heart for exposure may require verticalization for grafting the distal RCA and posterior descending artery) or only slight elevation with leftward displacement for the proximal RCA. Placement of a stabilizer on the RV decreases the RV chamber volume and impedes its filling leading to a rise in central venous pressure (CVP) and a compensatory tachycardia due to decreased LV filling. Management of haemodynamic compromise is similar to that as mentioned for verticalization of heart. Anastomosing the proximal RCA may lead to arrhythmias and complete heart block and therefore a pacemaker should be available in the operating room (22).

Anaesthetic management

Preoperative assessment

Preoperative assessment of patients for OPCAB requires the same thoroughness as for those undergoing on-pump CABG surgery (Chapter 19). Comorbidities like carotid artery stenosis, peripheral vascular disease (PVD) should be assessed by Doppler examination. A patient with carotid stenosis >70% has a higher perioperative neurological morbidity and mortality and may require carotid endarterectomy alone or as a combined procedure with OPCAB/CCABG (23). Similarly, a patient with PVD will have a difficulty in passage of IABC if required. Patients with diabetes, renal dysfunction, or pulmonary dysfunction have a higher perioperative morbidity and may require longer ICU and hospital stay (24). Therefore optimization of the patient by adequate preoperative measures like control of blood sugar levels, adequate hydration, and chest physiotherapy (lung recruitment manoeuvres, nebulization) helps in decreasing perioperative morbidity and mortality and also decreases ICU and hospital stay and costs (25).

Premedication

Adequate anxiolysis and analgesia achieved by the use of benzo-diazepines and opioids decreases the incidence of ischaemic pain as well as the pain of possible painful cannulation.Lorazepam (1–2 mg) given orally on the night before surgery and on the morning of surgery provides adequate sedation. The morning doses of antihypertensive and antianginal medication like beta-blockers, nitrates, and nicorandil should be administered. The morning dose of angiotensin-converting enzyme inhibitor (ACE-I) or angiotensin receptor blocker (ARB) should be omitted in view of possible hypotension during induction of anaesthesia (26). Alpha$_2$-agonists like clonidine and dexmedetomidine may be used but with caution because of a decrease in heart rate, contractility, mean BP and CO (27).

Anaesthetic induction and maintenance

Anaesthesia induction and maintenance for OPCAB has undergone a radical change in the past two decades with greater emphasis on enhanced recovery to improve patient outcome as well as to decrease ICU/hospital stay and overall costs. An important consideration in choosing anaesthetic induction and maintenance agents is LV function. Patients with poor LV function may have an exaggerated decrease in CO and mean arterial pressure (MAP) with normal doses of anaesthetic agents compared with those with good LV function who may require higher than normal doses to attenuate the stress response. For OPCAB, it is preferable to use shorter acting agents like propofol, etomidate, and remifentanil in order to achieve early recovery and tracheal extubation.

Enhance recovery

Anaesthesia for enhanced recovery from OPCAB depends on using titrated doses of shorter acting opioids, muscle relaxants, and inhalational agents, along with supplementation with regional techniques like epidural, intrathecal, or intrapleural opioids. Early tracheal extubation is one of the key parameters in fast track anaesthesia with various studies reporting mean time to extubation ranging from 4.1 to 10 hours with no appreciable increase in incidence of reintubation or ICU events but with a definite decrease in the duration of ICU stay and costs. Myles and colleagues (28) reviewed 10 studies with extubation times <10 hours and reported no significant difference in mortality and morbidity and a decrease in ICU stay by 5.4 hours. Ovrum and colleagues (29) studied 5658 patients extubated within five hours and reported only 1.1% reintubation rates.

Regional analgesia

Thoracic epidural analgesia (TEA) reduces haemodynamic correlates of the myocardial oxygen consumption, impaired regional (ischaemic zone) endocardial perfusion and reduce the extent of the MI in patients undergoing OPCAB. TEA provides good protection from stress response, ensures haemodynamic stability, allows early extubation, improves distribution of coronary blood flow and reduces demand for oxygen. Patients have better postoperative pulmonary function and less postoperative pain. It also reduces postoperative respiratory complications and perioperative arrhythmia such as supraventricular tachycardia (30,31).

Similarly, intrathecal morphine at a dose of 8 μg/kg for OPCAB is effective for excellent postoperative analgesia, preserves lung function with minimal undesirable effects, and facilitates early tracheal extubation (32).

Perioperative monitoring

Invasive blood pressure

Radial artery cannulation under local anaesthesia before anaesthetic induction is done for continuous monitoring of the systemic arterial pressure. Femoral arterial cannulation should also be done in patients with severe LV dysfunction and tight left main stenosis (diffuse disease) to facilitate quick insertion of an intra-aortic balloon catheter (IABC) in the event of myocardial ischaemia or haemodynamic instability. In addition, it also allows monitoring of the central to peripheral pressure gradient. The area under the arterial pressure trace curve gives a rough estimate of CO. The Flotrac/Vigileo system may be used to assess CO by connecting to the radial or femoral arterial line. It also provides stroke volume variation (SVV) which is a measure of fluid responsiveness (33).

Pulse oximetry

A pulse oximeter not only monitors SpO$_2$, but can be used in a modified Allen's test to assess palmar arterial collateral circulation before radial arterial cannulation and radial arterial conduit grafting. The area under the plethysmograph curve serves as a rough guide to CO (the principle behind the Masimo Technology device, Japan) (34).

Central venous pressure

A double or triple lumen central venous cannula is inserted usually in the right internal jugular vein before or after induction of anaesthesia. In patients with severe LV dysfunction, or tight left main stenosis then it is probably best inserted preinduction. CVP serves as a guide to filling pressures. The CVP trace also supplements the ECG for rhythm diagnosis for example an absent a-wave in atrial fibrillation and cannon a-waves in junctional rhythm. Continuous central venous oxygen saturation (ScVO$_2$) may be used to monitor tissue oxygen delivery (35). A ScVO2 <55% or a decrease by 20% suggests a decrease in CO and warrants measures to increase CO.

Pulmonary artery pressure

Of all the monitoring techniques, pulmonary artery catheters (PAC) remains the most controversial. A prospective cohort study by Connors and colleagues (36) that involved a mixed population of medical and surgical patients in ICUs found increased mortality, length of stay and costs associated with the use of the PAC, although none of these patients had undergone OPCAB. Sandham and colleagues performed a RCT, comparing goal-directed therapy guided by PAC with standard care without PAC (37). They found no benefit of therapy directed by PAC over standard care in elderly, high-risk, surgical patients requiring ICU. Therefore, PAC is more likely to be useful in patients undergoing OPCAB if they have depressed LV function, recent MI, renal dysfunction, or pulmonary hypertension. Indications for and complications of, PAC, as suggested by Kanchi and colleagues are listed in table 20.1 (38).

Table 20.1 Indications and complications of pulmonary artery catheters

Recommended Indication for PAC	Complications of PAC in 1000 Insertions
CABG with ↓ LV function	Arrhythmia: 12
Combined procedures	Coiling/knotting: 2
LV aneurysmectomy	Surgeon's stitch: 1
Recent MI (≤30 days)	Carotid puncture: 1
Renal dysfunction	Difficult flotation: 1
Pulmonary hypertension	Thrombocytopenia: 1
Diastolic dysfunction	Wedge infarct: 2
Acute VSD	Intrapulmonary bleeding: 2
LVAD	

PAC, pulmonary artery catheter; CABG, coronary artery bypass grafting; LV, left ventricle; MI, myocardial infarction; VSD, ventricular septal defect; LVAD, left ventricular assist device.

Cardiac output monitoring

Various techniques for CO monitoring are available and are discussed in detail in Chapter 3.

Transoesophageal echocardiography

Baseline regional wall motion abnormality (RWMA) and LV functional assessment can be done after induction of anaesthesia and insertion of a TOE probe. However, intraoperative detection of RWMAs as a monitor of myocardial ischaemia is difficult in the presence of pericardial swabs and verticalization impairs image acquisition. Postoperative persistence of RWMA predicts a poor long-term prognosis (39).

Temperature

Core body temperature may monitored by the PAC and should be maintained around 36°C using a forced air blanket or warming air mattress, an IV fluid warmer and by maintaining operating room temperature at around 24ºC. Hypothermia can delay tracheal extubation and cause coagulopathy.

Activated clotting time

Heparin 200 IU/kg should be administered before division of the internal mammary artery. The degree of anticoagulation during grafting should be monitored using the activated clotting time (ACT) (Chapter 17) aiming to maintain an ACT around 250–300 s. The ACT should be rechecked at hourly intervals. Heparin reversal with protamine following grafting is optional and an ACT maintained around 150 s in the postoperative period may improve graft patency.

Depth of anaesthesia monitoring

Bispectral index or entropy may be of value to monitor depth of anaesthesia as there is a common tendency amongst anaesthesiologists to reduce the concentration of inhalational agent that is being administered during hypotension, and which could result in awareness.

Intraoperative myocardial ischaemia and myocardial protection

During coronary anastomosis, brief periods of myocardial ischaemia as evidenced by RWMA with TOE, ST segment elevation on the ECG, or an increase in PAP may result in myocardial injury (40). The injury has been documented by rise in markers of myocardial injury (troponins, CPK-MB) but seem less than observed in cCABG surgery (41,42). Nevertheless, OPCAB also requires myocardial protection and this can be achieved by maintaining myocardial oxygen demand/supply balance, use of an intracoronary shunt and ischaemic and/or pharmacological preconditioning

Myocardial oxygen supply/demand balance

Myocardial oxygen demand can be reduced with by reducing heart rate and contractility using beta-adrenergic blockers. One should aim for heart rates of 50–60/min in patients with preserved LV function and between 80–90/min in patients with severe LV dysfunction. A short-acting beta-blocker like esmolol is ideal for these purposes (43). Oxygen supply should be maintained using a coronary perfusion pressure (CPP) of more than 50 mmHg or a MAP of 65–70 mmHg. Administration of a vasoconstrictor such as phenylephrine or norepinephrine (noradrenaline), and IV volume loading, is usually sufficient to maintain oxygen supply and limit myocardial ischaemia.

Intracoronary shunt

Intracoronary shunts provide a bloodless field for the surgeon and maintain coronary blood flow in the period during anastomosis. They decrease the incidences of RWMA and transient impairment of LV function during coronary anastomosis (43).

Preconditioning

The landmark observation by McMurry and colleagues (44) of ischaemic preconditioning in a canine heart model has been slow to translate into clinical practice. Brief periods of ischaemia followed by reperfusion renders the heart more resistant to a subsequent prolonged ischaemia (Chapter 15). However, preconditioning may also be induced pharmacologically by inhalational anaesthetics, opioids, and nitrates during OPCAB (45). Sevoflurane, isoflurane, desflurane all provide preconditioning (46,47). The common outcomes in studies investigating preconditioning are decreases in markers of myocardial injury, the incidence of arrhythmias, duration of stay, and ICU events. However, these do not translate into decreased mortality. So ischaemic preconditioning may be effective in reducing the infarct size in unprotected hearts but during cardiac surgery, it is stunning and not infarction that is important as the heart is near-optimally protected.

Conversion to on-pump CCABG

Recommendations by Chassot and colleagues for conversion from off- to on-pump CABG surgery are given in box 20.1 (2).

Minimally invasive coronary artery bypass grafting

Minimally invasive CABG is an increasingly popular technique for single- or double-vessel coronary artery disease (LAD and RCA). It is especially favoured in patients in whom other coronary arteries can be treated by percutaneous coronary intervention

Box 20.1 Indications for conversion from off- to on-pump coronary artery bypass grafting surgery

Persistence of the following for >15 min despite aggressive therapy

- Cardiac index <1.5 L/min/m^2
- SvO$_2$<60%
- MAP <50 mmHg
- ST-segment elevation >2 mV
- Large new RWMA or deterioration of LV function assessed by TOE
- Sustained malignant arrhythmias

SvO$_2$, mixed venous oxyhaemoglobin saturation with oxygen; MAP, mean arterial pressure; RWMA, regional wall motion artefact; LV, left ventricular function.

using a hybrid procedure, and in those with significant comorbidities. Surgically, it can be preformed through a small thoracotomy as minimally invasive direct coronary artery bypass (MIDCAB) or by totally endoscopic coronary artery bypass (TECAB).

Minimally invasive direct coronary artery bypass grafting

MIDCAB is performed through a left anterior short thoracotomy (LAST) in the fourth intercostal space for LIMA to LAD anastomoses. The patient is positioned supine with the left chest elevated by 30–40 degrees. A 6–10 cm thoracotomy is performed and the left lung is deflated then isolated by use of a double lumen tube or bronchial blocker (Chapter 33). The LIMA is then harvested and anastomosed to the LAD on the beating heart. Anaesthetic management is similar to OPCAB except for the use external defibrillator pads as limitation of space does not allow use of internal defibrillator paddles. For the RIMA to RCA anastomosis, a right thoracotomy is required. Enhanced MIDCAB consists of a robotically harvested LIMA with a small thoracotomy MIDCAB. Multivessel small thoracotomy (MVST) revascularization consists of a robotically harvested IMA and multiple vessel anastomoses.

Totally endoscopic coronary artery bypass

TECAB is done using a Da Vinci Telemanipulation system (Intuitive surgical,Inc.,Sunnyvale, CA), which allows precise control of endoscopic arms and instruments and provides a high resolution 3D image to the operating surgeon. TECAB is done in the same position as MIDCAB. A scope is inserted at the fourth intercostal space in the left anterior axillary line, and two additional ports in the third and seventh intercostal spaces are inserted for the endoscopic instruments. An additional port for CO$_2$ insufflation is required to create a retrosternal space for left internal mammary artery (LIMA) harvesting. Intrathoracic pressure should be maintained <10 mmHg so as to avoid a decrease in systemic venous return to the heart. After LIMA harvesting, an endoscopic epicardial stabilizer is inserted through the subxiphoid space. The learning curve for TECAB is steep and the indications are limited due to inability to access the posterior surface of heart.

Postoperative care

The most important benefit of OPCAB over on-pump cCABG is the increased likelihood of early tracheal extubation which is aided by anaesthesia aim for enhanced recovery. Mehta and colleagues (48) compared continuous thoracic epidural analgesia to paravertebral block in patients undergoing robotic-assisted OPCAB and reported comparable analgesia and postoperative pulmonary function. The overall outcome from OPCAB is a reduced durations of ICU and hospital stay (49), less blood loss and transfusion (11–13,50), lesser inotropic and IABC requirement, lower incidence of wound infection compared to cCABG surgery. The incidence of atrial fibrillation is comparable in patients undergoing OPCAB and CABG (51).

Conclusion

OPCAB is being done as a combined procedure with carotid endarterectomy, and non-cardiac procedures such as thyroidectomy (52) and cholecystectomy (53). OPCAB is expected to remain a genuine alternative to cCABG and anaesthetic techniques need to evolve to make it safer and better for the patient, particularly those with increased co-morbidities.

References

1. Thanikachalam M, Lombardi P, Tehrani HY, Katariya K, Salerno TA. The history and development of direct coronary surgery without cardiopulmonary bypass. *J Card Surg* 2004; **19**: 516–9
2. Chassot PG, Van Der Linden P, Zaugg M, Mueller XM, Spahn DR. Off-pump coronary artery bypass surgery: physiology and anaesthetic management. *Br J Anaesth* 2004; **92**: 400–13
3. Bergsland J, Karamanoukian HL, Soltoski PR, Salerno TA. 'Single suture' for circumflex exposure in off-pump coronary artery bypass grafting. *Ann Thorac Surg* 1999; **68**: 1428–30
4. Calafiore AM, Vitolla G, Mazzei V, et al. The LAST operation: techniques and results before and after the stabilization era. *Ann Thorac Surg* 1998; **66**: 998–1001
5. Ascione R, Lloyd CT, Underwood MJ, Gomes WJ, Angelini GD. On-pump versus off-pump coronary revascularization: evaluation of renal function. *Ann Thorac Surg* 1999; **68**: 493–8
6. Loef BG, Epema AH, Navis G, et al. Off-pump coronary revascularization attenuates transient renal damage compared with on-pump coronary revascularization. *Chest* 2002; **121**: 1190–4
7. Iaco AL, Contini M, Teodori G, et al. Off or on bypass: What is the safety threshold? *Ann Thorac Surg* 1999; **68**: 2237–42
8. Czerny M, Baumer H, Kilo J, et al. Inflammatory response and myocardial injury following coronary artery bypass grafting with or without cardiopulmonary bypass. *Eur J Cardiothorac Surg* 2000; **17**: 737–42
9. Diegeler A, Doll N, Rauch T, et al. Humoral immune response during coronary artery bypass grafting: a comparison of limited approach, 'off-pump' technique, and conventional cardiopulmonary bypass. *Circulation* 2000; **102**: 95–100
10. Reston JT, Tregear SJ, Turkelson CM. Meta-analysis of short-term and mid-term outcomes following off-pump coronary artery bypass grafting. *Ann Thorac Surg* 2003; **76**: 1510–5
11. Shroyer AL, Grover FL, Hattler B, et al. On-pump versus off-pump coronary-artery bypass surgery. *N Engl J Med* 2009; **361**: 1827–37
12. Hattler B, Messenger JC, Shroyer AL, et al.Off-pump coronary artery bypass surgery is associated with worse arterial and saphenous vein graft patency and less effective revascularization: results from the veterans affairs randomized on/off bypass (ROOBY) trial. *Circulation* 2012; **125**: 2827–35
13. Lamy A, Devereaux PJ, Prabhakaran D, et al. Off-pump or on-pump coronary-artery bypass grafting at 30 days. *N Engl J Med* 2012; **366**: 1489–97

14. Devereaux PJ, Bhandari M, Clarke M, et al. Need for expertise based randomised controlled trials. *Br Med J*2005; **330**: 88–91

15. Mehta Y, Juneja R. Off-pump coronary artery bypass grafting: new developments but a better outcome? *Curr Opin Anesthesisol* 2002; **15**: 9–18

16. Yakut N, Tulukoğlu E, Emrecan B, et al. Which is first: left anterior descending artery anastomosis or right coronary artery anastomosis in off-pump coronary artery bypass grafting? *Heart Surg Forum* 2009; **12**: E256–60

17. Mathison M, Edgerton JR, Horswell JL, Akin JJ, Mack MJ. Analysis of hemodynamic changes during beating heart surgical procedures. *Ann Thorac Surg* 2000; **70**: 1355–60

18. Nierich AP, Diephuis J, Jansen EW, Borst C, Knape JT. Heart displacement during off-pump CABG: how well is it tolerated? *Ann Thorac Surg* 2000; **70**: 466–72

19. George SJ, Al-Ruzzeh S, Amrani M. Mitral annulus distortion during beating heart surgery: a potential cause for hemodynamic disturbance: a three-dimensional echocardiography reconstruction study. *Ann Thorac Surg* 2002; **73**: 1424–30

20. Reuter DA, Felbinger TW, Schmidt C, et al. Trendelenburg positioning after cardiac surgery: effects on intrathoracic blood volume index and cardiac performance. *Eur J Anaesthesiol* 2003; **20**: 17–20

21. Nakajima Y, Mizobe T, Matsukawa T, et al. Thermoregulatory response to intraoperative head-down tilt. *Anesth Analg* 2002; **94**: 221–6

22. Omae T,Kakihana Y, Mastunaga A et al.Hemodynamic changes during off-pump coronary artery bypass anastomosis in patients with coexisting mitral regurgitation: improvement with milrinone. *Anesth Analg* 2005; **101**: 2–8

23. Meharwal ZS, Mishra A, Trehan N. Safety and efficacy of one stage off-pump coronary artery operation and carotid endarterectomy. *Ann Thorac Surg* 2002;**73**: 793–7.

24. Zhang X, Clough AR, Leavitt BJ, Morton J et al. The effect of comorbid illness on mortality outcomes in cardiac surgery. *Arch Surg* 2002; **137**: 428–33

25. Wu Z, Peng X, Wu A, et al. Prognosis of diabetic patients undergoing coronary artery bypass surgery compared with nondiabetics: A systematic review and meta-analysis. *J Cardiothorac Vasc Anesth* 2011; **25**: 288–98

26. Meersschaert K, Brun L, Gourdin M, et al. Terlipresin-ephedrine versus ephedrine to treat hypotension at induction of anesthesia in patients chronically treated with angiotensin converting enzyme inhibitors: A prospective, randomized double-blinded crossover study. *Anesth Analg* 2002; **94**: 835

27. Scheinin H, Jaakola ML, Sjovall S, et al. Intramuscular dexmedetomidine as premedication for general anesthesia. A comparative multi-center study. *Anesthesiology* 1993; **78**: 1065

28. Myles PS, Daly DJ, Djaiani G, et al. A systematic review of the safety and effectiveness of fast-track cardiac anesthesia. *Anesthesiology* 2003; **99**: 982

29. Ovrum E, Tangen G, Schiott C et al. Rapid recovery protocol applied to 5658 consecutive on-pump coronary bypass patients. *Ann Thorac Surg* 2000; **70**: 2000

30. Mehta Y, Vats M, Sharma M, Arora R, Trehan N. Thoracic epidural analgesia for off-pump coronary artery bypass surgery in patients with chronic obstructive pulmonary disease. *Ann Card Anaesth* 2010; **13**: 224–30

31. Vanek T, Straka Z, Brucek P, Widimsky P. Thoracic epidural anesthesia for off-pump coronary artery bypass without intubation. *Eur J Cardiothorac Surg* 2001; **20**: 858–60

32. Mehta Y, Kulkarni V, Juneja R et al. Spinal (subarachnoid) morphine for off-pump coronary artery bypass surgery. *Heart Surgery Forum* 2004; **7**: E205–10

33. Cannesson MH, Desebbe O, Boucau C, Simon R, Hénaine R, Lehot J. The ability of stroke volume variations obtained with Vigileo/FloTrac system to monitor fluid responsiveness in mechanically ventilated patients. *Anesth Analg*2009; **108**: 513–17

34. Forget P, Lois F, de Kock M. Goal-directed fluid management based on the pulse oximeter-derived pleth variability index reduces lactate levels and improves fluid management. *Anesth Analg* 2010; **111**: 910–4

35. Reinhart, K, et al. Continuous central venous and pulmonary artery oxygen saturation monitoring in the critically ill. *Intensive Care Med* 2004; **30**: 1572–8

36. Connors AF Jr, Speroff T, Dawson NV, et al. The effectiveness of right heart catheterization in the initial care of critically ill patients. *JAMA* 1996; **276**: 889–97

37. Sandham JD, Hull RD, Brant RF, et al. A randomized controlled trial of the use of pulmonary artery catheters in high-risk surgical patients. *N Engl J Med* 2003; **348**: 5–14

38. Kanchi M. Do we need a pulmonary artery catheter in cardiac anesthesia?—An Indian perspective. *Ann Card Anaesth* 2011; **14**: 25–9

39. Moises VA, Mesquita CB, Campos O, et al. Importance of intraoperative transesophageal echocardiography during coronary artery surgery without cardiopulmonary bypass. *J Am Soc Echocardiogr* 1998; **11**: 1139–44

40. Paparella D, Cappabianca G, Malvindi P, et al.Myocardial injury after off-pump coronary artery bypass grafting operation.*Eur J Cardiothorac Surg* 2007; **32**(3): 481–7

41. Brown JR, Hernandez F Jr, Klemperer JD, et al. Cardiac troponin T levels in on- and off-pump coronary artery bypass surgery. *Heart Surg Forum* 2007; **10**: E42–6

42. Chauhan S, Saxena N, Rao BH, Singh RS, Bhan A. A comparison of esmolol and diltiazem for heart rate control during coronary revascularisation on beating heart. *Indian J Med Res* 1999; **110**: 174–7

43. Yeatman M, Caputo M, Narayan P, et al.Intracoronary shunts reduce transient intraoperative myocardial dysfunction during off-pump coronary operations. *Ann Thorac Surg* 2002; **73**: 1411–17

44. Murry, CE, Jennings, RB, Reimer, KA. Preconditioning with ischemia: a delay of lethal cell injury in ischemic myocardium. *Circulation* 1986; **74**: 1124–36

45. Loveridge R, Schroeder F. Anaesthetic preconditioning. *Contin Educ Anaesth Crit Care Pain* 2010; **10**: 38–42

46. V. Piriou, J. Mantz, G. Goldfarb M, et al. Sevoflurane preconditioning at 1 MAC only provides limited protection in patients undergoing coronary artery bypass surgery: a randomized bi-centre trial. *Br J Anaesth* 2007; **99**: 624–31

47. Lange M, Roewer N, Kehl F. Anesthetic preconditioning as the alternative to ischemic preconditioning. *J Thorac Cardiovasc Surg* 2006; **131**: 252–3

48. Mehta Y, Swaminathan M, Mishra Y, Trehan N. A comparative evaluation of intrapleural and thoracic epidural analgesia for postoperative pain relief after minimally invasive direct coronary artery bypass surgery. *Ann Card Anaesth* 2008; **11**: 90–5

49. Al-Ruzzeh S, Ambler G, Asimakopoulos G, et al. Off-pump coronary artery bypass (OPCAB) surgery reduces risk-stratified morbidity and mortality: A United Kingdom multi-center comparative analysis of early clinical outcome. *Circulation* 2003; **108**[Suppl. II]: 1–8

50. Sellke FW, DiMaio JM, Caplan LR. AHA Scientific Statement. Comparing on-pump and off-pump coronary artery bypass grafting. *Circulation* 2005; **111**: 2858–64

51. Archbold RA, Curzen NP. Off-pump coronary artery bypass graft surgery: the incidence of postoperative atrial fibrillation. *Heart* 2003; **89**: 1134–7

52. Mehta YPS, Juneja R, Singh H, Sachdeva S, Trehan N. OPCAB and thyroidectomy in a patient with a severely compromised airway. *J Cardiothorac Vasc Anesth*2005; **19**:79–82

53. Masahiro R, Hiroshi I, Shinji T, et al. Combined operation in a patient with ischemic heart disease complicated by cholecystitis and idiopathic thrombocytopenic purpura. *J Japan Surg Assoc* 2007; **68**: 424–27

CHAPTER 21

Paediatric cardiac and thoracic anaesthesia

Marco Ranucci, Giuseppe Isgrò, and Anna Cazzaniga

Education and training in paediatric cardiothoracic anaesthesia

Anaesthesia for paediatric cardiac and thoracic surgery is a subspecialty within a subspecialty. Paediatric cardiac anaesthesiologists should follow a comprehensive training to correctly develop all the expertise that is needed for an adequate management of these complex patients. This training includes practical manual skills, as well as a deep knowledge of the pathophysiology of all the congenital heart defects and of the different technical aspects of the various operations that are performed to correct or palliate these defects. Moreover, a deep knowledge of the specific physiology of the newborn and infant patients is required, as well as their reaction to the anesthetic interventions in and to the drugs commonly used to induce and maintain anaesthesia, and to manage the haemodynamics before, during and after surgery.

At present, there are no training guidelines or certification processes for paediatric cardiac anaesthesia. In 2010, a working group of the Congenital Cardiac Anesthesia Society published a document suggesting the main steps for training in this sub-specialty (1). According to this consensus document, after a general anaesthesia basic training that is adequate to fulfill the local national training requirements, the applicants should spend a fellowship period of 12 months in adult cardiac anaesthesia, or 12 months in general paediatric anaesthesia, or 18 months in combined paediatric and paediatric cardiac anaesthesia. Subsequently, all the trainees should spend a 12-month period of clinical experience, with 9 months spent in the operating room, having a direct clinical experience on at least 50 patients in the first year of life and at least 25 in the first month of life.

Paediatric cardiothoracic anaesthesia training is presently differently structured in different Countries, sometimes including postoperative intensive care management, others being restricted to the intraoperative management. It should, however, include at least the minimal items reported in box 21.1.

Main patterns of congenital heart defects

This section addresses the main congenital heart defects including their anatomy, pathophysiology, and surgical or transcatheter interventions. The specific intraoperative problems related to the management of some of these clinical features will be addressed in specific sections later in this chapter.

Left-to-right shunt heart defects

Left-to-right shunt heart defects include a group of lesion characterized by a systemic to pulmonary shunt, with pulmonary overflow. This pattern, if left untreated, leads to pulmonary hypertension. When the pulmonary arterial pressure exceeds the systemic arterial pressure, the shunt is reversed to a right-to-left direction (Eisenmenger syndrome), and the heart defect is no longer amenable to surgical or interventional correction.

From the clinical point of view, patients with left-to-right shunt present with an X-ray pattern of cardiomegaly of the left heart chambers and increased pulmonary vascular markings. Due to the pulmonary overflow, they are particularly prone to respiratory tract infections, congestive heart failure, and delayed somatic growth.

Patent ductus arteriosus

The ductus arteriosus is a normal vessel in foetal life, connecting the main pulmonary/left pulmonary artery to the descending thoracic aorta. After birth, the ductus undergoes permanent closure between 48 hours to 6 weeks. A patent ductus arteriosus (PDA) may be found in pre-term newborns where it can be responsible for a diastolic systemic blood flow steal. However, the pathophysiological consequence of a PDA is a left-to-right shunt which, if left untreated, may lead to irreversible pulmonary hypertension. The treatment of PDA includes medical therapy (with non-steroidal anti-inflammatory drugs [NSAIDs]), interventional catheterization, and surgery (by mini-thoracotomy or thoracoscopy, without cardiopulmonary bypass [CPB]) depending on the age and the PDA size.

Atrial septal defects

Atrial septal defects (ASDs) are common congenital heart defects, presenting with different anatomical patterns, isolated or associated with other heart defects (figure 21.1). The ostium primum ASD is a failure of closure of the atrial septum at its base, in continuity with the atrioventricular valves. It is almost invariably associated with a mitral valve cleft of the anterior leaflet. This association is defined as partial atrioventricular septal defect) and represents about 10% of ASDs. The ostium secundum ASD is relatively central to the atrial septum and represents about 80% of the ASDs. The sinus venosus ASD accounts for the remaining 10% of

Box 21.1 Knowledge and skills required for a comprehensive paediatric training in cardiothoracic anaesthesia

- Basic knowledge of embryology of the cardiovascular system, inclusive of the morphological pattern of the congenital heart defects
- Pathophysiology of the congenital heart defects
- Technical aspects of the different surgical operation to correct or palliate the congenital heart defects
- Pharmacological and haemodynamic management of the paediatric patient with heart defects. Pharmacology of the medications used for the management of the paediatric patients with heart defects including anaesthetics, positive inotropes, and vasoactive drugs, in the context of each pathophysiological pattern.
- Electrocardiography and imaging including echocardiography, computerized tomography, magnetic resonance
- Invasive diagnostic procedures and invasive cardiac interventions undertaken in the cath lab.
- Electrophysiological procedures including pacemaker implantation
- Preanaesthetic evaluation, including fluid management, fasting rules, premedication, risk stratification.
- Monitoring of the patient: invasive (arterial and central venous cannulation) and noninvasive monitoring.
- Intraoperative transoesophageal echocardiography
- Cardiopulmonary bypass in newborns and infants
- Mechanical assist devices (ECMO, VADs)
- Postoperative pain management
- Mechanical ventilation in the setting of the specific heart defect and operation performed
- Postoperative haemodynamic management
- Ethical issues and how to deal with the patient's relatives

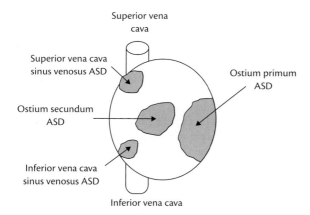

Fig. 21.1 Different types of atrial septal defect (ASD).

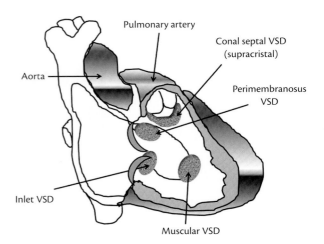

Fig. 21.2 Different types of ventricular septal defects (VSD).

the ASDs, and is placed in the high superior–posterior area of the septum, almost invariably associated with partial anomalous pulmonary venous return.

Closure of the ASDs may be performed by percutaneous transcatheter procedures (ostium secundum) if the size of the defect is not too large. Surgical closure is achieved with CPB and direct suture or pericardial patch (always in ostium primum and sinus venosus defects).

Ventricular septal defects

Ventricular septal defects (VSDs) represent about 20% of all the congenital heart defects (figure 21.2). According to Van Praagh's classification (2) they can be defined as: (i) inlet defect (atrioventricular canal type); (ii) muscular, which can be sub-classified as apical, central, marginal, or multiple depending on the position; (iii) conoventricular, which are subclassified into membranosus, perimembranosus, and malalignment, where the perimembranosus is the most common VSD, placed in the upper part of the septum; and (iv) conal, which are placed in the right ventricular outlet.

The surgical correction is based on patch closure using CPB. The approach is usually transatrial for the majority of the conoventricular, muscular, and inlet defects. Conal septal defects may be approach through the pulmonary valve or by infundibular right ventriculotomy. Apical muscular defects may require an apical ventriculotomy. Palliation of VSDs is based on pulmonary artery banding, to protect the pulmonary circulation from the effects of chronic overflow. It is presently restricted to critically ill patients.

Complete atrioventricular septal defects

Common associated with Down's syndrome, complete atrioventricular septal defects (CAVDs) represent about 3% of all the congenital heart defects. The definition of a CAVD requires the presence of an ASD (ostium primum), a VSD (inlet), and a common atrioventricular valve with valvular regurgitation and the resulting left-to-right shunt is severe. Surgical correction is performed by transatrial approach, with one or two patches using CPB. Palliative pulmonary artery banding is restricted to critically ill patients.

Right-to-left shunt heart defects

Right-to-left shunt is present when the deoxygenated blood from the systemic veins enters into the systemic circulation bypassing

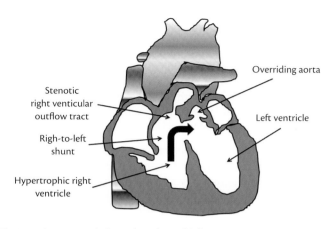

Fig. 21.3 Anatomopathology of tetralogy of Fallot.

the pulmonary circulation, through a heart defect. This leads to the pattern of cyanosis. Cyanosis is defined as subnormal arterial haemoglobin oxygen saturation SaO_2, and is a visible condition when SaO_2 falls below 85%, or below 75% in case of low haemoglobin concentration. A consequence of chronic cyanosis is the compensatory increase of the haematocrit, with increased blood viscosity. Chronic cyanotic patients may experience liver dysfunction and thrombocytopenia.

Transposition of the great arteries

Transposition of the great arteries (TGA) is the most common cyanotic congenital heart defect in newborns. There is a ventriculoarterial discordance in that the aorta rises from the right ventricle and the pulmonary artery from the left ventricle. An ASD, VSD, and PDA may be present, to guarantee adequate blood mixing and partial oxygenation.

Immediately after birth, the patient may be severely cyanotic and haemodynamically unstable if the PDA or the ASD are inadequate to guarantee an adequate blood mixing. The presence of a VSD usually (but not always) guarantees an adequate oxygenation. Whenever blood mixing is inadequate, PGE_1 must be initiated, and an atrial balloon septostomy performed. The surgical correction of choice is an arterial switch, which involves: (i) transection of both the great vessels; (ii) closure of the ASD and VSD; (iii) translocation of the pulmonary arteries anterior to the aorta; (iv) harvesting of the coronary arteries and re-implantation on the neo-aorta; (v) direct suture of the neoaorta to the native pulmonary root rising from the left ventricle and suture (with a patch) of the pulmonary arteries to the native aortic root rising from the right ventricle. Other TGA patterns, with associated VSD and pulmonary stenosis, require a different surgical management (1st step systemic-pulmonary shunt, 2nd step Rastelli operation or intraventricular repair).

Tetralogy of fallot

Tetralogy of Fallot (TOF) is one of the most common (15%) congenital heart defects. It includes four features: VSD, aorta overriding the VSD, right ventricular hypertrophy, and right ventricular outflow tract (RVOT) obstruction (figure 21.3). The most variable feature is the RVOT obstruction: being due to a muscular infundibular hypertrophy, it is a dynamic obstruction, with different degrees of severity depending on the hypertrophic muscle dimensions and on the haemodynamic conditions. Due to the RVOT obstruction, there is an intraventricular right-to-left shunt through the VSD, determining different degrees of cyanosis. Some patients, with mild RVOT obstruction, may be acyanotic.

Under specific haemodynamic conditions (catecholamine release due to pain and anxiety; hypovolaemia; a fall in the systemic resistance) the RVOT obstruction may become extremely severe, with profound cyanosis due to a dramatic decrease of the pulmonary blood flow and Q_p/Q_s. This cyanotic crises called 'Tet-spells', are fought by older children who assume a squatting position in the attempt to increase systemic vascular resistance and venous return.

In the 1990s many institutions treated cyanotic TOF infants with a palliative step as a systemic to pulmonary shunt and postponing the correction until about two years of age. Nowadays, with the only exception of severely cyanotic newborns, patients are treated with medical therapy (beta-blockers) and the total correction is planned for 2–6 months of age. Newborns with PDA and severe RVOT obstruction may experience severe cyanosis once the PDA closes. In these cases, alprostadil is used at a starting dose of 0.1 μg/kg/min followed by a lower dose of 0.01–0.05 μg/kg/min.

The surgical correction includes VSD closure and removal of the RVOT obstruction. While the VSD may be closed through a right atriotomy, the RVOT obstruction is accessed through the pulmonary artery and valve and the obstructive muscle bundles are resected. However, severe forms of RVOT obstruction require a right ventriculotomy that can also be used for the VSD closure. Pericardial patches are used to close the pulmonary artery and the right ventriculotomy. When the obstruction involves the pulmonary valve, a transannular patch is required.

Pulmonary atresia with an intact interventricular septum

Pulmonary atresia with an intact interventricular septum is characterized by an imperforate pulmonary valve, with various degrees of right ventriclar and tricuspid valve hypoplasia, often associated with coronary fistulas and sinusoids. Pulmonary blood flow is provided by a PDA. Systemic venous return may reach the left atrium through an ASD.

Ductal patency is maintained with prostaglandin E_1 (PGE_1) infusion before intervention and mechanical ventilation and IV infusion of vasoconstrictors are often necessary.

Currently, many institutions address this pathology with a transcatheter interventional approach to undertake radio-frequency-assisted valve perforation and balloon valvulotomy. Subsequently, the patient may require a stenting of the PDA, or the surgical placement of a Blalock–Taussig systemic-pulmonary shunt. As a second step, and depending on the right ventriclar size, the patient is treated with a two-ventricle repair (RVOT patch with or without additional shunt) or a single-ventricle repair (bidirectional Glenn and additional shunt). The third step is closure of the ASD and shunt for biventricular repair, and Fontan operation for single-ventricle repair.

Other congenital heart defects

Truncus arteriosus

Truncus arteriosus represents 0.7–1% of the congenital heart defects. In truncus arteriosus, there is a unique arterial trunk that provides blood flow to the coronary arteries and the pulmonary, and systemic circulations. A VSD is always present, and a single truncal valve. There are different types of truncus arteriosus depending on the pattern of pulmonary artery or arteries connection to the common trunk. The pathophysiology of this lesion is quite peculiar, with a distribution of blood flow to the systemic and pulmonary circulation that depends on the pulmonary and systemic arterial resistances. The ratio of pulmonary to systemic blood flow (Q_p/Q_s) varies according to the resistances. If there is a stenosis of the pulmonary arteries albeit very rare, it is decreased and the patient is cyanotic. Conversely, patients with normal pulmonary resistances have an increased Q_p/Q_s, with signs of cardiac failure and this is the most common form. This pathophysiology is of particular importance for the perioperative management before correction, because accidental hyperventilation may lead to catastrophic hypotension with a critical decrease in blood flow to the coronary arteries.

The surgical repair of isolated truncus arteriosus requires CPB and is based on the detachment of the pulmonary artery or arteries and their connection to the right ventricle with a valved conduit or a homograft.

Double-outlet right ventricle

Double-outlet right ventricle (DORV) includes a number of different anatomical forms which differ for the location of the VSD, the relationship between the great vessels and the ventricles, and the presence of RVOT obstruction. Depending on the previously reported patterns, cyanosis can be mild to severe. The surgical correction varies as well in the different anatomical conditions.

A preliminary palliation with a Blalock–Taussig shunt is considered in presence of RVOT obstruction and severe cyanosis, or a pulmonary artery banding in presence of an unrestricted VSD. The final repair may be complete, biventricular (closure of the VSD with a patch that is normally placed so as to direct the blood flow from the ventricles) with additional procedures (resection of RVOT or LVOT obstructions) when appropriate. Some patients with unfavorable anatomy are planned for univentricular repair (bidirectional Glenn and subsequently Fontan operation).

Hypoplastic left heart syndrome

Hypoplastic left heart syndrome (HLHS) accounts for about 1–2% of congenital heart defects and has a 95% mortality within the first month of life (3). HLHS includes different anatomical patterns, which have in common hypoplasia of the left ventricle and ascending aorta. The pathophysiology at birth is represented by a PDA-sustained systemic and coronary circulations, with the pulmonary venous blood that reaches the right atrium through a patent foramen ovale or ASD. The right ventricle is acting as the ventricle for both the systemic (through the PDA) and pulmonary circulations, with a Q_p/Q_s that depends on the ratio of systemic to pulmonary vascular resistances. Usually, the Q_p/Q_s is around 1 when the S_aO_2 is 70–80% (3). Closure of the PDA leads to cardiogenic shock and death, and maintaining the patency of the ductus arteriosus is mandatory using PGE_1 infusion.

There are different surgical approaches that all aim to obtain a single-ventricle correction with the right ventricle acting as systemic ventricle, and the pulmonary blood flow guaranteed by a Fontan circulation. There is the possibility of using a hybrid approach, with percutaneous stenting of the PDA, balloon septostomy if necessary, and surgical banding of both the pulmonary arteries. Subsequently, the patients undergo the aortic arch reconstruction and bidirectional superior vena cava to pulmonary artery connection, finally undergoing a transcatheter Fontan procedure

The classical surgical approach is the Norwood (or Sano-modified) procedure. This includes: (i) pulmonary blood flow provided by a Blalock–Taussig shunt (Norwood) or right ventricle-pulmonary artery conduit (Sano); (ii) reconstruction of the aortic arch and separation of the pulmonary arteries from the pulmonary trunk; (iii) suture of the pulmonary trunk to the proximal ascending aorta; (iv) atrial septectomy. Subsequently, the patient will undergo a bidirectional Glenn operation and a Fontan operation.

Anomalous pulmonary venous return

In partial and total anomalous pulmonary venous return (PAPVR and TAPVR), the pulmonary venous blood drain into the systemic veins either partially or totally causing a left-to-right shunt. In PAPVR, the left-sided pulmonary veins may drain into the coronary sinus or the left innominate vein, and the right-sided pulmonary veins into the superior or inferior vena cava.

TAPVR may be *supracardiac, cardiac, infradiaphragmatic,* or *mixed.* When the pulmonary venous return is obstructed, this represents a neonatal emergency for cardiac surgery. An ASD is necessary for survival and is part of the TAPVR pattern. The left heart chambers are loaded by a right-to-left shunt at the level of the ASD.

In patients with obstructed TAPVR there is a pulmonary venous hypertension and pulmonary oedema, with retrograde pulmonary arterial hypertension. Surgical repair of TAPVR requires CPB, and in newborns and small infants, hypothermic circulatory arrest may be necessary. Supracardiac and infracardiac TAPVR involves closure of the ASD and anastomosis of the pulmonary vein confluence with the left atrium. In the cardiac type, the anomalous pulmonary veins are funnelled into the left atrium with a pericardial patch, through the ASD, cutting the roof of the coronary sinus.

Pulmonary stenosis

Isolated valvular pulmonary stenosis is a relatively common (5–10%) congenital heart defect, whereas isolated subvalvular pulmonary stenosis is uncommon. Pulmonary artery stenosis may be present at the level of the main pulmonary artery and/or pulmonary artery branches. In all these conditions, there is a pressure gradient across the pulmonary blood flow, with right ventricular hypertrophy. This may lead, in the most severe cases, to a right-to-left shunt at the atrial level. The approach to valvular pulmonary stenosis is based on balloon valvuloplasty. Supravalvular obstructions may be treated with balloon pulmonary arterioplasty, stent implantation, or surgical pulmonary artery plasty.

Left ventricular outflow tract obstruction

Left ventricular outflow tract obstruction includes valvular, subvalvular, and supravalvular obstructions. The common pathophysiological pattern is the pressure overload of the left ventricle, with left ventricular hypertrophy. Aortic valve stenosis may be associated with monocuspid or bicuspid valve morphology. Severe stenosis in the newborn may require ductal patency preservation with PGE_1 and urgent balloon valvotomy. The surgical approach includes aortic valvotomy, aortic valve replacement with mechanical valve or aortic allografts, and the Ross procedure (pulmonary autograft on the left ventricle outflow and homograft on the right ventricle outflow).

Subaortic stenosis may be due to a subvalvular membrane, hypertrophic obstructive cardiomyopathy, or other rare causes of obstruction. The surgical approach is usually through the aorta, with removal of the obstructive tissue. Supra-aortic stenosis is a narrowing of the aortic root which requires a surgical plasty with an adequate enlargement patch.

Coarctation of the aorta

Coarctation of the aorta is a narrowing of the descending aorta at the level of the ductus implantation. In critical coarctation of the aorta, the flow distal to the narrowing is guaranteed by a PDA. Closure of the PDA determines cardiogenic shock and critical visceral organs perfusion. Surgical correction is the option of choice for coarctation of the aorta and is usually performed through a left thoracotomy without CPB. Depending on the anatomy of the lesion, the correction may include an end-to-end anastomosis, a prosthetic patch aortoplasty, or a subclavian flap aortoplasty. Transcatheter interventions (balloon dilatation with or without stenting) are restricted to older children and adolescents, or to post-surgical re-coarctation.

Preoperative assessment of the paediatric cardiac patient

According to the current standards, paediatric patients are defined as newborn (ages 0–1 month), infant (1 month–1 year), toddler (1–3 years), or child (4 years–13 years). Before being submitted to any procedure which require sedation or anaesthesia, the patient should receive a complete examination from an experienced anesthesiologist and preferably, the same one who will anaesthetize the child. This examination includes all the standard procedures of preoperative assessment in paediatric surgery, plus some specific items.

Physical examination

A physical examination is important to identify concomitant conditions which should cause the procedure to be postponed. Fever and upper respiratory tract infections are the most common reasons for postponement. However, some congenital heart defects (with left-to-right shunt) may predispose the patient to a chronic upper airways inflammation and secretions. In these cases waiting for a complete resolution of symptoms like cough and nasal secretions before operating may be unrealistic. In these cases, the patient should be evaluated using the chest X-rays and blood tests, including white cell count and C-reactive protein.

Important points to note are airway viability, dysmorphisms that may complicate tracheal intubation, access for the peripheral, central venous, and arterial catheters. Symptoms of cardiac failure including poor physical development, reduced exercise tolerance, tachycardia, tachypnoea, and hepatomegaly should be recorded, as well as cyanosis. The neurological status should be determined, and if deficits are found then a neurologist's opinion is valuable.

Blood tests

Standard blood tests should include a full blood count, coagulation screen (platelet count, activated partial thromboplastin time, prothrombin time with international normalized ratio), electrolytes, renal and liver function tests, and blood glucose levels. Additional tests may be required as, for example, when there is an abnormally long activated partial thromboplastin time in a patient who is not receiving heparin, which may indicate congenital thrombophilic patterns such as antiphospholipid syndrome.

In patients who have an arterial line in-situ then arterial blood-gas analysis is valuable.

Electrocardiograph and imaging

A recent 12-lead electrocardiograph should be examined. Imaging including chest X-ray, echocardiography, magnetic resonance imaging, computerized tomography, and angiography, is essential for the correct diagnosis of congenital heart defects. Not all these examinations are required but the available imaging should be sufficient to clearly diagnose the heart defect(s), and should always include chest X-rays and echocardiography. The anesthesiologist should be able to personally assess chest X-rays and to correctly interpret the reports from the other imaging procedures. In particular, he should identify additional pieces of information that may be relevant for the anaesthetic management, such as signs of tracheal obstruction or displacement on chest X-rays, dextroposition of the aortic arch on echocardiography and anomalous venous vessels on the angiogram.

Risk stratification

A thorough preoperative assessment is important as surgery may need to be postponed to improve the patient's conditions; to allow anaesthesia strategy to be planned; to ensure adequate amounts of concentrated red blood cells, fresh frozen plasma, and platelet concentrate are available; to ensure specific therapeutic measures such as inhaled nitric oxide; mechanical circulatory support are available; and so a risk stratification can be performed.

In contrast to adults, risk stratification in paediatric cardiac surgery is not a standardized because of the range of congenital heart defects and consequently, the wide range of cardiac surgery operations. The first attempts to stratify the mortality risk in paediatric cardiac surgery were based on a raw estimation of the operation complexity. The Risk Adjustment in Congenital Heart Surgery (RACHS-1) (4) and the Aristotle Basic Complexity (ABC) Score (5) measure the procedural complexity (table 21.1). Whilst the ABC Score includes no risk factors other than the surgery, the Aristotle Comprehensive Complexity (ACC) Score adds to the ABC Score a number of patient-related and procedure-independent factors.

Risk stratification is important for institutional databases to compare the complexity of the procedures over a number of years, and to enable audit of the surgical outcomes. In addition, it is a tool that allows adequate provision of information to the patient's parents about the severity and the risk of the procedure. However, a comprehensive explanation of the procedure with all the risks and benefits is better received by the parents and relatives than a crude number expressing the expected mortality rate. The perioperative period is enormously stressful for the family, and a frank and sympathetic contact between the attending physicians and the family is the best way to approach any kind of problem may occur during the hospitalization. Within this process, it is a good rule to allow the parents to accompany the child to the anaesthetic room together with a nurse, and possibly to stay with the patient until transfer to the operating room.

Preanaesthetic management

Fasting is required before anaesthesia for cath-lab procedures or surgery. However, and especially for patients with heart defects, prolonged fasting may lead to dehydration and hypovolaemia.

Table 21.1 Aristotle Basic Complexity Score for the common operations for congenital heart defects

Operation	Basic Score
Norwood procedure	14.5
Truncus arteriosus repair	11.0
Double outlet right ventricle intraventricular repair	10.3
Ross procedure	10.3
Arterial switch operation	10.0
Fontan operation	9.0
Total anomalous pulmonary venous return repair	9.0
Complete atrioventricular canal repair	9.0
Tetralogy of Fallot repair	7.5–11.0*
Bidrectional Glenn operation	7.0
Aortic coarctation repair	6.0–8.0*
Aortic stenosis (subvalvular) repair	6.3
Blalock–Taussig shunt	6.3
Pulmonary artery banding	6.0
Ventricular septal defect repair	6.0
Aortic stenosis (supravalvular) repair	5.5
Atrial septal defect repair	3.0
Patent ductus arteriosus closure	3.0

* Depending on the procedure type

This condition is particularly harmful in some specific congenital heart defects where the maintenance of an adequate cardiac output is strongly dependent on preload conditions. Hypovolaemia in TOF patients may trigger 'Tet-spells', In these and other severely ill patients, maintenance of an adequate hydration and euvolaemia may be achieved by administering intravenous (IV) fluids. Guidelines recommend that clear liquids such as water, fruit juices without pulp and tea are allowed up to 2 hours preoperatively; breast milk up to 4 hours preoperatively; infant formula up to 6 hours preoperatively; and solid food up to 6–8 hours preoperatively (6–8).

Before cardiac surgery or interventional transcatheter procedures, critically ill patients should be optimized to reach the operating room or cath lab in the best possible conditions (box 21.2).

Premedication

Premedication has a number of goals, including sedation, analgesia, and anti-cholinergic effects (9). However, premedication should be avoided in patients who are critically ill or weigh less than 3 kg. Anticholinergic drugs including atropine, scopolamine, and glycopyrrolate induce discomfort as they dry the mouth and so are avoided in many institutions (9). Sedative, hypnotic, and analgesic drugs include a wide number of agents and they can be used individually or more commonly, in combination (table 21.2).

Premedication with opioids may result in respiratory depression. Some conditions such as TOF, are prone to hypoxic events before and during induction of anaesthesia, and a heavy premedication may trigger 'Tet-spells' due to hypoxia and vasodilation.

Box 21.2 Main preoperative measures to stabilize critically ill patients

- Maintenance of ductus arteriosus patency in ductus-dependent congenital heart defects: prostaglandin E_1 infusion 0.01–0.05 µg/kg/min or higher starting dose if the ductus is closed.

- Tetralogy of Fallot with severe cyanosis: 100% oxygen, intubation, mechanical ventilation, sedation and paralysis. Correction of hypovolaemia with adequate crystalloid fluids administration and correction of metabolic acidosis. Beta-blockers (esmolol or propanolol). In Tet-spell crises refractory to these measures, phenylephrine or nor-epinephrine 2–5 µg/kg bolus followed by 0.1–0.2 µg/kg/min infusion.

- Neonatal critical aortic coarctation: maintenance of ductus arterious patency; fluid restriction to avoid pulmonary oedema; mechanical ventilation at ambient FiO_2 and $PaCO_2$ 40–45 mmHg, with positive end-expiratory pressure. Correction of metabolic acidosis. Reduction of systemic vascular resistances with vasodilators. Parenteral nutrition.

- Hypoplastic left heart syndrome: prevention of pulmonary blood overflow by addition of CO_2 to the inspired gas. When mechanically ventilated, balance the pulmonary and systemic blood flow through control of the $PaCO_2$, positive inotropes and vasodilators (milrinone).

- Truncus arteriosus: balance of the pulmonary/systemic blood flow (see text).

- Total anomalous pulmonary venous return: tracheal intubation and mechanical ventilation are mandatory. 100% oxygen with positive end expiratory pressure. Use of nitric oxide is controversial due to the risk of pulmonary oedema. In extreme cases, extracorporeal membrane oxygenation.

Additional preoperative measures

Whilst communication with the patient's family is important, children with sufficient comprehension to understand their situation also deserve information. So it is important to establish a sound rapport and to give them a good explanation of what they will experience on arrival in the operating room and during their recovery. If an inhalational induction of anaesthesia is anticipated, then investment of a few minutes to explain the procedure, showing them the face mask, and even simulating an induction is well worthwhile. Finally, anaesthetic creams should be applied to the skin of possible venipuncture sites to reduce or avoid pain.

Intraoperative management

Induction of anaesthesia

Anaesthesia may be induced using an inhalational or IV techniques and there are advantages and disadvantages to both. Inhalational induction avoids the possibly traumatic experience of venipuncture in the awake patient. Unsurprisingly, these children may be needle phobic because they have received previous surgical operations, angiographic examination and transcatheter procedures, or simply have been repeatedly submitted to venipuncture for collection of blood samples.

Table 21.2 Drugs for premedication

Drug and delivery route	Dose
Oral route	
Atropine	0.02 mg/kg (maximum 0.4 mg)
Meperidine	3 mg/kg (maximum 100 mg)
Diazepam	0.15 mg/kg (maximum 10 mg)
Fentanyl	10–20 µg/kg
Midazolam	0.5–1.0 mg/kg
Ketamine	6 mg/kg
Intramuscular route	
Atropine	0.02 mg/kg (maximum 0.4 mg)
Morphine	0,2 mg/kg (maximum 10 mg)
Meperidine	2 mg/kg
Fentanyl	5–10 µg/kg
Midazolam	0.8 mg/kg (maximum 5 mg)
Promethazine	1 mg/kg
Nasal route	
Midazolam	0.2–0.3 mg/kg
Ketamine	1–5 mg/kg
Sufentanil	0.3–3 µg/kg
Rectal route	
Midazolam	0.4 mg/kg
Diazepam	0.7 mg/kg

Reproduced from Lacour-Gayet F et al., 'The Aristotle score: a complexity-adjusted method to evaluate surgical results', *European Journal of Cardio-Thoracic Surgery*, 2004, **25**, 6, pp. 911–924, by permission of European Association for Cardio-Thoracic Surgery, European Society of Thoracic Surgeons and Oxford University Press

Mask induction usually requires two attending anesthesiologists. One takes care of induction and ventilation whilst the other establishes venous access to allow administration of neuromsucular blocking agents before tracheal intubation. Moreover, a lack of venous access may be dangerous when inducing anaesthesia in severely cyanotic tetralogy of Fallot because of the risk of 'Tet-spells' and in truncus arteriosus because hyperventilation may occur and cause steal of systemic and coronary blood flows.

As there is a risk of severe hypotension with halothane, sevoflurane is now used for inhalational induction (10,11). Desflurane and isoflurane are both unsuitable for inhalational induction because of their irritating properties that may trigger laryngospasm and coughing (12,13). Nitrous oxide may be added to the inhaled gas mixture but many patients with severe cyanotic lesions benefit from using 100% oxygen.

Even although many patients arrive in the operating room with an IV catheter already in place, induction of anaesthesia may require insertion of another peripheral venous catheter. Preparation of the skin with adequate anaesthetic cream limits the pain and venipuncture, may often be performed while the parents are still with the child in the preanesthetic room. However, some patients, and especially the cyanotic ones and those who have already experienced many venepunctures, may present a

challenge. In such cases, patients can be treated with intramuscular ketamine (5–7 mg/kg) 10–20 minutes before venipuncture.

IV induction of anaesthesia usually includes the use of a hypnotic and an analgesic drugs. Available hypnotics include diazepam, which is now rarely used, midazolam, pentobarbital, etomidate, ketamine, and propofol; the most commonly used are midazolam and propofol. Midazolam is a benzodiazepine that maintains cardiovascular stability (14,15), and is well tolerated even at doses as high as 0.6–0.8 mg/kg. Propofol (1–1.5 mg/kg) induces a considerable decrease of the systemic vascular resistance with consequent decrease of systemic arterial blood pressure (16). In contrast, ketamine (1 mg/kg) has the advantage of preserving heart rate, arterial blood pressure, and ejection fraction. Opioids are used during IV induction of anaesthesia for analgesia and fentanyl is commonly used (5 µg/kg up to a maximum of 100 µg).

The choice of drug for induction and maintenance of anaesthesia depends on the underlying cardiovascular disease. Some patients tolerate very poorly a sudden decrease of the systemic vascular resistance and in particular, those with right-to-left shunt that may be increased by reductions of pre-and after-load. Moreover, the anaesthetist should be aware of some specific challenges posed by some cardiovascular diseases. Induction of anaesthesia may trigger 'Tet-spells' in TOF patients, due to inadequate sedation, analgesia, hypovolaemia, and decrease of the systemic vascular resistance. Such crises must be promptly treated, because in the most severe cases they may lead to cardiac arrest. Pillars for the prevention and treatment of Tet-spell crises are listed in box 21.3.

Truncus arteriosus is another challenging condition as inadvertent hyperventilation decreases the P_aCO_2 and triggers an overflow of pulmonary blood, with consequent steal of systemic and coronary blood flow. During induction of anaesthesia and the pre-CPB period the P_aCO_2 should be maintained at normal or slightly supranormal values.

Maintenance of anaesthesia

Anaesthesia is usually maintained with a combination of hypnotic and analgesic drugs and inhalational anaesthetic agents. Continuous IV infusion of hypnotics and analgesics is useful to maintain a stable level of anaesthesia. Midazolam can be used at a dose of 1–3 µg/kg/min, and propofol at a dose of 3 mg/kg/hr. For IV infusions of opioids, the usual dose range is 2–4 µg/kg/min for fentanyl, 0.3–1 µg/kg/min for remifentanil, and 10–40 µg/kg/hr for morphine. Sufentanil and alfentanil are less commonly used.

Box 21.3 Prevention and treatment of 'Tet-spells'

- Hyperventilation at 100% oxygen
- Bolus administration of IV fluids (10 mL/kg)
- Opioids
- Beta-adrenergic blocker (esmolol or propranolol), noting that chronically beta-blocked patients may not respond
- Vasoconstrictors to increase the systemic vascular resistance and decrease the right-to-left shunt (phenylephrine 2–5 µg/kg or norepinephrine 2 µg/kg)
- Intravenous sodium bicarbonate administration (1–2 mEq/kg)

The adequacy of the anaesthesia level may be checked with the bi-spectral (BIS) monitoring. Except for remifentanil, deepening of the analgesia level may be obtained with supplemental bolus administration of opioids. A volatile agent such as sevoflurane, desflurane, or isoflurane, is usually added to the opioid anaesthesia, replacing or supplementing IV hypnotic drugs.

Neuromuscular blockade and tracheal intubation

Atracurium, cisatracurium, rocuronium, vecuronium, and mivacurium are the most commonly used neuromuscular blocking agents for tracheal intubation given at the usual doses for paediatric patients. Muscle relaxation may be maintained using a continuous IV infusion for some of these drugs (atracurium 5–10 µg/kg/min, rocuronium 0.6–1 mg/kg/hr, vecuronium 0.05–0.1 mg/kg/hr) (17).

For low-weight children, and whenever a prolonged postoperative intubation is anticipated, nasotracheal intubation should be used because there is a lower risk of tube displacement, accidental extubation, and better postoperative care of the airways. The size (internal diameter) of the tracheal tube (usually not-cuffed for small children) is 2.5–3.0 mm for 1–2 kg newborns and 3.0–3.5 mm for 0 to 3 months newborns. For the other infants and children, it may be calculated according to the formula: 4 + age/4.

Intravenous fluid administration

Before CPB, IV fluids are delivered to maintain normovolaemia. Some infants such as those with a left-to-right shunt because of a VSD arrive in the operating room particularly in need for IV fluid administration because of diuretic therapy. When 5% glucose solution is used, blood glucose should be carefully monitored to avoid hyperglycaemia. Alternatively, Hartmann's solution or 0.9% saline may be used and 5% albumin may be added to these solutions to avoid a decrease of colloid-osmotic pressure. Alternatively, in children more than 1 year, gelatins may be used.

Thermal management

Newborns and small infants are prone to heat loss and their core and surface temperatures should be monitored. Thermal management should include control of ambient temperature and active heating with a warming blanket, radiant heater and air warmer.

Monitoring during heart surgery

Except for simple operations such as closure of a PDA in a newborn, monitoring of the paediatric patient undergoing heart operations whether with or without CPB, should always include those listed in table 21.3, and in selected cases, additional monitoring may be required.

Electrocardiography

Intraoperative electrocardiography (ECG) using 12-leads is mandatory during every cardiac operation. The four peripheral leads plus a V_5 lead are usually monitored. The main indication is the detection of dysrhythmias. However, ST-segment changes are most important during the operation, and especially in surgical procedures which involve the coronary arteries such as switch operation for TGA. In addition, in open-heart procedures air may enter the left cardiac chambers and embolise into the coronary circulation and usually the right coronary artery. ST-segments changes in the V_2, V_3, aVF leads are suggestive for this event.

Table 21.3 Monitoring of the paediatric patient undergoing heart operations

STANDARD MONITORING	
Technique and materials	**Measurements**
5-leads electrocardiography on screen	Heart rate, arrhythmias, ST changes
Arterial catheterization	Invasive blood pressure
	$PaO_2 - SaO_2 - PaCO_2$
	Base excess
	Arterial blood lactates
	Blood glucose level
Central venous catheter	Central venous pressure
	$S_c\bar{v}O_2$
Pulse oxymetry	Arterial oxygen saturation
Capnography	End-tidal CO_2
Skin and core temperature probes	Peripheral and core temperature
ADDITIONAL MONITORING	
Left atrial catheter (surgically placed)	Left atrial pressure
Pulmonary artery catheter (surgically placed)	Pulmonary artery pressure
	$S\bar{v}O_2$
Oxymetric central venous catheters	Continuous $S_c\bar{v}O_2$
Near-infrared spectroscopy	rSO_2

Invasive arterial blood pressure

Arterial catheterization for measurement of the systemic arterial pressure is undertaken using dedicated arterial catheters or standard venous catheters. Possible sites of access are radial arteries, brachial arteries (a second choice due to the risk of arm ischaemia), and femoral arteries. Less commonly used sites include the axillary arteries, the dorsalis pedis and the posterior tibial arteries.

Central venous catheters

Central venous catheters (CVCs) can be inserted into the internal jugular (figure 21.4), subclavian, or femoral veins. The right internal jugular vein is the most direct approach to the superior vena cava. Caution should be taken when cannulating the left jugular vein as it is possible to perforate the vessel at junction between the jugular vein and anonymous venous trunk. The correct position of the tip of the CVC is the superior caval-atrial junction or inferior caval-atrial junction when inserted into femoral vein.

CVCs are important for administration of IV fluids and inotropic and vasoactive drugs. However, because of their length and small gauge most especially with double- and triple-lumen CVCs, they are inadequate for fast administration of large volumes of IV fluids. Positioning of a short venous catheter of adequate size inside another vessel such as an external jugular vein or a femoral vein, is required and could be life saving whenever a fast correction of acute hypovolaemia, as a result of major haemorrhage, is required.

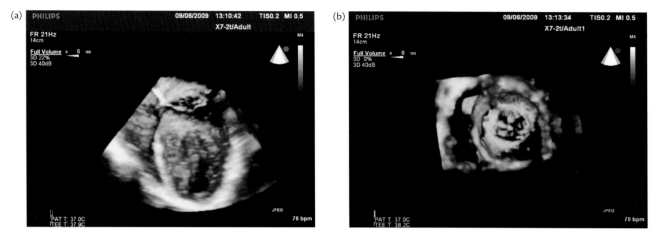

Fig. 2.2 Dilated left ventricle

(a) 3D echocardiography image illustrating a dilated left ventricle. (b) 3D transoesophageal echocardiography image demonstrating short axis view of a dilated left ventricle.

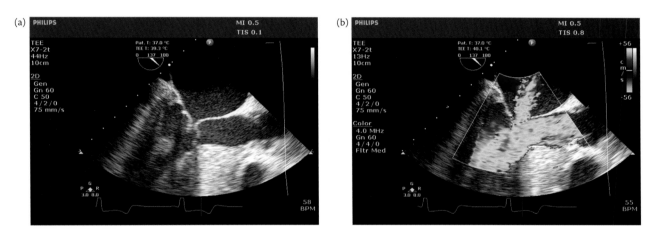

Fig. 2.3 Hypertrophic cardiomyopathy

(a) 2D Echo image of an obstructed left ventricular outflow tract in a patient with hypertrophic cardiomyopathy. (b) 2D colour flow Doppler image of the same left ventricular outflow tract obstruction demonstrating turbulence during systole, as well as mitral regurgitation.

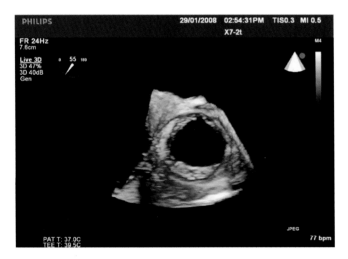

Fig. 2.5 Aortic valve

3D transoesophageal echocardiography image illustrating the normal triangular shape of the aortic valve in late systole.

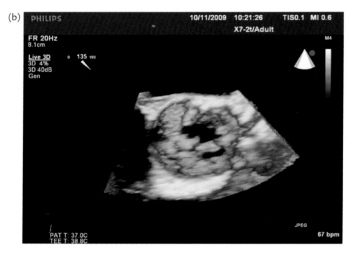

Fig. 2.6b Calcified aortic valve
3D echocardiography image clearly illustrating areas of calcification on a stenotic aortic valve.

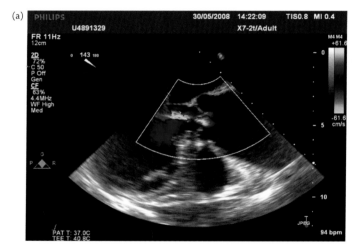

Fig. 2.9a Dilated aortic root
A 2D colour flow Doppler image illustrating a dilated aortic root and resultant functional aortic regurgitation.

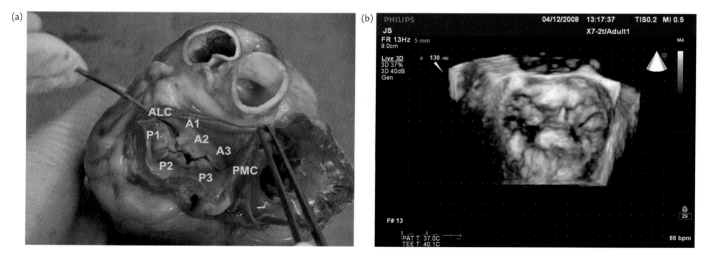

Fig. 2.11 Mitral valve
(a) Porcine heart illustrating normal arrangement of MV anatomy. (b) 3D echocardiography image of a normal MV, seen en-face from the atrial side.

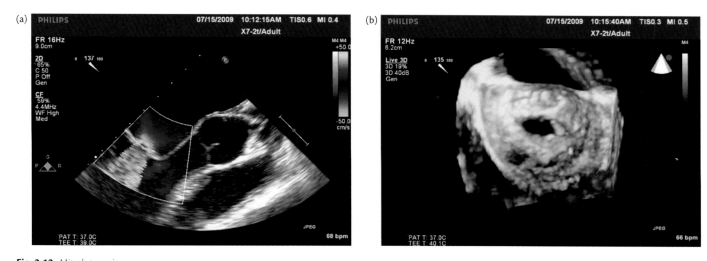

Fig. 2.12 Mitral stenosis

(a) 2D colour flow Doppler transoesophageal echocardiography image illustrating decreased inflow across a stenotic mitral valve. (b) 3D echocardiography image of a stenotic calcified mitral valve with fused commissures and consequent reduced MV area, seen again from the left atrial side.

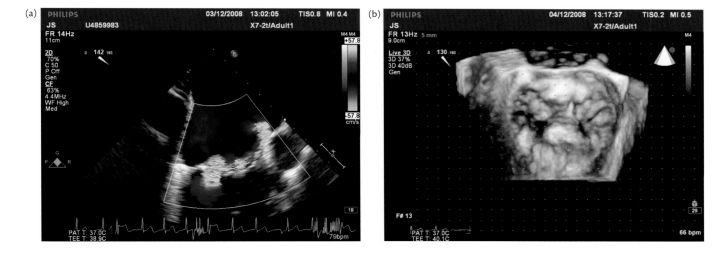

Fig. 2.15 Mitral regurgitation

(a) 2D colour flow Doppler image of an anteriorly directed eccentric regurgitant jet of mitral regurgitation. (b) 3D echocardiography image of mitral valve posterior leaflet prolapse seen from the atrial side.

(b)

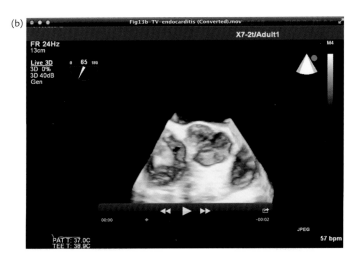

Fig. 2.18b Infective endocarditis
3D echocardiography image clearly demonstrating the same vegetations on the tricuspid valve.

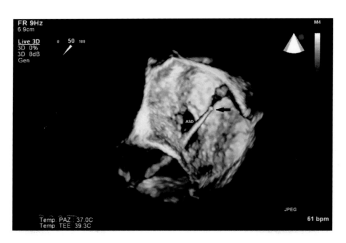

Fig. 9.2 RT3DTOE view of the atrial septum from the left atrial side. A catheter (arrow) is seen crossing the ASD

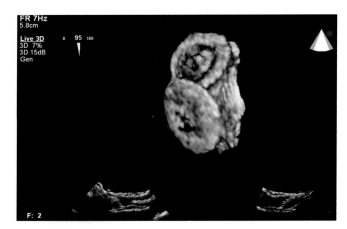

Fig. 9.3 Two devices have been implanted in two separate ASDs: RT3DTOE confirms their correct placement, with partial overlapping

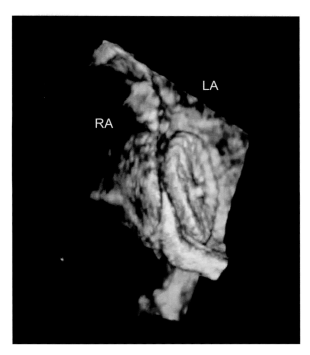

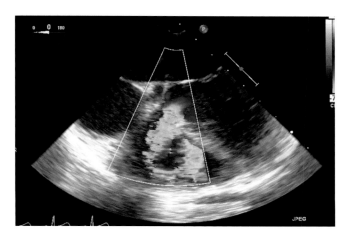

Fig. 9.6 2D Color TOE. Perimembranous VSD

Fig. 9.5 RT3DTOE: right and left disk of Amplatzer® PFO Occluder device, embracing the interatrial septum

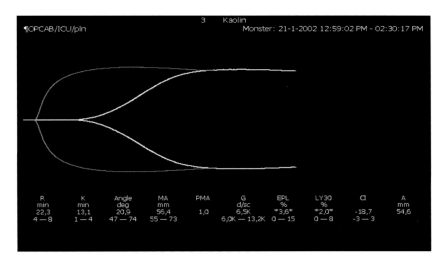

Fig. 11.12 Thromboelastographic tracing (with and without heparinase) of a patient with residual circulating heparin

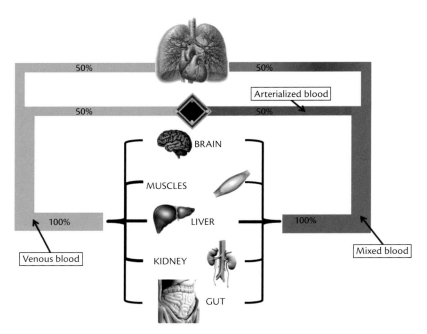

Fig. 12.1 Schematic representation of a veno-arterial ECMO circuit. For simplicity the case of a patient with complete pulmonary shunt is represented, i.e. a patient where the native lungs do not contribute to gas exchange

Venous blood is drained through a cannula placed in the venous system and pumped through the membrane lung. In figure, 50% of cardiac output is pumped through the artificial lung. Blood exiting from the membrane lung (in this case 50% of cardiac output) is completely oxygenated and cleared of CO_2. Thereafter it is delivered back to the arterial system, in this case through a cannula placed in the femoral artery. Here arterialized blood mixes with venous blood arriving from the failing lungs, and mixed blood perfuses the organs and tissues with retrograde flow. As can be noted, the retrograde flow does not assure an adequate oxygenation of the coronary arteries and of the brain. Moreover, the native lungs can be substantially underperfused, depending on the amount of blood shunted through the membrane lung. Blue represents venous blood, bright red represents arterialized blood exiting the artificial lung, while dark red represents mixed blood, i.e. a mixture of venous blood arriving from the native lungs and arterialized blood arriving from the artificial lung. Percentages represent percentages of circulating blood volume (for more details see the text).

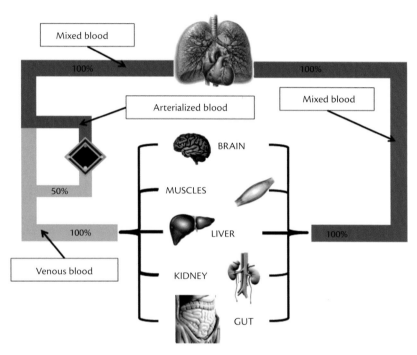

Fig. 12.2 Schematic representation of a venovenous ECMO circuit. For simplicity the case of a patient with complete pulmonary shunt is represented, i.e. a patient where the native lungs do not contribute to gas exchange

Venous blood is drained through a cannula placed in the venous system and pumped through the membrane lung. In the figure, 50% of cardiac output is pumped through the artificial lung. Blood exiting from the membrane lung (in this case 50% of cardiac output) is completely oxygenated and cleared from CO_2. Thereafter it is delivered back into the venous system (see Cannulation section for additional details). Here, arterialized blood mixes with venous blood and is pumped by the heart through the native, failing lungs. As can be noted, blood with high oxygen saturation passes through the lungs and is thereafter pumped by the heart in order to perfuse organs and tissues. An important difference compared to the veno-arterial approach is that 100% circulating volume reaches the native lungs (see figure 12.1 for comparison). Blue represents venous blood, bright red represents arterialized blood exiting the artificial lung, while dark red represents mixed blood, i.e. a mixture of venous blood arriving from the native lungs and arterialized blood arriving from the artificial lung. Percentages represent percentages of circulating blood volume (for more details see the text).

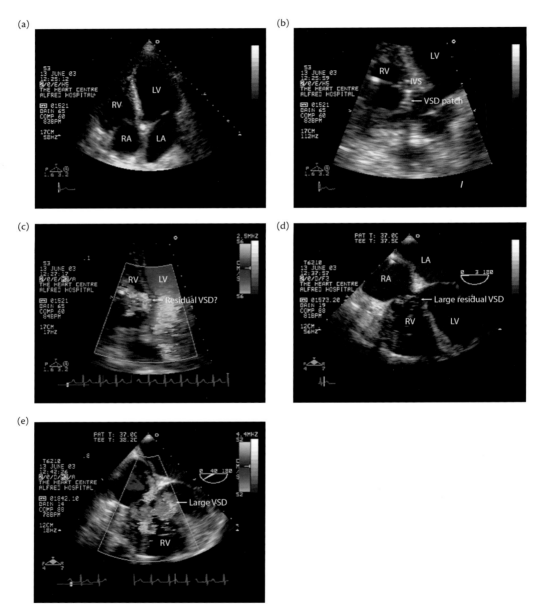

Fig. 28.5 Haemodynamic instability following elective repair of complex membranous ventricular septal defect (VSD)
(a and b) Urgent TTE assessment with patch repair of VSD identified on apical views. (c) Abnormal colour flow jet appearing in RV during systole. Consistent with residual VSD, but clinical significance unclear. (d) Subsequent TOE (mid-oesophageal views) reveals deficit in proximal IVS. (e) Colour flow Doppler demonstrates large flow abnormality consistent with failure of patch repair of VSD. Though TTE findings were consistent with residual VSD, TOE provided definitive evidence of large VSD secondary to failure of repair rather than residual small VSD. Patient returned to the operating room.
LA, left atrium; RA, right atrium; LV, left ventricle; RV, right ventricle; IVS, interventricular septum.

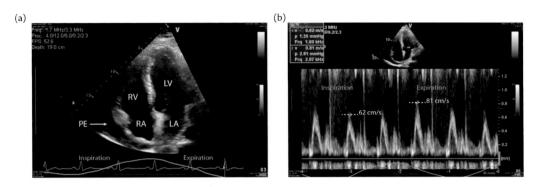

Fig. 28.6 Pericardial effusion with suspected cardiac tamponade
(a) Apical four-chamber view (TTE). Notice green respiratory signal derived from ECG. (b) PW Doppler of mitral inflow. Note inspiratory decrease in MVQ with respect to end-expiration. 25% change consistent with clinical diagnosis of tamponade in a spontaneously breathing patient.
LA, left atrium; RA, right atrium; LV, left ventricle; RV, right ventricle; PE, pericardial effusion.

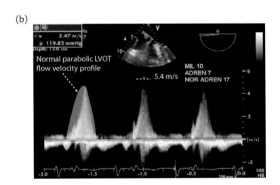

Fig. 28.7b Low cardiac output following cardiac surgery despite increasing inotropic support
CW Doppler of LVOT velocities. Normal CW profile of LVOT velocities is parabolic, with much lower velocities (<1 m/s). With dynamic LVOT obstruction LVOT CW profile becomes dagger shaped and with much higher velocities. Peak gradient across LVOT obstruction is 120 mmHg.

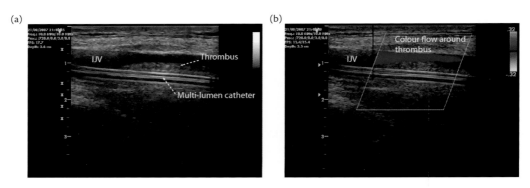

Fig. 28.9 Left IJV
(a and b) Multi-lumen central line in situ with adherent thrombus—confirmed with colour flow imaging
IJV, internal jugular vein.

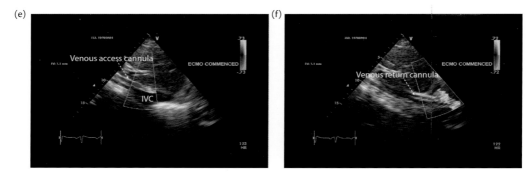

Fig. 28.12 Ultrasound guided venous cannulation for peripheral (venoarterial (VA) or venovenous (VV)) ECMO
(e) Peripheral VV ECMO Venous access cannula confirmed to be in IVC just distal to RA. (Subcostal TTE with colour Doppler). (f) Peripheral VV ECMO Venous return cannula confirmed to be in RA. (Subcostal TTE with colour Doppler).
IVC, inferior vena cava; RA, right atrium; LA, left atrium; SVC, superior vena cava.

(c)

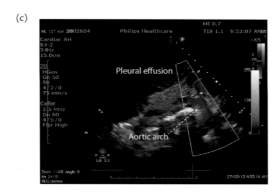

Fig. 28.13c Sudden onset of large pleural effusion and probable pneumothorax
Ultrasound from high posterior left (patient erect) demonstrating collapse of collapse of posterior segments. Note arch of aorta with systolic flow towards transducer.

(b)

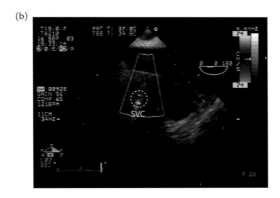

Fig. 28.15b Respiratory failure following aborted aborted right pneumonectomy (bronchogenic SCC)
Colour flow Doppler. Restricted turbulent flow demonstrated through subtotally occluded SVC.
SVC superior vena cava; RPA right pulmonary artery.

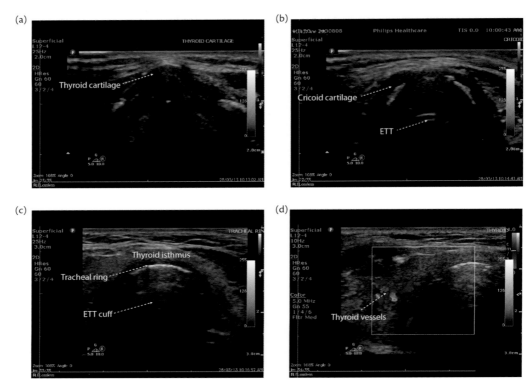

Fig. 28.17 Ultrasound airway assessment prior to tracheostomy (linear probe)
(a) Sharp angle of thyroid cartilage easily demonstrated. (b) Probe slid inferiorly, demonstrating thick round cricoid cartilage. Leading edge of ETT visible. (c) Probe slid further inferiorly demonstrating thinner tracheal ring and multiple reverberation artefact from inflated ETT cuff. Isthmus of thyroid seen anterior to tracheal ring. (d) Colour flow Doppler demonstrating thyroid vessels.
ETT, endotracheal tube.

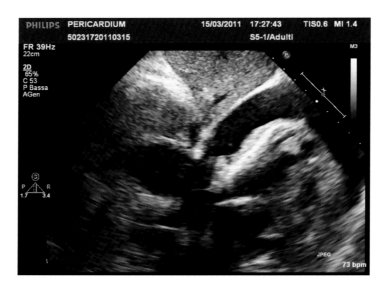

Fig. 29.1 Transthoracic subcostal view showing cardiac tamponade. The cardiac chambers are completely collapsed under by the intrapericardial overpressure.

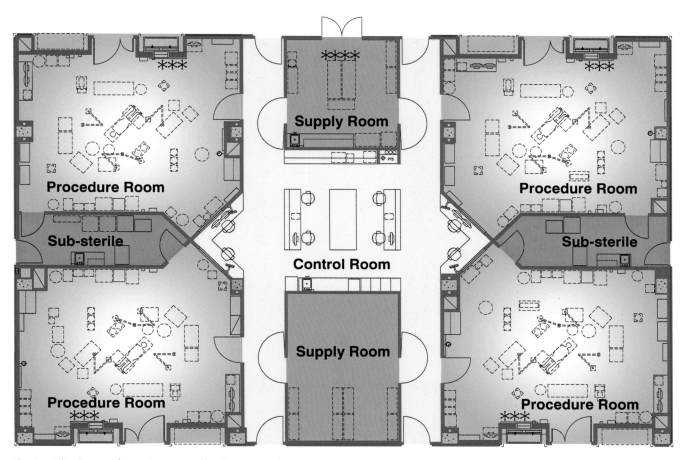

Fig. 40.5 Plan diagram of operating rooms with adjacent control room
Surgical tables placed diagonally within the operating room provide efficient utilization of the corners of the room and provide good visualization from the adjacent control room.

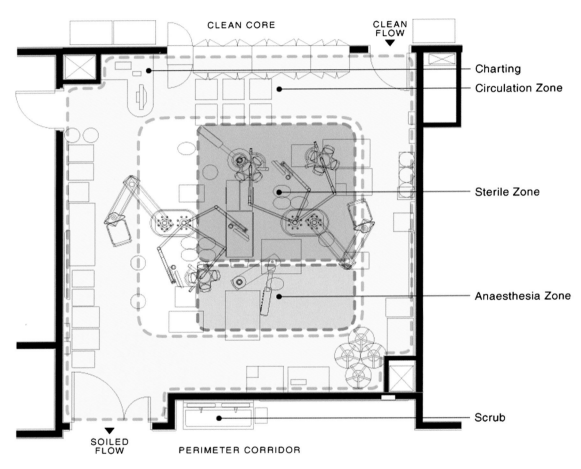

CLEAN CORE

CLEAN
FLOW ▼

Charting

Circulation Zone

Sterile Zone

Anaesthesia Zone

Scrub

SOILED
FLOW ▼

PERIMETER CORRIDOR

Fig. 40.6 Zoning within the surgical operating room
Floor plan showing demarcation of circulating, sterile and anesthesia zones.

(a)

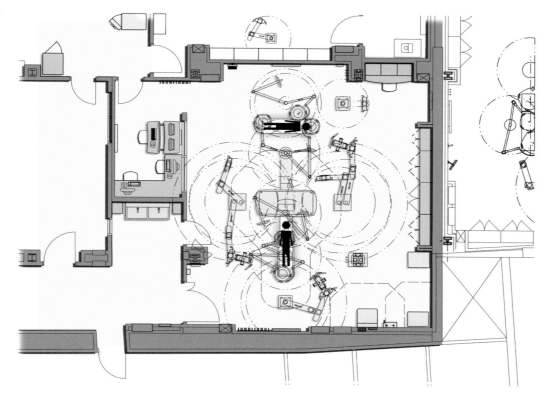

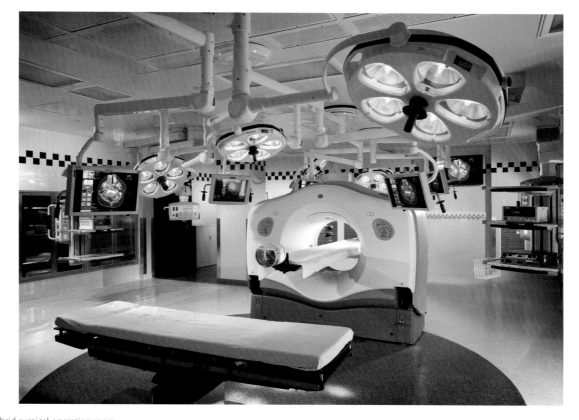

Fig. 40.7 Hybrid surgical operating room

(a) Floor plan and (b) photograph of hybrid surgical operating room with CT imaging capabilities.

(a) University of Pittsburgh Medical Center Hybrid OR # 12; floor plan, © 2007 Stantec Architecture. (b) Interior photograph of University of Pittsburgh Medical Center Hybrid OR 12, © 2007 Ed Massery.

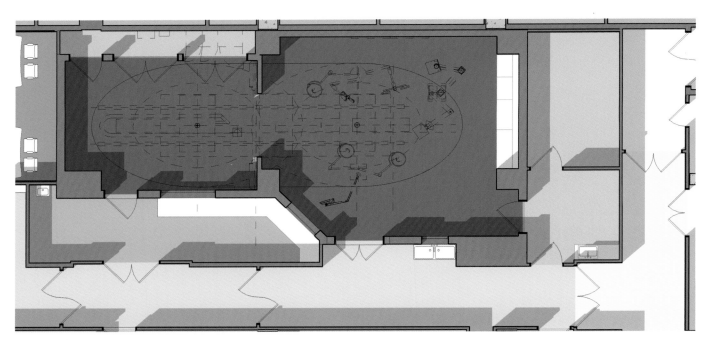

Fig. 40.8a Intraoperative MRI (I-MRI) suite

Intraoperative MR suite where magnet moves to and from patient (a) floor plan

Bostwick Design Partnership, Architect of Record; Anshen+Allen, a part of Stantec Architecture, Consulting Architect.

(a) © 2012 Bostwick Design Partnership..

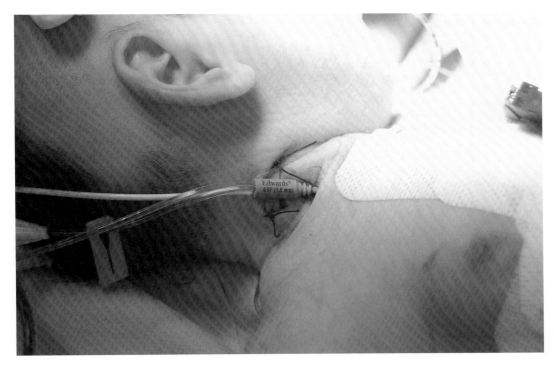

Fig. 21.4 Right internal jugular vein positioning of an oximetric central venous catheter.

CVCs allow continuous measurement of the central venous pressure (CVP). It can also be used to measure the oxyhaemoglobin saturation with oxygen in the superior vena cava ($S_c\bar{v}O_2$) using serial blood gas analyses. Intraoperatively, a low CVP (<10 mmHg) is generally related to hypovolaemia. Conversely, a high CVP (> 15 mmHg) may be caused by a number of different haemodynamic conditions including tricuspid regurgitation, primary systolic right ventricular dysfunction, right ventricular outflow obstruction, diastolic right ventricular dysfunction, pulmonary hypertension, pulmonary embolism, and cardiac tamponade when the chest is closed. The exact cause of elevated CVP may be diagnosed using additional investigations such as transoesophageal echocardiography (TOE).

$S_c\bar{v}O_2$ is indirectly related to the cardiac output. Whenever the oxygen delivery (DO_2) is inadequate to fulfill the systemic oxygen consumption (VO_2), the peripheral oxygen extraction rate (O_2ER) increases, and consequently, the $S_c\bar{v}O_2$ decreases. In paediatric patients, direct measurement of the cardiac output is technically challenging or impossible using pulmonary artery balloon catheters. Therefore, the $S_c\bar{v}O_2$ is commonly used as an estimate of the adequacy of cardiac output. However, the $S_c\bar{v}O_2$ may decrease below the normal (70–75%) range in presence of different hemodynamic and metabolic conditions, and its interpretation requires additional information (figure 21.5).

The $S_c\bar{v}O_2$ value during cardiac operations in paediatric patients has been used as the target of a 'goal-directed therapy' in stage 1 Norwood operations, with an associated reduction in operative morbidity and mortality (18,19). Recently, low values of $S_c\bar{v}O_2$ (<68%) during CPB have been found to be independent predictors of major morbidity following paediatric cardiac operations (20) and the nadir value of $S_c\bar{v}O_2$ has been associated with both increased risk of major morbidity and mortality. $S_c\bar{v}O_2$ can be continuously measured using oximetric CVCs that are currently commercially available (figure 21.6). These oximetric CVCs have an acceptable agreement with standard oximetry (21), and provide a continuous intraoperative $S_c\bar{v}O_2$ assessment which is extended to the postoperative stay in the ICU (figure 21.7).

Arterial blood lactate concentration

Serial measurements of arterial blood lactate concentration is another approach to the assessment of the adequacy of cardiac output. Hyperlactataemia may be a marker of poor organ perfusion, with anaerobic metabolism activated to provide energy to the cells, excessive pyruvate formation, pyruvate conversion to lactate. Many studies have established that hyperlactataemia is a marker of tissue hypoxia in circulatory shock, even if hyperlactataemia may have other causes. In paediatric cardiac surgery, hyperlactataemia at the end of the operation has been linked to poor outcome (22–26), and two studies (20,27) found that hyperlactataemia during CPB is associated with an increased major morbidity and mortality. The simultaneous presence of hyperlactataemia (> 3 mmol/L) and $S_c\bar{v}O_2$ < 68% during CPB has an 89% positive predictive value and 92% negative predictive value for major morbidity (20).

Intracardiac pressures

Pulmonary artery pressure (PAP) and left atrial pressure (LAP) may be measured directly using surgically placed catheters. Measurement of the PAP is useful in all patients at risk for pulmonary hypertension following surgery including CAVD, VSD, truncus arteriosus and TAPVR, and LAP for all the patients at risk of left ventricular failure (switch operation for TGA).

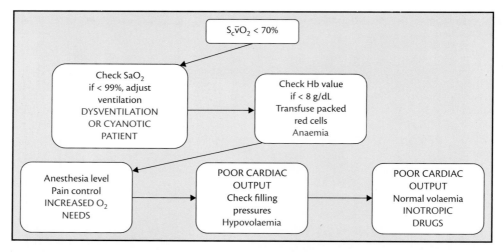

Fig. 21.5 Diagnostic and therapeutic algorithm based on central venous oxygen saturation ($S_c\bar{v}O_2$). Hb: haemoglobin; SaO_2: arterial oxygen saturation.

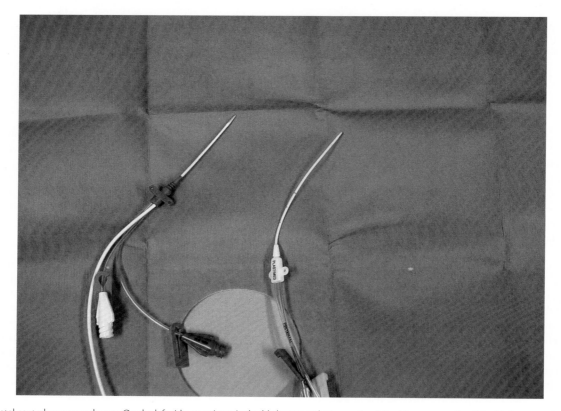

Fig. 21.6 Neonatal central venous catheters. On the left side, an oximetric double lumen catheter; on the right side, a conventional double lumen catheter.

Capnography

End-tidal capnography ($ETCO_2$) provides an assessment of the carbon dioxide (CO_2) exhaled by the lung. It is a complex index that may incorporate different factors and should be always evaluated in conjunction with arterial carbon dioxide tension ($PaCO_2$). When both the $ETCO_2$ and $PaCO_2$ are increased the most likely causes are hypoventilation, severe lung function impairment (respiratory distress syndrome) or hyperlactataemia (when lactate is buffered it produces CO_2). A decrease in $ETCO_2$ in presence of normal or increased $PaCO_2$ is suggestive for a reduced pulmonary blood flow due to a low cardiac output or pulmonary embolism, or simply indicative of a tracheal tube obstruction. Finally, if both the $ETCO_2$ and the $PaCO_2$ are decreased, a hyperventilation pattern is present.

Near-infrared spectroscopy

Near-infrared spectroscopy (NIRS) is a spectroscopic method that uses the near-infrared region of the electromagnetic spectrum. The probes are usually placed on the forehead, providing a continuous measurement of regional changes in cerebral oxygenation

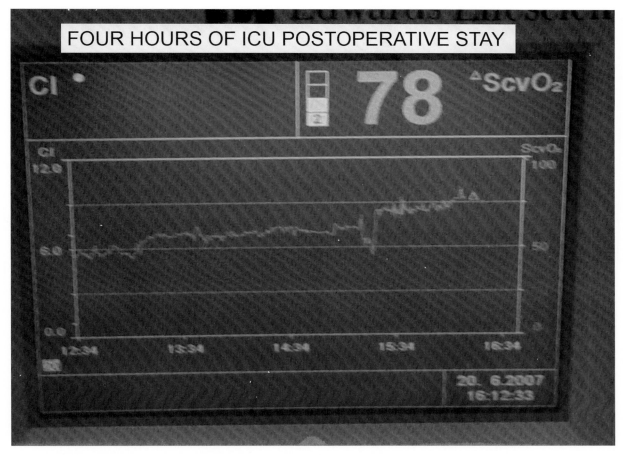

Fig. 21.7 Continuous $S_c\bar{v}O_2$ tracing during the first postoperative hours in a paediatric cardiac surgery patient.

(rSO$_2$) (figure 21.8). NIRS is particularly useful to monitor cerebral oxygenation during profound hypothermia (28).

Although the absolute values are generally different, rSO$_2$ also correlates well with $S_c\bar{v}O_2$ in a number of different conditions (29–33), including paediatric cardiac surgery (34). Somatic NIRS—that is when the probe is placed on the dorsal trunk at the level of the kidney—has been proposed as a means to separate cerebral from somatic rSO$_2$ (35).

Transesophageal echocardiography

TOE in children is a feasible technique if adequately small probes are used. Patients weighing less than 5 kg require a specific care to avoid complications of the probe insertions for example tracheal tube compression or displacement and oesophageal trauma. Specific mini-probes (36) or intravascular echocardiographic probes may be used in patients weighing less than 3 kg (37).

Intraoperative TOE is routinely used in many paediatric cardiac institutions. A specific training is required to correctly apply this technique (38). When correctly performed, intraoperative TOE offers a valuable piece of information. TOE before CPB, may confirm the diagnosis, discover additional defects, identify the site and mechanism of different congenital heart defects. The standard TOE views provide excellent anatomical definition (figure 21.9). After CPB, TOE may provide an important information about the quality of the repair, including the presence of residual defects (ASD or VSD) and the assessment of residual transvalvular gradients or valvular regurgitation. Additionally, haemodynamic measurements may be performed, including PAP and cardiac output. Finally, the right and left ventricular contractility may be checked, providing a useful guide for titration of inotropic and vasoactive drugs or, in the most severe cases, for mechanical assistance.

Indirect assessment of cardiac output

Intraoperatively, direct measurement of the cardiac output in paediatric patients is difficult and rarely performed. The gold-standard technique of thermodilution requires pulmonary artery catheters placement, is feasible only in larger patients, and difficult or impossible in almost all patients with right-sided congenital heart defects. The Fick method, using direct assessment of the systemic oxygen uptake across the lungs, requires specific devices and provides only intermittent measurements. Arterial pulse contour analysis has not been validated nor commonly used in paediatric patients. Finally, TOE measurement of the cardiac output is feasible, but requires a considerable skill, is strongly operator-dependent, and is biased by a certain degree of approximation. Physicians who take care of paediatric cardiac patients are more accustomed to indirectly assess the cardiac output using a number of signs and measurements listed in box 21.4. Whilst many of these signs are difficult to detect during surgery, a comprehensive evaluation should be undertaken before transferring the patient to the intensive care unit (ICU).

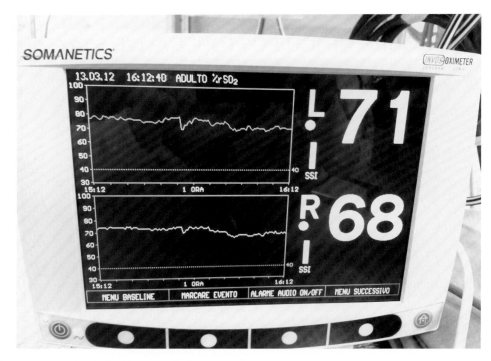

Fig. 21.8 Near-infrared spectroscopy tracing during 1 intraoperative hour.

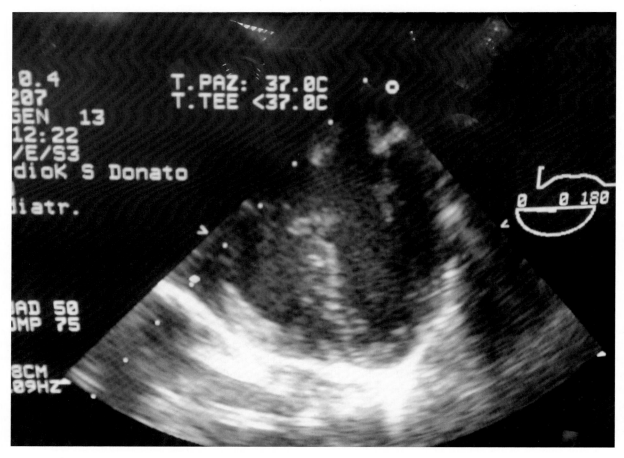

Fig. 21.9 Trans-oesophageal echocardiographic imaging in a complete atrioventricular canal.

Box 21.4 Indirect signs of poor cardiac output in paediatric patients

- Skin: cold, pallid, mottled
- Temperature: high central–peripheral gradient
- Peripheral vein refilling time: prolonged
- External jugular veins: dilated
- Liver: enlarged, stiff, sometimes pulsating
- Skull: interbone breach swollen, sometimes pulsating
- Peripheral pulses: faint or absent
- Urine output: poor
- Systemic blood pressure: low (but unreliable even if normal or high)
- Filling pressures: CVP, LAP: high
- $S_c\bar{v}O_2$: decreased (< 70% in acyanotic patients)
- Blood lactate: increased (> 3 mmol/L)

Cardiopulmonary bypass in paediatric patients

Circuit and oxygenator

Dedicated oxygenators exist for CPB in newborns, infants, and children (figure 21.10). The tubing in the circuit is a smaller diameter than used for adults and goes down to 1/4-inch venous tubing and 3/16-inch arterial tubing for newborns. These miniaturized circuits have oxygenators that require a small-volume to prime are intended to limit the major problem of CPB in small-sized patients, which is haemodilution.

Due to the disproportionately large prime compared to circulating blood volume, children experience a much greater degree of haemodilution than adults. This haemodilution leads to a decrease in colloid oncotic pressure and so fluid shift and oedema. In addition, it causes anaemia, which decreases systemic oxygen delivery, and dilution of coagulation factors and platelets with consequent coagulopathy. For these reasons, every attempt should be made to minimize the CPB circuit size.

Priming of the circuit

The composition priming is usually based on crystalloid solutions, with the addition of albumin to maintain the colloid-osmotic pressure. The use of fresh frozen plasma is an alternative; however, fresh frozen plasma contains coagulation factors that, during CPB, accelerate thrombin formation. The presence of anions in most crystalloid solutions requires balancing with the addition sodium bicarbonate.

During CPB, the target hematocrit should be 28–30%. A randomized controlled trial (RCT) of CPB at low or high haematocrit demonstrated that patients treated at low hematocrit (around 20%) had a worse psychomotor development at 1 year (39). A subsequent RCT found no difference in outcome whether the haematocrit was maintained at 25% or 35% (40). The target haematocrit should take into account the body temperature, with lower haematocrit values being allowed during hypothermia (Chapter 11). A lower value of 25% is acceptable in moderate hypothermia and values as low as 20% may be tolerated when using deep hypothermia. In small-sized and/or anaemic patients, achieving and maintaining

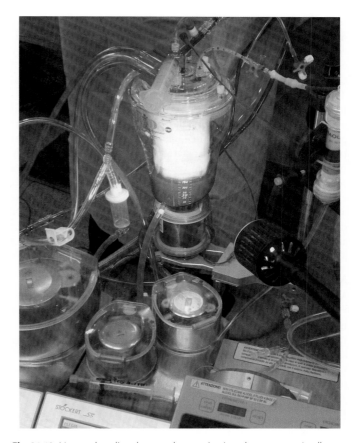

Fig. 21.10 Neonatal cardiopulmonary bypass circuit and oxygenator. A roller pump instead of a centrifugal pump is used to minimize the circuit size and the haemodilution.

these levels of haematocrit requires the addition of concentrated red blood cells to the priming solution in volumes that can be calculated using appropriate equations. However, there has been a recent report of the use of non-blood prime in specific miniaturized circuits even in patients who weigh less than 4 kg (41).

Pump flow rate

Pump flow rates that are used in paediatric patients varying greatly according to their weight and body temperature. In contrast to the adult perfusion, the pump flow rate is usually based on the weight rather than body surface area. Patients weighing less that 3 kg should be perfused with relatively high pump flow rates of 150–200 mL/kg. The flow rate should progressively decrease with increasing weight, to around 150 mL/kg from 3 to 10 kg, 130 mL/min from 10 to 15 kg, and 100 mL/min from 15 to 30 kg. Pump flow rates may be reduced during hypothermia.

Temperature and acid–base balance management

During deep (20–25°C) and profound (<20°C) hypothermia, the solubility of CO_2 in blood greatly increases, leading to an alkalosis. If the total blood CO_2 content is maintained unchanged, a $PaCO_2$ of 40 mmHg measured at 37°C corresponds to a P_aCO_2 <20 mmHg at 20–22°C, with a consequent pH that may reach 7.7–7.8. The cerebral circulation is regulated by the $PaCO_2$ even under hypothermic conditions, and therefore the pH management may have an important impact on cerebral perfusion when the temperature is lower than 28°C. Alpha-stat approach to acid–base management uses the blood gas values measured at 37°C without correcting for body temperature, whereas the pH-stat strategy corrects the values for body temperature requiring the addition of CO_2 to the sweep gas through the oxygenator during hypothermia. The optimal strategy in paediatric patients undergoing hypothermic CPB remains controversial. The only RCT comparing pH and alpha-stat acid–base management in infants and newborns undergoing heart surgery with deep hypothermic CPB found that pH-stat management was associated with a more favourable early postoperative outcome with a trend toward a lower incidence of seizures and shorter durations of mechanical ventilation and ICU and hospital stay, and lower mortality (42,43). However, at 1 year after surgery, there were no significant differences in psychomotor development and other indices of neurological deficit. Crossover strategies based on pH-stat management during cooling and alpha-stat management during rewarming have been proposed.

Modified ultrafiltration

Modified ultrafiltration (MUF) is widely used during paediatric cardiac surgery to remove fluids in excess and inflammatory mediators (44). MUF differs from conventional ultrafiltration as it is undertaken following CPB using a 'reverse flow' from the arterial cannula to one of the venous cannula. MUF may be terminated once a predetermined haematocrit is reached, or after a predetermined volume has been filtrated.

Perioperative pharmacological support

Some patients with severe congenital heart defects may require inotropic support and vasoactive drugs before CPB. In addition, pharmacological support is often required for weaning from and after CPB. Many drugs are available for assisting the cardiovascular system but none are specifically dedicated to the paediatric patient. However, the choice of drug or combinations of drugs should be based on the underlying cardiac pathology, the type of operation performed, and the haemodynamic assessment based on pressure measurements and imaging with TOE. Cathecolamines act on the cardiovascular system with different effects depending on their nature and dose (see Chapter 3). Some specific conditions before and after CPB suggest the pharmacological strategy.

Before CPB, the majority of the patients do not require inotropic or vasoactive treatment. However, inotropic support with a cathecolamine or milrinone, may be useful in patients with left ventricular output obstructions such as aortic stenosis and coarctation of the aorta. Heart rate should be maintained at a normal or supranormal level in aortic regurgitation, hypoplastic left heart syndrome, pulmonary valve stenosis, and TGA. The peripheral vascular resistance should be preserved in TOF and aortic stenosis, whereas a decrease in systemic vascular resistances is valuable for aortic regurgitation, coarctation of the aorta, and all the left-to-right shunt cardiac defects.

On weaning from CPB, many patients require some degree of pharmacological support, which may be provided with dopamine, dobutamine, milrinone, epinephrine (adrenaline), or isoproterenol. Depending on the type of operation, different strategies are suggested (table 21.4). However, the presence of residual defects after the operation may require different strategies from those recommended in table 21.4.

Table 21.4 Pharmacological support after different congenital heart operations

Operation	Desired effect	Suggested drugs
Atrio-ventricular canal	Decrease PVR	Dobutamine
		Milrinone
	Support contractility	Vasodilators
		Nitric oxide
Coarctation of the aorta	Decrease SVR	Vasodilators
Glenn or Fontan procedure	Decrease PVR with maintained preload	Nitric oxide
		Dopamine
		Epinephrine
Norwood operation	Balance of the systemic/pulmonary circulation	Dependent on the haemodynamic profile (see text)
Systemic-pulmonary shunt (without overflow)	Increase SVRs	Vasocontrictors
	Decrease PVRs	Nitric oxide
Tetralogy of Fallot	Support contractility	Milrinone
		Cathecolamines
TAPVR	Support contractility	Cathecolamines
	Decrease SVR	Milrinone
	Decrease PVR	Vasodilators
		Nitric oxide
TGA	Support contractility	Milrinone
	Decrease SVR	Low-dose cathecolamines + vasodilators
Truncus arteriosus	Support contractility	Milrinone
	Decrease PVR	Cathecolamines
		Nitric oxide
Ventricular septal defect	Support contractility	Cathecolamines
		Milrinone

PVR, pulmonary vascular resistance; SVR, systemic vascular resistance; TAPVR, total anomalous venous return; TGA, transposition of the great arteries.

After a Norwood operation for palliation of HLHS, the choice of the treatment varies greatly depending on the haemodynamics and a correct balance should be maintained between the two parallel circulations. Hypotension is a sign of increased Q_p/Q_s, which may be treated with ventilatory strategies (increase $PaCO_2$) and vasodilators when the systemic pressure allows it, whereas hypoxia is a sign of decreased Q_p/Q_s, which may be treated with hyperventilation and vasoconstrictors.

In patients undergoing a switch operation for correction of TGA, systemic vasoconstriction must be avoided. The afterload should be decreased to increase the left ventricular contractility.

A combination of inotropic support and systemic vasodilation is required which can be provided with either milrinone, or a combination of low-dose (0.01–0.03 µg/kg/min) epinephrine (adrenaline) and a systemic vasodilator.

Haemostasis and transfusion

As described for adult heart operations (Chapters 17 and 18), a number of factors contributes to impairment of haemostasis after CPB, including residual heparinization, platelet dysfunction and thrombocytopenia, coagulation factors consumption, fibrinolyisis activation. However, due to the particular effects of CPB in small-sized patients, some aspects of coagulation system dysfunction are specific of paediatric heart surgery. Haemodilution plays a central role in causing postoperative bleeding. Platelet function is impaired, but in contrast to the adult patients, this is rarely due to preoperative therapy with antiplatelet agents. Postoperative platelet dysfunction is not associated with postoperative bleeding (45), whereas a clear association is found for thrombocytopenia (45). The major factor underlying postoperative bleeding is dilution and consumption coagulation factors (46–48). Of the coagulation factors, a low fibrinogen level has been associated with postoperative bleeding (49).

Haemostatic agents including tranexamic acid, desmopressin, and recombinant factor VIIa, may be used in paediatric cardiac surgery (Chapter 17). However, whenever haemodilution and consumption of coagulation factors is anticipated such has with small-sized patients and prolonged CPB or low preoperative levels of coagulation factors as may occur with liver dysfunction, replenishment with fresh frozen plasma, prothrombin complexes, and fibrinogen is usually required. Near patient tests may provide useful information to guide therapy (Chapter 17). Prolonged CPB and severe haemodilution justify the use of platelet concentrate after CPB. Profound hypothermia during CPB increases the risk of dysfunction of the haemostatic system.

Concentrated red blood cells are used to maintain an adequate haematocrit during and after CPB. The use of freshly stored bank blood for CPB priming solution has been suggested by a recent study which highlights the association between prolonged blood storage time and adverse outcomes in paediatric cardiac surgery (50).

Anaesthesia for grown-up congenital heart (GUCH) patients

Due to the improvement in surgery and related technologies, congenital patients operated in the paediatric age are expected to grow-up to the adult age. Additionally, patients born in underdeveloped countries often fail to be recognized as congenital heart patients in paediatric age, and may face their first heart operation in adult age, under the conditions of the natural history of their disease. Finally, GUCH patients may need surgery for non-cardiac pathologies.

Overall, the GUCH patient population is increasing, and it has been estimated that it represents about 2800 patients per 1 million population (51).

GUCH patients represent a specific challenge for the surgeon and the anaesthesiologists, due to their peculiar pathophysiology.

Different kinds of GUCH patients

According to their clinical profile and history, GUCH patients belong to one of the following categories (52):

1. Patients with non-repaired heart defects: includes patients who reach the diagnosis in adult age, and who need a correction of palliation of their defect. ASD, VSD, TOF, Ebstein's disease, and other congenital defects may allow the patients to reach an adult age, of course with ongoing deterioration of their symptoms.

2. Patients with additional heart pathologies not related to the primary defect: coronary artery disease, aortic root dilation, and others.

3. Patients with previous complete repair of congenital defects, asymptomatic, needing non-cardiac surgery.

4. Patients with previous complete repair of congenital defects, with residual problems needing surgery. This is the case, for example, of TOF repair requiring a pulmonary valve implantation, or artificial valves/conduits substitution.

5. Patients with previous palliation of congenital heart defects, needing additional surgery. This is the case of patients with palliations like Fontan circulation, systemic to pulmonary shunts, and univentricular heart requiring Fontan conversion, conduits replacement, and others.

Specific issues in GUCH patients

Depending on the pathophysiology of the heart defect (untreated patients) and of the palliative surgery, different problems may be faced in anaesthesia management.

The cyanotic patient

Adult patients with untreated cyanotic heart defects, as well as patients who received a palliation with residual right-to-left shunt (cavopulmonary connection; systemic-pulmonary shunt; residual VSD and right ventricle obstruction after TOF repair) experience chronic hypoxaemia. Chronic hypoxaemia affects all the organs, and the heart function itself is severely depressed. At rest, the cardiac output is normal, but the patient has a very poor exercise tolerance. This depends to a number of myocardial cellular changes, including hypertrophy (53), down-regulation of beta-receptors due to increased levels of epinephrine (adrenaline) (54), or fibrosis.

The brain is another important target for chronic hypoxaemia. Motor and sensory systems are affected, and a delayed neurological development is often observed. The visceral organ function may be deteriorated as a direct or indirect consequence of chronic hypoxaemia. Kidney is particularly prone to low levels of oxygen tension; liver function may be deteriorated by venous hypertension due to a poor drainage of blood into the pulmonary circulation (Fontan operations), and/or the increased blood viscosity due to polycythaemia.

Polycythaemia is invariably present as a consequence of chronic hypoxaemia. It is a compensatory reaction mediated by erythropoietin released by the kidney, which stimulates the bone marrow for red blood cell production.

The increased haematocrit value determines a condition of hyperviscosity: a haematocrit of 60%, which can be found in these patients, corresponds to a blood viscosity that is almost double the normal. This, in turn, impairs both systemic and pulmonary blood flow. According to the Hagen–Poiseuille law, the pressure required to generate a fluid flow is linearly increased with increased levels of dynamic viscosity (Chapter 11). Blood stagnation in the right side of the circulation greatly increases the risk for venous thrombosis and thromboembolic events.

Finally, chronic hypoxaemia and hyperviscosity are both determinants of haemostasis and coagulation defects. The increased viscosity and blood stagnation cause a chronic liver dysfunction, with decreased levels of both coagulation factors and natural anticoagulants; additionally, polycythaemia is accompanied by thrombocytopenia, platelet dysfunction, and hyperfibrinolysis (55–57).

Increased pulmonary blood flow

Increased pulmonary blood flow is found in patients who have not undergone cardiac surgery (ASD, VSD, atrioventricular canal) and in patients who have undergone palliative surgery (systemic to pulmonary artery shunts with overflow; Damus–Kaye–Stansel operation with systemic–pulmonary shunt overflow).

Chronic excessive pulmonary blood flow leads to a progressive increase in pulmonary vascular resistance, anatomical changes of the pulmonary vessels, finally leading to pulmonary hypertension and right-to-left shunt (Eisenmenger's syndrome). In the early stages, pulmonary blood overflow increases the pulmonary venous return to the left heart, with left atrium enlargement and increased filling pressures. This may lead to an increase in extravascular lung water, interstitial and alveolar oedema. The lung compliance is decreased, and the airways resistance are increased.

Arrhythmias

Disorders of the conduction system are common in GUCH patients, as a result of previous injury during heart surgery, intrinsic pathologies, or chronic hypoxia (55). Supraventricular arrhythmias are more common in ASD, Ebstein's anomaly, Eisenmenger's syndrome, Fontan operation, Mustard and Senning operations. Ventricular arrhythmias are more common in Ebstein's anomaly, congenital coronary anomalies, VSD after patch correction, arterial switch operations. Finally, atrioventricular block may be found in non-corrected ASD, and after ASD, VSD, TOF correction, and arterial switch operation.

Endocarditis

Due to the presence of prosthetic materials (patches, conduits), mechanical or biological valve prostheses, and other specific conditions (cyanosis, hypertrophic cardiomyopathy), GUCH patients are particularly prone to the risk of infective endocarditis. In case of non-cardiac surgical operation, prophylaxis of the infective endocarditis is mandatory in high-risk patients (carriers of prosthetic cardiac valves, including homografts; previous bacterial endocarditis; complex cyanotic heart disease, systemic–pulmonary shunts or conduits). In the other cases, prophylaxis of bacterial endocarditis should be considered according to the different types of surgical procedures (58).

Anaesthetic considerations

Many GUCH patients require additional surgical heart procedures, and it is not usual the need for three or more re-sternotomies in the adult age. Additionally, some of these patients have artificial conduits placed in the previous operation(s). Under these

circumstances, the risk of damage to the heart, great vessels, and artificial conduits during the chest opening is high. The anaesthetist must be prepared for this, and be ready to tackle an acute haemorrhage. A high-flow intravenous catheter (i.e. an introducer plus multi-lumen device) should be placed in the right internal jugular vein or femoral vein. Adequate amounts of packed red cells should be readily available.

Hyperviscosity due to polycythaemia can be treated, in the most severe cases, with native blood removal (autologous predonation) immediately after the insertion of monitoring lines. Adequate amounts of blood can be removed and replaced with colloid solutions, 5% albumin, or fresh frozen plasma. The haematocrit is than restored to a more physiological value; replacement with fresh frozen plasma guarantees a recovery of the coagulation factors and natural anticoagulants that are usually decreased in polycythaemic patients.

The anesthesiological management should reflect the specific pathophysiological pattern of the patient. In particular, when dealing with decreased or increased pulmonary blood flow, adequate measures taken to avoid any further decrease or increase of the pulmonary blood flow.

When the pulmonary blood flow is critically decreased, systemic vasodilation should be avoided, and an adequate intravascular filling is mandatory, being the only driving force of venous blood to the lung in the case of single ventricle physiology. Mechanical ventilation should be set to avoid or limit an increase of pulmonary vascular resistance, avoiding excessive positive pressure, hypercapnia, and acidosis. Large differences between $PaCO_2$ and $ETCO_2$ are suggestive for a critically low pulmonary blood flow.

Patients with increased pulmonary blood flow are particularly prone to congestive heart failure due to chronic volume overload. Given the increased airways resistance and decreased lung compliance, adequate positive pressure should be applied during mechanical ventilation. These patients are at risk for acute pulmonary hypertension, especially as a reaction to specific stimuli, like pain, acidosis, hypoxia, hypercapnia, or tracheal suction. The sympathetic reactions to the noxious stimuli should be controlled with an adequate level of anaesthesia.

Pregnancy in GUCH patients

A recent survey in the USA (59) demonstrated that 0.07% of the births are delivered by GUCH patients (about 27 000 in 10 years of observation) with a maternal mortality rate of 0.09% (18-fold higher than in non-GUCH parturients). The main cardiac pathologies were VSD, aortic stenosis or insufficiency, pulmonary stenosis, and TOF. Patients with Eisenmenger's syndrome have a 50% mortality rate associated with pregnancy (60).

The main risk factors to be considered are the New York Heart Association (NYHA) class, pulmonary hypertension, congestive heart failure, and cyanosis (56).

In the majority of GUCH patients, vaginal delivery is preferred to caesarian section (unless for obstetric indications). However, an adequate haemodynamic monitoring is mandatory in case of potentially unstable haemodynamics (58). In case of caesarian section or during labour, the use of regional anaesthesia has been reported (61); however, caution should be applied in patients where a decrease in systemic vascular resistance should be avoided as it decreases pulmonary blood flow.

Both in general and epidural anaesthesia, caution must be taken to the consequences of a decreased sympathetic tone, and IV fluids or vasopressors should be used to compensate for a decreased pre- and after-load. These considerations particularly apply to cyanotic patients, where a sudden decrease in pre- and after-load may worsen hypoxaemia.

Anaesthesia for non-cardiac thoracic surgery

Paediatric thoracic surgery provides a considerable challenge for even the most experienced paediatric anaesthetist. Patients are often small-sized and may have significant respiratory diseases and surgery may compromise both the cardiovascular and respiratory systems. Moreover, the procedures can result in severe postoperative pain.

Thoracic surgical pathologies can generally be classified into congenital, infective, neoplastic, or traumatic. Patients may present at any age, from antenatal diagnosis (for example congenital lobar emphysema and diaphragmatic hernia), through the neonatal period (with a tracheoesophageal fistula or laryngotracheoesophageal cleft), on to infant age (with tracheal stenosis) and childhood (with pulmonary sequestration), and up to adolescent age (with vascular ring and vascular compression syndromes, mediastinal masses, and pectus excavatum). The following sections will separate thoracic lesions requiring surgical correction using cardiorespiratory support as CPB or ECMO from those requiring a sternal or thoracic surgical approach but without CPB.

Thoracic surgery requiring cardiorespiratory support

Laryngotracheoesophageal cleft

Laryngotracheoesophageal cleft (LTOC) is a rare congenital malformation which if not repaired, is fatal due to severe aspiration pneumonia and respiratory failure. LTOC arises as a result of embryogenetic arrest of the cranial advancement of the tracheo-oesophageal septum. There are four types of LTOC, and the most critical is Type IV, in which the cleft extends below the thoracic inlet to the tracheobronchial carina. This condition usually presents in the newborn or in the infant with the symptoms of stridor, cyanosis associated with feeding, and persistent aspiration. Endoscopic examination is essential to establish the diagnosis and chest X-ray may show signs of aspiration pneumonia. One challenge in treating this condition is managing the airways both during endoscopy and before surgery. Whenever feasible, the best approach is maintaining spontaneous ventilation and avoiding tracheal intubation. This last manoeuvre may be cumbersome due to the short length of the intact lower trachea that makes difficult to stabilize the tracheal tube. In some cases a preoperative stabilization with ECMO should be considered. The same problem is faced during surgery and most of these patients need CPB for the surgical treatment. Recently, the use of ECMO with peripheral cannulation has been proposed as a measure to maintain an adequate gas exchange during surgery (62). Any attempt to repair this defect carries a high mortality and morbidity, and usually involves a prolonged hospital stay.

Tracheal stenosis

Tracheal stenosis may be present as a single lesion or in association with vascular rings including double aortic arch, right aortic arch

with left sided ductus, or pulmonary artery sling. The first two types of vascular rings cause tracheal and oesophageal compression while the pulmonary sling causes only tracheal compression. The sling is created by anomalous origin of the left pulmonary artery, which arises from the right pulmonary artery. Tracheal stenosis and vascular rings usually present in infants with symptoms like stridor, cough (patients may be misdiagnosed as asthmatic), recurrent chest infections, or history of difficult tracheal intubation. When an oesophageal compression is present, difficulty feeding, vomiting, dysphagia, and failure to thrive may all occur. Chest X-ray may show air trapping or the typical cardiac profile, in case of double aortic arch. Bronchoscopy, echocardiography, and CT scan are useful for assessment of these lesions. Tracheal stenosis may be associated with cardiac defects like VSD and TOF. In such cases the majority of the authors suggest to correct both the defects at the same time even if the duration of CPB is longer.

Treatment of all these lesions requires surgery and the surgical approach depends on the precise anatomy of the ring. In most cases of double arch without tracheal stenosis, a left thoracotomy is used. Pulmonary artery sling is best managed through a sternotomy with or without CPB, according to the surgeon's preference, but in tracheal stenosis coexists, CPB is mandatory for surgical correction (63). Tracheal stenosis is secondary to the presence of complete cartilaginous tracheal rings and nowadays is treated with a slide tracheoplasty or tracheal resection for short segmental stenosis with the support of CPB. Bronchoscopy is mandatory during the operation to assess the size of tracheal lumen and its patency, after the repair.

All of these lesions involving surgery with CPB require the same intraoperative anaesthesiological management as previously described for cardiac surgery. Tracheal intubation in these patients may be difficult if the stenosis is very high or severe and the use of undersized tracheal tubes may be required. The tracheal tube is removed once CPB is started to permit surgery and repositioned at the end of surgery. The surgical repair is leak-tested under saline to an airway pressure of 35 cmH$_2$O. Postoperatively, a protective approach should be taken to mechanical ventilation using very low airway pressure to avoid dehiscence of the tracheal sutures. Nevertheless some air-leaking may be present in the first days producing pneumomediastinum or pneumothorax (64). Bronchial toilet must use gentle suctioning. Pulmonary infections are very common and the risk of mediastinitis is high, so that an aggressive antibiotic therapy is recommended.

Bronchoscopy should be performed before discharging home the patient to confirm the absence of tracheal stenosis. If there is residual tracheal stenosis then stenting of the trachea may be required (figure 21.11). Overall survival surgical correction of tracheal stenosis is excellent (95%) but the duration of hospital stay may be prolonged for many patients and associated with significant morbidity.

Thoracic surgery without cardiorespiratory support

Thoracic surgery without CPB may be undertaken for lung abscess, bronchiectasis, lung cysts, arteriovenous malformation, pulmonary sequestration, mediastinal masses, tracheoesophageal fistula, or congenital lobar emphysema (figure 21.12) and in the neonatal period, for congenital diaphragmatic hernia (CDH)

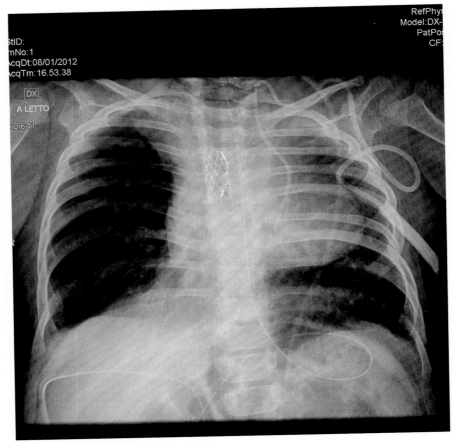

Fig. 21.11 Chest X-rays of a 10-month-old infant with a tracheal stent positioned for tracheal restenosis after corrective surgery for tracheal stenosis and tetralogy of Fallot.

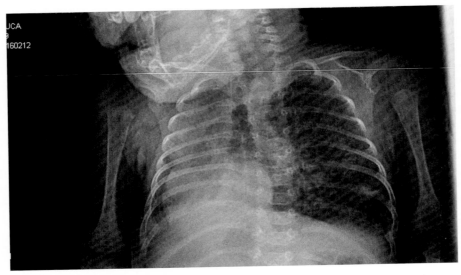

Fig. 21.12 Chest X-rays of a newborn of 10 days with congenital left lobar emphysema. Mediastinal shift to the right can be noted.

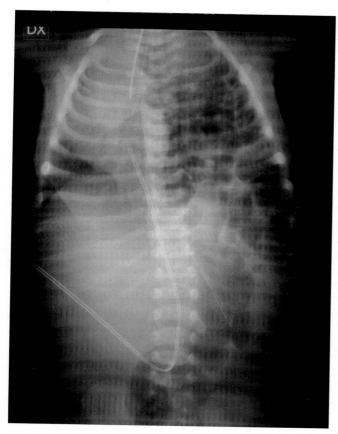

Fig. 21.13 Chest X-rays of a newborn of 1 day with congenital left diaphragmatic hernia (Bochdalek hernia). Bowel in the left hemithorax with deviation of the heart and mediastinum to the right can be noted.

(figure 21.13). Preoperative assessment should focus on the nature and degree of cardiopulmonary compromise. Important findings in the history and physical examination are respiratory symptoms and specifically, bronchospasm. Bronchial reactivity must be treated before surgery and an appropriate anaesthetic technique may be required to prevent its exacerbation. A CT scan must be performed and carefully evaluated.

Pulmonary function testing are available for children, but cooperation of the child is poor until they reach an age of 5–6 years. Preoperative treatments should include:

1. Achievement of positive caloric balance with sustained weight gain

2. Treatment of bronchial and pulmonary infection if present

3. Careful secretion clearance

4. Training on deep breathing and coughing exercise if the patient is old enough

5. Bronchospasm treatment

6. Cor pulmonae treatment (if present).

Monitoring should include direct measurement of arterial and central venous pressures in patients who are compromised and when the procedure is invasive. Anaesthesia is usually based on volatile agents, as they decrease the risk of bronchial spasm. Inhaled anaesthetic agents are the usual choice during maintenance of anaesthesia, although they inhibit hypoxic pulmonary vasoconstriction (HPV). Indeed, this action is of limited clinical significance. HPV may be a useful mechanism that redirects blood flow away from the hypoxic lung to well ventilated area during thoracic surgery especially when positioned in lateral decubitus position (LDP) as ventilation/perfusion (Va/Qc) mismatch occurs. The use of IV opioids may allow lower concentrations of inhaled anaesthetics to be used and thereby, limit HPV. Alternatively, total IV anaesthesia may be used with a variety of agents.

The combination of general anaesthesia with regional anaesthesia for postoperative analgesia is particularly valuable for thoracotomy. A combination of techniques is also beneficial for thoracoscopic procedures, especially when chest drains are used as these are a source of significant postoperative pain. A variety of regional anaesthetic techniques have been described.

Epidural anaesthesia

Thoracic epidural catheters may be safely placed in anaesthetized infants and children by anesthesiologists experienced in the technique and epidural kits for infants and children are available. The technique is very similar to the one for adults with some minor differences (65). It can be safely used intraoperatively to reduce the dose of anaesthetic drugs administered and in the postoperative period, to control pain and facilitate early spontaneous ventilation and tracheal extubation. Opioids can safely be used epidurally, to facilitate intraoperative anaesthesia in children as well to provide postoperative analgesia. Bupivacaine is a good choice for children and the recommended dose for the initial block is 1 mL/kg of 0.125% bupivacaine and then a maximum of 0.4 mg/kg/hr but the dose should be reduced by 30% in patients aged less than 6 months of age.

Physiology of the lateral decubitus position in children

Understanding the factors that influence the distribution of ventilation and perfusion in lateral decubitus position (LDP) is important, as the majority of thoracic surgical operations are performed in this position (Chapters 4 and 33). Va/Qc distribution is different in the awake compared to the anesthetized patient both when the chest is closed and open. Additional changes occur in small patients (aged < 1 year) compared to older children. In awake patients aged more than 1 year, ventilation is normally distributed preferentially to dependent regions of the lung, so that there is a gradient of increasing ventilation from the most nondependent to the most dependent lung segments. Because of gravitational effects, perfusion normally follows a similar distribution, with increased blood flow to dependent lung segments; therefore, ventilation and perfusion are normally well matched.

However, when ventilation is controlled under general anaesthesia there is decreased functional residual capacity and diaphragmatic contraction is absent and this results in a reverse distribution of ventilation. During thoracic surgery, these and other factors act to increase the ventilation/perfusion (Va/Qc) mismatch: compression of the dependent lung in the lateral decubitus position may cause atelectasis, and surgical retraction, single lung ventilation, or both, result in collapse of the operative lung. HPV, which acts by diverting blood flow away from underventilated lung regions, is a useful reflex response limiting the Va/Qc mismatch.

These factors similarly apply to infants, children, and adults, however, the overall effect of the LDP, is different in infants than in older children and adults.

In adults with unilateral lung disease, oxygenation is optimal when the patient is placed in the LDP, with the healthy lung in the dependent position (lower lung) and the diseased lung in the non-dependent (upper lung).

Gravity also causes a vertical gradient in pleural pressure, resulting in a less negative pleural pressure in the dependent lung. The non-dependent lung moves to the favourable portion of the compliance curve, while the dependent lung moves to the non-favourable portion of the curve.

The onset of mechanical positive pressure ventilation annihilates the favourable role of the dependent diaphragm and ventilation is distributed more to the non-dependent lung. As a result, the Va/Qc matching is deranged and hypoxaemia frequently occurs. The application of positive end-expiratory pressure (PEEP) usually improves the Va/Qc ratio, reverting each lung to the pre-mechanical ventilation position of the compliance curve. Opening the chest cavity exacerbates the Va/Qc mismatch and PEEP is mandatory under these conditions. A non-physiological, but clinically useful solution to this problem is often provided by the surgeon who retracts the non-dependent lung and redistributes ventilation to the better perfused dependent lung (66). These factors promote Va/Qc matching in the adult patient undergoing thoracic surgery in the LDP.

Infants have a soft and easily compressible ribcage, which cannot fully support the dependent lung. Functional residual capacity is closer to the residual volume, making airway closure likely to occur in the dependent lung. Finally, the infant's increased oxygen requirement, coupled with a small functional residual capacity, predisposes to hypoxaemia.

Infant normally has an oxygen requirement (6–8 mL/kg/min) greater than adult (2–3 mL/kg/min). For all these reasons, infant are at an increased risk of significant hypoxia during surgery in the LDP (67).

Lung isolation

The simplest way to provide to obtain lung isolation is to intentionally intubate the left or the right bronchus with a conventional tracheal tube. Due to its anatomy, intubation of the right bronchus is an easy procedure, whereas positioning a tube in the left bronchus requires bronchoscopy. This relatively simple procedure is suggested only in case of emergency intubation, for example massive haemoptysis. The main limitation of this approach is that it fails to protect the healthy lung from contamination by purulent material or blood coming from the other lung because the tube may not completely exclude the selected bronchus. An alternative technique is placement of a balloon-tipped bronchial blocker (68) or in children older than 6 years, a Univent tube. Important complications of all these techniques are dislodgment or occlusion of the tracheal tube.

Double-lumen tubes used for adults are only available for older children. Finally, another possible practice is to use a standard tracheal tube and achieve a partial single lung ventilation by compression of the lung by the surgeon. Once lung isolation the peak airways pressure should be no more than twice what the peak airway pressure was during two-lung ventilation when using the same tidal volume. Generally, smaller tidal volumes are used with an increased respiratory rate and permissive hypercapnia should be considered to avoid lung trauma. Hypocapnia should be avoided to preserve the HPV. A high inspired oxygen concentration is used in many cases as the potential benefits of a high inspiratory oxygen concentration that is vasodilatation of the dependent lung outweigh the potential disadvantage reabsorption atelectasis.

Intravenous fluid requirements during thoracic surgery

The usually applied rates for fluid replacement during thoracic surgery are:

- 4 mL/kg/hr in patients weighing < 10 kg
- 40 mL/hr + 2 mL/kg/hr in patients weighing 11–20 kg
- 60 mL/hr + 1 mL/kg/hr for each kg > 20 kg thereafter
- adding 3–4 mL/kg for insensible losses when the chest is open.

Whilst isotonic solutions are generally recommended, the use of glucose-containing solutions remains controversial as surgical trauma leads to hyperglycaemia, and whenever glucose 5% solution is used, strict control of blood glucose is recommended. As a rule, blood loss should be replaced with colloids (1 mL per each mL blood loss) or crystalloids (Hartmann's solution, 3 mL per each mL of blood loss) or packed red blood cells whenever transfusions are deemed to be necessary.

Congenital diaphragmatic hernia

Congenital diaphragmatic hernia (CDH) is a life-threatening condition that occurs in approximately 1 out 2000 live births. Failure of a portion of the fetal diaphragm to develop allows abdominal viscera to enter the thorax, interfering with the normal lung development.

The most common pattern is left diaphragmatic hernia through the posterolateral foramen of Bochdalek. In left diaphragmatic hernia there are both left lung and left ventricular hypoplasia. The reported survival rate for all cases of isolated CDH approaches 80% in those who do not require ECMO and is related to the grade of lung hypoplasia. Diagnosis is often made prenatally. In the newborn, it usually presents at birth with respiratory distress and X-ray examination confirms the diagnosis, showing abdominal viscera in the left hemithorax with shift of the mediastinum to the right. Pulmonary hypertension is usually present, due to the pulmonary hypoplasia, and TOE examination may show a patent foramen ovale with a right-to-left shunt and a PDA. In the past, ECMO was commonly used after birth and during the surgical correction. Nowadays it is more common practice to stabilise the patient with tracheal intubation, high frequency oscillatory ventilation (HFOV), nitric oxide (NO) and cathecolamines before performing the surgical operation.

Surgical correction of CDH is performed through a subcostal incision. High-dose opioid anaesthesia is recommended in these patients and surgery is usually feasible in the neonatal intensive care unit with ongoing HFOV, inhaled NO and catecolamines. The use of ECMO before and after surgery is nowadays controversial in these patients and the results are poor in ECMO runs performed for CDH probably because the prognosis depends on the extent of lung hypoplasia (69).

Conclusion

Anaesthesia and intensive care management of patients with congenital heart disease are still sub-specialties under evolution.

New surgical techniques like hybrid interventions have recently entered the scenario, and the number of adult patients with congenital heart disease is increasing, due to the success of surgical and interventional procedures in the early months or years of life. This poses new challenges and the need for an adequate training of physicians being involved in the treatment of these patients.

References

1. DiNardo JA, Andropoulos DB, Baum VC. A proposal for training in paediatric cardiac anaesthesia. *Anesth Analg* 2010; **110**: 1121–5

2. Van Praagh R, Geva T, Kreutzer J. Ventricular septal defects: how shall we describe, name, and classify them? *J Am Coll Cardiol* 1989; **14**: 1289–98

3. Domnina YA, Munoz RA, Kazmerski TM, Kreutzer J, Morell VO. Hypoplastic left heart syndrome. In: Munoz RA, Morell VO, da Cruz EM, Vetterly CG, eds. *Critical Care of Children with Heart Disease*. London: Springer-Verlag, 2010; 323–31

4. Jenkins KJ, Gauvreau K, Newburger JW, Spray TL, Moller JH, Iezzoni LI. Consensus-based method for risk adjustment for surgery for congenital heart disease. *J Thorac Cardiovasc Surg* 2002; **123**: 110–8

5. Lacour-Gayet F, Clarke D, Jacobs J, et al. The Aristotle score: a complexity-adjusted method to evaluate surgical results. *Eur J Cardiothorac Surg* 2004, **25**: 911–24

6. Ferrari LR, Rooney FM, Rockoff MA. Preoperative fasting practices in paediatrics. *Anesthesiology* 1999; **90**: 978–80

7. Splinter WM, Schreiner MS. Preoperative fasting in children. *Anesth Analg* 1999; **89**: 80–9

8. Smith I, Kranke P, Murat I, et al. Perioperative fasting in adults and children: guidelines from the European Society of Anaesthesiology. *Eur J Anaesthesiol* 2011; **28**: 556–69

9. Delphin E, Seckin AI, Moore RA. Preoperative evaluation. In: Lake CL, Booker PD eds. *Pediatric Cardiac Anaesthesia*. Philadelphia, PA: Lippincott Williams and Wilkins, 2005; 95–112

10. Redhu S, Jalwal GK, Saxena M, Shrivastava OP. A comparative study of induction, maintenance and recovery characteristics of sevoflurane and halothane anaesthesia in pediatric patients (6 months to 6 years). *J Anaesthesiol Clin Pharmacol* 2010; **26**:484–7

11. Russell IA, Miller Hance WC, Gregory G, et al. The safety and efficacy of sevoflurane anesthesia in infants and children with congenital heart disease. *Anesth Analg* 2001; **92**:1152–8

12. Friessen RH, Lichtor JL. Cardiovascular effects of inhalation induction with isoflurane in infants. *Anesth Analg* 1983; **62**: 411–4

13. Taylor RH, Lerman J. Induction, maintenance and recovery characteristics of desflurane in children and infants. *Can J Anaesth* 1992; **39**: 6–13

14. Nilson A, Lee P., Revenas B. Midazolam as induction agent prior to inhalational anesthesia: a comparison with thiopentone. *Acta Anesthesiol Scand* 1984; **28**: 249–51

15. Gamble J, Kawar P, Dundee J, Moore J, Griggs LP. Evaluation of midazolam as an intravenous induction agent. *Anaesthesia* 1981; **36**: 868–73

16. Aun CS, Sung RY, O'Meara ME, Short TG, Oh TE. Cardiovascular effects of intravenous induction in children: comparison between propofol and thiopentone. *Br J Anaesth* 1993; **70**: 647–53

17. Stokes MA. Anesthetic and peroperative management. In: Lake CL, Booker PD eds. *Pediatric cardiac anaesthesia*. Philadelphia, PA: Lippincott Williams and Wilkins, 2005; 174–90

18. Tweddel JS, Hoffman GM, Mussatto KA, et al. Improved survival of patients undergoing palliation of hypoplastic left heart syndrome: lessons learned from 115 consecutive patients. *Circulation* 2002; **106** (suppl I): I-829

19. Tweddel JS, Ghanayem NS, Mussatto KA, et al. Mixed venous oxygen saturation monitoring after satge 1 palliation for hypoplastic left heart syndrome. *Ann Thorac Surg* 2007; **84**: 1301–11

20. Ranucci M, Isgrò G, Carlucci C, De La Torre T, Enginoli S, Frigiola A. Central venous oxygen saturation and blood lactate levels during cardiopulmonary bypass are associated with outcome after pediatric cardiac surgery. *Crit Care* 2010; **14**: R149

21. Ranucci M, Isgrò G, De La Torre T, et al. Continuous monitoring of central venous oxygen saturation (Pediasat) in pediatric patients undergoing cardiac surgery: a validation study of a new technology. *J Cardiothorac Vasc Anesth* 2008; **22**: 847–52

22. Siegel LB, Hauser J, Hertzog JH, Hopkins RA, Hannah RL, Dalton HJ. Initial post-operative serum lactate predicts outcome in children after open heart surgery [abstract]. *Crit Care Med* 1995; **23**: A205

23. Shemie SD. Serum lactate predicts postoperative complications after pediatric cardiac surgery [abstract]. *Pediatr Res* 1996; **39**: 54A

24. Cheifetz IM, Kern FH, Schulman SR, Greeley WJ, Ungerleider RM, Meliones JN. Serum lactates correlate with mortality after operations for complex congenital heart disease. *Ann Thorac Surg* 1997; **64**: 735–38

25. Hatherill M, Sajjanhar T, Tibby SM, et al. Serum lactate as a predictor of mortality after paediatric cardiac surgery. *Arch Dis Child* 1997; **77**: 235–8

26. Duke T, Butt W, South M, Karl TR. Early markers of major adverse events in children after cardiac operations. *J Thorac Cardiovasc Surg* 1997; **114**: 1042–52

27. Munoz R, Laussen PC, Palacio G, Zienko L, Piercey G, Wessel DL. Changes in whole blood lactate levels during cardiopulmonary bypass for surgery for congenital cardiac disease: an early indicator of morbidity and mortality. *J Thorac Cardiovasc Surg* 2000; **119**: 155–62

28. DiNardo JA. Profound hypothermia and circulatory arrest. In: Lake CL, Booker PD eds. *Pediatric Cardiac Anesthesia*. Philadelphia, PA: Lippincott Williams and Wilkins, 2005; 253–66

29. Nagdyman N, Fleck T, Barth S, et al. Relation of cerebral tissue oxygenation index to central venous oxygen saturation in children. *Intens Care Med* 2004; **30**: 468–71

30. McQuillen PS, Nishimoto MS, Bottrell CL, et al. Regional and central venous oxygen saturation monitoring following pediatric cardiac surgery: concordance and association with clinical variables. *Pediatr Crit Care Med* 2007; **8**: 145–60

31. Weiss M, Dullenkopf A, Kolarova A, Schulz G, Frey B, Baenziger O. Near-infrared spectroscopy cerebral oxygenation reading in neonates and infants is associated with central venous oxygen saturation. *Paediatr Anaesth* 2005; **15**: 102–9

32. Tortoriello TA, Stayer SA, Mott AR, et al. A noninvasive estimation of mixed venous oxygen saturation using near-infrared spectroscopy by cerebral oximetry in pediatric cardiac surgery patients. *Paediatr Anaesth* 2005; **15**: 495–503

33. Abdul-Khaliq H, Troitzsch D, Berger F, Lange PE. Regional transcranial oximetry with near infrared spectroscopy (NIRS) in comparison with measuring oxygen saturation in the jugular bulb in infants and children for monitoring cerebral oxygenation. *Biomed Tech (Berl)* 2000; **45**: 328–32

34. Ranucci M, Isgrò G, De la Torre T, Romitti F, Conti D, Carlucci C. Near-infrared spectroscopy correlates with continuous superior vena cava oxygen saturation in pediatric cardiac surgery patients. *Paediatr Anaesth* 2008; **18**:1163–9

35. Horvath R, Shore S, Schultz SE, Rosenkranz ER, Cousins M, Ricci M. Cerebral and somatic oxygen saturation decrease after delayed sternal closure in children after cardiac surgery. *J Thorac Cardiovasc Surg* 2010; **139**:894–900

36. Zyblewski SC, Shirali GS, Forbus GA, et al. Initial experience with a miniaturized multiplane transesophageal probe in small infants undergoing cardiac operations. *Ann Thorac Surg* 2010; **89**:1990–4

37. Alabdulkarim N, Knudson OA, Shaffer E, Macheras J, Degroff C, Valdes-Cruz L. Three-dimensional imaging of aortic arch anomalies in infants and children with intravascular ultrasound catheters from a transesophageal approach. *J Am Soc Echocardiogr* 2000; **13**:924–31

38. Stevenson JG. Adherence to physician training guidelines for pediatric transesophageal echocardiography affects the outcome of patients undergoing repair of congenital cardiac defects. *J Am Soc Echocardiogr* 1999; **12**: 165–72

39. Jonas RA, Wypij D, Roth SJ, et al. The influence of hemodilution on outcome after hypothermic cardiopulmonary bypass: results of a randomized trial in infants. *J Thorac Cardiovasc Surg* 2003; **126**:1765–74

40. Newburger JW, Jonas RA, Soul J, et al. Randomized trial of hematocrit 25% versus 35% during hypothermic cardiopulmonary bypass in infant heart surgery. *J Thorac Cardiovasc Surg* 2008; **135**:347–54

41. Redlin M, Huebler M, Boettcher W, et al. Minimizing intraoperative hemodilution by use of a very low priming volume cardiopulmonary bypass in neonates with transposition of the great arteries. *J Thorac Cardiovasc Surg* 2011; **142**: 875–81

42. duPlessis AJ, Jonas RA, Wypij D, et al. Perioperative effects of alpha-stat versus pH-stat strategies for deep hypothermic cardiopulmonary bypass in infants. *J Thorac Cardiovasc Surg* 1997; **114**: 991–1000

43. Bellinger DC, Wypij D, duPlessis AJ, et al. Developmental and neurologic effects of alpha-stat versus pH-stat strategies for deep hypothermic cardiopulmonary bypass in infants. *J Thorac Cardiovasc Surg* 2001; **121**: 374–83

44. Groom RC, Froebe S, Martin J, et al. Update on pediatric perfusion practice in North America: 2005 survey. *J Extra Corpor Technol* 2005; **37**:343–50

45. Ranucci M, Carlucci C, Isgrò G, Baryshnikova E. A prospective pilot study of platelet function and its relationship with postoperative bleeding in pediatric cardiac surgery. *Minerva Anestesiol* 2012; **78**: 556–63

46. Williams GD, Bratton SL, Ramamoorthy C. Factors associated with blood loss and blood product transfusions: a multivariate analysis in children after open-heart surgery. *Anesth Analg* 1999; **89**: 57–64

47. Moganasundram S, Hunt BJ, Sykes K, et al. The relationship among thromboelastography, hemostatic variables, and bleeding after cardiopulmonary bypass surgery in children. *Anesth Analg* 2010; **110**: 995–1002

48. Miller BE, Guzzetta NA, Tosone R, Levy JH. Rapid evaluation of coagulopathies after cardiopulmonary bypass in children using modified thromboelastography. *Anesth Analg* 2000; **90**: 1324–30

49. Tirosh-Wagner T, Strauss T, Rubinshtein M, et al. Point of care testing in children undergoing cardiopulmonary bypass. *Pediatr Blood Cancer* 2011; **56**:794–98

50. Ranucci M, Carlucci C, Isgrò G, et al. Duration of red blood cell storage and outcomes in pediatric cardiac surgery: an association found for pump prime blood. *Crit Care* 2009;**13**: R207

51. Warnes CA, Liberthson R, Danielson GK, et al. Task force 1: The changing profile of congenital heart disease in adult life. *J Am Coll Cardiol*, 2001; **37**:1170–1175

52. Vouhé PR. Adult congenital surgery: current management. *Semin Thorac Cardiovasc Surg* 2011; **23**: 209–15

53. Perloff JK. The increase in and regression of ventricular mass. In: Perloff JK, Child JS, eds. *Congenital Heart Disease in Adults*. Philadelphia: WB Saunders, 1991; 313–22

54. Bernstein D, Voss E, Huang S, et al. Differential regulation of right and left ventricular β-adrenergic receptors in newborn lambs with experimental cyanotic heart disease. *J Clin Invest* 1990; **85**: 68–74

55. Frankville D. Anesthesia for noncardiac surgery in children and adults with congenital heart disease. In: Lake CL, Booker PD eds. *Pediatric Cardiac Anaesthesia*. Philadelphia, PA: Lippincott Williams and Wilkins, 2005; 601–32

56. Perloff JK, Rosove MH, Child JS, et al. Adults with cyanotic congenital heart disease: hematologic management. *Ann Intern Med* 1998; **109**: 406–13

57. Lill MC, Perloff JK, Child JS. Pathogenesis of thrombocytopenia in cyanotic congenital heart disease. *Am J Cardiol* 2006; **98**: 254–8

58. Deanfield J, Thaulow E, Warnes C, et al. Management of grown up congenital heart disease. *Eur Heart J* 2003; **24**: 1035–84

59. Karamlou T, Diggs BS, McCrindle BW, Welke KF. A growing problem: maternal death and peripartum complications are higher in women with grown-up congenital heart disease. *Ann Thorac Surg* 2011; **92**: 2193–8

60. Avila WS, Grinberg M, Snitcowsky R, et al. Maternal and fetal outcome in pregnant women with Eisenmenger's syndrome. *Eur Heart J* 1995; **16**: 460–4

61. Fong J, Druzin M, Gimbel AA, et al. Epidural anaesthesia for labour and caesarian section in a parturient with a single ventricle and transposition of the great arteries. *Can J Anaesth* 1990; **37**: 680–4

62. Mathur NN, Peek GJ, Bailey CM, Elliott MJ. Strategies for managing Type IV laryngotracheoesophageal clefts at Great Ormond Street Hospital for Children. *Int J Pediatr Otorhinolaryngol* 2006; **70**: 1901–10

63. Barron DJ, Brawn WJ. Vascular rings. In: Parikh DH, Crabb DCG, Auldist AW, Rothenberg SS Eds. *Pediatric Thoracic Surgery*. London: Springer-Verlag, 2009

64. Backer Cl, Mavroudis C, Gerber ME, Holinger LD. Tracheal surgery in children: an 18-year review of four techniques. *Eur J Cardiothorac Surg* 2001; **19**: 777–84

65. Polaner DM, Suresh S, Cotè CJ. Regional anesthesia. In: Cotè CJ, Lerman J, Todres D Eds. *A practice of Anesthesia*. Philadelphia PA: Saunders Elsevier, 2009

66. Hammer GB Anesthesia for thoracic surgery In: Cotè CJ, Lerman J, Todres D eds. *A Practice of Anesthesia*. Philadelphia PA: Saunders Elsevier, 2009

67. Heaf DP, Helms P, Gordon MB, Turner HM. Postural effects on gas exchange in infants. *N Engl J Med* 1983; **28**: 1505–8

68. Hammer GB, Harrison TK, Vricella LA, Black MD, Krane EJ. Single lung ventilation in children using a new pediatric bronchial blocker. *Paediatr Anaesth* 2002, **12**: 69–72

69. Morini F, Goldman A, Pierro A. Extracorporeal Membrane Oxygenation in infants with congenital diaphragmatic hernia: A sistematic review of the evidence. *Eur J Pediatr Surg* 2006; **16**: 385–91

CHAPTER 22

Anaesthesia for thoracic aortic surgery

Donna Greenhalgh

Introduction

Thoracic aortic disease is often asymptomatic and is often difficult to detect until it presents acutely, when a devastating complication, or death, may occur. By performing interventions and developing strategies, the anaesthetist plays an invaluable role in minimizing adverse outcomes (1,2). Therefore, the aim of this chapter is to provide an overview of the anaesthesia for thoracic aortic surgery.

Anatomy, pathology, and imaging of the thoracic aorta

Intimate knowledge of the aortic anatomy and awareness of how the disease processes may affect the relevant structures is essential to the anaesthetic management of thoracic aortic surgery (Chapter 2) (figure 22.1).

Pathology of the aorta can manifest as aneurysms or dissections and both may be present simultaneously or occur independently. A true aneurysm is defined as a permanent dilatation of an artery at least 50% greater than its original size, which involves all the layers of the wall of the aorta. A pseudoaneurysm is a rupture through all the layers but is held together by the inflammatory reaction to the blood and surrounding tissues. A dissection is a disruption of the media layer of the aorta with bleeding within the wall.

The aetiology of aortic diseases can be congenital or acquired. Common congenital conditions are usually associated with connective tissue diseases such as Marfan's and Ehlers–Danlos syndrome. Since syphilis became infrequent, acquired aneurysms are now most commonly due to atherosclerosis

Thoracic aortic disease may be diagnosed by utilizing various imaging modes. Each of these modalities has advantages and disadvantages, as indicated in table 22.1, the most important of which is the availability of personnel trained in their use. Whatever imaging technique is used, it is imperative to determine the extent of the lesion.

Preoperative management

Emergency surgery may limit the full evaluation of a patient. However, if time allows or when surgery is elective, then a full workup of all the major organ systems should be undertaken (3). Myocardial infarction, respiratory failure, renal failure, and stroke are all causes of mortality and morbidity resulting from thoracic aortic surgery and many diseases of the aorta are associated with old age, smoking, and hypertension.

Routine tests should include electrocardiograph (ECG), chest X-ray, full blood count, blood urea, creatinine and electrolytes, liver function tests, and a cardiac enzyme profile. Respiratory function tests, including arterial blood gases, are also valuable as many patients are former or current smokers and respiratory failure is a common co-morbidity.

Coronary angiography is valuable as myocardial revascularization may be indicated if the patient has unstable ischaemic heart disease, left main stem, or triple vessel disease. If the coronary artery disease is stable then revascularization is only recommended in ascending aortic surgery, as there is no evidence that it improves outcome for descending aortic surgery (2). Stents require antiplatelet therapy that is associated with excessive bleeding, so preoperative coronary stenting is not recommended. Echocardiography may also be valuable to assess aortic valvular involvement and ventricular function.

Pre-existing renal disease is the most important predictor of postoperative acute renal failure. Some centres advocate preoperative rehydration with 5% glucose/0.5% normal saline with potassium chloride and sodium bicarbonate⁻ 100–120 mL/hr. N-Acetylcysteine 600 mg nocte, repeated in the morning or 500 mg in 500 mL Normal saline three hours before surgery has also been recommended, although again there is no supporting evidence (2).

Duplex carotid angiography is also advisable, and in emergency situations may be performed at the time of coronary angiography. Carotid stenosis of greater than 50% increases the risk of stroke from 1.9% to 6.3% and complete occlusion increases the incidence to 15.6% (2). However, there is no evidence to support treating carotid disease before aortic surgery. Full cognitive testing has also been recommended to provide a baseline rather than to improve outcome (3).

Routine tests of coagulation should be undertaken (Chapter 17), as thoracic aortic surgery is associated with coagulopathy and haemorrhage. Related factors are the use of cardiopulmonary or left heart bypass, profound or moderate hypothermia, haemodilution and consumption of coagulation factors, fibrinolysis, as well as extensive surgical dissection.

Perioperative management

Anaesthetic management should be tailored to the individual patient and type of surgery. Standard anaesthetic monitoring

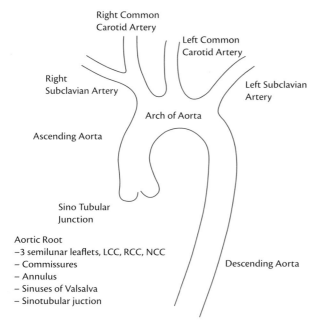

Fig. 22.1 Anatomy of the thoracic aorta.
LCC, left coronary cusp; RCC, right coronary cusp; NCC, non-coronary cusp.
Reproduced with kind permission from Kim Nishikawara.

Table 22.1 Diagnostic performance of imaging modalities in the evaluation of suspected dissection

Diagnostic performance	Angiography	CT	MRI	TOE
Sensitivity	++	++	+++	+++
Specificity	+++	+++	+++	++/+++
Site of intimal tear	++	+	+++	++
Presence of thrombus	+++	++	+++	+
Presence of aortic insufficiency	+++	_	+	+++
Pericardial effusion	-	++	+++	+++
Branch vessel involvement	+++	+	++	+
Coronary artery involvement	++	-	-	++

CT, computerized tomography, MRI, magnetic resonance imaging; TOE, transoesophageal echocardiography; +++ excellent; ++ good; +fair; - not detected.

Adapted from *New England Journal of Medicine*, Cigarro JE et al., 'Diagnostic imaging in the evaluation of suspected aortic dissection: old standards and new directions', 328, 1, pp. 35–43, Copyright © 1993 Massachusetts Medical Society. Reprinted with permission from Massachusetts Medical Society.

should be instituted, and at least one and preferably two, intravenous (IV) cannulae (≥16 gauge) should be placed before induction of anaesthesia for intravascular volume replacement. Urinary catheterization should be performed before surgery.

Central venous cannulation is usually by either of the internal jugular veins. The left subclavian vein may be used but it is close to the surgical field in thoracoabdominal aneurysms and may be inadvertently cross-clamped. A cannula in the right subclavian vein may kink when positioning the patient for surgery. The femoral veins are best avoided as they may be required for cardiopulmonary bypass (CPB) or be part of the surgical field.

Perioperative prophylactic placement of intra-aortic balloon pump (IABP) is of value in patients who are known to have coronary artery disease. Transoesophageal echocardiography (TOE) is extremely useful to monitor ventricular function and filling and has a Class 1 guideline recommendation (4). Additional advantages of TOE in dissections of the aorta include guided cannulation of the true lumen and evaluation of the involvement of aortic or other valves.

Neuroprotection
General methods of neuroprotection should be used (5).

Maintain cardiac output
Outcome is improved if the mean perfusion pressure is increased from 50 to 60 mmHg. The current trend is to allow higher perfusion pressures especially in patients with known end organ dysfunction.

Maintain cerebral perfusion pressure
Avoid both systemic hypotension and superior vena cava obstruction. During deep hypothermic circulatory arrest (DHCA), cerebral perfusion should be used and antegrade is preferable to retrograde

Decrease the numbers of emboli
Monitoring anticoagulation, limiting aortic manipulation and the use of epiaortic scanning may all reduce the number of emboli (5). TOE is useful in determining when the heart is completely de-aired before weaning from CPB. Additionally, the use of an arterial line filter and heparin bonded circuits along with limiting the use of cardiotomy suction, may also contribute to less cerebral emboli being generated.

Thermal management
Moderate (28°C) and deep (15–20°C) hypothermia are both used. Hyperthermia should be avoided during the rewarming phase of CPB, as this has been shown to be detrimental to the brain (5).

Glycaemic control
Hyperglycaemia above 10 mmol/L has been associated with poor neurological outcomes. However, despite no incidences of hypoglycaemia, tight glycaemic control of between 4–6 mmol/L has also been shown to have a poor outcome, including a higher incidence of stroke (6).

Acid–base management
Both hyper- and especially, hypocapnia are detrimental to cerebral blood flow. When CPB is initially instituted, the arterial carbon dioxide tension ($PaCO_2$) should be maintained within normal limits. Systemic hypothermia results from environmental or active cooling. As the body cools, the solubility of carbon dioxide increases and so, $PaCO_2$ decreases. If pH-stat acid–base management is used (measured at 37°C and corrected to patients temperature), then carbon dioxide has to be added to normalize the $PaCO_2$ to correct the apparent alkalosis. As a result, there is an increase in cerebral blood flow that is believed to increase the embolic load and so, is partly responsible for the poorer neurological outcomes associated with using pH-stat acid–base management. Consequently, for moderate hypothermia, α-stat acid–base management is commonly used (measured at 37°C and no temperature correction is applied) as neurological outcomes are better. However, DHCA is a different situation (5).

Cerebral monitoring

Near infrared spectroscopy (NIRS) and cerebral oximetry are emerging as valuable monitors that may improve cerebral outcome. A baseline figure is established and fluctuations in the oximetry reading allow manipulations of systolic blood pressure, haematocrit and maintaining $PaCO_2$ within normal parameters to maintain or improve a falling reading (7). NIRS has largely superseded transcranial Doppler ultrasound which records the embolic load received as it is happening. Jugular venous oximetry can be useful but is not in common practice.

Aortic root and ascending aorta

Perioperative management of dissections of the aortic root and ascending aorta is very similar to that for aortic valve surgery. Anaesthetic management of isolated replacement of the ascending aorta with an interposition graft is as described in Chapter 19 for adult cardiac surgery but the use of TOE has a Class 1 indication.

Root replacement with re-implantation of both coronary arteries depends on loss of normal anatomy with dilatation of the sinuses of Valsalva and/or sinotubular junction resulting in elongation of the coronaries allowing easier implantation.

TOE is indicated before CPB to assess the anatomy of the ascending aorta and then after CPB, to assess the valvular and ventricular function following re-implantation.

Hypertension after CPB should be actively controlled to minimize the risk of bleeding from suture lines in friable aortas. This can be achieved in a number of ways but most commonly using IV glycerol trinitrate (GTN) or sodium nitroprusside (SNP) titrated to effect (2,3).

Aortic dissections

The Stanford and DeBakey classifications are both in common use and they help delineate the need for urgent surgery (figure 22.2). The extent of the aortic pathology needs to be determined and the two main classification systems for dissections are defined on this basis: Stanford A and B and DeBakey I, II, and III. (Interestingly, DeBakey himself nearly died from an aortic dissection in 2005 at the age of 97.)

Only Stanford type A or DeBakey type I and II are considered for emergency surgery, as the incidence of rupture and death can be as high as 1% per hour increasing to an 80% mortality in the first two weeks.

TOE is invaluable in monitoring these patients, not only for confirmation of the diagnosis but also to identify aortic valve involvement, pericardial effusion, tamponade, and ventricular dysfunction. Mitral valve prolapse, which is common in connective tissue disorders, may also be diagnosed concurrently. Approximately 70% of dissections occur within the first 4 cm above the aortic valve, near the sinotubular junction and can be

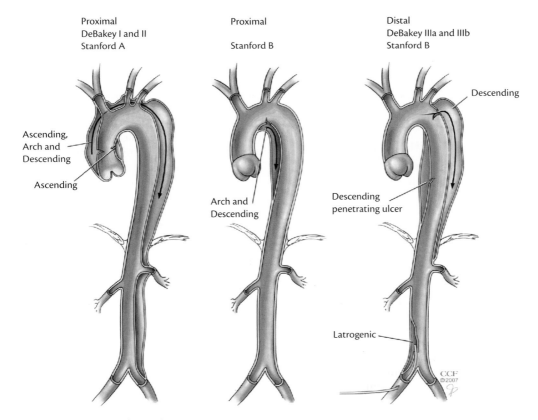

Fig. 22.2 Stanford and Debakey Classification of aortic dissections.
Reprinted with permission, Cleveland Clinic Center for Medical Art & Photography © 2007–2013. All Rights Reserved. Data from Daily PO, Trueblood HW, Stinson EB, Wuerflein RD, Shumway NE (1970) 'Management of acute aortic dissections', The Annuals of Thoracic Surgery, 10, 3, pp. 237–247; and DeBakey ME, Henly WS, Cooley DA, Morris GC Jr, Crawford ES, Beall AC Jr (1965) 'Surgical management of dissecting aneurysms of the aorta', The Journal of Thoracic Cardiovascular Surgery, 49, pp. 130–149.

imaged by TOE (2). Blood pressure control is essential during insertion of the TOE probe which should only be carried out in controlled conditions as rupture has occurred following insertion.

Hypertension, should be actively controlled to minimize the risk of rupture. This can be achieved with intravenous esmolol that has β-adrenergic blockade or labetolol, that has both α- and β-adrenergic blocking effects. One should aim for a target heart rate of 60 beats per minute and a target systolic blood pressure of <120 mmHg. Calcium channel blockers, like nifedipine, may be used if β-adrenergic blockers are contraindicated. If further reduction is needed then vasodilators like glyceral trinitrate (GTN) or sodium nitroprusside (SNP) can be used after β-adrenergic blockade is instituted to avoid reflex tachycardia.

The extent of the aortic dissection will affect the anaesthetic management. If a cross-clamp can be safely applied to the distal aorta to allow perfusion of the cerebral vessels, they can be managed as for aortic root and ascending aorta replacement. If this cannot be done then DHCA will be required (Chapter 14).

Arterial cannulation for CPB often uses the femoral or axillary arteries. Direct monitoring of arterial blood pressure should from the non-dominant radial artery. However, if the left subclavian artery is involved in the aneurysm then the left radial artery should be avoided. Similarly, the right radial artery should not be used if the right axillary is used for CPB. TOE can confirm placement of the arterial cannula within the true lumen of the aorta and that there is blood flow down the subclavian artery.

Stanford Type B and DeBakey III aortic dissections are managed either medically with blood pressure control or with an endovascular stent placement (TEVAR—thoracic endovascular aneurysm repair). Stenting is also used to treat some thoracoabdominal aneurysms (8). The mortality rates are initially lower with stenting compared to surgical treatment and there is less risk of paraplegia. However, the long-term outcome at 2 years is the same for both techniques and there are a different set of adverse events associated with stenting such as migration and leakage (9,10).

Aortic arch or hemi-arch surgery

DHCA is employed if the arch and distal aorta are diseased and a cross-clamp cannot be placed without compromising the cerebral vessels. Deep hypothermia (15 to 20°C) is used to minimise cerebral damage when circulation is arrested. Cerebral metabolic activity decreases by 7% for every degree Celsius cooled (11). Employing DHCA without any adjunct perfusion has been shown to be sufficient in improving neurological outcomes, especially if limited to less than 30 minutes (12). Antegrade and retrograde cerebral perfusion (ACP and RCP respectively) have both been shown to improve outcome, though ACP is superior to RCP providing more time to complete the anastomosis (13).

Gradual re-warming from hypothermia is required as too large a temperature differential between the patient and warming devices will result thermal damage to the skin. Avoiding hyperthermia is also important as this can worsen neurological outcome and even mild hyperthermia (38–39°C) increases excitotoxic neurotransmitter release (5,14).

Tracheal intubation with a single lumen tracheal tube is required. Central venous pressure monitoring is mandatory and TOE is frequently useful. Femoral or axillary arterial cannulation are usually employed for CPB with conventional atrial venous cannulation.

Acid–base management for DHCA should be the pH-stat during induction of hypothermia before stopping the circulation. This causes cerebral vasodilatation and increases cerebral blood flow so improving cooling of the brain especially to the subcortical areas. Additionally, it increases cerebral oxygen delivery and reduces the re-perfusion injury. Furthermore, there is faster recovery of cerebral ATP, the intracellular pH is more alkaline and cerebral oedema is reduced (5,15).

Conversely, during the rewarming phase of CPB, an α-stat acid–base management should be used, as theoretically, this should limit the cerebral embolic load as well as keep the brain cool to minimize the risk of cerebral hyperthermia. A best evidence study has stated that the particular blood gas management approach that should be employed depends on the age of the patient; pH-stat for paediatric patients and α-stat for adult patients (15).

Pharmacological cerebral protection

Thiopentone in a dose of 0.5 to 1.5 g IV has been used before circulatory arrest to decrease cerebral metabolic oxygen consumption (CM_RO_2) (5). While thiopentone is widely used, there is little evidence to support its efficacy but mortality figures are lower if used (16). Propofol also decreases CM_RO_2 and may exert its effects through GABA receptors (5). Cerebral blood flow is reduced so decreasing further embolic load. Calcium channel blockers and especially, nimodipine have been studied; however, an increase in bleeding has been associated with its use and the study was stopped due to adverse outcomes (5).

Aprotinin has been found to improve functional outcome from perioperative stroke in an animal model probably due to its anti-inflammatory properties (18). Glucocorticoids also decrease the inflammatory response but may worsen outcome (5,17). Other studies advocate their use though evidence is limited (19). Mannitol 12.5–225 g IV has also traditionally been used during CPB although little proof exists that it improves outcome (5). Remacemide is a competitive glutamate antagonist and has been implicated in improving outcome if given during cardiac surgery (5,18). In some studies it has been investigated as a neuroprotective agent along with magnesium sulphate 1–2 g IV (19). Acedesine an adenosine regulator substitute, and edavaone a free radical scavenger are all in clinical trials at present and awaiting publication of their results (5,20,21). Lidocaine has had two positive and two negative randomized clinical trials but a meta-analysis had concluded that its use as a neuroprotective agent cannot be ruled out (20). Erythropoietin given for three days starting the day before surgery appeared to result in a more rapid and complete recovery and confer benefit when given in a trial to pigs at 20°C (22).

Coagulopathy and blood loss

Profound hypothermia causes a coagulopathy but the extent of the procedure has a more profound effect on outcome (23). Augoustides and colleagues have reported less bleeding when using electroencephalograph (EEG) monitoring as this allowed circulatory arrest to be undertaken at higher temperatures following EEG silence and minimized the duration of CPB (23).

Many institutions routinely give fresh frozen plasma, platelets, and cryoprecipitate following termination of CPB. In extreme cases the patient may need to be packed with swabs or gauze roll to provide pressure. In these cases the skin is closed and then when the bleeding has stopped and the coagulopathy has been reversed,

Table 22.2 Predictors of prolonged (>72 hr) ventilation after aortic arch surgery using deep hypothermic circulatory arrest and antegrade cerebral perfusion

Increased duration of cardiopulmonary bypass
Increasing age
Emergency surgery
Elevated preoperative creatinine level

Table 22.3 Predictors of prolonged ICU stay (>5 days) in adults following thoracic aortic surgery and DHCA

Increasing age
Stroke
DHCA duration
Dependence on vasopressor support for longer than 72 hours
Renal dysfunction

ICU, intensive care unit; DHCA, deep hypothermic circulatory arrest.

Data from Givehchian M, Beschorner R, Ehmann C et al. Neuroprotective effects of erythropoietin during deep hypothermic circulatory arrest. Eur J Cardiothorac Surg 2010;37:662–8.

Augoustides JG, Pochettino A, Ochroch EA, Cowie D, McGarvey ML, Weiner J, Gambone AJ, Pinchasik D, Cheung AT, Bavaria JE. Clinical predictors for prolonged intensive care unit stay in adults undergoing thoracic aortic surgery requiring deep hypothermic circulatory arrest. J Cardiothorac Vasc Anesth 2006;20:8–13.

the patient can be formally closed. A change of packs before formal closure may often be needed.

Prolonged mechanical ventilation and stay in intensive care unit

Prolonged mechanical ventilation and stay in ICU are often required after deep hypothermic circulatory arrest (DHCA). All but the last of the variables in tables 22.2 and table 22.3 are both univariate and multivariate predictors of prolonged mechanical ventilation and stay in ICU (22,23).

Thoracoabdominal aneurysms

Pathophysiology of thoracoabdominal aneurysms

Thoracoabdominal aortic disease is associated with increasing age and with an ageing population, it will become more common. Understanding the extent and nature of the disease is paramount as to the conduct of the procedure. Crawford classified thoracoabdominal aortic aneurysms (TAAA) into four types according to the extent of the aneurysm (figure 22.3) and the different types are associated with different risk profiles for paraplegia. Other sources of morbidity associated with TAAA surgery are renal, myocardial and pulmonary dysfunction.

Anatomy of the blood supply to the spinal cord

Anaesthetic and surgical management has been directed at improving neurological outcome and in particular, minimizing paraplegia, which is a major source of morbidity. The incidence of paraplegia is presently reported to be between 2 and 6%, although it has been much higher (2). The blood supply to the spinal cord is unique in that there are few anastomoses so very little reserve. Perfusion is reliant on the anterior spinal artery which supplies the motor segment of the spinal cord. The posterior spinal artery supplies the sensory tracts and the intercostal arteries contribute little to the arterial blood supply of the spinal cord.

The upper spinal cord has no anterior arterial blood supply. In the majority of individuals, the spinal cord is supplied by the artery of Adamkiewicz that originates from the aorta about vertebral level T9–12. If the cross-clamp is applied below the origin of this artery then the chance of spinal cord ischaemia is reduced compared to when it is placed above its origin. Fortunately, in many patients with atherosclerosis and aortic aneurysms, the intercostal arteries are chronically occluded, which leads to the development of a collateral blood supply to the spinal cord.

Predictors of paraplegia

Risk factors that predict paraplegia are outlined in table 22.4. The duration of aortic cross-clamping is very important and a time of longer than 60 minutes has been associated with a poorer outcome, and although there are exceptions, durations less than 15–30 minutes are generally associated with better outcome (2,5,24). It has been postulated that spinal cord ischaemia is in part, a failed response to rewarming, with the development of hyperaemia when re-perfused, causing damage (25). Castraghi studied lactate levels in cerebrospinal fluid (CSF) as an early predictor of spinal cord injury and found that they were higher following aortic cross-clamping and, significantly higher before surgery in four patients who developed paraplegia (26).

Prevention of paraplegia

Maintenance of systemic arterial pressure

Spinal cord perfusion pressure (SCPP) is the mean arterial pressure minus the CSF pressure. The aim should be to maintain SCPP to minimize any ischaemic insult to the spinal cord. Left heart bypass is used during CPB with the arterial inflow usually into the femoral artery and the venous outflow by a pipe inserted in the left atrium. This approach optimizes perfusion of the spinal cord by maintaining the proximal and distal aortic pressure at about 60 mmHg.

Drainage of cerebrospinal fluid

Drainage of CSF reduces its pressure so increases the SCPP. A spinal drain is inserted into the CSF in the lumbar region and attached to a monitoring system, similar to a central venous pressure manometer. CSF is intermittently drained to maintain a low normal pressure of below 10 cmH$_2$O, as too low a pressure does not confer any further benefit (27). The drain is monitored and kept in situ for 48–72 hours following surgery, as paraplegia may occur in late postoperative period. Regarding the safety of drains associated with anticoagulation, Cheung studied 432 patients and had no haematological complication but 3.7% had catheter related problems (28). Side effects of spinal drains are as for any spinal puncture. CSF leaks usually resolve though a high proportion may need a blood patch (71% in Estrera's study) (29). A CSF drainage rate of greater than 10 mls per hour is associated with a higher incidence of intracranial haemorrhage and is thought to result from stretching of the dural veins. This is a serious complication that is associated with a high mortality so the presence

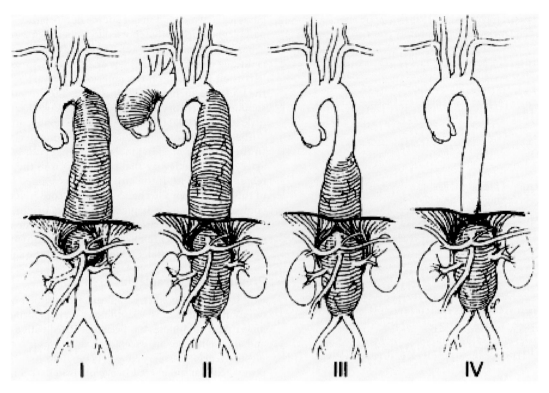

Fig. 22.3 Crawford's classification of thoracoabdominal aneurysms.
Type I extends from below the left subclavian down to above the renal arteries. Type II extends distal from the left subclavian artery down to the aortic bifurcation. Type III extends from the sixth intercostal space down to the aortic bifurcation. Type VI extends from the diaphragm to the aortic bifurcation. Crawford Type II is associated with the highest incidence of paraplegia and Type IV the lowest.
Reprinted from Journal of Vascular Surgery, 3, 3, ES Crawford et al., 'Thoracoabdominal aortic aneurysms: Preoperative and intraoperative factors determining immediate and long-term results of operations in 605 patients', pp. 389–404, Copyright 1986, Society for Vascular Surgery with permission from Elsevier.

Table 22.4 Risk factors for paraplegia following surgery for thoracoabdominal aneurysm surgery

Emergency surgery
Extensive disease (Crawford Type II)
Dissection
Age
Renal impairment
Perioperative hypotension
Prolonged aortic cross-clamp time

Table 22.5 Adjuncts to increase the tolerance of spinal cord to ischaemia

Moderate systemic hypothermia down to 32°C is tolerated with partial CPB
Irrigation of the epidural space with hypothermic fluids. Normal saline at 2–4°C has been associated with improved neurology despite increasing CSF pressure
High dose systemic glucocorticoids e.g. 30 mg/kg before and after aortic cross-clamping
Osmotic diuresis with mannitol and free radical scavenging.
Intrathecal papaverine, for arteriolar dilatation and reduction of arterial spasm

CPB, cardiopulmonary bypass; CSF, cerebrospinal fluid.

Data from: Hiratzka LF, Bakris GL, Beckman JA et al. Guidelines for the diagnosis and management of patients with thoracic aortic disease. Anesth Analg 2010;111:279-315; and Kahn RA, Stone ME, Moskowitz DM. Anesthetic consideration for descending thoracic aortic aneurysm repair. Semin Cardiothorac Vasc Anesth 2007;11:205-23.

These have Level B evidence (2,24).

of blood in the drain needs prompt investigation by a CT brain scan (27).

Monitoring evoked potentials

Monitoring of either somatosensory evoked potentials (SSEPs) or motor evoked potentials (MEPs) can determine which segmental arteries are critical to perfusion of the spinal cord and can also be used to assess the effectiveness of manoeuvres to improve SCPP (table 22.5). Generally a decrease in amplitude or an increase in latency indicate decreasing function that occurs physiologically with cooling or pathologically from ischaemia (25). However, both have limitations as they have strong negative predictive values in

that if there is no decrease in either SEP or MEP then it is unlikely that a neurological deficit will be present but the corollary is not necessarily true (fortunately) (25).

Control of hypertension

Control of the blood pressure in proximal aorta, ideally between 90–100 mmHg, during cross-clamping of the aorta helps reduce the incidences of left ventricular failure, myocardial infarction, and haemorrhagic cerebral events. SNP can be used to control blood pressure. However, at IV infusion rates of more than 5 µg/kg/min, SNP is also associated with decreased SCPP and cannot be compensated for by CSF drainage. GTN also decreases systemic arterial blood pressure and SCPP, although the fall in SCPP can be counteracted by CSF drainage. However both SNP and GTN have been associated with worse neurological outcome so their use is not advocated (25). Esmolol and isoflurane can also be used to control arterial blood pressure and both are associated with better spinal cord perfusion than either SNP or GTN (25,27). Perfluorocarbons infused into the subarachnoid space remains theoretical method of improving spinal cord perfusion. Draining blood into the cardiotomy reservoir decreases the preload and may be the best method of controlling proximal hypertension.

Hypotension

Hypotension during TAAA repair can be from a variety of causes. Whilst hypovolaemia is the commonest cause, myocardial depression from metabolites released when the lower limbs are re-perfused after aortic de-clamping, is another important factor. Additionally, these vasoactive metabolites also cause vasodilatation and consequently, also a relative intravascular hypovolaemia.

Renal impairment

Renal impairment is very common following TAAA with an incidence of about 25% and about 8% of patients will need renal replacement therapy. The risk factors failure are presented in table 22.6.

Selective renal artery perfusion has been shown to maintain urine output throughout and may contribute to decrease renal dysfunction postoperatively. Distal aortic perfusion may also help prevent dysfunction but studies are conflicting and it may depend on the position of the aortic cross-clamp.

Low dose dopamine 1–3 µg/kg/min increases renal blood flow and urinary sodium but its use has no advantage over intravascular volume loading (24). Mannitol 0.3 g/kg before aortic cross-clamping may decrease renal glomerular and tubular damage and although it causes a greater diuresis, there is no difference seen in the blood urea, creatinine or creatinine clearance during the first postoperative day. Mannitol is also a free radical scavenger and may decrease spinal cord oedema. Furosemide has not been shown to provide any renal protection (24).

Table 22.6 Risk factors for renal failure

Duration of renal ischaemia
Pre-existing renal impairment
Age ≥ 50 years
Extent of atherosclerotic disease
Transfusion ≥5 units of blood (donor or washed)

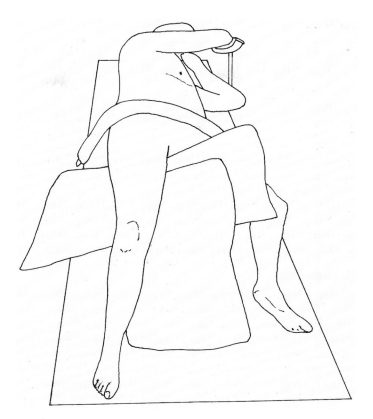

Fig. 22.4 Right lateral decubitus position.
Reproduced with kind permission from Kim Nishikawara.

Positioning and lung isolation

Surgical access for TAAA repair is usually through a large left thoracoabdominal incision with the patient in the right lateral decubitus position but the hips are flattened to allow access to both the femoral arteries for cannulation as well as the descending aorta (figure 22.4).

Isolation of the ipsilateral lung using either a double-lumen endobronchial tube or a bronchial blocker assists with surgical exposure and protects the contralateral lung from contamination during surgery. A double-lumen tube allows easier suctioning of the collapsed side, which may be important as bleeding into the lung can occur with protracted handling and prolonged heparinization.

Fibreoptic bronchoscopy should be used to confirm correct positioning of endobronchial tubes. Where there is a very large descending thoracic aneurysm distorting and/ or compressing the left main bronchus then a right-sided tube is preferable. A right-sided endobronchial tube is also preferable for ventilating the right lung. If a left double-lumen endobronchial tube is used then it should be inserted gently, as intubation has resulted in rupture of the aneurysm.

Changing a double-lumen tube at the end of the surgical procedure to a single-lumen is not advocated. Airway oedema is common and can convert a previously straightforward Grade 1 tracheal intubation into a much more difficult situation (30). Protection of the 'clean' lung may also be important, as previously discussed, as it is not uncommon for blood to be present in

Table 22.7 Factors in development of coagulopathy

Dilution and consumption of coagulation factors
Acquired platelet dysfunction from CPB and hypothermia
Heparin effects
Fibrinolysis

the left lumen of the tube at the end of the procedure. If changing to a single-lumen tracheal tube is required then the use of a tube exchanger is recommended.

Both radial and femoral artery monitoring are used, though it is possible to monitor the femoral pressure through the femoral line for left heart bypass. The right radial artery is the preferred side as the left may be involved in the aneurysm or cross-clamp.

Transfusion

Bleeding is common with all of these operations and because blood loss may be rapid and profound, at least one and preferably two large bore IV cannulas should be used, as well as central venous access to enable sufficient volume transfusion. Some kind of rapid transfusion device such Level One or Belmont® rapid infusor is essential as the ability to be able to warm as well as exchange transfuse may be life saving. In this situation, the turnaround of a mechanical cell saver to allow re-infusion of shed red cells, may be too slow.

Coagulopathy

There are a number of factors that lead to coagulopathy (table 22.7). In addition, endotoxaemia is associated with aortic clamping and peripheral ischaemia and can result in fibrinolysis as quickly as within 30 minutes of clamping. Endotoxaemia may be associated with visceral ischaemia as it doesn't occur with infrarenal clamping of the aorta. The use of antifibrinolytics is recommended (Chapter 17). Tranexamic acid 0.5 mg/kg is now recommended due to increased incidence of seizures (24). Fitting has been associated with higher doses. Aprotinin inhibits platelet activation of thrombin and glycoprotein receptors as well as non-specific serine proteases (31).

Conclusion

Anaesthesia for thoracic aortic surgery involves all the major systems and requires a detailed knowledge of the anatomy of the major blood vessels and their disease processes. Surgical treatment of the aorta can be extremely complex, prolonged, and cause massive physiological fluctuations. Neurological damage is a serious complication of surgery of the thoracic aorta and its prevention is an important part of the anaesthetic care. Most importantly, close communication between the anaesthetist, surgeon, and operating room team is paramount as teamwork is essential to the success of thoracic aortic surgery.

References

1. Cheung AT. An evolving role of anesthesiologists in the management of thoracic aortic diseases. *Anesth Analg* 2010; **111**: 259–60
2. Hiratzka LF, Bakris GL, Beckman JA et al. Guidelines for the diagnosis and management of patients with thoracic aortic disease. *Anesth Analg* 2010; **111**: 279–315
3. Silvay G, Stone ME. Repair of thoracic aneurysms, with special emphasis on the preoperative work-up. *Semin Cardiothorac Vasc Anesth* 2006; **10**: 11–5
4. Cheitlin MD, Armstrong WF, Aurigemma GP, et al. 2003 guideline update for the clinical application of echocardiography. *Circulation* 2003; **108**: 1146–62
5. Arrowsmith JE, Grocott HP, Reves JG, Newman MF. Central nervous system complications of cardiac surgery. *Br J Anaesth* 2000; **84**: 378–93
6. Farrokhi F, Smiley D, Umpierrez GE. Glycemic control in non-diabetic critically ill patients. *Best Pract Res Clin Endocrinol Metab* 2011; **25**: 813–24
7. Vohra HA, Modi A, Ohri SK. Does use of intra-operative cerebral regional oxygen saturation monitoring during cardiac surgery lead to improved clinical outcomes? *Interact Cardiovasc Thorac Surg* 2009; **9**: 318–22
8. Gilling-Smith GL, McWilliams RG, et al. Wholly endovascular repair of thoracoabdominal aneurysm. *Br J Surg* 2008; **95**: 703–8
9. Cheng D, Martin J, Shennib H, et al. Endovascular aortic repair versus open surgical repair for descending thoracic aortic disease a systematic review and meta-analysis of comparative studies. *J Am Coll Cardiol* 2010; **55**: 986–1001
10. See JJ, Lee CW, Lew TW. Anaesthetic management of planned or emergency endovascular stent graft surgery for thoracic aneurysms and dissections. *Anaesth Intensive Care* 2004; **32**: 510–8
11. Fukuda S, Warner DS. Cerebral protection. *Br J Anaesth* 2007; **99**: 10–7
12. Elefteriades JA. What is the best method for brain protection in surgery of the aortic arch? Straight DHCA. *Cardiol Clin* 2010; **28**: 381–7
13. Otani H, Imamura H. Cerebral protection during surgery for aortic arch aneurysms. *Ann Thorac Cardiovasc Surg* 2001; **7**: 4–10
14. Grocott HP. PRO: Temperature regimens and neuroprotection during cardiopulmonary bypass: does rewarming rate matter? *Anesth Analg* 2009; **109**: 1738–40
15. Abdul Aziz KA, Meduoye A. Is pH-stat or alpha-stat the best technique to follow in patients undergoing deep hypothermic circulatory arrest? *Interact Cardiovasc Thorac Surg* 2010; **10**: 271–82
16. Sinha AC, Cheung AT. Spinal cord protection and thoracic aortic surgery. *Curr Opin Anaesthesiol* 2010; **23**: 95–102
17. McIntosh LJ, Sapolsky RM. Glucocorticoids may enhance oxygen radical-mediated neurotoxicity. *Neurotoxicology* 1996; **17**: 873–82
18. Arrowsmith JE, Harrison MJ, Newman SP, Stygall J, Timberlake N, Pugsley WB. Neuroprotection of the brain during cardiopulmonary bypass: a randomized trial of remacemide during coronary artery bypass in 171 patients. *Stroke* 1998; **29**: 2357–62
19. Meloni BP, Zhu H, Knuckey NW. Is magnesium neuroprotective following global and focal cerebral ischaemia? A review of published studies. *Magnes Res* 2006; **19**: 123–37
20. Kellermann K, Jungwirth B. Avoiding stroke during cardiac surgery. *Semin Cardiothorac Vasc Anesth* 2010; **14**: 95–101
21. Hogue CW, Palin CA, Arrowsmith JE. Cardiopulmonary bypass management and neurologic outcomes: an evidence-based appraisal of current practices. *Anesth Analg* 2006; **103**: 21–37
22. Givehchian M, Beschorner R, Ehmann C, et al.. Neuroprotective effects of erythropoietin during deep hypothermic circulatory arrest. *Eur J Cardiothorac Surg* 2010; **37**: 662–8
23. Augoustides JG, Pochettino A, Ochroch EA, et al. Clinical predictors for prolonged intensive care unit stay in adults undergoing thoracic aortic surgery requiring deep hypothermic circulatory arrest. *J Cardiothorac Vasc Anesth* 2006; **20**: 8–13
24. Kahn RA, Stone ME, Moskowitz DM. Anesthetic consideration for descending thoracic aortic aneurysm repair. *Semin Cardiothorac Vasc Anesth* 2007; **11**: 205–23
25. Horiuchi T, Kawaguchi M, Inoue S, et al. Assessment of intraoperative motor evoked potentials for predicting postoperative paraplegia in thoracic and thoracoabdominal aortic aneurysm repair. *J Anesth* 2011; **25**: 18–28
26. Casiraghi G, Poli D, Landoni G, et al. Intrathecal lactate concentration and spinal cord injury in thoracoabdominal aortic surgery. *J Cardiothorac Vasc Anesth* 2011; **25**: 120–6

27. Fedorow CA, Moon MC, Mutch WA, Grocott HP. Lumbar cerebrospinal fluid drainage for thoracoabdominal aortic surgery: rationale and practical considerations for management. *Anesth Analg* 2010; **111**: 46–58

28. Cheung AT, Pochettino A, Guvakov DV, Weiss SJ, Shanmugan S, Bavaria JE. Safety of lumbar drains in thoracic aortic operations performed with extracorporeal circulation. *Ann Thorac Surg* 2003; **76**: 1190–6; discussion 6–7

29. Estrera AL, Sheinbaum R, Miller CC, et al. Cerebrospinal fluid drainage during thoracic aortic repair: safety and current management. *Ann Thorac Surg* 2009; **88**: 9–15; discussion

30. Augoustides JG, Floyd TF, McGarvey ML, et al. Major clinical outcomes in adults undergoing thoracic aortic surgery requiring deep hypothermic circulatory arrest: quantification of organ-based perioperative outcome and detection of opportunities for perioperative intervention. *J Cardiothorac Vasc Anesth* 2005; **19**: 446–52

31. Karkouti K, Beattie WS, Dattilo KM, et al. A propensity score case-control comparison of aprotinin and tranexamic acid in high-transfusion-risk cardiac surgery. *Transfusion* 2006; **46**: 327–38

CHAPTER 23

Anaesthesia for heart transplantation

Andy Gaunt and Nandor Marczin

Introduction

Anaesthetic management of cardiac transplantation is one of the greatest challenges facing an anaesthetist, but is also one of the most rewarding. It involves dealing with some of the most profound physiological alterations in perfusion and function of all organ systems in generally high-risk recipients, and frequently suboptimal donor organs.

The subspecialty is experiencing shifting indications for the procedure and management paradigms at the interphase of improved medical management, and a myriad of pharmacological and surgical technological developments. As a consequence, heart transplantation (HTX) demands much from the cardiac anaesthetist. Beyond the intraoperative period there is increasing anaesthetic involvement in transplant assessment, management of bridging to transplantation and as a continuity of care in the early postoperative period. Due to donor shortages worldwide (1,2), the majority of centres undertaking heart transplantation perform fewer than twenty cases per year (3), This represents new challenges in terms of developing and sustaining a pool of expertise and experience. Fortunately, experience gained from other forms of increasingly high-risk general cardiac surgery, routine use of intraoperative cardiac imaging such as echocardiography, widespread application of selective pulmonary vasodilation, and familiarity with short- and long-term mechanical support, are largely transferable to the heart transplant setting; this empowers the cardiac anaesthetist with novel opportunities to improve perioperative outcomes in heart transplantation. For these reasons, the aim of this chapter is review the anaesthetic management of patients undergoing heart transplantion.

Recipient and donor factors influencing transplant outcomes

The success of HTX in the late 20th century was predicated on ambulatory recipients (with end stage but stable heart failure and limited end organ dysfunction) receiving ideal donor hearts usually from young cadavers who died as a consequence of road traffic accidents (2). The current landscape has changed tremendously, both regarding functionality of recipients, and quality and performance of donor hearts. Despite these challenges, analysis of the International Society of Heart and Lung Transplantation (ISHLT) registry indicates that there has been a continued improvement in HTX survival over the past three decades (1). Interestingly, most of

this survival improvement is related to mortality reduction during the perioperative period and first post-transplant year, which vindicates anaesthetic and surgical commitment to ongoing development and refinement of techniques. The median survival of the entire ISHLT cohort of nearly 100 000 patients is approximately 10 years. Patients who survive the first postoperative year have a 63% likelihood of being alive 10 years post-transplant, and a 27% chance of being alive 20 years post-transplant (1).

While these achievements are remarkable, the procedure remains a high-risk medical treatment. There have been major efforts toward identification of recipient and donor related risk factors and incorporation of such knowledge into recipient selection, management on the waiting list and donor management. The anaesthetist should recognize these factors on an individual basis and should aim to mitigate these adverse risk mechanism throughout the entire perioperative period.

Recipient characteristics

Patients with advanced heart failure (HF) who are referred for transplantation are initially evaluated by a cardiology team followed by a multidisciplinary team discussion regarding severity of HF, suitability for transplant and best management options (4–6). With recent improved outcomes of medical management, stable HF patients are unlikely to have early survival benefit from transplants, but HTX may improve their quality of life. The majority of current listings, however, encompass patients who are positive inotrope dependent and deteriorating (5,6). Depending on the rate of the deterioration and future suitability of these patients to transplantation, they are generally bridged pending further management decisions by using a temporary or short-term mechanical support device, or considered for bridging to transplantation or destination therapy (Chapter 13). In these situation the time frame for consideration and implementation of mechanical cardiac support is dictated by the level of patient limitations and ranging from hours in patients with critical cardiogenic shock to weeks in those who can be stabilized but remain inotrope dependent (5).

The impact of mechanical support on survival on the waiting list is considerable. Analysis of waiting list mortality of a large (>33 000 heart transplant candidates) US cohort indicates that the introduction of continuous flow left ventricular assist devices (LVADs) as bridge to transplant since 2008 achieved favourable survival, which is similar to those (1.0% per month) with non-urgent status without LVADs (7). However, LVAD-related

Box 23.1 Indications and contraindications of heart transplantation

Indications for heart transplantation

- End-stage heart disease with life expectancy of 12–18 months
- New York Heart Association (NYHA) grade III or IV heart failure
- Pathophysiology refractory to medical or surgical therapy

Absolute contraindications to transplantation

- Irreversible secondary organ failure (combined organ transplant remains a possibility)
- Chronic systemic infection
- Continued smoking or excessive alcohol usage
- Malignant disease
- Cerebrovascular disease
- A psychiatric state likely to result in non-compliance
- Other condition likely to result in death within five years

Relative Contraindications to transplantation

- HIV or hepatitis B or C
- Obesity
- Pulmonary vascular resistance (PVR) > 4 Woods units
- Trans-pulmonary gradient (TPG) > 12 mmHg
- Chronic renal impairment (consider combined renal transplant)
- Diabetic end organ damage
- Amyloidosis

complications occur frequently (28%) and such events nearly double the mortality risk. Mortality risks increase fivefold if biventricular assist is required and highest (sevenfold) in patients with temporary device support.

Absolute and relative contraindications to heart transplant (box 23.1) are evolving and moving from personal and consensus opinion to evaluation of patient risks based on outcome analysis of large data sets (5,6). Singh and colleagues have developed a recipient related risk scoring model for early in hospital mortality by analysing a recent (2007–2009) US cohort of more than 4000 heart transplants (8). The best-fitting risk prediction model comprised factors related to age, diagnosis, type of mechanical support, ventilator support, estimated glomerular filtration rate, and total serum bilirubin. Older age at transplant (≥65 years) represented a nearly twofold risk when compared to younger recipients. Ischaemic cardiomyopathy had an odds ratio of 1.44 compared to dilated cardiomyopathy, whereas hypertrophic/restrictive cardiomyopathy [odds ratio: 2.16], and especially congenital heart disease [odds ratio: 4.18], represented the highest risk. Isolated LVAD support or total artificial heart or biventricular support, coupled with the presence of extracorporeal membrane oxygenation was

an incremental risk factor for in hospital mortality by a factor of 2.0–6.0. The odds ratios, for ventilator support and dialysis were 3.3 and 3.79. In addition, an estimated glomerular filtration rate of <30 mL/min and total serum bilirubin >2.5 mg/dL provided a more than twofold risk for in-hospital mortality (8).

A similar 50-point scoring system (IMPACT) incorporating 12 recipient-specific variables was introduced and validated in a large US cohort (>20 000 recipients) for 1 year mortality (9). Most recently, the IMPACT scoring was also validated for an international cohort of patients captured within the ISHLT registry (10).

In summary, in respect of recipient selection and presentation for heart transplantation, the landscape is changing dramatically. Currently, the greatest management paradigm is to define the role and type of mechanical support of the circulation. Short- and medium-term mechanical support is already playing an increased role in bridging patients to transplantation (see Chapter 13).

Donor characteristics

Organ donation relies upon acts of compassion by donors and their families. Organ donor registers are created to record people's wishes in advance regarding their desire to donate organs, and to help reduce the onus on families at a very stressful time. To date there are 18.6 million patients on the UK donor register.

Similarly to all other solid organs, the shortage of donor organs has long remained a major problem in cardiac transplantation. There are multiple components to this. First, not all reported donors could be considered for heart donation. Second, potential heart offers are scrutinized by the transplanting centres and clinicians frequently turn down the organ offer due to expertise-based perceived risk of unfavourable post-transplant outcome. Finally, the retrieval team may find additional physiological or clinical concerns to ultimately reject an accepted offer. These practices are vastly different in different regions. For instance, in the Eurotransplant zone, 39.2% of the reported donors were considered potential heart donors in in 2010, and of these 66.6% were ultimately used for heart transplantation (11). The situation in the UK is even worse, with reports of rejecting more than 80% of heart offers (2,4).

Different approaches have been used over the years to improve donor shortages. These have included attempts to increase the number of donors, to improve donor management and also accepting higher risk, so called 'marginal' donor organs. In order to standardize expert perceived risks for declining an offered heart, investigators from the Eurotransplant Zone have developed a more objective donor quality assessment tool (12). This incorporates multiple donor factors including age, cause of death, compromised history, hypertension, cardiac arrest; echocardiography, coronary angiogram, serum sodium, and level of inotropic support and have been shown to correlate with donor utilization in a recent validation cohort (12).

Similar scoring systems have been developed to better define donor risk factors for the development of postoperative graft failure and longer-term recipient survival. In a large (>22 000 heart transplants) retrospective study in the USA (1996 to 2007) Weiss and colleagues investigated the impact of 284 donor-specific variables on transplant outcomes (13). Ischaemic time, donor age, blood urea nitrogen/creatinine ratio, and donor–recipient gender mismatch (for male recipients only) were strongly associated with risk of 1-year mortality when combined in a multivariate model. A donor risk score based on these variables was predictive for both 30-day mortality and 5-year cumulative mortality (13).

While such scoring systems allow quantitative stratification of donor risks, there remains significant variability by region, centre, and surgeon in accepting or rejecting higher-risk organs. For instance, after some liberalization of donor criteria in the late 1990s in the USA, the recent trend has been in the opposite direction (14). Meanwhile, in the Eurotransplant zone, donor age continued to rise until recently (2,11,12).

The transplant process

Donor management, assessment, and organ retrieval

Organ donation in the United Kingdom (UK) is co-ordinated by a specialist donor co-ordinator. These highly trained specialists have extensive experience of dealing with grieving and distressed relatives, and also of donor management. They are an invaluable source of support and information for donating hospitals. Once brainstem death is confirmed and an offer of an organ is made to the UK transplant authorities, the organ is offered to the transplanting hospitals, depending upon clinical need. If there is no urgent recipient currently waiting for a heart in the donor's specific blood group, then the organ is offered to the transplanting centres in rotation. After being accepted by a transplanting hospital, a retrieval team is dispatched to procure the organs. At present, different specialist teams retrieve organs more or less simultaneously and the co-ordination of these teams is carried out by the donor co-ordinator.

Assessment of the donor heart

- The electrocardiograph (ECG) is examined for evidence of acute or chronic ischaemia or conduction abnormalities. T-wave changes may occur acutely depending upon the donor's pathology.

- Basic haemodynamics such as arterial blood and central venous pressures are interpreted taking into account the positive inotropic/pressor requirements to provide a basic assessment of circulation and heart function.

- A pulmonary artery balloon catheter allows estimation of pulmonary artery pressure, left ventricular filling pressure, cardiac output and systemic vascular resistance (SVR).

- Transoesophageal echocardiography (TOE) can be used to assess left ventricular (LV) function and dimensions (fractional area change, ejection fraction, transmitral E/A ratio and pulmonary venous flow patterns), right ventricular (RV) function (ventricular dimensions and tricuspid annulus plane systolic excursion), valve function and structural abnormalities. Regional wall motion abnormalities can give insight into previous ischaemic damage and TOE is invaluable in assessing a heart for donation (15,16). It must be born in mind that some common pathologies in donors (i.e. subarachnoid haemorrhage) can cause regional wall motion abnormalities.

- A visual inspection is carried out to identify obvious areas of infarction, coronary artery pathology and structural abnormalities.

Brain death is associated with dramatically changing haemodynamic and whole body responses, which triggers multiple mechanisms of donor organ injury. There are widespread efforts to minimize or reverse these injuries by appropriate intensive care treatment and active donor management (17–19).

Once a decision has been made to accept the heart and continue with donation, the aorta is cross-clamped, the left ventricle is vented to prevent distension by cardioplegia and cold cardioplegia is administered. The ischaemic time begins when the aorta is cross-clamped. The choice of cardioplegia solution depends upon the harvesting centre's preference, the authors centre uses HTK-Bretschneider's solution, but most solutions have been used successfully. 1–2 litres of cold solution (4–8°C) is administered and the organ is sealed in cold cardioplegia solution under ice. The heart is then dispatched to the implanting hospital.

Minimizing ischaemic time

Ischaemic time can be reduced in the following ways:

- Careful recipient co-ordination to ensure that organ implantation can occur as soon as the donated heart arrives in the implanting hospital. This can require two clear hours of operating theatre time, prior to the organ arriving, in cases requiring a redo-sternotomy or VAD explantation.

- Aorta, left atrium and Pulmonary artery is followed by cross clamp removal to reperfuse the heart. The remaining anastamosis is performed with a perfused heart (20,21).

- The Transmedics Organ Care System® is a new development aimed at minimising the ischaemic time for donated organs (see figure 23.1) (22). It pumps oxygenated blood and nutrients through the heart once harvested, thus reducing the need for long ischaemic times.

Once the heart is excised from the donor the great vessels are anastomosed to connectors that allow the heart to be attached to the machine. The system allows manipulation of oxygenation, positive inotropic support, and pre- and afterload to maintain the beating heart in optimal condition. The heart is then monitored and transported, still beating, to the implanting hospital. The initial study was carried out on 20 consecutive patients and reported a 100% organ and 30 day patient survival. Ischaemic time was reduced to around 60 min. Further studies are underway to fully evaluate the efficacy of this exciting development.

Preparation of the heart transplant recipient

Once a heart has been offered to a transplanting centre, the recipient is identified by the implanting team. Matching is done on the basis of ABO blood group compatibility and the size ratio of donors and recipients. There is some evidence that hearts that are harvested from slightly larger recipients may perform better particularly in the setting of elevated pulmonary artery pressure (1).

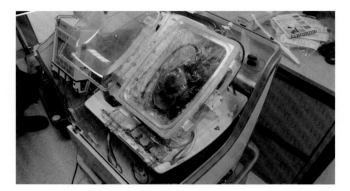

Fig. 23.1 The TransMedics Organ Care System.

Some 46% of the recipients in the 2002–2010 recipient cohort were already hospitalized at the time of transplant (1) indicating the frequent poor health of these patients, or the need for specialist inpatient care in those with mechanical circulatory support. The un-hospitalized recipient is then asked to attend at the implanting hospital; a back-up candidate is often identified at the same time in case the health of the recipient has deteriorated significantly in ways that might require suspension from the active waiting list. Upon arrival the recipient is prepared for theatre.

Anaesthetic pre-assessment of the heart transplant recipient

Beyond the usual anaesthetic evaluation, the anaesthetic assessment on the night of the HTX should particularly focus on the following issues:

- Anaesthetic history including previous complications including airway issues and previous postoperative problems.

- Medication history—transplant patients often have complicated drug regimes, and frequently develop allergies or intolerances to medications. Systemic anticoagulation is common and has implications for the anaesthetic and surgical conduct. A history of corticosteroid use is important as steroid supplementation may be required to prevent an Addisonian crisis.

- Pathology, including the latest echocardiography report and catheter study findings, particularly RV function and the presence of pulmonary hypertension or a high transpulmonary gradient.

- Intercurrent pathologies such as liver or renal impairment.

- The presence of pacemakers, automatic implantable cardioverter defibrillators (AICDs) or cardiac re-synchronization therapy (biventricular pacing systems). AICDs should have their defibrillator therapy turned off before surgery, and all devices may have implication for central venous line placement during anaesthesia.

- Dental condition and airway scoring.

- Fasted time, as patients can often arrive un-fasted, necessitating a rapid sequence induction.

- Latest available blood analysis results.

- The blood group.

- Blood and blood product availability.

- Any risks or likely procedures discussed, for example invasive vascular lines and possible complications, risks of TOE placement, etc.

- Those undergoing resternotomy and those with VADs in situ should have undergone preoperative computerized tomography scanning to document proximity of the RV to the underside of the sternum and the location of VAD outflow pipes. These are not infrequently damaged during resternotomy.

Premedication for heart transplant recipients is generally unnecessary. Judicious intravenous short-acting sedation (e.g. midazolam) in the closely monitored setting of the operating room is possibly preferable to oral sedatives. Immunosuppressant therapy is often given orally prior to commencement of anaesthesia.

Monitoring of heart transplant patients

The following monitors are recommended for heart transplant recipients (23).

- ECG—leads II and V5 as a minimum.

- Peripheral oxygen saturation.

- Arterial blood pressure monitoring. Recipients who have axial flow VAD support have no pulsation in their arterial circulation, and in these patients arterial cannulation is best achieved by ultrasound-guided puncture of the radial or brachial artery. It is equally feasible to cannulate the femoral artery, but these are often required for femoral cannulation in the case of re-sternotomy, of for balloon pump support.

- Central venous pressure (CVP) gives an index of RV function and volume status.

- Pulmonary artery catheters (PACs) are sited following weaning from cardiopulmonary bypass (CPB) for the purpose of evaluation of pulmonary haemodynamics, cardiac output, left atrial filling pressure, systemic vascular resistance, and mixed venous oxygen saturation.

- Left atrial pressure can be measured directly using a left atrial pressure line, and provides a more directly measured index of LV end-diastolic pressure.

- Temperature monitoring is mandatory for cases on CPB and moderate hypothermia (30–32°C) is usually employed.
- TOE provides monitoring of de-airing, LV and RV function, volume status, and valve function and is invaluable throughout the course of heart transplantation.

Induction of anaesthesia

Strict asepsis must be observed to reduce the risk of line infections in immunocompromised patients. The decision to site central venous access prior to induction is an individual choice. Additional sheaths can be placed to facilitate PAC insertion, but this may best be achieved after induction of anaesthesia. Preoxygenation for a short period is advisable, as a hypoxic spell immediately after induction is best avoided. Induction should be extremely slow and careful, and titrated to the patient's conscious level. In all but the obviously volume overloaded patient, giving the induction drugs via a fast flowing drip line can minimize the dose and create a faster, smoother induction. However, it is important to remember to decrease the flow rate immediately after induction, accidental fluid overload should be avoided in patients requiring heart transplantation.

The choice of induction drugs is dictated by individual preference. All the current induction drugs can be used safely if given carefully and in controlled circumstances. High dose opioid induction is still a viable option for heart transplantation, as so called 'fast tracking' of HTX patients is not yet considered a desirable aim.

Coagulation management

Blood loss following heart transplantation can be quite profound (24). Many centres recommend the use of antifibrinolytic agents of some description, prior to sternotomy. Aprotinin and tranexamic acid have been used successfully. There have been recent concerns regarding the effects of aprotinin on organ function and outcome; however, the adverse effects of both blood and blood product transfusion on factors such as the pulmonary circulation, renal function and circulating volume cannot be ignored.

Patients anticoagulated with warfarin will need supplementary factors post transplant. Both fresh frozen plasma and factor concentrates are useful in correcting warfarin effects; warfarinization to an INR of less that 1.5 prior to CPB is currently recommended by the ISHLT. A single dose of intravenous vitamin K prior to anaesthesia will begin the process of warfarin reversal. Thromboelastography provides a useful guide to factor and platelet replacement while heparinized, and is a simply accomplished near-patient test where available.

Maintenance of anaesthesia

The period following induction of anaesthesia, which includes transfer to the operating room (if an induction room is used), preparation, and surgery including cannulation is a time of frequent haemodynamic disruption. CVP, PA pressure, and estimation of cardiac output, along with TOE are invaluable in both diagnosing the cause of, and dealing with haemodynamic disturbance.

Total intravenous anaesthesia (TIVA), using agents such as propofol and remifentanil, and vapour-based inhalation anaethetics have all been used safely in cardiac transplantation. Often the balanced approach of a combination of these is used.

Once cannulation is achieved and the patient is ready for CPB, the donated heart is inspected and prepared for implantation by trimming all the necessary anastomotic sites (aorta, left and right atria, and PA) and by looking for common congenital anomalies prior to commencement of CPB in order to minimize the bypass time.

Excision of the native heart and implantation

When CPB is commenced, the native heart is excised, and there are surgical options available depending on local policy. The standard Lower–Shumway technique involves leaving a significant proportion of native left and right atrium around the pulmonary veins and superior and inferior vena cava (20,21). This entails fewer anastomoses and a potential quicker implantation time, and it may also reduce the risk of iatrogenic venous stenosis as the atrial anastomoses are larger and more forgiving. Unfortunately, this technique does create somewhat large and anatomically abnormal atria, which have been linked to complications such as valve regurgitation (25) and arrhythmias (26). The superior and inferior vena cavae can be anastomosed separately to preserve the shape and function of the donor right atrium (27). Also, the pulmonary veins can be implanted as separate left and right islands to preserve as much of the donor left atrium as possible. In the authors unit, if a bicaval anastomosis is planned, it is policy to site a central venous line in a femoral vessel to facilitate estimation of inferior vena cava pressure to try to rule out venous hypertension secondary to a narrowed anastomosis. Alternatively, the venous pressures proximal and distal to the anastomoses can be measured directly using a needle connected to a pressure transducer.

During implantation there are a number of steps for the anaesthetist (box 23.2). Preparing for weaning of CPB is key to success, and discussion of the necessary positive inotropic support should take place between anaesthetist and surgeon, if it is not dictated by departmental protocol.

Inotropes, chronotropes, and pressor agents

There is no clear consensus on the correct positive inotropes and chronotropes to use following cardiac transplantation. There is a wealth of anecdotal evidence but very little convincing data from randomized controlled clinical trials (23). It is likely that the true path to success lies in consistency of management, early recognition

---

Box 23.2 Check list for preparation for weaning

1. Positive inotropes for weaning are connected and running at low levels (this avoids having to wait for inotropic effect while the central line dead space is run through).

2. All drugs likely to be required are to hand. Weaning of a heart transplant from CPB is no time to be rifling through the drug cupboard.

3. Nitric oxide, if required, needs to be calibrated and set up.

4. A dual chamber pacing box is available.

5. Pressure transducers for PA and left atrial pressures are set up if not already available.

and treatment of evolving graft dysfunction, and consistent multi-disciplinary intensive care.

Epinephrine, dopamine, dobutamine, and phosphodiesterase inhibitors, including enoximone and milrinone, have all been used successfully to maintain/augment cardiac output following transplantation (28). Noradrenaline, phenylephedrine, and vasopressin have been used to treat vasoplegic syndrome following cardiac surgery (29). Isoprenaline infusions are routinely employed in some institutions to increase heart rate and reduce afterload in the donor heart. Nitric oxide, inhaled prostacyclin and sildenafil have been used to reduce RV afterload in cases of right heart impairment/reversible pulmonary hypertension (30–33).

Reperfusion

Once three of the four anastomoses are finished the aortic cross-clamp can be removed and the final anastomosis completed using the pump suckers to remove blood from the field, which gives the heart a shorter ischaemic time. There then follows a period of reperfusion and de-airing. Pacing wires should be sited on the ventricle in the first instance and pacing commenced at 90–100 bpm to prevent ventricular distension, particularly if the LV vent has been removed. Faster pacing rates limit diastolic filling time and reduce wall stress in the same way as tachycardia is a compensatory mechanism in heart failure.

TOE should be carried out to assess the adequacy of de-airing; air tends to accumulate in the apex of the LV, the atrial appendage, and pulmonary veins, and de-airing must be rigorous. Reperfusion is continued until the ECG trace has normalized (or at least no longer changing), there is complete de-airing, and there is visible indication of vigorous contraction. Reperfusion is often continued for a period dictated by the CPB or ischaemic time. The aim is to reduce ischaemic time to under 3 hours. There is an adverse correlation with outcome beyond 4 hours ischaemic time.

The process of weaning from CPB depends on local policy (box 23.3) but the best approach is slowly. Stepwise weaning to 75%,

---

Box 23.3 Check list for commencement of weaning from CPB

1. Ventilation is resumed.

2. 'Warm' blood gases show K$^+$, haemoglobin, and pH are within acceptable limits.

3. Heart rhythm is acceptable, VVI pacing as a minimum, DDD, or AAI is preferable.

4. TOE has assessed de-airing, we recommend the 4/5 chamber views for weaning.

5. Inotropes/chronotropes/pressors are connected and running at the required rates.

6. Nitric oxide is running if required.

7. A intra-aortic balloon pump (IABP) should be available, if not used routinely.

8. We recommend the siting of a left atrial line to assess LV filling pressure. We also utilize a fibreoptic thermodilution PAC to estimate cardiac output, PA pressure and mixed venous oxygen saturation. It may only be possible to site this once cardiac output has been restored.

50%, and 25% of full flow allows for identification of potential problems such as ventricular distension or rhythm disturbances. Poor ventricular function whilst still on CPB necessitates increases in positive inotrope provision or mechanical support (IABP in the first instance, progression to left/right VAD or biventricular assistance) (23,34,35). Primary graft failure can manifest itself in a variety of ways from complete failure of contraction to early right or left ventricular failure which progresses rapidly to biventricular failure (36). Prompt diagnosis allows early intervention, and obvious ventricular failure should be treated by increasing supportive CPB whilst therapeutic measures are commenced.

Once CPB is successfully weaned, there are other physiologically challenging times that can lead to a deterioration in graft function. These are:

1. Protamine administration—both vasodilatation secondary to rapid administration and acute RV failure have been attributed to protamine. Administration should be slow and careful with close monitoring of RV function and systemic blood pressure.

2. Blood product administration—platelet administration in particular seems to adversely affect the pulmonary circulation. This may be due to vasoactive substance release, volume overload or just co-incidental with a deterioration in graft function as loading of the newly transplanted heart takes its toll.

3. Chest closure—compression of a distended under-functioning RV can cause rapid decompensation. If the surface of the RV is compressed by the sternal wires then a trial of chest closure by limited tightening of one wire should be carried out. If chest closure causes a marked deterioration in graft function or haemodynamic parameters which is not easily treated, stenting of the chest is recommended. Twenty-four hours with a stented chest is preferable to worsening right heart failure.

Intensive care of the heart transplant recipient

Characteristically, graft function can worsen in the 4–24 hr post transplant period. This is thought to be due to manifestations of reperfusion injury. Intensive care is therefore focused on monitoring of graft function and the primary aim must be early definitive therapy for organ dysfunction (24,34–36). Heart failure is more difficult to treat once it becomes established. Up to 50% of all post-heart transplant complications are due to RV failure, therefore careful fluid management to avoid exacerbating RV dysfunction can be key.

The following is a summary of most common early postoperative complications and management considerations.

Hypotension/low output states

There is a wide variety of causes including hypovolaemia, ventricular failure, systemic vasodilatation secondary to drugs or systemic inflammatory response syndrome/sepsis. A flow chart is presented in figure 23.2 to guide differential diagnosis and main management principles.

Acute heart failure

- Defined largely on TOE with evidence of ventricular dilatation with falling cardiac output / rising CVP.

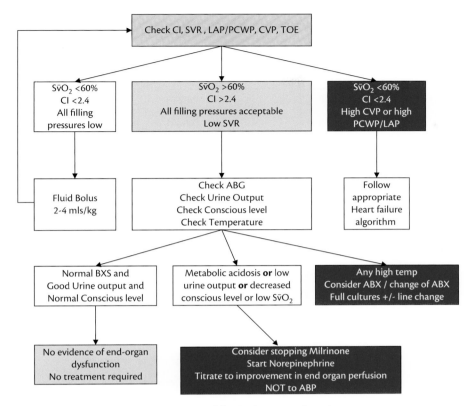

Fig. 23.2 Evaluation of hypotension and associated low cardiac output state following heart transplantation.

CI, cardiac index; SVR, systemic vascular resistance; CVP, central venous pressure; LAP, left atrial pressure; PCWP, pulmonary capillary wedge pressure; TOE, transoesphageal echocardiography; VAD, ventricular support device; ABG, arterial blood gases; ABP, arterial blood pressure; BXS, base excess; ABX, antibiotics.

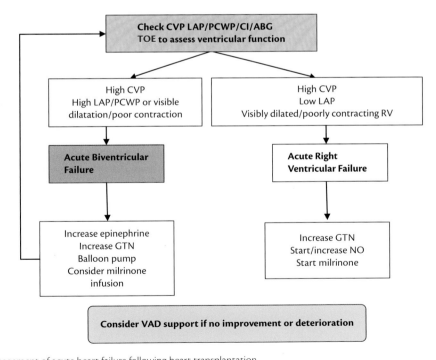

Fig. 23.3 Evaluation and management of acute heart failure following heart transplantation.

GTN, glyceryl trinitrite; NO, nitric oxide; VAD, ventricular assist device; NO, nitric oxide; CI, cardiac index; CVP, central venous pressure; LAP, left atrial pressure; PCWP, pulmonary capillary wedge pressure; GTN, glyceral trinitrate; VAD, ventricular support device

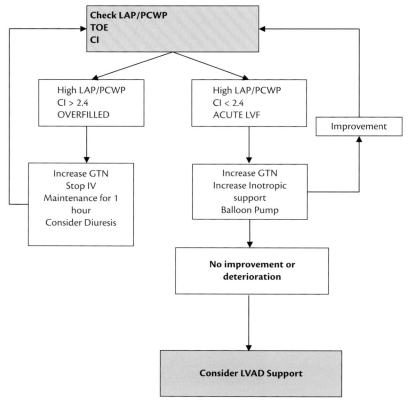

Fig. 23.4 Evaluation and management of acute left ventricular failure.

- Increasing discrepancy between CVP and LA pressure (LAP) i.e. an increasing CVP but LAP remaining constant or falling.

- RV failure can occur secondary to acute LV failure.

- May be a cause for oliguria in the presence of high CVP.

- May be a sign of rejection.

- Figure 23.3 depicts a flow chart for differential diagnosis and management principles for acute heart failure.

Acute left ventricular failure

- Rising LAP/pulmonary capillary wedge pressure (PCWP) with falling cardiac output.

- Rising LAP/PCWP in the presence of an unchanged cardiac output represents a patient at the top of their starling curve and further filling is inappropriate.

- Figure 23.4 depicts a flow chart to evaluate and manage acute left ventricular failure.

Conclusion

Over and above the standard understanding of cardiac anaesthesia, the management of patients undergoing heart transplantation requires the anaesthetist to have a continuum of knowledge from assessment of the donor heart and preoperative management of the recipient through anaesthesia to postoperative critical care. Armed with this knowledge, cardiac anaesthesiologists can make

a major contribution to the long-term survival of patients undergoing heart transplantation.

References

1. Stehlik J, Edwards LB, Kucheryavaya AY, et al. International Society of Heart and Lung Transplantation. The Registry of the International Society for Heart and Lung Transplantation: 29th official adult heart transplant report–2012. *J Heart Lung Transplant* 2012; **31**: 1052–64

2. Thekkudan J, Rogers CA, Thomas HL, van der Meulen JH, Bonser RS, Banner NR, Steering Group, UK Cardiothoracic Transplant Audit. Trends in adult heart transplantation: a national survey from the United Kingdom Cardiothoracic Transplant Audit 1995–2007. *Eur J Cardiothorac Surg* 2010; **37**: 80–6

3. Kilic A, Weiss ES, Allen JG, et al. Should orthotopic heart transplantation using marginal donors be limited to higher volume centers? *Ann Thorac Surg* 2012; **94**: 695–702

4. Banner NR, Bonser RS, Clark AL, et al. UK guidelines for referral and assessment of adults for heart transplantation. *Heart* 2011; **97**: 1520–7

5. Mancini D, Lietz K. Selection of cardiac transplantation candidates in 2010. *Circulation* 2010; **122**: 173–83

6. Kinkhabwala MP, Mancini D. Patient selection for cardiac transplant in 2012. *Expert Rev Cardiovasc Ther* 2013; **11**: 179–91

7. Wever-Pinzon O, Drakos SG, Kfoury AG, et al. Morbidity and mortality in heart transplant candidates supported with mechanical circulatory support: is reappraisal of the current United network for organ sharing thoracic organ allocation policy justified? *Circulation* 2013; **127**: 452–62

8. Singh TP, Almond CS, Semigran MJ, Piercey G, Gauvreau K. Risk prediction for early in-hospital mortality following heart transplantation in the United States. *Circ Heart Fail* 2012; **5**: 259–66

9. Weiss ES, Allen JG, Arnaoutakis GJ, et al. Creation of a quantitative recipient risk index for mortality prediction after cardiac

transplantation (IMPACT). *Ann Thorac Surg* 2011; **92**: 914–21; discussion 921–2

10. Kilic A, Allen JG, Weiss ES. Validation of the United States-derived Index for Mortality Prediction After Cardiac Transplantation (IMPACT) using international registry data. *J Heart Lung Transplant* 2013; **32**: 492–8

11. Smits JM, van der Bij W, Van Raemdonck D, et al. Defining an extended criteria donor lung: an empirical approach based on the Eurotransplant experience. *Transpl Int* 2011; **24**: 393–400

12. Smits JM, De Pauw M, de Vries E, et al. Donor scoring system for heart transplantation and the impact on patient survival. *J Heart Lung Transplant* 2012; **31**: 387–97

13. Weiss ES, Allen JG, Kilic A, Russell SD, Baumgartner WA, Conte JV, Shah AS. Development of a quantitative donor risk index to predict short-term mortality in orthotopic heart transplantation. *J Heart Lung Transplant* 2012; **31**: 266–73

14. Nativi JN, Brown RN, Taylor DO, Kfoury AG, Kirklin JK, Stehlik J. Cardiac Transplant Research Database Group. Temporal trends in heart transplantation from high-risk donors: are there lessons to be learned? A multi-institutional analysis. *J Heart Lung Transplant* 2010; **29**: 847–52

15. Gilbert EM, Krueger SK, Murray JL, et al. Echocardiographic evaluation of potential cardiac transplant donors. *J Thorac Cardiovasc Surg* 1988; **95**: 1003–7

16. Venkateswaran RV, Townend JN, Wilson IC, Mascaro JG, Bonser RS, Steeds RP. Echocardiography in the potential heart donor. *Transplantation* 2010; **89**: 894–901

17. Wheeldon DR, Potter CD, Oduro A, Wallwork J, Large SR. Transforming the 'unacceptable' donor: outcomes from the adoption of a standardized donor management technique. *J Heart Lung Transplan* 1995; **14**: 734–42

18. Murali B, Vuylsteke A, Latimer RD. Anaesthetic management of the multi-organ donor. *Ann Card Anaesth* 2003; **6**: 31–4

19. Ullah S, Zabala L, Watkins B, Schmitz ML. Cardiac organ donor management. *Perfusion* 2006; **21**: 93–8

20. Lower RR, Stofer RC, Shumway NE. Homovital transplantation of the heart. *J Thorac Cardiovasc Surg* 1961; **41**: 196–204

21. Shumway NE, Lower RR, Stofer RC. Transplantation of the heart. *Adv Surg* 1966; **2**: 265–84

22. Ghodsizad A, Bordel V, Ungerer M, Karck M, Bekeredjian R, Ruhparwar A. Ex vivo coronary angiography of a donor heart in the organ care system. *Heart Surg Forum* 2012; **15**: E161–3

23. Costanzo MR, Dipchand A, Starling R, et al. International Society of Heart and Lung Transplantation Guidelines. The International Society of Heart and Lung Transplantation Guidelines for the care of heart transplant recipients. *J Heart Lung Transplant* 2010; **29**: 914–56

24. Chee YL, Crawford JC, Watson HG, Greaves M. Guidelines on the assessment of bleeding risk prior to surgery or invasive procedures. British Committee for Standards in Haematology. *Br J Haematol* 2008; **140**: 496–504

25. Angermann CE, Spes CH, Tammen A, et al. Anatomic characteristics and valvular function of the transplanted heart: transthoracic versus transesophageal echocardiographic findings. *J Heart Transplant* 1990; **9**: 331–8

26. Jacquet L, Ziady G, Stein K, et al. Cardiac rhythm disturbances early after orthotopic heart transplantation: prevalence and clinical importance of the observed abnormalities. *J Am Coll Cardiol* 1990; **16**: 832–7

27. Sarsam MA, Campbell CS, Yonan NA, Deiraniya AK, Rahman AN. An alternative surgical technique in orthotopic cardiac transplantation. *J Card Surg* 1993; **8**: 344–9

28. Chen EP, Bittner HB, Davis RD, Van Trigt P. Hemodynamic and inotropic effects of milrinone after heart transplantation in the setting of recipient pulmonary hypertension. *J Heart Lung Transplant* 1998; **17**: 669–78

29. Byrne JG, Leacche M, Paul S, et al. Risk factors and outcomes for 'vasoplegia syndrome' following cardiac transplantation. *Eur J Cardiothorac Surg* 2004; **25**: 327–32

30. Theodoraki K, Tsiapras D, Tsourelis L, et al. Inhaled iloprost in eight heart transplant recipients presenting with post-bypass acute right ventricular dysfunction. *Acta Anaesthesiol Scand* 2006; **50**: 1213–7

31. Ardehali A, Hughes K, Sadeghi A, et al. Inhaled nitric oxide for pulmonary hypertension after heart transplantation. *Transplantation* 2001; **72**: 638–41

32. Germann P, Braschi A, Della Rocca G, et al. Inhaled nitric oxide therapy in adults: European expert recommendations. *Intensive Care Med* 2005; **31**: 1029–41

33. De Santo LS, Mastroianni C, Romano G, et al. Role of sildenafil in acute posttransplant right ventricular dysfunction: successful experience in 13 consecutive patients. *Transplant Proc* 2008; **40**: 2015–8

34. Tenderich G, Koerner MM, Stuettgen B, et al. Mechanical circulatory support after orthotopic heart transplantation. *Int J Artif Organs* 1998; **21**: 414–6

35. Hetzer R, Delmo Walter EM. Rescue mechanical circulatory support for failing transplanted hearts. *Eur J Cardiothorac Surg* 2012; **42**: 702–3

36. Siniawski H, Dandel M, Lehmkuhl HB, et al. Clinical, haemodynamic and echocardiographic features of early cardiac graft dysfunction. *Kardiol Pol* 2012; **70**: 1010–6

CHAPTER 24

Anaesthesia for adult patients with acquired heart disease for non-cardiac surgery

Alastair F. Nimmo and Matthew T. Royds

Introduction

Many more patients with heart disease undergo non-cardiac surgery than cardiac surgery. Cardiac disease increases the risk of perioperative death and complications; the risk depending on the nature and severity of cardiac disease, and the type and magnitude of non-cardiac surgery.

This chapter discusses the assessment and management of patients with coronary artery disease, cardiac failure, and valvular heart disease presenting for non-cardiac surgery.

The literature in this field can appear complex, and useful starting references are the comprehensive consensus guidelines of the American College of Cardiology Foundation/American Heart Association (ACCF/AHA), and the European Society of Cardiology (ESC). These documents, which are revised periodically, are recommended for further reading (1,2).

Nature and urgency of the non-cardiac surgery

Table 24.1 shows the risk of cardiovascular death or myocardial infarction within 30 days of different types on non-cardiac surgery (2).

It can be seen that for some types of surgery the risk of these complications is low, and additional investigations or changes to management are not usually required unless the patient has an 'active' cardiac condition (table 24.2). The ACCF/AHA Guidelines (1) state that 'The presence of one or more active cardiac conditions mandates intensive management and may result in delay or cancellation of surgery unless the surgery is emergent'.

On the other hand, some vascular surgical procedures are associated with a much higher risk of cardiac complications, so that additional preoperative investigation and/or additional treatment of the cardiac disease before surgery may be appropriate.

When surgery has to be undertaken urgently there may be little or no opportunity for investigation or management of cardiac disease before the operation. However, attention to the appropriate continuation of chronic cardiovascular medical therapy and perioperative management will be important.

Preoperative risk assessment

Assessment before surgery enables the patient and surgeon to be better informed about the risks of surgery, and for options such as non-operative management or a less major operation to be considered. The management of the patient before, during, and after surgery may be modified as a result of the preoperative assessment.

Risk assessment typically involves the calculation of a clinical risk score, plus or minus further investigations.

Clinical risk scoring

Clinical risk scores are calculated from the patient's history and the results of routinely performed preoperative investigations. Lee's Revised Cardiac Risk Index (RCRI) (3) is the most widely used risk score in non-cardiac surgery and has been incorporated into the ESC and ACCF/AHA guidelines. One point is allocated for each risk factor shown in table 24.3.

In a validation cohort in the original study, the incidence of major cardiac complications was 0.4%, 0.9%, 7%, and 11% for patients with a score of 0, 1, 2, or ≥ 3, respectively. A systematic review concluded that the RCRI had moderate performance at discriminating patients at high or low risk following mixed major non-cardiac surgery, with sensitivity 0.65 and specificity 0.76, but that it did not perform well at predicting cardiac events after vascular surgery or at predicting death (4).

Functional status

Functional status or exercise capacity may be expressed in terms of metabolic equivalents (METS; i.e. multiples of resting energy expenditure). The ability to perform more than 4 METS (walking up two flights of stairs, heavy housework, running a short distance) without symptoms is considered in both the ESC and ACCF/AHA guidelines to be associated with acceptable perioperative risk. In a prospective study of 600 patients undergoing

Table 24.1 Risk of myocardial infarction and cardiac death

Low risk <1%	Intermediate risk 1–5%	High risk >5%
Breast	Abdominal	Aortic and major vascular surgery
Dental Endocrine	Carotid	Peripheral vascular surgery
Eye	Peripheral arterial angioplasty	
Gynaecology	Endovascular aneurysm repair	
Reconstructive	Head and neck surgery	
Orthopaedic-minor (knee surgery)	Neurologic/ orthopaedic-major (hip and spine surgery)	
Urologic-minor	Pulmonary/ renal/liver transplant	
	Urologic-major	

Estimated risk of myocardial infarction and cardiac death within 30 days after different types of surgery.

Adapted from *The American Journal of Medicine*, **118**, 10, E Boersma et al., 'Perioperative cardiovascular mortality in noncardiac surgery: Validation of the Lee cardiac risk index', pp. 1134–1141, Copyright 2005, with permission from the Alliance for Academic Internal Medicine and Elsevier

Table 24.2 Patients who should undergo evaluation and treatment before surgery Active cardiac conditions for which the patient should undergo evaluation and treatment before non-cardiac surgery.

Condition	Examples
Unstable coronary syndromes	Unstable or severe angina (CCS class III or IV)
	Recent MI (within 30 days)
Decompensated HF (NYHA functional class IV; worsening or new-onset HF)	
Significant arrhythmias	High-grade atrioventricular block
	Mobitz II atrioventricular block
	Third-degree atrioventricular heart block
	Symptomatic ventricular arrhythmias
	Supraventricular arrhythmias (including atrial fibrillation) with uncontrolled ventricular rate (heart rate >100 bpm at rest)
	Symptomatic bradycardia
	Newly recognized ventricular tachycardia
Severe valvular disease	Severe aortic stenosis (mean pressure gradient >40 mmHg, aortic valve area <1.0 cm^2, or symptomatic)
	Symptomatic mitral stenosis (progressive dyspnoea on exertion, exertional presyncope, or HF) or MVA <1.5 cm^2

Reproduced from Fleisher LA et al., 'ACCF/AHA focused update on perioperative beta blockade incorporated into the ACC/AHA 2007 guidelines on perioperative cardiovascular evaluation and care for noncardiac surgery', *Circulation*, **120**, 21, pp. e169–276, copyright 2009, with permission from American Heart Association Available online and an updated version may be available: http://my.americanheart.org/professional/StatementsGuidelines/ByTopic/TopicsA-C/ACCAHA-Joint-Guidelines_UCM_321694_Article.jsp(accessed 10 September 2013)

bpm, beats per minute; CCS, Canadian Cardiovascular Society; HF, heart failure; MI, myocardial infarction; MVA, mitral valve area; NYHA, New York Heart Association.

Table 24.3 Lee's revised cardiac index risk, from reference (3)

Risk factor
High-risk type of surgery
Ischaemic heart disease/history of ischaemic heart disease
Congestive cardiac failure/history of congestive cardiac failure
History of cerebrovascular disease
Insulin therapy for diabetes
Preoperative serum creatinine >2.0mg/dl (> 177 µmol/l)

Reproduced from Lee TH et al., 'Derivation and prospective validation of a simple index for prediction of cardiac risk of major noncardiac surgery', *Circulation*, **100**, 10, pp. 1043–1049, copyright American Heart Association

major non-cardiac surgery, poor self-reported exercise tolerance (defined as the inability to walk up two flights of stairs) was associated with increased postoperative complications, odds ratio (OR) (95% CI) 2.13 (1.33–3.42). The age-adjusted OR for peroperative myocardial ischaemia was 4.68 in this group (5).

Cardiopulmonary exercise testing

Cardiopulmonary exercise testing (CPET) provides an objective assessment of cardiorespiratory function (6) (Chapter 8). During CPET, oxygen consumption, carbon dioxide production, 12 lead electrocardiograph (ECG), blood pressure, and oxygen saturation are measured as the subject performs work against a progressively braked static cycle ergometer. The peak oxygen consumption is determined as well as the anaerobic threshold (AT) after which CO_2 production increases out of proportion to O_2 consumption. The AT is thought to represent the onset of sustained lactate production supplementing aerobic respiration. This occurs at submaximal exercise and is not influenced by patient effort or motivation.

Studies in patients undergoing major abdominal surgery have found that a low AT is associated with increased postoperative morbidity and mortality. Three studies have found that an AT < 11 mL/kg/min identifies patients at increased risk of hospital mortality (7–9). A further study (10) found the threshold value of 10.1 mL/kg/min to predict postoperative complications with good sensitivity (88%) and specificity (79%). Before elective abdominal aortic aneurysm repair (11), combining the results of the RCRI with results from CPET provided better prediction of survival after surgery than did either result alone (figure 24.1).

Serum biomarkers

Brain natriuretic peptide (BNP) is secreted from myocytes in response to cardiac wall stress. An elevated preoperative plasma BNP (or N-terminal pro-hormone of BNP) concentration is an independent predictor of adverse cardiovascular outcomes after non-cardiac surgery (12).

Stress testing for inducible myocardial ischaemia

Stress testing techniques include dobutamine-atropine stress echocardiography (DSE), radionucleotide myocardial perfusion imaging, and exercise electrocardiography. CPET also usually includes

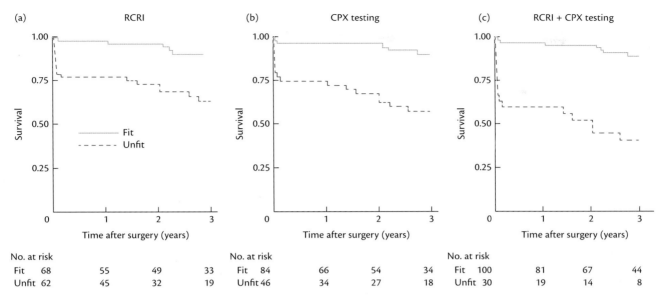

Fig. 24.1 Kaplan–Meier overall survival curves for 130 patients who underwent open abdominal aortic aneurysm repair categorized as 'fit' or 'unfit' respectively by (a) a Revised Cardiac Risk Index (RCRI) of 1 (no comorbidities) or > 1 (at least one comorbidity), (b) ventilatory equivalent for carbon dioxide ($\dot{V}E/\dot{V}CO_2$) below 43 or above 42 on cardiopulmonary exercise (CPX) testing, and (c) no comorbidity (or comorbidity and a $\dot{V}E/\dot{V}CO_2$ below 43) or comorbidity with a $\dot{V}E/\dot{V}CO_2$ above 42 (RCRI + CPX testing). (a) $\chi^2 = 16.2$, $p < 0.001$, (b) $\chi^2 = 19.7$, $p < 0.001$, (c) $\chi^2 = 44.5$, $p < 0.001$ (log rank test)..

Reproduced with permission from Carlisle J and Swart M, 'Mid-term survival after abdominal aortic aneurysm surgery predicted by cardiopulmonary exercise testing', British Journal of Surgery, 94, 8, pp. 966–969, published by Wiley, © 2007 British Journal of Surgery Society Ltd.

an exercise electrocardiography test. A meta-analysis suggested that DSE may be better at predicting perioperative cardiac death and non-fatal myocardial infarction than the other tests (13).

During DSE an incremental infusion of dobutamine is used to increase the heart rate towards the predicted maximum while echocardiography monitors for areas of new or worsening regional wall motion abnormality (RWMA) indicative of ischaemia.

Preoperative DSE has a high negative predictive value (93–100%) for cardiac death or myocardial infarction (MI), so a negative test indicates a low risk of perioperative cardiac complications. The positive predictive value is much lower (0–33%) (1). In this regard the extent of inducible ischaemia may be prognostically important. A multicentre cohort study including 1097 patients who underwent DSE before major vascular surgery found that those who had extensive new RWMA (≥5 segments) suffered a higher cardiac event rate (36%) compared to those with more limited inducible RWMA (2.8%) (14). Likewise, the heart-rate at which RWMA occurred (known as the ischaemic threshold) has been shown to be important. A retrospective study including 530 patients, who were unable to exercise and underwent DSE before non-vascular surgery, found that subjects with an ischaemic threshold less than 60% of their maximum predicted heart rate had a perioperative cardiac event rate of 43%, compared to 9% for those where the ischaemic threshold was >60% maximum predicted heart rate, and 0% where the test was negative (15).

A retrospective cohort study (16) concluded that preoperative non-invasive cardiac stress testing was associated with improved 1 year survival and length of hospital stay in patients undergoing elective intermediate to high risk non-cardiac surgery. These benefits principally applied to patients with risk factors for perioperative cardiac complications.

Coronary angiography

Coronary angiography may be undertaken after positive results have been obtained in a stress test. In vascular surgery patients there is a high incidence of significant coronary artery disease. Hertzer et al (17) performed routine coronary angiography in 1000 patients being considered for elective vascular surgery. Using greater than 70% stenosis as the criterion, significant coronary artery disease (CAD) involved one coronary artery in 27%, two vessels in 19%, and three vessels in 11%, while 4% of patients had a left main stem stenosis of over 50%.

A strategy of routine preoperative coronary angiography may be appropriate in patients having extremely major vascular surgery such as thoracoabdominal aortic aneurysm repair. Computed tomography coronary angiography (CTCA) is an alternative to conventional catheter angiography but in some patients extensive coronary artery calcification may make it difficult or impossible to determine the severity of coronary stenosis from the CT scan.

Echocardiography

When the presence of heart valve disease is known or suspected a resting echocardiogram may be useful to confirm its presence and severity. Echocardiography may also be used to assess left ventricular function. However, 'routine' preoperative assessment of left ventricular function has not been shown to be of value (18).

Coronary artery disease

CAD increases the risk of perioperative myocardial ischaemia, infarction, and cardiac death. Chest pain is often absent in patients suffering a perioperative MI and ST segment depression rather than elevation is the commonest ECG abnormality. Perioperative

MI may result from the rupture or erosion of coronary artery plaque and subsequent thrombus formation, or from oxygen supply–demand imbalance in an area of myocardium supplied by a severely stenosed or chronically occluded coronary artery (19). When an MI is caused by thrombotic occlusion of a coronary artery, endogenous fibrinolysis commonly results in spontaneous dissolution of the clot after the MI has occurred (20), so that the thrombus may not be present at the time of a subsequent coronary angiogram or autopsy. It has also been suggested that after surgery low flow in stenosed coronary arteries and platelet activation could result in the formation of thrombus in the absence of plaque rupture or erosion (21). The inflammatory response to surgery increase the risk of plaque rupture or erosion whilst the prothrombotic state that typically occurs after surgery increases the risk of thrombus formation. Tachycardia is associated with perioperative ischaemia and infarction (19).

Unstable angina and recent MI (within 30 days) are two of the active cardiac conditions associated with very high risk of perioperative cardiac events.

Risk modification strategies

Drug therapies that might be expected to reduce the risk of perioperative MI are those which stabilize coronary plaque (statins), reduce the tendency to thrombus formation in the coronary arteries (antiplatelet drugs), or prevent perioperative tachycardia (beta-blockers, the non-dihydropyridine calcium channel blockers verapamil and diltiazem, centrally acting α_2 adrenergic agonists such as clonidine, and the selective If current inhibitor ivabradine). Preoperative coronary revascularization might also be expected to reduce the risk of perioperative MI. We consider the evidence for some of these interventions next.

Statins

In addition to their lipid-lowering effects, statins have plaque-stabilizing and anti-inflammatory properties, which may reduce the risk of perioperative MI (22). Retrospective studies in non-cardiac and vascular surgery have reported lower mortality in statin users. Two double-blind placebo-controlled trials of perioperative statins in patients having vascular surgery have been published. Durazzo randomized 100 patients to receive atorvastatin 20 mg or placebo for 45 days, started on average 30 days before surgery (23). At follow-up after 6 months four patients in the statin group had suffered a cardiovascular event compared to 13 in the placebo group ($p = 0.031$). Schouten randomized 497 patients to receive extended-release fluvastatin 80 mg, commenced a median of 37 days before vascular surgery and continued for at least 30 days postoperatively, or placebo (24). Postoperative myocardial ischaemia occurred in 10.8% of the statin group and 19% of the placebo group (HR 0.55, CI 0.34–0.88). There were fewer deaths in the fluvastatin group and the composite secondary outcome of death or non-fatal MI was significantly reduced from 10.1% in the placebo group to 4.8% in the fluvastatin-treated group.

Withdrawal of chronic statin therapy in the perioperative period may be harmful. In an observational study including nearly 700 patients undergoing aortic surgery, statin withdrawal was found to be an independent predictor of myocardial necrosis as diagnosed by a rise in troponin (OR 2.9 CI 1.5–5.6) (25).

Patients with cardiovascular disease should already be taking a statin (26). If a patient scheduled for, or being assessed for, vascular surgery is not taking a statin it is recommended that statin treatment be commenced, unless there is a contraindication. Statin therapy should be continued perioperatively. There are no parenteral statins available but statins may be given nasogastrically after surgery. The use of extended release statin formulations before surgery has been suggested in order to provide a more prolonged effect in case a postoperative dose is omitted or not absorbed from the gut.

Antiplatelet agents

Antiplatelet drugs are given to patients with coronary, cerebral, and peripheral vascular disease to reduce the risk of death, MI, and stroke (Chapter 16). Perioperative antiplatelet therapy may increase bleeding. The bleeding risk can be reduced by drug withdrawal but this may increase the risk of thrombotic complications such as MI.

Aspirin withdrawal may result in a rebound thrombogenic state with increased platelet activation (27). A meta-analysis of studies in cardiology and cardiac surgery found aspirin withdrawal to be associated with a threefold increase in major adverse cardiac events (28). A review and meta-analysis of studies of aspirin-related bleeding risk in non-cardiac surgery (29) concluded that the number of bleeding complications was increased by a factor of 1.5 in patients taking aspirin, but there was no increase in the severity of bleeding complications, with the possible exception of intracranial surgery and transurethral prostatectomy.

However, a recently published double blind trial has not found perioperative aspirin therapy to be beneficial. The POISE 2 trial (30) randomised 10 010 patients who were about to undergo noncardiac surgery and were deemed "at risk" for vascular complications to receive either aspirin or placebo. There was no difference between the aspirin and placebo groups in the primary outcome–a composite of death and non-fatal MI at 30 days. This was the case both for patients who had previously been taking aspirin and those who had not. Major bleeding was more common in the aspirin group than the placebo group but the incidence of life-threatening bleeding was similar. Patients who had undergone insertion of a bare-metal coronary stent less than 6 weeks before surgery or a drug-eluting coronary stent less than 1 year before surgery were excluded from the study.

In non-surgical patients clopidogrel is a slightly more effective antiplatelet drug than aspirin but is not associated with more bleeding complications (31). However, there appears to be greater variability in response between patients to clopidogrel than to aspirin, with platelet function testing showing little or no platelet inhibition in some patients and very marked inhibition in others. Clopidogrel is usually regarded as causing more bleeding complications than aspirin in surgical patients but many of the reports of excessive bleeding on clopidogrel turn out on closer examination to be reports of patients receiving both aspirin and clopidogrel. It is uncertain whether or not the overall risk of bleeding during surgery is significantly higher in patients receiving clopidogrel alone than in patients receiving aspirin alone. No randomized trials have addressed this question. The authors of two observational studies in vascular surgery (32,33) concluded that surgery may be safely undertaken in patients on clopidogrel.

Randomized trials of perioperative dual antiplatelet therapy with both aspirin and clopidogrel versus aspirin alone in carotid surgery (34) and lower limb arterial surgery (35) do show increased bleeding with dual therapy, but also potential beneficial effects on reducing perioperative thrombotic complications. The decision as to whether to stop clopidogrel before surgery will depend on a judgement of the relative risks of thrombotic and bleeding complications. As is the case with aspirin, if it is desired that the anti-platelet effect wears off completely before surgery then the drug should be stopped 5–7 days before surgery.

Beta-blockers

The role of beta-blockers in reducing the risk of cardiac complications and death in patients having non-cardiac surgery has been the subject of much controversy in recent years. Large observational studies using propensity-score matching have found that total mortality and perioperative cardiac events are lower in patients taking a beta-blocker if the RCRI is 2 or higher but that in 'low risk' patients with an RCRI score of 0 or 1 beta-blocker therapy was associated with no benefit and with possible harm (36,37). The study by London (38) found a significantly lower rate of mortality in patients receiving atenolol than those receiving metoprolol. The cardioprotective effect of beta-blockers has sometimes been regarded as a class effect with the choice of beta-blocker being of little importance. However, other observational studies in the perioperative setting (38) and in patients with heart failure (39) have also reported lower mortality in patients receiving atenolol than those receiving metoprolol.

Randomized trials in which beta-blocker therapy was started before non-cardiac surgery have produced conflicting results. Studies from Poldermans' group in high-risk vascular surgery patients with positive DSE results (40) and intermediate risk non-cardiovascular surgery patients (41), in which bisoprolol was started a median of 5 weeks before surgery, and the dose increased if required to achieve satisfactory heart rate control, reported a reduction in cardiac death and MI. All-cause mortality was also reduced, but this reduction was statistically significant only in the study of high-risk vascular surgery patients.

In contrast, the POISE study (42), a double-blind study in which extended release metoprolol was started 2–4 hours before non-cardiac surgery, reported a reduction in MIs in the beta-blocker group, but an increase in overall mortality and in stroke. It was suggested that the higher incidence of stroke resulted from there being more hypotension in the beta-blocker group.

The validity of the data in Poldermans' studies has been questioned following findings of research misconduct (43). The POISE study has been criticized for the use of a relatively large dose of metoprolol and for starting it shortly before surgery. A meta-analysis (44) of nine randomized studies, which excluded studies from Poldermans' group, concluded that starting beta-blockers before non-cardiac surgery resulted in an increase in all-cause mortality. This meta-analysis was heavily influenced by the POISE trial, which was much larger than the other studies. In the other eight studies the combined number of deaths in the beta-blocker groups was not higher than in the control groups. At the time of writing (in 2013) both the ESC/ESA and the ACCF/AHA guidelines on the management of patients with cardiac disease having non-cardiac surgery are in the process of being revised.

Our practice is to prescribe beta-blockers in patients having high-risk (vascular) surgery if they have a high clinical risk score or positive preoperative stress test for myocardial ischaemia. However, we take steps to reduce the incidence and severity of perioperative hypotension if beta-blockers are started (table 24.4).

Table 24.4 Strategies to reduce the incidence and severity of perioperative hypotension in patients started on a beta-blocker before surgery

Start the beta-blocker at least a week before surgery, preferably earlier.
Start with a low dose, e.g. bisoprolol 2.5 mg daily or atenolol 25 mg daily (dose may be increased or an extra dose given if heart rate is inadequately controlled).
If the patient is taking another antihypertensive or anti-anginal drug consider stopping it when starting the beta-blocker.
Consider omitting other antihypertensive drugs at the time of surgery and during postoperative analgesia with epidural local anaesthetic.
Avoid or correct hypovolaemia during and after surgery.
Consider the use of a low-dose vasoconstrictor infusion during postoperative analgesia with epidural local anaesthetic.
Monitor blood pressure closely after surgery.
Specify a minimum acceptable postoperative arterial pressure and have a protocol for the management of blood pressure below this limit.
Omit a dose of beta-blocker if the heart rate is below a predefined limit or if the blood pressure remains lower than desired despite the above management.

Where patients are already on a beta-blocker, observational studies suggest that perioperative withdrawal results in increased cardiac events and mortality. Therefore, beta blockade should be continued perioperatively (1,2).

Other classes of drug that reduce heart rate may reduce perioperative myocardial ischaemia and infarction. However, the POISE 2 trial (45), a double blind trial in which 10 010 patients who were about to undergo noncardiac surgery and were at risk for vascular complications were randomised to receive either clonidine or placebo (and either aspirin or placebo) did not show a benefit from perioperative clonidine administration. In the clonidine group there was no reduction in death or non-fatal MI at 30 days and there was an increased rate of clinically significant hypotension and nonfatal cardiac arrest. The dihydropyridine calcium channel blockers amlodipine, nifedipine, and felodipine, which increase heart rate, were independently associated with increased mortality in an observational study of 1000 aortic aneurysm patients (46).

Preoperative coronary revascularization

Revascularization refers to two very different procedures—surgical coronary artery bypass grafting (CABG), and percutaneous coronary intervention (PCI), with angioplasty and the insertion of coronary stents.

Observational studies suggest that patients who have undergone CABG have a lower incidence of death and MI after intermediate or high-risk surgery than patients whose coronary artery disease is managed medically (47). However, performing CABG before non-cardiac surgery adds the risks of the cardiac surgical procedure to that of the non-cardiac surgery, and delays the non-cardiac surgery.

Prophylactic revascularization has been addressed by two studies. In the Coronary Artery Revascularization Prophylaxis (CARP) trial, 510 patients were randomized to revascularization or medical therapy before elective vascular surgery (48). There was no difference in the rate of MI within 30 days of surgery, or mortality at 2.7 years. Patients were excluded from the study if they had a stenosis of the left main stem of at least 50%, a left ventricular ejection fraction of less than 20%, or severe aortic stenosis. Most patients had significant stenosis of only one or two coronary arteries, and most revascularization procedures were by PCI rather than CABG. The Dutch Echocardiographic Cardiac Risk Evaluation Applying Stress Echocardiography V (DECREASE-V) study (49) included 101 patients with severe CAD who were randomized to revascularization or medical therapy. Revascularization did not improve the composite outcome of death and MI at 30 days or 1 year. Again, most revascularization procedures were PCI rather than CABG. The validity of the data in the DECREASE-V study has been questioned following findings of research misconduct (43).

Biccard analysed the results of the CARP and DECREASE-V studies according to the type of revascularization performed (50). Preoperative PCI was associated with a worse 30-day and late composite outcome of death and non-fatal MI than medical therapy. Comparing CABG with medical therapy, there was no significant difference in the composite outcome but there was a trend towards better longer-term outcome in the CABG group.

Monaco (51) randomized 208 vascular surgery patients to a strategy of either routine or selective preoperative angiography. The routine angiography group had a higher rate of preoperative myocardial revascularization, a higher proportion of revascularization by CABG rather than PCI, and significantly lower mortality.

It seems clear that preoperative PCI with insertion of coronary stents in patients with stable cardiac disease before non-cardiac surgery does not improve, and may worsen, outcome. The role of preoperative CABG is less certain and may depend on the severity of the coronary disease, the nature and magnitude of the proposed surgery and the consequences of delaying the non-cardiac surgery.

Surgery in patients with coronary stents

Non-cardiac surgery soon after coronary stent insertion carries a high risk of death or non-fatal MI caused by stent thrombosis. This is due to the thrombogenic nature of the stent, coupled with the prothrombotic response to surgery. The risk decreases with time as the stent endothelializes, but this process is delayed in drug-eluting stents (DES). Continuing antiplatelet therapy perioperatively may provide partial protection against stent thrombosis.

Patients typically remain on dual antiplatelet therapy (aspirin and clopidogrel) for three months after insertion of bare metal stents (BMS) and for 12 months after DES, and premature discontinuation is associated with a large increase in the risk of stent thrombosis. In a prospective observational cohort study of 2229 consecutive patients with DES (52), five of 17 patients with premature antiplatelet therapy discontinuation had stent thrombosis.

The incidence of cardiac complications in patients undergoing non-cardiac surgery in the first 6 weeks following coronary stenting is as high as 35–50% despite antiplatelet therapy being continued (53,54). It is recommended that elective surgery be avoided for at least 6 weeks and preferably for 3 months after insertion of a BMS and for a year after insertion of a DES. After these times elective surgery may be undertaken but at least aspirin therapy should be continued perioperatively (2).

Patients presenting for urgent surgery within these time periods are at increased risk of cardiac complications. Dual antiplatelet therapy may be continued, accepting increased bleeding risk, or clopidogrel stopped and only aspirin continued with a probable increased risk of cardiac complications. The decision should be a consensus between surgeon, anaesthetist, and cardiologist, and surgery should ideally be undertaken in a centre with PCI availability.

Heart failure

Approximately 1–2% of the adult population in developed countries have heart failure, with the prevalence rising to ≥10% in the elderly (55). Decompensated cardiac failure is one of the active cardiac conditions which are major predictors of adverse perioperative outcome (1) and a history of cardiac failure increases the risk of perioperative complications and mortality after major non-cardiac surgery (3). In a retrospective study of 30 000 patients with heart failure undergoing major non-cardiac surgery the adjusted mortality ratio for patients with a previous diagnosis of heart failure compared with controls was 1.63 (95% CI 1.52–1.74) (56). The risk is, however, likely to depend on the severity of the heart failure.

In heart failure patients with a reduced left ventricular (LV) ejection fraction mortality can be reduced by treatment with angiotension-converting enzyme (ACE) inhibitors, beta-blockers, and aldosterone antagonists (57). It is appropriate for symptomatic status to be optimized with these medications preoperatively, and there is limited evidence that outcome is improved in this population if they are continued throughout the perioperative period (58). ACE inhibitors and angiotensin receptor blockers (ARBs) may be associated with perioperative hypotension, and this may be more severe if other drugs and techniques that lower blood pressure (e.g. beta-blockers and epidural analgesia) are also used. The balance of risks and benefits of omitting ACE inhibitors or ARBs before surgery in this situation is uncertain in patients with heart failure.

There are no specific perioperative interventions that have been shown to improve prognosis in heart failure patients having non-cardiac surgery.

Valvular heart disease

There is significant risk of morbidity and mortality in patients with valvular heart disease (VHD) undergoing non-cardiac surgery, especially patients with severe aortic stenosis (AS) (59). The ESC and European Association for Cardio-Thoracic Surgery (EACTS) Guidelines on the management of valvular heart disease (60) includes recommendations on management of patients presenting for non-cardiac surgery; the anaesthetic management of these patients has been reviewed by Mittnacht (61) and Brown (62).

Before non-cardiac surgery patients with AS should undergo a detailed clinical and echocardiographic evaluation to fully assess the nature and severity of the lesion. Associated symptoms (typically dyspnoea, angina, and syncope) should be sought, as should the presence of arrhythmias, left ventricular dysfunction, pulmonary hypertension, and co-existing CAD.

The decision as to whether to proceed with non-cardiac surgery in a patient with severe AS must be decided on an individual basis taking into account the importance and urgency of the non-cardiac surgery, but a framework for guidance is illustrated in figure 24.2, taken from the ESC/EACTS Guidelines (60).

Where patients are symptomatic from severe AS, serious consideration of valve replacement must take place, even before

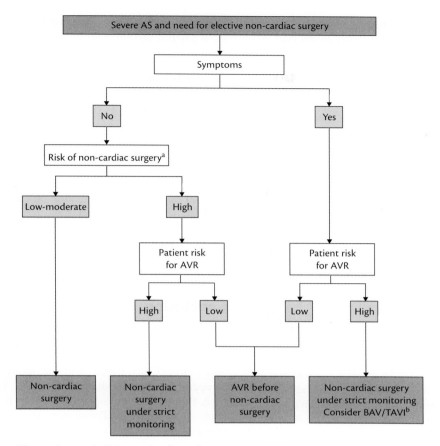

AS = aortic stenosis; AVR = aortic valve replacement; BAV = balloon aortic valvuloplasty;
TAVI = transcatheter aortic valve implantation.
[a]Classification into three groups according to the risk of cardic complications (30-day death and
myocardial infarction) for non-cardiac surgery (227) (high risk >5%; intermediate risk 1–5%; low risk <1%.
[b]Non-cardiac surgery performed only if strictly needed. The choice between balloon aortic valvuloplasty
and transcatheter aortic valve implantation should take into account patient life expectancy.

Fig. 24.2 Management of severe aortic stenosis and elective non-cardiac surgery according to patient characteristics and the type of surgery.
Reproduced from Vahanian A, et al., 'Guidelines on the management of valvular heart disease: The Joint Task Force on the Management of Valvular Heart Disease of the European Society of Cardiology (ESC) and the European Association for Cardio-Thoracic Surgery (EACTS)', European Heart Journal, 2012, 33, 19, pp. 2451–2496, by permission of the European Society of Cardiology.

non-cardiac surgery considered only low or intermediate risk. Where preoperative valve replacement is not appropriate percutaneous valvuloplasty warrants consideration as a bridging intervention (63). Transcatheter aortic valve implantation (TAVI) may also be considered in centres where expertise exists. In patients with severe AS who are asymptomatic the risk associated with the non-cardiac surgical procedure will strongly influence management decisions.

The pathophysiology of AS involves chronic pressure overload leading to LV hypertrophy and increased myocardial oxygen demand (Chapter 2). This coupled with reduced aortic diastolic pressures and elevated LV diastolic pressures (due to the pressure gradient across the narrowed valve orifice) can result in precarious myocardial oxygen supply-demand balance and ischaemia, even in the presence of normal coronary arteries. Additionally, the resistance to flow offered by the reduced valve orifice area eventually limits the ability of the ventricle to increase cardiac output. Tachycardia, loss of sinus rhythm, and reductions in preload and afterload are poorly tolerated with the risk of a vicious cycle of reduced cardiac output and myocardial ischaemia developing.

The haemodynamic goals in managing a patient with severe AS include maintaining normovolaemia and avoiding significant reductions in preload and afterload due to vasodilation. It is important to maintain sinus rhythm, while aiming for a low normal heart rate. Continuous invasive arterial blood pressure monitoring should be used perioperatively. Local anaesthetic spinal or epidural block is commonly avoided because of the potential for profound vasodilation, but carefully titrated spinal or epidural anaesthesia can be employed.

Anaesthetic techniques and management

There is little evidence that particular anaesthetic techniques such as regional versus general anaesthesia, or controlled versus spontaneous ventilation, should be chosen because a patient has cardiac disease. Nor is there good evidence that one anaesthetic agent is better than another in regard to cardiac complications.

Nevertheless, the anaesthetist's perioperative management of the patient may be of great importance in reducing the risk of complications. For example, outcome may be improved by ensuring that medical therapy for cardiac disease is appropriately continued perioperatively, maintaining normovolaemia and normothermia, avoiding both sever anaemia and unnecessary allogeneic red cell transfusion, and appropriate monitoring for, and prompt management of cardiac complications.

Monitoring

ECG monitoring should as a minimum be five-lead, with V5 and II displayed along with continuous display of ST segment deviation. The addition of ST monitoring of V4 increases the sensitivity for the detection of myocardial ischaemia (64). The development of new ST segment depression during surgery may represent the occurrence of an intraoperative MI or a high risk of postoperative MI and is an indication for admission to a critical care unit after surgery.

About 10% of patients with peripheral vascular disease have a difference in systolic BP of >45 mmHg between the left and right arms (65), usually as the result of a subclavian artery stenosis causing a falsely low BP reading in one arm. The BP should be compared in both arms before surgery. Where there is a significant difference, only the arm with the higher pressure should be used for monitoring. Whether invasive haemodynamic monitoring is used will depend both on the nature of the proposed surgery and the severity of the cardiac disease. An arterial cannula enables, not only continuous arterial pressure monitoring, but also the use of pulse contour analysis monitors. These monitors can be used to calculate the change in stroke volume in response to an intravenous fluid challenge and also, in ventilated patients with a closed chest and regular cardiac rhythm, the variation in pulse pressure variation and stroke volume over the respiratory cycle and provide a better guide to appropriateness of fluid administration than measurement of central venous pressure. An alternative is to use oesophageal Doppler monitoring.

Transoesophageal echocardiography may be useful during major non-cardiac surgery for the assessment of ventricular filling and function, the detection of wall motion abnormalities resulting from myocardial ischaemia and as an aid to the diagnosis of the cause of episodes of marked hypotension (66).

Postoperative management

Most cardiac complications of non-cardiac surgery occur, or at least become apparent, after rather than during surgery. Continued ECG and arterial blood pressure monitoring, with early detection and treatment of myocardial ischaemia, arrhythmias, marked hypotension or hypertension, may prevent the development of more serious complications. A study of ECG monitoring and troponin concentrations in 185 patients after vascular surgery (67) found that in all 12 patients suffering an MI the troponin rise occurred during or immediately after a prolonged period of ST depression. All documented ischaemic events culminating in perioperative MI were preceded by an increase in heart rate.

Postoperative management in a critical care unit (high-dependency or intensive care unit) permits the closer monitoring of ECG and blood pressure and may also facilitate early detection and management of hypoxia, hypovolaemia, or evidence of inadequate organ perfusion, and better pain control. A case-controlled study of critical care or surgical ward care after elective open colorectal surgery in patients who had a low anaerobic threshold on preoperative cardiopulmonary exercise testing found that there were fewer cardiac events in the patients allocated to critical care than to ward care (68).

Longer-term management

The goal of most surgical operations is to prolong life or improve the quality of a patient's life. In a patient with cardiac disease, the optimal management of that disease after surgery may be at least as important in achieving these objectives as the surgical procedure itself. Patients who suffer perioperative MI are at high risk of future cardiac events. It is important that they are discharged on appropriate therapy for cardiac disease treatment and secondary prevention. Any new information on the presence or severity of cardiac disease obtained during assessment for surgery or the hospital admission, and also details of any perioperative cardiac complications should be given to the physicians who will be caring for the patient in future. Cardiology referral for further management may be appropriate.

Conclusion

A sound understanding of the pathophysiology of the heart disease is a good basis for the anaesthetic management of these patients. However, management also requires understanding of how to assess, investigate, and risk stratify patients, as well as perioperative use of cardiovascular drugs. With this core knowledge, the great number of patients who have heart disease can safely undergo non-cardiac surgery, anaesthetized by non-cardiac anaesthetists.

References

1. Fleisher LA, Beckman JA, Brown KA et al (2009). ACCF/AHA focused update on perioperative beta blockade incorporated into the ACC/AHA 2007 guidelines on perioperative cardiovascular evaluation and care for noncardiac surgery. Circulation, 120, e169–276 Available online and an updated version may be available: http://my.americanheart.org/professional/StatementsGuidelines/ByTopic/TopicsA-C/ACCAHA-Joint-Guidelines_UCM_321694_Article.jsp (accessed 10 September 2013)
2. Poldermans D, Bax JJ, Boersma E, et al. The Task Force for Preoperative Cardiac Risk Assessment and Perioperative Cardiac Management in Non-cardiac Surgery of the European Society of Cardiology (ESC) and endorsed by the European Society of Anaesthesiology (ESA). (2009). Guidelines for preoperative cardiac risk assessment and perioperative cardiac management in non-cardiac surgery. Eur Heart J, 30, 2769–2812 Available online and an updated version may be available: http://www.escardio.org/guidelines-surveys/esc-guidelines/Pages/GuidelinesList.aspx (accessed 10 September 2013)
3. Lee TH, Marcantonio ER, Mangione CM, et al. Derivation and prospective validation of a simple index for prediction of cardiac risk of major noncardiac surgery. *Circulation* 1999; **100**(10): 1043–9
4. Ford MK, Beattie WS, Wijeysundera DN. Systematic review: prediction of perioperative cardiac complications and mortality by the revised cardiac risk index. *Ann Intern Med* 2010; **152**(1): 26–35
5. Reilly DF, McNeely MJ, Doerner D, et al. Self-reported exercise tolerance and the risk of serious perioperative complications. *Arch Intern Med* 1999; **159**: 2185–92
6. Hennis PJ, Meale PM, Grocott MP. Cardiopulmonary exercise testing for the evaluation of perioperative risk in non-cardiopulmonary surgery. *Postgrad Med J* 2011; **87**: 550–7
7. Older P, Smith, R, Courtney P, Hone R. Preoperative evaluation of cardiac failure and ischaemia in elderly patients by cardiopulmonary exercise testing. *Chest* 1993; **104**: 701–4

8. Older P, Hall A, Hader R. Cardiopulmonary exercise testing as a screening test for perioperative management of major surgery in the elderly. *Chest* 1999; **116**: 355–62

9. Wilson RJT, Davies S, Yates D, Redman J, Stone M. Impaired functional capacity is associated with all-cause mortality after major elective intra-abdominal surgery. *Br J Anaesth* 2010; **105**(3): 297–303

10. Snowden CP, Prentis JM, Anderson HL, et al. Submaximal cardiopulmonary exercise testing predicts complications and hospital length of stay in patients undergoing major elective surgery. *Ann Surg* 2010; **251**(3): 535–41

11. Carlisle J, Swart M. Mid-term survival after abdominal aortic aneurysm surgery predicted by cardiopulmonary exercise testing. *Br J Surg* 2007; **94**(8): 966–9

12. Karthikeyan G, Moncur RA, Levine O, et al. Is a pre-operative brain natriuretic peptide or N-terminal pro-B-type natriuretic peptide measurement an independent predictor of adverse cardiovascular outcomes within 30 days of noncardiac surgery? A systematic review and meta-analysis of observational studies. *J Am Coll Cardiol* 2009; **54**(17): 1599–606

13. Kertai MD, Boersma E, Bax JJ. et al. A meta-analysis comparing the prognostic accuracy of six diagnostic tests for predicting perioperative cardiac risk in patients undergoing major vascular surgery. *Heart* 2003; **89**: 1327–334

14. Boersma E, Poldermans D, Bax JJ, et al. Predictors of cardiac events after major vascular surgery: Role of clinical characteristics, dobutamine echocardiography, and beta-blocker therapy. *JAMA* 2001; **285**(14): 1865–73

15. Das MK, Pellikka PA, Mahoney DW, et al. Assessment of cardiac risk before nonvascular surgery: dobutamine stress echocardiography in 530 patients. *J Am Coll Cardiol* 2000; **35**(6): 1647–53

16. Wijeysundera DN, Beattie WS, Austin PC, Hux JE, Laupacis A. Non-invasive cardiac stress testing before elective major non-cardiac surgery: a population based cohort study. *Br Med J* 2010; **340**: b5526

17. Hertzer NR, Bever EG, Young JR, et al. Coronary artery disease in peripheral vascular patients: a classification of 1000 coronary angiograms and results of surgical management. *Ann Surg* 1984; **199**: 223–33

18. Wijeysundera DN, Beattie WS, Karkouti K, Neuman MD, Austin PC, Laupacis A. Association of echocardiography before major elective non-cardiac surgery with postoperative survival and length of hospital stay: population based cohort study. *Br Med J* 2011; **342**: d3695

19. Landesberg G, Beattie WS, Mosseri M, Jaffe AS, Alpert JS. Perioperative myocardial infarction. *Circulation* 2009; **119**: 2936–44

20. Newby DE. Triggering of acute myocardial infarction: beyond the vulnerable plaque. *Heart* 2010; **96**: 1247–51

21. Biccard BM, Rodseth RN. The pathophysiology of perioperative myocardial infarction. *Anaesthesia* 2010; **65**(7): 733–41

22. Biccard BM. A peri-operative statin update for non-cardiac surgery. Part II: Statin therapy for vascular surgery and perioperative statin trial design. Anaesthesia, (2008). 63(2), 162–71

23. Durazzo AE, Machado FS, Ikeoka DT, et al. Reduction in cardiovascular events after vascular surgery with atorvastatin: a randomised trial. *J Vasc Surg* 2004; **39**: 967–76

24. Schouten O, Boersma E, Hoeks SE, et al. Fluvastatin and perioperative events in patients undergoing vascular surgery. *N Eng J Med* 2009; **361**(10): 980–9

25. Le Manach Y, Godet G, Coriat P, et al. (2007). The impact of postoperative discontinuation or continuation of chronic statin therapy on cardiac outcome after major vascular surgery. *Anesth Analg* **104**(6): 1326–33

26. National Institute for Health and Care Excellence. Statins for the prevention of cardiovascular events. Technology appraisal 94. Available at: http://www.nice.org.uk/page.aspx?o=TA094guidance (accessed 10 September 2013)

27. Chassot PG, Delabays A, Spahn DR. Perioperative antiplatelet therapy: the case for continuing therapy in patients at risk of myocardial infarction. *Br J Anaesth* 2007; **99**(3): 316–28

28. Biondi-Zoccai GGL, Lotrionte M, Agostoni P, et al. A systematic review and meta-analysis on the hazards of discontinuing or not adhering to aspirin among 50279 patients at risk for coronary artery disease. *Eur Heart J* 2006; **27**: 2667–74

29. Burger W, Chemnitius JM, Kneissl GD, Rucker G. Low-dose aspirin for secondary cardiovascular prevention—cardiovascular risks after its perioperative withdrawal versus bleeding risks with its continuation—review and meta-analysis. *J Intern Med* 2005; **257**(5): 399–414

30. Devereaux PJ, Mrkobrada M, Sessler DI, et al. The POISE-2 Investigators (2014). Aspirin in patients undergoing noncardiac surgery. *N Engl J Med*. 2014 Mar 31. [Epub ahead of print]

31. CAPRIE Steering Committee. A randomised, blinded, trial of clopidogrel versus aspirin in patients at risk of ischaemic events (CAPRIE). *Lancet* 1996; **348**: 1329–39

32. Stone DH, Goodney PP, Schanzer A. et al. Vascular Study Group of New England. Clopidogrel is not associated with major bleeding complications during peripheral arterial surgery. *J Vasc Surg* 2011; **54**: 779–84

33. Saadeh C, Sfeir J. Discontinuation of preoperative clopidogrel is unnecessary in peripheral arterial surgery. *J Vasc Surg* 2013; S0741-5214(13)01124-5. doi: 10.1016/j.jvs.2013.05.092. [Epub ahead of print]

34. Payne DA, Jones CI, Hayes PD, et al. Beneficial effects of clopidogrel combined with aspirin in reducing cerebral emboli in patients undergoing carotid endarterectomy. *Circulation* 2004; **109**: 1476–81

35. Burdess A, Nimmo AF, Garden OJ, et al. Randomized controlled trial of dual antiplatelet therapy in patients undergoing surgery for critical limb ischemia. *Ann Surg* 2010; **252**: 37–42

36. Lindenauer PK, Pekow P, Wang K, Mamidi DK, Gutierrez B, Benjamin EM. Perioperative beta-blocker therapy and mortality after major noncardiac surgery. *N Engl J Med* 2005; **353**: 349–61

37. London MJ, Hur K, Schwartz GG, et al. Association of perioperative-blockade with mortality and cardiovascular morbidity following major noncardiac surgery. *JAMA* 2013; **309**: 1704–13

38. Redelmeier D, Scales D, Kopp A. Beta-blockers for elective surgery in elderly patients: population based, retrospective cohort study. *Br Med J* 2005; **331**: 932A–4A

39. Lazarus DL, Jackevicius CA, Behlouli H, Johansen H, Pilote L. Population-based analysis of class effect of β blockers in heart failure. *Am J Cardiol* 2011; **107**(8): 1196–202

40. Poldermans D, Boersma E, Bax JJ, et al. The effect of bisoprolol on perioperative mortality and myocardial infarction in high-risk patients undergoing vascular surgery. *N Engl J Med* 1999; **341**(24): 1789–94

41. Dunkelgrun M, Boersma E, Schouten O, et al. Bisoprolol and fluvastatin for the reduction of perioperative cardiac mortality and myocardial infarction in intermediate-risk patients undergoing noncardiovascular surgery: a randomized controlled trial (DECREASE-IV). *Ann Surg* 2009; **249**(6): 921–6

42. Devereaux PJ, Yang H, Yusuf S, et al. Effects of extended-release metoprolol succinate in patients undergoing non-cardiac surgery (POISE trial): a randomised controlled trial. *Lancet* 2008; **371**: 1839–47

43. Erasmus Medical Centre. Report on the 2012 follow-up investigation of possible breaches of academic integrity. Available at: http://cardiobrief.files.wordpress.com/2012/10/integrity-report-2012-10-english-translation.pdf (accessed 11 July 2014)

44. Bouri S, Shun-Shin MJ, Cole GD, Mayet J, Francis DP. Meta-analysis of secure randomised controlled trials of β-blockade to prevent perioperative death in non-cardiac surgery. *Heart* 2014; **100**(6): 456–64

45. Devereaux PJ, Sessler DI, Leslie K, et al. The POISE-2 Investigators (2014). Clonidine in patients undergoing noncardiac surgery. *N Engl J Med*. 2014 Mar 31. [Epub ahead of print]

46. Kertai MD, Westerhout CM, Varga KS, Acsady G, Gal J. Dihydropiridine calcium-channel blockers and perioperative mortality in aortic aneurysm surgery. *Br J Anaesth* 2008; **101**: 458–65

47. Eagle KA, Rihal CS, Mickel MC, Holmes DR, Foster ED, Gersh BJ. Cardiac risk of noncardiac surgery: influence of coronary disease and type of surgery in 3368 operations. *Circulation* 1997; **96**(6): 1882–7

48. McFalls EO, Ward HB, Moritz TE, et al. Coronary-artery revascularization before elective major vascular surgery. *N Engl J Med* 2004; **351**: 2795–804

49. Poldermans D, Schouten O, Vidakovic R, et al. A clinical randomised trial to evaluate the safety of a noninvasive approach in high-risk patients undergoing major vascular surgery: the DECREASE-V Pilot Study. *J Am Coll Cardiol* 2007; **49**: 1763–9

50. Biccard BM, Rodseth RN. A meta-analysis of the prospective randomised trials of coronary revascularisation before noncardiac vascular surgery with attention to the type of coronary revascularisation performed. *Anaesthesia* 2009; **64**(10): 1105–13

51. Monaco M, Stassano P, Di Tommaso L, et al. Systematic strategy of prophylactic coronary angiography improves long-term outcome after major vascular surgery in medium- to high-risk patients: a prospective, randomized study. *J Am Coll Cardiol* 2009; **54**: 989–96

52. Iakovou I, Schmidt T, Bonizzoni E, et al. Incidence, predictors, and outcome of thrombosis after successful implantation of drug-eluting stents. *JAMA* 2005; **293**(17): 2126–30

53. van Kuijk JP, Flu WJ, Schouten O, et al. Timing of noncardiac surgery after coronary artery stenting with bare metal or drug-eluting stents. *Am J Cardiol* 2009; **104**: 1229–34

54. Cruden NL, Harding SA, Flapan AD, et al. Previous coronary stent implantation and cardiac events in patients undergoing noncardiac surgery. *Circ Cardiovasc Interv* 2010; **3**: 236–42

55. Mosterd A, Hoes AW. Clinical epidemiology of heart failure. *Heart* 2007; **93**: 1137–46

56. Hammill BG, Curtis LH, Bennett-Guerrero E, et al. Impact of heart failure on patients undergoing major noncardiac surgery. *Anesthesiology* 2008; **108**(4): 559–67

57. McMurray JJ, Adamopoulos S, Anker SD, et al. ESC Guidelines for the diagnosis and treatment of acute and chronic heart failure 2012. *Eur Heart J* 2012; **33**(14): 1787–847. Available online and an updated version may be available: http://www.escardio.org/guidelines-surveys/esc-guidelines/Pages/GuidelinesList.aspx (accessed 10 September 2013)

58. Feringa HH, Bax JJ, Schouten O, Poldermans D. Protecting the heart with medication in patients with left ventricular dysfunction undergoing major noncardiac vascular surgery. *Semin Cardiothorac Vasc Anesth* 2006; **10**(1): 25–31

59. Kertai MD, Bountioukos M, Boersma E, et al. Aortic stenosis: an underestimated risk factor for perioperative complications in patients undergoing noncardiac surgery. *Am J Med* 2004; **116**: 8–13

60. Vahanian A, Alfieri O, Andreotti F, et al. Guidelines on the management of valvular heart disease (version 2012). Joint Task Force on the Management of Valvular Heart Disease of the European Society of Cardiology (ESC); European Association for Cardio-Thoracic Surgery (EACTS). *Eur Heart J* 2012; **33**(19): 2451–96. Available online and an updated version may be available: http://www.escardio.org/guidelines-surveys/esc-guidelines/Pages/GuidelinesList.aspx (accessed 10 September 2013)

61. Mittnacht AJ, Fanshawe M, Konstadt S. Anaesthetic considerations in the patient with valvular heart disease undergoing noncardiac surgery. *Semin Cardiothorac Vasc Anesth* 2008; **12**(1): 33–59

62. Brown J, Morgan-Hughes NJ. Aortic stenosis and non-cardiac surgery. *Contin Educ Anaesth Crit Care Pain* 2005; **5**(1): 1–4

63. Levine MJ, Berman AD, Safian RD, Diver DJ, McKay RG. Palliation of valvular aortic stenosis by balloon valvuloplasty as preoperative preparation for noncardiac surgery. *Am J Cardiol* 1988; **62**: 1309–10

64. London MJ, Hollenberg M, Wong M, et al. Intraoperative myocardial ischemia: localization by continuous 12-lead electrocardiography. *Anesthesiology* 1988; **69**: 232–41

65. Frank SM, Norris EJ, Christopherson R, Beattie C. Right- and left-arm blood pressure discrepancies in vascular surgery patients. Anesthesiology 1991; **75**: 457–63

66. American Society of Anesthesiologists and Society of Cardiovascular Anesthesiologists Task Force on Transesophageal Echocardiography. Practice guidelines for perioperative transesophageal echocardiography. *Anesthesiology* 2010; **112**(5): 1084–96

67. Landesberg G, Mosseri M, Zahger D, et al. Myocardial infarction after vascular surgery: the role of prolonged stress-induced, ST depression-type ischemia. *J Am Coll Cardiol* 2001; **37**(7): 1839–45

68. Swart M, Carlisle JB. Case-controlled study of critical care or surgical ward care after elective open colorectal surgery. *Br J Surg* 2012; **99**(2): 295–9

CHAPTER 25

Anaesthesia for cardiac electrophysiological interventions

Bodil Steen Rasmussen

Introduction

As an understanding of the of heart's electrophysiology and pathophysiology is fundamental to the practice of cardiothoracic anaesthesia, this chapter will review the conduction system of the heart, its abnormalities and their treatment.

The cardiac conduction system

The cardiac conduction system consists of specialized myocytes with specific capacities for impulse formation and impulse propagation. The anatomy of the cardiac conduction system was clarified more than a century ago (1–4). The new era of molecular biology and immunohistochemistry has validated this early anatomic definition of myocardial tissue that generates and disseminates the cardiac impulse (5–8). Complexity is a key feature of the conduction tissue consisting of the sinus node, the atrioventricular node, the bundle of His, the left and right bundles, and the Purkinje fibres (figure 25.1).

Anatomy of the conduction system

The sinus node is an intramural structure with its head located subepicardially at the junction of the right atrium and the superior vena cava and its tail extending along the crista terminalis (9). There is no specific conductive tissue located towards the atrioventricular node, however, studies have shown a complex and heterogeneous pattern of expression of ion channels in the sinus node as well as in the paranodal area and right atrium (6). The atrioventricular node is located subendocardially in the right side of the artrial septum just above the fibrous arterioventricular ring. Reaching the atrioventricular node, the impulse is delayed giving atrial contraction the time to fill the ventricles before the impulse is transmitted rapidly through the central fibrous bundle of His emerging into the left ventricular outflow tract at the crest of the muscular ventricular septum with bifurcation into the right and left branches splitting up into interlinked fascicles and the Purkinje network to trigger simultaneous ventricular contraction from apex to base.

Physiology of the conduction system

The cardiac conduction system initiates and conducts the sinus impulse, ensuring an appropriate rate and timing of contraction in the different cardiac chambers (5). The pacemaker cells cardiac conduction system has the capacity of pacing and activating the heart, thus having an autorhythmicity. The sinus node is the primary cardiac pacemaker generating the cardiac impulse, which is conducted in a non-uniform anisotropic fashion through the atrial myocardium to the atrioventricular node (10). Due to its high inherent discharge rate, the sinus node activates and resets the other pacemakers in the heart bringing those to have the physiological role of acting as back-ups pacemakers. The atrioventricular node has a multiple of functions, such as providing a critical delay between atrial and ventricular systole, protecting against life-threatening rapid supraventricular rates, and providing contingent pacemaking in the event of failure of the sinus node (5,7,9). The sinus node possess the fastest and most robust pacemaker activity, while the atrioventricular node is slower and the His–Purkinje system weakest. The working myocardium does not have pacemaker activity, but all myocytes within the myocardium have the capacity to conduct the cardiac impulse.

Action potential of myocytes

The cardiac conduction system generates and conducts electrical signals, action potentials, throughout the heart to trigger and coordinate the heart beat. The membrane of a resting myocardial muscle cell is polarized with positive charges on the outside and negative charges within, and with a resting negative membrane potential of 60–90 mV the source for contraction must be capable of reducing the membrane potential of the myocytes (figure 25.2). Reduction of the membrane potential beyond the critical level, the threshold, activates the myocytes to contract. This depolarization of the myocytes with a rapid increase towards a positive membrane potential up to 30 mV is called phase 0 and is succeeded by a brief period of rapid repolarization towards the zero potential (phase 1), a plateau period (phase 2), and terminated by rapid repolarization (phase 3) followed by a diastolic period with consistent membrane potential. This entire sequence is named the action potential of the myocytes. This electrical activity is highly dependent on the expression of ion channels in myocytes of the conduction system with influx of sodium and calcium ions into the cells during depolarization and a transport of potassium out of the cells during depolarization. Ion channel expression in the cardiac conduction

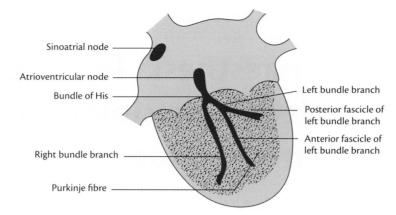

Fig. 25.1 The conduction system of the heart.
Reproduced with kind permission from Dr. Bjarne Mühldorff Sigurd
Sandøe E and Sigurd B (1984). Arrhythmia, diagnosis and Management: A clinical electrographic guide, 1st edn. Fachmed AG, St. Gallen, Switzerland

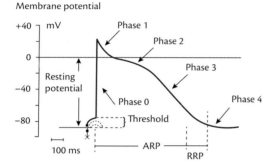

Fig. 25.2 The action potential of the myocardial cell.
ARP, absolute refractory period; RRP, reactive refractory period.
Reproduced with kind permission from Dr. Bjarne Mühldorff Sigurd.
Sandøe E and Sigurd B (1984). Arrhythmia, diagnosis and Management: A clinical electrographic guide, 1st edn. Fachmed AG, St. Gallen, Switzerland

system has been shown to be fundamentally different from that in the working myocardium (6–8). The expression of ion channels in the specialized myocytes is described in details in recent studies investigating the sinus node and the atrial musculature (6), and the conduction axis from the atrioventricular node through the His-Purkinje system (7,8). The working myocytes have the capacity for propagating impulses from one cell to the next as the action potential of the more proximal cells activate the adjoining more distal cells. Backward conduction of the impulse is hindered by the non-responsiveness of already activated cells divided up to an absolute and a relative refractory period.

Blood supply to sinus and atrioventricular nodes

The blood supply of the pulse generating nodes is important knowledge during open heart surgery performed via the right atrium and catheter-based interventional cardiology. A large study using multidector computerized tomography has confirmed earlier results from cadaver and angiographic studies (11) by visualizing that the sinoatrial nodal artery and the atrioventricular node artery originates primarily from the right coronary artery with a minority arising from the left circumflex artery.

Electrocardiograph

The sequence of electrical activation in the myocardium, initiated and coordinated by the cardiac conduction tissue, is registered in the normal electrocardiograph (ECG) (figure 25.3). The ECG is the technique used for recording the cardiac electrical activity at the skin surface and as such the graphic recording of changes in voltage related to activation and subsequent repolarization of the myocardium. The impulse formation in the sinus node is recorded as an isoelectric line in the electrocardiogram, the activation of the atrial myocardium is depicted as a small blunt wave, the P wave, and during activation of the atrioventricular node and the bundle of His, the electrocardiogram returns to an isoelectrical line, the activation of all parts of the ventricular myocardium forms the ORS complex and is followed by an isoelectric line, the ST segment, and finally the repolarization of the ventricular myocardium is recorded as a T wave, which may be followed by a U wave during late repolarization of some regions of the ventricular myocardium (figure 25.4).

A 12-lead electrocardiogram is often used as a standard. Figure 25.5 shows the orientation of the twelve leads to the various parts of the right and left ventricles. Differences in the ORS pattern are seen with right-sided and left-sided hypertrophy of the ventricles (figure 25.6). It is important to be aware of anatomic location and the electrophysiology of all the cardiac conduction tissue, as this provides not only the basis for understanding the function of the normal cardiac conduction system but also the genesis of abnormal rhythms.

Abnormalities of the cardiac conduction system

Diseases of the cardiac conduction system have been identified as alteration of impulse generation, impulse propagation, or both. Cardiac conduction system dysfunction is primarily due to acquired conditions such as myocardial ischaemia or infarction, age-related degeneration, procedural complications, and drug toxicity. Inherited forms of cardiac conduction system dysfunction are rare, with gene families being implicated in human cardiac conduction system disease of rhythm, conduction block, accessory conduction, and development being elucidated (12).

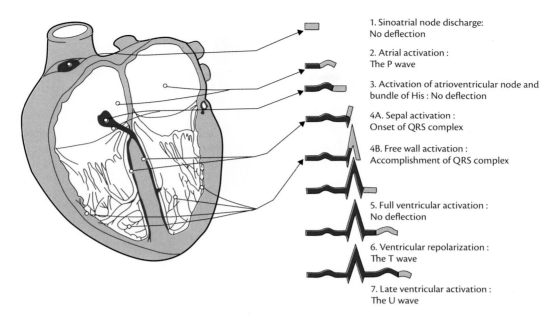

1. Sinoatrial node discharge:
No deflection

2. Atrial activation :
The P wave

3. Activation of atrioventricular node and
bundle of His : No deflection

4A. Sepal activation :
Onset of QRS complex

4B. Free wall activation :
Accomplishment of QRS complex

5. Full ventricular activation :
No deflection

6. Ventricular repolarization :
The T wave

7. Late ventricular activation :
The U wave

Fig. 25.3 Formation of the major deflections in the electrocardiograph.
Reproduced with kind permission from Dr. Bjarne Mühldorff Sigurd.
Sandøe E and Sigurd B (1984). Arrhythmia, diagnosis and Management: A clinical electrographic guide, 1st edn. Fachmed AG, St. Gallen, Switzerland

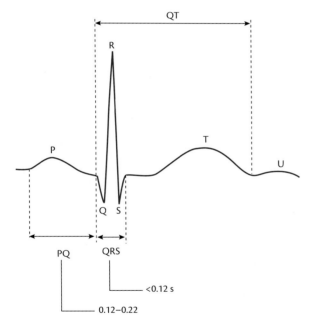

Fig. 25.4 Normal impulse conduction and length of systole.
Reproduced with kind permission from Dr. Bjarne Mühldorff Sigurd.
Sandøe E and Sigurd B (1984). Arrhythmia, diagnosis and Management: A clinical
electrographic guide, 1st edn. Fachmed AG, St. Gallen, Switzerland

Definition and diagnosis of arrhythmias

Arrhythmia is an overall term for any cardiac rhythm that deviates from normal sinus rhythm. Thus, arrhythmia is a label for abnormal impulse formation and/or conduction, not a designation of irregular heart activity. Arrhythmia is a symptom and should always be considered as such. To classify an arrhythmia, it is important to evaluate the origin of impulse formation, the type and

sequence of impulse formation and the mode of impulse conduction. Most types of arrhythmias can be diagnosed correctly on the basis of a conventional 12-lead ECG. Interestingly, the biology of arrhythmia is now largely quantifiable, which allows for systematic analysis that could transform treatment strategies that are often still empirical into management based on molecular medicine (13).

Impulse formation may be either sinus or ectopic, the rhythm regular or irregular and the rate fast, normal or low. Supraventricular arrhythmias are defined as impulse formations in the upper part of the heart above the bifurcation of the bundle of His leading to narrow QRS complexes visualized on the ECG. In ventricular arrhythmias, impulse formation arises in the bundle branches distal to the bifurcation of the bundle of His or in the Purkinje fibres, or rarely in the ordinary working myocardium of the ventricles. Thus the impulse conduction takes place without support of the normal intraventricular conduction system leading to a completely altered and prolonged activation and contraction of the ventricles with a consequently wide QRS complex recorded on the electrocardiogram. Arrhythmias due to abnormal impulse formation/generation are presented in figure 25.7.

Atrial fibrillation and atrial flutter is the most common arrhythmia following cardiac, as well as non-cardiac surgery, and is associated with increased morbidity and mortality (14,15). In general, atrial fibrillation is age-related, with a life-time risk estimated at 25% for a 40-year-old person (16).

Conduction block

Conduction block can occur at any level of the conduction system and can manifest as sinoatrial exit block, atrioventricular block, infra-Hisian block, or bundle branch block. Impaired conduction can be caused by ion channel defects that alter action potential shape or by defective coupling between myocytes, or pre-excitation of ventricular myocardium via an accessory pathway that bypasses the normal slow conduction through the atrioventricular node

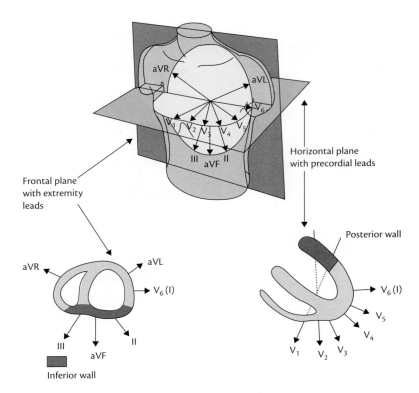

Fig. 25.5 The orientation of the 12 leads electrocardiograph to the various parts of the ventricles.
Reproduced with kind permission from Dr. Bjarne Mühldorff Sigurd.
Sandøe E and Sigurd B (1984). Arrhythmia, diagnosis and Management: A clinical electrographic guide, 1st edn. Fachmed AG, St. Gallen, Switzerland

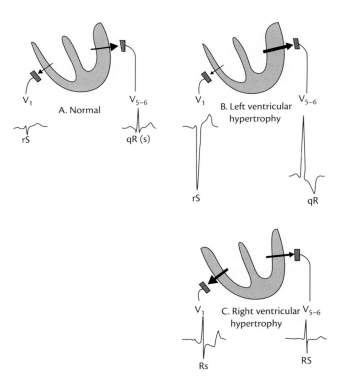

Fig. 25.6 ECG changes in left and right ventricular hypertrophy.
Reproduced with kind permission from Dr. Bjarne Mühldorff Sigurd.
Sandøe E and Sigurd B (1984). Arrhythmia, diagnosis and Management: A clinical electrographic guide, 1st edn. Fachmed AG, St. Gallen, Switzerland

(12). Sinoatrial block is an exit block located around the normal pacemaker of the heart, the sinus node. A sinoatrial block may lengthen impulse propagation from the sinus node to the surrounding atrial myocardium or completely stop impulse conduction. Atrioventricular block is a delay or failure of impulse conduction from the atria to the ventricles and is classified as blocks of first, second, and third degree. First degree atrioventricular block is characterized by a prolonged PR interval >0.23 seconds always followed by a QRS complex. Second-degree atrioventricular block is an irregular failure of pulse conduction with drop-outs of QRS complexes, and is subdivided into two types of block. Mobitz type I block (Wenckeback) is characterized with a progressive lengthening of the PR interval until drop-out of a QRS complex, while Mobitz II is defined as an occasional block of the impulse propagation with drop-out of a QRS complex, or the drop-out of two or more QRS complexes in a row. Third degree atrioventricular block, or complete atrioventricular block, is characterized by a complete cessation of impulse conduction from the atrial to the ventricular myocardium. The sinus node usually continues its normal impulse formation and the ventricular rhythm will often be of a slower rate triggered by an ectopic atrioventricular junctional or ventricular pacemaker. Blocks of the right or left bundle branches, including hemi-blocks of the leftsided branches, will also alter the ventricular synchronicity. Arrhythmias due to abnormal pulse conduction (i.e. heart blocks) are presented in figure 25.8. Failure of any of the three major parts of the cardiac conduction system, sinus node, atrioventricular node or His–Purkinje system, is potentially life threatening, and treatable only with an electronic pacemaker.

Atrioventricular impulse conduction disorders are common after aortic or mitral valve surgery, primarily leading to temporary

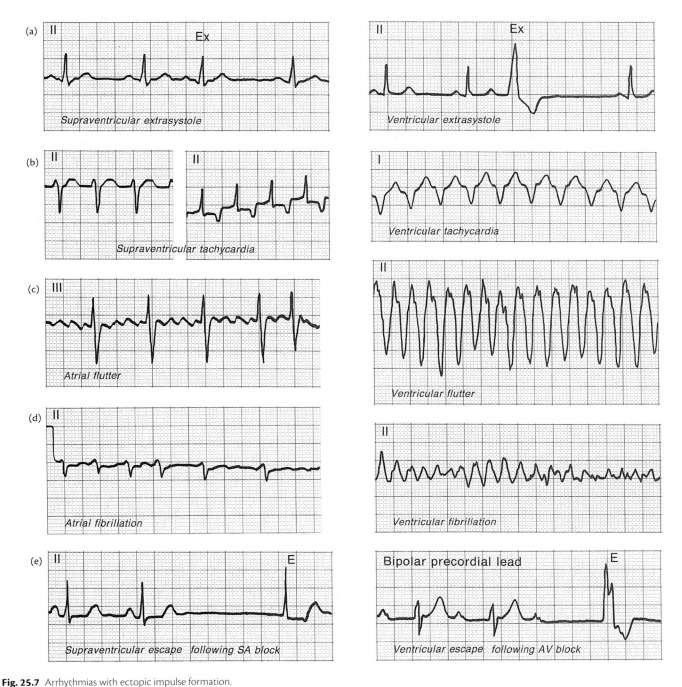

Fig. 25.7 Arrhythmias with ectopic impulse formation.

Reproduced with kind permission from Dr. Bjarne Mühldorff Sigurd.

Sandøe E and Sigurd B (1984). Arrhythmia, diagnosis and Management: A clinical electrographic guide, 1st edn. Fachmed AG, St. Gallen, Switzerland

pacing in the early postoperative period, with a minority of patients having need for a permanent pacemaker system (17,18).

Cardiac pacing

Permanent cardiac pacemakers

The first pacemakers were developed in the early 1950s and their use in the management of symptomatic bradyarrhythmias has become well established. Efforts towards a strict code system, last reviewed in 2002 (19), have lead to a uniform nomenclature of the different modalities of external pacing. Table 25.1 shows The North American Society of Pacing and Electrophysiology (NASPE) and British Pacing and Electrophysiology Group (BPEG) Generic Code (the NPG Code) for antibradycardia pacing (19).

The heart is paced artificially by delivering a very short (<1.0 ms), low voltage (<3.0 V) electrical current rhythmically to the endocardium or the myocardium of the ventricles (ventricular pacing), or the atria (atrial pacing), or to both chambers (dual chamber pacing). The stimulating electrical pacemaker impulse is generated by a pulse generator and a lithium iodine battery with a

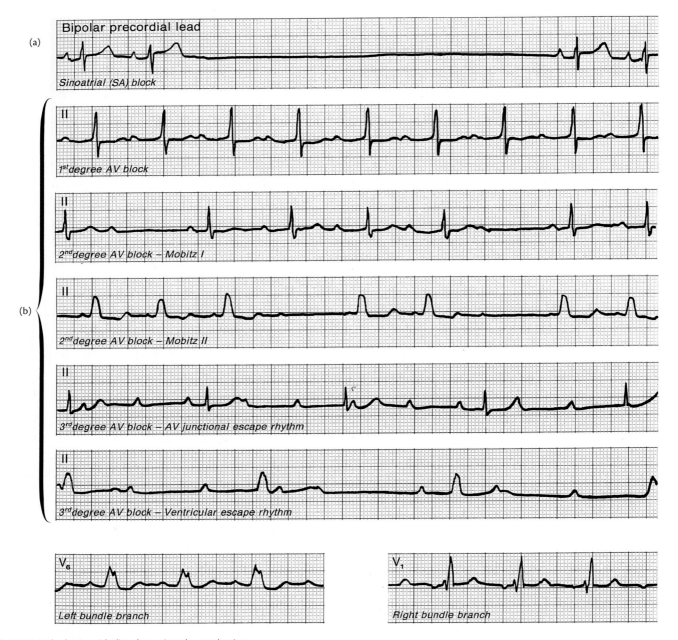

Fig. 25.8 Arrhythmias with disturbance in pulse conduction.
Reproduced with kind permission from Dr. Bjarne Mühldorff Sigurd.
Sandøe E and Sigurd B (1984). Arrhythmia, diagnosis and Management: A clinical electrographic guide, 1st edn. Fachmed AG, St. Gallen, Switzerland

battery life to well over 10 years (20). The preferable mode is dual chamber pacing, both atrial and ventricular—called the physiological pacemaker—as the physiological heart rate regulation is preserved and the atrial contribution to the ventricular diastolic filling is leading to an optimal stroke volume (21,22).

Biventricular pacing, named cardiac resynchronization therapy (CRT), aims to improve the haemodynamic function in patients with moderate to severe heart failure having a higher incidence of both interventricular and intraventricular asynchrony resulting from altered conduction throughout the His–Purkinje system; it uses additional leads to pace multiple sites within the cardiac chambers (23). CRT with pacemaker function is recommended

to reduce morbidity in patients in New York Heart Asscoiation (NYHA) III–IV class who are symptomatic despite optimal medical therapy, and who have a reduced left ventricular ejection fraction (LVEF) ≤35% and QRS prolongation (QRS width ≥120 ms) (24,25). Additionally, CRT has been shown to reduce mortality in patients undergoing coronary artery bypass surgery with pre-existing ischemic heart failure and dyssynchrony (26).

Temporary epicardial pacing

Knowledge of epicardial pacing is required for the intra- and postoperative management of patients undergoing cardiac surgery (27,28). The majority of cardiac centres prophylactically implant

Table 25.1 The NASPE/BPES codes for antibradycardia, adaptive rate, and multisite pacing

Position I	Position II	Position III	Position IV	Position V
Chamber(s) Paced	Chamber(s) Sensed	Response to Sensing	Rate Modulation	Multisite Pacing
O = None	**O** = None	**O** = None	**O** = None	O = None
A = Atrium	**A** = Atrium	**T** = Triggered	**R** = Rate modulation	A = Atrium
V = Ventricle	**V** = Ventricle	**I** = Inhibited		V = Ventricle
D = Dual (A + V)	**D** = Dual (A + V)	**D** = Dual (T + I)		D = Dual (A + V)

The NASPE/BPEG codes for antibradycardia, adaptive rate, and multisite pacing (19). All five positions are used exclusively to describe antibradycardia pacing (18). The first three positions are always required to describe the mode in which a pacemaker is functioning. Positions I, II, and III indicate the chambers in which pacing and sensing occur, and the effect of each instance of sensing on the triggering or inhibition of subsequent pacing stimuli. Position IV is used to indicate the presence (R) or absence (O) of an adaptive-rate pacing (rate modulation). Position V is used to indicate whether multisite pacing is present in (O) none of the cardiac chambers, (A) one or both of the atria, (V) one or both of the ventricles, or (D) any combination of A or V.

Reproduced from Bernstein AD et al., 'The revised NASPE/BPEG generic code for antibradycardia, adaptive-rate, and multisite pacing', *Pacing and Clinical Electrophysiology*, 25, 2, pp. 260–264, © Futura Publishing Company, Inc. 2002, with permission

at least ventricular epicardial wires in all patients during cardiac surgery to manage bradycardia and/or conduction blocks that might arise. However, many patients undergoing cardiac surgery, in particular those with reduced ventricular compliance, benefit from dual chamber pacing (atrial and ventricular). Atrial or atrial–ventricular sequential pacing is associated with a 25% increase in cardiac output with compared to ventricular pacing alone (29). The nomenclature used for epicardial pacemakers is the first three positions listed in table 25.1. The DDD mode is the most commonly used in patients with both atrial and ventricular wires, and AOO mode or AAI mode in patients with normal impulse conduction through the atrioventricular node (28). The need for epicardial pacing have to be regularly assessed during surgery and in the postoperative period, with persistent attention to the wires sensitivity, the capture thresholds, the pacemaker output to stimulate an action potential and the heart rate (27).

Automatic implantable cardioverters/defibrillators

Implantable cardioverters are devices capable of detecting ventricular tachyarrhythmias and of delivering defibrillator shocks. Automatic implantable cardioverters defibrillators (AICDs) combined with CRT have become standard of care in modern treatment of heart failure (24). These relative new devices have had a steadily increase in growth rate of implantation worldwide (30). In patients with ventricular tachyarrhythmias, AICDs clearly reduce deaths, and are prognostically superior to antiarrhythmic drug therapy (31).

AICD therapy for secondary prevention was introduced in the 1980s (32), and is today recommended for survivors of ventricular fibrillation, and for patients with documented haemodynamically unstable ventricular tachycardia and/or with syncope, a LVEF ≤40%, on optimal medical therapy, and with an expectation of survival with good functional status for >1 year (25). AICD for primary prevention is recommended to reduce mortality in patients with left ventricular dysfunction due to prior myocardial infarction or in patients with non-ischaemic cardiomyopathy having a

LVEF ≤35%, in NYHA functional class II or III, receiving optimal medical therapy, and who have a reasonable expectation of survival with good functional status for >1 year (25).

Anaesthetic requirements during non-theatre cardiac interventions

There is a broad discussion worldwide about the need for an anaesthetist to be continuously on site during cardiologic interventions. The patient population varies from young healthy patients scheduled for catheter ablation for supraventricular arrhythmias to the majority of patients receiving AICDs or RCT having multiple comorbidities, including a history of ventricular tachyarrhythmias, a LVEF ≤40%, and often, coronary artery disease, as these conditions are indicators for implantable cardiac device (ICD) placement (25).

Most of the implantable devices are inserted using infiltration of local anaesthetic by the cardiologists and often supplemented with mild to moderate sedation, while testing of an AICD typically is performed twice at the end of the procedure and requires deep sedation or general anaesthesia (33). Anaesthetists are uniquely trained to care for the complex patient population, allowing the cardiologist to focus on completing the interventional procedure successfully (33). However, in a recent published survey handling of deep sedation during electrophysiological interventions were exclusively performed by anaesthetists in only 16% of the cases (34). Moreover, intravenous sedation administrated by non-anaesthesia personnel has been shown to be safe and cost-effective (35). It is, however, important to notice that need for tracheal intubation may not be solely related to sedation but to circumstances like cardiac decompensation or procedure-related complications (36).

With the increasing number of implantable devices, the need for lead extraction is growing. Percutaneous lead extraction has become the preferred method for removal, however, the procedure involve significant risks, including cardiac tamponade, haemothorax, pulmonary embolism, lead migration, and death, even in experienced hands (37,38). Thus, the performance of these

Box 25.1 Preoperative planing for a patient with an implantable cardiac device

- ◆ Type and location of surgical procedure
- ◆ Patient position during the surgical procedure
- ◆ Type of electrosurgery (monopolar or bipolar)
- ◆ Need for other types of electromagnetic interference during the surgical procedure
- ◆ Need for cardioversion or defibrillation during the surgical procedure
- ◆ Special circumstances: cardiothoracic and chest wall surgical procedure with risk of impairment or damage of the leads, anticipated large blood loos, operation in close proximity to the pulse generator
- ◆ Availability of members from the specific cardiology team during surgery

Data from: Stone ME, Salter B, Fischer A (2011). Perioperative management of patients with cardiac implantable electronic devices. Br J Anaesth, 107(S1): i16–26; Crossley GH, Poole JE, Rozner MA, et al (2011). The heart rhythm society (HRS)/American Society of Anesthesiologists (ASA) expert consensus statement on the perioperative management of patients with implantable defibrillators, pacemakers and arrhytmia monitors: facilities and patient management: executive summary. Heart Rhythm, 8(7): 1114–54; Apfelbaum JL, Belott P, Connis RT, et al (2011), for the American Society of Anesthesiologists Committee on Standards and Practice parameters. Practice advisory for the perioperative management of patients with cardiac implantable electronic devices: pacemakers and implantable cardioverter-defibrillators. Anesthesiology 114: 247–61.

Box 25.2 Monitoring of patients with implantable cardiac electronic devices

- ◆ Cardiac rate and rhythm must be carefully monitored, and the peripheral pulse must be continuously assessed due to the risk of pulseless electrical activity
- ◆ External defibrillation equipment immediately available in the operating room. Some patients may need to have defibrillation/pacing pads placed prophylactically during surgery in the upper part of the body
- ◆ Keep a magnet immediately available
- ◆ Tight communication with the surgeon during the procedure as any changes in electrical activity or haemodynamic instability that seems to be related to electrocoagulation

Data from: Stone ME, Salter B, Fischer A (2011). Perioperative management of patients with cardiac implantable electronic devices. Br J Anaesth, 107(S1): i16–26; Crossley GH, Poole JE, Rozner MA, et al (2011). The heart rhythm society (HRS)/American Society of Anesthesiologists (ASA) expert consensus statement on the perioperative management of patients with implantable defibrillators, pacemakers and arrhytmia monitors: facilities and patient management: executive summary. Heart Rhythm, 8(7): 1114–54; Apfelbaum JL, Belott P, Connis RT, et al (2011), for the American Society of Anesthesiologists Committee on Standards and Practice parameters. Practice advisory for the perioperative management of patients with cardiac implantable electronic devices: pacemakers and implantable cardioverter-defibrillators. Anesthesiology 114(?): 247–61.

procedures should be limited to centres with the appropriate facilities, with direct availability of cardiothoracic surgery on site to provide backup in the event of complications. General anaesthesia with intraarterial pressure monitoring is recommended for complicated percutaneous lead extractions.

Collaboration and planning between cardiologists and anaesthetists is mandatory for both patient safety and procedural success during cardiological interventions. There are no established guidelines for anaesthesia consultation, but many emergencies can be avoided by preprocedure planning of patient sedation or advising that general anaesthesia should be considered, based either on patient factors or procedure complexity.

Perioperative management of patients with implantable cardiac devices

Consensus statements have provide recommendations that promotes safe management of patients with ICD throughout the perioperative period and reduce the likelihood of adverse outcomes (39–41). Anaesthetists will encounter patients with ICDs frequently. It is of great importance to have a good understanding of device function and management in the operating room setting, particularly with the advent of newer devices with more complex technology. Collaboration with cardiologists, surgeons and anaesthetists is essential to obtain an optimal preoperatively planning, which preferable should be done at least for elective procedures (box 25.1).

It is essential to determine the dependence on the ICD, pacing for bradyarrhythmias or defibrillation for tachyarrhythmias, and to determine whether preoperatively reprogramming is necessary (39–41). Exposure to significant electromagnetic interference can result in inhibition of pacing due to over sensing and/or in an inappropriate delivery of a defibrillator shock (42).

The potentially hazardous interaction can be reduced by placing the indifferent electrode of the cautery unit as far as possible or at least 8 cm from the ICD (monopolar configuration), and by using the electrocautery in brief bursts rather than continuously (39,40). Other strategies to minimize the risk are to use bipolar electrosurgery (42).

However, placement of a magnet on the ICD has become the standard approach to perioperative management. Application of a magnet to a modern pacemaker produces a reliable asynchronous fixed-rate mode of pacing (AOO, VOO, and DOO) depending on the programming configuration of the ICD and thereby protecting the patient from electromagnetic interference (39–41). Removal of the magnet results in quickly reversion to baseline device programming. A magnet placed on an AICD suspends the arrhythmia detection function and prevent discharge, and removal of the magnet promptly reactivates the AICD (39–41).

The recommendations for peroperative monitoring of with and the indications for postoperative interrogation of, implantable cardiac devices are presented in box 25.2 and box 25.3. The recommendations emphasize the need for an individualized approach in patients with an implantable cardiac devices scheduled for surgery (39–41). Multidiscplinary management of these patients scheduled

Box 25.3 Postoperative interrogation of implantable cardiac devices

◆ Appropriately monitoring with immediate availability of external pacing/defibrillation until settings are restored

◆ Resetting of the implantable cardiac electronic device before discharge from recovery or intensive care unit

◆ After cardiac and vascular surgery, inclusive use of pulmonary catheters in the setting of recently implanted leads (<6 weeks)

◆ Following significant intraoperative events including cardiac arrest

◆ Emergent surgery where the site of electromagnetic interference were above the umbilicus

Data from: Stone ME, Salter B, Fischer A (2011). Perioperative management of patients with cardiac implantable electronic devices. Br J Anaesth, 107(S1): i16–26; Crossley GH, Poole JE, Rozner MA, et al (2011). The heart rhythm society (HRS)/American Society of Anesthesiologists (ASA) expert consensus statement on the perioperative management of patients with implantable defibrillators, pacemakers and arrhytmia monitors: facilities and patient management: executive summary. Heart Rhythm, 8(7): 1114–54; Apfelbaum JL, Belott P, Connis RT, et al (2011), for the American Society of Anesthesiologists Committee on Standards and Practice parameters. Practice advisory for the perioperative management of patients with cardiac implantable electronic devices: pacemakers and implantable cardioverter-defibrillators. Anesthesiology 114: 247–61.

for surgical procedures is most preferable and should include the time period from admission to discharge. However, in emergency situation this is not always possible and it is therefore decisive that the anaesthetists are familiar with the current recommendations.

Conclusion

Many patients presenting for heart surgery have abnormalities of their cardiac conduction system and some will have implantable electronic cardiac devices. Many more patients will develop abnormalities all be they short lived, of their conduction system during heart surgery that because of the severe haemodynamic adverse effects, require the use of pacemakers. A sound knowledge of the physiology and and electropathophysiology of the heart's conduction system enables cardiothoracic anaesthesiologists to safely manage these patients before, during and after surgery.

References

1. Tawara S. The conduction system of the mammalian heart, in Suma K, Shimada M (eds) An anatomico-histological study of the atrioventricular bundle and the Purkinje fibers. Imperial College Press, London, 2000; 8–160

2. Keith A, Flack M. The form and nature of the muscular connections between the primary divisions of the vertebrate heart. *J Anat Physiol* 1907; **41**(Pt 3): 172–89

3. Aschoff L. Referat über die hertzstorungen in ihren beziehungen zu den spezifischen muskelsystem des hersens. *Verh Dstch Pathol Ges* 1910; **14**: 3–35

4. Möckenberg JG. Beitrage zur normalen und pathologischen anatomie des herzens. *Verh Dtsch Pathol Ges* 1910; **14**: 64–71

5. Moorman AF, Christoffels VM, Anderson RH. Anatomic substrates for cardiac conduction. *Heart Rhythm* 2005; **2**(8): 875–86

6. Chandler NJ, Greener ID, Tellez JO, et al. Molecular architecture of the human sinus node. Insight into the function of the cardiac pacemaker. *Circulation* 2009; **119**(12): 1562–75

7. Greener ID, Monfredi O, Inada S, et al. Molecular architecture of the human specialised atrioventricular axis. *J Mol Cell Cardiol* 2011; **50**(4): 642–51

8. Atkinson A, Inada S, Li J, et al. Anatomical and molecular mapping of the left and right ventricular His-Purkinje conduction networks. *J Mol Cell Cardiol* 2011; **51**(5): 689–701

9. Anderson KR, Ho SY, Anderson RH. Location and vascular supply of sinus node in human heart. *Br Heart J* 1979: **41**(1): 28–32

10. Spach MS, Kootsey JM. The nature of electrical propagation in cardiac muscle. *Am J Physiol* 1983; **224**(1): H3–22

11. Cezlan T, Senturk S, Karcaaltincaba M, Bilici A. Multidetector CT imaging of arterial supply to sinuatrial and atrioventricular nodes. *Surg Radiol Anat* 2012; **34**(4): 357–65

12. Park DS, Fishman GI. The cardiac conduction system. *Circulation* 2011; **123**(8): 904–15

13. Grace AA, Roden DM. Cardiac arrhythmia 1 System biology and cardiac arrthytmias. *Lancet* 2012; **380**(9852): 1498–508

14. Saxena A, Dinh DT, Smith JA, Shardey GC, Reid CM, Newcomb AE. Usefulness of postoperative fibrillation as an independent predictor for worse early and late outcomes after isolated coronary artery bypass grafting (multicenter Australian study of 19,497 patients). *Am J Cardiol* 2012; **109**(2): 219–25

15. Bhave PD, Goldman LE, Vittinghoff E, Maselli J, Auerbach A. Incidence, predictors, and outcomes associated with postoperative atrial fibrillation after major noncardiac surgery. *Am Heart J* 2012; **164**(6): 918–24

16. Magnani JW, Rienstra M, Lin H, et al. Atrial fibrillation: current knowledge and future directions in epidemiology and genomics. *Circulation* 2011; **124**(18): 1982–93

17. Dawkins S, Hobson AR, Kalra PR, Tang AT, Monro JL, Dawkins KD. Permanent pacemaker implantation after isolated aortic valve replacement: incidence, indications, and predictors. *Ann Thorac Surg* 2008; **85**(1): 108–12

18. Berdajs D, Schurr UP, Wagner A, Seifert B, Turina MI, Genoni M. Incidence and pathophysiology of atrioventricular block following mitral valve replacement and ring annuloplasty. *Eur J Cardiothorac Surg* 2008; **34**(1): 55–61

19. Bernstein AD, Daubert JC, Fletcher RD, et al. The revised NASPE/BPEG generic code for antibradycardia, adaptive-rate, and multisite pacing. North American Society of Pacing and Electrophysiology/British Pacing and Electrophysiology Group. *Pacing Clin Electrophysiol* 2002; **25**(2): 260–4

20. Allen M. Pacemakers and implantable cardioverter defibrillators. *Anaesthesia* 2006; **61**(9): 883–90

21. Lamas GA, Lee KL, Sweeny MO, et al. Ventricular pacing or dual-chamber pacing for sinus-node dysfunction. *N Engl J Med* 2002; **346**(24): 1854–62

22. Kerr CR, Connolly SJ, Abdollah H, et al. Canadian trial of physiological pacing: effects of physiological pacing during long-term follow-up. *Circulation* 2004; **109**(3): 357–62

23. Holzmeister J, Leclercq C. Implantable cardioverter defibrillators and cardiac resynchronisation therapy. *Lancet* 2011; **378**(9792): 722–30

24. Rivero-Ayerza M, Theuns DA, Garcia-Garcia HM, Boersma E, Simoons M, Jordaens LJ. Effects of cardiac resynchronization therapy on overall mortality and mode of death: a meta-analysis of randomized clinical trials. *Eur Heart J* 2006; **27**(22): 2682–8

25. McMurray JJ, Adamopoulus S, Anker SD, et al. ESC guidelines for the diagnosis and treatment of acute and chronic heart failure 2012: the task force for the diagnosis and treatment of acute and chronic heart failure 2012 of the European Society of Cardiology. Developed in collaboration with the Heart Failure Association (HFA) of the ESC and endorsed by the European Society of Intensive Care Medicine. *Eur J Heart Fail* 2012; **14**(8): 803–69

26. Pokushalov E, Romanov A, Porhorova D, et al. Coronary artery bypass grafting with concomitant cardiac recynchronisation therapy in patients with ischaemic heart failure and left ventricular dyssynchrony. *Eur J Cardiothorac Surg* 2010; **38**(6): 773–80

27. Reade MC. Temporary epicardial pacing after cardiac surgery: a practical review: part 1: general considerations in the management of epicardial pacing. *Anaesthesia* 2007; **62**(3): 264–71

28. Reade MC. Temporary epicardial pacing after cardiac surgery: a practical review: part 2: selection of epicardial pacing modes and troubleshooting. *Anaesthesia* 2007; **62**(4): 364–73

29. Curtis J, Maloney JD, Barnhorst DA, Pluth JR, Hartzler GO, Wallace RB. A critical look at temporary ventricular pacing following cardiac surgery. *Surgery* 1977; **82**(6): 888–93

30. Camm AJ, Nisam S. European utilization of the implantable defibrillator: has 10 years changed the 'enigma'? *Europace* 2010; **12**(1): 1063–9

31. Buxton AE, Lee KL, Fisher JD, et al. A randomized study of the prevention of sudden death in patients with coronary artery disease. Multicenter Unsustained Tachycardia Trial Investigators. *N Engl J Med* 1999; **341**(25): 1882–90

32. Mirowski M, Reid PR, Mower MM, et al. Termination of malignant ventricular arrhythmias with an implanted automatic defibrillator in human beings. *N Engl J Med* 1980; **303**(6): 322–4

33. Shook DC, Savage RM. Anesthesia in the cardiac catheterization laboratory and electrophysiology laboratory. *Anesthesiol Clin* 2009; **27**(1): 47–56

34. Gaitan BD, Trentman TL, Fassett SL, Mueller JT, Altemose GT. Sedation and analgesia in the cardiac electrophysiology laboratory: a national survey of electrophysiologists investigation the who, how and why? *J Cardiothorac Vasc Anesth* 2011; **25**(4): 647–59

35. Kezerashvili A, Fisher JD, DeLaney J, et al. Intravenous sedation for cardiac procedures can be administrated safely and cost-effectively by non-anesthesia personnel. *J Interv Card Electrophysiol* 2008; **21**(1): 43–51

36. Letter to the editor. Should an anesthesiologist be present on site during cardiologic interventions. *J Cardiothorac Vasc Anesth* 2011; **25**(6): e51–7

37. Jones SO 4th, Eckart RE, Albert CM, Epstein LM. Large, single-center, single-operator experience with transvenous lead extraction: outcomes and changing indications. *Heart Rhythm* 2008; **5**(4): 520–5

38. Smith MC, Love CJ. Extraction of transvenous pacing and ICD leads. *Pacing Clin Electrophysiol* 2008; **31**(6): 736–52

39. Stone ME, Salter B, Fischer A. Perioperative management of patients with cardiac implantable electronic devices. *Br J Anaesth* 2011; **107**(S1): i16–26

40. Crossley GH, Poole JE, Rozner MA, et al. The heart rhythm society (HRS)/American Society of Anesthesiologists (ASA) expert consensus statement on the perioperative management of patients with implantable defibrillators, pacemakers and arrhytmia monitors: facilities and patient management: executive summary. *Heart Rhythm* 2011; **8**(7): 1114–54

41. Apfelbaum JL, Belott P, Connis RT, et al. for the American Society of Anesthesiologists Committee on Standards and Practice parameters. Practice advisory for the perioperative management of patients with cardiac implantable electronic devices: pacemakers and implantable cardioverter-defibrillators. *Anesthesiology* 2011; **114**: 247–61

42. Misiri J, Kusumoto F, Goldschlager N. Electromagnetic interference and implanted cardiac devices: the medical environment (Part II). *Clin Cardiol* 2011; **35**(6): 321–8

CHAPTER 26

Critical care following cardiac surgery

Lisen Hockings, Deirdre Murphy, and Carlos Scheinkestel

Introduction

Initial recovery of the cardiothoracic patient takes place in the Intensive Care Unit (ICU). ICUs are complex environments in which care is provided by a multidisciplinary team led by an ICU specialist. The team members include ICU medical and nursing staff, pharmacists, nutritionists, physiotherapists, ward support staff, reception staff, social work, occupational therapy staff, and equipment support staff. ICU staffing varies between countries. It is common in many units for ventilated patients to require 1:1 patient: nurse ratio and patients who do not require invasive support (ventilator, haemofilter, high dose inotropes etc.) to require a 1:2 nurse: patient ratio. Minimal standards for ICUs are published by relevant governing bodies, such as the College of Intensive Care Medicine in Australia (1), and these cover many aspects of the ICU structure, staffing, monitoring requirements, equipment and physical environment.

Routine care of patients after cardiac surgery

Advances in percutaneous coronary intervention and medical management of chronic cardiovascular and other diseases coupled with the aging population have resulted in older and more medically complex patients presenting for cardiac surgery. Consequently, the duration of ICU stay has increased by 10% in the last 4 years (2).

Handover

The ICU management of the cardiac surgical patient commences with handover from the anaesthetic-surgical team. During this period of time the patient's tracheal tube, ventilator and ventilator tubing, multiple infusions and pumps, monitoring lines, transducers and displays, temporary epicardial pacing, pleural/mediastinal drains, and urinary catheter (amongst other potential devices such as an intra-aortic balloon pump) have to be safely transported from the operating room to the ICU. In addition, vital information about events over the previous several hours in the operating room needs to be communicated without error or omission of important details. This is a vulnerable period for the patient. An ideal handover will be succinct and structured, ensuring continuity of care during and after the exchange of information. Human factors' research in recent years has recognized the importance of good handover to ensure adequate ongoing patient care (3). A standard approach to handover can be very useful to prevent loss of critical information. One interesting approach described utilizing expertise from areas outside of medicine—Formula 1 pit stop teams and aviation medicine—to streamline this process. The authors described an impressive reduction in errors and a shortening of the time required for handover when they focused on each stage of the handover and adopted a structured approach with clear leadership, well-defined task sequence and task allocation, discipline, composure of the team, and no interruptions during the handover of information (4) (figure 26.1).

An initial history must cover the patients major past medical, surgical and anaesthetic history. Specific issues to be covered are listed in table 26.1. The initial clinical assessment of the post-cardiac surgical patient focuses on the haemodynamics and current infusions of inotropic, vasopressor, and vasodilator agents; other infusions, respiratory function and ventilator settings; mediastinal/pleural and urinary catheter drainage and a focused clinical examination. Suggested early priorities are listed in table 26.2.

Standardizing management

Routine postoperative care of the cardiac surgical patient is an area of intensive care medicine in which use of evidence-based protocols and checklists to guide management have been shown be very successful. Many units utilize some form of clinical pathway to achieve this. A clinical pathway is a means by which evidence-based guidelines and protocols can be adapted to link evidence to management of patients in a local environment (5). A well-considered clinical pathway can improve cost-effectiveness as well as leading to improvements in clinical outcomes.

As the intensive care unit environment becomes increasingly complex it can be difficult for clinicians to consistently remember the multitude of routine tasks necessary for excellent care of each patient. Checklists, or care bundles, can be used to ensure that routine measures that are known to improve outcomes in intensive care patients are applied to all. One of the first descriptions of the power of utilizing daily checklists for setting routine

Phase 0: prehandover	The Patient Transfer Form is completed by the anaesthetist and collected operating room at least 30 min before the patient is transferred to the ICU.
	The receiving nurse ensures the bed space is set up according to the monitoring, ventilation and other requirements specified on the Patient Transfer Form.
	The receiving doctor ensures that all appropriate paperwork as ready.
Phase 1: equipment and technology handover	On arrival the team transfers the patient ventilation, monitoring and support from portable system used during the transfer to the ICU systems.

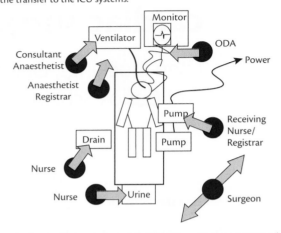

Phase 2: information handover	Safety check: the anaesthetist checks the equipment and that the patient is appropriately ventilated and monitored and is stable. The receiving nurse and doctor are identified and confirm their readiness.
	The anaesthetist, then the surgeon, speck alone and uninterrupted, providing the relevant information about the case, using the *Information Transfer Aid Memoir*.
	Safety check: the receiving nurse and doctor should use the *Information Transfer Aid Memoir yo check* that all necessary information has been obtained, and ask appropriate questions.
Phase 3: discussion and plan	The surgeon, anaesthetist and receiving team discuss the case as a group. The receiving physician manages the discussions, identifies anticipated problems, and anticipated recovery is discussed.
	The ICU team now has responsibility for patient care, and confirms the plans for the patient.

Fig. 26.1 Handover of care in the intensive care unit after heart surgery.

ODA, operating department assistant.

Reproduced from Catchpole KR, et al., 'Patient handover from surgery to intensive care: using Formula 1 pit-stop and aviation models to improve safety and quality', Paediatric Anaesthesia, 17, 5, pp. 470–478, © 2007 Wiley, with permission

ICU goals of care was Pronovost's landmark 2003 paper, which described the implementation of a checklist with a 50% reduction in ICU duration of stay 6).

An example of a checklist is provided in table 26.3. The headings are deliberately broad and non-specific. They are designed to prompt the memory to ensure completeness in dealing with all aspects of daily patient care in the ICU.

Ventilation and respiratory management

The use of modern anaesthesia techniques means that the majority of cardiac surgical patients can safely have tracheal extubation in the hours following the procedure. The median duration of mechanical ventilation following cardiac surgery with fast track anaesthesia is 6 hours (IQR 3–16) (7). However, given the patients are older and more complex, the duration of mechanical ventilation that is required, is usually longer. Having guidelines for postoperative respiratory weaning from mechanical ventilation helps avoid unnecessary delays in tracheal extubation (8).

A small proportion of patients will need prolonged mechanical ventilation. In one recent study 6% of patients required ventilation beyond 72 hours. These patients had a 30-day mortality risk of 33% (9). Factors associated with requirement for prolonged mechanical ventilation include combined valve and CABG surgery, aortic surgery, female sex, age more than 70 years, ejection fraction less than 30%, hypertension, peripheral vascular disease, chronic obstructive pulmonary disease (COPD), and diabetes mellitus (8).

Analgesia

Acute pain following cardiac surgery is common and multifactorial in origin. Nociceptive inputs may arise from the tissue trauma caused by sternotomy, from sternal retraction, from chest drains or other irritation of the parietal pleura or pericardium. Pain is typically worst on the first postoperative day at the site of sternotomy, and is amplified by coughing or movement. However, significant pain can continue for up to a week after surgery (10). Adequate analgesia helps to achieve excellent clinical outcomes and reduce complications associated with poor pain control such as respiratory failure, cardiac ischaemia, arrhythmias, and increased wound infection rates. It is important to exclude occult or recurrent ischaemia as a cause of pain as may occur due to graft failure, inadequate flow in an ungrafted coronary vessel, or to complications from heart valve surgery with inadvertent coronary artery occlusion (e.g. from suture material). Analgesic regimens include both non-opioid and opioid-based agents, and occasionally regional anaesthetic techniques. For a detailed discussion please refer to Chapter 38.

Table 26.1 Key issues to be discussed at handover

Surgical:

♦ Nature of surgery—elective, urgent or emergent

♦ Revascularization strategy employed +/− valvular interventions if appropriate

♦ Any intraoperative surgical complications and how they were overcome

♦ Location of mediastinal/pleural drains and epicardial pacing wires

♦ Any major surgical concerns

Anaesthesia:

♦ Airway management issues, adjuncts used and any complications encountered

♦ Ventilator settings

♦ Allergies

♦ Haemodynamic stability intraoperatively and post-bypass and trends over time

♦ Echocardiography: Baseline ventricular and valvular performance, intraoperative findings and any postprocedural changes

♦ Transfusions and other medications administered

♦ Coagulation status perioperatively (including post-protamine ACT and drain outputs since insertion)

♦ Current infusions

Past medical and drug history

♦ Major cardiovascular risk factors and any previous interventions

♦ Chronic health conditions that may influence perioperative care

♦ Other chronic health conditions

♦ Current medications

Social history

♦ Baseline functional status and next of kin

Sedation

Short-acting sedative agents such as propofol are used in the immediate postoperative phase. Once cardiorespiratory status has been stabilized, normothermia achieved, and neuromuscular blockade has worn off, these agents are weaned for assessment of neurological function and with a view to tracheal extubation. In unstable patients where prolonged mechanical ventilation may be required, a switch to a longer-duration agent such as midazolam may be required. Daily interruptions of sedation and a trend towards lower sedation targets have been associated with reduced durations of ICU and hospital stay (11–13), but this rarely applies to the cardiac population, in whom the majority have tracheal extubation promptly and within 24 hours. The use of alternative sedative agents such as dexmedetomidine, particularly to reduce the incidence and duration of delirium (14–16) may be appropriate when mechanical ventilation becomes prolonged.

Fluid management

Postoperative fluid management aims to maintain euvolaemia, to avoid over-distension of the right heart, and to maintain adequate intravascular volume to ensure optimal end organ function. Fluid

overload can lead to respiratory failure, tissue and interstitial oedema, and poor wound healing. The paradigm of fluid management has recently been challenged with some landmark publications outside of cardiac surgery (17,18). Our understanding of the effects and distribution of colloid and crystalloid fluid resuscitation is similarly being challenged (19). A better understanding of cardiorespiratory interactions has led to an interest in the monitoring of dynamic rather than static parameters to assess volume responsiveness; for example pulse pressure and stroke volume variability.

Temperature management

Postoperative hyperthermia is associated with worsened cognitive dysfunction at six weeks following surgery and needs to be avoided (19). Conversely, ongoing hypothermia may contribute to bleeding and coagulopathy and may also lead to problems with temporary epicardial pacing. Following cardiopulmonary bypass (CPB), there is an after-drop in temperature. A large database review has demonstrated that up to 66% of patients have transient hypothermia in the first 24 hours following cardiac surgery. Persistent postoperative hypothermia that is not corrected in the first 24 hours is rare (0.3%) but when present is associated with a marked increase in mortality (OR 6.3, 95% CI: 3.3–12.0) (21).

Metabolic management

Metabolic derangements are common following CPB. They may reflect preoperative medications or underlying medical conditions such as chronic renal impairment; occur as a result of the blood and extracorporeal surface interaction; drugs or blood product administration intraoperatively; post-CPB diuresis (cold diuresis, mannitol/other diuretic therapy on CPB); or may reflect a new complication (e.g. acute kidney injury (AKI)). The metabolic response to cardiac surgery and CPB includes hyperglycaemia, hyperlactataemia, and hypokalaemia, with an increase in pro-inflammatory cytokine production. Dysnatraemia (both hyper- and hypo-), hypomagnesaemia, hyperkalaemia, and hypophosphataemia may also be seen. Hypocalcaemia is common in patients who have received massive transfusion and in particular large volumes of fresh frozen plasma (FFP). Treating low ionized blood calcium levels may help in treatment of coagulopathy as well as improving myocardial performance. Maintaining normal electrolyte balance is helpful in preventing postoperative arrhythmias and at least daily electrolyte monitoring is recommended whilst patients remain in the ICU.

Glucose control

The ideal target for blood glucose has been extensively investigated in the last two decades. Previously, hyperglycaemia was seen as a 'normal' response to surgical stress or critical illness. Early, small trials and retrospective reviews suggested that intensive insulin therapy to control hyperglycaemia was associated with a reduced mortality. More recently, larger, single and multi-centre (including multinational) randomized controlled trials have demonstrated that targeting a 'tight' blood glucose control level (4.5–6 mmol/L (81–108 mg/dL) as opposed to interventions to keep blood glucose less than 10mmol/L) is associated with an increase in mortality mostly due to cardiovascular events (22–24). Given the high percentage of cardiac patients who are diabetic, the need to control glucose postoperatively is now common and treatment should be titrated to achieve a blood sugar less than 10 mmol/L (180 mg/dL).

Table 26.2 Initial priorities following handover

	AIM	TASKS
VENTILATION	Ensure initial settings adequate	Check PIP waveforms, patient ventilator synchrony
		Check ETT size and position at teeth
MONITOR	Display all relevant information	Zero all pressures to phlebostatic axis
		Ensure correct channel display
		Set up cardiac output monitoring for PAC if required
		Check pressure waveforms for fidelity of pressure traces (damping) and evidence of volume depletion
CLINICAL EXAMINATION	Rapid assessment of:	Pupils
	hemodynamic stability	GCS
	respiratory function	Temperature
	blood loss	Peripheral perfusion (capillary refill, any mottling?)
	level of sedation	Neck veins
	exclude major neurological complications	Breath sounds
		Heart sounds (often difficult)
		Mediastinal/pleural drain outputs
		Urine output
INFUSIONS	Infusions commenced in OR connected and running at an appropriate rate	Check all infusion pumps
		Ensure adequate volume remaining and make up any infusions due to run out shortly
INVESTIGATIONS	Establish baseline post-operative laboratory values and confirm line/tube positions	Initial blood gas
		Formal bloods: FBP, UEC, coagulation profile
		CXR
FLUIDS AND ELECTROLYTES	Euvolaemia	Chart any bolus fluids and type
DRUGS	Haemodynamic stability	Chart antiemetic and analgesia regimen
	Analgesia	Consider stress ulcer prophylaxis
	Secondary prophylaxis	electrolyte replacement to avoid any gross abnormalities that may predispose to arrhythmia (aim $Mg^{2+} \geq 1.0$; $K^+ \geq 4.5$)
	Ensure important medications restarted at an appropriate time	
PACING	Safe temporary epicardial pacing mode	Avoid VOO
		Perform pacing check when temperature above 35°C
GLUCOSE	Normoglycaemia	Commence insulin/glucose infusion in accordance with unit protocols if required
DOCUMENTATION	Facilitate communication	Clear, accurate, concise medical records and instructions

ETT, endotracheal tube; FBP, full blood profile; GCS, Glasgow Coma Score; PIP, peak inspired pressure; UEC, urea electrolytes, creatinine.

Feeding

Most routine cardiac surgical patients can safely have tracheal extubation within hours of their surgery. In the event that perioperative issues necessitate prolonged mechanical ventilation, enteral feeding should be commenced. Enteral nutrition is generally well tolerated in this patient group and is preferred over parenteral nutrition. Prokinetic agents can be utilized to promote gastric emptying. Recent, unintended weight loss, or poor food intake prior to surgery, is a marker for worse outcome after surgery.

Pacing

For a detailed description of temporary epicardial pacing see Chapter 25.

A pacing check algorithm is provided in figure 26.2.

Chest drains

Mediastinal, pericardial and pleural drains are frequently inserted to minimize the effects of occult bleeding into confined spaces postoperatively. Many different modes of manipulating chest drains to prevent blockage have been advocated—milking, rolling, fanfolding, and tapping. It is unknown if intervention is required, nor if one technique is superior. Some of these techniques may have potentially adverse side effects such as increased patient discomfort (25). Drains can usually be removed when output is consistently less than 20 ml/h. Routine chest X-ray (CXR) following removal of these drains is probably unwarranted. Clinically significant pneumothorax is uncommon and when present is likely to cause symptoms leading to radiological investigation.

Table 26.3 A proposed checklist

√	*Please review each item daily*	
	Sedation/analgesia/sleep	ICU
	Falls/injury risk? restraints	Chart
	Ventilator weaning	Review
	Glucose 4–10 mmol/L?	
	Feeding/bowels	
	Fluid balance	
	Lines? correct setup? remove	Daily
	Head up 30 degrees	Examination
	Pressure area problems?	
	X-ray review: ETT, Lines, NG tube	Radiology
	Antibiotics/Micro r/v/Stop date	Drug
	Prophylaxis/DVT/peptic ulcer	Chart
	Daily goals completed on blue chart	Planning
	Treatment limitations required?	
	Can patient sit out of bed?	
	Discharge planning required?	
	Family/parent unit contact required?	

Practicalities

In our institution, routine, uncomplicated cardiac patients are 'warmed, weaned, woken, and extubated'. Formal bloods are sent on admission to the ICU and daily thereafter. Potassium levels are checked more frequently using arterial blood gas analysis. A CXR is performed on admission and on the first postoperative day. Subsequent imaging is dictated by clinical condition and is not routine. Thromboprophylaxis is with intermittent pneumatic compression devices and chemical thromboprophylaxis with subcutaneous enoxaparin, which is usually commenced on the first postoperative day. Pulmonary artery catheters are removed when patients have been haemodynamically stable on minimal inotropic/vasopressor supports for more than six hours. Central venous and arterial lines are removed as soon as possible to minimize the risk of catheter-related bloodstream infection. When there has been no requirement for temporary epicardial pacing for 24 hours in a back-up mode, the pacing wires are isolated. Prophylactic enoxaparin is withheld the following morning and they are removed before 1400 h and after the coagulation profile is confirmed to be normal. Indwelling urinary catheters are usually removed on the second postoperative day.

Secondary prophylaxis after coronary revascularization

Intensive care management of the post-cardiac surgical patient encompasses the acute physiological support of the perioperative patient, and also the beginning of the process of recovery, rehabilitation, and secondary prevention of atherosclerosis. In cases of urgent or emergent cardiac surgery the hospital admission may represent the first opportunity for cardiac risk factor intervention. In elective cases it allows for inpatient optimisation of comorbid conditions.

Patients who have undergone coronary revascularization remain at risk from progressive coronary artery disease (CAD)—in both their native coronary vessels and within the bypass grafts. Conduit selection and other surgical factors play an important role in minimizing both early and late graft occlusion (26–28). Cardiac risk factor modification and appropriate medical therapy are an integral part of secondary prevention of atherosclerosis and have been shown to improve outcomes when commenced in the early postoperative period (29–31).

Antiplatelet therapy

Antiplatelet agents should be commenced as soon as possible after CABG surgery to improve both short- and long-term outcomes (30,32–35). Current international guidelines make a Class I/Level A recommendation to commence aspirin 100 mg within six hours of surgery. This treatment should continue indefinitely (35–37). The decision to start aspirin in the early post-CABG period in an individual patient should be based around a clinical assessment of bleeding risk. Outcome benefits have been demonstrated when aspirin is commenced up to 48 hours postoperatively (30). In patients who are intolerant or allergic to aspirin, clopidogrel has been recommended in the face of very limited specific postoperative data (35,37).

The competing risk of bleeding and the protective antithrombotic effects of antiplatelet therapy in the perioperative period are likely to become more challenging if large prospective trials of hybrid revascularization (percutaneous coronary intervention combined with CABG) techniques prove the technique to be beneficial (40). Large-scale trials continue to examine the role of maintaining aspirin therapy throughout the perioperative period (39,40).

Lipid-lowering agents

Treatment of hyperlipidaemia to achieve levels of low-density lipoprotein (LDL) cholesterol less than 2.5 mmol/dL (100 mg/dL) is associated with improved long-term outcomes in patients with CAD (41). Statin therapy has been shown to reduce long-term complications in the post-CABG cohort and is recommended in all patients unless a specific contraindication exists (31,34,35,42–45). Moreover, withdrawal of statin therapy in previously treated patients is associated with increased in-hospital mortality after CABG (46). Statin therapy should be reintroduced when patients resume enteral intake postoperatively, in the absence of specific contraindications such as acute liver dysfunction and myositis. High-dose statin therapy should be instituted in patients who were not on preoperative lipid-lowering treatment and do not have a contraindication. If statins are initiated postoperatively then careful monitoring for potential side effects including reversible memory loss, is required (47). Alternative lipid-lowering agents may be considered if statins are contraindicated or not tolerated.

Beta-blockers

Preoperative beta-adrenergic blockade is now recommended in all patients without contraindication, to reduce the incidence of post-CABG atrial fibrillation (AF). The role of routine

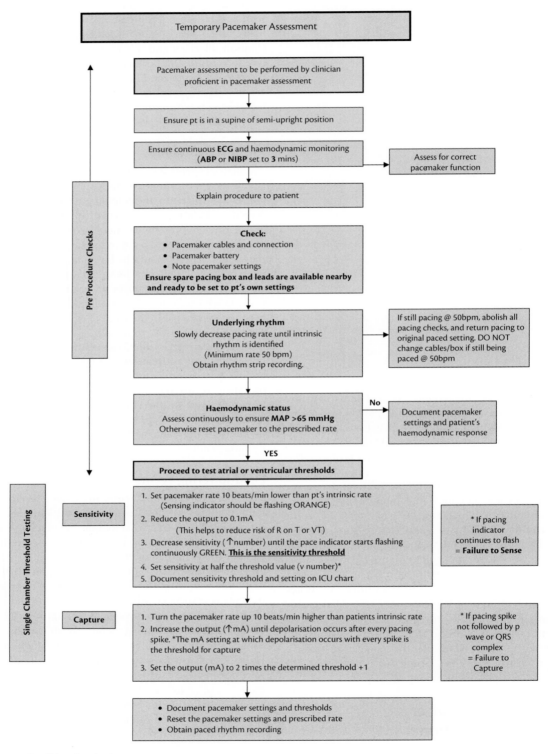

Temporary Pacemaker Assessment

Pacemaker assessment to be performed by clinician proficient in pacemaker assessment

Ensure pt is in a supine of semi-upright position

Ensure continuous **ECG** and haemodynamic monitoring (**ABP** or **NIBP** set to **3** mins)

Assess for correct pacemaker function

Explain procedure to patient

Check:
- Pacemaker cables and connection
- Pacemaker battery
- Note pacemaker settings

Ensure spare pacing box and leads are available nearby and ready to be set to pt's own settings

Underlying rhythm
Slowly decrease pacing rate until intrinsic rhythm is identified
(Minimum rate 50 bpm)
Obtain rhythm strip recording.

If still pacing @ 50bpm, abolish all pacing checks, and return pacing to original paced setting. DO NOT change cables/box if still being paced @ 50bpm

Haemodynamic status
Assess continuously to ensure **MAP >65 mmHg**
Otherwise reset pacemaker to the prescribed rate

No → Document pacemaker settings and patient's haemodynamic response

YES

Proceed to test atrial or ventricular thresholds

Pre Procedure Checks

Single Chamber Threshold Testing

Sensitivity

1. Set pacemaker rate 10 beats/min lower than pt's intrinsic rate
   (Sensing indicator should be flashing ORANGE)
2. Reduce the output to 0.1mA
   (This helps to reduce risk of R on T or VT)
3. Decrease sensitivity (↑number) until the pace indicator starts flashing continuously GREEN. **This is the sensitivity threshold**
4. Set sensitivity at half the threshold value (v number)*
5. Document sensitivity threshold and setting on ICU chart

* If pacing indicator continues to flash
= **Failure to Sense**

Capture

1. Turn the pacemaker rate up 10 beats/min higher than patients intrinsic rate
2. Increase the output (↑mA) until depolarisation occurs after every pacing spike. *The mA setting at which depolarisation occurs with every spike is the threshold for capture
3. Set the output (mA) to 2 times the determined threshold +1

* If pacing spike not followed by p wave or QRS complex
= Failure to Capture

- Document pacemaker settings and thresholds
- Reset the pacemaker settings and prescribed rate
- Obtain paced rhythm recording

Fig. 26.2 Temporary epicardial pacing check.

beta-adrenergic blockade in the acute postoperative period is less certain where acute physiological disturbances including bradycardia and reduced myocardial contractility frequently render a patient dependent upon inotropes and pacing. Beta-blockers should be reinstituted on an individual patient basis in the ICU or as soon as practicable in the postoperative period. Beta-adrenergic blockade is recommended on discharge from hospital for all patients after CABG (35).

Angiotensin-converting enzyme inhibitors and angiotensin ii receptor blockers

Angiotensin-converting enzyme inhibitors (ACEI) and angiotensin II receptor blockers (ARB) should be considered in all patients without contraindication following CABG (35). The timing of their postoperative introduction must be balanced around perioperative haemodynamic stability and the known risks of AKI following CABG. Non-steroidal anti-inflammatories are not recommended in patients on ACEI/ARB.

Common complications after cardiac surgery

A systematic approach is required to the unstable patient after cardiac surgery. A suggested approach is presented in table 26.4.

Haemodynamic instability

Haemodynamic instability after cardiac surgery is common and may be multifactorial. A reasonable approach may include an

Table 26.4 A suggested approach to the unstable post-cardiac surgical patient

History
Confirm pre- and perioperative history

Look and listen

Monitor
◆ Heart rate and rhythm
◆ Blood pressure and CVP—values and waveform
◆ PA pressures (if PAC *in situ*)
◆ ETCO$_2$ trace—absolute value, slope and trend (confirms ETT position and presence of cardiac output)
◆ SpO$_2$ trace O$_2$—saturation and peripheral perfusion
◆ Temperature
◆ If monitored parameters and pulse check confirm the absence of cardiac output proceed to ACLS algorithm

Inspection/examination

Airway
◆ Ensure ETT appropriately positioned, secured and patent (pass suction catheter)
◆ Exclude cuff leak (listen)

Breathing
◆ Ensure that the ventilator is set appropriately
◆ Look at peak pressure (VCV—exclude pressure limiting as a cause of hypoventilation) or volumes being delivered (PCV and CPAP/pulmonary stenosis modes)
◆ Ventilator waveforms—exclude airway obstruction/dynamic hyperinflation/dys-synchrony.
◆ Palpate the trachea and ensure it is midline
◆ Examine the chest for obvious unilateral expansion, subcutaneous emphysema, or signs of PTx/HTx

Circulation
◆ Correlate monitored parameters with clinical examination:
◆ Look at degree of neck vein distension and the adequacy of peripheral perfusion
◆ If a PAC is *in situ* perform thermodilution assessment of cardiac output and/or measure mixed venous saturation

Mediastinal/pleural drains
◆ Look at the outputs from the drains and the trends—ensure that they are patent (no output may mean they are blocked)

Abdomen
◆ Examine for complications from mediastinal/pleural drain and/or attempted IABP insertion

(Continued)

Table 26.4 (Continued)

Urine output

♦ Surrogate marker of the adequacy of cardiac output

Infusions/medications

♦ Confirm appropriately prepared and definitively being delivered at appropriate rates.

♦ Recheck allergies

♦ Exclude missed doses of medications

Investigations

ECG

Confirm rhythm and adequate temporary pacemaker function (if present/required)

Exclude ischaemia from acute graft occlusion, air embolus or other cause

Look at voltage of QRS (tamponade?)

Arterial blood gas

Adequacy of oxygenation and ventilation

Major metabolic and electrolyte derangements—particularly metabolic acidosis, hyper/hypokalaemia, and hypocalcaemia (especially in the setting of significant transfusion)

Lactate as a marker of adequacy of systemic perfusion (increased anion gap)

Confirm glucose maintained between 4–120mmol/L

Haemoglobin concentration

ACT/TEG

Consider if the major problem is bleeding.

CXR

Confirm position of lines/ETT

Look for PTx, HTx, effusion and atelectasis

Examine the cardiac contour

Exclude pneumoperitoneum (erect/semi-erect CXR)

Chest ultrasound

May be more useful and more readily available to differentiate the aetiology of respiratory dysfunction.

Transthoracic(TTE)/transoesophageal (TOE) echocardiography

Reasonable TTE images can be obtained in a large proportion of post-operative patients in the setting of acute instability. TOE is indicated if TTE windows are inadequate or for specific questions (eg prosthetic valve evaluation).

In the acutely unstable patient the diagnoses that should be looked for include:

Pericardial effusion causing echocardiographic features of tamponade (although this can be very difficult in the perioperative setting and tamponade remains a clinical diagnosis)

New regional wall motion abnormalities consistent with acute graft occlusion

Acute valvular dysfunction

Cardiorespiratory interactions

Fluid responsiveness

Assessment of biventricular performance

The presence of dynamic outflow tract or mid-cavity obstruction

Full blood picture

Formal assessment of haemoglobin level

Platelet count (especially if bleeding—quantitative analysis does not indicate platelet function)

White cell count may be raised post-operatively in the absence of sepsis.

Coagulation profile

Particularly in the bleeding patient (don't wait for results to begin treatment.)

Consider further investigations as clinically indicated

algorithm to work through likely precipitants. For example, an algorithm based around the determinants of cardiac output (see table 26.5):

Cardiac output = Heart rate (and rhythm) × cardiac output (preload, afterload, contractility)

Volume resuscitation, inotropes, vasopressors and vasodilators (systemic and pulmonary) +/– mechanical supports including intra-aortic balloon counterpulsation (IABP), and extracorporeal membrane oxygenation should be considered to support cardiac output during resuscitation (please see Chapters 12 and 13 for detailed discussion of mechanical cardiovascular supports). Reversible causes must be sought and addressed as soon as possible. For detailed discussion of the management of postoperative complications after cardiac surgery, see Chapters 30–32.

Elderly patients undergoing cardiac surgery

The population of patients older than 80 years of age is increasing worldwide—both in terms of absolute number and as a proportion of the population. Several large cohort studies have demonstrated that the rate of ICU admission of very old patients increased over the period of study observation. These increased rates of admission are predicted to accelerate over time. Elderly patients admitted to intensive care have prolonged ICU and hospital LOS, lower short-term survival, and survivors who are more likely to be discharged to rehabilitation or long-term care facilities. However, mortality rates in this cohort have been improving. Furthermore, elderly patients undergoing elective surgery have improved outcomes compared with emergency admissions (48–52). Comorbidity and preoperative functional status may be better predictors of long-term survival than age (53). Age has been associated with an increase in the duration of stay in ICU after cardiac surgery and with increased mortality (49,54). The potential confounders in these studies as well as the ethical and economic implications of offering progressively more complicated surgery to older patients are beyond the scope of this chapter. Future planning of hospital, ICU, and long-term care facilities should figure in cost analyses when the scope of cardiac surgical interventions is evaluated.

End of life issues

Cardiac surgery and intensive care treatment are undertaken with the intention of improving both quantity and quality of life. However, not all patients have an improvement in quality of life after surgery (55). Significant morbidity and mortality affect a small proportion of the surgical cohort. There is increasing recognition of the importance of advanced care planning to improve end of life care—in all patients and specifically in those about to undergo major surgery. Knowledge of patients' wishes in the event of significant perioperative complications and acceptable outcomes from proposed interventions can improve patient and family satisfaction and psychological outcomes in surviving relatives (56–59). The ethical principles of autonomy, beneficence, non-maleficence, justice and patient consent must inform all discussions and decisions with respect to end of life care in the ICU.

Table 26.5 An algorithm for the causes of haemodynamic instability post-CABG

Determinant of cardiac output	Issue	Potential cause
Heart rate and rhythm	Tachydysrhythmia	Pacing malfunction
		Electrolyte imbalance
	Bradydysrhythmia	Pacing malfunction
		Electrolyte imbalance
		Ischaemia
Preload	Hypovolaemia	Bleeding
		Diuretic therapy (especially on CPB)
		Rewarming or excessive vasodilator therapy (causing relative hypovolaemia)
		Note: diastolic dysfunction will accentuate the effects of hypovolaemia
	Increased intrathoracic pressure	Excessive PEEP Pneumothorax
	Increased intra-pericardial pressure	Cardiac tamponade
	RV failure (causing LV preload reduction)	See causes of RV contractility failure and increased RV afterload
Afterload	Increased LV afterload	Aortic valve dysfunction
		Excessive vasoconstrictor therapy
		Dynamic outflow tract or mid-cavity obstruction
	Decreased LV afterload	SIRS
		Post CPB vasoplegia
		Anaphylaxis
		Excessive vasodilator therapy
	Increased RV afterload	Acidosis
		Hypoxia
		Excessive PEEP
		Thromboembolism
Contractility	Ischaemia	Acute graft dysfunction
		Air embolus (particularly in RCA)
	Inadequate myocardial protection on CPB	Inadequate cardioplegia or ventricular dilatation
	Pre-existing ventricular dysfunction	

PEEP, positive end-expiratory pressure; SIRS, systemic inflammatory response.

Conclusion

Critical care of the cardiac surgical patient requires a clear understanding of the surgery undertaken and the underlying pathophysiological processes, aiming to optimize recovery with early detection and treatment of complications. Effective coordinated care is underpinned by clear communication and teamwork. Critical care is expensive, demanding consideration of cost-effectiveness and appropriateness of care in this complex hospital environment.

References

1. College of Intensive Care Medicine Australia. Policy Document on Minimum Standards for Australian Intensive Care units. http://www.cicm.org.au/policydocs.php (accessed 27 May 2014)

2. Tran L, Chand V, Newcomb A, Billah B, Shardey G, Reid C. Cardiac surgery in Victorian public hospitals, 2010–11. http://www.health.vic.gov.au/surgicalperformance/cardiac.htm. p. 1–28 (accessed 27 May 2014)

3. Kalkman CJ. Handover in the perioperative care process. *Curr Opin Anaesthesiol* 2010; **23**(6): 749–53

4. Catchpole KR, de Leval MR, McEwan A, et al. Patient handover from surgery to intensive care: using Formula 1 pit-stop and aviation models to improve safety and quality. *Paediatr Anaesth* 2007; **17**(5): 470–8

5. Rotter T, Kinsman L, James EL et al. *Cochrane Database of Systematic Reviews*. The Cochrane Collaboration, Rotter T, editor. Chichester, UK: John Wiley & Sons, Ltd, 1996.

6. Pronovost P, Berenholtz S, Dorman T, Lipsett PA, Simmonds T, Haraden C. Improving communication in the ICU using daily goals. *J Crit Care* 2003; **18**(2): 71–5.

7. Svircevic V, Nierich AP, Moons KGM, Brandon Bravo Bruinsma GJ, Kalkman CJ, van Dijk D. Fast-track anesthesia and cardiac surgery: a retrospective cohort study of 7989 patients. *Anesthes Analg* 2009; **108**(3): 727–33

8. Filsoufi F, Rahmanian PB, Castillo JG, Chikwe J, Adams DH. Predictors and early and late outcomes of respiratory failure in contemporary cardiac surgery. *Chest* 2008; **133**(3): 713–21

9. Trouillet J-L, Combes A, Vaissier E, et al. Prolonged mechanical ventilation after cardiac surgery: Outcome and predictors. *J Thorac Cardiovasc Surg* 2009; **138**(4): 948–53

10. Mazzeffi M, Khelemsky Y. Poststernotomy pain: a clinical review. *J Cardiothorac Vasc Anesthes* 2011; **25**(6): 1163–78

11. Kress JP, Pohlman AS, O'Connor MF, Hall JB. Daily interruption of sedative infusions in critically ill patients undergoing mechanical ventilation. *N Engl J Med* 2000; **342**(20): 1471–7

12. Girard TD, Kress JP, Fuchs BD, et al. Efficacy and safety of a paired sedation and ventilator weaning protocol for mechanically ventilated patients in intensive care (Awakening and Breathing Controlled trial): a randomised controlled trial. *Lancet* 2008; **371**(9607): 126–34

13. Strøm T, Martinussen T, Toft P. A protocol of no sedation for critically ill patients receiving mechanical ventilation: a randomised trial. *Lancet* 2010 ; **375**(9713): 475–80

14. Ruokonen E, Parviainen I, Jakob SM. Dexmedetomidine versus propofol/midazolam for long-term sedation during mechanical ventilation. *Intens Care Med* 2009; **35**(2): 282–90.

15. Riker RR, Shehabi Y, Bokesch PM, et al. Dexmedetomidine vs midazolam for sedation of critically ill patients: a randomized trial. *JAMA* 2009; **301**(5): 489–99

16. Herr DL, Sum-Ping STJ, England M. ICU sedation after coronary artery bypass graft surgery: dexmedetomidine-based versus propofol-based sedation regimens. *J Cardiothorac Vasc Anesthes* 2003; **17**(5): 576–84

17. Maitland K, Kiguli S, Opoka RO, et al. Mortality after fluid bolus in African children with severe infection. *N Engl J Med* 2011; **364**(26): 2483–95

18. The RENAL Replacement Therapy Study Investigators. An observational study fluid balance and patient outcomes in the randomized evaluation of normal vs. augmented level of replacement therapy trial. *Crit Care Med* 2012; **40**(6): 1753–60.

19. Woodcock TE, Woodcock TM. Revised Starling equation and the glycocalyx model of transvascular fluid exchange: an improved paradigm for prescribing intravenous fluid therapy. *Br J Anaesth* 2012; **108**(3): 384–94

20. Grocott HP. Postoperative hyperthermia is associated with cognitive dysfunction after coronary artery bypass graft surgery. *Stroke* 2002; **33**(2): 537–41

21. Karalapillai D, Story D, Hart GK, et al. Postoperative hypothermia and patient outcomes after elective cardiac surgery. *Anaesthesia* 2011; **66**(9): 780–4

22. Van Den Berghe G, Wouters P, Weekers F, et al. Intensive insulin therapy in critically ill patients. *N Engl J Med* 2001; **345**(19): 1359–67

23. NICE-SUGAR Study Investigators, Finfer S, Chittock DR, Su SY-S, et al. Intensive versus conventional glucose control in critically ill patients. *N Engl J Med* 2009; **360**(13): 1283–97

24. Gandhi GY, Nuttall GA, Abel MD, et al. Intensive intraoperative insulin therapy versus conventional glucose management during cardiac surgery: a randomized trial. *Ann Intern Med* 2007; **146**(4): 233–43

25. Wallen M, Morrison A, Gillies D, O'Riordan E, Bridge C, Stoddart F. Mediastinal chest drain clearance for cardiac surgery. *Cochrane Database Syst Rev* 2004; **4**: CD003042.

26. Mehta RH, Ferguson TB, Lopes RD, et al. saphenous vein grafts with multiple versus single distal targets in patients undergoing coronary artery bypass surgery: one-year graft failure and five-year outcomes from the Project of Ex-Vivo Vein Graft Engineering via Transfection (PREVENT) IV Trial. *Circulation* 2011; **124**(3): 280–8

27. Ruttmann E, Fischler N, Sakic, A et al. Second internal thoracic artery versus radial artery in coronary artery bypass grafting: a long-term, propensity score-matched follow-up study. *Circulation* 2011; **124**(12): 1321–9

28. Van Domburg RT, Kappetein AP, Bogers AJ. The clinical outcome after coronary bypass surgery: a 30-year follow-up study. *Eur Heart J* 2008; **30**(4): 453–8

29. Okrainec K, Platt R, Pilote L, Eisenberg MJ. Cardiac medical therapy in patients after undergoing coronary artery bypass graft surgery: a review of randomized controlled trials. *J Am Coll Cardiol* 2005; **45**(2): 177–84

30. Mangano DT, Multicenter Study of Perioperative Ischemia Research Group. Aspirin and mortality from coronary bypass surgery. *N Engl J Med* 2002; **347**(17): 1309–17

31. Goyal A, Alexander JH, Hafley GE, et al. Outcomes associated with the use of secondary prevention medications after coronary artery bypass graft surgery. *Ann Thorac Surg* 2007; **83**(3): 993–1001

32. Gavaghan TP, Gebski V, Baron DW. Immediate postoperative aspirin improves vein graft patency early and late after coronary artery bypass graft surgery. A placebo-controlled, randomized study. *Circulation* 1991; **83**(5): 1526–33

33. Stein PD, Dalen JE, Goldman S, Theroux P. Antithrombotic therapy in patients with saphenous vein and internal mammary artery bypass grafts. *Chest* 1998; **114**(5 Supplement): 658S–65S

34. Developed with the special contribution of the European Association for Percutaneous Cardiovascular Interventions (EAPCI), Authors/ Task Force Members, Wijns W, Kolh P, Danchin N, Di Mario C, et al. Guidelines on myocardial revascularization: The Task Force on Myocardial Revascularization of the European Society of Cardiology (ESC) and the European Association for Cardio-Thoracic Surgery (EACTS). *Eur Heart J* 2010; **31**(20): 2501–55

35. Hillis LD, Smith PK, Anderson JL, et al. 2011 ACCF/AHA Guideline for Coronary Artery Bypass Graft Surgery: A Report of the American College of Cardiology Foundation/American Heart Association Task Force on Practice Guidelines. *Circulation* 2011; **124**(23): e652–735

36. Ferraris VA, Ferraris SP, Moliterno DJ, et al. The Society of Thoracic Surgeons Practice Guideline Series: Aspirin and other antiplatelet agents during operative coronary revascularization (Executive Summary). *Ann Thorac Surg* 2005; **79**(4): 1454–61

37. Becker RC, Meade TW, Berger PB, et al. The primary and secondary prevention of coronary artery disease: American College of Chest Physicians Evidence-Based Clinical Practice Guidelines (8th Edition). *Chest* 2008; **133**(6 suppl): 776S–814S

38. Reicher B, Poston RS, Mehra MR, et al. Simultaneous 'hybrid' percutaneous coronary intervention and minimally invasive surgical bypass grafting: Feasibility, safety, and clinical outcomes. *Am Heart J* 2008; **155**(4): 661–7

39. Myles PS, Smith J, Knight J, et al. Aspirin and Tranexamic Acid for Coronary Artery Surgery (ATACAS) Trial: Rationale and design. *Am Heart J* 2008; **155**(2): 224–30

40. Jacob M, Smedira N, Blackstone E, Williams S, Cho L. Effect of timing of chronic preoperative aspirin discontinuation on morbidity and mortality in coronary artery bypass surgery. *Circulation* 2011; **123**(6): 577–83

41. Grundy SM. Implications of recent clinical trials for the National Cholesterol Education Program Adult Treatment Panel III Guidelines. *Circulation* 2004; **110**(2): 227–39

42. Shah SJ, Waters DD, Barter P, et al. Intensive lipid-lowering with atorvastatin for secondary prevention in patients after coronary artery bypass surgery. *J Am Coll Cardiol* 2008; **51**(20): 1938–43

43. Kulik A, Brookhart MA, Levin R, Ruel M, Solomon DH, Choudhry NK. Impact of statin use on outcomes after coronary artery bypass graft surgery. *Circulation* 2008; **118**(18): 1785–92

44. Pan W. Statins are associated with a reduced incidence of perioperative mortality after coronary artery bypass graft surgery. *Circulation* 2004; **110**(11 suppl 1): II-45–II-49

45. Liakopoulos OJ, Choi Y-H, Haldenwang PL, et al. Impact of preoperative statin therapy on adverse postoperative outcomes in patients undergoing cardiac surgery: a meta-analysis of over 30 000 patients. *Eur Heart J* 2008; **29**(12): 1548–59

46. Collard CD, Body SC, Shernan SK, Wang S, Mangano DT. Preoperative statin therapy is associated with reduced cardiac mortality after coronary artery bypass graft surgery. *J Thorac Cardiovasc Surg* 2006; **132**(2): 392–400.e1

47. Drug Safety and Availability > FDA Drug Safety Communication: Important safety label changes to cholesterol-lowering statin drugs [Internet]. fda.gov. Available from: http://www.fda.gov/Drugs/DrugSafety/ucm293101.htm (accessed 27 May 2014)

48. Boumendil A, Somme D, Garrouste-Orgeas M, Guidet B. Should elderly patients be admitted to the intensive care unit? *Intens Care Med* 2007; **33**(7): 1252–62

49. Scott BH, Seifert FC, Grimson R, Glass PSA. Octogenarians undergoing coronary artery bypass graft surgery: resource utilization, postoperative mortality, and morbidity. *J Cardiothorac and Vasc Anesthes.* 2005; **19**(5): 583–8.

50. Bagshaw SM, Webb SAR, Delaney A, et al. Very old patients admitted to intensive care in Australia and New Zealand: a multi-centre cohort analysis. *Crit Care* 2009; **13**(2): R45

51. Nguyen Y-L, Angus DC, Boumendil A, Guidet B. The challenge of admitting the very elderly to intensive care. *Ann Intens Care* 2011; **1**(1): 29

52. Ihra GC, Lehberger J, Hochrieser H, et al. Development of demographics and outcome of very old critically ill patients admitted to intensive care units. *Intens Care Med* 2012; **38**(4): 620–6

53. Somme D, Maillet J-M, Gisselbrecht M, Novara A, Ract C, Fagon J-Y. Critically ill old and the oldest-old patients in intensive care: short- and long-term outcomes. *Intens Care Med* 2003; **29**(12): 2137–43

54. Hein OV, Birnbaum J, Wernecke K, England M, Konertz W, Spies C. Prolonged intensive care unit stay in cardiac surgery: risk factors and long-term-survival. *Ann Thorac Surg* 2006; **81**(3): 880–5

55. Myles PS, Hunt JO, Fletcher H, Solly R, Woodward D, Kelly S. Relation between quality of recovery in hospital and quality of life at 3 months after cardiac surgery. *Anesthesiology* 2001; **95**(4): 862–7

56. Truog RD, Campbell ML, Curtis JR, et al. Recommendations for end-of-life care in the intensive care unit: A consensus statement by the American Academy of Critical Care Medicine. *Crit Care Med* 2008; **36**(3): 953–63

57. Song M-K, Kirchhoff KT, Douglas J, Ward S, Hammes B. A randomized, controlled trial to improve advance care planning among patients undergoing cardiac surgery. *Med Care* 2005; **43**(10): 1049–53

58. Detering KM, Hancock AD, Reade MC, Silvester W. The impact of advance care planning on end of life care in elderly patients: randomised controlled trial. *Br Med J* 2010; **340**(1): c1345–5

59. Silvester W, Detering K. Advance directives, perioperative care and end-of-life planning. *Best Pract Res Clin Anaesthesiol* 2011; **25**(3): 451–60

CHAPTER 27

Enhanced recovery from heart surgery

Stefan Probst and Jörg Ender

Introduction

Requirements in cardiac anaesthesia have changed in the last two decades. In the 1970s and 1980s, high dose opioid anaesthesia was shown to be cardiovascularly stable and to improve patient outcome and safety (1–3). However, the price paid for improved stability was prolonged respiratory depression, as a result of the very high dosage of opioid that were used, and which led to mandatory postoperative mechanical ventilation. The 1990s were characterized by increasing age and comorbidity of the patients presenting for cardiac surgery, the introduction of new surgical techniques, an outstripping of intensive care unit (ICU) capacities, and cost containment processes in most of the developed world. So, the prolonged duration of ICU stay became an obvious target. As a result, the requirements for anaesthesia moved from providing a haemodynamically stable patient during surgery to being a key stakeholder in development and introduction of fast-track or enhanced recovery (4). The aim of this chapter is to describe the different aspects that are important to establish for enhanced recovery of cardiac surgery patients in individual centres. As it involves the whole of the patient journey and not just the durations of tracheal intubation and ICU stay, this chapter will use the term 'enhanced recovery' rather than 'fast-track'.

Milestones of the development of enhanced recovery from heart surgery

- 1977: Prakash and colleagues reported extubation of a small patient group within one hour after cardiac surgery (5).

- 1986: Aps and co-workers described the first treatment of cardiac surgery patient in a postoperative anaesthesia care unit (6).

- 1993: Chong and colleagues reduced the duration of tracheal intubation in cardiac surgery patients from 7 to 2 hours by changing their management during anaesthesia and introducing a specialized recovery (7).

- 1994: Massey and Meggit showed that a specialized recovery unit for patients undergoing cardiac surgery reduced the duration of mechanical ventilation and costs without compromising patient outcome (8). They concluded that a specialized postoperative care unit be the future for patients undergoing cardiac surgery.

- 1998: Cheng and colleagues demonstrated that a fast-track concept of postoperative care, including early tracheal extubation, was both safe and economical for patients undergoing cardiac surgery when compared to conventional treatment (9).

Management of the patient for enhanced recovery

Commonly, tracheal extubation times up to six hours and a duration of ICU stay less than 24 hours are recognized as enhanced recovery in cardiac anaesthesia (box 27.1). Several centres have developed their own concepts for enhanced recovery to decrease the duration of stay in intensive care unit and reduce treatment costs. This may be achieved using short-acting hypnotics and analgesics or even with high thoracic epidural anaesthesia in the conscious patient (10–15). Establishing enhanced recovery needs re-organization of the whole patient flow within the hospital (box 27.1). There are three parts of this re-organization that have to be considered: the pre-, intra- and postoperative management.

Preoperative management

In contrast to non-cardiac surgery, there are some specific points that have to be considered when implementing enhanced recovery in patients undergoing cardiac surgery such as advanced age, higher incidence of comorbidities and the use of cardiopulmonary bypass (CPB) with associated haemodilution and hypothermia.

Identifying patients for enhanced recovery

In principle, nearly every patient presenting for cardiac surgery may be considered for enhanced recovery. Even high-risk patients may benefit from early recovery and shortened durations of stay in ICU and hospital. However, readmission to the ICU is associated with higher mortality. Depending on the definition of enhanced recovery of the individual institutions, the incidence of failure of enhanced recovery varies in the literature from 3.3–63%.

Risk factors for failure of enhanced recovery may be classified into three categories, which are procedure related, patient, or management related. Procedure related factors are prolonged durations of CPB and aortic cross-clamping, the use of a intra-aortic balloon pump (IABP) or ventricular assist device as well as re-do operations or re-thoracotomy, combined and/or complex surgery, and emergency operations (16). Patient-related factors include advanced age, female gender, renal impairment,

---

Box 27.1 Objectives for enhanced recovery

- Anaesthesia technique that allows early tracheal extubation
- Early tracheal extubation within 6 hours
- Decreasing duration of ICU of stay
- Decreasing postoperative morbidity and enhancing recovery
  - Avoiding cardiopulmonary complications
  - Decreasing intra- and post-operative stress
- Adequate pain management
- Prophylaxis and therapy for nausea and vomiting
- Early postoperative mobilization
- Early enteral nutrition

References 9–11 16–20

Box 27.2 Inclusion criteria for enhanced recovery

- Elective surgery
- Pre- and post-operative cardiopulmonary stability without or with only minimal inotropic support
- Surgical procedures undertaken with normothermia, mild or moderate hypothermia
- No risk factors for postoperative bleeding, e.g. endocarditis, complex coagulation disorders, redo- operation.
- No complex surgery (i.e. not multiple valve replacement in combination with coronary surgery or major aortic surgery)

Box 27.3 Exclusion criteria for enhanced recovery

- Emergency cases
- High intraoperative blood loss
- High risk of excessive postoperative bleeding
- Mechanical assist devices pre- or post-operatively
- Complex surgery
- Endocarditis
- Psychiatric and/or neurological disorders
- Postoperative cardiovascular instability (high inotropic support, increased lactate, Horowitz index <200)
- Re-do operation (relative)
- Intraoperative hypothermia <32°C (relative)
- Ejection fraction <30% (relative)
- Renal impairment (relative)

Box 27.4 Drugs recommended for enhanced recovery

Hypnotics

- Sevoflurane, desflurane 0.8–1.0 MAC
- Propofol $\geq$ 3 mg/kg/hr during surgery

Opioids

- Sufentanil 5–10 µg/kg cumulative dose during surgery
- Fentanyl 5–15 µg/kg cumulative dose during surgery
- Remifentanil 0.2–0.75 µg/kg/min as continuous infusion (dose adapted to follow the stress level during surgery)

Neuromuscular blocker

- Rocuronium 0.6–1 mg/kg as initial dose and 0.075–0.15 mg/kg for repetition
- Cis-Atracurium 0.1–0.4 mg/kg as initial dose and 0.03 mg/kg for repetition

---

poor left ventricular function (ejection fraction <30%), recent myocardial infarction, pulmonary hypertension ($\geq$60 mmHg), respiratory distress, deep sedation, confusion, excessive bleeding, and high inotropic support. Management-related factors are: missing standard operation procedures or protocols for anaesthesia, weaning, analgesia or discharge criteria; unfavourable ratio in the ICU the bed numbers of the ICU (increasing the number of beds increases the risk failure) and whether the ICU is a general one or specifically for cardiac surgery (16–20).

Patient- and procedure-related factors account for two-thirds of the risk of prolonged durations of mechanical ventilation and ICU stay and management-related factors for the remaining third of the risk (11,17–20). Accurate patient selection is ensured by undertaking a thorough assessment and work-up of patients followed by discussion between surgical and anaesthetic teams. Inclusion of patients in enhanced recovery is an individual decision that should account for individual risk factors, hospital related processes and structures and it is helpful to define criteria for inclusion (box 27.2) or exclusion (box 27.3) of patients in enhanced recovery (17–19).

Intraoperative management

Intraoperative management to ensure enhanced recovery includes adapting drug and fluid therapy as well as thermal control.

Drugs

The choice of anaesthetic agents for cardiac anaesthesia is a key factor for a successful enhanced recovery. Short-acting anaesthetic and analgesic drugs that do not accumulate in the body are recommended (box 27.4).

Hypnotics

Sevoflurane, desflurane, and propofol are commonly used hypnotic agents in anaesthetic techniques for enhanced recovery. In off-pump cardiac surgery that is without CPB, volatile anaesthetic agents are widely used because they have little accumulation. In some studies, a cardioprotective effect has been described, resulting from myocardial preconditioning by volatile anaesthetic agents (21). In on-pump surgery, most workers recommend the use of propofol as the hypnotic agent of choice. However, administration of volatile anaesthetic agents during CPB requires a specially equipped CPB machine, and if high sweep gas flow rates are used, can be expensive.

Opioids

An opioid needs to be part of the anaesthetic technique to reduce the intraoperative stress response and postoperative opioid consumption. Intermediate-acting opioids like fentanyl, alfentanil, and sufentanil can be used (Chapter 6). The risk of accumulation and prolonged mechanical ventilation due to the use of intermediate-acting opioids can be decreased by reducing the dose of these opioids. However, this could increase the endocrine stress response during cardiac surgery (10,22–25). Remifentanil is an ultra-short-acting opioid as it is metabolized by unspecific plasma esterases, so its metabolism is not affected by organ failures, duration, or amount of administration (Chapter 6). The context-sensitive half time of remifentanil is 3.7 minutes. Therefore it is important to administer postoperative pain therapy 20–30 minutes before stopping a continuous intravenous (IV) infusion of remifentanil.

Several authors have shown that using remifentanil in an enhanced recovery protocol is of similar effectiveness as fentanyl or sufentanil. Remifentanil reduces stress response to surgery more effectively than fentanyl, sufentanil, and alfentanil and results in less haemodynamic responses to surgical stimuli (22,24,26–30). There is an on-going discussion about cardiac protection by pre- and post-conditioning effects of remifentanil (31–33).

Neuromuscular blockers

Continuous neuromuscular blockade throughout cardiac surgery is not required (34). Even a single administration of the long-acting neuromuscular blocker pancuronium can produce a sustained neuromuscular blockade, which can significantly prolong the duration of postoperative mechanical ventilation (35). Rocuronium and cis-atracurium, with their favourable side effect profiles and predictable durations of action, should be used instead.

Management of the body temperature

Optimization of the thermal management of patients undergoing cardiac surgery is essential for enhanced recovery. In most centres, mild to moderate hypothermia is induced during CPB to increase the tolerance of organs to ischaemia. Pronounced hypothermia during cardiac surgery and in the postoperative period is associated with adverse outcomes including impaired immune function and drug metabolism, coagulopathy, increased cardiac morbidity, shivering, reduced cognitive functions and awareness, respiratory distress, and increased use of hospital resources (36). Sufficient rewarming is essential and the core body temperature should reach at least 36°C before weaning from CPB. To avoid after-drop of body temperature, patient and IV fluid warming systems and an increased operating room temperature should be used (37,38). Patients having cardiac surgery off-pump should be kept normothermic (≥36°C).

Different patient warming systems are available and most are based on convective warming by forced air or conductive warming by heated water. The effectiveness of patient warming systems depends on their capacity to transfer heat to the patient and the energy transfer per square metre body of surface is lower with convecting than conducting systems. However, forced air systems are more effective than just a water mattress under the back of the patient, but less effective than circulating water garments. Fluid warmers are only effective if a substantial amount of IV fluid is given to the patient (36,39).

Fluid management

Adequate IV fluid loading is the *sine qua non* for haemodynamic optimization of patients having cardiac surgery. Optimal management in cardiac anaesthesia is impaired by inadequate IV fluid administration, resulting in hypovolaemia and end-organ hypoperfusion, and excessive administration of IV fluids with the risk of congestive heart failure and the adverse effects of oedema formation. The composition of IV fluids that should be used remains controversial and not specific to enhanced recovery.

Regional anaesthesia

Different regional anaesthesia techniques usually in combination with general anaesthesia, have been used for enhanced recovery (40,41). Some centres prefer regional anaesthesia alone for selected patient groups (14,15,42,43). Commonly used regional anaesthetic techniques in cardiac surgery are thoracic epidural anaesthesia (TEA), intrathecal opioid injection (with or without clonidine), intercostal catheter, and paravertebral or parasternal injection of local anaesthetics.

TEA is the mostly commonly used regional anaesthesia technique in cardiac anaesthesia and it provides a segmental sympathetic block, which is assumed to be the mediator of its perioperative effects (44). However, TEA has some serious adverse effects, including epidural haematoma and abscess and infarction of the spinal cord, resulting in paraplegia. There is insufficient data to determine the incidence of epidural haematoma after TEA when used for cardiac surgery. Systematic review and meta-analyses of studies were unable to estimate the risk of severe neurologic sequelae (45,46). One estimation of maximal risk of epidural haematoma is 1 in 1528 after epidural catheter techniques and 1 in 3610 for single shot spinal puncture technique after cardiac surgery (47). The incidence of an epidural abscess after TEA is reported as 1:10 000–24 000 (48).

Several studies have shown reductions in the duration of postoperative ventilation time and pain scores to be associated with the use of regional anaesthesia, but a superiority over enhanced recovery from general anaesthesia alone has not yet been shown (14,15,40–43,46).

Postoperative management

For postoperative management, several different pathways have been described (figure 27.1). It has to be tailored to the structure of the individual hospital and resources of human staff that is nurses and physicians. Generally, tracheal extubation in the operating room is feasible but does not reduce the duration of stay in ICU (27,49). Implementation of a step-down unit allows discharge of patient from ICU on the day of surgery (50). Essential for a successful enhanced recovery protocol are a high nurse to patient ratio, staff trained in the protocol (i.e. weaning, pain therapy), designated patient rooms with reduced acoustic level, and non-invasive mechanical ventilation (13,50).

Post-anaesthesia care unit

Conventionally, patients following cardiac surgery were transferred to the ICU for postoperative treatment (Chapter 26). Several studies have shown that the postoperative treatment of a selected group of patients in a separate unit on an ICU or in a post-anaesthesia

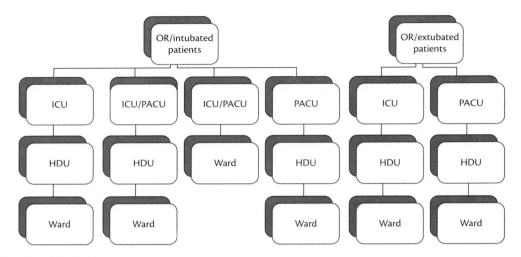

Fig. 27.1 Pathways for patients following heart surgery.
ICU, intensive care unit; PACU, post-anaesthesia care unit; HDU, high dependency unit; OR, operating room.

Box 27.5 Requirement for the equipment of a post-anaesthesia care unit

- Fully invasive and non-invasive cardiopulmonary monitoring
- Mechanical ventilators with invasive and non-invasive modes
- Point of care diagnostics: i.e blood gas analysis, electrolytes, lactate, glucose
- Ultrasound imaging (TTE, TOE, abdominal ultrasonography)
- Access to all patient relevant information (laboratory results, X-rays, etc.)
- X-ray examination
- Availability of blood products
- Close connection to the operating room
- Possibility to pass on patients to the ICU
- Full equipment for cardiopulmonary resuscitation

TTE, transthoracic echocardiography; TOE, transoesophageal echocardiography; ICU, intensive care unit.

---

care unit (PACU) may be beneficial (6,11,51). Equipment recommended for such a PACU is listed in box 27.5.

Pain therapy

The management of pain following cardiac surgery is discussed in detail in Chapter 39. However, as effective pain relief is essential for enhanced recovery it merits some additional consideration in this chapter. Postoperative pain following cardiac surgery is moderate to severe, but unfortunately, pain therapy is often based on the belief that pain is mild and alleviated quickly (52). Maximum pain intensity occurs in the first two postoperative days, declining between the second and third postoperative day. The location of pain is in the first day is related to the sternotomy and later, moves to the back and shoulders. Patients younger than the age of 60 and females have higher pain scores (53,54). Effective control of postoperative pain is mandatory to facilitate enhanced recovery

and so it is important to establish guidelines for the treatment of postoperative pain. The objective of such guidelines should be pain scores below 4 on a numeric or visual analogue scale of 1 to 10. Following the World Health Organization (WHO) guidelines (www.who.int) for pain treatment a non-opioid analgesic should be combined with an opioid analgesic.

In principle, regional anaesthesia techniques can provide an excellent quality of analgesia. An intrathecal single-shot of morphine can significantly reduce pain scores and opioid consumption in the first 24 hr after surgery (22,55–57). TEA delivers an excellent quality of pain control after cardiac surgery and it reduces the overall systemic opioid consumption and reduces opioid related side effects (58–60). However, in an ICU setting using guidelines for treatment of pain, discomfort and agitation, IV administration of opioids provided a similar quality of pain relief as did TEA (61). In addition, as discussed earlier in this chapter, regional anaesthesia techniques should be used with caution because of their potential adverse effects.

Economic considerations

ICU treatment is the major cost factor in postoperative treatment of the cardiac surgical patient. When compared to conventional treatment following coronary artery bypass grafting surgery, a possible 25% cost reduction can be achieved by using an enhanced recovery approach (10). Unsurprisingly, early tracheal extubation alone did not show any cost reduction, as long as duration of stay in ICU was not reduced. Decreasing the duration of ICU stay reduces resource utilization and costs without compromising patient safety (13,62). Transfer of appropriate patients from ICU to a step-down unit on the same day is safe and allows intensive care beds to be used by more than one patient each day (50). With implementation of a PACU for immediate postoperative treatment of selected patients and the transfer to a step down unit on the same day then a relevant amount of costs can be saved without affecting patient safety (63).

Conclusion

There are many different ways to establish an enhanced recovery progamme. However, the most important factors for the success of enhanced recovery are patient selection, good patient and physician, and patient to nurse ratios, and a protocol that is customized to fit the individual circumstances in each hospital.

References

1. Bennett GM, Stanley TH. Cardiovascular effects of fentanyl during enflurane anesthesia in man. *Anesth Analg* 1979; **58**: 179–82

2. Prakash O, Verdouw PD, de Jong JW, et al. Haemodynamic and biochemical variables after induction of anaesthesia with fentanyl and nitrous oxide in patients undergoing coronary artery by-pass surgery. *Can Anaesth Soc J* 1980; **27**: 223–9

3. Stanley TH, Webster LR. Anesthetic requirements and cardiovascular effects of fentanyl-oxygen and fentanyl-diazepam-oxygen anesthesia in man. *Anesth Analg* 1978; **57**: 411–6

4. Krier C, Martin J. [Process remodeling DRG's, SOP's, clinical pathways and the role of the physician]. *Anasthesiol Intensivmed Notfallmed Schmerzther* 2006; **41**: 135–6

5. Prakash O, Jonson B, Meij S, et al. Criteria for early extubation after intracardiac surgery in adults. *Anesth Analg* 1977; **56**: 703–8

6. Aps C, Hutter JA, Williams BT. Anaesthetic management and postoperative care of cardiac surgical patients in a general recovery ward. *Anaesthesia* 1986; **41**: 533–7

7. Chong JL, Grebenik C, Sinclair M, Fisher A, Pillai R, Westaby S. The effect of a cardiac surgical recovery area on the timing of extubation. *J Cardiothorac Vasc Anesth* 1993; **7**: 137–41

8. Massey D, Meggit G. Recovery units: the future of postoperative cardiac care. Intensive Crit Care Nurs 1994;**10**: 71–4

9. Cheng DC. Impact of early tracheal extubation on hospital discharge. *J Cardiothorac Vasc Anesth* 1998; **12**(Suppl 2): 35–40

10. Cheng DC, Karski J, Peniston C, et al. Early tracheal extubation after coronary artery bypass graft surgery reduces costs and improves resource use. A prospective, randomized, controlled trial. *Anesthesiology* 1996; **85**: 1300–10

11. Ender J, Borger MA, Scholz M, et al. Cardiac surgery fast-track treatment in a postanesthetic care unit: six-month results of the Leipzig fast-track concept. *Anesthesiology* 2008; **109**: 61–6.

12. van Mastrigt GA, Maessen JG, Heijmans J, Severens JL, Prins MH. Does fast-track treatment lead to a decrease of intensive care unit and hospital length of stay in coronary artery bypass patients? A meta-regression of randomized clinical trials. *Crit Care Med* 2006; **34**: 1624–34

13. Svircevic V, Nierich AP, Moons KG, Brandon Bravo Bruinsma GJ, Kalkman CJ, van Dijk D. Fast-track anesthesia and cardiac surgery: a retrospective cohort study of 7989 patients. *Anesth Analg* 2009; **108**: 727–33

14. Noiseux N, Prieto I, Bracco D, Basile F, Hemmerling T. Coronary artery bypass grafting in the awake patient combining high thoracic epidural and femoral nerve block: first series of 15 patients. *Br J Anaesth* 2008; **100**: 184–9

15. Watanabe G, Tomita S, Yamaguchi S, Yashiki N. Awake coronary artery bypass grafting under thoracic epidural anesthesia: great impact on off-pump coronary revascularization and fast-track recovery. *Eur J Cardiothorac Surg* 2011; **40**: 788–93

16. Constantinides VA, Tekkis PP, Fazil A et al. Fast-track failure after cardiac surgery: development of a prediction model. *Crit Care Med* 2006; **34**: 2875–82

17. Toraman F, Senay S, Gullu U, Karabulut H, Alhan C. Readmission to the intensive care unit after fast-track cardiac surgery: an analysis of risk factors and outcome according to the type of operation. *Heart Surg Forum* 2010; **13**: E212–E217

18. Constantinides VA, Tekkis PP, Fazil A, et al. Fast-track failure after cardiac surgery: development of a prediction model. *Crit Care Med* 2006; **34**: 2875–82

19. Akhtar MI, Hamid M. Success and failure of fast track extubation in cardiac surgery patients of tertiary care hospital: one year audit. *J Pak Med Assoc* 2009; **59**: 154–6

20. Lassnigg A, Hiesmayr MJ, Bauer P, Haisjackl M. Effect of centre-, patient- and procedure-related factors on intensive care resource utilisation after cardiac surgery. *Intensive Care Med* 2002; **28**: 1453–61

21. Van Der Linden PJ, Daper A, Trenchant A, De Hert SG. Cardioprotective effects of volatile anesthetics in cardiac surgery. *Anesthesiology* 2003; **99**: 516–7

22. Latham P, Zarate E, White PF, et al. Fast-track cardiac anesthesia: a comparison of remifentanil plus intrathecal morphine with sufentanil in a desflurane-based anesthetic. *J Cardiothorac Vasc Anesth* 2000; **14**: 645–51

23. Engoren M, Luther G, Fenn-Buderer N. A comparison of fentanyl, sufentanil, and remifentanil for fast-track cardiac anesthesia. *Anesth Analg* 2001; **93**: 859–64

24. Howie MB, Cheng D, Newman MF, et al. A randomized double-blinded multicenter comparison of remifentanil versus fentanyl when combined with isoflurane/propofol for early extubation in coronary artery bypass graft surgery. *Anesth Analg* 2001; **92**: 1084–93

25. Winterhalter M, Brandl K, Rahe-Meyer N, et al. Endocrine stress response and inflammatory activation during CABG surgery. A randomized trial comparing remifentanil infusion to intermittent fentanyl. *Eur J Anaesthesiol* 2008; **25**: 326–35

26. Cheng DC, Newman MF, Duke P, et al. The efficacy and resource utilization of remifentanil and fentanyl in fast-track coronary artery bypass graft surgery: a prospective randomized, double-blinded controlled, multi-center trial. *Anesth Analg* 2001; **92**: 1094–102

27. Straka Z, Brucek P, Vanek T, Votava J, Widimsky P. Routine immediate extubation for off-pump coronary artery bypass grafting without thoracic epidural analgesia. *Ann Thorac Surg* 2002; **74**: 1544–7

28. Cartwright DP, Kvalsvik O, Cassuto J et al. A randomized, blind comparison of remifentanil and alfentanil during anesthesia for outpatient surgery. *Anesth Analg* 1997; **85**: 1014–9

29. Knapik M, Knapik P, Nadziakiewicz P, et al. Comparison of remifentanil or fentanyl administration during isoflurane anesthesia for coronary artery bypass surgery. *Med Sci Monit* 2006; **12**: I33–I38

30. Pleym H, Stenseth R, Wiseth R, Karevold A, Dale O. Supplemental remifentanil during coronary artery bypass grafting is followed by a transient postoperative cardiac depression. *Acta Anaesthesiol Scand* 2004; **48**: 1155–62

31. Wong GT, Huang Z, Ji S, Irwin MG. Remifentanil reduces the release of biochemical markers of myocardial damage after coronary artery bypass surgery: a randomized trial. *J Cardiothorac Vasc Anesth* 2010; **24**: 790–6

32. Wong GT, Li R, Jiang LL, Irwin MG. Remifentanil post-conditioning attenuates cardiac ischemia-reperfusion injury via kappa or delta opioid receptor activation. *Acta Anaesthesiol Scand* 2010; **54**: 510–8

33. Wong GT, Ling LJ, Irwin MG. Activation of central opioid receptors induces cardioprotection against ischemia-reperfusion injury. *Anesth Analg* 2010; **111**: 24–8

34. Gueret G, Rossignol B, Kiss G et al. Is muscle relaxant necessary for cardiac surgery? *Anesth Analg* 2004; **99**: 1330–3

35. Thomas R, Smith D, Strike P. Prospective randomised double-blind comparative study of rocuronium and pancuronium in adult patients scheduled for elective 'fast-track' cardiac surgery involving hypothermic cardiopulmonary bypass. *Anaesthesia* 2003; **58**: 265–71

36. Insler SR, Bakri MH, Nageeb F, Mascha E, Mihaljevic T, Sessler DI. An evaluation of a full-access underbody forced-air warming system during near-normothermic, on-pump cardiac surgery. *Anesth Analg* 2008; **106**: 746–50

37. Hofer CK, Ganter MT, Zollinger A. Evaluation of a modified ThermoWrap for the Allon warming system in patients undergoing elective off-pump coronary artery bypass grafting. *J Thorac Cardiovasc Surg* 2006; **131**: 929–30

38. Kiessling AH, Isgro F, Lehmann A, Piper S, Blome M, Saggau W. Evaluating a new method for maintaining body temperature during OPCAB and robotic procedures. *Med Sci Monit* 2006; **12**: MT39–42

39. Moola S, Lockwood C. Effectiveness of strategies for the management and/or prevention of hypothermia within the adult perioperative environment. *Int J Evid Based Healthc* 2011; **9**: 337–45

40. Chaney MA. Intrathecal and epidural anesthesia and analgesia for cardiac surgery. *Anesth Analg* 2006; **102**: 45–64

41. Hemmerling TM, Prieto I, Choiniere JL, Basile F, Fortier JD. Ultra-fast-track anesthesia in off-pump coronary artery bypass grafting: a prospective audit comparing opioid-based anesthesia vs thoracic epidural-based anesthesia. *Can J Anaesth* 2004; **51**: 163–8.

42. Picozzi P, Lappa A, Menichetti A. Mitral valve replacement under thoracic epidural anesthesia in an awake patient suffering from systemic sclerosis. *Acta Anaesthesiol Scand* 2007; **51**: 644

43. Bottio T, Bisleri G, Piccoli P, Negri A, Manzato A, Muneretto C. Heart valve surgery in a very high-risk population: a preliminary experience in awake patients. *J Heart Valve Dis* 2007; **16**: 187–94

44. Clemente A, Carli F. The physiological effects of thoracic epidural anesthesia and analgesia on the cardiovascular, respiratory and gastrointestinal systems. *Minerva Anestesiol* 2008; **74**: 549–63

45. Svircevic V, van Dijk D, Nierich AP, Passier MP, Kalkman CJ, van der Heijden GJ, et al. Meta-analysis of thoracic epidural anesthesia versus general anesthesia for cardiac surgery. *Anesthesiology* 2011; **114**: 271–82

46. Djaiani G, Fedorko L, Beattie WS. Regional anesthesia in cardiac surgery: a friend or a foe? *Semin Cardiothorac Vasc Anesth* 2005; **9**: 87–104

47. Ho AM, Chung DC, Joynt GM. Neuraxial blockade and hematoma in cardiac surgery: estimating the risk of a rare adverse event that has not (yet) occurred. *Chest* 2000; **117**: 551–5

48. Freise H, Van Aken HK. Risks and benefits of thoracic epidural anaesthesia. *Br J Anaesth* 2011; **107**: 859–68

49. Montes FR, Sanchez SI, Giraldo JC, et al. The lack of benefit of tracheal extubation in the operating room after coronary artery bypass surgery. *Anesth Analg* 2000; **91**: 776–80

50. Flynn M, Reddy S, Shepherd W, et al. Fast-tracking revisited: routine cardiac surgical patients need minimal intensive care. *Eur J Cardiothorac Surg* 2004; **25**: 116–22

51. Novick RJ, Fox SA, Stitt LW et al. Impact of the opening of a specialized cardiac surgery recovery unit on postoperative outcomes in an academic health sciences centre. *Can J Anaesth* 2007; **54**: 737–43

52. Watt-Watson J, Stevens B. Managing pain after coronary artery bypass surgery. *J Cardiovasc Nurs* 1998; **12**: 39–51

53. Mueller XM, Tinguely F, Tevaearai HT, Revelly JP, Chiolero R, von Segesser LK. Pain location, distribution, and intensity after cardiac surgery. *Chest* 2000; **118**: 391–6

54. Meehan DA, McRae ME, Rourke DA, Eisenring C, Imperial FA. Analgesic administration, pain intensity, and patient satisfaction in cardiac surgical patients. *Am J Crit Care* 1995; **4**: 435–42

55. Turker G, Goren S, Bayram S, Sahin S, Korfali G. Comparison of lumbar epidural tramadol and lumbar epidural morphine for pain relief after thoracotomy: a repeated-dose study. *J Cardiothorac Vasc Anesth* 2005; **19**: 468–74

56. Mukherjee C, Koch E, Banusch J, Scholz M, Kaisers UX, Ender J. Intrathecal morphine is superior to intravenous PCA in patients undergoing minimally invasive cardiac surgery. *Ann Card Anaesth* 2012; **15**: 122–7

57. Bowler I, Djaiani G, Abel R, Pugh S, Dunne J, Hall J. A combination of intrathecal morphine and remifentanil anesthesia for fast-track cardiac anesthesia and surgery. *J Cardiothorac Vasc Anesth* 2002; **16**: 709–14

58. Priestley MC, Cope L, Halliwell R, et al. Thoracic epidural anesthesia for cardiac surgery: the effects on tracheal intubation time and length of hospital stay. *Anesth Analg* 2002; **94**: 275–82

59. Hansdottir V, Philip J, Olsen MF, Eduard C, Houltz E, Ricksten SE. Thoracic epidural versus intravenous patient-controlled analgesia after cardiac surgery: a randomized controlled trial on length of hospital stay and patient-perceived quality of recovery. *Anesthesiology* 2006; **104**: 142–51

60. Royse C, Royse A, Soeding P, Blake D, Pang J. Prospective randomized trial of high thoracic epidural analgesia for coronary artery bypass surgery. *Ann Thorac Surg* 2003; **75**: 93–100

61. Fillinger MP, Yeager MP, Dodds TM, Fillinger MF, Whalen PK, Glass DD. Epidural anesthesia and analgesia: effects on recovery from cardiac surgery. *J Cardiothorac Vasc Anesth* 2002; **16**: 15–20

62. Silbert BS, Myles PS. Is fast-track cardiac anesthesia now the global standard of care? *Anesth Analg* 2009; **108**: 689–91

63. Hantschel D, Fassl J, Scholz M, et al. [Leipzig fast-track protocol for cardio-anesthesia. Effective, safe and economical]. *Anaesthesist* 2009; **58**: 379–86

CHAPTER 28

Ultrasound imaging in critical care

Andrew Hilton

Introduction

Eliciting and interpreting physical signs is often difficult when clinically assessing the critically ill patient. Impaired patient communication, constraints on their positioning in bed, and presence of mechanical cardiorespiratory supports impede traditional clinical examination techniques and may render the presence or absence of signs inconclusive. Hence, imaging technology is required to provide information additional to sparse and sometimes confusing clinical data. However, the cost, size, and expertise required to both operate and interpret imaging technology has presented significant barriers to optimal management of the intensive care unit (ICU) patient. Such equipment is often centralized in an imaging department (e.g. Radiology) outside the ICU, necessitating transfer of a potentially unstable patient to a clinically 'hostile' environment; urgent imaging can be difficult to organize out of normal working hours; serial imaging of patients is often impractical; and examination is often performed or interpreted by imaging technicians or specialists who may be unfamiliar with the clinical context of the study.

The portability of ultrasonography has overcome many of these problems. Ultrasonography cannot always substitute for other imaging modalities, but when indicated, can be performed in the ICU with little or no risk to the patient, and in the very unstable patient may be the only practical imaging modality available. Furthermore, apart from diagnostic use ultrasonography can guide and improve the safety of invasive procedures (e.g. central venous access, pleural drainage, pericardiocentesis) (1).

Until recently ultrasonography has been predominantly performed and interpreted by imaging services and relevant specialists outside the ICU (e.g. Radiology and Cardiology). These services have and continue to provide valuable anatomic or pathologic information that may be crucial to patient management. However, critically ill patients present at any time of day or night, can deteriorate rapidly, and may need immediate and repeated imaging. Furthermore, they may require urgent, sometimes risky invasive procedures. The ultrasound examination required might not necessarily be a full diagnostic study but one tailored to answering or facilitating the specific question or invasive procedure relevant to the immediate management and needs of the patient (2,3). Imaging services outside the ICU cannot always satisfy these demands. Hence, though specialist ultrasound imaging remains necessary particularly when rare or complex pathology is involved, critical care physicians themselves are more frequently performing point-of-care echocardiographic and ultrasound examinations in order to satisfy these more timely requirements (figure 28.1).

Equipment

Machines capable of meeting the ultrasound imaging requirements of ICU patients range from large multifunctional platforms capable of many imaging modes (echocardiography, vascular access, thoracic and general abdominal imaging) through to small simple to use single applications machines (figure 28.2). Though all relying on common physical principles, the various modes of clinical ultrasonography each have particular technological features and requirements. The type of ultrasound probe to be used and its supporting hardware and software differ widely between the various ultrasound-imaging modalities (figure 28.3). When a specific ultrasound examination is referred to imaging specialists outside the ICU then the choice of ultrasound equipment for ICU imaging will simply be restricted to the range of equipment available in their own individual department, a range dictated by their expert imaging needs, experience and budgetary constraints.

However, with the increasing use of point-of-care ultrasonography, intensivists are deciding the choice of ultrasound equipment. This decision needs to be commensurate with the anticipated range and quality of ultrasound imaging and will have to take into account the range of probes required, and features of the platform itself including ergonomic design, ease of use and disinfection, image quality, data management, purchase and maintenance costs, and vendor support.

Ultrasound probes and platforms have been identified as potential sources of nosocomial infection—a risk that appears greater if the same equipment is used sequentially on many ICU patients. Individual equipment vendors have disinfection guidelines for their machines and probes. Importantly, these should be adhered to and performed after every patient examination. For ICU-based machines this is clearly very important and appears advisable to keep a log book that documents every patient use and disinfection afterwards, and can be used to both enforce appropriate cleaning but also track machine use especially during bouts of severe nosocomial infection.

Echocardiography

Traditionally cardiovascular and haemodynamic assessment of the cardiothoracic ICU patient has relied on physical examination,

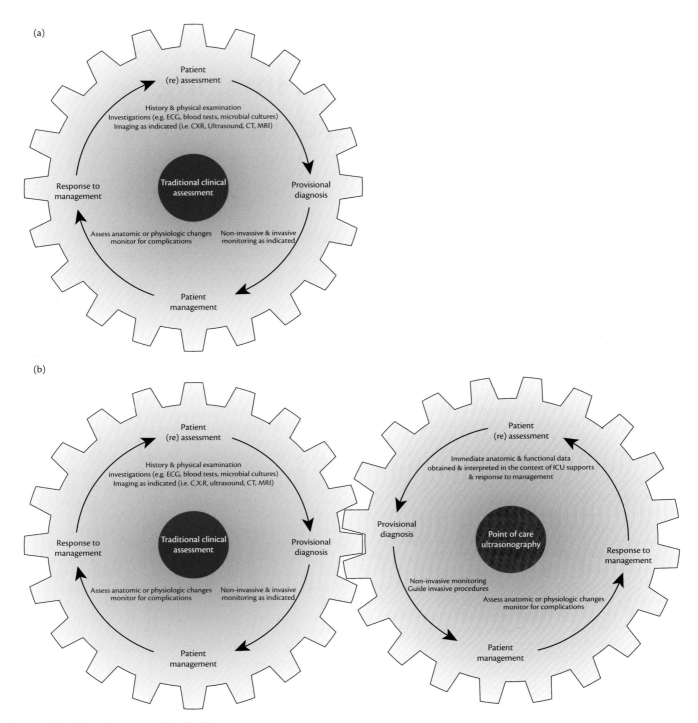

Fig. 28.1 Point of care ultrasonography in the ICU.

(a) Traditional clinical assessment of the critically ill patient is an iterative process cycling between patient assessment, establishing a provisional diagnosis or problem list, deciding upon and instituting a management plan, assessing response to management, and in that assessment refining or altering the diagnosis of problem list according to response and any other new clinical data. Delays in this process in the critically ill can be due to inaccurate or incomplete history and physical examination, delays in acquiring supplemental imaging data, time required to establish invasive monitoring without distracting monitoring related patient complications, inaccurate interpretation of physiologic data, and limitations in clinical response to management. (b) 'Point-of-care' ultrasonography is performed by the medical team managing the patient. It is not a substitute for traditional clinical assessment but an additional potentially synergistic process. It facilitates the complex iterative process of ICU management by accelerating many of its components:

i. Provides immediate anatomic imaging and physiologic information at the bedside without potential delays awaiting the services of other imaging specialists.

ii. Imaging data interpreted more accurately in the known context of ICU supports and interventions.

iii. Repeated imaging as required.

iv. Ultrasound-guided invasive procedures potentially minimize patient complications with their intendant delays and morbidity.

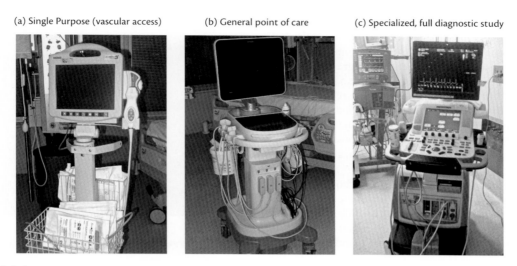

Fig. 28.2 Ultrasound platforms.
(a) Single purpose ultrasound platform used for vascular access. (b) Point of care ultrasound machine with extended range of transducers and clinical applications. (c) Advanced echocardiography platform capable of all echocardiography imaging modes including three-dimensional imaging. With appropriate transducers and software it can also perform vascular and general ultrasound imaging.

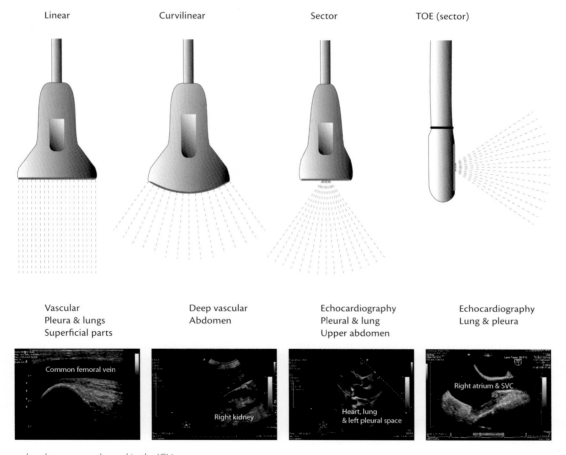

Fig. 28.3 Ultrasound probes commonly used in the ICU.
Most ultrasound platforms can operate a broad range of transducer types depending on the imaging required. These are the most common types of transducers used in the cardiothoracic ICU and a brief, but not exclusive list of their imaging capabilities. Note also that in cardiothoracic patients other types of transducers may occasionally be used by imaging specialists (e.g. bronchoscopic endobronchial ultrasound, intravascular echocardiography catheters).

electrocardiography, chest X-ray, and invasive haemodynamic monitoring. All of these have diagnostic utility, but in the ICU their performance may be limited, or their results misleading, uninterpretable or inaccurate (2). Echocardiography provides real-time bedside imaging of cardiac structure and function, and Doppler assessment of intracardiac blood flow echocardiography, which may facilitate interpretation of traditional data (5). In particular, data obtained via invasive haemodynamic monitoring can be interpreted in the context of directly observed cardiac pathology and function, and estimates of intracardiac volume and flows.

Compelling evidence supporting the use of echocardiography in the ICU is provided by studies that include cardiothoracic patients where echocardiographic diagnostic utility is inferred by the hard end-point of indicated surgical re-exploration (4). The majority of these reports are over 10 years old and describe the then emerging ICU use of transoesophageal echocardiography (TOE) in comparison to transthoracic echocardiography (TTE). At that time TTE did not produce consistent image quality in ICU patients due to older beam forming technology, which could not always overcome the limited transthoracic 'acoustic windows' of the cardiothoracic ICU patient. The latter are due to the effects of positive pressure ventilation and positive end-expiratory pressure (PEEP), restricted patient positioning, and presence of chest drains and injuries. TOE utilizes an acoustic window that obviates these TTE limitations, and provides the ability to better examine posterior cardiac structures and the thoracic aorta, all of particular relevance in the cardiothoracic ICU patient (e.g. evaluation of prosthetic mitral valve; aortic dissection).

Recent technological improvements in TTE, especially harmonic imaging, now make it possible to satisfactorily image at least 70% of ICU patients obviating the need and possible risks of TOE (5,6). In our experience TTE, performed by a well-trained operator using modern equipment, is very useful in the assessment of cardiothoracic patients especially following acute haemodynamic deterioration (see figure 28.4 and figure 28.5). Not all standard TTE views are usually possible, but the information required can be quickly obtained and is often sufficient to guide initial management in the majority of cardiothoracic patients. However, TOE remains an important option as it may be preferable or necessary pending the clinical question to be answered, feasibility of TTE or results of an initial TTE examination, and the probability of contingent surgical intervention (see table 28.1 and table 28.2).

Practical considerations

The performance of echocardiography in cardiothoracic intensive care patient often differs significantly from that performed elsewhere in the hospital due to limitations and challenges imposed by the ICU environment, the acutely ill patient, and urgent simultaneous medical and surgical management.

Transthoracic echocardiography

Patient positioning

Attention to patient positioning can make a significant difference to the ease and quality of TTE imaging. The patient is ideally positioned for TTE when placed on their left side, with the left arm abducted and externally rotated at the shoulder, elbow flexed, and the hand placed underneath the patient's head. This position

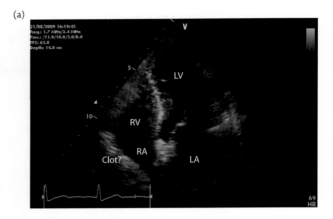

(a)

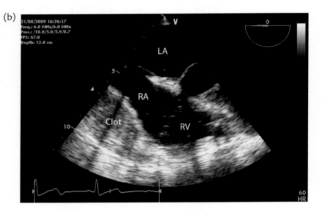

(b)

Fig. 28.4 Low cardiac output and elevated CVP following cardiac (CABG) surgery.
(a) Urgent TTE assessment performed but only apical views available. Right atrium has triangular rather than rounded appearance and right ventricle appears relatively small. Findings consistent with probable 'clot' compression of RA and possibly RV. (b) TOE performed in order to confirm TTE finding. Foreshortened mid-oesophageal view of right heart demonstrates definite 'clot' compression of right atrium extending inferiorly over anterior right ventricle.
LA, left atrium; RA, right atrium; LV, left ventricle; RV, right ventricle.

facilitates better imaging by improving acoustic windows with less interference by sternum, ribs, and lung. The heart tends to come out laterally from beneath the sternum and lie closer to the chest wall; and the positioning of the arm widens rib spaces laterally, further improving apical windows. However, some patients cannot be easily or safely changed to a more left lateral position in their bed (e.g. chest and mediastinal drains; severe haemodynamic instability; open sternum); and in the elderly patient, or any patient with left upper limb disease or injury it may not be possible to position the left arm optimally. In this case subcostal views may provide better imaging, or at times the only useful views.

In some patients, despite all positioning attempts and optimization of echocardiographic settings, satisfactory imaging remains impossible. If TOE is contraindicated or unavailable a potential solution is the use of ultrasound contrast. This appears to be a safe option in critically ill patients but does require greater operator expertise and specific echocardiography platform capabilities (7). Ultrasound contrast enhances endocardial border identification allowing the visualization of LV wall motion and intracavitary pathology and devices (e.g. left ventricular assist device inflow cannulae).

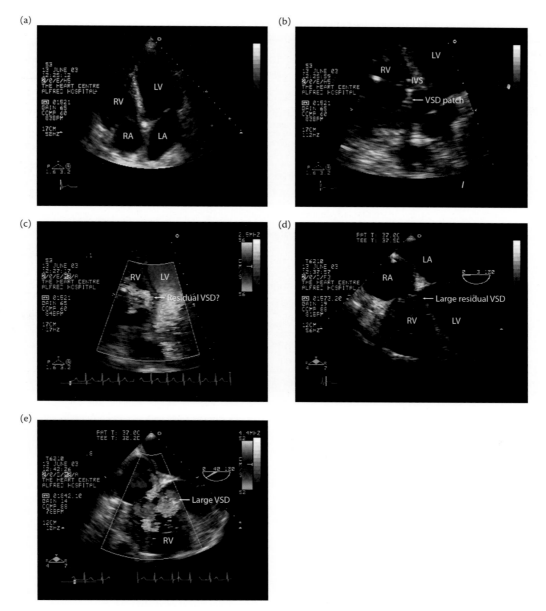

Fig. 28.5 Haemodynamic instability following elective repair of complex membranous ventricular septal defect (VSD).
(a and b) Urgent TTE assessment with patch repair of VSD identified on apical views. (c) Abnormal colour flow jet appearing in RV during systole. Consistent with residual VSD, but clinical significance unclear. (d) Subsequent TOE (mid-oesophageal views) reveals deficit in proximal IVS. (e) Colour flow Doppler demonstrates large flow abnormality consistent with failure of patch repair of VSD. Though TTE findings were consistent with residual VSD, TOE provided definitive evidence of large VSD secondary to failure of repair rather than residual small VSD. Patient returned to the operating room. (See also figure in colour plates section)
LA, left atrium; RA, right atrium; LV, left ventricle; RV, right ventricle; IVS, interventricular septum.

Operator and machine positioning

Whether to perform the examination from the patient's left or right side depends on the operator's training and preference. Our preference is to perform TTE from the left side as it can be challenging to image from the right side a large patient positioned on their left side in a wide ICU bed. Irrespective of the usual side from which the patient is examined, in an unstable cardiothoracic patient the echocardiographer and equipment should be positioned on the patient's side that best allows access to ventilator, intravenous resuscitation fluids, vasopressor and inotropic infusions, and other circulatory supports (e.g. intra-aortic balloon pump (IABP), extracorporeal membrane oxygenation (ECMO)) so that any necessary changes to these supports can be made during the course of the examination. Hence, in the urgent situation an acquired degree of ambidexterity in a well-trained echocardiographer is very useful.

Technical consideration

Except in the most urgent situations an electrocardiogram (ECG) trace should be displayed with the echocardiographic images. A practical and time saving solution is to have echocardiographic equipment that can obtain an ECG signal via a slave cable

Table 28.1 Echocardiography for haemodynamic monitoring in cardiothoracic ICU patients (47)

Haemodynamic parameter	Comments
Cardiac output and stroke volume	PW Doppler of LVOT (or RVOT). Good agreement with thermodilution methods. Easily done with either TTE or TOE.
	New generation of 3D echo technology can directly calculate volumetric estimates of SV.
Left ventricular ejection fraction	Qualitative estimates by experienced echocardiographers demonstrate good agreement—adequate for clinically relevant decisions re haemodynamic management.
	Calculated using modified Simpson method. New generation of 3D echo technology can directly calculate volumetric estimates of EF.
Other measures of left ventricular performance	S′ : peak systolic tissue velocity velocity using tissue Doppler at mitral annulus.
	MR dP/dT using CW Doppler of MR jet.
Estimates of LVEDP/LAP	Size of left atrium. Displacement of IAS to either left or right.
	E/E′ : Ratio of peak early diastolic mitral inflow (PW Doppler—E) to peak early diastolic tissue velocity at mitral annulus (Tissue Doppler—E′).
Right ventricular ejection fraction	Difficult to estimate qualitatively.
	2D quantitative methods may be inaccurate because of geometric assumptions
	New generation of 3D echo technology can directly calculate volumetric estimates of RVEF.
Other measures of right ventricular performance	TAPSE: Tricuspid annular plane systolic excursion by M Mode.
	S′ : peak systolic tissue velocity velocity using tissue Doppler at tricuspid annulus.
	TR dP/dT using CW Doppler of TR jet.
Pulmonary artery pressure	CW Doppler of TR jet. RVESP = TR peak gradient + RAP
	CW Doppler of PR jet. PAD = PR end diastolic gradient + RAP
	PW Doppler PV. PA acceleration time (start of RV ejection to peak) inversely proportional to MPAP (likely increase if acceleration time < 100ms)
Volume responsiveness	Increased respiratory variation in IVC diameter (TTE or TOE) or SVC (TOE) in fully mechanically ventilate patients—not validated if breathing spontaneously.

PW, pulse wave; LVOT,left ventricular outflow tract; RVOT, right ventricular outflow tract; TTE, transthoracic echocardiography; TOE, transoesophageal echocardiography; SV, stroke volume; EF, ejection fract; S′ , S prime-tissue Doppler systolic velocity; MR, mitral regurgitation; dP/dT, rate of pressure rise in early systole; CW, continuous wave; IAS, interatrial septum; E/E′ , ratio of early mitral inflow and tissue Doppler velocities; RVEF, right ventricular ejection frcation; TAPSE, tricuspid annular plane systolic excursion; TR, tricuspid regurgitation; RVESP, right ventricular end-systolic pressure; RAP, right atrial pressure; PR,pulmonary regurgitation; PAD, pulmonary artery diastolic pressure; MPAP, mean pulmonary artery pressure; IVC, inferior vena cava; SVC, superior vena cava.

Data from Romero-Bermejo, F.J., et al., Echocardiographic hemodynamic monitoring in the critically ill patient. Current Cardiology Reviews, 2011. 7(3): p. 146–156.

connection to a compatible ICU monitor. This avoids the necessity of connecting another set of ECG electrodes to the patient.

Though echocardiographic loops can be recorded according to pre-set time intervals (often the default mode when no ECG signal is present), loops gated to the ECG R wave contain complete cardiac cycles, have smoother play back on review, and also provide a record of the patient's heart rate and rhythm—all of which may facilitate the interpretation of the study. Echo loop length (number of cardiac cycles or time duration) depends on personal preference, machine storage capacity, and clinical questions to be answered. Echocardiographic views or measurements accompanied by significant respiratory variation or irregular rhythms may be best represented or averaged by several cycle length capture. With respect to the former, an ECG derived respiratory plethysmograph signal is clinically useful when respiratory phasic changes are of diagnostic interest: e.g. tamponade and respiration induced intracardiac flow variation in the spontaneously breathing patient (figure 28.6).

Recording and interpreting study

Prior to performing the echo study the patient's relevant demographic data should be entered and identified with the study.

However, most machines have an emergency mode that allows the performance and recording of an exam with subsequent retrospective entering of patient demographic data. Also, as patient supports may be changed or titrated during the course of the study it is useful to annotate these changes on the echo display so that that on subsequent review the study can be interpreted in the context of these changes (figure 28.7). It is important to be able to share and review images with all involved medical specialties (e.g. Cardiology, Cardiothoracic Surgery) particularly for the diagnosis of complex pathologies or if surgical intervention is likely to be necessary.

Furthermore, whether via on screen annotation or by written report, it is desirable to document relevant ICU organ supports that may influence or limit the interpretation of echo findings. For example, the interpretation or significance of echocardiographic cardiorespiratory interactions depends on the mode of ventilation. Thus, increased respiratory mitral flow variation in a spontaneously patient with a pericardial effusion may support the presence of cardiac tamponade, but is of no proven utility in the patient receiving intermittent positive pressure ventilation (PEEP) (8). The presence and magnitude of mechanical and pharmacologic circulatory supports need to be recorded and the findings

Table 28.2 Common indications for diagnostic use of echocardiography in cardiothoracic ICU patients

Clinical state	Cardiac status	Echocardiographic information
Hypotension and shock	LV function RV function	TTE may provide adequate views for global estimates of ventricular systolic function but more subtle SWMAs may be easier seen with TOE.
	Valvular function	TTE may be sufficient for native valves (depending on available acoustic windows). TOE preferred to evaluate significant eccentric valvular regurgitant jet, prosthetic valvular dysfunction suspected, or if uncertainty remains,
	Cardiac tamponade	Early postoperative tamponade usually due to localized chamber compression by haematoma—may be difficult to visualize with TTE (48). TOE usually more definitive especially for posterior haematoma compression (e.g. left atrium).
	Dynamic LVOT obstruction	Very difficult diagnosis to make clinically. Echocardiography invaluable—may be adequately diagnosed with either TTE or TOE. Requires careful 2D imaging and CW Doppler of LVOT velocities.
Respiratory Failure	Ventricular function	Echocardiographic evidence of increased LA pressure (e.g. increased LA size; increase E:E' ratio > 15 with PW and tissue Doppler). Possible with either TTE or TOE. RV systolic dysfunction may be secondary to cause (e.g. PE) or therapies (e.g. IPPV with high inspiratory pressures and PEEP). (49)
	Valvular function	As for Hypotension and shock.
	Suspected PE	Indirect evidence: acute RV dilatation, flattening and shift of IVS to left and decreased systolic function (decreased RV wall motion, TAPSE or tricuspid valve annular S'). TTE may be adequate. Direct evidence: Thrombosis seen in transit through right heart and into proximal pulmonary arteries. More likely to be seen with TOE.
	Intracardiac shunt	ASD or VSD can be diagnosed with either TTE or TOE, though TOE generally superior. May require contrast study (e.g. 'agitated' saline).
Source of sepsis	Endocarditis	Large vegetations may be easily seen with TTE. TOE provides more definitive study especially if prosthetic valve, or complications need to be evaluated (e.g. extension of infection into valve annulus and abscess formation).
Source of systemic embolization	Intracavity thrombosis Aortic atheroma	LV apical thrombus may be best seen with TTE (especially if ultrasound contrast used). Otherwise TOE superior especially for left atrial examination, and examination of thoracic aorta for severe atheromatous disease with or without adherent thrombus.
Assess MCS	IABP ECMO VAD	Echocardiographic positioning of devices and cannulae; intravascular/intra-cardiac thrombus formation; obstruction of cannulae, especially inflow (LVAD) or access cannulae (ECMO); monitor for LV cavity 'suck down' (continuous flow LVAD). 2D imaging may be sufficient though Doppler useful to confirm/diagnose cannulae obstruction. (19,50) Possible with TTE but TOE often easier.
Post lung and heart transplantation	Primary graft dysfunction	As for assessment of LV and RV function.
	Pulmonary venous anastomoses	TOE required. Can be difficult to diagnose. PW Doppler may provide confirmatory evidence—absent or accelerated PV flow velocities.
	Acute rejection	Systolic or diastolic dysfunction; pericardial effusion. May be diagnosed with either TTE or TOE.
Other	Alveolar lavage	TOE can provide excellent images of lung; assess for possible acute RV dysfunction.
	Arrhythmia	Evidence of atrio-ventricular dissociation on PW Doppler of mitral and pulmonary venous inflow.

ASD, atrial septal defect; LVAD, left ventricular assist device; SWMA, segmental wall motion abnormality; TAPSE, tricuspid annular plane systolic excursion; VSD, ventricular septal defect.

Data from: Price, S., et al., Tamponade following cardiac surgery: terminology and echocardiography may both mislead. European journal of cardio-thoracic surgery, 2004. 26(6): p. 1156–1160; Vieillard-Baron, A., et al., Echo-Doppler demonstration of acute cor pulmonale at the bedside in the medical intensive care unit. American Journal of Respiratory and Critical Care Medicine, 2002. 166(10): p. 1310–1319; Sidebotham, D., et al., Extracorporeal membrane oxygenation for treating severe cardiac and respiratory failure in adults: part 2-technical considerations. Journal of cardiothoracic and vascular anesthesia, 2010. 24(1): p. 164–172; Kirkpatrick, J.N., S.E. Wiegers, and R.M. Lang, Left ventricular assist devices and other devices for end-stage heart failure: utility of echocardiography. Current Cardiology Reports, 2010. 12(3): p. 257–264.

interpreted accordingly. Some echocardiographic studies may involve the weaning of these supports. Ideally, appropriate annotated images should be provided with each change in level of circulatory support, and documented in the report.

Transoesophageal echocardiography

This shares many of the same considerations as per TTE performed in the ICU, and intraoperative TOE. Exceptions include:

Patient positioning and preparation

Most patients in the ICU who have acute haemodynamic deterioration before or after cardiothoracic surgery will have an endotracheal tube (ETT) in situ. It will often be desirable in these patients to provide deep sedation with muscle relaxation, the selection and dosing of which is dictated by the drugs available, clinician preference, and patient's haemodynamic state. However, in some patients with an artificial airway (ETT or tracheostomy) muscle relaxation may be not desirable or necessary, and sedation with, or without

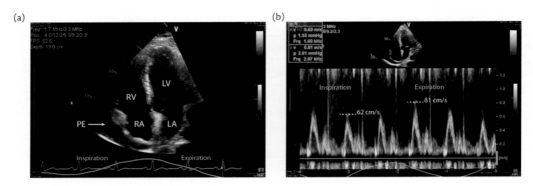

Fig. 28.6 Pericardial effusion with suspected cardiac tamponade.
(a) Apical four-chamber view (TTE). Notice green respiratory signal derived from ECG. (b) PW Doppler of mitral inflow. Note inspiratory decrease in MVQ with respect to end-expiration. 25% change consistent with clinical diagnosis of tamponade in a spontaneously breathing patient. (See also figure in colour plates section)
LA, left atrium; RA, right atrium; LV, left ventricle; RV, right ventricle; PE, pericardial effusion.

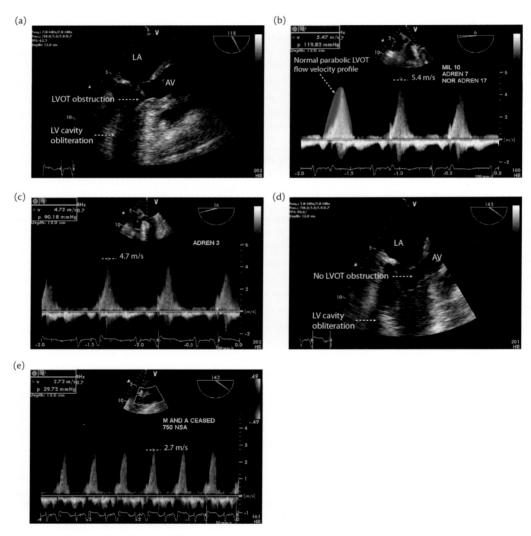

Fig. 28.7 Low cardiac output following cardiac surgery despite increasing inotropic support.
(a) Mid-oesophageal long axis view (TOE). Mid-systolic LVOT outflow obstruction by mitral valve leaflets demonstrated. Patient supported with adrenaline (7 μg/min), norepinephrine (noradrenaline) (17 μg/min), and milrinone (10 μg/min). Note also LV cavity obliteration. (b) CW Doppler of LVOT velocities. Normal CW profile of LVOT velocities is parabolic, with much lower velocities (<1 m/s). With dynamic LVOT obstruction LVOT CW profile becomes dagger shaped and with much higher velocities. Peak gradient across LVOT obstruction is 120 mmHg. (c) Milrinone ceased and epinephrine (adrenaline) decreased to 3. LVOT gradient decreased to 90 mmHg. (d) Mid-oesophageal LV long axis view (TOE). Milrinone, epinephrine (adrenaline) and norepinephrine (noradrenaline) ceased, and 750 mL of colloid given. No obvious LVOT obstruction, but LV cavity obliteration still present. (e) LVOT gradient decreased to 30 with less concave upstroke. Residual gradient coming remaining LV mid cavity obstruction. (See also figure in colour plates section)
LA, left atrium; LV, left ventricle; AV, aortic valve; LVOT, left ventricular outflow tract.

local anaesthetic topicalization of the pharynx may be sufficient. Less commonly, an ICU patient without an artificial airway will require TOE. In the unstable patient it is often safer to intubate first. However, if tracheal intubation is not safe, indicated or necessary then 'awake' sedation with pharyngeal local anaesthetic topicalization of the pharynx will be required, preferably by an operator skilled in performing TOE in patients without artificial airways.

Vascular ultrasound

Vascular ultrasonography is a common procedure in the critically ill patient that broadly serves two purposes: ultrasound-guided vascular access; and diagnosis of vascular disease and vascular complications occurring in the ICU patient. See table 28.3 (9).

Ultrasonography for vascular access

Percutaneous placement of intravascular catheters and devices is a very common procedure in the cardiothoracic ICU patient. This is performed in order to gain venous vascular access for the delivery of drugs or fluids, and provide continuous renal replacement therapy; or the monitoring of haemodynamic indices derived from central venous and right heart placement of catheters. Similarly, intra-arterial placement of devices may also be required for haemodynamic monitoring (direct blood pressure and cardiac output) and therapeutic support (IABP and peripheral ECMO).

Vascular access can be difficult or present significant risk of vascular or other complications. These may arise because of: anatomic variation not accounted for in traditional anatomic landmark methods; abnormalities of the vessels themselves, which prevent blind cannulation or contribute to increased post-cannulation risk of complications; or the nature of the intervention (e.g. insertion of IABP) or clinical context (e.g. severe coagulopathy), presenting increased patient risk if vascular access is unsuccessful or complicated even though vascular anatomy may be normal. In these situations vascular ultrasound may decrease risk to the patient.

Table 28.3 Vascular ultrasonography

	Clinical problem	Comments
Venous ultrasonography	Central venous cannulation	Recommended by many authorities in order to decrease complications, number of unsuccessful attempts, and time required for the procedure. Requires training and simultaneous use of both the techniques of ultrasound and central venous cannulation and may introduce other errors especially in beginners.
		Most published evidence pertains to IJV cannulation—less evidence for femoral and subclavian routes. (9)
	Peripheral venous cannulation	Not extensively studied. Useful for peripheral insertion of central lines (PICC lines). Aim is more to increase success rate rather than avoid complications, though incidence of site infection may be reduced.
	Lower limb deep vein thrombosis (51)	Prevalence in ICU unknown but averages 10%.
		Direct compressibility of imaged veins 'gold standard' sign. Thrombus may be visualized but is distinguished from artefact by incompressibility of venous segment containing thrombus. Doppler techniques (PW and colour flow) can be used to access venous flow and corroborate findings. Pelvic veins may be difficult to image and not compressible. Lack of respiratory variation on PW Doppler of more distal venous flow (common femoral vein) supportive of pelvic venous obstruction. Subcostal imaging with a sector scanner can assess IVC and SVC venous flow with sector scanner. TOE is particularly useful for assessing the SVC.
	Upper limb deep vein thrombosis (52)	Upper limb DVT may be responsible for 18% of DVT. Presence of central venous catheter or pacemaker wires increases risk.
		More difficult examination to perform than that for lower limbs—not all veins are directly compressible (subclavian and axillary veins) and may have to rely on Doppler PW and Colour flow (with respiratory variation) to establish patency in these vessels.
Arterial ultrasonography	Arterial cannulation for arterial access (10)	Only small number of studies directly support use of ultrasound—particularly useful if vessels small or pulsatility difficult to ascertain. Techniques used similar to that for venous puncture.
	Acute arterial insufficiency	Not uncommon but serious complication secondary to ICU interventions and supports such as insertion of arterial lines and IABP. Other causes include peripheral embolization of thrombus (e.g. atrial fibrillation) or complication of surgical disease (e.g. aortic dissection). May be particularly difficult to diagnose clinically in the absence of a pulsatile circulation with mechanical circulatory support (e.g. VA ECMO, continuous flow VAD).
		Requires 2D visualization of luminal patency and Doppler analysis with PW and Colour flow.
	Acute aortic syndromes	Aortic aneurysm and dissection may be diagnosed surface ultrasound (surface abdominal imaging for abdominal AAA, transthoracic imaging for thoracic aneurysm or dissection; TOE for thoracic aortic disease and ascertain cardiac complications). Peripheral complications assessed as in previous entry. Pleural and pericardial spaces for haemorrhage.
	Insertion of IABP	Paucity of published literature. Vascular ultrasound to assess artery (vessel calibre and patency; presence of disease); guide arterial puncture and placement of balloon just distal to SCA (TOE) and above mesenteric vessels (TTE and TOE).

IVC, inferior vena cava; SCA, superior carotid artery; SVC, superior vena cava.

Data from: Lamperti, M., et al., International evidence-based recommendations on ultrasound-guided vascular access. Intensive Care Medicine, 2012. 38(7): p. 1105–1117; Hamper, U.M., M.R. DeJong, and L.M. Scoutt, Ultrasound evaluation of the lower extremity veins. Radiologic Clinics of North America, 2007. 45(3): p. 525–47–ix; Weber, T.M., M.E. Lockhart, and M.L. Robbin, Upper extremity venous Doppler ultrasound. Radiologic Clinics of North America, 2007. 45(3): p. 513–24–viii–ix; Shiloh, A.L., et al., Ultrasound-guided catheterization of the radial artery: a systematic review and meta-analysis of randomized controlled trials. Chest, 2011. 139(3): p. 524–529.

Most of the evidence that supports ultrasound-guided vascular access has come from studies of central venous cannulation and have demonstrated increased success rates, decreased the number of attempts, and less overall complications (9). A smaller and limited number of published studies also support ultrasound-guided arterial cannulation (10). However, it is important to note that improper use of ultrasound can also result in vascular complications (11,12).

Practical considerations

There are many reviews and texts that describe the use and problems of ultrasound for vascular access (13,14). The following is a generic description of the equipment required and general principles of its use.

♦ *Machine*: The machine should be positioned so that in lies in the operator's direct line of site whilst performing the procedure itself. This ensures that vascular access needle manipulation and its ultrasound visualization are simultaneous, thereby avoiding the necessity of the operator having to repeatedly turn their body or head during the procedure. Occasionally, another person is required to adjust or operate the machine.

♦ *Probe*: A linear probe with a wide frequency bandwidth provides the best image resolution in relation to depth of structures being visualized. Various probe sizes are available—those with a small footprint are best utilized for identifying small vascular structures (e.g. peripheral arterial or venous cannulation), whereas larger transducers are better for deeper and larger vessels (e.g. femoral). Curvilinear transducers are useful for very deep vessels (e.g. femoral vessels in a large patient). Sterile probe covers/sheaths are necessary if imaging is performed during a sterile procedure.

♦ *Imaging*: Image depth is adjusted in order to have both the best and largest view of the vessel of interest. Demonstrating expected anatomic relationships, and assessing wall thickness and echogenicity, vessel compressibility, and pulsatility aids in identifying observed vascular structures (figure 28.8). The vessels should be imaged in both transverse and longitudinal planes in order to assess the vessels' diameter, depth, direction, and relationship to other structures. If available, colour flow imaging and pulse wave Doppler facilitates the correct identification of vascular structure by helping to delineate venous as opposed to arterial flow. Furthermore, it will confirm abnormal or absent flow consistent with vascular obstruction figure 28.9).

Diagnostic vascular ultrasound in the ICU

Common indications for diagnostic vascular ultrasonography in cardiothoracic ICU patients include diagnosis of deep vein thrombosis (DVT), arterial sufficiency following insertion of IABP (or other intra-arterial devices), and acute aortic syndromes. The latter may involve TOE in order to assess the thoracic aorta when aortic dissection or aneurysm is suspected. Most of these studies

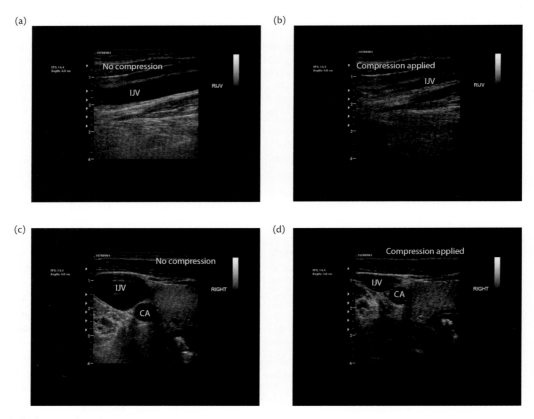

Fig. 28.8 Ultrasound of right internal jugular vein.
(a) Long axis view of right IJV. No transducer compression applied. (b) IJV compressed by applied pressure from linear transducer. (c) Transverse view of right IJV and common carotid artery. (d) IJV compressed by applied pressure from linear transducer. Note no change in shape of right carotid artery.
IJV, internal jugular vein; CA, carotid artery.

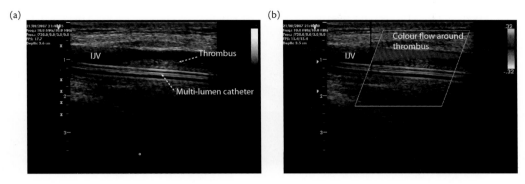

Fig. 28.9 Left IJV.
(a and b) Multi-lumen central line in situ with adherent thrombus—confirmed with colour flow imaging. (See also figure in colour plates section)
IJV, internal jugular vein.

have traditionally been performed by specialist imaging services outside the ICU. Evidence supporting intensivist-performed diagnostic vascular ultrasound is inferred from the description and study of point of care vascular ultrasound performed in the Emergency Department for the screening of DVT and diagnosis of aortic aneurysms (15). Furthermore, one study suggests that the minimal training requirements for competency in ultrasound imaging for diagnosis of peripheral arterial disease may be as small as 15 studies (16).

Specific uses of vascular ultrasound in the cardiothoracic ICU

Placement of IABP

Insertion and management of an IABP is common practice in the cardiothoracic ICU. Unfortunately, IABP-related vascular complications are not uncommon. Though ultrasound guided IABP placement may decrease the known risks of this procedure, there is surprisingly little published evidence to support this practice.

Bleeding and ischaemic complications may be avoided by correctly identifying the common femoral artery below the inguinal ligament, excluding significant femoral arterial disease, and confirming intravascular placement of the guide-wire. The presence of the guide-wire in the abdominal aorta can be confirmed by subcostal TTE imaging; and in the thoracic aorta by either TTE or TOE. Correct IABP positioning just distal to origin of left subclavian artery can be established with surfacing scanning from a left supraclavicular window, but is more easily and reliably established with TOE. Ultrasound can also be used to minimize the risk of occlusion at the origin of the coeliac and superior mesenteric arteries (figure 28.10) (17).

Vascular ultrasound is invaluable for the diagnosis of ischaemic complications post-IABP insertion. Complete, or near complete, absence of arterial flow may be easily diagnosed with Doppler ultrasound. However, more subtle changes to peripheral arterial flow, or complex pathology (e.g. peripheral arterial dissection), are best investigated by the experienced vascular sonographer

Peripheral ECMO

Percutaneous cannulation for peripheral ECMO using femoral vessels and/or internal jugular access is now an excepted and increasingly common procedure. However, given the sizes of the cannulae, the need for careful positioning of venous access cannulae, and the time-critical emergency context of the intervention, vascular complications are a significant risk and likely to result in patient death. A number of case reports and reviews support the use of ultrasound in order to safely cannulate patients for peripheral ECMO and to optimize intravascular cannula positioning (18,19). A linear or curvilinear ultrasound probe can be used to identify femoral vessels, establish their patency, and assess size relative to that of the cannulae (figure 28.11).

In peripheral venoarterial ECMO, if backflow cannulation of the superficial femoral artery is necessary, then the superficial femoral artery can be ultrasonically identified and anterograde cannulation guided accordingly. With subcostal TTE imaging or TOE, guide wire positioning in either the inferior vena cava (IVC) or abdominal/thoracic aorta can be confirmed before proceeding with further dilation of the cannulated vessel. This will importantly confirm whether either the femoral vein or artery has been punctured—something not always easy to immediately determine in the possibly hypotensive, hypoxic patient. Final placement of venous cannula in IVC or right atrium (RA) can also be guided with TTE (subcostal views) or TOE. If internal jugular vein cannulation is required then this can be guided with combination of surface ultrasound and final positioning with TTE or TOE (figure 28.12).

Lung ultrasound

Chest X-rays are the most common diagnostic modality used for imaging the lungs in the ICU. However, their limitations are well known and described, and even when definitely indicated (e.g. suspicion of tension pneumothorax) can be difficult to arrange urgently. Chest computerized tomography (CT) is the gold standard for imaging the lungs for pneumothorax, pleural disease, parenchymal disease, and pulmonary vascular disease (20). However, it requires transport of the patient out of the ICU, and in emergent situations may not be possible to perform quickly. Ultrasound has been used for the diagnosis of pulmonary and pleural pathology for many years and can, in many situations, provide valuable diagnostic information without moving the patient from the ICU (21). Furthermore, if point of care ultrasonography is available in the ICU a suitably trained critical care physician

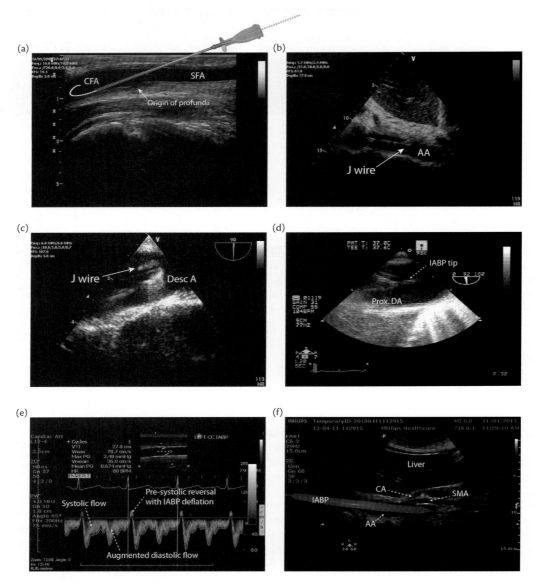

Fig. 28.10 Ultrasound guide IABP placement.

(a) Ultrasound of right femoral artery using linear transducer. The common femoral, superficial femoral and profunda arteries are identified. Significant peripheral vascular disease is excluded and the common femoral artery is of sufficient size to accept an IABP. The femoral artery is is penetrated by the needle below the inguinal ligament and above origin of profunda artery. Intra-arterial placement of guide wire can be confirmed by ultrasound, establishing that the femoral artery rather than femoral vein was accessed, and that the wire has not followed an extravascular course, making subsequent vessel dilatation and passage of the balloon safer. (b) J wire seen in abdominal aorta with subcostal imaging (sector scanner). (c) J wire seen in descending thoracic aorta (TOE). (d) IABP sited just distal to aortic arch with TOE. TTE can be used but requires suprasternal imaging which is difficult in the ICU patient. (e) PW Doppler can be used to confirm unobstructed flow to left carotid and subclavian arteries. Note biphasic forward flow—first due to unobstructed systolic flow, and the second due to IABP inflation (distal to origin of left carotid artery) and augmented diastolic pressure. Also a transient systolic reversal of flow is presented with IABP deflation. (f) The inferior positioning of the IABP can be identified. In particular, the origin of SMA and coeliac arteries can be identified (curvilinear probe) and mesenteric arterial flow can be assessed. However, in practice this can be difficult because of IABP related ultrasound artefact.

CFA, common femoral artery; SFA, superficial femoral artery; AA, abdominal aorta; Prox DA, proximal descending aorta; IABP, intra-aortic balloon pump; CA, coeliac artery; SMA, superior mesenteric artery.

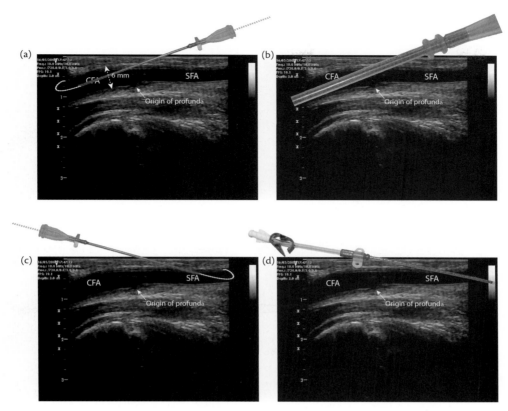

Fig. 28.11 Ultrasound guided arterial cannulation for peripheral venoarterial ECMO.
(a and b) Assessing femoral artery, guiding arterial puncture, and confirming guide wire position are the same as for insertion of IABP (see figure 28.10). Confirming J wire position is particularly important given the size of the ECMO arterial return cannula (usually 15 to 21F) and the sequential dilation required for its placement. (c and d) The arterial return cannula can obstruct distal flow to the lower limb. It is common practice to prevent leg ischaemia by anterograde 'backflow' cannulation of the SFA. This cannula is connected to a side-port of the arterial return cannula and provides perfusion of the distal limb with oxygenated blood.
It is important that the profunda artery is identified and not cannulated by mistake. The profunda itself will be perfused by any flow that continues around the arterial return cannula and that provided by the arterial 'back flow' cannula.
CFA, common femoral artery; SFA, superficial femoral artery.

can rapidly diagnose important pleural and lung pathology (22) (table 28.4).

Practical considerations

♦ *Probes and machine*: Either linear or sector probe can be used, though a linear probe gives better near field definition (23).

♦ *Patient position*: The patient can be either supine or erect. A systematic approach is required, imaging from multiple rib spaces on both sides of the chest from parasternal, mid-clavicular, and axillary lines.

Ultrasonography for pleural and lung disease

Various techniques are used including surface ultrasound with either a sector or linear probe, TOE, and endobronchial ultrasound (24). The techniques most commonly available to the intensivist are surface ultrasonography (sector or linear probe) and TOE. Furthermore, ultrasound can help estimate the size, and composition of the pleural effusion, and differentiate between complex

and simple effusions (figure 28.13 and figure 28.14) (25–27). Also, ultrasound-guided insertion of pleural drains may possibly decrease associated complications especially in the case of loculated effusions with pleural septa and adhesions between the lung and chest wall (28).

There is increasing evidence for the use of lung ultrasound to diagnose pneumothorax (29,30). In the normal lung, ultrasound signs, such as the sliding pleural sign or presence of B lines (comet tail artefact), are easily demonstrable. When these are visualized pneumothorax can be excluded with a very high degree of certainty, with diagnostic utility at least equal to portable chest X-ray. Ultrasound signs that positively include the presence of pneumothorax are less commonly seen (e.g. lung point), but appear to be specific when present.

Parenchymal lung pathology can also be diagnosed with ultrasound. Interstitial oedema can be diagnosed with surface ultrasound and may be a possible guide to the limits or appropriateness of volume therapy (31,32). Lung consolidation and air–fluid levels can easily be demonstrated. TOE can provide some very dramatic pictures of these pathologies (figure 28.15, figure 28.16, and figure 28.17), including pulmonary abscess and metastatic cancer.

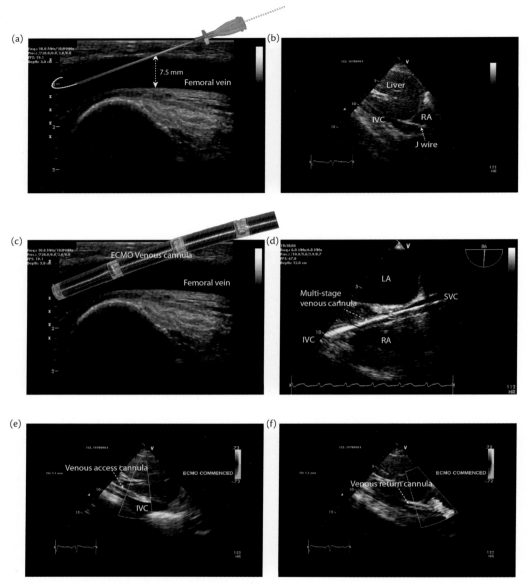

Fig. 28.12 Ultrasound guided venous cannulation for peripheral (venoarterial (VA) or venovenous (VV)) ECMO.
(a) Ultrasound of right femoral vein using linear transducer. The common femoral vein and its tributaries (long saphenous and profunda veins) are identified. The ECMO venous cannula can be sized according to the diameter of the femoral vein. The needle penetrates the common femoral vein just below the inguinal ligament.
(b and c) Intravenous placement of guide wire can be confirmed by ultrasound. In this example the j wire is imaged by subcostal view (sector scanner) demonstrating passage of wire through the IVC into the right atrium. This establishes that the femoral vein rather than femoral artery was accessed, and that the wire has not followed an extravascular course. Given the large sizes of venous ECMO cannula (19 to 27 F) subsequent vessel dilatation and passage of the venous cannula is potentially safer.
(d) Peripheral VA ECMO. Multi-stage venous access cannula positioned in RA with tip in proximal SVC (TOE bi-caval view). (e) Peripheral VV ECMO Venous access cannula confirmed to be in IVC just distal to RA. (Subcostal TTE with colour Doppler). (f) Peripheral VV ECMO Venous return cannula confirmed to be in RA. (Subcostal TTE with colour Doppler). (See also figure in colour plates section)
IVC, inferior vena cava; RA, right atrium; LA, left atrium; SVC, superior vena cava.

Ultrasonography of the upper airway

Ultrasound has been used to assess the upper airway prior to extubation, especially to measure subglottic diameter, and positioning of the endotracheal tube (ETT) post-intubation (34). There is also increasing interest in the use of ultrasound for percutaneous tracheostomy (35,36). The airway anatomy can be ascertained, particularly the level of the cricoid cartilage and first tracheal ring. The ETT can be visualized though with some difficulty. If seen, it is

possible to determine the level of the ETT cuff, especially when the ETT is partially withdrawn prior to percutaneous puncture of the trachea (figure 28.18). The ETT cuff is easier to visualize if water is used to inflate the cuff. Aberrant midline neck vessels can be identified in order to minimize bleeding by a percutaneous technique by directing site for percutaneous puncture; or to indicate an open surgical technique instead. Needle puncture of the trachea can be guided in real time, analogous to the technique used for vascular access.

Table 28.4 Thoracic ultrasonography

	Clinical problem	Comments
Upper airway (34)	Pre-intubation assessment	Epiglottis, larynx, subglottic trachea, and anterior neck easily imaged though require some experience for interpretation. May help predict difficult intubation. May be able to visualize ETT directly post-extubation especially if ETT cuff inflated with fluid and air mixture
Lower airway	Consolidation and atelectasis	May be more sensitive and specific than CXR. Continuum of appearance from ill-defined hypo-echogenic areas to well-defined areas of solid organ like density. Air and fluid bronchograms may be present. Dynamic changes in bronchograms may differentiate consolidation from atelectasis. Lung vasculature identified with colour Doppler
	Pulmonary oedema	Multiple B lines or comet tail artefacts more than 7 mm apart diagnostic of interstitial oedema; less than 3 mm apart diagnostic of pulmonary oedema. Signs seen in main dependent part of lung suggests cardiogenic oedema. If seen in non-dependent areas and heterogeneous in distribution & appearance suggests acute lung injury
	Pulmonary abscess	Rounded hypoechogenic areas, with irregular walls. May demonstrate fluid air interface with hyperechoic signal. Can demonstrate lung vasculature around margin of abscess with colour Doppler Possible to differentiate peripheral lung abscess from empyema
Pleural space	Pneumothorax	Demonstration of sliding pleural sign excludes presence of pneumothorax—better than CXR. However, absence of sliding pleural sign not specific for pneumothorax. Absence of B-lines & lung pulse supportive of pneumothorax. Lung point sign a very specific positive sign for pneumothorax but is not sensitive (30)
	Pleural effusion and empyema	Simple pleural effusions (transudates) appear as an anechoic space between visceral and parietal pleura with respiratory movement of lung within this space. Complex effusions (exudates) and some transudates have increased internal echogenicity, secondary to suspended particles or septa (e.g. haemothorax and empyema) Ultrasound more accurate than CXR and near accurate as CT. Volume of effusion can be estimated
Ultrasound-guided procedures	Pleurocentesis	Evidence supports the increased safety of ultrasound-guided pleural drainage including patients on positive pressure ventilation (28)
	Lung recruitment	PEEP-induced changes in dependent lung density can be observed on TOE. Systematic evaluation of regional lung aeration scores can be determined by chest wall ultrasonography—may enable optimal PEEP to be determined in ALI. Note that over expanded areas of lung cannot be determined by ultrasound (53)
	Ventilator weaning	Respiratory changes in diaphragmatic thickness can be used as an estimate of diaphragmatic function and workload (54) Decreased (<25 mm) diaphragmatic inspiratory excursion diagnostic of severe diaphragmatic dysfunction post cardiac surgery; and may predict weaning difficulty in ventilated medical patients (55) Ultrasound determined loss of lung aeration with a weaning trial may be predictive of extubation failure (56)
	Percutaneous tracheostomy	Thyroid cartilage, cricoid cartilage, and tracheal rings can be identified, guiding level & depth of needle puncture of the trachea. Real-time guidance (analogous to vascular access) of trachea possible. Potential decrease in percutaneous tracheostomy related complications (35,36)

ALI, acute lung injury; CXR, chest X-ray.

Data from various sources, see reference numbers.

Abdominal ultrasound

Intra-abdominal and renal complications following cardiothoracic surgery are not uncommon. Abdominal ultrasound is a well-established imaging modality that can be used to diagnose both intra-abdominal and retroperitoneal pathology (table 28.5). Its ability to aid in the diagnosis of many acute pathologies is similar to abdominal CT (37). The diagnostic utility of abdominal ultrasound in the critically ill has long been recognized, particularly as it may obviate the risk associated with patient transport out of the ICU (38,39). However, abdominal sonography requires time, patience, and experience. In the critically ill patient this is further complicated by poor imaging, due to restrictions in patient positioning, and the lack of acoustic windows due to bowel gas, and the presence of surgical incisions and drains. Hence, when definite diagnosis is required in a critically ill patient, abdominal CT is often preferred especially when combined with a request for CT of other body regions (e.g. brain, chest); or in conditions where CT may be the preferred modality (e.g. pancreatic disorders). However, even if abdominal CT is preferred it is not always available; patient transport may be impossible; ultrasound may be a better initial diagnostic modality (e.g. hepatobiliary disease); or CT may be relatively contraindicated (e.g. pregnancy, risk of contrast nephropathy, or anaphylaxis). Thus, abdominal ultrasound remains a valuable technique in the assessment of the critically ill patient.

Intensivist performed abdominal ultrasonography has the support of international consensus but the experience and training required remains poorly defined (40). Few studies have addressed the feasibility or diagnostic utility of intensivist-performed

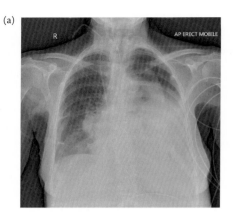

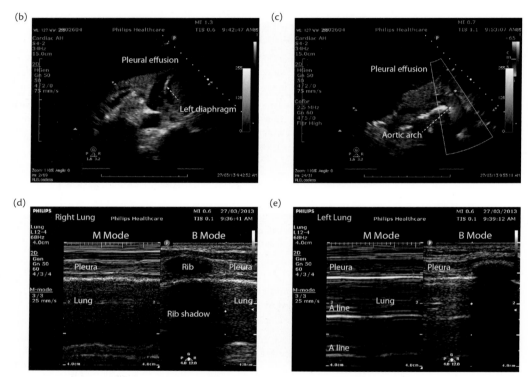

Fig. 28.13 Sudden onset of large pleural effusion and probable pneumothorax.
(a) CXR findings consistent with very large large left pleural effusion and probable pneumothorax. (b) Ultrasound (sector scanner) at base of left lung demonstrating pleural effusion and collapsed left lower lobe. (c) Ultrasound from high posterior left (patient erect) demonstrating collapse of collapse of posterior segments. Note arch of aorta with systolic flow towards transducer. (d) B-mode (2D) and M mode imaging of right chest. A single bright pleural reflection is evident. On M-mode, the pleural reflection separates the linear appearance of the components of the chest wall from the granular appearance of the right lung due to respiratory movement ('sea-shore sign'). This M-mode finding excludes pneumothorax in the right chest. (e) B-mode (2D) and M mode imaging of left chest. Multiple bright pleural reflections are evident on M-mode (A lines). On M-mode, above the pleural reflection the linear appearance of the components of the chest wall is unchanged. However, left lung does not have a granular appearance because of the absence of respiratory movement and instead appears has many linear echos ('stratosphere sign'). This is consistent with pneumothorax, but can be due to any cause that limits respiratory lung movement (e.g. lobar collapse, pleural adhesions). Insertion of chest tube drained both gas and serous fluid. Subsequent diagnosis of oesophageal rupture was made. (See also figure in colour plates section)

abdominal ultrasound. However, similar to diagnostic vascular ultrasonography, there is a well established and successful precedent in the practice of 'focused' abdominal ultrasound performed by Emergency Department physicians and it seems reasonable to expect that ICU physicians could be equally proficient (41,42).

The possible indications for abdominal ultrasound in the ICU are broad and varied, and include both intraperitoneal and retroperitoneal solid organ pathology and the gastrointestinal tract.

(table 28.5: Abdominal ultrasound) The more common indications, such as the diagnosis of: peritoneal fluid, blood, or ascites (and ultrasound guidance for drainage); biliary tract disease especially cholecystitis; and acute obstructive renal disease, especially ureteric obstruction, all lend themselves to focused training of intensivists in the diagnosis of these pathologies (43) (figure 28.18). It is also feasible that an enthusiastic critical care ultrasonographer could screen for many more pathologies including

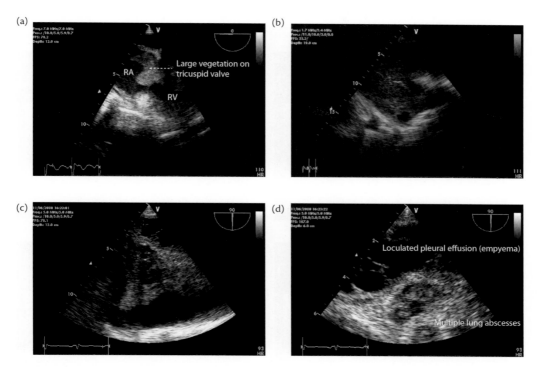

Fig. 28.14 Tricuspid valve endocarditis and respiratory failure.
(a) Mid-oesophageal four chamber view of tricuspid valve demonstrating very large vegetation on septal leaflet (TOE). (b) Complex left pleural effusion with increased echogenicity and linear densities consistent with empyema (sector scanner). (c) TOE of left lung demonstrating complex effusion and lung abscess. (d) TOE of left lung (close up view) demonstrating complex effusion and lung abscess.

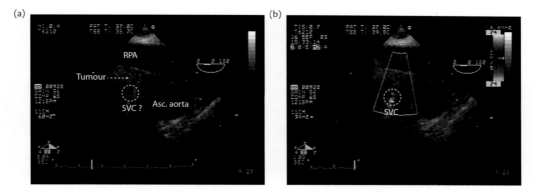

Fig. 28.15 Respiratory failure following aborted aborted right pneumonectomy (bronchogenic SCC).
(a) High oesophageal short axis view of great vessels (TOE). Mass seen between right pulmonary artery and ascending aorta. SVC not clearly visible. (b) Colour flow Doppler. Restricted turbulent flow demonstrated through subtotally occluded SVC. (See also figure in colour plates section)
SVC superior vena cava; RPA right pulmonary artery.

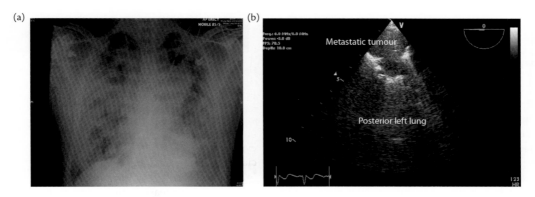

Fig. 28.16 Respiratory failure and metastatic germ cell tumour.
(a) CXR demonstrating widespread discrete opacities in both lungs. (b) Mid-oesophageal view of posterior mediastinum (TOE). Metastatic tumour adjacent to oesophagus.

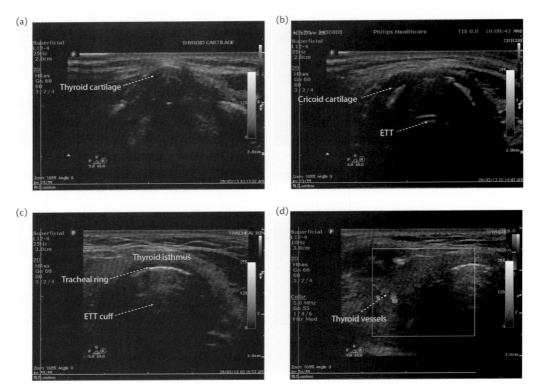

Fig. 28.17 Ultrasound airway assessment prior to tracheostomy (linear probe).
(a) Sharp angle of thyroid cartilage easily demonstrated. (b) Probe slid inferiorly, demonstrating thick round cricoid cartilage. Leading edge of ETT visible. (c) Probe slid further inferiorly demonstrating thinner tracheal ring and multiple reverberation artefact from inflated ETT cuff. Isthmus of thyroid seen anterior to tracheal ring. (d) Colour flow Doppler demonstrating thyroid vessels. (See also figure in colour plates section)
ETT, endotracheal tube.

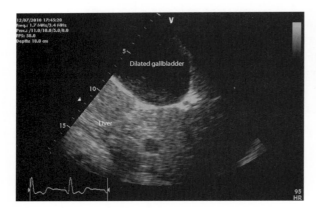

Fig. 28.18 Shock 10 days following heart transplant.
Markedly dilated gallbladder was an incidental finding while performing TTE. Percutaneous drainage of the gall bladder was performed. Enterococcus was isolated on culture of the bile.

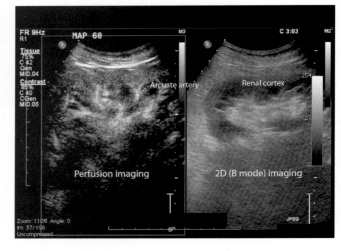

Fig. 28.19 Ultrasound contrast perfusion imaging of kidney.
On right is 2D (B mode) image of right kidney. On the left is the simultaneously acquired perfusion image obtained with continuous infusion of ultrasound contrast, and immediately following 'flash destruction' of microbubbles with a high intensity ultrasound burst.

those not routinely performed by Radiology (e.g. mesenteric ischaemia, small bowel obstruction, inflammatory bowel disease), but this would require considerable training, time, and expertise (44). Continuing development in ultrasound contrast perfusion imaging could potentially allow the real-time evaluation of visceral perfusion, and its response to therapeutic intervention (figure 28.19) (45).

Practical considerations

There are now many reviews and texts that describe the use abdominal ultrasound in the critically ill (3,46).

Table 28.5 Abdominal ultrasonography

	Clinical problem	Comments
Upper GIT	Assess gastric volume and risk of aspiration	Pre-intubation assessment may help prevent pulmonary aspiration of gastric contents (57)
	Cholelithiasis, biliary obstruction, or acute cholecystitis.	Ultrasonography first line investigation (46)
	Ischaemic hepatitis	Patency of portal and hepatic veins can be assessed. Hepatic arterial flow can be assessed with Doppler ultrasound.
		Ultrasound contrast may aid Doppler signal and provide perfusion imaging of liver—mainly experimental at present.
	Dilatation of hepatic veins and IVC	Confirm pericardial disease (tamponade and constriction), severe tricuspid regurgitation and congestive heart failure.
	Splenic abscess and infarction	May be secondary to bacterial endocarditis or systemic embolization.
	Acute pancreatitis	CT usually preferred; associated paralytic ileus may make ultrasound imaging difficult.
Lower GIT (44,58)	Small bowel obstruction	Ultrasound determined bowel dilatation and decreased peristalsis could be more sensitive and specific than plain AXR.
	Acute mesenteric ischaemia	May be difficult because of ileus. Proximal obstruction of SMA may be demonstrable. However, no consensus on Doppler criteria for diagnosis stenosis
		Ultrasound contrast may aid Doppler signal and provide perfusion imaging of small bowel—mainly experimental at present
	Pseudomembranous colitis	Symmetrical bowel thickening supportive but non-specific finding
GIT other	Haemoperitoneum and ascites	Well-established indications
	Pneumoperitoneum	Ring down artefact from non-dependent areas of abdominal wall that shifts with changes in patient positioning and dynamic imaging. Useful if erect CXR or CT not possible
Renal tract (59)	Acute renal failure	Normal sized kidneys with increased parenchymal echogenicity and hypoechoic papillae. Small kidneys supportive of chronic renal disease. Hydronephrosis, ureteric obstruction, and bladder distension can be excluded.
		Renal perfusion can be confirmed and assessed with Doppler ultrasound. High resistance intrarenal arterial consistent with acute tubular necrosis
		Ultrasound contrast may aid Doppler signal and provide perfusion imaging of kidney—mainly experimental at present
Ultrasound-guided procedures	Positioning of gastric tubes	High positive predictive value. Sensitivity limited by amount of interposed bowel gas (60)
	Abdominal paracentesis	Easily learned procedure that may minimize complication rate

AXR, abdominal X-ray; GIT, gastrointestinal tract.

Data from: Perlas, A., et al., Validation of a mathematical model for ultrasound assessment of gastric volume by gastroscopic examination. Anesthesia Analgesia, 2013. 116(2): p. 357–363; Wang, H.-P. and S.-C. Chen, Upper abdominal ultrasound in the critically ill. Critical Care Medicine, 2007. 35(5 Suppl): p. S208–15; Nylund, K., et al., Sonography of the small intestine. World Journal of Gastroenterology, 2009. 15(11): p. 1319–1330; Dietrich, C.F., M. Jedrzejczyk, and A. Ignee, Sonographic assessment of splanchnic arteries and the bowel wall. European Journal of Radiology, 2007. 64(2): p. 202–212.

Probes and machine: Either curvilinear or sector probes can be used. A sector scanner is particularly useful for subcostal and intercostal imaging. A curvilinear probe is better for deeper imaging or large patients.

Patient position: The patient can be either supine, or placed in a more lateral position, in order to displace bowel artefact from obscuring imaging of solid organs, and to image kidney.

Conclusion

Ultrasonography is a valuable imaging modality in the cardio-thoracic ICU. It facilitates rapid, safe diagnosis in the critically ill, can provide an immediate assessment of patient response to therapeutic interventions, and potentially improve the safety of many invasive procedures. Ultrasound contrast imaging can improve image acquisition (e.g. transthoracic imaging in ventilated patients), and potentially provide real-time evaluation of organ perfusion.

Point-of-care ultrasonography presents the critical care physician with both great opportunity and significant responsibility. He or she is uniquely situated to simultaneous perform and interpret the study in the familiar context of pharmacological and mechanical organ supports, diagnose and initiate management accordingly, and repeat the examination as necessary in order to assess response to treatment and refine diagnosis. However, this requires adequate ICU physician training sufficient to the scope of managing a patient in the ICU; selection and use of equipment appropriate to ICU needs; and the experience, knowledge and confidence to know when the specific ultrasound imaging demands are exceeding either the capabilities of the ICU physician or the equipment available, and that specialist referral and imaging is required.

References

1. Nicolaou S, Talsky A, Khashoggi K, Venu V. Ultrasound-guided interventional radiology in critical care. *Crit Care Med* 2007; **35**(5 Suppl): S186–97

2. Kirkpatrick A, Šustic A, Blaivas M. Introduction to the use of ultrasound in critical care medicine. *Crit Care Med* 2007; **35**(5): S123.

3. Moore CL, Copel JA. Point-of-care ultrasonography. *N Engl J Med* 2011; **364**(8): 749–57

4. Royse, CF, Canty DJ, Faris J, Haji DL, Veltman M, Royse A. Core review: physician-performed ultrasound: the time has come for routine use in acute care medicine. *Anesth Analg* 2012; **115**(5): 1007–28

5. Becher H, Tiemann K, Schlosser T, et al. Improvement in endocardial border delineation using tissue harmonic imaging. *Echocardiography* 1998; **15**(5): 511–8

6. Orme RML, Oram MP, McKinstry CE. Impact of echocardiography on patient management in the intensive care unit: an audit of district general hospital practice. *Br J Anaesth* 2009; **102**(3): 340–4

7. Platts DG, Fraser JF. Contrast echocardiography in critical care: echoes of the future? A review of the role of microsphere contrast echocardiography. *Crit Care Resusc* 2011; **13**(1): 44–55

8. Appleton CP, Hatle LK, Popp RL. Cardiac tamponade and pericardial effusion: respiratory variation in transvalvular flow velocities studied by Doppler echocardiography. *J Am Coll Cardiol* 1988; **11**(5): 1020–30

9. Lamperti, M, Bodenham AR, Pittiruti M, et al. International evidence-based recommendations on ultrasound-guided vascular access. *Intens Care Med* 2012; **38**(7): 1105–1710.

10. Shiloh A.L, Savel RH, Paulin LM, Eisen LA. Ultrasound-guided catheterization of the radial artery: a systematic review and meta-analysis of randomized controlled trials. *Chest* 2011; **139**(3): 524–9

11. Theodoro D, Krauss M, Kollef M, Evanoff B. Risk factors for acute adverse events during ultrasound-guided central venous cannulation in the emergency department. *Acad Emerg Med* 2010; **17**(10): 1055–61

12. French JLH, Raine-Fenning NJ, Hardman JG, Bedforth NM. Pitfalls of ultrasound guided vascular access: the use of three/four-dimensional ultrasound. *Anaesthesia* 2008; **63**(8): 806–13

13. Kumar A, nd Chuan A. Ultrasound guided vascular access: efficacy and safety. *Best Pract Res Clin Anaesthesiol* 2009; **23**(3): 299–311

14. Maecken T, Grau T. Ultrasound imaging in vascular access. *Crit Care Med* 2007; **35**(5 Suppl): S178–S185

15. Burnside PR, Brown MD, Kline JA. Systematic review of emergency physician-performed ultrasonography for lower-extremity deep vein thrombosis. *Acad Emerg Med* 2008; **15**(6): 493–8

16. Eiberg JP, Hansen MA, Grønvall Rasmussen JB, Schroeder TV. Minimum training requirement in ultrasound imaging of peripheral arterial disease. *Eur J Vasc Endovasc Surg* 2008; **36**(3): 325–30

17. Meco M, Caratti A, Cirri S. A new and simple method for the correct localization of the intra-aortic balloon: the celiac artery Doppler ultrasound. *Acta Anaesthesiol Scand* 2011; **55**(10): 1284–5

18. Platts DG, Sedgwick JF, Burstow DJ, Mullany DV, Fraser JF. The role of echocardiography in the management of patients supported by extracorporeal membrane oxygenation. *J Am Soc Echocardiogr* 2012; **25**(2): 131–4119.

19. Sidebotham D, McGeorge A, McGuinness S, Edwards M, Willcox T, Beca J. Extracorporeal membrane oxygenation for treating severe cardiac and respiratory failure in adults: part 2-technical considerations. *J Cardiothorac Vasc Anesth* 2010; **24**(1): 164–72

20. Hill JR, Horner PE, Primack SL. ICU imaging. *Clin Chest Med* 2008; **29**(1): 59–76-vi

21. Yu CJ, Yang PC, Chang DB, Luh KT. Diagnostic and therapeutic use of chest sonography: value in critically ill patients. *Am J Roentgenol* 1992; **159**(4): 695–701

22. Tutino L, Cianchi G, Barbani F, Batacchi S, Cammelli R, Peris A. Time needed to achieve completeness and accuracy in bedside lung ultrasound reporting in intensive care unit. *Scand J Trauma Resusc Emerg Med* 2010; **18**: 44

23. Bouhemad B, Zhang M, Lu Q, Rouby JJ. Clinical review: Bedside lung ultrasound in critical care practice. *Crit Care* 2007; **11**(1): 205

24. Mathis G, Lessnau K-D, eds. *Atlas of Chest Sonography*. Berlin: Springer-Verlag, 2003

25. Balik M, Plasil P, Waldauf P, Pazout J, Fric M, Otahal M, et al. Ultrasound estimation of volume of pleural fluid in mechanically ventilated patients. *Intens Care Med* 2006; **32**(2): 318–21

26. Remérand F, Dellamonica J, Mao Z, et al. Multiplane ultrasound approach to quantify pleural effusion at the bedside. *Intens Care Med* 2010; **36**(4): 656–64

27. Yang PC, Luh KT, Chang DB, et al. Value of sonography in determining the nature of pleural effusion: analysis of 320 cases. *Am J Roentgenol* 1992; **159**(1): 29–33

28. Liang S-J, Tu CY, Chen HJ, et al. Application of ultrasound-guided pigtail catheter for drainage of pleural effusions in the ICU. *Intens Care Med* 2009; **35**(2): 350–54

29. Ding W, Shen Y, Yang J, He X, Zhang M. Diagnosis of pneumothorax by radiography and ultrasonography: a meta-analysis. *Chest* 2011; **140**(4): 859–66

30. Volpicelli G. Sonographic diagnosis of pneumothorax. *Intens Care Med* 2011; **37**(2): 224–32

31. Lichtenstein DA. Mezière GA, Lagoueyte JF, Biderman P, Goldstein I, Gepner A. A-lines and B-lines: lung ultrasound as a bedside tool for predicting pulmonary artery occlusion pressure in the critically ill. *Chest* 2009; **136**(4): 1014–20

32. Volpicelli G Elbarbary M, Blaivas M, et al. International evidence-based recommendations for point-of-care lung ultrasound. *Intens Care Med* 2012; **38**(4): 577–91

33. Sustić A. Role of ultrasound in the airway management of critically ill patients. *Crit Care Med* 2007; **35**(5 Suppl): S173–7

34. Lakhal K, Delplace X, Cottier J-P, et al. The feasibility of ultrasound to assess subglottic diameter. *Anesth Analg* 2007; **104**(3): 611–4

35. Flint AC, Midde R, Rao VA, Lasman TE, Ho PT. Bedside ultrasound screening for pretracheal vascular structures may minimize the risks of percutaneous dilatational tracheostomy. *Neurocrit Care* 2009; **11**(3): 372–6

36. Rajajee V. Fletcher JJ, Rochlen LR, Jacobs TL. Real-time ultrasound-guided percutaneous dilatational tracheostomy: a feasibility study. *Crit Care* 2011; **15**(1): R67

37. van Randen A. Laméris W, van Es HW, et al A comparison of the accuracy of ultrasound and computed tomography in common diagnoses causing acute abdominal pain. *Eur Radiol* 2011; **21**(7): 1535–45

38. Schacherer D. Klebl F, Goetz D, et al. Abdominal ultrasound in the intensive care unit: a 3-year survey on 400 patients. *Intens Care Med* 2007; **33**(5): 841–4

39. Slasky BS, Auerbach D, Skolnick ML. Value of portable real-time ultrasound in the ICU. *Crit Care Med*, 1983; **11**(3): 160–4

40. International expert statement on training standards for critical care ultrasonography. *Intens Care Med* 2011; **37**(7): 1077–83

41. Bassler D, Snoey ER, Kim J. Goal-directed abdominal ultrasonography: impact on real-time decision making in the emergency department. *J Emerg Med* 2003; **24**(4): 375–8

42. Gaspari RJ, Dickman E, Blehar D. Learning curve of bedside ultrasound of the gallbladder. *JEM* 2009; **37**(1): 51–6

43. Chalumeau-Lemoine L, Baudel J-L, Das V, et al. Results of short-term training of naïve physicians in focused general ultrasonography in an intensive-care unit. *Intens Care Med* 2009; **35**(10): 1767–71

44. Nylund K, Ødegaard S, Hausken T, et al. Sonography of the small intestine. *World J Gastroenterol* 2009; **15**(11): 1319–30

45. Nicolau C, Ripollés T. Contrast-enhanced ultrasound in abdominal imaging. *Abdominal Imaging* 2012; **37**(1): 1–19

46. Wang H-P, Chen S-C. Upper abdominal ultrasound in the critically ill. *Crit Care Med* 2007; **35**(5 Suppl): S208–15

47. Romero-Bermejo FJ, Ruiz Bailén M, Guerrero-De-Mier M, Lopez-Alvaro J. Echocardiographic hemodynamic monitoring in the critically ill patient. *Curr Cardiol Rev* 2011; **7**(3): 146–56

48. Price S, Prout J, Jaggar SI, Gibson DG, Pepper JR.Tamponade following cardiac surgery: terminology and echocardiography may both mislead. *Eur J Cardio-Thorac Surg* 2004; **26**(6): 1156–60

49. Vieillard-Baron A, Prin S, Chergui K, Dubourg O, Jardin F.Echo-Doppler demonstration of acute cor pulmonale at the bedside in the medical intensive care unit. *Am J RespirCrit Care Med* 2002; **166**(10): 1310–9

50. Kirkpatrick JN, Wiegers SE, Lang RM. Left ventricular assist devices and other devices for end-stage heart failure: utility of echocardiography. *Curr Cardiol Rep* 2010; **12**(3): 257–64

51. Hamper UM, DeJong MR, Scoutt LM. Ultrasound evaluation of the lower extremity veins. *Radiol Clin N Am* 2007; **45**(3): 525–47-ix

52. Weber TM, Lockhart ME, Robbin ML. Upper extremity venous Doppler ultrasound. *Radiol Clin N Am* 2007; **45**(3): 513–24, viii–ix

53. Arbelot C, Ferrari F, Bouhemad B, Rouby J-J.Lung ultrasound in acute respiratory distress syndrome and acute lung injury. *Curr Opin Crit Care* 2008; **14**(1): 70–4

54. Kim WY, Suh HJ, Hong S-B, Koh Y, Lim C-M. Diaphragm dysfunction assessed by ultrasonography: Influence on weaning from mechanical ventilation. *Crit Care Med* 2011; **39**(12): 2627–30

55. Lerolle N, Guérot E, Dimassi S, et al.Ultrasonographic diagnostic criterion for severe diaphragmatic dysfunction after cardiac surgery. *Chest* 2009; **135**(2): 401–7

56. Soummer A, Perbet S, Brisson H, et al.Ultrasound assessment of lung aeration loss during a successful weaning trial predicts postextubation distress. *Crit Care Med* 2012; **40**(7): 2064–72

57. Perlas A, Mitsakakis N, Liu L, et al.Validation of a mathematical model for ultrasound assessment of gastric volume by gastroscopic examination. *Anesth Analg* 2013; **116**(2): 357–63

58. Dietrich CF, Jedrzejczyk M, Ignee A. Sonographic assessment of splanchnic arteries and the bowel wall. *Eur J Radiol* 2007; **64**(2): 202–12

59. Barozzi L, Valentino M, Santoro A, Mancini E, Pavlica P.Renal ultrasonography in critically ill patients. *Crit Care Med* 2007; **35**(5 Suppl): S198–205

60. Chenaitia H, Brun P-M, Querellou E, et al.Ultrasound to confirm gastric tube placement in prehospital management. *Resuscitation* 2012;**83**(4): 447–51

CHAPTER 29

Cardiovascular complications of cardiac surgery

Fabio Guarracino and Rubia Baldassarri

Introduction

The morbidity and mortality associated with cardiac surgery has progressively decreased in the recent years, but cardiovascular complications still significantly impact on the clinical outcome. Although most of the cardiovascular complications of cardiac surgery depend on the surgical procedures, the improvement of both surgery and perioperative care has allowed patients who are very high risk because they are older and have significant comorbidities, to undergo surgery (1,2).

Predisposing factors for developing cardiovascular complications are the type of surgery, patient risk factors, and critically, the preoperative clinical condition (3,4). Considering the high morbidity and mortality associated with the major cardiovascular complications of cardiac surgery, all efforts to reduce the perioperative risk should be undertaken. Despite the limited surgical approach, minimally invasive cardiac surgery is also prone to cardiovascular complications, as well as conventional surgery (5). For these reasons, the aim of this chapter is to review the major cardiovascular complications of heart surgery.

Cardiovascular complications

Perioperative life-threatening cardiovascular events require both a prompt diagnosis and immediate treatment. The main cardiovascular complications of cardiac surgery are:

♦ Cardiac tamponade

♦ Low cardiac output and organ dysfunction

♦ Perioperative myocardial infarction

♦ Arrhythmias

♦ Stroke

♦ Peripheral and mesenteric ischaemia.

Cardiac tamponade

Cardiac tamponade is one of the most serious complications of heart surgery occurring in 0.5–6% of the patients within the first 24–48 postoperative hours (6). The rapid accumulation of blood around the heart increases intrapericardial pressure and compresses the cardiac chambers, leading to obstructive acute heart failure (Chapter 2). In some cases, localized compression on a single chamber or vessel can depend on limited blood collection.

After heart surgery either an excessive postoperative bleeding or the occlusion of the chest drainages by clots, may lead to the accumulation of the blood around the heart.

Diagnosis

On the basis of a strong clinical suspicion based on signs including hypotension, tachycardia, elevated central venous pressure, reduced urine output, pulsus paradoxus, dyspnea, and mental confusion in awake patients, and of a characteristic haemodynamic profile of equalization of pressures in the right and the left heart chambers and a low cardiac output (CO), both transthoracic (TTE) and transoesophageal echocardiography (TOE) can immediately detect the presence of circumferential pericardial effusion compressing the cardiac chambers (7) (figures 2.12 and 29.1). However, clinical signs may be blunted when localized tamponade is present.

Prevention

Current strategies to limit the postoperative bleeding in cardiac surgery are based on the administration of prophylactic drugs to reduce the risk of bleeding and on the use of prohaemostatic agents to ameliorate the coagulation pattern (8,9). Surgical approach based on posterior pericardiotomy has been employed in recent years. Frequent and adequate suction of the chest tubes to avoid clot formation and consequent occlusion reduces the risk of postoperative cardiac tamponade.

Treatment

The only therapeutic management of cardiac tamponade is the evacuation of the pericardial space. Percutaneous (pericardiocentesis) or surgical (resternotomy) approach should be performed according to either the clinical conditions (severe haemodynamic instability, urgency) and the feasibility of the manoeuvre (10). Meanwhile, an adequate volume replacement with allogenic blood units and colloids allows the maintenance of the haemodynamics, while the cardiac function may be sustained with positive inotropic and vasoactive agents

Heart failure

Heart failure can acutely complicate cardiac surgery in about 20% of the cases, impairing the weaning from cardiopulmonary bypass (CPB) in 1% of patients (11). Severe cardiac impairment and cardiogenic shock acutely decrease CO leading to systemic hypoperfusion and organs dysfunction (table 29.1). Both left ventricle (LV) and right ventricle (RV) function can acutely decompensate during cardiac surgery (12).

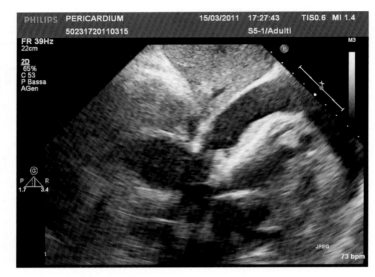

Fig. 29.1 Transthoracic subcostal view showing cardiac tamponade. The cardiac chambers are completely collapsed under by the intrapericardial overpressure. (See also figure in colour plates section)

Table 29.1 Perioperative heart failure: causes and mechanisms

Causes	Mechanism of heart failure
Pre-existing poor cardiac function	Intolerance to cardioplegic standstill, ischaemic–reperfusion injury
Ischaemic–reperfusion injury	Inadequate myocardial protection
	Hypovolaemia
	CPB haemodynamic impairment
	Coronary artery spasm, thrombi, embolism
	Occlusion of the bypass graft (kinking, thrombi, low flow)
Injury to the conductive pathway	Rhythm alterations
Gas-exchange impairment	Hypoxia, hypercapnia acidosis
Uncorrected heart diseases	Valve dysfunction, intracardiac shunt, myocardial hypertrophy
Surgical defects	Prosthetic heart valve dysfunction
	Incomplete revascularization
	Occlusion of the bypass graft

Left ventricular dysfunction

LV systolic function is a main determinant of the CO by providing an adequate stroke volume (SV). Since LV systolic function depends on the myocardial contractility, the LV performance is affected by any alteration of the contractile function. Considering that myocardial contractility is an energy-dependent mechanism, the mismatch of the myocardial oxygen supply–demand balance can acutely decompensate LV systolic function leading to low CO and systemic hypoperfusion. The most common mechanisms of the acute LV systolic dysfunction are myocardial ischaemia, acute myocardial infarction (AMI), and myocardial stunning (13).

During cardiac surgery, different mechanisms can predispose to perioperative myocardial ischaemia altering either the myocardial oxygen delivery (DO_2) or oxygen consumption (VO_2). The contractile myocardial dysfunction leads to regional wall motion abnormalities. According to the distribution of the coronary arteries flow, contractile dysfunction can either extend to one or more ventricular walls or be limited to some segments of them. The extension of the ischaemic injury determines the severity of the LV systolic dysfunction.

Myocardial stunning occurs in about 45% of the patients undergoing elective cardiac surgery. It is represented by viable myocardium that has suffered from prolonged coronary hypoperfusion during heart surgery. Therefore, the causal mechanism of stunning is the ischaemic reperfusion injury. The systolic dysfunction correlated with myocardial stunning is generally transient and responsive to positive inotropes with a complete recovery of the heart function in the early postoperative hours (14).

Perioperative myocardial infarction

AMI occurs when the ischaemic injury leads to myocardial necrosis and definitive damage of the contractile function of the LV in the territory the culprit lesion. Although the main mechanisms of the myocardial infarction is a mismatch between the myocardial oxygen supply and demand and ischaemia–reperfusion injury, thrombosis of the coronary grafts should be suspected when AMI acutely occurs in cardiac surgery patients (15) (table 29.2).

Diagnosis

Depending on the extent of the ischaemic injury and on the regional wall motion abnormalities, acute LV systolic dysfunction can either be completely asymptomatic or lead to cardiogenic shock. Post-cardiac surgery patients should be adequately monitored for myocardial ischaemia and LV systolic dysfunction using:

• continuous electrocardiography (ECG) monitoring, which allows both the analysis of the ST-segment and of the heart rhythm in order to recognize any acute variation;

• basic haemodynamic monitoring providing information about systemic blood pressure, central venous pressure and arterial oxygenation;

Table 29.2 Myocardial ischaemia and blood flow

a) Myocardial ischaemia		
Mismatch DmO_2/VmO_2	Pre-existing critical stenosis	Detectable by preoperative tests
Plaque rupture or thrombosis	No pre-existing critical stenosis	Non detectable
b)	Blood flow through left coronary artery	
	At rest	Exercise
Healthy people	Mainly diastolic	Diastolic and systolic increase
Coronary artery disease	Systolic reversal	No increase

(a) Myocardial oxygen supply demand uncoupling is the most frequent mechanism o myocardial ischaemia especially in patients with pre-existing coronary artery critical stenosis. The other cause of myocardial ischaemia is represented by either the rupture of an atherosclerotic plaque or by the formation of intracoronary thrombi without critical stenosis; (b) distribution of the blood flow through the left coronary artery at rest and during exercise.

- advanced haemodynamic monitoring can be required in patients with clinical manifestation of low CO and systemic hypoperfusion. Despite pulmonary artery catheterization (PAC) being the gold standard for measurement of CO, many less or completely non-invasive monitoring systems have been widely employed in the clinical practice (16). PAC also provides the continuous monitoring of the pulmonary pressures and the mixed venous blood oxygenation (SvO_2).

- both TTE and TOE are extremely helpful to recognize regional wall motion abnormalities detecting myocardial dysfunction (17).

- biochemical markers of myocardial necrosis (troponin-I) should be routinely measured although their elevation is generally delayed respect with the onset of myocardial injury (18).

Prevention

Risk stratification is commonly used to identify the population of cardiac surgery patients that are at risk to develop perioperative cardiac dysfunction. The EuroSCORE is the most used score system in cardiac surgery (3). Other predictors of postoperative cardiac dysfunction are preoperative brain natriuretic peptide (BNP), the amino-terminal fragment of pro-BNP (NT pro-BNP) levels and a preoperative low LV ejection fraction, EF of less than 35% (19,20). Considering that the intraoperative myocardial ischaemia and ischaemic-reperfusion damage are the major causes of perioperative LV systolic failure, every effort to increase myocardial oxygen delivery and to reduce consumption, should be undertaken. Different strategies to induce myocardial protection have been proposed:

- Cardioplegia: hypothermic cardioplegia is commonly employed in cardiac surgery to provide heart standstill (Chapter 15). It reduces the VmO_2 and it reverses the ischaemic injury-carrying oxygen and metabolic substrates. Cold blood cardioplegia is the most commonly employed in adult heart surgery: it provides a good oxygen supply and induces hypothermia. Antegrade and both antegrade and retrograde administration are considered the best strategies for cardioprotection (21).

- Myocardial conditioning: myocardium seems to be protected from ischaemic injury when it is submitted to brief episodes of ischaemia–reperfusion before the potential ischaemic damage occurs. Strategies of ischaemic preconditioning, postconditioning, and remote conditioning have been proposed. The application of this strategy seems to reduce the myocardial ischaemic injury.
  - Ischaemic preconditioning: ischaemic preconditioning can limit the myocardial ischaemic–reperfusion injury, as clearly demonstrated by the postoperative reduction of troponin-I release, by the decreased need for positive inotropic support, by the evidence of higher CO, and shorter intensive care unit (ICU) length of stay (22). The preconditioning action of alogenates has been largely demonstrated in cardiac surgery patients, although the beneficial effects on the clinical outcome are still debated (23).
  - Ischaemic postconditioning: interventional or pharmacological strategies applied when the ischaemic injury occurs is able to reduce the myocardial damage and the extension of the infarct area (24). Intraoperative coronary angioplasty and/or the performance of new coronary bypass grafting can restore the blood flow in the ischaemic territory.
  - Remote ischaemic conditioning: the application of brief ischaemic–reperfusion episodes at the upper limb skeletal muscle seems provide a general myocardial protection. The cardioprotective action of remote conditioning has been demonstrated by different studies (25).

- Hypothermia: it has been largely considered an important strategy to reduce the ischaemic–reperfusion myocardial injury. At very low temperature the VmO_2 is significantly decreased and the heart is less sensitive to the ischaemic damage. Despite the beneficial effects on myocardial protection, systemic hypotermia is associated with high risk of neurological complications and its use is controversial (26).

- Drugs: pharmacological prevention of perioperative ischaemic injury has been clearly demonstrated. The cardioprotective action of anaesthetic drugs, especially the volatile agents, have been widely reported (27,28). Levosimendan infusion ameliorates the LV systolic function by the beneficial effects on the arterial–ventricular coupling. The perioperative administration of levosimendan significantly reduces the myocardial ischaemic injury, improves cardiac performance, and impacts on the clinical outcome (29).

- Surgery: off-pump coronary artery bypass grafting (OPCABG) and minimally invasive heart surgery have been proposed to reduce the ischaemic–reperfusion injury correlated either with CPB or with high surgical stress. Despite the avoidance of cardioplegia and cardiac standstill, OPCABG also predisposes for myocardial ischaemia (30), because of either the surgical manipulation of the heart or of the increased myocardial VO_2. The surgical stress, and the alteration of the relationship between the coronary artery blood flow and vascular resistance typically present in patients with coronary artery disease, are important mechanisms of ischaemic injury during off-pump surgery.

- IABP: the intra-aortic balloon pump (IABP) reduces the left ventricle afterload and improves diastolic coronary artery perfusion by the mechanism on intra-aortic counterpulsation. IABP

Table 29.3 Perioperative heart failure: the severity of the heart dysfunction and the clinical manifestations direct the appropriate treatment

Severity of the heart dysfunction	Clinical scenario	Treatment
Mild to moderate heart failure	Difficult weaning from CPB	Volaemic assessment, low doses of positive inotropes and/or vasopressors to maintain SBP>80 mmHg and/or CI >1.8 L/min/m^2
Cardiogenic shock	Low cardiac output syndrome (SBP < 80 mmHg and/or CI < 1.8 L/min/m^2)	Volaemic assessment, high doses of positive inotropes and/or vasopressors, eventual mechanical support (IAPB) to maintain SBP >80 mmHg and/or CI >1.8 L/min/m^2
Refractory cardiogenic shock	Low cardiac output syndrome. Haemodynamic instability non-responsive to maximal treatment (SBP < 80 mmHg and/or CI <1.8 L/min/m^2)	Volaemic assessment, increasing doses of positive inotropes and/or vasopressors, mechanical support (IAPB) to maintain SBP >80 mmHg and/or CI >1.8 L/min/m^2. ECMO, VAD
Cardiac arrest		CPR

SPB, systolic blood pressure; CI, cardiac index; CPB. cardiopulmonary bypass; IAPB, intraortic balloon pump; VAD, ventricular assist device; ECMO, extracorporeal membrane oxygenation; CPR, cardiopulmonary resuscitation.

significantly decreases the heart work, restoring an adequate balance between the oxygen supply and demand. For all these reasons the employment of IABP is particularly indicated when coronary hypoperfusion is either documented or suspected (31).

Treatment

Post-cardiac surgery patients who develop clinical evidence of myocardial ischaemia complicated by low CO syndrome (systemic hypotension, tachycardia, metabolic acidosis, and decreased urine output) and haemodynamic instability, generally require either pharmacological treatment or mechanical support (table 29.3). According to the clinical conditions and to the TOE data on LV systolic function, the persistence of low cardiac output (cardiac index less than 1.8 L/min/m^2), despite the optimization of the loading conditions and under pharmacological therapy with positive inotropes and vasoconstrictors, generally requires mechanical support. Adult postcardiotomy cardiogenic shock potentially requiring mechanical support (IAPB, LV assist devices) occurs in 0.5% to 1.5% of cases (32).

♦ Cardiac preload should be adequately assessed before the administration of positive inotropes and vasopressors. Assessing a dynamic index of preload using the concept of fluid responsiveness seem to better reflect the volaemic state than simply using the filling pressures (33).

♦ Positive inotropic agents should be considered in a stepwise fashion:

  • mild heart dysfunction; low dose of dopamine to both improve LV ejection and increase heart rate so increasing CO (34)
  • moderate to severe heart dysfunction impairing weaning from CPB: low to moderate doses of inodilators such as enoximone or milrinone are generally provide an adequate SV and reduce pulmonary artery pressure (35)
  • severe heart dysfunction: the administration of levosimendan should be considered either to increase the SV and restoration of the arterial-ventricular coupling (36); low-dose epinephrine support should be considered
  • use vasopressors such as norepinephrine or vasopressin to maintain adequate perfusion pressure when vasoplegia and low systemic blood pressure are present.

♦ Consider rescue coronary angioplasty or surgical reintervention when the thrombosis of one or more of the coronary artery bypass grafts is suspected or confirmed.

♦ About 2–6% of the patients submitted to elective cardiac surgery develop refractory cardiogenic shock and some require extracorporeal membrane oxygenation (ECMO) support (37). In recent years the usage of ECMO has progressively increased, because of both the improvement of technologies and the advancements in cardiorespiratory support (Chapter 12). ECMO is associated with serious complications. Bleeding and thromboembolic events can occur in patients on ECMO, often leading to dramatic consequences. The balance between the anticoagulation required for ECMO and the coagulation needed for the postoperative hemostasis is the real challenge for the management of these patients (8).

Right ventricular dysfunction

RV failure can acutely complicate heart surgery (38). The most common cause of RV impairment is ischaemic–reperfusion injury in the area of the right coronary artery (myocardial stunning and/or AMI), or of the circumflex artery in patients who have a dominant left coronary blood flow, and the acute increase of the afterload secondary to pulmonary embolism, acute mitral valve insufficiency, or severe LV dysfunction.

Diagnosis

The acute decompensation of the RV should be suspected in cardiac surgery patients with severe haemodynamic instability and clinical signs of RV overload including jugular veins distention, high CVP and peripheral oedema. Difficulty weaning from mechanical ventilation should also suggest investigation of RV function. Electrocardiograph (ECG) and chest X-ray may be either normal or nonspecifically altered. TOE is the most useful diagnostic tool for the evaluation of the RV failure because it allows evaluation of both RV morphology and function (39).

Prevention

Protect myocardial contractility: any effort to preserve myocardial contractility from the ischaemic–reperfusion injury should be performed. Antegrade cardioplegia is preferable because the coronary sinus primarily drains the left portion of the coronary flow (40).

Preload: an adequate preload should be provided to maintain a sufficient RV ejection, also in the presence of increased afterload.

Increased pulmonary vascular resistance (PVR) and pulmonary hypertension: CPB, mechanical ventilation, LV dysfunction occurring in open-heart operations can independently increase the PVR leading to pulmonary hypertension. Adequate ventilatory pattern employing low inspiratory pressures and providing good oxygenation is mandatory. Inhaled nitric oxide may be considered.

The most common cause of RV myocardial infarction is the occlusion of the right coronary artery because of graft thrombosis or air embolism (41). Intraoperative TOE is fundamental to promptly reveal sudden alterations of the RV walls' kinesis and the passage of air bubbles into the right coronary artery at the separation from the CPB. Any effort to either avoid or reduce the increase in PVR should be undertaken.

Mechanical ventilation and the respiratory parameters can contribute to increase the PVR leading to pulmonary hypertension. For this reason, the employment of a ventilatory pattern with low inspiratory pressures is fundamental to reduce the RV afterload. Adequate ventilatory pattern to maintain a good gas-exchange (PaO_2, $PaCO_2$, and pH) is also required.

Maintenance of sinus rhythm is of paramount importance.

Treatment

RV dysfunction following cardiac surgery often requires aggressive management (42). Once all the strategies to minimize RV impairment have been unsuccessfully employed, pharmacological and/or mechanical support can be necessary to restore RV function (43).

Positive inotropes are indicated when poor myocardial contractility is the first mechanism of RV dysfunction. As afterload is one of the main factors influencing RV ejection, inodilators such as the phosphodiesterase inhibitors including enoximone, amrinone, milrinone or the calcium sensitizer, levosimendan that both increase myocardial contractility and reduce PVR by pulmonary vasodilatation are employed when RV dysfunction occurs (44).

Alpha-adrenergic agonists, such as norepinephrine (noradrenaline), to maintain a normal systemic arterial pressure play a major role in providing adequate coronary flow to the right ventricle wall. Importantly, it should be kept in mind that while left coronary flow occurs mainly during diastole, the right coronary flow depends on mean systemic arterial pressure.

Specific drugs can be used to reduce PVR and RV afterload when severe pulmonary hypertension occurs. Nitric oxide (NO) induces pulmonary vasodilatation by acting on the smooth muscle of the pulmonary vessels. It can be used for short-term treatment of perioperative pulmonary hypertension in mechanical ventilated patients. Prostaglandin E_1 has been employed for the powerful vasodilatation induced in the pulmonary vessels. Because the systemic vasodilatation and hypotension associated with the usage of IV prostaglandin E_1, inhalatory prostacycline has been recommended (45).

The use of mechanical support as RV-assisted devices are indicated when RV dysfunction is refractory to the common therapy and leads to severe cardiogenic shock.

Organ failure

Low CO leads to systemic hypoperfusion and tissue oxygen supply demand mismatch, so that multiorgan failure may occur. The peripheral organs that are most sensitive to hypoperfusion include kidney, the brain and the splanchnic organs, quickly decompensate.

Acute kidney injury

Acute kidney injury (AKI) can complicate elective cardiac surgery, even in patients with normal renal function, in about 30% of the surgical population. However, only 1–5% of the AKI patients develop chronic renal failure requiring dialysis (46). Postoperative AKI is strongly associated with an increasing morbidity and mortality (47). However, according to the literature, the incidence of postoperative AKI is extremely variable because of the different definitions used to identify the disease. AKI following cardiac surgery is more extensively reviewed in Chapter 31.

Mesenteric infarction

Mesenteric infarction is one of the most serious complications of cardiac surgery. Although its incidence is quite low (<0.5%), the associated mortality rate is >50% (48). Predisposing risk factors for the development of postoperative intestinal ischaemia have been identified: advanced age, prolonged CPB, haemodynamic instability, heart failure requiring IABP employment and/or high positive inotropic support, peripheral vascular disease, emergency cardiac surgery, and postoperative AKI are the most important.

Intestinal ischaemia arises from the low perfusion in the territory of the mesenteric arteries. It can be due either to systemic hypotension and consequent organ hypoperfusion as happens in low CO syndrome, or to the thrombosis of the mesenteric vessel consequently to the mobilization of thrombi from the cardiac chambers, as can occur in patients with atrial fibrillation. Mesenteric ischaemia following cardiac surgery is more extensively reviewed in Chapter 31.

Acute lower limb ischaemia

Acute lower limb ischaemia is a life-threatening disease, generally due to the acute arterial occlusion, with consequent ischaemic injury of the limb. Following cardiac surgery, acute lower limb ischaemia may be embolic or thrombotic. Embolic sources are intracardiac thrombi, including atrial fibrillation, congestive heart failure, cardiac masses, and endocarditic vegetations (49). Thrombotic occlusion of the lower limb arteries may be caused by coagulopathy. Low CO and poor heart function can be complicated by peripheral ischaemia because of systemic hypoperfusion. Peripheral arterial cannulation for mechanical devices predisposes to acute arterial occlusion and consequent lower limb ischaemia (50).

Arrhythmias

Atrial fibrillation (AF), with an incidence from 20 to 40%, is one of the most common rhythm disturbances occurring after cardiac surgery (51). AF generally onsets acutely in the second or third postoperative day, although it may present earlier or later. Although AF is a benign and self-limited event in most cases, sometimes it causes a severe reduction of the CO, haemodynamic instability, and organ dysfunction. Because of its associated complications, AF impacts on both short- and long-term morbidity and mortality (52). It seems likely that postoperative AF affects long-term survival in patients undergoing isolated CABG surgery, whereas late mortality after heart valve surgery and combined procedures is less influenced by the onset of postoperative AF (53).

Table 29.4 Predisposing factors (left) and perioperative mechanisms of atrial fibirillation (right)

Predisposing factors	Perioperative mechanisms
◆ History of AF	◆ Surgical trauma
◆ Age	◆ Inadequate cardioprotection
◆ Preoperative electrocardiographic alterations (P-wave duration >110 ms)	◆ Incomplete cooling of the atrium
	◆ Withdraw of preoperative beta-blockers therapy
◆ Systemic hypertension	◆ Increased sympathetic tone
◆ Chronic obstructive pulmonary disease	
◆ Preoperative use of digoxin	
◆ Mitral valve surgery	

The most significant complications of AF are thromboembolic events including stroke, peripheral ischaemia, AMI, AKI, and low CO syndrome.

Diagnosis

The diagnosis of new onset AF is generally easy and immediate because of the continuous ECG monitoring provided to all post-cardiac surgery patients in the first postoperative days. Basic haemodynamic monitoring can promptly reveal both the rhythm variation and the haemodynamic impairment. Awake patients can experience symptoms as palpitation, mental confusion, and dyspnoea when systemic hypotension and heart failure occur. AF can acutely decompensate pre-existing poor heart function especially in heart valve surgery patient.

Echocardiography is the best diagnostic tool to asses heart function in patients with haemodynamic instability. TOE is also particularly useful to evaluate the presence of thrombi in the left appendage when an electrical cardioversion is required

Prevention

Postoperative AF impacts on short- and long-term morbidity and mortality, increases hospital stay, and the incidence of ICU readmission, with consequent additional cost of care (54). Perioperative risk stratification for postoperative AF would be favourable. The most largely recognized predicting factors for the developing of postoperative AF are reported in table 29.4 (55).

The new onset of postoperative AF has been correlated to the kind of cardiac surgery. CABG is more often associated with new onset AF than both heart valve surgery and combined surgery. Despite the lack of randomized controlled trials, recent investigations have reported that OPCAB grafting significantly reduces the incidence of postoperative AF (56).

Preoperative beta-blockers seem reduce the incidence of postoperative AF in cardiac surgery (57).

The prevention of postoperative stroke related to new onset AF requires adjusted oral anticoagulation therapy. Many trials have recently demonstrated the superiority of warfarin in reducing the incidence of postoperative stroke with respect to the administration of both aspirin alone and the association between aspirin and clopidrogel (58). Despite the risk of bleeding is increased in cardiac surgery patients, target-controlled oral anticoagulants is strongly recommended.

Treatment

Current guidelines recommends electrical cardioversion for the management of new onset AF with haemodynamic instability. Beta-adrenergic blockers are the first choice in haemodynamically stable patients, and amiodarone is recommended when beta-blockers are contraindicated. The high incidence of postoperative stroke in patients with AF suggests the early administration of anticoagulant therapy. The adequate balance between the risk of bleeding and the risk of thromboembolic events should be individually assessed (59). Intraoperative procedures as the closure of the left appendage and the maze procedure can be effective in reduce the postoperative incidence of AF (60). Electrical cardioversion should be considered in AF refractory to pharamacologi treatment.

Stroke

Postoperative stroke causing severe neurological dysfunction, and invalidating peripheral neurological diseases, can complicate cardiac surgery and impact on the clinical outcome. The incidence of postoperative stoke ranges from 1 to 8%, while there is a significant variability of the incidence of postoperative cognitive impairment that actually persists. The risk of postoperative stroke is highly increased, up to fivefold, by the occurrence of AF. Stroke in cardiac surgery is extensively reviewed in Chapter 32.

Conclusion

Some of the most serious complications that occur after cardiac surgery are cardiovascular. Indeed, they can be life threatening or cause permanent disability. Therefore, a sound understanding of the cardiovascular complications that may arise after cardiac surgery is essential for their prevention, diagnosis and treatment.

References

1. Landoni G, Rodseth RN, Santini F, et al. Randomized evidence for reduction of perioperative mortality. *J Cardiothorac Vasc Anesth* 2012; **26**: 764–72
2. Society of Thoracic Surgeons: 2006 Adult Cardiac Database Executive Summary. Available from http://www.sts.org Accessed April 2007.
3. Nashef SA, Roques F, Michel P, Gauducheau E, Lemeshow S, Salamon R. European system for cardiac operative risk evaluation (EuroSCORE). *Eur J Cardiothorac Surg* 1999; **16**: 9–13
4. Deiwick M, Tandler R, Möllhoff T, et al. Heart surgery in patients aged eighty years and above: determinants of morbidity and mortality. *Thorac Cardiovasc Surg* 1997; **45**: 119–26
5. Holzhey DM, Cornely JP, Rastan AJ, Davierwala P, Mohr FW. Review of a 13-year single-center experience with minimally invasive direct coronary artery bypass as the primary surgical treatment of coronary artery disease. *Heart Surg Forum* 2012; **15**: E61–8
6. Bodson L, Bouferrache K, Vieillard-Baron A. Cardiac tamponade. *Curr Opin Crit Care* 2011; **17**: 416–24
7. Guarracino F, Baldassarri R Transesophageal echocardiography in the OR and ICU. *Minerva Anestesiol* 2009; **75**: 518–29
8. Ranucci M, Baryshnikova E, Colella D. Monitoring prohemostatic treatment in bleeding patients. *Semin Thromb Hemost* 2012; **38**: 282–91
9. Levy JH, Sniecinski RM. Prohemostatic treatment in cardiac surgery. *Semin Thromb Hemost* 2012; **38**: 237–43
10. Seferović PM, Ristić AD, Imazio M, et al. Management strategies in pericardial emergencies. *Herz* 2006; **31**: 891–900
11. Widyastuti Y, Stenseth R, Berg KS, Pleym H, Wahba A, Videm V. Preoperative and intraoperative prediction of risk of cardiac dysfunction following open heart surgery. *Eur J Anaesthesiol* 2012; **29**: 143–51

12. Dickstein K, Cohen-Solal A, Filippatos G, et al. ESC Committee for Practice Guidelines (CPG).ESC Guidelines for the diagnosis and treatment of acute and chronic heart failure 2008: the Task Force for the Diagnosis and Treatment of Acute and Chronic Heart Failure 2008 of the European Society of Cardiology. Developed in collaboration with the Heart Failure Association of the ESC (HFA) and endorsed by the European Society of Intensive Care Medicine (ESICM). *Eur Heart J* 2008; **29**: 2388–442

13. Buja LM. Myocardial ischemia and reperfusion injury. *Cardiovasc Pathol* 2005; **14**: 170–5

14. Rudiger A, Businger F, Streit M, Schmid ER, Maggiorini M, Follath F. Presentation and outcome of critically ill medical and cardiac-surgery patients with acute heart failure. *Swiss Med Wkly* 2009; **139**: 110–6

15. Landesberg G, Beattie WS, Mosseri M, Jaffe AS, Alpert JS. Perioperative myocardial infarction. *Circulation* 2009; **119**: 2936–44

16. Vincent JL, Rhodes A, Perel A, et al. Clinical review: Update on hemodynamic monitoring—a consensus of 16. *Crit Care* 2011; **15**: 229

17. Cheitlin MD, Armstrong WF, Aurigemma GP, et al. ACC; AHA; ASE. ACC/AHA/ASE 2003 Guideline Update for the Clinical Application of Echocardiography: summary article. A report of the American College of Cardiology/American Heart Association Task Force on Practice Guidelines (ACC/AHA/ASE Committee to Update the 1997 Guidelines for the Clinical Application of Echocardiography). *J Am Soc Echocardiogr* 2003; **16**: 1091–110

18. Kociol RD, Pang PS, Gheorghiade M, Fonarow GC, O'Connor CM, Felker GM. Troponin elevation in heart failure prevalence, mechanisms, and clinical implications. *J Am Coll Cardiol* 2010; **56**: 1071–8

19. Eliasdottir SB, Klemenzson G, Torfason B, Valsson F. Brain natriuretic peptide is a good predictor for outcome in cardiac surgery. *Acta Anaesthesiol Scand* 2008; **52**: 182–7

20. Venugopal V, Ludman A, Yellon DM, Hausenloy DJ. 'Conditioning' the heart during surgery. *Eur J Cardiothorac Surg* 2009; **35**: 977–87

21. Weisel RD. Blood or crystalloid cardioplegia: which is better? *Eur J Cardiothorac Surg* 2013; **43**: 532–3

22. Yu CH, Beattie WS. The effects of volatile anesthetics on cardiac ischemic complications and mortality in CABG: a meta-analysis. *Can J Anaesth* 2006; **53**: 906–18

23. Thibault H, Piot C, Ovize M. Postconditioning in man. *Heart Fail Rev* 2007; **12**: 245–8

24. Thibault H, Piot C, Staat P, et al. Long-term benefit of postconditioning. *Circulation* 2008; **117**: 1037–44

25. Mansour Z, Charles AL, Bouitbir J, et al. Remote and local ischemic postconditioning further impaired skeletal muscle mitochondrial function after ischemia-reperfusion. *J Vasc Surg* 2012; **56**: 774–82

26. Todaro MC, Oreto L, Gupta A, Bajwa T, Khandheria BK. Hypothermia: a double-edged sword. *Cardiology* 2012; **122**: 126–8

27. De Hert S, Cromheecke S, ten Broecke P. Effects of propofol, desflurane, and sevoflurane on recovery of myocardial function after coronary surgery in elderly high-risk patients. *Anesthesiology* 2003; **99**: 314–23

28. Conzen PF, Fischer S, Detter C, Peter K. Sevoflurane provides greater protection to the myocardium than propofol in patients undergoing offpump coronary artery bypass surgery. *Anesthesiology* 2003; **99**: 826–33

29. De Hert SG, Lorsomradee S, Cromheecke S, Van der Linden PJ. The effects of levosimendan in cardiac surgery patients with poor left ventricular function. *Anesth Analg* 2007; **104**: 766–73

30. Møller CH, Penninga L, Wetterslev J, Steinbrüchel DA, Gluud C. Off-pump versus on-pump coronary artery bypass grafting for ischaemic heart disease. *Cochrane Database Syst Rev* 2012; **3**: CD007224

31. Cheng JM, den Uil CA, Hoeks SE, et al. Percutaneous left ventricular assist devices vs. intra-aortic balloon pump counterpulsation for treatment of cardiogenic shock: a meta-analysis of controlled trials. *Eur Heart J* 2009; **30**: 2102–8

32. Rastan AJ, Dege A, Mohr M, et al. Early and late outcomes of 517 consecutive adult patients treated with extracorporeal membrane oxygenation for refractory postcardiotomy cardiogenic shock. *J Thorac Cardiovasc Surg* 2010; **139**: 302–11, 311

33. Cavallaro F, Sandroni C, Antonelli M. Functional hemodynamic monitoring and dynamic indices of fluid responsiveness. *Minerva Anestesiol* 2008; **74**: 123–35

34. Tarr TJ, Moore NA, Frazer RS, Shearer ES, Desmond MJ. Haemodynamic effects and comparison of enoximone, dobutamine and dopamine following mitral valve surgery. *Eur J Anaesthesiol Suppl* 1993, **8**: 15–24

35. Boldt J, Knothe C, Zickmann B, et al. The role of enoximone in cardiac surgery. *Br J Anaesth* 1992; **69**: 45–50

36. Guarracino F, Cariello C, Danella A, et al. Effect of levosimendan on ventriculo-arterial coupling in patients with ischemic cardiomyopathy. *Acta Anaesthesiol Scand* 2007; **51**: 1217–24

37. Pokersnik JA, Buda T, Bashour CA, Gonzalez-Stawinski GV. Have changes in ECMO technology impacted outcomes in adult patients developing postcardiotomy cardiogenic shock? *J Card Surg* 2012; **27**: 246–52

38. Kevin LG, Barnard M. Right ventricular failure. *Contin Educ Anaesth Crit CarePain* 2007; **7**: 89–94

39. Ahmad H, Mor-Avi V, Lang RM, et al. Assessment of right Vventricular function using echocardiographic speckle tracking of the tricuspid annular motion: comparison with cardiac magnetic resonance. *Echocardiography* 2011; **29**: 19–24

40. Honkonen EL, Kaukinen L, Pehkonen EJ, Kaukinen S. Myocardial cooling and right ventricular function in patients with right coronary artery disease: antegrade vs. retrograde cardioplegia. *Acta Anaesthesiol Scand* 1997; **41**: 287–96

41. Chen YL, Hang CL, Fang HY, et al. Comparison of prognostic outcome between left circumflex artery-related and right coronary artery-related acute inferior wall myocardial infarction undergoing primary percutaneous coronary intervention. *Clin Cardiol* 2011; **34**: 249–53

42. Lahm T, McCaslin CA, Wozniak TC, et al. Medical and surgical treatment of acute right ventricular failure. *J Am Coll Cardiol* 2010; **56**: 1435–46

43. Boeken U, Feindt P, Litmathe J, Kurt M, Gams E. Intraaortic balloon pumping in patients with right ventricular insufficiency after cardiac surgery: parameters to predict failure of IABP Support. *Thorac Cardiovasc Surg* 2009; **57**: 324–8

44. Toller W, Algotsson L, Guarracino F, et al. Perioperative use of levosimendan: best practice in operative settings. *J Cardiothorac Vasc Anesth* 2013; **27**: 361–6

45. Tritapepe L, Voci P, Cogliati AA, Pasotti E, Papalia U, Menichetti A. Successful weaning from cardiopulmonary bypass with central venous prostaglandin E1 and left atrial norepinephrine infusion in patients with acute pulmonary hypertension. *Crit Care Med* 1999; **27**: 2180–3

46. Doddakula K, Al-Sarraf N, Gately K, et al. Predictors of acute renal failure requiring renal replacement therapy post cardiac surgery in patients with preoperatively normal renal function. *Interact Cardiovasc Thorac Surg* 2007; **6**: 314–8

47. Rosner MH, Okusa MD. Acute kidney injury associated with cardiac surgery. *Clin J Am Soc Nephrol* 2006; **1**: 19–32

48. Pang PYK, Sin YK, Lim CH, Su JW, Chua YL. Outcome and survival analysis of intestinal ischaemia following cardiac surgery. *Interact Cardiovasc Thorac* 2012; **15**: 215–8

49. Pepi M, Evangelista A, Nihoyannopoulos P, et al. European Association of Echocardiography. Recommendations for echocardiography use in the diagnosis and management of cardiac sources of embolism: European Association of Echocardiography (EAE) (a registered branch of the ESC). *Eur J Echocardiogr* 2010; **11**: 461–76

50. Foley PJ, Morris RJ, Woo EY,et al. Limb ischemia during femoral cannulation for cardiopulmonary support. *J Vasc Surg* 2010; **52**: 850–3

51. Jongnarangsin K, Oral H. Postoperative atrial fibrillation. *Cardiol Clin* 2009; **27**: 69–78

52. Bramer S, Ter Woorst FJ, van Geldorp MW, et al. Does new-onset postoperative atrial fibrillation after coronary artery bypass grafting affect postoperative quality of life? *J Thorac Cardiovasc Surg* 2012; **146**: 114–8

53. Shantsila E, Watson T, Lip GY. Atrial fibrillation post-cardiac surgery: changing perspectives [review]. *Curr Med Res Opin* 2006; **22**: 1437–41

54. Amar D, Shi W, Hogue CW, Jr., et al. Clinical prediction rule for atrial fibrillation after coronary artery bypass grafting. *J Am Coll Cardiol* 2004; **44**: 1248–53

55. Mariscalco G, Engström KG. Postoperative atrial fibrillation is associated with late mortality after coronary surgery, but not after valvular surgery. *Ann Thorac Surg* 2009; **88**: 1871–6

56. Zhu J, Wang C, Gao D, et al. Meta-analysis of amiodarone versus beta-blocker as a prophylactic therapy against atrial fibrillation following cardiac surgery. *Intern Med J* 2012; **42**: 1078–87

57. Camm AJ, Kirchhof P, Lip GY, et al. Guidelines for the management of atrial fibrillation: the Task Force for the Management of Atrial Fibrillation of the European Society of Cardiology (ESC). *Eur Heart J* 2010; **31**: 2369–429

58. Cairns JA, Connolly S, McMurtry S, et al. CCS Atrial Fibrillation Guidelines Committee. Canadian Cardiovascular Society Atrial Fibrillation Guidelines 2010: prevention of stroke and systemic thromboembolism in atrial fibrillation and flutter. *Can J Cardiol* 2011; **27**: 74–90

59. Malaisrie SC, Lee R, Kruse J, et al. Atrial fibrillation ablation in patients undergoing aortic valve replacement. *J Heart Valve Dis* 2012; **21**: 350–7

60. Leal S, Moreno R, de Sousa Almeida M, Silva JA, Lopez-Sendon JL. Evidence-based percutaneous closure of the left atrial appendage in patients with atrial fibrillation. *Curr Cardiol Rev* 2012; **8**: 37–42

CHAPTER 30

Pulmonary complications after cardiac surgery

Rainer Thell and Michael Hiesmayr

Introduction

Pulmonary dysfunction remains a potential complication after cardiac surgery that can lead to increases in durations of stay in intensive care unit (ICU) and hospital, the cost of health care and mortality. Pulmonary complications significantly contribute to extracardiac early postoperative morbidity. Post-mortem studies have shown that 5–8% of deaths after cardiac surgery can be attributed to pulmonary reasons (1). The risk of pulmonary complications is associated with preoperative chronic lung disease, smoking, higher age, and frailty, in addition to intraoperative factors such as physical manipulation of the lungs, cardiopulmonary bypass (CPB) associated inflammation, fluid management, and postoperative factors such as weaning strategy, cardiac function, mobilization, and pain control. The aim of this chapter is to describe risk factors and a comprehensive preventive and treatment strategy. In addition, we will attempt to link clinical symptoms, understanding of aetiology, and therapeutic decisions.

Risk factors

Chronic obstructive lung disease

Chronic obstructive lung disease (COPD) is a major independent risk factor for mortality post cardiac surgery (2). COPD that requires treatment with either bronchodilators or steroids is included in the new EuroScore II, a scoring system to evaluate 30-day mortality (3). Based on this system, COPD increases the relative risk of death by 20% and is equivalent to being 7 years older. One third of patients with a history of COPD have no signs of obstruction in pulmonary function tests.

Smoking

The risk of pulmonary complications of smokers was found to be twice as high as in non- or ex-smokers who had quit smoking for at least 6 months (4).

Pulmonary hypertension

Chronic pulmonary disease may be associated with pulmonary hypertension. Moderately raised systolic pulmonary artery pressures from 31 to 55 mmHg increases the risk of death to a similar extent as COPD, whereas severe hypertension >55 mmHg increases the risk twice as much.

Obstructive sleep apnoea

Obstructive sleep apnoea, a condition associated with upper airway obstruction during sleep, is often undiagnosed but may increase the risk of postoperative hypercapnia and hypoxia, and thus of acute right heart failure.

Malnutrition

Acute and chronic malnutrition is associated with a high risk of pulmonary complications. Starvation for a few days decreases the responsiveness of the respiratory system to hypoxia and to increases in metabolic demand (5,6).

Congestive heart failure

Heart failure is a strong predictor of pulmonary complications because of a higher risk of pulmonary oedema. Pulmonary oedema increases work of breathing and impairs oxygenation. Heart failure is often associated with loss of appetite and signs of malnutrition.

Cardiopulmonary bypass

A profound systemic inflammatory response to cardiac surgery is considered to arise from contact of blood with the surface of the CPB bypass circuit, contact of blood with air in the cardiotomy reservoir, reperfusion injury, and operative tissue injury (Chapter 5). Activated white blood cells are largely sequestered in the lung during reperfusion. The inflammatory response in off-pump coronary artery bypass grafting (CABG) surgery is less pronounced, with decreased induction of cytokine response, complement activation as well as lower neutrophil and monocyte count but virtually no effect on pulmonary gas exchange (7–10). In addition, the lung is prone to suffer from interruption of blood flow through the pulmonary artery. The consequence is partial ischaemia, liberation of vasoactive agents like thromboxane, and adhesion of leukocytes to endothelial cells. On partial CPB compared to total CPB these effects are much less pronounced (11,12).

Age

Older age is a risk factor that cannot be modified and will become more and more prevalent with the ongoing demographic development in many developed countries. With aging, the lung undergoes profound changes such as decrease of alveolar surface, decrease in capillary density, loss of elastic fibres, and increased airway collapse but also increased stiffness of the chest wall and decreased force of the diaphragm and intercostal muscles (13). Age effects are best appraised with a frailty assessment score, which usually includes spirometry (14).

Diaphragmatic atrophy

Mechanical ventilation induces a diaphragmatic atrophy caused by an increased protein breakdown, while protein synthesis is also decreased (15).

Swallowing disorders

Dysphagia is relatively common even after few days of ventilation and favours aspiration and pulmonary complications (16). Several risk factors such as higher age, diabetes, malnutrition, and use of transoesophageal echocardiography may explain the higher incidence after cardiac surgery.

Signs and symptoms

Early detection and treatment of pulmonary complications is essential for patient outcome. Key symptoms are hypoxia, hypercapnia, and abnormal respiratory rate that are linked with frequent and rare complications (see figure 30.1). The diagnostic categories that need to be considered depend on the severity of the clinical symptoms and the rate of change. Respiratory symptoms that are accompanied by a sudden change in circulatory conditions should prompt immediate diagnostic and therapeutic action (see figure 30.1). Haemoptysis is observed sometimes in patients on ventricular assist device or extracoporeal membrane oxygenation (ECMO). The combination of chronic anticoagulant use, often low-molecular weight heparins (LMWHs) in the initial phase, and depletion of coagulation factors such as factor XIII favours spontaneous bleeding from the lungs or the intestine.

Pulmonary complications

Atelectasis

Atelectasis is diagnosed by chest X-ray in the majority of patients. They occur through artificial ventilation, manual compression during the operative procedure, and lung collapse during CPB. Harvesting of the internal mammary artery, opening the pleura, prolonged duration of CPB, fluid overload, or poor pain relief increase the risk of atelectasis, but specific diagnostic steps are only necessary for extensive atelectasis that does not respond to treatment. Atelectasis may not have a large effect on arterial blood gas analysis, when the pulmonary vascular reactivity to local hypoxia is preserved. Nevertheless, atelectasis indicates an increased risk of lung collapse, hypoxia, and pneumonia. Major therapeutic measures are early spontaneous breathing and extubation, mobilisation, sufficient positive end-expiratory pressure (PEEP) levels, and use of alveolar recruitment manoeuvres.

Haemothorax and pleural effusions

Accumulation of blood or fluid in the thorax is common after cardiac surgery. Haemothorax typically develops early after surgery when adequate drainage from chest tubes is not obtained, but also occurs later. Most cardiac surgery patients will develop postoperative pleural effusions to some degree. They are most commonly left-sided, and in the majority of patients they are small and resolve spontaneously. When diagnosed with chest X-ray, the incidence is 50%, and even higher when ultrasonic imaging is used. Pleural effusions result from bleeding, chest infection, atelectasis, pulmonary oedema, lesions of the lymphatic system, intraoperative hypothermia, and the postpericardiotomy syndrome (17).

Ultrasound is used to confirm effusion and to identify the best site of puncture. Larger effusions hindering a proper expansion of the lung may have a detrimental effect on respiratory efficiency.

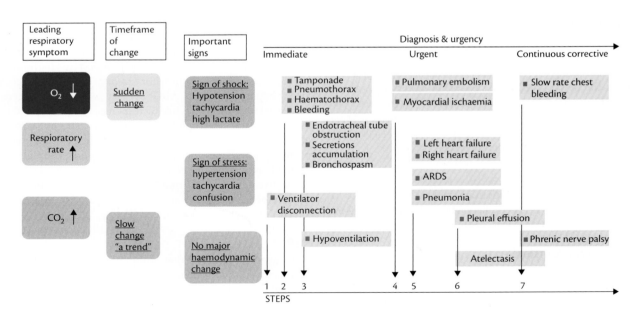

Fig. 30.1 Seven steps differential diagnostic work scheme leading from clinical respiratory signs to diagnosis and urgency: Severity decreases from top left to bottom right. ARDS, adult respiratory distress syndrome.

Postpericardiotomy syndrome

The postpericardiotomy syndrome affects 10 to 40% of patients. Symptoms and signs include fever without an alternative origin, pleuritic chest pain, friction rub, pleural effusion, and pericardial effusion, and at least two of the criteria are required for the diagnosis (18). Generally, the postpericardiotomy immune-mediated inflammatory process occurs later than 5 days after surgery. However, it is occasionally diagnosed after 3 months postoperatively. Usually, it is associated with mild symptoms and an overall good outcome but it can lead to hospital readmission and, rarely, to pericardial tamponade. Treatment includes anti-inflammatory drugs and colchicine.

Chylothorax

Chylothorax is found in 0.1 to 1.5% of cardiac surgery patients and can appear on either side, and occur mostly after lesions of the thoracic duct. Diagnostic criteria are the drainage of more than 1 L of milky fluid with a high fat content. If triglycerides are >110 mg/dL the chance that the fluid is chyle is 99%, whereas the chance is <5% if triglycerides are <50 mg/dL. The first therapeutic step is an absolutely fat-free oral diet for several days and parenteral nutrition is usually necessary to maintain energy balance. The second step is the use of subcutaneous octreotide, a long-acting somatostatin analogue. Octreotide acts on vascular somatostatin receptors, minimizing lymph fluid excretion, and also decreases intestinal blood flow, so reducing lymphatic flow. The final step, thoracic duct ligation or, in rare extremes, a pleuroperitoneal shunt is an alternative if all conservative methods fail.

Pneumothorax

Pneumothorax results from direct injury of the lung through surgery, central venous cannulation, spontaneous rupture of alveoli, or from mechanical ventilation. Underlying conditions that promote the development of pneumothoraces include emphysema in COPD, antitrypsin deficiency, leioangiomyomatosis, congenital bullae, and especially in male adolescents, an asthenic habit. A life-threatening complication is tension pneumothorax with haemodynamic instability due to decreased venous return and compression of the heart chambers. Pneumothorax may manifest as subcutaneous or interstitial emphysema, pneumopericardium, pneumomediastinum, or in rare chronic cases as bronchopleural fistula. A contemporary, and very accurate, diagnostic tool is ultrasonic imaging of the chest (figure 30.2a and b).

Pneumonia

Pneumonia is the complication of cardiac surgery with the highest morbidity and mortality. Its incidence ranges from 2 to 22% following cardiac surgery. This wide range results from different study populations and definitions of pneumonia. In a multicentre European study, 3.8% of the studied population developed ventilation-associated pneumonia (VAP) (19). VAP is diagnosed in patients who have been mechanically ventilated for at least 2 days. The diagnostic criteria recommended by the European Centre for Disease Control (ECDC) include clinical, radiographic and bacteriological criteria (20). Antibiotic administration during the first eight days reduces early-onset pneumonia rates, but increases the risk of VAP through selection of resistant pathogens (21). In uncomplicated cardiac surgery without signs of preoperative infection, antibiotics should never be administered prophylactically after admission to ICU.

Pulmonary congestion and oedema

Pulmonary congestion is seen in every chest radiograph of a patient in supine position. This finding might have no clinical impact if the patient is clinically well, but might need intervention if signs of increased respiratory efforts are observed. Low cardiac output with left heart failure may induce cardiogenic pulmonary oedema, increased work of breathing that may even lead to exhaustion of the respiratory muscles. Treatment includes the use of PEEP, invasive or non-invasive ventilation, inotropic agents, pharmacological afterload reduction and, ultimately, ECMO or left ventricular assist devices.

Adult respiratory distress syndrome

The incidence of adult respiratory distress syndrome (ARDS) after cardiac surgery is between 0.4% and 4%. Physical compression of the lungs, discontinuation of ventilation, blood transfusion and, more important, CPB may cause the syndrome. The pathogenesis of ARDS includes an activated inflammatory process with lesions of the alveolar epithelium and the endothelium. The definition of ARDS has been recently revised and no longer includes a

(a)

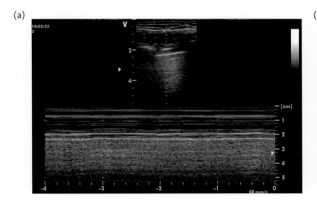

(b)

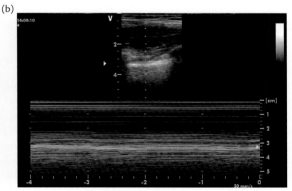

Fig. 30.2 (a) Normal M-mode ultrasound of the chest—'the shore on top, the beach below'. (b) Abnormal M-mode ultrasound of the chest with pneumothorax—'the barcode sign: no beach visible!'.

pulmonary capillary wedge pressure less than 18 mmHg as criterion since ARDS and signs of heart failure may coexist (22).

Ventilation strategies aim to avoid a ventilator-induced lung injury (VILI) as a result of barotrauma, volutrauma or collapse trauma by means of PEEP and limiting plateau pressures. Reducing tidal volumes are often required so blood carbon dioxide (CO_2) tension will rise, which is a widely accepted strategy. Hypercapnia may be associated with further worsening of pulmonary hypertension and thus should be used cautiously in patients with ARDS and impaired right ventricular (RV) function. In severe ARDS, higher plateau pressure, namely above 27 mmHg, increases (RV after load further (23). The RV plays a pivotal role in survival of patients with ARDS, so its function should be regularly assessed.

Pulmonary embolism

Pulmonary embolism (PE) is a relatively rare but potentially fatal complication after cardiac surgery accounting for 1–4% of all deaths. PE should always be considered if sudden unexplained circulatory collapse occurs. The major risk factor is deep venous thrombosis, which is a relatively common condition (13–18%) even if systemic thromboprophylaxis has been used (24,25). DVTs are not limited to the leg where veins are harvested from for CABG, and a major risk factor is prolonged immobilization and mechanical ventilation.

The first diagnostic step should usually be echocardiography with a focus on new signs of RV dysfunction such as dilatation, tricuspid regurgitation, and paradoxical movement of the interventricular septum. Imaging of a thrombus, in the part of the pulmonary artery that is visible to echocardiography, is rare. Monitoring may show a widened gap between arterial and end-tidal CO_2 on capnography, whereas an increased pulmonary artery or central venous pressures may not be present if the cardiac output is substantially decreased. Laboratory tests such as D-dimer are useless in the perioperative setting and ventilation/perfusion scanning is technically not feasible in ventilated patients. European guidelines (26) recommend prophylactic treatment with LMWH whereas American College of Chest Physicians (ACCP) guidelines suggest compression stockings unless patients have had a prolonged hospital stay.

Phrenic nerve palsy

A lesion of the phrenic nerve should always to be excluded if ventilation is asymmetric or large atelectasis occurs despite using a systematic lung recruitment strategy. Unilateral phrenic nerve lesion presents with pulmonary embarrassment and elevated diaphragm but is usually not life threatening. However, bilateral diaphragmatic paralysis is potentially fatal. The left is more commonly affected than the right phrenic nerve.

Causes of phrenic nerve palsy after cardiac surgery include cold saline for myocardial preservation, ice slush in cardiac transplantation, mechanical irritation, and direct surgical trauma. Diagnosis is made using the sniff test which is fluoroscopic imaging of diaphragm during a rapid inspiration. Also, phrenic nerve conduction studies can be obtained with an oesophageal electrode to record nerve activity and percutaneous stimulation. Further, ultrasonic imaging allows using a subcostal view to identify a flattened hemidiaphragm and a paradoxical motion of the diaphragm away from the probe (17).

In a unilateral lesion, which is accompanied by transient dyspnoea or is often asymptomatic, respiratory physiotherapy should be performed. Eighty percent of phrenic nerve injuries will heal within 6 to 12 weeks. However, the risk of atelectasis and chest infections is increased. Diaphragmatic plication for unilateral palsy may be necessary if significant respiratory dysfunction is persistent. In bilateral lesions, the respiratory insufficiency may require implantation of a phrenic nerve pacemaker.

Management and preventive strategies

Optimization of pulmonary outcome after cardiac surgery is based on a four-step approach addressing patient preparation, minimizing intraoperative lung injury, decreasing duration of artificial ventilation, and early mobilization, as well as timely discharge from ICU (figure 30.3).

Postoperative ventilation

Mechanical ventilation after cardiac surgery is common but is often unnecessary. A lung protective strategy, similar to that recommended for ARDS, should be routine because the lungs after CPB must be considered as lungs at risk. The protective strategy will include appropriate recruitment to minimize non-aerated lung areas, keeping the lung open with PEEP, using small tidal volumes (5–7 mL/kg body weight), and allowing spontaneous breathing as early as possible. Weaning from intermittent positive pressure ventilation should be commenced immediately after ICU admission.

The level of PEEP used should be that required to maintain functional residual capacity and adequate levels of oxygenation. The targeted level of oxygenation should take into account the preoperative oxygenation capacity of the lung, which decreases with increasing age (13). The haemodynamic effects of increasing PEEP are an instantaneous decrease in venous return and an afterload increase for the right ventricle. Thus PEEP is used as a first line treatment of acute left ventricular failure with pulmonary congestion. Patients with left heart failure experience a nearly immediate reduction in ventilatory distress, improved oxygenation and systemic arterial pressure and stroke volume can be maintained or even improved.

Weaning should be attempted immediately after verification of the responsiveness and cooperation from the patient, adequacy of oxygenation and spontaneous ventilation. A comprehensive checklist should include also several non-pulmonary categories to improve patient safety (box 30.1), but should not prolong ventilation any longer than absolutely necessary. If initial weaning fails, a strategy with daily sedation interruption and a spontaneous breathing trial, according to a protocol is mandatory (27).

Enhanced recovery

Enhanced recovery following heart surgery is more than just swift tracheal extubation. It is an interaction of surgical concepts, CPB technique, anaesthetic concepts, and postoperative ICU management. It can be applied to reduce the duration of ICU stay and costs but does not necessarily reduce mortality or the duration of hospital stay (28). Systematic sedation after cardiac surgery is not necessary in uncomplicated patients. Enhanced recovery is discussed in detail in Chapter 27.

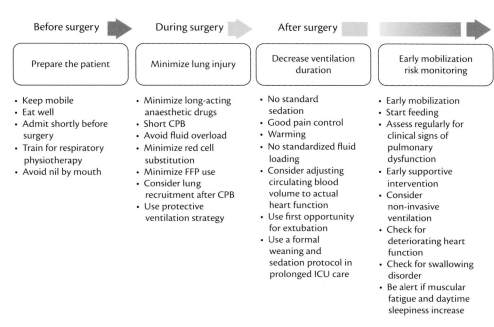

Fig. 30.3 How to prevent pulmonary complications with specific measures at each stage of the perioperative course.

Box 30.1 Patient safety checklist before early extubation:	
Surgical site	bleeding controlled
Haemodynamics	stable, no volume overload
Pulmonary function	pO_2 & pCO_2 as preoperative respiratory rate >12 & <25 coughing adequate
Brain/Nerve/Muscles	adequate response to commands
Pain	well controlled
Drugs	no residual relaxants or sedatives
Temperature	skin warm, no shivering
Lab values	K+ >4, PO4– >0.8, lactate

Surgical concepts

Several variations of surgical techniques have been developed to reduce tissue trauma and minimize impairment of pulmonary function. The aims are to avoid CPB and sternotomy or to reduce the surgical field exposed with an associated decrease in inflammation and bleeding. The drawbacks to such approaches are increased complexity, poorer visualisation of the field and longer duration of surgery. However, the duration of mechanical ventilation is shorter and blood loss is reduced, although overall outcome is unchanged (29).

Cardiopulmonary bypass

Modified CPB techniques aim to reduce the proinflammatory stimulus that is created by the contact to foreign surfaces and to reduce haemodilution by using smaller priming volumes.

Heparin-coated circuits

Heparin increases biocompatibility of cardiopulmonary circuits by inhibiting activation of inflammatory cells and factors. The use of heparin-coated cardiopulmonary circuits reduced (in one trial)

the amount of blood transfused, re-sternotomy and duration of mechanical ventilation, ICU, and hospital stay (30).

Miniaturized cardiopulmonary bypass systems

Closed extracorporeal circulation is designed to reduce priming volume of the CPB circuit, diminish blood–air interface, and is performed without suctioning cardiotomy blood. A reduction of blood loss and in postoperative stroke rate with miniaturized systems has been demonstrated (31).

Lung protection during CPB

Supplementary pulmonary perfusion with either arterial or venous blood is a possibility to impede the side-effects of partial ischaemia of the collapsed lung during CPB. Additional experimental approaches include applying cardioplegic solutions to the lung, use of leucocyte depletion filters on CPB circuits and inhaled carbon monoxide but none are used routinely in clinical practice. Minimal ventilation or the application of continuous positive airway pressure (CPAP) during CPB to reduce fluid accumulation associated with lung collapse have not been found to be effective (32).

Off- versus on-pump coronary artery bypass grafting surgery

Although the evidence is clear that CPB increases the risk of pulmonary dysfunction, there is no clear benefit of off- compared to on-pump CABG surgery, on outcome (33,34).

Ultrafiltration

Ultrafiltration was initially used with the aim of removing the priming volume of the CPB circuit, to reduce fluid overload and thus to improve pulmonary compliance and gas exchange. However, zero-balanced ultrafiltration, where the amount of withdrawn ultrafiltrate is replaced by crystalloids or colloids, has not been found to have significant benefits on outcome (35).

Postoperative analgesia

Effective pain relief is essential not only to improve patient comfort but also to permit deeper breathing and to allow effective expectoration of sputum. Moreover, effective pain treatment is essential for early mobilization. Postoperative analgesia is discussed in detail in Chapter 38.

Corticosteroids

Using corticosteroids to prevent inflammation resulting from CPB remains attractive. Results of two meta-analyses show a reduction in postoperative new onset of atrial fibrillation and trends towards a reduced length of ventilation, reduced bleeding, shortened durations of stay in ICU and hospital. Concerns regarding optimal dose and adverse effects remain (36,37). In a large multi-centre trial of high-dose dexamethasone versus placebo in more than 4000 patients a non-significant effect with an absolute risk reduction of 1.5% (95% confidence interval (CI) –3.0% to +0.1%) on the composite outcome death, myocardial infarction, stroke, renal failure, or respiratory failure was found (38). In the secondary analysis of the individual components of the composite endpoint only respiratory failure was reduced (RR 0.69 (95%CI 0.51–0.94)). There was also a significant trend that dexamethasone is beneficial in younger patients but harmful in the oldest patients' quartile. Any effect on rate of atrial fibrillation, as suggested by the meta-analysis, could not be confirmed.

Blood transfusion

Transfusion of red blood cells can be associated with signs of pulmonary inflammation even when the criteria for transfusion related lung injury are not fulfilled (39). A restrictive transfusion strategy was found to yield similar outcome as a liberal strategy (40). Increasing rates of transfusion were associated with more frequent complications. Mounting evidence suggests a relationship between the administration of fresh frozen plasma and an inflammatory reaction of the lung, potentially resulting in an acute lung injury, called transfusion related acute lung injury (TRALI) (see Chapter 18) (41).

Physiotherapy in the context of cardiac surgery

Physiotherapy for prevention of pulmonary complications after cardiac surgery is widely used to improve patients' oxygenation and prevent pneumonia by means of increasing removal of pulmonary secretions, reducing atelectasis and enhancing pulmonary function (42). Unfortunately, the effect of physiotherapy on outcome remains unclear (43,44).

Failure to wean from mechanical ventilation and tracheal reintubation

Tracheal reintubation is necessary in 2 to 25% of patients in ICU. Risk factors for re-intubation include: upper airway obstruction, cardiac failure, excessive mucus, ineffective expectoration of sputum, prolonged mechanical ventilation, long-acting sedatives, haemoglobin concentration of less than 10 mg/dL, age older than 70 years, hypercaloric nutrition, and encephalopathy (45). Understanding the reasons for failure of tracheal extubation is essential to be able to create better conditions for the next extubation. Cardiac failure may be precipitated by tracheal extubation when the heart cannot support the increased blood flow demand from the work of the diaphragm (46). In cases of failure to wean from mechanical ventilation in patients where a relatively high minute-ventilation (>150 mL/kg/min) is required to maintain a normal arterial carbon dioxide tension, over-nutrition should be considered and a new weaning trial be performed after reducing caloric intake by 30–50%.

Ventilatory fatigue is a frequent observation in patients with decreased muscle mass, older age and chronic inflammation when an increased airway resistance or decreased pulmonary compliance are present. Elevated levels of bronchial secretions that need to be cleared and increased stiffness of the lung with heart failure are the most frequent factors that drive fatigue.

Readmission to intensive care and pulmonary complications

Readmission rates to ICU after cardiac surgery range from 2.2 to 7.8% and the main cause is respiratory failure which accounts for 50% of readmissions. Further causes are cardiovascular instability, renal failure, cardiac tamponade/bleeding, gastrointestinal complications, and sepsis. An alert and aggressive mindset is therefore required for early diagnosis and treatment of respiratory problems on normal wards (47–49).

Conclusion

Pulmonary complications are some of the most frequent complications that occur after cardiac surgery that may, prolong hospital stay, contribute to postoperative morbidity and, increase mortality. The most important approach is to systematically apply a bundle of measures at each stage of the surgical process, such as patient preparation, minimizing intraoperative lung injury, decreasing duration of mechanical ventilation, and early mobilization, as well as timely discharge from the ICU (figure 30.3). When clinical signs are found, early diagnosis and prompt intervention in a stepwise manner (figure 30.1) can minimize the impact of pulmonary complications on outcome from cardiothoracic surgery.

References

1. Goodwin AT, Goddard M, Taylor GJ, Ritchie AJ. Clinical versus actual outcome in cardiac surgery: a post-mortem study. *Eur J Cardiothorac Surg* 2000; **17**(6): 747–51
2. Wu C, Camacho FT, Wechsler AS, et al. Risk score for predicting long-term mortality after coronary artery bypass graft surgery. *Circulation* 2012; **125**(20): 2423–30
3. Nashef SA, Roques F, Sharples LD, et al. EuroSCORE II. *Eur J Cardiothorac Surg* 2012; **41**(4): 734–44
4. Ngaage DL, Martins E, Orkell E, et al. The impact of the duration of mechanical ventilation on the respiratory outcome in smokers undergoing cardiac surgery. *Cardiovasc Surg* 2002; **10**(4): 345–50
5. Baier H, Somani P. Ventilatory drive in normal man during semistarvation. *Chest* 1984; **85**(2): 222–5
6. Weissman C, Goldstein S, Askanazi J, Rosenbaum SH, Milic-Emili J, Kinney JM. Semistarvation and exercise. *J Appl Physiol* 1986; **60**(6): 2035–9
7. Ascione R, Lloyd CT, Underwood MJ, Lotto AA, Pitsis AA, Angelini GD. Inflammatory response after coronary revascularization with or without cardiopulmonary bypass. *Ann Thorac Surg* 2000; **69**(4): 1198–204
8. Bayram H, Erer D, Iriz E, Zor MH, Gulbahar O, Ozdogan ME. Comparison of the effects of pulsatile cardiopulmonary bypass, non-pulsatile cardiopulmonary bypass and off-pump coronary artery

bypass grafting on the inflammatory response and S-100beta protein. *Perfusion* 2012; **27**(1): 56–64

9. Cox CM, Ascione R, Cohen AM, Davies IM, Ryder IG, Angelini GD. Effect of cardiopulmonary bypass on pulmonary gas exchange: a prospective randomized study. *Ann Thorac Surg* 2000; **69**(1): 140–5

10. Hall RI, Smith MS, Rocker G. The systemic inflammatory response to cardiopulmonary bypass: pathophysiological, therapeutic, and pharmacological considerations. *Anesth Analg* 1997; **85**(4): 766–82

11. Friedman M, Sellke FW, Wang SY, Weintraub RM, Johnson RG. Parameters of pulmonary injury after total or partial cardiopulmonary bypass. *Circulation* 1994; **90**(5 Pt 2): II262–8

12. Chai PJ, Williamson JA, Lodge AJ, et al. Effects of ischemia on pulmonary dysfunction after cardiopulmonary bypass. *Ann Thorac Surg* 1999; **67**(3): 731–5

13. Janssens JP, Pache JC, Nicod LP. Physiological changes in respiratory function associated with ageing. *Eur Respir J* 1999; **13**(1): 197–205

14. Sundermann S, Dademasch A, Praetorius J, et al. Comprehensive assessment of frailty for elderly high-risk patients undergoing cardiac surgery. *Eur J Cardiothorac Surg* 2011; **39**(1): 33–7

15. Jaber S, Jung B, Matecki S, Petrof BJ. Clinical review: ventilator-induced diaphragmatic dysfunction—human studies confirm animal model findings. *Crit Care* 2011; **15**(2): 206

16. Skoretz SA, Flowers HL, Martino R. The incidence of dysphagia following endotracheal intubation: a systematic review. *Chest* 2010; **137**(3): 665–73

17. Balaji S, Kunovsky P, Sullivan I. Ultrasound in the diagnosis of diaphragmatic paralysis after operation for congenital heart disease. *Br Heart J* 1990; **64**(1): 20–2

18. Imazio M, Brucato A, Ferrazzi P, Spodick DH, Adler Y. Postpericardiotomy syndrome: a proposal for diagnostic criteria. *J Cardiovasc Med* 2013;**14**(5): 351–3

19. Bouza E, Hortal J, Munoz P, et al. Infections following major heart surgery in European intensive care units: there is room for improvement (ESGNI 007 Study). *J Hosp Infect* 2006; **63**(4): 399–405

20. ECDC. HAIICU Protocol V1.01. Secondary HAIICU Protocol V1.01 2012. http://www.ecdc.europa.eu/en/aboutus/calls/Procurement%20 Related%20Documents/5_ECDC_HAIICU_protocol_v1_1.pdf (accessed 29 May 2014)

21. Trouillet JL. Ventilator-associated pneumonia: a comprehensive review. *Hosp Pract* 2012; **40**(2): 165–75

22. Force ADT, Ranieri VM, Rubenfeld GD, et al. Acute respiratory distress syndrome: the Berlin Definition. *JAMA* 2012; **307**(23): 2526–33

23. Jardin F, Vieillard-Baron A. Is there a safe plateau pressure in ARDS? The right heart only knows. *Intens Care Med* 2007; **33**(3): 444–7

24. Ambrosetti M, Salerno M, Zambelli M, Mastropasqua F, Tramarin R, Pedretti RF. Deep vein thrombosis among patients entering cardiac rehabilitation after coronary artery bypass surgery. *Chest* 2004; **125**(1): 191–6

25. Schwann TA, Kistler L, Engoren MC, Habib RH. Incidence and predictors of postoperative deep vein thrombosis in cardiac surgery in the era of aggressive thromboprophylaxis. *Ann Thorac Surg* 2010; **90**(3): 760–6; discussion 66–8

26. Prevention of venous thromboembolism. Secondary Prevention of venous thromboembolism 2010. http://www.leitlinien.de/mdb/downloads/dgch/prophylaxe-vte-kurz.pdf (accessed 29 May 2014) (in German)

27. Luetz A, Goldmann A, Weber-Carstens S, Spies C. Weaning from mechanical ventilation and sedation. *Curr Opin Anaesthesiol* 2012; **25**(2): 164–9

28. Zhu F, Lee A, Chee YE. Fast-track cardiac care for adult cardiac surgical patients. *Cochrane Database Syst Rev* 2012; **10**: CD003587

29. Brown ML, McKellar SH, Sundt TM, Schaff HV. Ministernotomy versus conventional sternotomy for aortic valve replacement: a systematic review and meta-analysis. *J Thorac Cardiovasc Surg* 2009; **137**(3): 670–79 e5

30. Mangoush O, Purkayastha S, Haj-Yahia S, et al. Heparin-bonded circuits versus nonheparin-bonded circuits: an evaluation of their effect on clinical outcomes. *Eur J Cardiothorac Surg* 2007; **31**(6): 1058–69

31. Biancari F, Rimpilainen R. Meta-analysis of randomised trials comparing the effectiveness of miniaturised versus conventional cardiopulmonary bypass in adult cardiac surgery. *Heart* 2009; **95**(12): 964–9

32. Schreiber JU, Lance MD, de Korte M, Artmann T, Aleksic I, Kranke P. The effect of different lung-protective strategies in patients during cardiopulmonary bypass: a meta-analysis and semiquantitative review of randomized trials. *J Cardiothorac Vasc Anesth* 2012; **26**(3): 448–54

33. Raja SG, Dreyfus GD. Current status of off-pump coronary artery bypass surgery. *Asian Cardiovasc Thorac Ann* 2008; **16**(2): 164–78

34. Hattler B, Messenger JC, Shroyer AL, et al. Off-pump coronary artery bypass surgery is associated with worse arterial and saphenous vein graft patency and less effective revascularization: Results from the Veterans Affairs Randomized On/Off Bypass (ROOBY) trial. *Circulation* 2012; **125**(23): 2827–35

35. Zhu X, Ji B, Liu J, Long C, Wang G. The effects of zero-balance ultrafiltration on postoperative recovery after cardiopulmonary bypass: a meta-analysis of randomized controlled trials. *Perfusion* 2012; **27**(5): 386–92

36. Ho KM, Tan JA. Benefits and risks of corticosteroid prophylaxis in adult cardiac surgery: a dose-response meta-analysis. *Circulation* 2009; **119**(14): 1853–66

37. Whitlock RP, Chan S, Devereaux PJ, et al. Clinical benefit of steroid use in patients undergoing cardiopulmonary bypass: a meta-analysis of randomized trials. *Eur Heart J* 2008; **29**(21): 2592–600

38. Dieleman JM, Nierich AP, Rosseel PM, et al. Intraoperative high-dose dexamethasone for cardiac surgery: a randomized controlled trial. *JAMA* 2012; **308**(17): 1761–7

39. Tuinman PR, Vlaar AP, Cornet AD, et al. Blood transfusion during cardiac surgery is associated with inflammation and coagulation in the lung: a case control study. *Crit Care* 2011; **15**(1): R59

40. Hajjar LA, Vincent JL, Galas FR, et al. Transfusion requirements after cardiac surgery: the TRACS randomized controlled trial. *JAMA* 2010; **304**(14): 1559–67

41. Nascimento B, Callum J, Rubenfeld G, Neto JB, Lin Y, Rizoli S. Clinical review: Fresh frozen plasma in massive bleedings—more questions than answers. *Crit Care* 2010; **14**(1): 202

42. Haeffener MP, Ferreira GM, Barreto SSM, Arena R, Dallago P. Incentive spirometry with expiratory positive airway pressure reduces pulmonary complications, improves pulmonary function and 6-minute walk distance in patients undergoing coronary artery bypass graft surgery. *Am Heart J* 2008; **156**(5); 900.e1–900.e8

43. Pasquina P, Tramer MR, Walder B. Prophylactic respiratory physiotherapy after cardiac surgery: systematic review. *Br Med J* 2003; **327**(7428): 1379

44. Freitas ER, Soares BG, Cardoso JR, Atallah AN. Incentive spirometry for preventing pulmonary complications after coronary artery bypass graft. *Cochrane Database Syst Rev* 2012; **9**: CD004466

45. Epstein SK. Decision to extubate. *Intens Care Med* 2002; **28**(5): 535–46

46. Lemaire F, Teboul JL, Cinotti L, et al. Acute left ventricular dysfunction during unsuccessful weaning from mechanical ventilation. *Anesthesiology* 1988; **69**(2): 171–9

47. Vohra HA, Goldsmith IR, Rosin MD, Briffa NP, Patel RL. The predictors and outcome of recidivism in cardiac ICUs. *Eur J Cardiothorac Surg* 2005; **27**(3): 508–11

48. Joskowiak D, Wilbring M, Szlapka M, et al. Readmission to the intensive care unit after cardiac surgery: a single-center experience with 7105 patients. *J Cardiovasc Surg* 2012; **53**(5): 671–6

49. Litmathe J, Kurt M, Feindt P, Gams E, Boeken U. Predictors and outcome of ICU readmission after cardiac surgery. *Thorac Cardiovasc Surg* 2009; **57**(7): 391–4

CHAPTER 31

Renal, hepatic, and gastrointestinal complications of cardiac surgery

Sara Jane Allen and David Sidebotham

Introduction

Cardiogenic and other shock states threaten vital organ perfusion and function. Although tissue/organ autoregulation can mitigate the risk of injury, these mechanisms may be impaired in patients undergoing cardiac surgery, particularly the elderly and those with hypertension and other atherosclerotic disease. Non-pulsatile cardiopulmonary bypass is probably an additional aggravating factor. This chapter outlines the pathophysiology, clinical manifestations and management of renal and mesenteric organ injury associated with cardiac surgery.

Renal complications

Cardiac surgery-associated acute kidney injury

The Acute Dialysis Quality Initiative published consensus criteria for diagnosing acute kidney injury (AKI) in 2004. These criteria consist of three stages of kidney injury (*Risk*, *Injury*, *Failure*) and two clinical outcomes (*Loss* and *End-stage kidney disease*) (table 31.1) (1). These RIFLE criteria were modified in 2007 by the Acute Kidney Injury Network to produce the AKIN consensus criteria (2). Using these criteria, the incidence of AKI following cardiac surgery is 20–30%, with approximately 2–3% of patients requiring renal replacement therapy (RRT) (3,4).

Mortality associated with AKI is directly related to the severity of the kidney injury, being over 40% in patients requiring RRT (4). Even mild forms of AKI are associated with significantly increased mortality risk (4). In one study, even a modest creatinine rise (<45 μmol/L, or 0.5 mg/dL) after cardiac surgery was associated with a three-fold increased mortality (5).

Pathophysiology

The terms prerenal azotaemia (elevated levels of nitrogen wastes in the blood due to renal hypoperfusion) and acute tubular necrosis have traditionally been used to describe the early and late states of AKI. However, the terms do not describe distinct clinical entities and are not reliably distinguished by standard biochemical tests of kidney function. More recently, the concepts of 'volume-responsive' and 'non-volume-responsive' have been introduced to describe the early and late phases of AKI.

Volume-responsive AKI describes a condition of reduced glomerular filtration rate (GFR) resulting from renal hypoperfusion without histopathological changes within the kidney. Volume-responsive AKI is characterized by a series of adaptive physiological responses that include tubuloglomerular feedback, renin release by the kidney, aldosterone release from the adrenal gland, and vasopressin release by the posterior pituitary. These physiological responses act to maintain GFR and result in the production of concentrated, salt-poor urine. Within limits, these changes can be reversed by volume administration and restoration of renal perfusion pressure.

However, a sustained fall in renal blood flow leads to histopathological changes in the renal microvasculature and tubules due to ischaemia and inflammation that is not reversed by fluid administration. Tubular damage is associated with loss of the hypertonic medullary interstitium and an inability to generate concentrated urine. Failure of tubular reabsorption leads to increased urinary sodium loss. The serum concentrations of substances dependent on filtration and tubular secretion, such as potassium, hydrogen ions, and phosphate, increase. Oliguria may progress to anuria.

Depending on the severity of the injury and the degree of renal reserve, renal function may stabilize and recover or progress to irreversible renal failure. During the recovery phase the ability to generate concentrated urine may be impaired, leading to the production of a large volume of solute-poor urine.

Characteristic biochemical changes associated with volume-responsive and non-volume-responsive AKI are shown in table 31.2.

While the concept of volume-responsiveness is clinically useful for most forms of AKI, it is less so for cardiac surgery-associated AKI, in which the primary mechanism of renal injury is only rarely hypoperfusion. The mechanism of cardiac surgery-associated AKI is complex and involves endogenous toxin production,

Table 31.1 RIFLE and AKIN criteria for acute kidney injury

	RIFLE			AKIN		
Stage	**Creatinine/GFR**	**Urine output**	**Stage**	**Creatinine/GFR**	**Urine output**	
Risk	Increased Cr × 2 or GFR decreased 25%	<0.5 mL/kg/hr × 6 hrs	I	Increased Cr × 1.5 or > 25 μmol/L	< 0.5 mL/kg/hr × 6 hr	
Injury	Increased Cr × 2 or GFR decreased 50%	<0.5 mL/kg/hr × 12 hr	II	Increased Cr × 2	<0.5 mL/kg/hr × 12 hr	
Failure	Increased Cr × 3 or GFR decreased 75% Or Creatinine >350 μmol/L with acute rise 45 μmol/L	< 0.3 mL/kg/hr × 24 hr or anuria × 12 hours	III	Increased Cr × 3 Or Creatinine >350 μmol/L with acute rise 45 μmol/L	< 0.3 mL/kg/hr × 24 hr or anuria × 12 hours	
Loss	Loss of renal function > 4 weeks					
End-stage disease	End-stage disease					

GFR = glomerular filtration rate.

Reproduced with permission from the Acute Kidney Injury Network (AKIN) guidelines, 2007, adapted from the RIFLE Criteria (Risk, Injury, Failure, Loss, End-stage), 2004 also copyright of the Acute Kidney Injury Network.

Table 31.2 Biochemical changes associated with acute kidney injury

Test	Volume responsive AKI	Non-volume responsive AKI
Serum urea/creatinine ratio	15:1 to 20:1	<10:1
Urine osmolality (mOsmol/L)	>500	<350
Urine sodium (mmol/L)	<20	>40
Fractional excretion of sodium (%)	<1	>1

AKI = acute kidney injury. The fractional excretion of sodium (FE_{Na}) can be estimated from the urinary (U) and plasma (P) concentrations of sodium (Na) and creatinine (cr):

$$FE_{Na} = \left(\frac{[U_{cr}]}{[P_{Na}]} \right) \cdot \left(\frac{[P_{LT}]}{[U_{cr}]} \right)$$

ischaemia–reperfusion, inflammation, and oxidative stress, largely from the effects of cardiopulmonary bypass (6).

Biochemical tests of acute kidney injury (7–9)
Creatinine and creatinine clearance
Creatinine, the most widely used marker of kidney function, is released from skeletal muscle at a fairly constant rate, is freely filtered by the glomerulus, and, unlike urea, does not undergo tubular reabsorption. Creatinine does undergo tubular secretion, however, accounting for 10–40% of creatinine clearance. There are several limitations of using creatinine as a measure of GFR. GFR must decline approximately 50% before creatinine increases significantly. Thus, a rise in creatinine from 50 to 100 μmol/L represents a much greater proportional reduction in GFR than a rise from 200 to 250 μmol/L. Creatinine rise is delayed 48–72 hours from the initiation of renal injury. Serum creatinine is influenced by body size, muscle mass, protein intake, gender, volume of distribution, and catabolic state. In older patients, reduced muscle mass is matched by reduced GFR, resulting in little change in serum creatinine. Thus, creatinine does not reflect age-related decline in GFR. The normal range for serum creatinine is 50–120 μmol/L (0.6–1.4 mg/dL) for males and 40–100 μmol/L (0.5–1.1 mg/dL) for females.

Creatinine clearance (in mL/min) is a more accurate method of evaluating GFR than creatinine concentration, particularly in the elderly and patients with abnormal body mass index. Creatinine clearance (C_{cr}) can be measured from the plasma (P_{cr}) and urinary (U_{cr}) concentrations of creatinine and the 24-hour urine volume (V), as:

$$C_{cr} = \frac{U_{cr} \times V}{P_{cr}}$$

Several empiric formulae are available for estimating creatinine clearance, such as that of Cockcroft and Gault:

$$C_{cr} = \frac{(140 - age) \times weight[kg]}{P_{cr}|\mu mol| \times 0.8136} (\times 0.85[females])$$

Empiric formulae are useful for estimating creatinine clearance preoperatively but are not valid in oliguric patients, and should not be used during evolving AKI. The normal range for creatinine clearance is 120 ± 25 mL/min for males and 95 ± 20 mL/min for females.

Novel biomarkers
Because of the limitations of existing tests of kidney function, there has been considerable interest in novel biomarkers of AKI (7–9). Biomarkers investigated include cystatin C, neutrophil gelatinase-associated lipocalin (NGAL), interleukin-18 (IL-18), kidney injury molecule-1 (KIM-1), and liver-type fatty acid binding protein (L-FABP). An ideal biomarker would rapidly increase following the initiation of AKI and be able to distinguish between volume and non-volume responsive AKI. Novel biomarkers are either physiologic or pathologic. Cystatin C, a protein released from nucleated cells, is a physiologic marker, similar to creatinine. Cystatin C is freely filtered by the glomerulus and is almost completely reabsorbed and catabolized in the proximal tubule; it does not undergo tubular secretion. Plasma and (particularly) urinary concentrations of cystatin C reflect changes in GFR and tubular function. Cystatin C increases within 12-hours of the initiation of AKI.

NGAL, KIM-1, and IL-18 are all immunological proteins, whereas L-FABP is a fatty-acid binding and transport protein found in the proximal renal tubule. The expression of all four substances is dramatically increased by tubular injury, and as such they are considered pathologic biomarkers. NGAL is the most widely studied. The plasma concentration of NGAL increases early, within 2 hours, of renal injury, and has been shown to be predictive of the duration and severity of AKI and the need for RRT (10,11). Consensus guidelines continue to recommend serum creatinine as the primary biomarker in assessing patients with evolving AKI (8).

Aetiology and prevention of cardiac surgery-associated acute kidney injury

Factors associated with cardiac surgery-associated AKI are listed in table 31.3. Of all these factors by far the most important is pre-existing renal impairment. In a cohort of over 10 000 cardiac surgical patients, a preoperative GFR of 30–60 mL/min was associated with threefold increased odds of requiring RRT, (odds ratio) OR 3.58 (95% confidence interval [CI] 2.45–5.26), whereas a GFR less than

Table 31.3 Factors associated with acute kidney injury during cardiac surgery

Preoperative
Pre-existing renal dysfunction
ACEi/ARB therapy
Heart failure
Diabetes mellitus
Age > 70 years
Systolic hypertension (>140 mmHg) and wide pulse pressure (>40 mmHg)
Inotrope administration preoperatively
Hepatic disease
Intraoperative
Anaemia/haemodilution
Blood transfusion
Haemodynamic instability
Prolonged CPB (>2–3 hr)
On-pump CABG (versus off-pump CABG)
Valvular or aortic surgery (versus CABG surgery)
Use of multiple inotropic drugs
Use of IABP
Use of aprotinin
Postoperative
Hypotension
Sepsis
Use of aminoglycosides or vancomycin
Prolonged mechanical ventilation
High APACHE score
Use of IABP
Use of multiple inotropic drugs

ACEi = angiotensin converting enzyme inhibitor. ARB = angiotensin receptor blocker. CPB = cardiopulmonary bypass. CABG = coronary artery bypass graft. IAPB = intra-aortic balloon pump. APACHE = acute physiology and chronic health evaluation; a scoring system for patients admitted to intensive care.

Data from Table 2, Weir et al, Acute Injury following Cardiac Surgery. *American Journal of Nephrology* 2011; **33**:438–452 (6).

30 mL/min was associated with a 16-fold increased odds of requiring RRT, (odds ratio) OR 16.35 (95% CI 9.34–28.02) (3).

Several factors associated with cardiac surgery contribute to postoperative AKI, including impaired autoregulation during CPB (12), non-pulsatile flow during CPB (13), CBP-induced systemic inflammation, haemolysis (14), anaemia (15), blood transfusion (16,17), prolonged CPB (18), and haemodynamic instability (19).

With respect to anaemia, a haematocrit less than 0.24 during CPB is associated with an increased likelihood of developing AKI (15). The association between blood transfusion and AKI is significantly greater in anaemic patients than in non-anaemic patients (16). Thus, strategies to minimize the likelihood of both anaemia and blood transfusion are likely to be beneficial. Such strategies include correcting anaemia preoperatively, minimizing fluid administration during surgery, using autologous retrograde priming of the circuit, using small-volume circuits, using cell saving devices, and administering an antifibrinolytic such as tranexamic acid (not aprotinin). If blood transfusion is necessary, avoiding over transfusion (i.e., a haemoglobin concentration >80 g/L), and using fresh (i.e. <14 days old), leukocyte-depleted blood is probably beneficial (17,20).

Systolic hypertension (>140 mmHg), particularly that associated with a wide pulse pressure (>40 mmHg) or labile blood pressure, is a risk factor for postoperative AKI, but diastolic hypertension (>90 mmHg) is not (21,22). It is unclear whether treating hypertension or controlling blood pressure lability intraoperatively ameliorates AKI (17,23–25).

For most patients, maintaining a mean arterial pressure (MAP) above 60–70 mmHg during the pre- and post-CPB periods and above 50–60 mmHg during CPB are reasonable targets. Higher targets may be appropriate in patients with severe hypertension or flow limiting atherosclerosis. During the postoperative period, once intravascular volume has been optimized, hypotension should be treated with vasoactive drugs, targeting a MAP above 65 mmHg (8). Augmenting cardiac output or blood pressure to supraphysiological levels to prevent AKI is not recommended (8).

A recent large multicentre randomized trial comparing fluid resuscitation with 0.9% saline or 6% hydroxyethylstarch in intensive care demonstrated an increased need for RRT in the starch treated patients (26).

Numerous pharmacological agents have been studied for their potential to ameliorate cardiac surgery-associated AKI, including dopamine, frusemide, nesiritide (B-type natriuretic peptide), fenoldopam, diltiazem, *N*-acetylcysteine, atrial natriuretic peptide, and corticosteroids (19,27). There are few data supporting a nephroprotective effect for any of these drugs, and current guidelines do not support the routine use of specific nephroprotective agents (8).

Frusemide may convert oliguric AKI to polyuric AKI, which is much easier to manage clinically. Frusemide can be used to treat hyperkalaemia, but if brisk diuresis does not occur frusemide should be discontinued as it is renally eliminated and high blood levels can cause deafness. There are limited data from non-randomized case series that tight perioperative glucose control (i.e. targeting a blood glucose 4.5–6.1 mmol/L) reduces the incidence and severity of AKI in cardiac surgical patients (28). Countered against this is the fact that tight glycaemic control increases the risk of hypoglycaemia (29,30). In the absence of further data, targeting a blood glucose less than 10 mmol/L during the intraoperative period is reasonable.

A recent systematic review documented a renoprotective effect of off-pump surgery in observational studies, but data from randomized trials were insufficient to reach a consensus recommendation (31). This issue is unresolved.

Considerations in patients with acute kidney injury undergoing cardiac surgery

Patients may present for cardiac surgery with established or evolving AKI. Common causes in this circumstance include heart failure (cardiorenal syndrome), administration of nephrotoxic agents (e.g. contrast media, gentamicin, vancomycin), and sepsis (e.g. endocarditis). Several issues must be addressed in patients with severe AKI presenting for cardiac surgery. First, can surgery be delayed until kidney function has returned to baseline? Second, whichstrategies should be employed to minimize further kidney injury associated with cardiac surgery and CPB? Third, what are the metabolic consequences of severe AKI? Fourth, is RRT indicated prior to, or likely immediately following, surgery? Finally, what are the implications for pharmacotherapy?

The indications for initiating RRT are listed in box 31.1. If RRT is thought likely to be required in the early postoperative period it is helpful for the anaesthetist to place a temporary dialysis catheter following induction of anaesthesia. Catheter length should be tailored to the access site: 15 cm in the right internal jugular vein; 20 cm in the left internal jugular vein; 25 cm in the femoral vein.

Metabolic consequences of severe acute kidney injury

The important clinical consequences of severe AKI are listed in box 31.2.

Hyperkalaemia

Hyperkalaemia can cause life-threatening cardiac arrhythmias, and requires urgent intervention. A potassium concentration above 6.5–7.0 mmol/L is an indication for urgent RRT; RRT should also be considered for a potassium concentration of 6.0–6.5 mmol/L.

For life-threatening hyperkalaemia (potassium >6.5 mmol/L) the following treatments reduce the risk of arrhythmias and acutely lower the serum potassium concentration:

+ modest hyperventilation
+ intravenous (IV) calcium chloride (3–6 mmol)
+ IV sodium bicarbonate (50–100 mmol of 8% solution, in a separate IV line to the calcium)
+ IV insulin/dextrose (25 units of rapidly acting insulin + 50 mL of 50% dextrose).

Box 31.1 Indications for urgent renal replacement therapy

Potassium >6.5 mmol/L
Severe metabolic acidosis (pH < 7.1, base deficit > 10)
Severe oliguria (urine volume <50 mL/12 hr)
Pulmonary oedema not responsive to diuretics
Uraemic encephalopathy (typically associated with urea >30 mmol/L)
Sodium concentration < 115 or > 155 mmol/L

Box 31.2 Important clinical consequences of severe acute kidney injury

Oliguria or anuria
Intravascular volume overload
Hyperkalaemia
Hypernatraemia or hyponatraemia
Hyperphosphataemia
Hypermagnesaemia
Hypocalcaemia
Depressed level of consciousness
Hypertension
Pulmonary oedema

Less severely elevated potassium (5.5–6.5 mmol/L) may be treated with nebulized salbutamol (5 mg every 15 minutes) and intravenous frusemide (40 mg IV). Potassium and glucose concentrations should be checked at least every 30 minutes following dextrose/insulin therapy and when the potassium concentration is above 6.5 mmol/L. Note that, of the treatments listed, only frusemide and RRT actually remove potassium from the patient; the other treatments stabilize the myocardium (calcium chloride) or increase potassium entry into cells (hyperventilation, sodium bicarbonate, insulin), and thus are only temporizing measures.

Metabolic acidosis

AKI typically results in an elevated anion gap acidosis due to the build up of organic acids, mainly arising from protein metabolism. Rarely, AKI causes a non-anion gap acidosis (i.e. renal tubular acidosis) due to renal bicarbonate wasting. As a temporizing measure, modest hyperventilation and sodium bicarbonate administration will increase pH, but should not delay institution of RRT; 0.9% saline solution, which has an acidifying effect, should be avoided.

Sodium and water balance

Patients with severe AKI typically have an expanded extracellular volume with total body water and sodium overload. The serum sodium concentration may be high or low depending on sodium and water intake and diuretic administration. Mild hyponatraemia is common due to the oral intake or intravenous administration of hypotonic fluids.

Frusemide can cause both hypo- and hypernatraemia. Administration of IV frusemide leads to the production of hypotonic urine (urinary sodium ≈75 mmol/L), which, in the absence of water replacement, leads to hypernatraemia. However, chronically, fluid losses due to frusemide are usually replaced with hypotonic fluids (e.g. tap water), which can lead to hyponatraemia.

Adding a haemofilter to the CPB machine intraoperatively can be used to treat hyperkalaemia, acidosis, and volume overload intraoperatively. For volume overload the ultrafiltrate is not replaced and the device functions as a haemoconcentrator. However, bolus doses of 50–100 mmol (8.4% solution) sodium bicarbonate are typically needed to prevent acidosis due to bicarbonate loss in the ultrafiltrate. For hyperkalaemia and acidosis, the ultrafiltrate is replaced with an equal amount of bicarbonate containing balanced salt solution.

Calcium and phosphate

Impaired renal excretion of phosphate leads to hyperphosphataemia, and the formation of insoluble calcium phosphate salts, which in turn leads to (ionized) hypocalcaemia and secondary hyperparathyroidism. Ionized hypocalcaemia is exacerbated by alkalosis (e.g. due to hyperventilation or bicarbonate administration), blood transfusion (due to citrate chelation), CPB, and heparin and protamine administration. Mild ionized hypocalcaemia (<1 mmol/L) can contribute to myocardial dysfunction and arrhythmias; severe hypocalcaemia is associated with tetany and seizures.

Uraemic encephalopathy

With severe AKI, acidosis and hyperkalaemia have usually necessitated institution of RRT prior to the development of uraemic symptoms. Uraemia may contribute to delayed extubation in patients with chronic renal failure. Treatment of uraemic encephalopathy is RRT, targeting a urea concentration less than 20 mmol/L.

Alterations to pharmacotherapy

Ideally, nephrotoxic drugs should be avoided in patients with AKI (box 31.3). Some nephrotoxic agents—such as gentamicin, vancomycin, and cyclosporine—may otherwise be clinically indicated, in which case dose-adjustment and therapeutic drug monitoring are required.

Box 31.3 Drugs that should be avoided or be used with caution in patients with AKI

Nephrotoxic drugs
ACEi/ARB
NSAIDs
Iodinated contrast media
Aminoglycosides
Amphotericin (non-liposomal form)
Vancomycin
Aprotinin
Cyclosporine

Excessive side-effects
Suxamethonium
ACEi/ARB
Spironolactone
Metformin
Sucralfate

Renally eliminated: dose adjustment required
Digoxin
Aminoglycosides
Vancomycin
Most β-lactam antibiotics
Fluoroquinolone antibiotics
Pancuronium
Frusemide

Renally eliminated active metabolites
Diazepam
Midazolam
Morphine

Altered protein binding (increased clinical effect)
Warfarin
Phenytoin
Midazolam

ACEi, angiotensin converting enzyme inhibitor; ARB, angiotensin receptor blocker; NSAIDs, non-steroidal anti-inflammatory drugs.

The side effects of certain drugs may be exacerbated with AKI, notably hyperkalaemia with angiotensin converting enzyme inhibitors, angiotensin receptor blockers, and potassium sparing diuretics. The risk of lactic acidosis with metformin is increased with AKI, and this drug should be avoided in patients with a creatinine above 150 μmol/L. Most beta-lactam antibiotics require dose adjustment in patients with severe kidney injury. AKI affects the protein binding of warfarin and phenytoin, increasing their pharmacological effect.

Most drugs used for balanced cardiac anaesthesia are lipid soluble and hepatically metabolized and can be used safely in patients with severe AKI. Exceptions are pancuronium, which is eliminated unchanged by the kidney, and morphine, midazolam, and diazepam, which have renally eliminated active metabolites. Suxamethonium should be avoided in patients with hyperkalaemia.

Considerations for patients receiving haemodialysis undergoing cardiac surgery

Patients with dialysis-dependent end-stage kidney disease have several potential problems that are of concern prior to cardiac surgery (box 31.4).

Ideally, surgery should occur when the patient is at their euvolaemic (dry) weight and their serum potassium concentration is at the lower end of the normal range. These goals are best achieved by performing dialysis on the day prior to surgery. Patients who are hypovolaemic at the time of surgery are at risk of developing severe hypotension on induction of anaesthesia. Angiotensin-converting enzyme inhibitors and angiotensin receptor antagonists should be withheld on the morning of surgery. Severe hypotension should be treated with a vasopressor rather than aggressive fluid administration. As most patients receiving chronic dialysis produce little or no urine, a restrictive approach to fluid and potassium administration is warranted. Hypo- and hyperkalaemia are well tolerated; nevertheless, dialysis patients are at increased risk of cardiac arrhythmias compared to other cardiac surgical patients, particularly with manipulation of guide wires during placement of central venous catheters. A urinary catheter is not required for anuric or severely oliguric patients.

It is essential venous and arterial catheters are not placed into or adjacent to surgically created arteriovenous (AV) fistulae, and that AV fistulae sites are carefully protected during surgery.

Cardiovascular disease is a common and well-recognized accompaniment to end-stage kidney disease. However, one complication—pulmonary hypertension—is often overlooked, despite occurring in up to 40% of dialysis patients (32). Pulmonary hypertension is an independent predictor of outcome in patients receiving haemodialysis, with a 5-year survival of only 25% compared to an overall survival of 39% (32). The presence and severity of pulmonary hypertension, along with any accompanying right ventricular dysfunction should be specifically sought on a preoperative echocardiogram.

Gastrointestinal and hepatic complications

Gastrointestinal (GI) and hepatic complications are uncommon following cardiac surgery; however, they are associated with increased hospital length of stay and cost, and significant

Box 31.4 Anaesthetic considerations in chronic dialysis patients presenting for cardiac surgery

Care of dialysis fistula or catheter
Increased susceptibility to infection
Pharmacological considerations
Haematological problems
Anaemia
Platelet dysfunction
Fluid and metabolic disturbance
Hypervolaemia/hypovolaemia
Hypokalaemia/hyperkalaemia
Acidosis
Hyperglycaemia (in diabetic patients)
Calcium and phosphate disturbance
Secondary hyperparathyroidism (high phosphate/low calcium)
Tertiary hyperparathyroidism (high phosphate/high calcium)
Cardiovascular disease
Arterial hypertension and left ventricular hypertrophy
Arrhythmias
Pulmonary hypertension
Coronary artery disease
Heart failure
Peripheral vascular disease
Cerebrovascular disease
Other comorbidities
Diabetes
Collagen vascular disease

morbidity and mortality. Diagnosis of GI complications following cardiac surgery is often difficult, as patients may have atypical symptoms and signs, altered responses to clinical examination, underlying comorbidities, and concurrent drug therapies (e.g. sedatives, neuromuscular blocking agents, opioid analgesics, immunosuppressants), which interfere with clinical assessment. A high index of clinical suspicion and a low threshold for further investigation are necessary to allow early intervention and appropriate treatment, and thus optimize outcomes.

Incidence

The reported incidence of GI complications following cardiac surgery varies considerably, with an average incidence of approximately 1% and average mortality of approximately 30% (33–35). The most common GI complications reported are bleeding, mesenteric ischaemia, pancreatitis, cholecystitis, and peptic ulcer disease (35). Diverticulitis, ileus, intestinal obstruction and perforation, and hepatic dysfunction are less commonly reported. Other rarely reported complications include drug-induced hepatotoxicity, iatrogenic injury to intra-abdominal organs, pseudomembranous colitis, and peritonitis (34).

Pathogenesis

Whilst the pathogenesis is complex, and likely multifactorial, the majority of complications are ischaemic in origin. Splanchnic hypoperfusion, impaired mucosal oxygenation, and the systemic inflammatory response syndrome (SIRS) appear to have important roles in causing ischaemia (36). Inflammation also has an important role in the alteration of normal absorptive and barrier functions of the GI tract.

Contributors include reduced systemic MAP, reduced or altered distribution of blood flow or cardiac output, and vasoconstriction due to inflammatory mediator release, hypothermia, or drug therapy (36). Non-pulsatile flow during CPB may also contribute, by causing renal release of renin secretion of angiotensin II. Angiotensin II is a potent vasoconstrictor with high affinity for mesenteric vascular smooth muscle, which reduces splanchnic flow. The splanchnic and renal circulations are unable to effectively autoregulate perfusion at the extremes of blood pressure and flow, therefore reduced MAP or flow (e.g. during CPB, haemorrhage, or arrhythmia) results in reduced perfusion. The association between GI complications and AKI supports the role of hypoperfusion in the pathogenesis of complications following cardiac surgery. Interestingly, renal dysfunction may also reduce jejunal motility and shorten colonic transit time (37).

Cardiac surgery also results in activation of vasoactive inflammatory mediators and the complement and cytokine cascades via the surgical stress response and contact with the CPB circuit. Thromboxane A_2 and B_2, leukotrienes, and C5a have mesenteric vasoconstrictor actions, while cytokines are implicated in vascular endothelial dysfunction and damage (36). Ischaemia itself may activate and sustain SIRS and is associated with free radical production during reperfusion, further contributing to endothelial dysfunction, maldistribution of blood flow, and impaired mucosal oxygen delivery.

Additional contributors include macro- and microemboli, and haemodilution during CPB, which impairs oxygen delivery. Prolonged mechanical ventilation is associated with GI complications, possible mechanisms include sympathetic nervous system activation, ventilator-associated lung injury with inflammatory cascade activation and decreased cardiac output, as well as underlying association with worse illness severity (38). Non-ischaemic mechanisms of GI complications include adverse drug reactions, pre-existing GI pathology, excess anticoagulation, and mechanical organ injury (e.g. malpositioned intercostal drains).

Risk factors

Patients with significant comorbidities, and those with prolonged or complicated recovery are at high risk of GI complications (39,40). Specific risk factors are summarized in box 31.5. Importantly, whilst prolonged duration of CPB is a risk factor for GI complications, studies have failed to demonstrate a difference in incidence or mortality of GI complications between on-pump or off-pump CABG (41).

Prevention

Identification of high-risk patients preoperatively may allow specific preventative strategies to be used, and earlier investigation, diagnosis and management of complications to occur postoperatively (35).

Preoperative optimisation of haemodynamic state, including correction of hypovolaemia or anaemia, and optimization of cardiac output and respiratory function is recommended. Intraoperative monitoring and maintenance of adequate cardiac output and oxygenation is important; however, mucosal ischaemia may occur despite global adequacy of oxygen delivery, due to local

Box 31.5 Risk factors for GI complications after cardiac surgery

Preoperative risk factors
Age > 70 years
Reoperation
Chronic renal failure
Peripheral vascular disease
Diabetes mellitus
Chronic obstructive pulmonary disease
IABP or inotrope therapy
Congestive heart failure (NYHA class III or IV)

Intraoperative risk factors
Prolonged CPB duration
Valve surgery
Emergency surgery
Re-operation for bleeding
Blood transfusion
Non-pulsatile CPB flow
IABP

Postoperative risk factors
Arrhythmias (particularly atrial fibrillation)
Prolonged mechanical ventilation (>24 hours)
AKI
Low cardiac output state
Sepsis
Deep sternal wound infection

Data from Huddy SPJ, Joyce WP, Pepper JR. Gastrointestinal complications in 4473 patients who underwent cardiopulmonary bypass surgery. Br J Surg 1991;78:293–6; Rodriguez R, Robich MP, Plate JF, Trooskin SZ, Sellke FW. Gastrointestinal complications following cardiac surgery: A comprehensive review. J Card Surg 2010;25:188–97; Perugini RA, Orr RK, Porter D, Dumas EM, Maini BS. Gastrointestinal complications following cardiac surgery. An analysis of 1477 cardiac surgery patients. Arch Surg 1997;132:352–7.

NYHA, New York Heart Association.

alterations in metabolic demand and perfusion. Intraoperative prevention strategies have focused on optimizing perfusion, and reducing the inflammatory response to surgery and CPB.

Drug therapies
Several drug therapies have been investigated for prevention of GI complications.

Aspirin administration within 48 hours postoperatively was associated with reduced incidence of both GI ischaemia/infarction and mortality due to GI complications (42). Dobutamine may increase splanchnic blood flow and oxygen delivery; however, it has a variable effect on gastric mucosal pH, with several studies reporting decreased pH consistent with mucosal ischaemia (43,44). Dopamine has a possible detrimental effect on mucosal oxygenation and GI motility (45). Studies of milrinone have shown inconsistent results. (46) Vasopressin probably impairs gastric mucosal perfusion (45).

Modification of cpb
Maintaining a normal cardiac index and MAP is advocated to allow adequate GI perfusion; however, the use of vasopressors

to achieve this has been associated with decreased splanchnic flow and worsened mucosal perfusion. Minimizing the use of pure vasoconstrictors, and administration of inotropes or inodilators may reduce abdominal complications. Significant haemodilution (i.e. haematocrit <25) is associated with reduced splanchnic oxygen delivery, and increased mortality in some studies (47). Thus, avoidance of severe anaemia is also prudent. The use of pulsatile rather than nonpulsatile flow during CPB has been associated with improved mucosal oxygenation and perfusion in some but not all trials (48). Hypothermia has been postulated to be protective against ischaemic injury to the GIT; however, normothermic temperature management on bypass has not been demonstrated to alter the incidence of complications (49). Intravascular filters reduce microemboli; however, these have not been shown to reduce the incidence of GI complications. Nonetheless, an approach that seeks to minimize the risk of emboli by careful selection of aortic cannulation site, echo assessment of the aorta, avoidance of IABP in patients with severe atheroma, and meticulous de-airing of circuit and connectors, is warranted. Off-pump surgery has not been demonstrated to reduce the incidence of GI complications (45). Methods to reduce the inflammatory response to CPB have been used, including minimization of circuit surface area and volume, reduction of blood–air interfaces, and use of biocompatible surfaces in the CPB circuit; however, evidence to support these strategies is so far lacking.

Other strategies
Gastric acid suppression and avoidance of over-anticoagulation are recommended to reduce the risk of peptic and duodenal ulceration and GI bleeding, but high level supportive evidence is lacking.

Diagnosis

Diagnosis of GI pathology is difficult in the cardiac surgical patient. Sedative and analgesic drugs alter symptoms and signs, and may make the patient entirely inaccessible. Haemodynamic and metabolic derangements or multiorgan failure due to any cause are non-specific, and may mask signs of abdominal pathology, leading to delay or failure in diagnosis. Clinical presentation is variable according to pathology, and no single clinical, laboratory or radiological test reliably diagnoses all abdominal complications. A high index of suspicion and a low threshold for investigation is recommended for patients with non-routine postoperative course.

Investigation is directed by patient presentation, and may include biochemical and haematological blood analysis, plain abdominal radiography, abdominal ultrasound, computerized tomography (CT) scanning, upper and lower endoscopy, and early diagnostic and interventional laparotomy. Early investigation and diagnosis is vital to facilitate management, as delayed diagnosis and management is associated with worse outcome (34,35). Table 31.4 summarizes suggested diagnostic investigations for specific GI complications.

Treatment

Treatment is determined by the specific complication, with the important principle that treatment should not be withheld because of recent cardiac surgery.

Table 31.4 Specific GI complications and investigations

Gastrointestinal haemorrhage	Haemoglobin ↓
	LDH↑
	Upper GI endoscopy
	Lower GI endoscopy
Mesenteric ischaemia	Abdomen X-ray
	Computerized tomography (CT) scan abdomen
	CT mesenteric angiography
	Colonoscopy
	Laparotomy
Pancreatitis	Pancreatic amylase↑
	Lipase↑
	Abdominal ultrasound
	CT abdomen
	Magnetic resonance imaging
Cholecystitis	White cell count↑
	Alkaline phosphatase↑
	Bilirubin↑
	Abdominal ultrasound
	Radionuclide scan
	CT abdomen
Diverticulitis	CT abdomen
Ileus	Abdomen X-ray
Intestinal obstruction/ perforation	Abdomen X-ray
	CT abdomen
	Laparotomy
Hepatic dysfunction	Bilirubin↑
	AST, ALT↑
	Albumin↓
	INR↑
	Ultrasound scan abdomen

AST, aspartate transaminase; ALT, alanine transaminase.

Specific complications

Haemorrhage

Bleeding is the most common GI complication reported after cardiac surgery, accounting for approximately 30–35% of GI complications (35,40,45). Most frequently, bleeding occurs in the upper GI tract, presenting as altered blood or melaena passed per rectum. Upper GI bleeding is commonly due to gastric or duodenal ulceration and erosion. Lower GI bleeding presents as haematochezia, and is usually due to diverticulitis, although may occur with arteriovenous malformations, colitis, or neoplasms. Accurate diagnosis requires endoscopy, which frequently allows therapeutic intervention with clipping or sclerotherapy to bleeding vessels. Management also includes fluid resuscitation, transfusion of blood products as required, correction of coagulopathy, and treatment with proton pump inhibitors. Bleeding from the lower GI tract may be difficult to localize with endoscopy, and may require angiography. Bleeding, uncontrolled by endoscopy,

requires surgical intervention and resection. Mortality associated with GI haemorrhage after cardiac surgery is 19% (35).

Mesenteric ischaemia

Mesenteric ischaemia causes between 14–20% of GI complications (35,40,45). Two types of ischaemia occur: occlusive ischaemia (due to emboli or thrombus) and non-occlusive ischaemia, or NOMI (due to mesenteric hypoperfusion). Clinical signs include abdominal pain and distension, intolerance of enteral nutrition, and lower GI bleeding. Other features may include leucocytosis and metabolic lactic acidosis, but the absence of an elevated lactate is non-reassuring. CT mesenteric angiography may demonstrate abnormalities in the arterial tree, along with bowel wall thickening, stranding, distension, and necrosis. Treatment includes IV resuscitation and circulatory support, antibiotics, and early surgical referral and resection of affected bowel. Endovascular stenting may be possible for occlusive disease. Mesenteric ischaemia is associated with a high mortality of 50–76% (35,49).

Peptic ulcer disease

Gastric or duodenal ulcer perforation constitutes 6–8% of GI complications (35). The incidence is reduced with the prophylactic use of proton pump inhibitors. Typical clinical features include abdominal pain, distension, peritonism, and possibly shock. Diagnosis can be confirmed by abdominal X-ray or CT scan. Treatment includes aggressive resuscitation and early laparotomy. Ongoing treatment with a proton pump inhibitor is recommended. Mortality associated with perforation is approximately 30% (35,40).

Pancreatitis

Hyperamylasaemia is common, occurring in 25–35% of patients after cardiac surgery, whilst acute pancreatitis is rare, occurring in only 0.5–1.0% of cases. Early postoperative isolated hyperamylasaemia is usually due to salivary isoenzyme of amylase. Patients with isolated salivary hyperamylasaemia require no specific therapy and are usually asymptomatic. A smaller number of patients have an associated elevated lipase, but remain asymptomatic, consistent with subclinical pancreatitis. These patients must be monitored closely for symptoms or signs of pancreatitis. Presentation may include back and epigastric pain, nausea and vomiting, abdominal distension, and prolonged or unexplained SIRS. Amylase levels are typically elevated more than four times normal levels, and lipase is also elevated. CT scan enables diagnosis and prognostication, and is helpful in determining the extent of inflammation and necrosis. Management is with enteral rest, no oral intake and a nasogastric tube placed for drainage. Jejunal or total parenteral nutrition is usually required. Prophylactic antibiotic therapy is not recommended. The presence of collections, extensive necrosis, or pseudocyst formation on CT scan necessitates further surgical review and may require antibiotics, percutaneous drainage, or surgical debridement. Mortality occurs in 20–50% (35).

Cholecystitis

Causes 6–11% of GI complications, with a high associated mortality. Presentation is typically 5–15 days after surgery, with right upper quadrant pain, fever, and leucocytosis; haemodynamic instability and SIRS. Cholecystitis is frequently (35–50%) acalculous in this population, and gangrenous cholecystitis is also common. The diagnosis can be made with abdominal ultrasound or CT, radionuclide studies, or even diagnostic laparoscopy. A cholecystectomy is usually required for calculous cholecystitis, but acalculous cholecystitis may be initially managed with fluid resuscitation and intravenous antibiotics, with percutaneous cholecystostomy or surgical intervention if no improvement occurs over 24–48 hours.

Hepatic dysfunction

Transient increases in hepatic enzymes occur in up to 40% of cardiac surgical patients, but acute hepatic dysfunction and failure are rare, occuring in 0.02–0.4% of cases; mortality associated with hepatic failure is over 50% (35,45). Hyperbilirubinaemia is most common and is usually asymptomatic, but liver transaminase (AST, ALT) enzyme elevation suggests hepatic ischaemia. Risk factors for hepatic injury include prolonged bypass time, complex surgery, hypotension, hypoxia, and elevated right atrial pressure, especially due to right heart failure. Drugs and toxins, in particular amiodarone and antibiotics, may be implicated. Management includes treating the underlying cause, stopping hepatotoxic drugs, and optimising cardiac output and perfusion. Abdominal ultrasound should be performed to exclude biliary obstruction, thrombosis, or abscess.

Impaired perfusion, inflammation, and possibly embolism associated with CPB and cross-clamping threaten vital organ function in cardiac surgery. Efforts to minimize these sources of organ injury, perhaps more than any specific therapy, are likely to be most helpful in improving outcome.

Conclusion

Critical care of the cardiac surgical patient requires a clear understanding of the surgery undertaken and the underlying pathophysiological processes, aiming to optimize recovery with early detection and treatment of complications. Effective co-ordinated care is underpinned by clear communication and teamwork. Critical care is expensive, demanding consideration of cost-effectiveness and appropriateness of care in this complex hospital environment.

References

1. Bellomo R, Ronco C, Kellum JA, Mehta RL, Palevsky P. Acute renal failure—definition, outcome measures, animal models, fluid therapy and information technology needs: the Second International Consensus Conference of the Acute Dialysis Quality Initiative (ADQI) Group. *Crit Care* 2004; **8**: R204–12

2. Mehta RL, Kellum JA, Shah SV, et al. Acute Kidney Injury Network: report of an initiative to improve outcomes in acute kidney injury. *Crit Care* 2007; **11**: R31

3. Englberger L, Suri RM, Li Z, et al. Clinical accuracy of RIFLE and Acute Kidney Injury Network (AKIN) criteria for acute kidney injury in patients undergoing cardiac surgery. *Crit Care* 2011; **15**: R16

4. Wijeysundera DN, Karkouti K, Dupuis JY, et al. Derivation and validation of a simplified predictive index for renal replacement therapy after cardiac surgery. *JAMA* 2007; **297**: 1801–9

5. Lassnigg A, Schmidlin D, Mouhieddine M, et al. Minimal changes of serum creatinine predict prognosis in patients after cardiothoracic surgery: a prospective cohort study. *J Am Soc Nephrol* 2004; **15**: 1597–605

6. Bellomo R, Auriemma S, Fabbri A, et al. The pathophysiology of cardiac surgery-associated acute kidney injury (CSA-AKI). *Int J Artif Organs* 2008; **31**: 166–78

7. Hudson C, Hudson J, Swaminathan M, Shaw A, Stafford-Smith M, Patel UD. Emerging concepts in acute kidney injury following cardiac surgery. *Semin CardiothoracVasc Anesth* 2008; **12**: 320–30

8. Brochard L, Abroug F, Brenner M, et al. An Official ATS/ERS/ESICM/SCCM/SRLF Statement: Prevention and Management of Acute Renal Failure in the ICU Patient: an international consensus conference in intensive care medicine. *Am J Respir Crit Care Med* 2010; **181**: 1128–55

9. Soni SS, Ronco C, Katz N, Cruz DN. Early diagnosis of acute kidney injury: the promise of novel biomarkers. *Blood Purif* 2009; **28**: 165–74

10. Haase-Fielitz A, Bellomo R, Devarajan P, et al. Novel and conventional serum biomarkers predicting acute kidney injury in adult cardiac surgery—a prospective cohort study. *Crit Care Med* 2009; **37**: 553–60

11. Haase-Fielitz A, Bellomo R, Devarajan P, et al. The predictive performance of plasma neutrophil gelatinase-associated lipocalin (NGAL) increases with grade of acute kidney injury. *Nephrol Dial Transplant* 2009; **24**: 3349–54

12. Andersson LG, Bratteby LE, Ekroth R, et al. Renal function during cardiopulmonary bypass: influence of pump flow and systemic blood pressure. *Eur J Cardiothorac Surg* 1994; **8**: 597–602

13. Onorati F, Presta P, Fuiano G, et al. A randomized trial of pulsatile perfusion using an intra-aortic balloon pump versus nonpulsatile perfusion on short-term changes in kidney function during cardiopulmonary bypass during myocardial reperfusion. *Am J Kidney Dis* 2007; **50**: 229–38

14. Haase M, Haase-Fielitz A, Bagshaw SM, Ronco C, Bellomo R. Cardiopulmonary bypass-associated acute kidney injury: a pigment nephropathy? *Contrib Nephrol* 2007; **156**: 340–53

15. Huybregts RA, de Vroege R, Jansen EK, van Schijndel AW, Christiaans HM, van Oeveren W. The association of hemodilution and transfusion of red blood cells with biochemical markers of splanchnic and renal injury during cardiopulmonary bypass. *Anesth Analg* 2009; **109**: 331–9

16. Karkouti K, Wijeysundera DN, Yau TM, et al. Influence of erythrocyte transfusion on the risk of acute kidney injury after cardiac surgery differs in anemic and nonanemic patients. *Anesthesiology* 2011; **115**: 523–30

17. Haase M, Bellomo R, Story D, et al. Effect of mean arterial pressure, haemoglobin and blood transfusion during cardiopulmonary bypass on post-operative acute kidney injury. *Nephrol Dial Transplant* 2012; **27**: 153–60

18. Kumar AB, Suneja M, Bayman EO, Weide GD, Tarasi M. Association between postoperative acute kidney injury and duration of cardiopulmonary bypass: a meta-analysis. *J Cardiothorac Vasc Anesth* 2011; **26**: 64–9

19. Weir MR, Aronson S, Avery EG, Pollack CV, Jr. Acute kidney injury following cardiac surgery: role of perioperative blood pressure control. *Am J Nephrol* 2011; **33**: 438–52

20. Sanders J, Patel S, Cooper J, et al. Red blood cell storage is associated with length of stay and renal complications after cardiac surgery. *Transfusion* 2011; **51**: 2286–94

21. Aronson S, Fontes ML, Miao Y, Mangano DT. Risk index for perioperative renal dysfunction/failure: critical dependence on pulse pressure hypertension. *Circulation* 2007; **115**: 733–42

22. Aronson S, Dyke CM, Levy JH, et al. Does perioperative systolic blood pressure variability predict mortality after cardiac surgery? An exploratory analysis of the ECLIPSE trials. *Anesth Analg* 2011; **113**: 19–30

23. Fischer UM, Weissenberger WK, Warters RD, Geissler JH, Allen SJ, Mehlhorn U. Impact of cardiopulmonary bypass management on postcardiac surgery renal function. *Perfusion* 2002; **17**: 401–6

24. Sirvinskas E, Andrejaitiene J, Raliene L, et al. Cardiopulmonary bypass management and acute renal failure: risk factors and prognosis. *Perfusion* 2008; **23**: 323–7

25. Urzua J, Troncoso S, Bugedo G, et al. Renal function and cardiopulmonary bypass: effect of perfusion pressure. *J Cardiothorac Vasc Anesth* 1992; **6**:299–303

26. Myburgh JA, Finfer S, Bellomo R, et al. Hydroxyethyl starch or saline for fluid resuscitation in intensive care. *N Engl J Med* 2012; **367**: 1901–11

27. Patel NN, Rogers CA, Angelini GD, Murphy GJ. Pharmacological therapies for the prevention of acute kidney injury following cardiac surgery: a systematic review. *Heart Fail Rev* 2011; **16**: 553–67

28. Lecomte P, Van Vlem B, Coddens J, et al. Tight perioperative glucose control is associated with a reduction in renal impairment and renal failure in non-diabetic cardiac surgical patients. *Crit Care* 2008; **12**: R154

29. Lazar HL, McDOnnell MM, Chipkin S, Fitzgerald C, Bliss C, Cabral H. Effects of aggressive versus moderate glycaemic control on clinical outcomes in diabetic coronary artery bypass graft patients. *Ann Surg* 2011; **254**: 458–63

30. Finfer S, Chittock DR, Su SY, et al. Intensive versus conventional glucose control in critically ill patients. *N Engl J Med* 2009; **360**: 1283–97

31. Nigwekar SU, Kandula P, Hix JK, Thakar CV. Off-pump coronary artery bypass surgery and acute kidney injury: a meta-analysis of randomized and observational studies. *Am J Kidney Dis* 2009; **54**: 413–23

32. Yigla M, Nakhoul F, Sabag A, et al. Pulmonary hypertension in patients with end-stage renal disease. *Chest* 2003; **123**: 1577–82

33. McSweeney ME, Garwood S, Levin J, et al. Adverse gastrointestinal complications after cardiopulmonary bypass: Can outcome be predicted from preoperative risk factors? *Anesth Analg* 2004; **98**: 1610–17

34. Huddy SPJ, Joyce WP, Pepper JR. Gastrointestinal complications in 4473 patients who underwent cardiopulmonary bypass surgery. *Br J Surg* 1991; **78**: 293–6

35. Rodriguez R, Robich MP, Plate JF, Trooskin SZ, Sellke FW. Gastrointestinal complications following cardiac surgery: A comprehensive review. *J Card Surg* 2010; **25**: 188–97

36. Ohri SK, Velissaris T. Gastrointestinal dysfunction following cardiac surgery. *Perfusion* 2006; **21**: 215–23

37. Asimakopoulas G, Taylor KM. The effect of cardiopulmonary bypass on neutrophil and endothelial adhesion molecules. *Ann Thorac Surg* 1998; **66**: 2135–44

38. Mutlu GM, Mutlu EA, Factor P. GI complications in patients receiving mechanical ventilation. *Chest* 2001; **119**: 1222–41

39. Perugini RA, Orr RK, Porter D, Dumas EM, Maini BS. Gastrointestinal complications following cardiac surgery. An analysis of 1477 cardiac surgery patients. *Arch Surg* 1997; **132**: 352–7

40. Andersson B, Nilsson J, Brandt J, Hoglund P, Andersson R. Gastrointestinal complications after cardiac surgery. *Br J Surg* 2005; **92**: 326–33

41. Musleh GS, Patel NC, Grayson AD, et al. Off-pump coronary artery bypass surgery does not reduce gastrointestinal complications. *Eur J Cardiothorac Surg* 2003; **23**: 170–4

42. Mangano DT. Aspirin and mortality from coronary bypass surgery. *N Engl J Med* 2002; **347**: 1309–17

43. Parviarnen I, Ruokonen E, Takala J. Dobutamine-induced dissociation between changes in splanchnic blood flow and gastric intra-mucosal pH after cardiac surgery. *Br J Anaesth* 1995; **54**: 277–82

44. Uusaro A, Ruokonen E, Takala J. Splanchnic oxygen transport after cardiac surgery: Evidence for inadequate tissue perfusion after stabilization of hemodynamics. *Intens Care Med* 1996; **22**: 26–33

45. Hessel EA. Abdominal organ injury after cardiac surgery. *Semin Cardiothorac Anesth* 2004; **8**: 243–63

46. Mollhoff T, Loick HM, van Aken H, et al. Milrinone modulates endotoxemia systemic inflammation and subsequent acute phase response after cardiopulmonary bypass. *Anesthesiology* 1999; **90**: 72–80

47. De Foe GR, Ross CS, Olmstead EM, et al. Lowest hematocrit on bypass and adverse outcomes associated with coronary artery bypass grafting. *Ann Thorac Surg* 2001; **71**: 769–76

48. Ohri SK, Bowles CW, Mathie RT, et al. Effect of cardiopulmonary bypass perfusion protocols on gut tissue oxygenation and blood flow. *Ann Thorac Surg* 1997; **64**: 163–70

49. Edwards M, Sidebotham D, Smith M, Leemput JV, Anderson B. Diagnosis and outcome from suspected mesenteric ischaemia following cardiac surgery. *Anaesth Intens Care* 2005; **33**: 210–7

CHAPTER 32

Cerebral complications of heart surgery

Thomas H. Ottens and Diederik van Dijk

Classification of cerebral complications

Introduction

Cerebral complications are a major concern for patients undergoing heart surgery. These complications can be classified in several ways. Based on a study of coronary artery bypass grafting (CABG) surgery patients from 24 institutions in the United States of America (USA) by Roach, cerebral complications are classified into Type I outcomes, defined as focal neurological injury, stupor, or coma and Type II outcomes, defined as deterioration in intellectual function, disorientation, or seizures (1). In this chapter, cerebral complications of heart surgery will be categorized into stroke, cognitive decline, and delirium. There is little doubt that stroke is a devastating complication, which is associated with an increased risk of mortality, high costs, and a decreased quality of life. However, severe cognitive decline may also prevent a patient's return to employment, whilst delirium can be a major burden during an often prolonged hospital stay. The signs of stroke and delirium may already be apparent in the first hours after surgery. Subtle changes in cognitive function may only become evident after weeks or months (2).

Stroke

In the USA, CABG surgery is the leading cause of iatrogenic stroke (3). The risk of stroke is increased in elderly patients undergoing heart surgery. Other risk factors include poor left ventricular function, atrial fibrillation, carotid or aortic atherosclerosis, and previous stroke (1,4–6). Stroke after cardiac surgery is more common in women than in men (7). Imaging studies show that about one-half of strokes after cardiac surgery are caused by macroemboli (1,5). Most ischaemic events occur during surgery, but over 20% of strokes occur in the postoperative period (1,8). Most strokes are clinically detected within the first two days of surgery (9).

Despite the increasing age of patients undergoing elective CABG surgery, the incidence of clinically relevant stroke has declined over the past two decades. Prospective studies in the last decades of the 20th century reported incidences of 3 to 5% (2,9). More recent publications report incidences around 2% (4). Magnetic resonance imaging studies in patients who underwent cardiac surgery consistently report much higher rates of new infarctions, which are often not accompanied by clinical deficits (5,10). The incidence of new ischaemic brain lesions after CABG surgery was 31 to 45% and after valve replacement the rate was 38 to 47% (5,10,11). Moreover, studies in elderly patients show that 50% of patients who undergo CABG surgery have ischaemic brain lesions before their surgery, which are typically asymptomatic (5).

Stroke not only has a great impact on the patient's quality of life, it is also expensive. Direct medical costs for the first 30 days after a mild ischaemic stroke are on average $13 000, and over $20 000 for severe stroke (6).

Postoperative cognitive decline

Postoperative cognitive decline (POCD) can be defined as a decrease in performance on neuropsychological tests, beyond natural variation in test performance, from preoperatively to postoperatively (12). Clinically, the patient may suffer from memory loss, decreased attention and slow information processing. Relatives may identify the signs of POCD more accurately than patients themselves, who may not be aware of the changes (8). Severe POCD reduces quality of life of both patients and relatives, and is associated with increased health resource consumption and costs (1,2,13).

Depending on the timing of neuropsychological assessment and the definition of POCD, the reported incidence of POCD after CABG surgery varies between 3 and 70% (4,12). There is currently no widely accepted clinical definition of POCD and there is no doubt that arbitrarily chosen definitions have resulted in substantial overestimation of the incidence of the problem (14). Treatment is not available, but most patients will recover spontaneously within the first months after surgery. The estimation of the incidence of long-term POCD is difficult, as normal ageing and dementia interfere with such studies in elderly populations (14–16).

Delirium

Delirium is an acute, fluctuating disturbance of consciousness and attention that presents either with or without agitation (17). It is very common in elderly postoperative patients, in particular after cardiac surgery. Delirium after cardiac surgery typically presents on the second postoperative day. Risk factors include advanced age, long duration of surgery, and sleep deprivation. Patients who develop delirium after cardiac surgery are at increased risk of death as well as prolonged durations stay in intensive care unit and hospital (17,18).

Causes of cerebral complications

Cardiopulmonary bypass, emboli, and inflammation

Cerebral complications of cardiac surgery have often been attributed to the use of cardiopulmonary bypass (CPB) (1,2). Indeed, many studies have demonstrated potentially harmful side effects of CPB on the brain. Cannulation and cross-clamping of the ascending aorta may induce atheromatous macroemboli, which are usually held responsible for perioperative stroke (19). The CPB itself and cardiotomy suction are sources of solid and gaseous microemboli, especially when unprocessed cardiotomy blood is recirculated (20,21). These microemboli can be detected in the middle cerebral arteries with transcranial Doppler (TCD) ultrasonography (22). A post-mortem study on the brains of patients who died after cardiac surgery have demonstrated so-called small capillary and arteriolar dilatations (23).

The CPB circuit brings the blood into contact with large synthetic surfaces and this induces a profound inflammatory response (1,24). Surgical trauma also contributes to the inflammatory response. The pathophysiology of the CPB-induced inflammatory response involves complement activation, activation of the coagulation and fibrinolytic pathways, platelets and leukocytes (Chapter 5). The subsequent release of endotoxins and cytokines leads to increased permeability of the blood–brain barrier. Brain swelling can be observed in patients who undergo magnetic resonance imaging immediately after on-pump CABG surgery surgery (25). Serum concentrations of S-100 protein, a biochemical marker of cerebral injury, are elevated after on-pump CABG surgery (26). Because of all these potentially negative effects of CPB on the brain, many regard the use of CPB as the culprit in cerebral complications following cardiac surgery. However, randomized controlled trials (RCTs) carried out so far indicate no favourable effect of off-versus on-pump CABG surgery on stroke rate or long-term cognitive outcome (4).

Hypoperfusion

During and after CPB, episodes of low blood pressure may occur, to a degree that is usually not considered acceptable in patients undergoing non-cardiac surgery. Imaging studies of patients who had a clinical stroke after cardiac surgery have shown that a lower mean arterial pressure (MAP) during surgery is associated with a higher risk of watershed infarctions (27). Cerebral hypoperfusion may also aggravate the damage caused by microemboli due to reduced washout (2,4). The role of cerebral hypoperfusion in the pathogenesis of cognitive decline remains uncertain, as the results of studies on the association between mean arterial pressure (MAP) and the incidence of POCD conflict (2,4,28,29). The assumption that cerebral autoregulation will keep the patients brain adequately perfused during episodes of low blood pressure may be false in patients who presents for cardiac surgery, especially in those with a history of hypertension.

Anaesthesia

In the authors' experience, most patients simply point towards the 'heavy anaesthetic' when experiencing cognitive problems after their cardiac surgery. The neurotoxicity of anaesthetic agents is subject of great controversy. The incidence of POCD does not depend on the type of anaesthesia, and POCD also occurs after non-cardiac surgery with neuraxial anaesthesia (30,31). It is currently unclear whether anaesthetic agents contribute to the pathogenesis of cognitive decline after cardiac surgery.

Patient related factors

Major risk factors for stroke after on-pump CABG surgery are advanced age, atherosclerosis of the ascending aorta, carotid artery stenosis and a history of cerebrovascular disease. Other risk factors include diabetes mellitus, a history of peripheral vascular disease and hypertension (1,4,8,29). A stroke risk index can be used preoperatively to estimate the risk of stroke in a patient undergoing CABG surgery (32). Patient risk factors for POCD are largely comparable to those for stroke. A higher level of education protects against POCD (13,28).

Strategies to improve cerebral outcome

Monitoring

Transcranial doppler

TCD ultrasonography can be used to monitor blood flow velocity in the middle cerebral artery. TCD also allows quantification of the number of emboli transiting the middle cerebral artery. The usefulness of this technique is limited by its reliability: a usable flow signal cannot be obtained in up to 25% of patients (33). There is currently no evidence to support the use of TCD as a tool to prevent cerebral complications of cardiac surgery. There is no relation between numbers of emboli detected with TCD, and cerebral outcome (2,34).

Cerebral oximetry

Near-infrared spectroscopy (NIRS) is a non-invasive technique of monitoring oxygen saturation in a small part of the frontal lobes, using visible and near-infrared light. Commercially available monitors display separate oxygen saturation readings for the left and right hemisphere. In 2007, Denault and colleagues proposed an algorithm that can be used to optimize cerebral saturation using NIRS (figure 32.1) (35). Studies that used such management algorithms suggested a reduction of perioperative morbidity, including a trend towards a reduced incidence of stroke (33,35). Reduction of the incidence of POCD has not been demonstrated. NIRS appears to be a safe and user-friendly monitor that may warn the anaesthetist and cardiac surgeon for impeding disaster. However, normal NIRS readings do not guarantee overall adequate cerebral oxygenation and may give a false sense of safety during episodes of low blood pressure.

Anaesthesia and perfusion

Temperature management

Hypothermia may have neuroprotective effects in patients with stroke and traumatic injury and it is considered a proven strategy for reducing cerebral injury after cardiac arrest. There is no evidence that mild or moderate hypothermia during CPB reduces cerebral complications. Concurrently, there is no doubt that deep hypothermia protects the brain and other organs during procedures that require complete circulatory arrest (36).

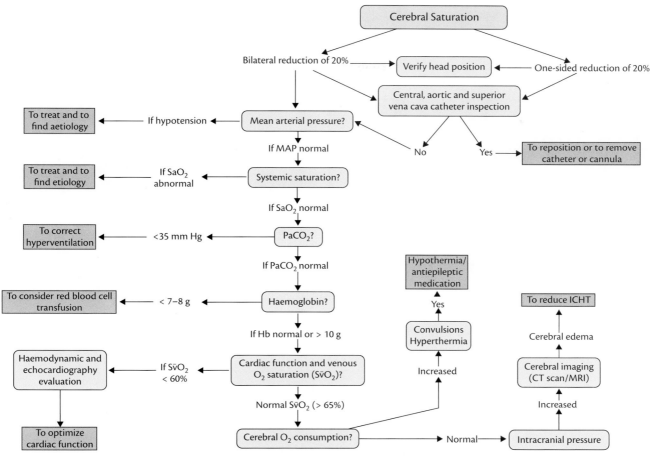

Fig. 32.1 Proposed algorithm in the use of brain oximetry.

CT, computerized tomography; ICHT, intracranial hypertension; MAP, mean arterial pressure; MRI, magnetic resonance imaging; MAP, mean arterial pressure; SaO_2, arterial oxyhaemoglobin saturation with oxygen; $PaCO_2$, arterial carbon dioxide tension; Hb, haemoglobin concentration; $S\bar{v}O_2$, mixed venous oxyhaemoglobin saturation with oxygen; CT, computerised tomography; MRI, magnetic resonance imaging.

A. Denault, A. Deschamps and J. M. Murkin; A Proposed Algorithm for the Intraoperative Use of Cerebral Near-Infrared Spectroscopy; Semin Cardiothorac Vasc Anesth. December 2007 11: 274-281; Sage Publications.

Hyperthermia, on the other hand, may aggravate injury sustained from other sources. Hyperthermia can be induced when patients are rapidly rewarmed (overshoot), but it can also be caused by inflammation in the postoperative period. Hyperthermia increases neurotransmitter release, oxygen-derived free radical production, and intracellular acidosis (36). In studies of stroke, hyperthermia increased ischaemic depolarization in the peri-infarct region, leading to increased infarct size (5). Both peak body temperature and the speed of rewarming have been demonstrated to affect the rate of POCD after cardiac surgery (36).

The temperature management recommendations from a literature review by Grigore et al (36) are shown in figure 32.2. Method A uses passive cooling (drifting) to 34–35°C, and slow rewarming to 37°C, resulting in normothermia in the postoperative phase, and is recommended for patients at low risk for developing cerebral injury. Method B uses active cooling to 28–30°C, followed by slow rewarming to 37°C, again resulting in postoperative normothermia. This method is advised for patients at high risk for cerebral injury. This method is more time consuming, but is perhaps useful when longer CPB time is acceptable. Method C involves active cooling to 32°C, followed

by slow rewarming. The patients is weaned of CPB at 34–35°C. This method reduces CPB time compared with method B, and results in mild postoperative hypothermia that is further corrected slowly during the ICU-stay. Method C could be used in patients at high risk for cerebral injury, when prolonged CPB time is undesirable (36). There is no evidence yet that these temperature management recommendations based on the risk of cerebral injury improve outcomes.

In general, patients should be rewarmed slowly, and intra- and postoperative hyperthermia should be avoided. Tympanic temperature may estimate brain temperature more accurately than conventional temperature probes, but even tympanic temperature may underestimate the true brain temperature during rewarming (5).

Acid–base management

A decrease of body temperature leads to decreased arterial carbon dioxide tension ($PaCO_2$) and increased pH. Cerebral blood flow is linearly related to $PaCO_2$, and therefore the decreased $PaCO_2$ during hypothermia leads to a reduced cerebral blood flow. Adding carbon dioxide to the CPB circuit to keep blood pH at 7.4 and $PaCO_2$ at 40 mmHg (pH-stat acid–base management) keeps cerebral

(a)

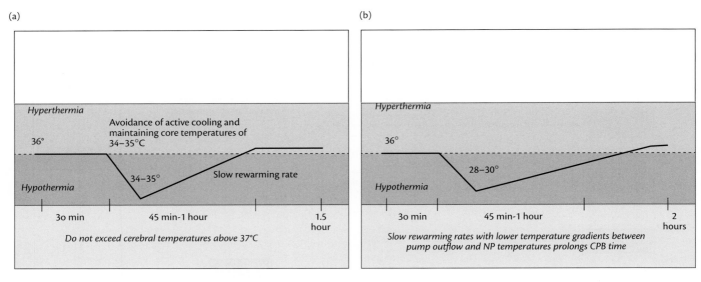

(b)

(c)

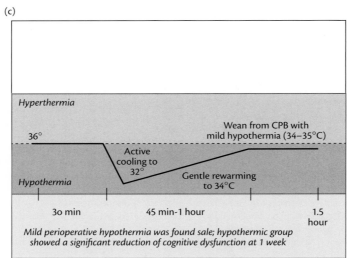

Fig. 32.2 Temperature regimens. (A) Avoided active cooling, mild hypothermia, slow rewarming rates followed by normothermia. (B) Active cooling, slow rewarming rates, followed by normothermia. (C) Active cooling, slow rewarming to mild hypothermia, and weaned off cardiopulmonary bypass (CPB). NP, nasopharyngeal.
Reproduced from Grigore AM, et al., 'A Core Review of Temperature Regimens and Neuroprotection During Cardiopulmonary Bypass: Does Rewarming Rate Matter?', Anesthesia Analgesia, 109, 6, pp. 1741–1751, Copyright 2009, with permission from International Anesthesia Research Society.

blood flow at a normal level despite the hypothermia. However, the cerebral metabolic rate for oxygen ($CMRO_2$) is reduced during hypothermic CPB. Thus, pH-stat blood gas management results in uncoupling of blood supply and demand ('luxury perfusion') to the brain. This may lead to increased cerebral microembolic load and cerebral arterial steal, but evidence for this phenomenon is sparse.

In the 1980s, alpha-stat acid–base management was introduced. This strategy keeps pH and $PaCO_2$ at 7.4 and 40 mmHg respectively, if measured at 37°C. This means that the hypothermic patient is hypocapnic and therefore, has a reduced cerebral blood flow. Blood supply and demand theoretically remain coupled, and cerebral blood flow may be reduced as much as 40% at 26°C. In adult patient, alpha-stat acid–base management may improve cerebral outcomes by avoiding steal and reducing embolic load. However, the studies that have compared the effect of pH- and alpha-stat acid–base management on cerebral outcomes have had inconclusive results (8,12,37).

Blood pressure management

The healthy brain vasculature has an intrinsic ability to maintain cerebral blood flow stable between a mean arterial pressure of 60 and 150 mmHg (38). This mechanism is commonly known as cerebral autoregulation, and a similar mechanism is found in the kidneys. Using alpha-stat pH acid–base management, cerebral autoregulation is assumed to remain functionally intact with CPB flows of 1.6 to 2.4 L/min/m² (37). However, as previously mentioned, the assumption of functionally intact cerebral autoregulation at the lower (and higher) ends of the MAP scale may not hold for patients with common conditions, such as hypertension, diabetes or cerebrovascular disease. In such patients, it may not be appropriate to allow the MAP to fall to 50–60 mmHg. Some studies suggest that stroke rates may be reduced when a MAP of 80–100 mmHg is maintained, especially in elderly patients (12).

Different vasopressors can be used to increase MAP during cardiac surgery, including norepinephrine, vasopressin, and phenylephrine. The use of the latter is subject of debate, because although phenylephrine increases MAP, it may decrease cerebral oxygenation measured with NIRS (38).

Preoperative assessment

Preoperative screening of patients presenting for cardiac surgery is needed to identify risk factors for cerebral complications such as advanced age, pre-existing cerebrovascular disease or cognitive deficits, diabetes, and hypertension (4,32). Ultrasonography of the carotid arteries can be performed to identify carotid stenosis, but is unclear how the results of this screening should modify the surgical management of patients presenting for CABG surgery (39). It is also still uncertain whether perioperative statin use reduces the risk of stroke (40). Aspirin reduces the risk of stroke when given during the first 48 hrs after CABG surgery (41), but the use of aspirin before CABG surgery is controversial. After induction of anaesthesia and before aortic cannulation, transoesophageal echocardiography can be used to screen the descending aorta and the visible part of the ascending aorta for the presence of atheroma, which is an important risk factor for stroke (4,6).

Surgery

Off-pump surgery

The use of CPB is associated with microemboli, macroemboli, episodes of hypotension, and a profound inflammatory response (2,19,22–24). Cerebral complications of CABG surgery have therefore been attributed to the use of CPB. CABG surgery without CPB was reintroduced when cardiac stabilizing devices became available in the late 1990s, and it was expected that this would significantly reduce the risk of cerebral complications. Several RCTs comparing off- and on-pump CABG surgery have been performed, but often without adequate randomisation procedure and without blinded outcome assessment (42). The methodological quality of the RCTs appears to be inversely associated with the effect size of off-pump surgery on stroke rate. Figure 32.3 shows a

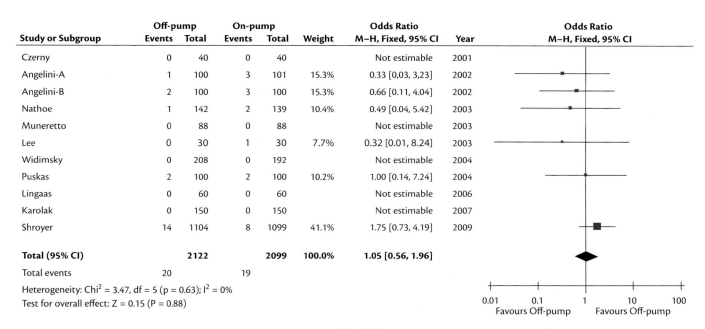

Study or Subgroup	Off-pump Events	Off-pump Total	On-pump Events	On-pump Total	Weight	Odds Ratio M–H, Fixed, 95% CI	Year
Czerny	0	40	0	40		Not estimable	2001
Angelini-A	1	100	3	101	15.3%	0.33 [0,03, 3,23]	2002
Angelini-B	2	100	3	100	15.3%	0.66 [0.11, 4.04]	2002
Nathoe	1	142	2	139	10.4%	0.49 [0.04, 5.42]	2003
Muneretto	0	88	0	88		Not estimable	2003
Lee	0	30	1	30	7.7%	0.32 [0.01, 8.24]	2003
Widimsky	0	208	0	192		Not estimable	2004
Puskas	2	100	2	100	10.2%	1.00 [0.14, 7.24]	2004
Lingaas	0	60	0	60		Not estimable	2006
Karolak	0	150	0	150		Not estimable	2007
Shroyer	14	1104	8	1099	41.1%	1.75 [0.73, 4.19]	2009
Total (95% CI)		**2122**		**2099**	**100.0%**	**1.05 [0.56, 1.96]**	
Total events	20		19				

Heterogeneity: Chi^2 = 3.47, df = 5 (p = 0.63); I^2 = 0%
Test for overall effect: Z = 0.15 (P = 0.88)

Fig. 32.3 Forest plot of 11 high quality randomized clinical trials: intervention effect of off-pump versus on-pump coronary artery bypass grafting on the risk of stroke. CI denotes confidence interval; M-H denotes Mantel–Haenszel odds ratio.

Czerny M, Baumer H, Kilo J, et al. Complete revascularization in coronary artery bypass grafting with and without cardiopulmonary bypass. Ann Thorac Surg 2001; 71: 165–9.

Angelini GD, Taylor FC, Reeves BC, Ascione R. Early and midterm outcome after off-pump and on-pump surgery in Beating Heart Against Cardioplegic Arrest Studies (BHACAS 1 and 2): a pooled analysis of two randomised controlled trials. Lancet 2002; 359: 1194–9.

Nathoe HM, van Dijk D, Jansen EWL, et al. A comparison of on-pump and off-pump coronary bypass surgery in low-risk patients. N Engl J Med 2003; 348: 394–402.

Muneretto C, Bisleri G, Negri A, et al. Off-pump coronary artery bypass surgery technique for total arterial myocardial revascularization: a prospective randomized study. Ann Thorac Surg 2003; 76: 778–82.

Lee JD, Lee SJ, Tsushima WT, et al. Benefits of off-pump bypass on neurologic and clinical morbidity: a prospective randomized trial. Ann Thorac Surg 2003; 76: 18–25.

Straka Z, Widimsky P, Jirasek K, et al. Off-pump versus on-pump coronary surgery: final results from a prospective randomized study PRAGUE-4. Ann Thorac Surg 2004; 77: 789–93.

Puskas JD, Williams WH, Duke PG, et al. Off-pump coronary artery bypass grafting provides complete revascularization with reduced myocardial injury, transfusion requirements, and length of stay: a prospective randomized comparison of two hundred unselected patients undergoing off-pump versus conventional coronary artery bypass grafting. J Thorac Cardiovasc Surg 2003; 125: 797–808.

Lingaas PS, Hol PK, Lundblad R, et al. Clinical and angiographic outcome of coronary surgery with and without cardiopulmonary bypass: a Prospective Randomized Trial. Heart Surg Forum 2004; 7: 37–41.

Karolak W, Hirsch G, Buth K, Légaré JF. Medium-term outcomes of coronary artery bypass graft surgery on pump versus off pump: results from a randomized controlled trial. Am Heart J 2007; 153(4): 689–95.

Shroyer AL, Grover FL, Hattler B, et al; Group VAROOBRS. On-pump versus off-pump coronary-artery bypass surgery. N Engl J Med 2009; 361: 1827–37.

forest plot of an up-to-date meta-analysis of 11 high quality RCTs comparing strokes rates after off- and on-pump CABG surgery. In a pooled sample of 4121 patients randomized to off- versus on-pump CABG surgery, the incidence of stroke was 0.94% and 0.91%, respectively (relative risk 1.05; 95% CI 0.56–1.96). Although this meta-analysis suggests that there is not even a trend towards a lower stroke rate after off-pump CABG surgery, the confidence interval is wide and it is still possible that an adequately powered RCT would show a benefit (or harm) of off-pump CABG surgery on stroke rate. It would require a sample size of around 5000 patients to demonstrate a statistically significant reduction in the incidence of stroke from 2% after on-pump CABG surgery to 1% after off-pump CABG surgery. It is obvious that such a large RCT would be difficult to perform as the largest trial conducted thus far included only 2203 patients (43).

The assessment of POCD requires the administration of neuropsychological tests before and after the operation. Therefore, the sample size of studies evaluating the incidence of POCD is usually smaller than the sample size of studies evaluating the incidence of stroke. The first large RCT comparing cognitive outcomes after off- versus on-pump CABG surgery study was the Octopus trial, which included 281 patients (44). A post-hoc analysis of the 3-month cognitive performance using a reliable and conservative definition of POCD showed that the incidence of POCD was 3.9% after off-pump and 11.7% after on-pump surgery (relative risk 0.34; 95% CI 0.12–0.90) (14). However, at 1- and 5-year follow-up, there was no difference between the two groups, regardless of the definition applied (44). A study in 120 elderly patients undergoing CABG surgery failed to demonstrate a difference in the incidence of POCD (45). The ROOBY trial completed a cognitive assessment in 1156 of the 2203 randomized patients, and again failed to demonstrate a difference POCD at 1-year follow-up (43).

Several other RCTs have been performed, but because all trials conducted differ in the composition the neuropsychological test battery, the timing of assessment, and definitions of POCD, a valid meta-analysis of the data from these trials is impossible. Taking all the evidence into account that is currently available, it must be concluded that there is probably some benefit of off-pump CABG surgery on cognitive outcome in the first months after surgery. However, there seems to be no measurable effect of off-pump versus on-pump CABG surgery on long-term cognitive outcome (4,44).

Techniques to reduce embolization of aortic atheroma

Significant atherosclerosis of the ascending aorta is present in approximately 10–15% of patients undergoing cardiac surgery. Atheromatous plaques that are manipulated (due to palpation, clamping, and cannulation) or exposed to aortic cannula flow (sandblasting effect) are prone to release emboli, which may result in stroke. There are several techniques that may help to reduce the risk of embolization.

Epiaortic ultrasound scanning can guide the surgeon to select cannulation and cross-clamping sites free of atheroma (6). When severe atheroma is detected, the surgeon may use techniques involving less aortic manipulation, such as axillary or femoral cannulation, the use of a single cross-clamp technique, converting

to off-pump surgery or even replacement of the ascending aorta. Observational studies suggest that surgical decision making guided by epiaortic ultrasound may result in a lower risk of stroke (4). However, the use of epiaortic ultrasound varies widely across centres.

Transoesophageal echocardiography can be performed before sternotomy, which enables the surgeon to make strategic decisions at a more appropriate time. However, visualization of the distal part of the ascending aorta is hindered by the interposition of the trachea. Atheroma in the descending aorta, however, does predict the presence of atheroma in the ascending aorta (5,6).

Other strategies to improve cerebral outcome

Prevention and treatment of delirium

In cardiac surgery patients, strategies to prevent delirium have not been extensively studied. Simple measures to improve sleep quality, such as ear plugs, noise reduction, and frequent orientation will do no harm, but there is no evidence that such measures are effective (17,18).

Treatment of delirium should start with an investigation into possible treatable underlying causes, such as infection, hypoxaemia, withdrawal from substances or medication, or anticholinergic medication. Orientation aides (clock, calendar) should be provided and noise reduced where possible. Pharmacological intervention is usually based on antipsychotic drugs, most commonly haloperidol, olanzapine, or quetiapine. Benzodiazepines and opioids may prolong the duration of delirium, whereas sedation with dexmedetomidine may reduce the incidence of delirium in intensive care patients. The treatment of hypoactive delirium is difficult, as antipsychotic drugs also have a sedative effect (17,18).

Prevention of atrial fibrillation

New onset atrial fibrillation after cardiac surgery is common, and poses a risk of cerebral embolization. The reported incidence of new onset atrial fibrillation after cardiac surgery varies between 20 and 50%. Postoperative prophylactic drugs to decrease the risk of new onset atrial fibrillation include low doses of metoprolol, sotalol, amiodarone and hydrocortisone (46).

Conclusion

In conclusion, cerebral complications of heart surgery range from clinically apparent stroke to more subtle cognitive changes and transient postoperative delirium. Cerebral complications are still common, but the incidence of stroke due to cardiac surgery has decreased over the last decades. Cerebral complications of heart surgery have been attributed to the use of CPB, but RCTs in patients undergoing CABG surgery indicate no favourable effect of off-pump versus on-pump surgery on stroke rate or long-term cognitive outcome. Preoperative and intraoperative screening can be used to identify patients with an increased risk for cerebral complications. Surgical and perfusion techniques can be modified according to the results of this screening to improve cerebral outcomes.

References

1. Roach GW, Kanchuger M, Mangano CM et al. Adverse cerebral outcomes after coronary bypass surgery. Multicenter study of Perioperative Ischemia Research Group and the Ischemia Research and Education Foundation Investigators. *N Engl J Med* 1996; **335**: 1857–63

2. Newman MF, Mathew JP, Grocott HP et al. Central nervous system injury associated with cardiac surgery. *Lancet* 2006; **368**: 694–703

3. Stamou SC, Hill PC, Dangas G et al. Stroke after coronary artery bypass: incidence, predictors, and clinical outcome. *Stroke* 2001; **32**: 1508–13

4. Selnes OA, Gottesman RF, Grega MA, Baumgartner WA, Zeger SL, Mckhann GM. Cognitive and neurologic outcomes after coronary-artery bypass surgery. *N Engl J Med* 2012; **366**: 250–7

5. Grogan K, Stearns J, Hogue CW. Brain protection in cardiac surgery. *Anesthesiol Clin* 2008; **26**: 521–38

6. Van Zaane B, Zuithoff NPA, Reitsma JB, Bax L, Nierich AP, Moons KGM. Meta-analysis of the diagnostic accuracy of transesophageal echocardiography for assessment of atherosclerosis in the ascending aorta in patients undergoing cardiac surgery. *Acta Anaesthesiol Scand* 2008; **52**: 1179–87

7. Hogue CW, Barzilai B, Pieper KS et al. Sex differences in neurological outcomes and mortality after cardiac surgery: a society of thoracic surgery national database report. *Circulation* 2001; **103**: 2133–7

8. Newman SP, Harrison MJG (2002). Coronary-artery bypass surgery and the brain: persisting concerns. *Lancet Neurol* **1**: 119–25

9. Mckhann GM, Grega MA, Borowicz LM, Baumgartner WA, Selnes OA. Stroke and encephalopathy after cardiac surgery: an update. *Stroke* 2006; **37**: 562–71

10. Leary MC, Caplan LR. Technology insight: brain MRI and cardiac surgery—detection of postoperative brain ischemia. *Nat Clin Pract Cardiovasc Med* (2007). **4**: 379–88

11. Bendszus M, Stoll G. Silent cerebral ischaemia: hidden fingerprints of invasive medical procedures. *Lancet Neurol* 2006; **5**: 364–72

12. Van Dijk D, Keizer AMA, Diephuis JC, Durand C, Vos LJ, Hijman R. Neurocognitive dysfunctions following coronary artery bypass surgery: a systematic review. *J Thorac Cardiovasc Surg* 2000; **120**: 632–9

13. Newman MF, Kirchner JL, Phillips-Bute B, et al. Longitudinal assessment of neurocognitive function after coronary-artery bypass surgery. *N Engl J Med* 2001; **344**: 395–402

14. Keizer AMA, Hijman R, Kalkman CJ, Kahn RS, Van Dijk D, Octopus Study Group. The incidence of cognitive decline after (not) undergoing coronary artery bypass grafting: the impact of a controlled definition. *Acta Anaesthesiol Scand* 2005; **49**: 1232–5

15. Selnes OA, Pham L, Zeger S, Mckhann GM. Defining cognitive change after CABG: decline versus normal variability. *Ann Thorac Surg* 2006; **82**: 388–90

16. Lewis MS, Maruff P, Silbert BS, Evered LA, Scott DA. Detection of postoperative cognitive decline after coronary artery bypass graft surgery is affected by the number of neuropsychological tests in the assessment battery. *Ann Thorac Surg* 2006; **81**: 2097–104

17. van Eijk MMJ, Slooter AJC. Delirium in intensive care unit patients. *Semin Cardiothorac Vasc Anesth* 2010; **14**: 141–7

18. Gottesman RF, Grega MA, Bailey MM, et al. Delirium after coronary artery bypass graft surgery and late mortality. *Ann Neurol* 2010; **67**: 338–44

19. Hartman GS, Yao FS, Bruefach M 3rd et al. Severity of aortic atheromatous disease diagnosed by transesophageal echocardiography predicts stroke and other outcomes associated with coronary artery surgery: a prospective study. *Anesth Analg* 1996; **83**: 701–8

20. Djaiani G, Fedorko L, Borger MA et al. Continuous-flow cell saver reduces cognitive decline in elderly patients after coronary bypass surgery. *Circulation* 2007; **116**: 1888–95

21. Rubens FD, Boodhwani M, Mesana T, et al. The cardiotomy trial: a randomized, double-blind study to assess the effect of processing of shed blood during cardiopulmonary bypass on transfusion and neurocognitive function. *Circulation* 2007; **116**(11 Suppl): I89–97

22. Martin KK, Wigginton JB, Babikian VL, Pochay VE, Crittenden MD, Rudolph JL. Intraoperative cerebral high-intensity transient signals and postoperative cognitive function: a systematic review. *Am J Surg* 2009; **197**: 55–63

23. Moody DM, Brown WR, Challa VR, Stump DA, Reboussin DM, Legault C. Brain microemboli associated with cardiopulmonary bypass: a histologic and magnetic resonance imaging study. *Ann Thorac Surg* 1995; **59**: 1304–7

24. Moat NE, Shore DF, Evans TW. Organ dysfunction and cardiopulmonary bypass: the role of complement and complement regulatory proteins. *Eur J Cardiothorac Surg* 1993; **7**: 563–73

25. Harris DN, Bailey SM, Smith PL, Taylor KM, Oatridge A, Bydder GM. Brain swelling in first hour after coronary artery bypass surgery. *Lancet* 1993; **342**: 586–7

26. Lloyd CT, Ascione R, Underwood MJ, Gardner F, Black A, Angelini GD. Serum S-100 protein release and neuropsychologic outcome during coronary revascularization on the beating heart: a prospective randomized study. *J Thorac Cardiovasc Surg* 2000; **119**: 148–54

27. Gottesman RF, Sherman PM, Grega MA et al. Watershed strokes after cardiac surgery: diagnosis, etiology, and outcome. *Stroke* (2006). **37**: 2306–11

28. Moller JT, Cluitmans P, Rasmussen LS, et al. Long-term postoperative cognitive dysfunction in the elderly ISPOCD1 study. ISPOCD investigators. International Study of Post-Operative Cognitive Dysfunction. *Lancet* 1998; **351**: 857–61

29. Selnes OA, Mckhann GM. Neurocognitive complications after coronary artery bypass surgery. *Ann Neurol* 2005; **57**: 615–21

30. Evered L, Scott DA, Silbert B, Maruff P. Postoperative cognitive dysfunction is independent of type of surgery and anesthetic. *Anesth Analg* 2011; **112**: 1179–85

31. Crosby G, Culley DJ. Surgery and anesthesia: healing the body but harming the brain? *Anesth Analg* 2011; **112**: 999–1001

32. Newman MF, Wolman R, Kanchuger M, et al. Multicenter preoperative stroke risk index for patients undergoing coronary artery bypass graft surgery. Multicenter Study of Perioperative Ischemia (McSPI) Research Group. *Circulation* 1996; **94**: II74–80

33. Fedorow C, Grocott HP. Cerebral monitoring to optimize outcomes after cardiac surgery. *Curr Opin Anaesthesiol* 2010; **23**: 89–94.

34. Rodriguez RA, Rubens FD, Wozny D, Nathan HJ. Cerebral emboli detected by transcranial Doppler during cardiopulmonary bypass are not correlated with postoperative cognitive deficits. *Stroke* 2010; **41**: 2229–35

35. Denault A, Deschamps A, Murkin JM. A proposed algorithm for the intraoperative use of cerebral near-infrared spectroscopy. *Semin Cardiothorac Vasc Anesth* 2007; **11**: 274–81

36. Grigore AM, Murray CF, Ramakrishna H, Djaiani G. A core review of temperature regimens and neuroprotection during cardiopulmonary bypass: does rewarming rate matter? *Anesth Analg* 2009; **109**: 1741–51

37. Hogue CW Jr, Palin CA, Arrowsmith JE. Cardiopulmonary bypass management and neurologic outcomes: an evidence-based appraisal of current practices. *Anesth Analg* 2006; **103**: 21–37

38. Nissen P, Brassard P, Jørgensen TB, Secher NH. Phenylephrine but not ephedrine reduces frontal lobe oxygenation following anesthesia-induced hypotension. *Neurocrit Care* 2009; **12**(1): 17–23

39. Li Y, Walicki D, Mathiesen C, et al. Strokes after cardiac surgery and relationship to carotid stenosis. *Arch Neurol* 2009; **66**: 1091–6

40. Bouchard D, Carrier M, Demers P, et al. Statin in combination with beta-blocker therapy reduces postoperative stroke after coronary artery bypass graft surgery. *Ann Thorac Surg* 2011; **91**: 654–9

41. Mangano DT. Aspirin and mortality from coronary bypass surgery. *N Engl J Med* 2002; **347**: 1309–17

42. Møller CH, Penninga L, Wetterslev J, Steinbrüchel DA, Gluud C. Clinical outcomes in randomized trials of off- vs. on-pump coronary

artery bypass surgery: systematic review with meta-analyses and trial sequential analyses. *Eur Heart J* 2008; **29**: 2601–16

43. Shroyer AL, Grover FL, Hattler B, et al. On-pump versus off-pump coronary-artery bypass surgery. *N Engl J Med* 2009; **361**: 1827–37

44. Van Dijk D, Spoor M, Hijman R, et al. Cognitive and cardiac outcomes 5 years after off-pump vs on-pump coronary artery bypass graft surgery. *JAMA* 2007; **297**: 701–8

45. Jensen BØ, Hughes P, Rasmussen LS, Pedersen PU, Steinbrüchel DA. Cognitive outcomes in elderly high-risk patients after off-pump versus conventional coronary artery bypass grafting: a randomized trial. *Circulation* 2006; **113**: 2790–5

46. Dieleman JM, van Paassen J, Van Dijk D, et al. Prophylactic corticosteroids for cardiopulmonary bypass in adults. *Cochrane Database Syst Rev* 2011; **5**: CD005566

CHAPTER 33

Anaesthesia for thoracic surgery

Jean S. Bussières and Annie Rousseau

Introduction

Thoracic surgery and anaesthesia have a long and thrilling history (Chapter 1). The pioneer period of thoracic anaesthesia began at the onset of the 20th century and ended in the 1930s. The first thoracic surgeries were performed for empyema and tuberculosis. Control of the airway and the possibility of lung isolation with one lung ventilation (OLV) led to the first pneumonectomy for bronchiectasis in 1931. The development period extended until the late 1960s, beginning with the introduction of bronchial blockers (BB), then single-lumen endobronchial tubes, and with the first double-lumen endobronchial tube (DLT) used in 1949 (Chapter 1). The Copenhagen poliomyelitis epidemic of 1952 was associated with the invention of volumetric ventilators that led to major progress in this period. During the 1950s, a declining need for surgery for infective lung disease was associated with the emergence of lung resection for malignant tumours.

In the 1970s, during the innovative period, new concepts were introduced such as epidural analgesia and fibreoptic bronchoscopy (FOB). The 1980s saw a golden age for thoracic anaesthesia, the refinement period. Polyvinyl chloride DLTs and ready access to FOB simplified lung isolation. Greater understanding of the differential positive end-expiratory pressure (PEEP) and continuous positive airway pressure (CPAP) effects and the demonstration of the utility of CPAP on the non-dependent lung increased the safety of OLV. Pulse oximetry, end-tidal capnography, and the use of continuous spirometry added to the efficacy and safety of OLV. The marketing of specific BBs, initially inserted in the wall of a single-lumen tube (SLT), and then followed by single BBs with a multiport adaptor allowing easier insertion via a standard SLT, led to the rebirth of this type of lung isolation.

Finally, with the new century began the non-invasive surgery period. Widespread use of video-assisted thoracoscopic surgery (VATS), precluding application of CPAP on the non-dependant lung, but highlighting the value of PEEP on the dependent lung was confirmed as a useful adjunct during OLV. Epidural analgesia lost its popularity with VATS, favouring paravertebral blockade. The sickest patients which were previously denied surgery by thoracotomy may now have a pulmonary resection through minimally invasive surgery.

Open thoracotomy and video-assisted thoracoscopy

Open thoracotomy

The standard postero-lateral thoracotomy is still the most commonly used surgical approach but others can be used according to specific indications (table 33.1).

Thoracotomy incisions are associated with variable degrees of postoperative pain and all have the potential for chronic post-thoracotomy pain (Chapter 39). Posterolateral thoracotomy has the worse reputation, anterior incisions provoke less pain. Muscle-sparing thoracotomies are thought to induce less postoperative pain because the chest wall muscles are retracted as opposed to being divided.

Video-assisted thoracoscopy

Technologic developments in video imaging systems and instrumentation have led to the increasing popularity of VATS since the early 1990s. A large variety of medical and surgical procedures, involving pleura, lung, mediastinum, and oesophagus, are now routinely performed by VATS. Other procedures such as sympathectomy, spinal surgery, or post-trauma procedures may be also done with VATS. Many patients who could not tolerate thoracic surgery by a traditional open approach may now undergo their surgery by VATS. The benefits are a reduction in severity and duration of postoperative pain, less respiratory dysfunction, shorter hospital stay, and faster recovery (1).

Medical thoracoscopy

Medical thoracoscopy is done for diagnostic purposes, mainly for pleural effusion of unknown aetiology or malignant pleural disease. It is done by a pulmonologist in the endoscopy suite and involves a single entry port into the thoracic cavity under local anaesthesia. Thoracoscopy can be safely done in an awake, spontaneously breathing subject using supplemental oxygen with conscious sedation and analgesia. In spontaneously breathing patients, although the lung is partially deflated during the procedure, there is little change in arterial oxygen (PaO_2) and carbon dioxide ($PaCO_2$) tension, or cardiac rhythm (2,3).

Table 33.1 Surgical approaches used in cardiothoracic surgery

Approaches	Usual indications
Antero superior approaches	
Cervical transverse	Tracheal surgery
	Thyroid surgery
Supraclavicular	Surgery of tumours located in the thoracic inlet (Pancoast tumours)
Transverse cervical (Mediastinoscopy)	Staging of lung cancer
Anterior thoracic incisions	
Median sternotomy	Cardiac surgery
Partial sternotomy	Resection of mediastinal tumours
	Thyroid, thymus
	Tracheal (middle) resection
Transverse sternotomy (Clamshell, hemi-clamshell)	Resection of mediastinal tumours
	Lung transplant
Parasternal (Mediastinotomy)	Staging lung cancer
Anterolateral thoracic incisions	Surgery of bullous lung diseases
	Lung biopsy
Axillary thoracic incisions	Surgery for pneumothorax
Posterior thoracic incisions	
Posterolateral thoracotomy	Pulmonary resection
	Tracheal (lower) and carinal resection
Lateral muscle-sparing thoracotomy	Pulmonary resection
Thoraco-abdominal incision	Extensive aortic surgery
	Oesophageal surgery
Abdominal	
Upper midline incision	Access to oesophageal hiatus

When the nondependent hemithorax is opened during thoracoscopy, the negative pleural pressure causes air to enter into the pleural cavity, creating a pneumothorax. The open-chest lung, exposed to the atmospheric pressure, tends to collapse because of unopposed elastic recoil. During spontaneous ventilation, this collapse is accentuated by the inspiration, because of increased negative pleural pressure, and is decreased during expiration. This reversal of lung movement during respiration has been named pendelluft or paradoxical respiration (4). Around the dependent, closed-chest lung, pleural pressure is also negative during inspiration, creating an imbalance between the two sides of the mediastinum which shifts toward the dependant lung during inspiration. The tidal volume of the closed-chest lung is thus reduced by the mediastinal shift. This mediastinal shift can also decrease venous return to the right heart, with concomitant activation of the sympathetic system. These changes have surprisingly little effect on the physiological and clinical parameters measured during the procedure, partly owing to the fact that the dependent lower lung is better perfused and ventilated and compensates for its open-chest counterpart.

Surgical video-assisted thoracoscopy

VATS is performed in the operating room by a thoracic surgeon and entails multiple small incisions in the chest wall, allowing introduction of a video camera and surgical instruments into the thoracic cavity through access ports. VATS is usually performed in the lateral decubitus position, as with posterolateral thoracotomy. PEEP, rather than CPAP, can be used to optimize oxygenation during OLV (5). Paravertebral block (PVB), either as a single injection or as a continuous infusion, is ideally suited to VATS. Chronic post-thoracotomy pain is reported in at least 40–80% of open thoracotomy patients, and a similar incidence has been reported post-VATS (Chapter 39) (6).

Mediastinoscopy

Mediastinoscopy is usually done to obtain tissue samples to establish the operability of intrathoracic tumours (7). The mediastinoscope is introduced through a small suprasternal incision and advanced by blunt dissection into the superior mediastinum, between the trachea and the aortic arch. An alternative procedure is the anterior (or parasternal) mediastinotomy, made through a small incision in the interchondral space or via an excised second costal cartilage. Left parasternal mediastinotomy may be used for staging left upper lobe lesions.

Prior to these procedures, a large-bore intravenous cannula should be inserted because of the risk of major haemorrhage. If the patient presents with a superior vena cava (SVC) syndrome, the cannula should be placed in the lower limb. In patients with compromized cerebral perfusion, such as cerebrovascular disease, the use of an arterial line in the right arm may be useful to diagnose intermittent obstruction of the innominate artery by the mediastinoscope, impairing right common carotid artery blood flow. This obstruction may cause cerebral hypoperfusion and transient or permanent cerebral damage. If persistent compression occurs, the surgeon should be advised to reposition the mediastinoscope. The patient is positioned with a rolled cushion under the shoulders to obtain maximal cervical extension. A head ring may be used to stabilize the head. The tracheal tube should be carefully secured as it might be dislodged by the surgeon's manipulations.

Bleeding from surgical trauma to a great vessel in the mediastinum is an infrequent but major complication. Mild haemorrhage may be controlled by conservative measures such as head-up position, controlled hypotension and wound tamponade with surgical sponges. Catastrophic bleeding requires emergency sternotomy or lateral thoracotomy. Additional intravenous access should be obtained in the lower limbs if the SVC is traumatized.

Airway compression may occur during induction of anaesthesia, during the mediastinoscopy and also postoperatively, secondary to surgery-related oedema. It is important to review prior radiological and bronchoscopic evaluations to detect any potential risk of airway compression. A local anaesthetic technique may be preferable in some circumstances.

Air embolism through an open mediastinal vein is a risk associated with mediastinoscopy. Positive pressure ventilation and avoiding the head down position are useful to minimize this complication. Other complications include pneumothorax, paresis of the laryngeal nerve, phrenic nerve injury, oesophageal injury, and chylothorax. All these events are usually diagnosed in the immediate postoperative period.

Pulmonary resection

Pulmonary resection is most often done for malignant tumours. The vast majority of these resections require lung isolation and OLV, now most often with VATS.

Monitoring

In addition to basic monitoring, non-invasive respiratory monitoring should be considered. As significant episodes of desaturation might occur during OLV, the role of pulse oximetry is magnified. In addition, intermittent measurements of arterial blood gases are needed to estimate the margin of safety above desaturation compared with oximetry. Continuous measurement of the inspired oxygen fraction (FiO_2) is essential as during the OLV, it should be minimized to limit potential oxygen toxicity to the lung. Capnometry ($ETCO_2$) is a less reliable indicator of $PaCO_2$ during OLV, as the $PaCO_2$-$ETCO_2$ gradient is usually increased. During OLV, $ETCO_2$ reflects the lung perfusion in each lung (8). During OLV, the dependent lung with a higher $ETCO_2$ tends to have a better PaO_2, as the perfusion is higher in this lung. Regardless, the $ETCO_2$ trend may be useful to detect modifications in minute ventilation. Continuous spirometry loops are useful to detect the loss of lung isolation, highlighted by a sudden decrease in expiratory volume or a failure to close the loop at the end of the expiration, and to assess and manage pulmonary air leak during or after pulmonary resection (9). Finally, during OLV, the development of a persistent end-expiratory flow on the flow-volume loop correlates with the existence of auto-PEEP (10).

Invasive monitoring with an arterial line is essential for the vast majority of intrathoracic procedures. Beat-to-beat assessment of systemic blood pressure is a practical mean to detect transient severe hypotension that may happen frequently during intrathoracic intervention from surgical compression of the heart or of the great vessels. Moreover, it allows intermittent blood gases analysis perioperatively. Central venous pressure monitoring is usually reserved for pneumonectomy, where fluid status is critical. In patients having lesser resections, the presence of some concomitant diseases may nevertheless necessitate the insertion of a central venous catheter. A pulmonary artery catheter is rarely helpful.

Transoesophageal echocardiography (TOE) has a limited role in thoracic surgery but may be valuable where there is cardiac involvement by the tumour during pulmonary thrombo-endarterectomy, lung transplantation, and for some thoracic trauma. However, imaging may poor in the lateral position because of mediastinal shift.

Positioning

The vast majority of intrathoracic surgeries require lateral positioning of the patient to access the thoracic cavity, whether via open thoracotomy or thoracoscopy. General anaesthesia is usually induced with the patient in the supine position. The patient is then positioned on its side, with the operative lung in the non-dependent position.

Cervical spine

Special attention needs to be paid to the cervical spine as it needs to be kept in a neutral position to avoid vascular occlusion and neuromuscular trauma. In addition, extension of the cervical spine may dislodge the lung isolation device, and flexion may lead to lobar obstruction. For this reason, after the patient is positioned laterally, FOB is mandatory to verify and if required, reposition the device.

Neurovascular complications

Eyes and ears should be protected against pressure injury. The cervical spine should be carefully positioned and stabilized, as excessive lateral flexion may cause a 'whiplash' syndrome. Padding or a pillow should be used under the thorax to keep the weight of the upper body off the dependent brachial plexus. Attention should be paid to avoid stretch lesion or vascular compression of the upper non-dependent arm when placed on the arm support. The dependent leg should be slightly flexed, and padding used to protect the lateral peroneal nerve and avoid vascular compression. Finally, to avoid sciatic nerve compression, it is essential to not use excessively tight strapping at the level of the buttocks.

Respiratory changes

The application of PEEP to the dependent lung usually improves gas exchange by restoring functional residual capacity (FRC) and compliance.

Anaesthetic management

Although regional anaesthesia is widely used (10–15), many general anaesthetic regimens can be used for thoracic surgery. Specific skills include lung isolation techniques, OLV, and regional anaesthesia. IV fluids should be minimized to avoid postpneumonectomy pulmonary oedema (16), but judicious replacement is unlikely to cause harm (17–19). Body temperature is frequently difficult to maintain during thoracotomy as the hemithorax is wide open and favours heat loss. Lower body forced-air warming is useful to prevent hypothermia (20). Heated intravenous fluids are helpful if confronted with significant haemorrhage.

Following pneumonectomy, many surgeons use intrathoracic aspiration, with both a syringe and needle, to balance the mediastinum and prevent excessive mediastinal shift. Throughout this manoeuvre, the anaesthetist must monitor the arterial blood pressure closely.

Early tracheal extubation is recommended to prevent positive pressure putting undue stress on parenchymal or bronchial suture lines. A portable chest radiograph is always obtained to rule out pneumothorax, atelectasis, haemothorax, or other problems. Postoperative analgesia should be optimized before the patient is discharged from the recovery room.

Lung isolation techniques

DLT are most commonly used to obtain lung isolation but some anaesthesiologists favour BBs, and single lumen endobronchial tubes are now rarely used (21–23).

Absolute indications

- For protection against spillage of pus (abscess, bronchiectasis), liquid (cyst, lung lavage), or blood (massive haemoptysis) from the contralateral lung.
- To control ventilation to each lung if rupture of a major airway such as bronchopleural fistula, or traumatic lesion of parenchyma, for example giant bullae or pneumothorax.

Table 33.2 Relationship between dimensions of some fibreoptic bronchoscopes and lung isolation bronchial tubes

'FOB Olympus'	BFQ-180	LVF-180	BFXP-160F
External diameter (mm)	5.5	4.1	2.8
Inner diameter (mm)	2.0	1.2	1.2
Vision angle (degrees)	120	120	90
Curvature angle (degrees)	180–130	120–120	180–130
DLT*		**Fr**	**Fr**
Double lumen tube* (DLT)	X	41–39–37–35	32–28–26
BB**	**mm**	**mm**	**mm**
Simple lumen tube (SLT)	7.5	5.0	3.5
SLT + BB** Cook (9 Fr)	9.0	7.5	6.5
SLT + BB** Cook (7 Fr)	X	7.0	5.5
SLT + BB** Fuji (9 Fr)	9.0	7.5	6.5
SLT + Fogarty (8 Fr)	9.0	7.0	6.0
BB + DLT	**Fr**	**Fr**	**Fr**
DLT + BB** Cook (9 Fr)	X	41–39	41–39–37–35
DLT + BB** Cook (7 Fr)	X	41–39–37	41–39–37–35
DLT + BB** Fuji (9 Fr)	X	41–39	41–39–37–35
DLT + Fogarty (7 Fr)	X	41–39–37	41–39–37–35
Suction + exchanger			
DLT	37–39–41	35	32
Suction	#14	#12	#10
Exchanger Cook (green)	5 mm (14 Fr)	4 mm (11 Fr)	

* DLT: Mallinckrodt **BB: bronchial blocker

Relative indications

• To keep the lung immobile for thoracic, mediastinal, oesophageal, cardiac, vascular, or vertebral surgery.

Radiological imaging

When planning lung isolation, it is essential to review the radiographic imaging to determine what type and size of device should be chosen. New modalities such as 3-D reconstitution can be helpful to anticipate and prevent difficulties in lung isolation.

Fibreoptic bronchoscopy

Results of preoperative bronchoscopic imaging can be very useful, but FOB examination performed during the actual anaesthetic is frequently more helpful (24,25). A modern thoracic operating room needs infrastructure such as two separate, but interrelated, towers of video equipment, one for the surgical team and the other for the anaesthesia team. The imaging from one tower should be exportable on the screen of the other system when one team needs

to present or to discuss a particular view. The anaesthesia tower should have at least two FOBs: one of regular size (5.2 mm) for airway examination and bronchial toilet through an endotracheal tube (ETT) of 7.0 mm or more, and one of smaller size (3.8–4.2 mm) for DLT positioning. In addition, an even smaller FOB (2.8 mm) may be useful in some special circumstances such as the placement of a BB into a small ETT or DLT (26, 28, 32 Fr). An adult-size regular FOB is the only one with suction channels large enough (2 mm) to provide adequate suctioning. The suction channels of smaller FOBs are too small (1.2 mm; see table 33.2). They can be used for light suction but the blind use of a suction catheter is often more efficacious when used in conjunction with FOB.

Anatomy of the tracheobronchial tree

The knowledge of the normal anatomy of the tracheobronchial tree is essential to manipulate lung isolation devices, such as FOB, DLT, and BB (figure 33.1). Thoracic anaesthesiologists should be able to identify every lobar bronchus and the number of segmental bronchi originating from each lobar bronchus.

Double-lumen tube

DLTs are available from many manufacturers in left and right versions. There is no noticeable difference between the products of each company for the left-sided DLT (L-DLT) (figure 33.2) but

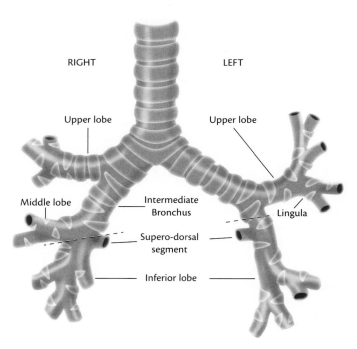

Fig. 33.1 Anatomy of the bronchial tree.
On the right main stem bronchus (MSB), the right upper lobe is originating from less than 2.5 cm of the tracheal carina, showing the classical image of the three segmental bronchi. Looking down, the intermediate bronchus follows and the *view* consists of, from left to right: 1—the middle lobe bronchus 2—the basal pyramid of the lower lobe with four segments and 3- the apical segment of the lower lobe with three sub segments.
The left MSB is longer (up to 5.0 cm) compared to the right MSB. The left upper lobe presents two superior segmental bronchi and a lingular segmental bronchus which separates into two segmental bronchi. The left lower lobe bronchus presents an apical segmental bronchus and a pyramid of three segmental bronchi.

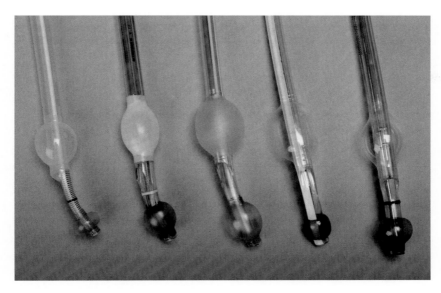

Fig. 33.2 Left-sided double lumen tubes.
From left to right: Phycon SilBroncho tube, Fuji System Corporation, Japan; Hudson RCI Sheridan Sher-I-Bronch® endobronchial tube, Teleflex Medical Research, Triangle Park, NC, USA; Portex® Blue Line endobronchial tube, Smiths Medical International Ltd; Keene, NH, USA; Bronchopart® double lumen bronchial tube, Laboratoires Pharmaceutiques Rusch France; Broncho-Cath®, Mallinckrodt™ endobronchial tube, Covidien, Mansfield, MA, USA.

there are significant differences between the right-sided DLT (R-DLT), as shown in figure 33.3.

Different sizes are available: 26, 28, 32, 35, 37, 39, and 41 French (Fr). Some studies suggest measuring the tracheal diameter on the posteroanterior chest radiograph (25) or CT image reconstruction (26) to predict optimal DLT size, but these measurements are not universally used. In the authors' practice, 39 and 41 Fr are frequently used for men and 35 and 37 Fr are chosen for women.

Insertion of double-lumen tubes

The insertion of left- and right-sided DLT should be considered differently since the anatomy differs for each main bronchus (figure 33.1). Because of the origin of the right upper lobe (RUL) bronchus, situated at 1.5–2 cm from the carina, the manufacturers incorporated a specially designed endobronchial cuff and an opening to allow ventilation of the RUL (figure 33.4).

Left-sided lumen tubes

A left-sided DLT (L-DLT) should be inserted with the malleable guide supplied by the manufacturer inserted into the bronchial lumen, with the assistance of a laryngoscope. After the tip of the DLT passes through the vocal cords, the stylet is removed and the L-DLT is rotated 90° to the left and advanced blindly until a small level of resistance is encountered. The tracheal cuff is inflated and ventilation initiated. At this point, auscultation may be used but FOB will ensure rapid and accurate positioning of the L-DLT. This blind technique is more effective and rapid for initial insertion of L-DLT than a completely directed FOB approach (27). Hybrid use of auscultation and FOB has been recently suggested and this may give the best results (28). If repositioning of the DLT is necessary, it is essential to deflate the tracheal cuff.

The authors' sequence is described next and illustrated in figure 33.5. The right bronchial tree is initially explored to confirm that the L-DLT is properly positioned into the left main bronchus, and to visualize any pathological lesion that may need to be looked over during the surgery. The relative position of the black radio-opaque line, the tracheal carina, and the bronchial cuff are then noted. Additional information, obtained by the introduction of the FOB in the bronchial lumen, is needed to finely position the L-DLT. The L-DLT is optimally positioned when the origin of the superior and the inferior left lobe bronchus are visualized by FOB. Withdrawing the FOB, a rapid look by transparency allows visualization of the tracheal carina by FOB through the transparent wall of the bronchial lumen of the DLT and the evaluation of its relative position between the black radiopaque line and the superior portion of the bronchial cuff (29). This position may add a margin of safety, up to 10 mm, for any distal displacement of the L-DLT during the patient's positioning. In some patients, this view is obscured by the humidity generated during the expiratory phase, but it should clear itself during inspiration. Unfortunately, some commercial designs of L-DLTs have characteristics such as an opaque bronchial-lumen wall, precluding use of this technique (30). Once the L-DLT extremity is properly positioned, the bronchial cuff may be inflated, or left deflated until the patient is positioned in LDP.

Right-sided double lumen tube

Indications for a right-DLT (R-DLT) include anatomical distortion of the left main bronchus by an endobronchial mass or extrinsic compression, left pneumonectomy, and sleeve resection. Many thoracic anaesthesiologists choose to use R-DLT as frequently as they can to increase their ability to use it when it becomes mandatory (31,32).

As for L-DLT, R-DLTs are inserted with a malleable guide. The stylet is removed when the tip of the DLT passes through the glottis, then the R-DLT is turned 90° to the right. Unlike L-DLT, the R-DLT is only advanced for a few centimetres to position its bronchial extremity just above the tracheal carina. Even if the tracheal cuff is not inflated, ventilation may be initiated at that moment with a high flow of 100% O_2. The FOB is then introduced into the bronchial lumen, according to the sequence illustrated

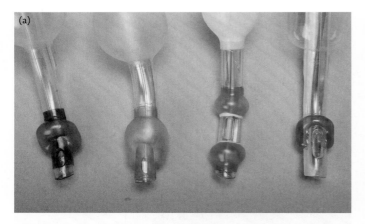

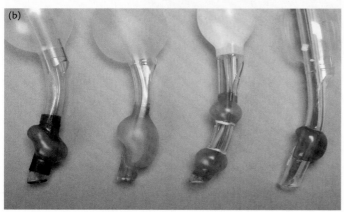

Fig. 33.3 Right-sided double lumen tubes.
(a) Anterior view; (b) Lateral view. From left to right: Broncho-Cath® Mallinckrodt™ endobronchial tube, Covidien, Mansfield, MA, USA; Portex® Blue Line endobronchial tube, Smiths Medical International Ltd, Keene, NH, USA; Hudson RCI Sheridan Sher-I-Bronch® endobronchial tube, Teleflex Medical Research, Triangle Park, NC, USA; Bronchopart® double lumen bronchial tube, Laboratoires Pharmaceutiques Rusch, France.

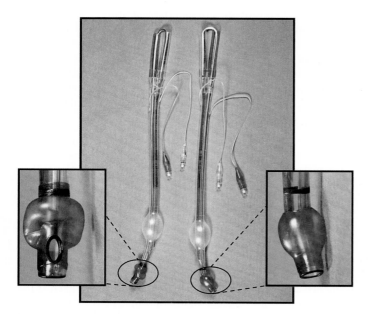

Fig. 33.4 Right and left-sided double lumen tubes.
Note the difference between the right and the left endobronchial blue cuff.

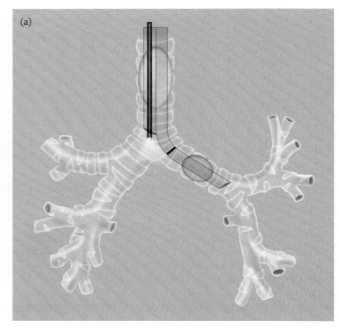

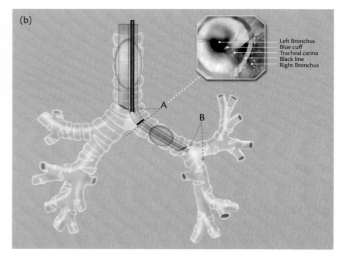

Left Bronchus
Blue cuff
Tracheal carina
Black line
Right Bronchus

Fig. 33.5 Positioning left-sided double lumen tube.
(a) Following the blind introduction of a left-sided double lumen tube into the left main stem bronchus, the fibreoptic bronchoscope is inserted into the right tracheal lumen to visualize the carina, the radiopaque line and possibly the top of the blue bronchial cuff of the left sided double lumen tube. Finally, the right sided bronchial tree is rapidly examined. (b) The fibreoptic bronchoscope is then introduced into the bronchial lumen. Going down, a look-by transparency through the wall of the bronchial lumen of the double lumen tube allows visualization of the tracheal carina. Its relative position between the black radiopaque line and the superior portion of the bronchial cuff can be then evaluated (B). Progressing distally, the superior and inferior lobar bronchus should be clearly identified (A). Withdrawing the FOB, a final view by transparency (B) is done.

in figure 33.6. Initially, the origin of the right upper lobe (RUL) bronchus as well as the anatomy of the right bronchial tree are identified prior the insertion of the R-DLT into the right main bronchus. The R-DLT is then inserted over the FOB positioned in front of the RUL bronchus origin, allowing insertion of the R-DLT in front of the lateral opening. An alternative technique of blindly-inserting the R-DLT and looking through the RUL's should then be used. A R-DLT tube with a double RUL opening has recently been introduced on the market. This design could be useful when the RUL bronchus is higher than usual (33).

Once the R-DLT's extremity is positioned, the bronchial cuff may be inflated immediately, or later when the patient is positioned in LDP. Sometimes, a compromise needs to be made between a partial alignment of the RUL bronchus origin to the lateral opening of the R-DLT and the seal of the bronchial cuff at the origin of the right main bronchus. A final look should be taken in the intermediate bronchus to confirm non-obstruction of the middle and inferior bronchi. Finally, the FOB should be reintroduced in the tracheal lumen to inspect the bronchial cuff, which may offer an adequate seal of the right main bronchus even if it is slightly herniated across the carina.

A modification of the R-DLT has been described, with an enlargement of the distal opening directed toward the RUL (figure 33.7). This facilitates the alignment between the R-DLT opening and the origin of the RUL bronchus (34).

FOB should be done every time the patient is repositioned, and should be available during the course of surgery. Another way to monitor DLT position and function during OLV is to use the volume-pressure loop (9,10). Any leak will be reflected by this curve well before it becomes clinically noticeable, allowing for quick correction of the problem before it interferes with the surgery.

Complications of double-lumen tubes

The major complication associated with a DLT is airway injury. The majority are associated with smaller DLTs (35). The trauma is most often in the membranous part of the trachea, occurring at any stage of anaesthesia and surgery.

Malposition is usually secondary to outward displacement of the endobronchial extremity into the trachea. The main causes are overinflation of the bronchial cuff, excessive surgical manipulation of the bronchus, and extension of the cervical spine during lateral positioning (36,37). On the left side, to minimize the occurrence of herniation of the bronchial cuff, the DLT should be secured with the black radio-opaque line aligned with tracheal carina level, this position adds around 10 mm of margin of security (28,29).

Bronchial blocker

A BB is an excellent alternative to a DLT, and for many anaesthesiologists it is their first choice for lung isolation. The introduction of the Univent tube, with an enclosed BB in 1988 (38,39), triggered a regained interest for BBs (figure 33.8). The introduction of the Arndt BB in 1998 (40), followed by the Cohen BB (41), and then the Uniblocker (42), convinced sceptics that BBs can be easily used and reliable (table 33.3).

BBs have a long catheter of at least 65 cm, long enough to allow the blockade of a main stem bronchus or a lobar bronchus, with an inner lumen varying between 1.3 mm and 2.0 mm. The balloon of a modern adult BB (9 Fr) is spherical, needing about 8 mL of air at low pressure.

BBs are used to occlude a mainstem bronchus to obtain lung collapse. They can also be used to selectively block lobar bronchi. BBs are all inserted inside a regular SLT and require a multiport connector (figure 33.9). The first port connects with the respiratory circuit, the second with the SLT, the third allows insertion of a FOB

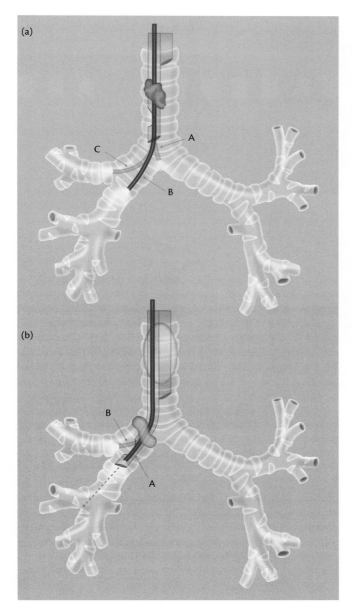

Fig. 33.6 Positioning right-sided double lumen tube.
(a) Following the blind introduction of a right-sided double lumen tube into the trachea, the FOB is inserted into the bronchial lumen. The tracheal bifurcation is visualized (A), followed by the bronchus intermedius (B), and the origin of the right upper lobe bronchus (C). The tip of the fibreoptic bronchoscope should be fixed in front of the right upper lobe bronchus' origin (B). (b) Right-sided double lumen tube is then inserted over the fibreoptic bronchoscope, positioned at the level of the right upper lobe bronchus (A), keeping the distal carina at a constant distance (arrow). When the extremity of the right-sided double lumen tube is seen through the fibreoptic bronchoscope, the insertion of the right-sided double lumen tube is stopped and the fibreoptic bronchoscope is flexed allowing visualization of the right upper lobe bronchus through the lateral orifice of the right-sided double lumen tube (B).

orifice, searching for the RUL bronchus, is more difficult and time consuming.

If the origin of the RUL bronchus is too close to the tracheal carina, the R-DLT cannot be used because the bronchial cuff will occlude the left main bronchus if properly positioned. A L-DLT

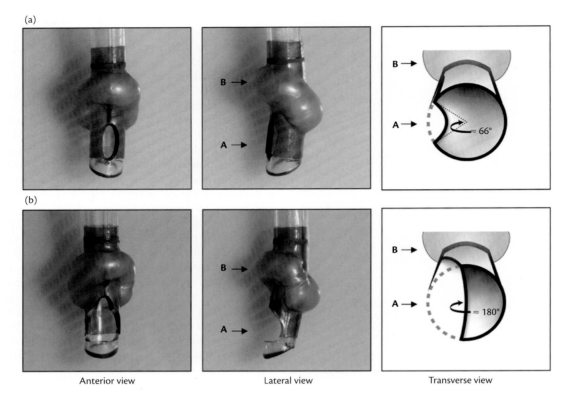

Anterior view   Lateral view   Transverse view

Fig. 33.7 Modified right-sided double lumen tube orifice.
Left: Modified right-sided Broncho-Cath® Mallinckrodt™ endobronchial tube; right: Regular right-sided Broncho-Cath® Mallinckrodt™ endobronchial tube. Note the enlarged right upper lobe orifice, which assures a better alignment with the right upper lobe bronchus' origin.

Reproduced from Springer and Canadian Anesthesiologists Society, Canadian Journal of Anaesthesia, 54, 4, pp. 276–282, 'Modified right-sided Broncho-CathTM double lumen tube improves endobronchial positioning: a randomized study', Bussières JS, et al., Copyright 2007, with kind permission from Springer Science and Business Media.

Table 33.3 Characteristics of commonly used bronchial blockers

Bronchial Blockers	Arndt			Cohen	Uniblocker	
Manufacturer	Cook			Cook	Fuji	
Year of release	1999			2005	2007	
Size (F)	**5**	**7**	**9**	**9**	5	**9**
Lenght (cm)	50	65	78	65	40	66,5
Effective length (cm)	45	57	70	57	30	51
Smallest ETT (FOB 4.2 mm)	nd	7	8	8	4.5	8
Smallest ETT (monography)	4.5	6	7.5	7,5	na	na
Balloon max vol. (cc)	2	6	**8**	**8**	3	**8**
Ballon pressure	low			low	< 30 mmHg	
Ballon shape	spherical			spherical	spherical	
Ballon length (mm)	8	20	20	23	8	22
Inner diam.(mm)	0,7	1,3	1,3	1,6	nd	2
Connector	multiport			multiport	swivel multiport	
Movement	Nylon wire loop coupled to FOB			Tip-deflecting (30°) wheel-turning device and torque control	Preshaped tip (25°) and torque control	
Miscellaneous	guide loop assembly may be re-inserted (9 Fr only)			1/4 turn max	0	
Other	side holes of 9 F			side holes	0	
Color	yellow			green	light blue	
Latex	free			free	free	

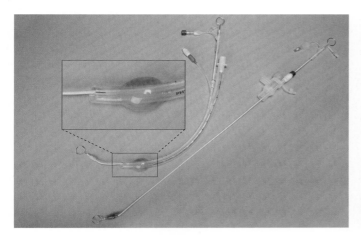

Fig. 33.8 Fuji System Corporation bronchial blockers.
Upper: the TBC Univent® tube and its enclosed bronchial blocker; lower: the Uniblocker®, which is an independent and a longer version of the enclosed bronchial blocker of the Univent®.

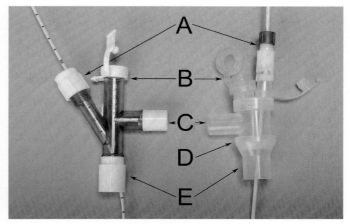

Fig. 33.9 Multi-Port Airway Adapter.
Cook Medical Inc. (left) and Fuji System Corporation (right). (A) Bronchial blocker port and locking system; (B) Fibreoptic broncoscope port; (C) Respiratory circuit port; (D) Swivel mechanism; (E) Endotracheal tube port.

through a swivel port, and the fourth is designed for inserting and locking the BB. The limiting factor is the inner diameter of the SLT, which has to accommodate at the same time the BB (usually 9 Fr or 3 mm) and the FOB (up to 4.2 mm)—see table 33.1.

Insertion of bronchial blockers

Following review of radiological imaging and the bronchoscopic report, and taking into account the planned surgery, the operative side, the localization of the BB and the diameter of SLT should be decided. The balloon should be completely deflated, as there is always a small quantity of air inside the balloon during the storage, to avoid the inner lining to stick over the main shaft of the BB. The BB and fibrescope should both be well lubricated to facilitate progression inside the SLT, taking care not to obstruct the distal end and side holes of the BB with the lubricating gel. Following tracheal intubation with a sufficiently large SLT and using a multiport connector to ventilate the patient at a FiO_2 of 1.0 ± PEEP at 5 cmH$_2$O, the BB is introduced in the upper part of the SLT along with the FOB slightly above the cuff of the BB. Balloon integrity should be checked after passing through the multiport adaptor, by inflating it until it reaches its maximal volume (see table 33.2). Care should be taken to avoid perforation of the balloon by the FOB. When the FOB is ahead of the BB in small SLTs, its movement may induce friction inside the relatively small lumen and thus may damage the balloon.

The FOB is kept above the BB until its cuff is out of the SLT. The FOB is then advanced alongside the balloon to allow viewing of the tracheal carina. A quick look inside both major bronchi may help confirm which side the BB will be directed. It is important that the extremity of the SLT is as far as possible from the carina, because it allows a wider range of motion and eases the BB's positioning under direct vision (see the next section for specific instruction for every BB). Following inflation of the balloon, the superior part of the balloon should be located between 5 to 10 mm below the level of the tracheal carina (figure 33.10 and figure 33.11). The balloon should be kept deflated. It should be reinflated under direct vision with the FOB when the patient is positioned in lateral decubitus position.

When the trachea is distorted, it is sometimes impossible to insert the BB into the desired bronchus. A solution to this problem

is to insert, under FOB guidance, the extremity of the SLT directly at the origin of the desired main bronchus. Then, the BB is pushed into position and the ETT is pulled back to the standard tracheal position.

Specific bronchial blockers
Arndt bronchial blocker

The Arndt BB has an inner lumen in which a retractable guide with a distal loop wire is inserted. (figure 33.12 A) This loop should be secured over the FOB once the two devices are passed

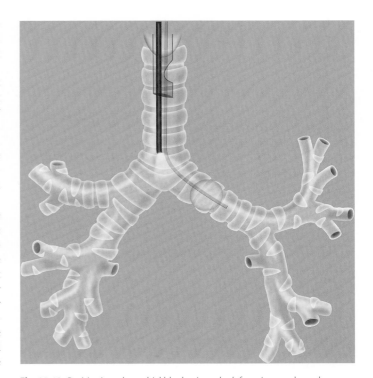

Fig. 33.10 Positioning a bronchial blocker into the left main stem bronchus
The cuff of a bronchial blocker may be positioned 10 mm down to the tracheal carina in the left main stem bronchus.

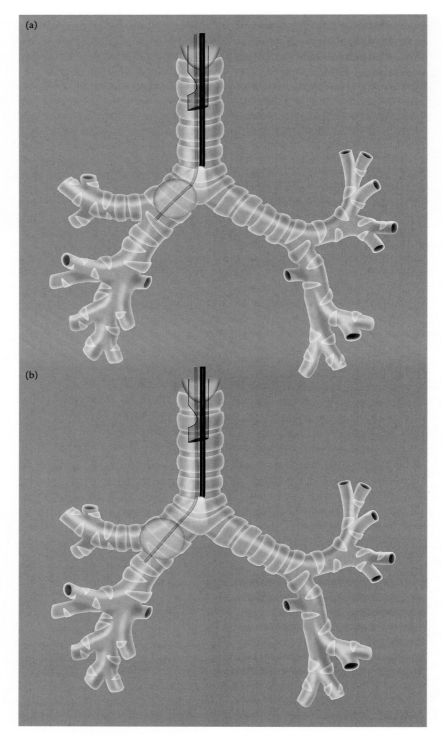

Fig. 33.11 Positioning a bronchial blocker into the right main stem bronchus.
Positioning the bronchial blocker into the right main stem bronchus is difficult because of the short right upper lobe bronchus. When the bronchial blocker is inserted to the right upper lobe bronchus, it is usually positioned near the tracheal carina and may be easily dislodged (a). Many anaesthesiologists prefer to insert the cuff of the bronchial blocker deeply as it herniates into the origin of the right upper lobe bronchus. At that time, the cuff is at approximately 10 mm down to the tracheal carina (b).

through their specific orifices of the multiport connector. This assemblage is then inserted into the SLT and its port is connected to it. At this point, the FOB is in front of the BB. Resistance to the progression of FOB and BB in smaller SLTs can be observed and consequently damaging to the cuff may occur. After identification of each main bronchus, the FOB guides the extremity of the BB in the chosen side. When the BB is in a good position, the loop is released, and the FOB is pulled back into the trachea. The balloon is then inflated under direct vision. Only with the 9 Fr BB, the loop may be retracted completely as it can be easily re-inserted. Once

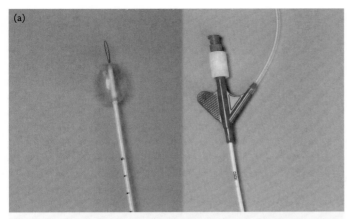

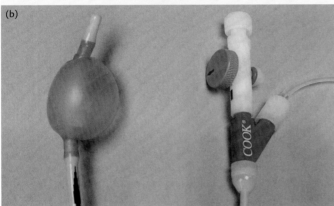

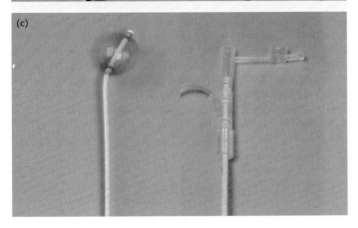

Fig. 33.12 Modern independent bronchial blockers.
(a) Arndt Endobronchial Blocker® from Cook Medical Inc, Bloomington IN, USA; wire loop and proximal extremity control; (b) Cohen Tip Deflecting Endobronchial Blocker® from Cook Medical Inc, Bloomington IN, USA; Fibreoptic like with angle up to 30°; (c) Uniblocker® BB from Fuji System Corporation, Japan, preshaped extremity at 25° and torque control.

the loop is completely retracted, suction may be applied via the inner channel to accelerate the isolated lung's deflation, or oxygen or PEEP may be delivered to this lung. There are reported cases of the loop being inadvertently trapped in the suture line when not retracted completely. Inadvertent contralateral bronchial blockade is possible at any time. If this occurs, it is preferable to completely remove the BB and repeat the entire insertion procedure.

Cohen bronchial blocker

The Cohen BB is inserted as previously described for the Arndt BB, but without the wire loop (figure 33.12 B). The tip of this BB is controlled with a wheel-turning device, under visual guidance using FOB. The presence of a torque grip at 55 cm allows easy mobilization of the distal end to orient it toward the targeted bronchus.

Univent bronchial blocker

The Univent BB is inserted in the same way as for the Cohen blocker (figure 33.12 C). With its preshaped tip with an angle of 25° and torque-control incorporated into the shaft, the extremity of this BB is easily guided into the desired bronchus.

Collapsing the lung with a bronchial blocker

Several approaches can be taken to lung deflation. The first is when the inner channel of the BB is opened to atmosphere, allowing spontaneous loss of gas from the lung. An apnoeic period helps to accelerate lung deflation (42). If lung collapse remains inadequate with this approach, suction may be applied to the inner channel (43,44). However, this suction should not be applied for a prolonged duration because of the risk of developing negative pressure pulmonary oedema (45). Lung collapse can be facilitated by administration of 100% oxygen before inflation of the balloon to denitrogenate the airways and so promote absorption atelectasis (43,46). A final pragmatic approach is to stop mechanical ventilation and open the airway to atmospheric pressure, when the chest is opened, then in inflate the bronchial blocker's balloon once the lung has collapsed, then resume mechanical ventilation

Selective lobar isolation

Lobar bronchus blockade is feasible and may be indicated in some circumstances (figure 33.13): for example, a patient with a previous right pneumonectomy and needing a VATS for a wedge resection of the left upper lobe (LUL) (47). Selective lobar bronchus blockade is easy to achieve in all bronchi except for the right upper lobe (RUL), where the angulation poses a special challenge. In this circumstance a SLT could be pushed into the intermediate bronchus, bypassing the RUL and allowing ventilation of the middle and inferior lobes, taking care not to obstruct the apical segment of the lower lobe.

Indications for bronchial blockers

Compared to DLTs, BBs provide clinically similar surgical exposure during thoracotomy or VATS, but take a longer time to deflate the isolated lung adequately and require more repositioning during the surgery (48). In cases of difficult intubation or in the presence of a tracheotomy, a BB is an excellent means to manage lung isolation. Another indication for a BB is severe pulmonary bleeding when a DLT cannot be inserted or is unavailable (49).

Complications of bronchial blockers

Complications are less frequent with BBs than with DLTs. However, stapling of the BB in the suture line of the resected bronchus has been occasionally reported. In addition, displacement of the endobronchial balloon back into the tracheal lumen may occur causing complete tracheal obstruction.

Endobronchial single lumen tube

First used in 1931, the endobronchial SLT has very limited indications (figure 33.14). The Phycon tube (Fuji Systems Corporation,Tokyo, Japan; North American distributor is

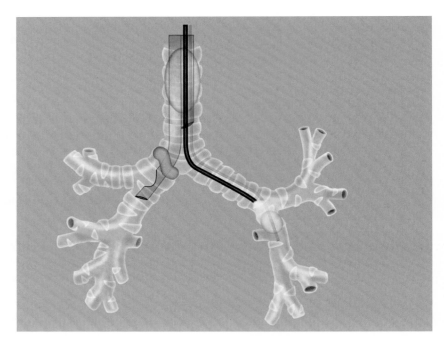

Fig. 33.13 Selective lung isolation.
Selective left inferior lobe isolation with a BB inserted through the tracheal lumen of a R- DLT.

Vitaid, Toronto, ON,Canada) is 40 cm in length, compared to 30 cm for the 6.5 mm SLT, and comes in incremental sizes from 5.5 to 7.5 mm ID. Its outer diameter (9 mm for the 6.5 mm) is similar to the endobronchial extremity of DLT but far smaller than the endotracheal part (13 mm for a 35 Fr) of the DLT. In addition to being very flexible compare, it has a short cuff and a small extremity without a bevel or a Murphy eye and can provide a seal in either the trachea or a bronchus. The short extremity helps to avoid obstruction or trauma of a distal lobar bronchus (50).

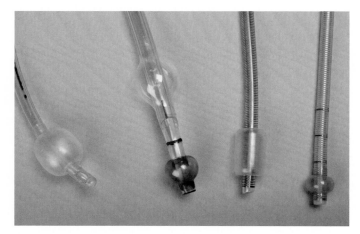

Fig. 33.14 Alternatives for endobronchial intubation.
From left to right: Mallinckrodt™ tracheal tube, Covidien, Mansfield, MA, USA with large cuff, long endobronchial tip, and stiff tube; Broncho-Cath®, Mallinckrodt™ endobronchial tube, Covidien, Mansfield, MA, USA with small cuff, short tip but very stiff and very large tube; RüschFlex armoured tracheal tube with large cuff, middle tip, middle tube, and very flexible; Wire reinforced endotracheal tube, Fuji System Corporation, Japan, with small cuff, small tip and very flexible middle tube.

Carinal sleeve or sleeve pneumonectomy resection, and repair of bronchopleural fistula are the main indications for an endobronchial SLT. Additionally, it may be also be used for tracheal resection and in emergency situations when no others lung isolation devices are available.

As this type of tube is used when a lesion is present in the tracheobronchial tree, it is imperative that FOB is used to guide the endobronchial SLT into position and when the tube needs to be withdrawn. In addition, the tube may also be manipulated by the surgeon to directly intubate the distal part of the trachea or a bronchus. When insertion is not guided by FOB, there is some risk of trauma to the airway or to worsen any lesion present in the tracheobronchial tree, introducing blood and tissue fragments in the distal bronchus.

Lung isolation in difficult airways

Ideally, a difficult airway should be diagnosed before induction of anaesthesia. The wide variety of devices available for lung isolation allows the anaesthetist to achieve safe lung isolation for most subglottic lesions. Upper airway abnormalities are more frequent in practice, and these can be dealt with in various traditional ways. The presence of natural upper teeth may limit intubation with a DLT and the tracheal cuff is at risk of a tear as the DLT is passed through the glottis. An easier option may be to use a BB and SLT. However, alternatives include use of a tube exchanger that is longer and stiffer than that used for SLT, for DLT (figure 33.15). Alternatively, if the SLT is long enough, it can be introduced under FOB guidance deeper into a main bronchus.

Videolaryngoscopy has a useful role in some circumstances, with a specially designed DLT guide that can resolve some difficult situations (figure 33.16) (51). Moreover, it allows visualization of the progression of the DLT over the tube exchanger through the glottis so limits trauma (51). Finally, a BB is probably the best

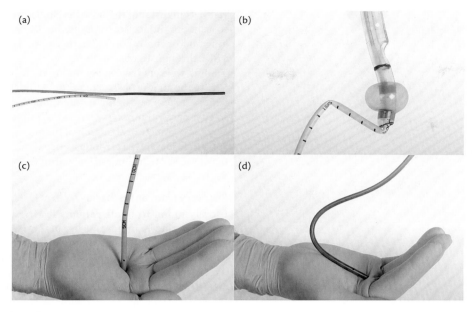

Fig. 33.15 Double lumen tube exchangers.
Cook Medical Inc.: (a) The shortest exchanger for single lumen tube is yellow; (b) The yellow exchanger is too flexible for double lumen tube exchange; (c) The original green exchanger too stiff and presenting a risk for airway traumatism or perforation; (d) The purple end of the green exchanger, without risk for the airway.

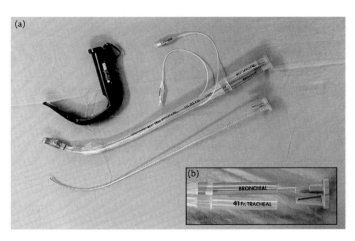

Fig. 33.16 Videolaryngoscopy double lumen tube stylet.
(a) Upper left: GlideScope®, Center: GlideRite Double Lumen Tube Stylet® inserted in a 41Fr left double lumen tube, Lower right: GlideRite Double Lumen Tube Stylet®, Verathon Medical Canada ULC, Vancouver, Canada. (b) Adequate insertion of the handle of the GlideRite Double Lumen Tube Stylet® in a double lumen tube.
Reproduced from Springer and Canadian Anaesthesiologists Society, Canadian Journal of Anaesthesia, 59, 4, pp. 424–425, 'A customized stylet for GlideScope® insertion of double lumen tube', Bussières JS, et al., Copyright 2012, with kind permission from Springer Science and Business Media.

technique when confronted with a nasal SLT, tracheostomy or laryngeal mask (figure 33.17).

Mediastinal masses

Patients with mediastinal masses, particularly those located in the anterior or superior mediastinum, present unique problems for the anaesthetist when undergoing diagnostic and/or therapeutic procedures because general anaesthesia may exacerbate major airway and vascular compression. In particular, these complications may arise when the patient is supine and in some cases, the risk of surgery is too high (52–58).

Anaesthesia for patients with airway obstruction

In patients with anterior mediastinal masses, the trachea or main bronchi can be compressed or partially obstructed. More commonly and dangerously, this occurs in infants and small children (59–61). General anaesthesia decreases FRC, and thus decreases expending forces acting on the tracheobronchial tree acting to decrease airway diameter. In addition, loss of chest wall tone and active inspiration can worsen obstruction. Complete obstruction can occur during tracheal intubation, during surgical manipulations of the tumour that may produce oedema and bleeding, or during postoperative recovery.

Evaluation and preparation of the patient with airway obstruction

Before induction of anaesthesia, the size of the mediastinal mass and its relation to the tracheobronchial tree and major cardiovascular structures should be established. The simplest and most useful piece of information is to ask the patient if its symptoms worsen when lying down. Pulmonary function testing has been recommended but flow-volume loops correlate poorly with the degree of airway obstruction (62).

The anaesthetist must review the results of imaging of the airway to determine the diameter of the airway proximal to and at the level of, the maximal obstruction. Previous diagnostic FOB may also be valuable as it may have identified dynamic airway obstruction. Transthoracic echocardiography can be considered if there is any suspicion of invasion of cardiac structures or pericardial effusion. Consideration should be given as to whether

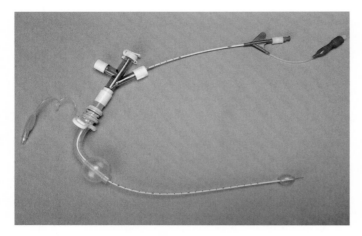

Fig. 33.17 Bronchial blocker and tracheostomy.
Arndt Endobronchial Blocker® from Cook Medical Inc, Bloomington, IN, USA, inserted into a tracheostomy via a multi-port airway adapter.

preoperative treatment with steroids, chemotherapy, and radio-therapy might decrease the size of the mass.

Anaesthetic management of the patient with airway obstruction

When possible, diagnostic procedures, whether percutaneous CT guided needle biopsy, biopsy of an extrathoracic mass, anterior mediastinoscopy or –tomy, or endobronchial ultrasound-guided transbronchial needle aspiration, should be done under local anaesthesia. However, most mediastinal masses will require surgical resection and general anaesthesia. Before induction of anaesthesia, all equipment for a difficult intubation, including rigid bronchoscopes, should be available. In all instances the surgeon must be in the room at induction should intervention with rigid bronchoscopy be required. In addition to standard monitoring, it is essential to establish large-bore intravenous access and invasive arterial pressure monitoring. If there is SVC obstruction, inferior limb venous access should be used. Sometimes, a central venous access or TOE may be also be valuable.

The method chosen for induction depends on the preoperative evaluation and likelihood of respiratory obstruction. The standard of care should be the use of a reversible technique that can be aborted at any point. An inhalation anaesthetic induction with spontaneous breathing has the advantage that the transpulmonary pressure gradient tends to distend the airway so maintaining its patency, even in the presence of significant airway obstruction. Occasionally, a mixture of helium and oxygen (Heliox 70–30%) may help to overcome obstruction-related flow restriction. Changes to the positioning of the patient may be necessary to alleviate obstruction after induction of anaesthesia (63).

Intubation of the airway may have to be carried out with the patient in the sitting position or with the use of FOB. Again, maintenance of spontaneous respiration and avoidance of neuromuscular blockers are important until the anaesthetist has full control of the airway. Should airway obstruction occur, its management may require advancing the endotracheal tube beyond the lesion often into a main bronchus, or changing the patient's position from supine to prone or lateral decubitus. Additionally, a rigid bronchoscope may be passed through the obstruction to enable jet ventilation distal to the obstruction. However, care must be taken so as not to induce air trapping that leads to hyperinflation of the lung and pneumothorax. Furthermore, FOB may also help guide a SLT through an obstruction.

Some workers have suggested that all patients with more than 50% of the airway obstructed should undergo cannulation of their femoral artery and veing before induction of general anaesthesia so that cardiopulmonary bypass (CPB), can be instituted in the event of complete obstruction of the airway (64–66). However, this approach may be hazardous as heparinization required for CPB may exacerbate haemorrhage within the tumour and increase the degree of obstruction.

Recovery from anaesthesia

Closely monitoring all patients during the immediate postoperative period is important because airway obstruction secondary to oedema or haemorrhage caused by surgical manipulations or unsuccessful decompression of the mediastinum may occur. Anxiety, tachypnoea, cough, and pain during emergence from anaesthesia, may also cause turbulence within the airway and worsen obstruction. Tracheomalacia may be present after an extended period of tracheal compression, which only becomes apparent after the tumour has been resected. If any of these complications occurs, rigid bronchoscopy may be the only way to regain control of the airway.

Anaesthesia of patient with compression of major vascular structures

Pathophysiology of vascular compression related to anaesthesia

SVC obstruction is almost always due to malignant tumour that can directly invade the vein causing extrinsic compression, or cause a narrowing with the lumen by the formation of a mural thrombus. General anaesthesia in chronic SVC obstruction is usually not a problem because there is invariably extensive collateral circulation. By contrast, acute SVC obstruction may create laryngeal and upper airway oedema as well as intracranial venous hypertension with secondary cerebral oedema. Subclinical SVC obstruction often becomes significant when the patient assumes a supine position. Moreover, the syndrome can also be exacerbated by excessive administration of fluid.

The pulmonary arteries are less vulnerable than the SVC to compression and obstruction. When it does occur, it may cause a significant reduction in cardiac output and consequently, haemodynamic compromize. Compression of the pulmonary arteries may also cause significant hypoperfusion of the lungs with secondary hypoxia. Like SVC obstruction, these haemodynamic irregularities often relate to posture being made worse in the supine position. Compression of the pericardium and so tamponade of the heart will restrict of diastolic filling. Syncope during a forced Valsalva manoeuvre is characteristic of right heart and pulmonary vascular compression. Furthermore, tumour infiltration of the cardiac muscle may cause impairment of systolic ventricular function.

Preanaesthetic evaluation and preparation of patients with vascular obstruction

Although the diagnosis of SVC syndrome can usually be made on clinical grounds by the presence of dilated collateral veins in the upper body, useful imaging techniques include contrast-enhanced CT scanning, venous angiography, and TOE, to determinate whether the mechanism of obstruction is compression, thrombus or both. Patients with masses compressing the pulmonary artery are often asymptomatic, but it can be diagnosed preoperatively by contrast-enhanced CT, magnetic resonance imaging, or TOE whilst cardiac invasion is best imaged by contrast-enhanced CT.

It is important to have a clear plan for anaesthesia and surgery; the surgeon and anaesthetist must meet to discuss the indication for surgery, the risk of the operation, and its conduct including SVC resection and need for CPB.

Anaesthetic management of patients with vascular obstruction

The patient should be brought into the operating room in the sitting position and throughout induction of anaesthesia, the supine position should be avoided because it reduces the pressure gradient across the obstruction. Central venous catheterization of the SVC is generally contraindicated because of the dangers of perforation. However, a short jugular venous catheter can be extremely useful to estimate the intracerebral venous pressure and the cerebral perfusion pressure in patients in whom the surgeon expects to resect the SVC.

Manipulations of the airway should be done gently to avoid mucosal trauma, increased oedema, or haemorrhage because patients with SVC obstruction often have some degree of laryngeal oedema. Pre- or intraoperative administration of steroids may decrease the oedema and improve symptoms. Diuretics may also be valuable but excessive diuresis may further decrease preload and consequently, cardiac output causing hypotension.

The choice between spontaneous and controlled ventilation in the presence of SVC obstruction is unclear. However, coughing, bucking, and straining are to be avoided because they may exacerbate the obstruction or cause an increase in intracranial pressure. Again, patients should be positioned head-up and with avoidance of cervical flexion or rotation. Intravenous fluid infusion into the upper extremities should be avoided because it may aggravate pre-existent airway oedema or further increase in intracranial pressure.

Resection of the SVC involves the vein being cross-clamped for 15 to 30 minutes. Before clamping, the patient is fully heparinized, and 1500 to 2000 mL of intravenous fluid must be administered to prevent low-output status during cross-clamping. In these situations, it is extremely useful to monitor the venous pressure proximal to the site of clamping. If the venous pressure does not rise above 30 to 35 cmH$_2$O, cross-clamping time can be prolonged without danger. Should the venous pressure rises to 50 cmH$_2$O or more, the duration of cross-clamping must be as short as possible because permanent brain damage may occur. Clamp placement that occludes less than 50% of the circumference of the SVC is usually not associated with significant abnormalities in cerebral perfusion. Systemic arterial blood pressure should be augmented in order to maintain cerebral perfusion pressure.

Recovery from anaesthesia of patients with vascular obstruction

On occasion, the patient with SVC obstruction will develop oedema of the upper airway, including the larynx, during the immediate postoperative period. This may happen when the tumour has not been resected or if a graft used for caval reconstruction

has become suddenly occluded. Close observation is mandatory because severe obstruction can occur acutely and rapid tracheal re-intubation or even tracheotomy may be lifesaving.

Risk factors

Risk factors for perioperative complications include patients presenting with severe symptoms of orthopnoea, stridor, cyanosis, jugular vein distension, or SVC syndrome. Postoperative respiratory complications are associated with tracheal compression of more than 50% on CT scan and combined obstructive and restrictive pattern in pulmonary function tests (56).

Alternatives to general anaesthesia

Occasionally, the patient with a mediastinal mass is at a high or prohibitive risk from general anaesthesia. As most patients require only tissue diagnosis, other strategies should be considered including avoidance of surgery altogether. In particular, this applies to tumours for which treatment can be started on the basis of elevated tumour markers in the blood. However, it also applies to other anterior mediastinal masses when a tissue diagnosis can be achieved with percutaneous fine-needle or core biopsy done under local anaesthesia. Mediastinoscopy should never be done under local anaesthesia even if the patient is at extremely high risk for general anaesthesia as the additional pressure created by the mediastinoscope, bleeding, or patient agitation is likely to lead to catastrophic complications.

Anaesthetic management during tracheal resection

Diseases of the major airways requiring diagnostic or therapeutic interventions are not uncommon, and they present a challenge to the anaesthetist and surgeon because of the necessity of a shared airway. Experience and a thorough knowledge of tracheal anatomy (Chapter 3) and surgical techniques are prerequisite for this type of work (67,68).

Preanaesthetic evaluation and management of the patient for tracheal resection

The anaesthetist must review all bronchoscopic and imaging studies that were used to determine the location, nature, and extent of the tracheal lesion and know the planned surgical approach. In general, lesions of the upper third of the trachea are approached through a cervical incision with or without full or partial median sternotomy whereas lesions of the lower third and those of the carina are best approached through a right posterolateral thoracotomy or through a median or transverse (clamshell incision) sternotomy.

Preoperative administration of steroids may decrease the severity of tracheal oedema but this has to be balanced with possible detrimental effect on the healing of the tracheal anastomosis. Furthermore, the beneficial effects of premedication must be also be balanced against the potentially detrimental results of oversedation, with significant narrowing of the airway. In general, premedication should not be administered until the patient is under the direct supervision of the anaesthetist in the operating room.

Anaesthetic equipment of the patient for tracheal resection

A number of specialized pieces of equipment must be available before induction of anaesthesia, including a selection of standard tracheal tubes, armoured tubes, ventilating catheters, and perhaps microlaryngeal tubes. Sterile anaesthesia corrugated tubing, connectors, and armoured tracheal tubes must be on the surgical operating table and ready to be used by the surgeon during reconstruction of the airway. An anaesthesia work station capable of delivering high-flow oxygen of approximately 20 L per minute, is desirable, especially during rigid bronchoscopy or when the airways are open. Under such conditions, the air leak with low flow equipment may be associated with inadequate ventilation. Jet injectors and high frequency positive pressure ventilators able to deliver respiratory rates of 60 to 120 breaths per minute are valuable options. As the open airway precludes the effective administration of inhalational anaesthetics, it is essential to use total intravenous anaesthesia (TIVA).

Monitoring of the patient for tracheal resection

Because the innominate artery lies anterior to the trachea and sometimes has to be retracted, the arterial line is usually inserted on the left arm. For the same reason, venous access is generally obtained through central venous cannulation installed on the left side of the neck, through the left antecubital vein, or less commonly through a femoral vein. Following intubation, an oesophageal stethoscope can be inserted to monitor breath and heart sounds. Moreover, its insertion is also useful to the surgeon to facilitate identification of the oesophagus by palpation. Capnometry and pressure–volume curves are also useful monitors.

Positioning of the patient of the patient for tracheal resection

Patients with compromised respiration often breathe more effectively in the sitting position. Once the airway is controlled the patient may be placed in a supine position if a cervical or sternotomy approach is to be used. An inflatable bag is then placed transversely underneath the scapulae so that flexion or extension of the neck is permitted. It is important that the anaesthetist has unrestricted access to the patient's head and neck areas at all times. For the reconstruction period the neck should be maximally flexed and sometime the chin can be fixed to the sternum with a stitch to prevent inadvertent cervical extension and stretch of the anastomosis.

Induction and maintenance of anaesthesia of the patient for tracheal resection

An inhalation anaesthetic technique is often helpful. If a benign stenosis or a tumour narrows the airway to a diameter of 5 mm or less then dilatation must be performed before a tracheal tube is advanced beyond the lesion and this is best accomplished with rigid bronchoscopy done during induction. It is important that a sufficient level of anaesthesia is achieved to prevent coughing or bucking that can result in endoluminal trauma with secondary oedema or haemorrhage. Following bronchoscopy and dilatation, tracheal intubation is carried out with a reinforced tube.

With modern techniques of anaesthesia, it is seldom necessary to perform an awake intubation under topical anaesthesia. If it is necessary, however, it can be done with a small tracheal tube under the guidance of FOB. The laryngeal mask airway can also be used for the same purpose as it allows FOB with little increase in the airway resistance. Once intubation has been safely performed and the tracheal obstruction bypassed by the SLT, neuromuscular blockers may be used and anaesthesia is converted to TIVA.

Ventilation techniques during reconstruction of the airway

Orotracheal intubation

A standard technique that is recommended when the severity of airway obstruction is minimal is as follows. After induction of anaesthesia, a reinforced tracheal tube is positioned proximal to the stenotic area of the trachea. Once the surgeon has dilated the airway, the tube is advanced under direct vision into the distal trachea. The surgeon then completes the resection and performs the anastomosis around the tube. The two main disadvantages of this technique are that the surgical field is intermittently obstructed and the tip of the tube may traumatize the lesion causing bleeding or dislodgement of some tissue.

Distal tracheal intubation and intermittent apnoea

The following technique is the most widely used and reliable one for providing adequate oxygenation during tracheal reconstruction. After rigid bronchoscopy and tracheal dilation is done as needed, the patient is intubated with a small tracheal tube that is advanced beyond the lesion (figure 33.18A). Once the trachea (cervical or thoracic) has been fully mobilized and before surgical resection, anaesthesia tubing and connectors are passed from the surgical field to the anaesthetist so that they can be connected to the anaesthesia ventilator. The trachea is then transected at a point below the obstruction and the tracheal tube is pulled back into the proximal trachea. A stitch is often sewn to the distal tip of the tracheal tube so that it can be retrieved if necessary. The distal trachea is then intubated with the operative tube, from the surgical field and ventilation resumed (figure 33.18B). If tracheal resection is performed near the carina, the operative tube is advanced into the left main bronchus and OLV instituted. Before the anastomosis is performed, an inflatable bag that has been placed beneath the scapula is deflated so that the neck can be maximally flexed to reduce tension at the level of the anastomosis.

Interrupted sutures are then placed through both tracheal ends; short periods of apnoea with the operative tube pulled out of the distal trachea generally facilitate the placement of these sutures (figure 33.18C). Once all sutures are in place, the operative tube is withdrawn from the distal trachea and the original oral tracheal tube is re-advanced through the anastomosis under direct vision. Ventilation is then restarted through the oral tube as the sutures are tied (figure 33.18D). While performing the reconstruction, the surgeon must make sure that the tracheal tube is in the distal trachea rather than being in a main bronchus, and that blood and other debris are regularly aspirated from the distal airway.

Short and intermittent periods of apnoea are usually well tolerated by the patient. Often preoxygenation of the patient with 100% oxygen and added PEEP will allow longer periods of apnoea of up to 6 to 7 minutes. After completion of the tracheal anastomosis, the tracheal tube is pulled back to lie well above the anastomosis (figure 33.18 E).

Catheter ventilation

Ventilation through a small catheter can be valuable during airway surgery (figure 33.19). The small size of the catheter provides

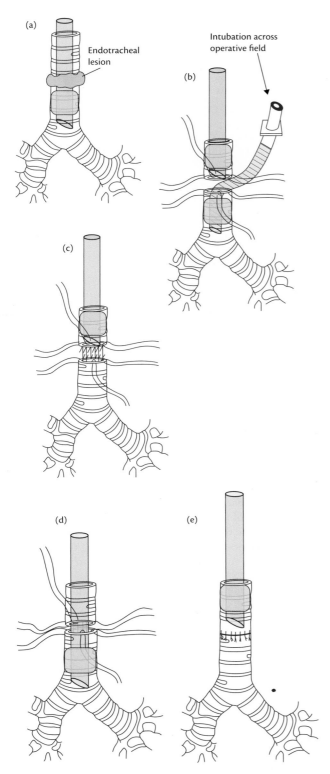

Fig. 33.18 Distal tracheal intubation and intermittent apnoea. (a) Placement of a small oral endotracheal tube beyond the lesion. (b) The oral endotracheal tube is pulled back, and the distal airway is intubated with a tube from the operative field. (c) Intermittent periods of apnea facilitate surgical reconstruction and suture placement. (d) Anaesthesia is restarted through the original oral endotracheal tube as the sutures are tied. (e) After completion of the anastomosis, the oral endotracheal tube is pulled back well above the anastomosis.

This figure was published in *Handbook of Perioperative Care in General Thoracic Surgery*, Deslauriers J. and Mehran R., pp. 183–184, Copyright Elsevier 2005.

optimal surgical access to the circumferences of transected airways and facilitates the uninterrupted reconstruction. These catheters, such as a nasogastric tube (69), are inserted into the distal airway through the tracheal tube or laryngeal mask (70,71). Two different modes of catheter ventilation can be used during airway reconstruction.

High-flow jet ventilation

Manual injector jet ventilation delivers a large tidal volume of 500 to 1500 mL at a respiratory rate of 10 to 30 breaths.per min. The technique achieves adequate gas exchanges by bulk flow similar to conventional positive-pressure ventilation. Jet insufflation also generates a negative pressure around the tip of the catheter, which causes entrainment of air by the Venturi effect and provides an enlarged tidal volume necessary for adequate ventilation. Potential disadvantages of the technique include barotrauma to the lung, pneumothorax, sub-cutaneaous emphysema, air embolism, and aspiration of blood, and mucus or other debris in the open airway because of the Venturi effect.

Low-flow, high-frequency ventilation

This technique delivers small tidal volumes (50 to 250 mL/min) at a rapid respiratory rate of 50 to 150 breaths/min, achieving gas exchange by a combination of convective flow and acceleration of gas diffusion. The repeated insufflations of small volumes at high velocity may also generate a continuously positive airway pressure, which increases FRC, improves gas mixing and distribution, and reduces the risk of alveolar collapse (72). Other advantages include minimal lung and mediastinal movements as well as less entrainment of blood or mucus in the open airway (73).

Cardiopulmonary bypass

CPB is rarely required for tracheal reconstruction. The main disadvantages of using CPB are its complexity and need for systemic heparinization with the potential of intrapulmonary haemorrhage.

Recovery and complications following tracheal resection

At the conclusion of the procedure, resumption of spontaneous respiration and early tracheal extubation are important as the tracheal tube has the potential to cause direct trauma to the suture line. An infusion of propofol during the final stages of the procedure often allows rapid emergence to a wakeful state without agitation. At this stage, the surgeon will often use flexible bronchoscopy to inspect the anastomosis and aspirate blood or mucus that might still be in the airway. Patients will likely have their neck extremely flexed at the end of operation and therefore will be prone to have some inability to clear secretions. Aspiration can also be a significant early problem after tracheal surgery, especially in those patients who have had a laryngeal release as part of the operation.

If there is concern about the patency of the reconstructed trachea or upper airway or glottic oedema, most surgeons will insert a tracheotomy tube or a silicone Montgomery T-tube that facilitate safe emergence from the anaesthesia.

Serial measurements of arterial blood gases are mandatory. A chest X-ray must also be obtained in the immediate postoperative period to rule out pneumothorax. Patients will sometimes experience some degree of respiratory difficulties after tracheal extubation. Because this is most likely due to local oedema, nebulized racemic epinephrine (adrenaline) 1:200 (0.5 mL in 2 mL saline)

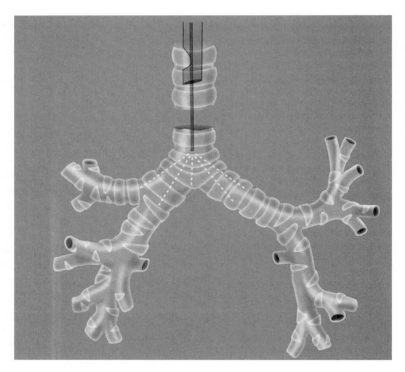

Fig. 33.19 High frequency jet ventilation during tracheal resection.
Small catheter for high frequency jet ventilation introduced through a single lumen tube and passing through the tracheal transection, allowing ventilation of the distal airway with minimal interference with the surgical intervention.

may be helpful. In addition, the administration of Heliox by a face mask and/or dexamethasone (4 to 10 mg) IV may be valuable.

Should tracheal reintubation be required, this is best accomplished under direct vision with FOB and the orotracheal or nasotracheal tube should be positioned well away from the anastomosis. Whenever possible, the tube proximal rather than distal to the anastomosis because this location has less potential for suture line damage. Chest physical therapy and routine nursing procedures may be difficult if not impossible when the head is maintained in an extreme flexed position.

The acute relief of airway obstruction may result in a marked increase in transpulmonary pressure inducing acute pulmonary oedema. Treatment is supportive and most patients will require reintubation for a short time. Alternative management includes non-invasive ventilation and/or oxygen supplementation and administration of diuretics.

One of the most significant but underestimated problems that often occur after tracheal surgery relates to dysphagia and microaspiration. Although there may be many potential causes for dysphagia, it is usually secondary to an incoordination between swallowing, initiation of the pharyngeal motor wave, and relaxation of the cricopharynx. Treatment of this condition must be supportive and often the patient should not be allowed to drink or eat for several days postoperatively, and occasionally, bronchoscopy may be required for removal of particulate matter.

Airway management during bronchial sleeve resection

Bronchial sleeve resection involves resection of main bronchus for neoplasm or benign stricture. Sleeve lobectomy involves parenchyma-sparing techniques in patients with limited pulmonary reserve and who cannot tolerate a pneumonectomy. Patients undergoing sleeve pneumonectomy require lung isolation with a contralateral DLT. Sleeve resection of the carina with or without associated pneumonectomy or right upper lobectomy implies complete transection of the trachea to remove the carina. Following complete resection, the reconstruction necessitates an end-to-end anastomosis of one main bronchus and an end-to-side anastomosis of the other main bronchus onto the first to recreate a new functional carina. Such surgical intervention requires the use of the same ventilation techniques as describe earlier for tracheal resection.

Emergency surgery

Emergency anaesthesia for thoracic surgery is usually for chest trauma that may be blunt or penetrating. The spectrum of chest injuries ranges from isolated rib fractures to complex tracheobronchial disruption and exsanguinating cardiovascular rupture.

Blunt trauma

Blunt trauma is more often the result of motor vehicle accidents, followed by falls from a height, then assaults, and sports-related crush injuries, and is its immediate management is often related to the mechanism of injury.

Direct impact over the chest wall may result in rib fractures, flail chest, and lung and cardiac contusion. Forceful anteroposterior compression increases the transverse diameter of the thoracic cavity and may lead to a tracheobronchial tear. In these cases, the negative intrapleural pressure pulls the lungs away from the fixed carina, and main bronchial disruption may occur. In head-on car accidents, an unrestrained occupant with no seat belt may be thrust forward, and the direct impact of the steering wheel or the dashboard over the hyperextended neck may cause significant laryngotracheal injuries.

Rapid deceleration results in shearing forces on the airway and aorta and may thus contribute to the high incidence of bronchial or aortic rupture observed in motor vehicle accidents. Vertical deceleration, such as falling from a height, may be associated with rupture of the ascending aorta, whereas longitudinal deceleration is more likely to result in aortic rupture distal to the aortopulmonary ligament.

Blunt impact to the chest occurring with a closed glottis often produces a sudden rise in airway pressure that may contribute to tracheobronchial disruption. Similarly, a rapid increase in intra-abdominal pressure may be a precursor of diaphragmatic rupture.

Initial evaluation and management of blunt trauma

Important information to gather includes the mechanism and time of injury, which can inform the patient's stability post-trauma and fasting period. Airway, breathing, and circulation (ABC) constitute the priorities of both the initial assessment and management. Because many patients with severe blunt thoracic injuries also have head injuries or fracture of the cervical spine, these must be looked for during the initial evaluation. If these are suspected, manual cervical spine alignment must be maintained throughout the initial resuscitation and evaluation.

The first priority is to secure the airway, which may have become obstructed by blood, secretions, or foreign bodies such as teeth or dentures. This can often be done by simple manoeuvres, such as manual removal of foreign bodies, suctioning of secretions, lifting the jaw anteriorly (lifts up the epiglottis and brings it forward), and use of a nasopharyngeal or oropharyngeal airway tube.

Ultimately, tracheal intubation is the best method of airway control. It can be done through the nose or over a flexible bronchoscope if a cervical spine injury is suspected. Repeated attempts at intubation should, however, be avoided because they may exacerbate mucosal injuries or transform a partial airway disruption into a complete one. In such cases, emergency tracheostomy should be performed quickly and without hesitation. One must avoid excessive neck manipulations until a cervical spine fracture has been ruled out.

Respiratory failure

Acute, life-threatening respiratory failure can be caused by severe lung contusion, flail chest, tension pneumothorax, tracheobronchial rupture, or any combination of these injuries.

Pulmonary contusion is often associated with multiple rib fractures or flail chest. In severe cases, respiratory failure can develop quickly as it is related to multiple factors including the flail segment, severe pain, lung damage with alveolar haemorrhage and interstitial oedema, and reflex diaphragmatic paralysis. If initial supportive care consisting of oxygen supplementation, pain control, and chest physiotherapy including suctioning does not relieve the problem, tracheal intubation and mechanical ventilation may become necessary.

Tension pneumothoraces are caused by a valvular mechanism that allows air to enter the pleural space during inspiration but prevents its escape during expiration. Eventually, the positive pleural pressure will cause mediastinal displacement, compression of the opposite lung, and distortion of the vena cavae with secondary decrease in venous return and cardiac output. Immediate treatment involves space decompression either with a needle attached to a water seal or with thoracoscomy tube drainage.

Most tracheobronchial ruptures occur within 2.5 cm of the carina, and the most common injury is a complete avulsion of the right main bronchus off the trachea. Because associated injuries are common, the majority of these patients do not reach the hospital alive.

Penetrating trauma

Approximately 15% to 20% of penetrating trauma victims will require emergency or immediate thoracotomy and they are among the most challenging problems in the practice of thoracic anaesthesia and surgery. In urban centres, they are usually caused by low-velocity missiles such as a bullet from a handgun, whereas in war zones, bomb fragments and high-velocity missiles are the main sources of injury. Although less frequent, industrial accidents or high-speed motor vehicle accidents can also be associated with penetrating chest injuries.

Pathophysiology and mechanism of injury of penetrating trauma

In cases of firearm injuries, the amount of tissue destruction suffered during traumatic penetration of the chest depends on the type of weapon used as well as the velocity and mass of the missile. Stab wounds and low-velocity (<300 m/s) missiles from handguns have low-impact kinetic energy that generally causes no major tissue destruction beyond the trajectory of the missile. By contrast, high-velocity (750 to 850 m/s) missiles, such as those from automatic rifles or machine guns, have high-impact kinetic energy that creates an explosion-like effect causing laceration and cavitation of tissues adjacent to the missile's trajectory (collateral damage). In high-velocity injuries, the extent of tissue damage is also related to the range of shooting and characteristics of the tissue being injured. Short-range (<5 m) shots, for example from shotguns, cause more massive tissue destruction than long-range shots. Commonly injured thoracic structures in penetrating trauma are listed in table 33.4.

Initial assessment of patients with penetrating chest injury

The initial assessment of patients with penetrating chest trauma must include a brief record of the nature of the incident: for example, the length of knife blade, calibre of firearm and range of shooting, position of the victim during the injury, and what happened afterward. If the patient is in cardiac arrest or imminent cardiac arrest, he/she may need immediate thoracotomy in the emergency department.

Table 33.4 Commonly injured thoracic structure in penetrating trauma

Structure	Incidence (%)
Chest wall	100
Lung	90
Diaphragm	20–30
Heart and great vessels	10
Airway	<5
Oesophagus	<2

Management of the patient with penetrating chest injury

Patients with severe respiratory difficulties and those in profound shock should be intubated and mechanically ventilated. During the initial assessment period, all patients should have two large intravenous lines inserted, and blood should be sent for typing and crossmatching. Patients with severe hypotension but not in immediate danger of cardiac arrest should initially be given crystalloids followed by packed red cells as necessary.

The next step is to decide whether the patient requires immediate thoracotomy. A large amount of initial bleeding (>1500 mL) associated with an unstable blood pressure or a continuous high drainage (> 250 to 300 mL/hr) for 2 to 3 hours is generally considered an indication for emergency explorative surgery. This is particularly true if the penetration has occurred in the cardiac proximity or cardiac box that is defined as an anatomic territory bounded superiorly by the clavicles, inferiorly by the costal margins, and laterally by the midclavicular lines, or if the entrance wound is in the thoracic inlet or supraclavicular regions with possible great vessel injury. Immediate surgery may also be indicated in unstable patients with a pericardial tamponade that is most likely to be due to cardiac penetration.

Emergency department thoracotomy is usually performed in moribund patients presenting with profound hypotension as a result of pericardial tamponade, or massive thoracic or thoracoabdominal bleeding. The patient who has suffered a cardiac arrest shortly after arrival may also benefit of an emergency department thoracotomy. The chest is opened anteriorly through a left fourth interspace incision. A left anterior thoracotomy provides the most rapid exposure to the heart and allows excellent access to most of the cardiac surfaces, left hilum, and aorta. Effective open cardiac massage may be performed. Lifesaving direct pressure can be applied to the site of major blood vessel penetration, and in cases of extensive lung injury, a vascular clamp can be placed across the entire pulmonary hilum. Midthoracic aortic cross-clamping for periods of 10 to 20 minutes may temporarily improve cerebral and coronary blood flow. If the injury requires access to the right chest, the incision can be extended to the right across the sternum. The incision can also be extended posteriorly for access to the descending thoracic aorta. To be successful, emergency department thoracotomies must be performed by experienced teams operating in a well-equipped trauma centre. Under such circumstances, survival is approximately 30% for patients with stab wounds and less than 10% for those with high-velocity bullet wounds. A significant proportion of survivors will suffer from permanent neurologic sequelae.

A median sternotomy can also be used for transmediastinal gunshot wounds, wounds to the right side of the sternum, or injuries to vessels of the thoracic inlet including the innominate, subclavian, and carotid arteries. Although cardiopulmonary bypass is seldom required, the surgical team should be ready to use it if necessary. Once the site of penetration has been identified, which is most commonly the right ventricle, digital pressure is applied until suture control can be accomplished.

Management of stable patients and possible indications for early operation in penetrating trauma

More than half of patients who are stable on admission or have become stable with fluid resuscitation will never require surgery. Penetration of the chest wall may require surgery to control injuries to the intercostal vascular bundle or internal mammary artery.

High-velocity missiles or shotgun blasts can also cause extensive loss of chest wall tissues, creating an open chest wound that must be completely debrided. Most surgeons agree that if large amounts of blood clots are retained in the pleural space despite thoracostomy drainage, they should be evacuated usually through the use of videothoracoscopy, as it may prevent the occurrence of late empyema.

In civilian practice, less than 5% of patients with penetrating chest trauma will require operative treatment of lung injuries, and in the majority of those cases, the indication is based on haemorrhage from pulmonary blood vessels rather than air leakage. Most lung injuries can be repaired by direct suturing. Extensive lung destruction may require lobectomy or pneumonectomy, but the latter procedure is associated with significant mortality. Penetrating trauma to the airway is usually associated with other major mediastinal injury. Once diagnosed, the site of injury should be primarily repaired during immediate thoracotomy. Surprisingly, many of these patients will be stabilized both haemodynamically and from a respiratory point of view, and the lesion will have been found under bronchoscopy done for any haemoptysis, subcutaneous emphysema, or stridor. This is because tracheobronchial injuries associated with penetrating trauma are almost always partial ruptures as opposed to the usually complete ruptures associated with blunt trauma.

The incidence of diaphragmatic injury is high at 40–50% in patients with penetrating trauma to the left lower chest, or in those with thoracoabdominal injuries. In the acute setting, these patients are often asymptomatic. If there is still a high suspicion of diaphragmatic injury, VATS surgery is useful to identify or to rule out such injuries. Small lacerations can be repaired through this approach but larger defects may require conversion to open thoracotomy. Diaphragmatic defects should be repaired as soon as possible because they can result in diaphragmatic herniation with potential for incarceration and strangulation of abdominal viscera. Diaphragmatic penetration can also be assessed laparoscopically and by laparotomy.

Airway trauma

Tracheobronchial injuries have been recognized as a source of intrathoracic trauma for many years, but their true incidence is still unknown because many patients will die before reaching the hospital. Although the estimated mortality of patients with tracheobronchial injuries is 30%, 90% of patients reaching the hospital alive can anticipate full recovery. Successful outcome depends on early diagnosis, accurate assessment of the extent of the injury, and appropriate treatment.

Laryngotracheal trauma

Because of the protected position of the larynx and cervical trachea in the neck surrounded by the mandible, sternum and spine, penetrating or non-penetrating injuries to these structures are uncommon. Most penetrating injuries of the larynx or upper trachea are due to knife or bullet wounds. Blunt injuries are produced by localized blows over the hyperextended neck often related to a steering wheel or dashboard impact. Indeed, the classic dashboard airway injury involves an unrestrained driver with no seat belt, or front seat passenger whose hyperextended neck strikes the dashboard during a head-on collision. Another mechanism of blunt injury is strangulation. This includes seat belt injury with a compressive force to the neck during a head-on collision. Yet another typical example of this type of injury is the snowmobile or motorbike rider who hits an unseen rope while travelling at high speed.

Initial airway management of laryngotracheal trauma

Securing the airway is the most important initial step in managing such trauma victims. In patients with severe distress, tracheal intubation can be attempted but repeated attempts should be avoided. In many cases, intubation will be facilitated by the guidance of a flexible bronchoscope, which will direct the tube beyond the injury. If any difficulties are encountered during bronchoscopy or in patients with severe maxillofacial trauma, an emergency tracheostomy may be required. If the distal segment has retracted into the mediastinum, it is best found by inserting a finger in the mediastinum, palpating the trachea, and grasping it with a clamp to bring it back out to the neck.

Definitive management of laryngotracheal trauma

Early surgical exploration, best achieved by a low cervical collar incision, and primary repair of most laryngotracheal injuries will provide the best results. When the cervical trachea has been transected transversely, a primary anastomosis is easily achieved, and a tracheostomy is usually not necessary. In cases of upper airway injuries, the otorhinolaryngologist may also be involved in the diagnosis and management.

Disruption of the intrathoracic trachea

Rupture of the intrathoracic trachea is the least common of airway injuries. The usual mechanism is a burst disruption due to a sudden increase in intracheal pressure against a closed glottis. Laceration of the intrathoracic trachea can also result from difficult or forceful intubation. Management requires tracheal intubation and prompt primary repair.

Bronchial rupture

Most bronchial tears are the result of severe crush injury suffered in automobile accidents. Rupture occurs when the elasticity of the tracheobronchial tree is exceeded. If the glottis is closed moments before the impact, the crushing of the chest will result in sudden increase of intrabronchial pressure, producing a shearing or explosive force within the airway. Rapid deceleration may also generate shearing forces at points of fixation, causing bronchial disruption. Eighty percent of all tears occur within 2.5 cm of the carina and the lobar or segmental bronchi are seldom affected.

Free communication with the pleural space

With free communication between ruptured bronchus and pleural space, typical clinical features are those of respiratory distress, subcutaneous emphysema, and haemoptysis. The major clues to diagnosis are pneumothorax either on the side of rupture or bilaterally, persistent lung collapse despite tube drainage, and large air leak through the chest tube. There is often increased respiratory distress or even suffocation when suction is applied to the chest tube because most of the inspired air will be sucked away from the functioning lung.

Little or no communication with pleural space

In this group, the site of disruption is within the mediastinum. The symptoms are more subtle because bronchial continuity is often maintained by apposition of peribronchial soft tissues, and the tear is sealed by fibrin or blood clot. Pneumothorax may or may not be present, but in most cases, the lung expands readily with tube drainage.

Definitive diagnosis of bronchial rupture

Bronchoscopy is the most useful procedure to confirm the diagnosis of bronchial rupture, to determine its location and extent, and to plan the repair. It should be done under operating room conditions in the event that the injury is aggravated by endobronchial manipulations. Although there is often an abundance of blood in the airway, we prefer the use of flexible bronchoscopy under local anaesthesia and light sedation over rigid bronchoscopy. The rupture can often clearly be seen, although the full extent of injury may not be apparent. If the disruption is not clearly visualized, indirect endoscopic signs, such as local bleeding, air bubbling, and local oedema may suggest the diagnosis.

Resuscitation and early management of bronchial rupture

Contrary to what one might expect, the airway of patients with bronchial rupture is seldom obstructed. It is thus possible to manage most of these patients without intubation, until such time as bronchoscopy and surgical repair can be carried out. If intubation is deemed necessary, blind insertion of a tracheal tube can be extremely hazardous and should probably be avoided if one is not ready to proceed immediately with bronchoscopy or thoracotomy. Under those circumstances, especially if the trauma victim is far from a specialized centre, emergency tracheotomy may be preferred to blind tracheal intubation. The most significant advantage of a tracheotomy is the easy access given to the airway for aspiration of blood while the patient is transported from a peripheral medical centre to a major trauma unit. Tracheostomy also provides an opening by which trapped mediastinal air can be released, and it considerably reduces intratracheal pressures. Thoracostomy tubes should be inserted bilaterally and connected to underwater seal drainage systems without suction.

Definitive management of bronchial rupture

Although excellent results can be expected with early reconstruction, there must be an important coordination and cooperation among the surgeon, the anaesthetist, and the operating room personnel. All major bronchial disruptions require immediate repair, and the procedure should be carefully planned between the surgeon and anaesthetist at the time of endoscopy. Intubation with a DLT in optimal position, verified with FOB, and OLV during the repair is routine.

The main goal of surgery is primary repair of the bronchial tear without sacrificing healthy lung. In general, pulmonary resection is almost never required other than in rupture involving smaller bronchi, where reconstruction may be difficult and parenchymal damage more difficult to assess.

Conclusion

Anaesthesia for thoracic surgery has greatly progressed in recent decades. Advances in techniques and equipment allow delivery of safe and efficacious anaesthesia in sicker patients. Lung isolation is easier to achieve, even in the face of a difficult airway. The management of patients with mediastinal masses, tumours of the airway, or victims of thoracic trauma, is now better understood and provides excellent clinical outcomes.

Acknowledgement

The authors wish to thanks Professor Jean Deslauriers for his inspiration and revision of the text.

References

1. Cattaneo SM, Park BJ, Wilton AS, et al. Use of video-assisted thoracic surgery for lobectomy in the elderly results in fewer complications. *Ann Thorac Surg* 2008; **85**(1): 231–5; discussion 5–6

2. Faurschou P, Madsen F, Viskum K. Thoracoscopy: influence of the procedure on some respiratory and cardiac values. *Thorax* 1983; **38**(5): 341–3

3. Oldenburg FA, Jr., Newhouse MT. Thoracoscopy. A safe, accurate diagnostic procedure using the rigid thoracoscope and local anesthesia. *Chest* 1979; **75**(1): 45–50

4. Horswell JL. Anesthetic techniques for thoracoscopy. *Ann Thorac Surg* 1993; **56**(3): 624–9

5. Cohen E, Eisenkraft JB. Positive end-expiratory pressure during one-lung ventilation improves oxygenation in patients with low arterial oxygen tensions. *J Cardiothorac Vasc Anesth* 1996; **10**(5): 578–82

6. Steegers MA, Snik DM, Verhagen AF, van der Drift MA, Wilder-Smith OH. Only half of the chronic pain after thoracic surgery shows a neuropathic component. *J Pain* 2008; **9**(10): 955–61

7. Khoo KL, Ho KY. Endoscopic mediastinal staging of lung cancer. *Respir Med* 2011; **105**(4): 515–8

8. Fujii S, Kikura M, Takada T, Katoh S, Aoyama N, Sato S. A noninvasive partial carbon dioxide rebreathing technique for measurement of pulmonary capillary blood flow is also a useful oxygenation monitor during one-lung ventilation. *J Clin Anesth* 2004; **16**(5): 347–52

9. Bardoczky GI, Levarlet M, Engelman E, deFrancquen P. Continuous spirometry for detection of double-lumen endobronchial tube displacement. *Br J Anaesth* 1993; **70**(5): 499–502

10. Bardoczky G, d'Hollander A, Yernault JC, Van Meuylem A, Moures JM, Rocmans P. On-line expiratory flow-volume curves during thoracic surgery: occurrence of auto-PEEP. *Br J Anaesth* 1994 Jan;72(1):25–8.

11. Joshi GP, Bonnet F, Shah R, et al. A systematic review of randomized trials evaluating regional techniques for postthoracotomy analgesia. *Anesthes Analg* 2008; **107**(3): 1026–40.

12. Daly DJ, Myles PS. Update on the role of paravertebral blocks for thoracic surgery: are they worth it? *Curr Opin Anaesthesiol* 2009; **22**(1): 38–43

13. Conlon NP, Shaw AD, Grichnik KP. Postthoracotomy paravertebral analgesia: will it replace epidural analgesia? *Anesthesiol Clin* 2008; **26**(2): 369–80, viii

14. Gottschalk A, Cohen SP, Yang S, Ochroch EA. Preventing and treating pain after thoracic surgery. Anesthesiology. 2006; **104**(3): 594–600

15. Horlocker TT. Regional anaesthesia in the patient receiving antithrombotic and antiplatelet therapy. *Br J Anaesth* [2011; **107**(Suppl 1): i96–106

16. Zeldin RA, Normandin D, Landtwing D, Peters RM. Postpneumonectomy pulmonary edema. *J Thorac Cardiovasc Surg.* 1984; **87**(3): 359–65

17. Chong PC, Greco EF, Stothart D, et al. Substantial variation of both opinions and practice regarding perioperative fluid resuscitation. *Can J Surg* 2009; **52**(3): 207–14

18. Jackson TA, Mehran RJ, Thakar D, Riedel B, Nunnally ME, Slinger P. Case 5–2007 postoperative complications after pneumonectomy: clinical conference. *J Cardiothorac Vasc Anesth.* 2007; **21**(5): 743–51

19. Jordan S, Mitchell JA, Quinlan GJ, Goldstraw P, Evans TW. The pathogenesis of lung injury following pulmonary resection. *Eur Respir J* 2000; **15**(4): 790–9

20. Bussieres JS, Tremblay D. Does warming the inferior limbs reduce body calorie loss during posterolateral thoracotomy? In: SCA, editor. SCA Annual Meeting; 1997; Baltimore, USA, 1997; SCA124

21. Campos JH. Which device should be considered the best for lung isolation: double-lumen endotracheal tube versus bronchial blockers. *Curr Opin Anaesthesiol* 2007; **20**(1): 27–31

22. Bjork VO, Carlens E. The prevention of spread during pulmonary resection by the use of a double-lumen catheter. *J Thorac Surg* 1950; **20**: 151–7

23. Campos JH. Update on tracheobronchial anatomy and flexible fiber-optic bronchoscopy in thoracic anesthesia. *Curr Opin Anaesthesiol* 2009; **22**(1): 4–10

24. Campos JH, Hallam EA, Van Natta T, Kernstine KH. Devices for lung isolation used by anesthesiologists with limited thoracic experience: comparison of double-lumen endotracheal tube, Univent torque control blocker, and Arndt wire-guided endobronchial blocker. *Anesthesiology* 2006; **104**(2): 261–6, discussion 5A

25. Brodsky JB, Macario A, Mark JB. Tracheal diameter predicts double-lumen tube size: a method for selecting left double-lumen tubes. *Anesthes Analg* 1996; **82**(4): 861–4

26. Eberle B, Weiler N, Vogel N, Kauczor HU, Heinrichs W. Computed tomography-based tracheobronchial image reconstruction allows selection of the individually appropriate double-lumen tube size. *J Cardiothorac Vasc Anesth* 1999; **13**(5): 532–7

27. Boucek CD, Landreneau R, Freeman JA, Strollo D, Bircher NG. A comparison of techniques for placement of double-lumen endobronchial tubes. *J Clin Anesth* 1998; **10**(7): 557–60

28. Bussières JS, Slinger P. Correct positioning of double-lumen tubes. *Can J Anaesth* 2012; **59**(5): 431–6

29. Fortier G, Cote D, Bergeron C, Bussieres JS. New landmarks improve the positioning of the left Broncho-Cath double-lumen tube-comparison with the classic technique. *Can J Anaesth* 2001; **48**(8): 790–4

30. Lohser J, Brodsky JB. Silbronco double-lumen tube. *J Cardiothorac Vasc Anesth* 2006; **20**(1): 129–31

31. Campos JH, Gomez MN. Pro: right-sided double-lumen endotracheal tubes should be routinely used in thoracic surgery. *J Cardiothorac Vasc Anesth* 2002; **16**(2): 246–8

32. Ehrenfeld JM, Walsh JL, Sandberg WS. Right- and left-sided Mallinckrodt double-lumen tubes have identical clinical performance. *Anesthes Analg* 2008; **106**(6): 1847–52

33. Hagihira S, Takashina M, Mashimo T. Application of a newly designed right-sided, double-lumen endobronchial tube in patients with a very short right mainstem bronchus. *Anesthesiology* 2008; **109**(3) :565–8

34. Bussières JS, Lacasse Y, Cote D, et al. Modified right-sided Broncho-Cath double lumen tube improves endobronchial positioning: a randomized study. *Can J Anaesth* 2007; **54**(4): 276–82

35. Fitzmaurice BG, Brodsky JB. Airway rupture from double-lumen tubes. *J Cardiothorac Vasc Anesth* 1999; **13**(3): 322–9

36. Saito S, Dohi S, Naito H. Alteration of double-lumen endobronchial tube position by flexion and extension of the neck. *Anesthesiology* 1985; **62**(5): 696–7

37. Seo JH, Hong DM, Lee JM, Chung EJ, Bahk JH. Double-lumen tube placement without a headrest in supine position minimizes displacement during lateral positioning. *Can J Anaesth* 2012; **59**(5): 437–41.

38. Ginsberg RJ. New technique for one-lung anesthesia using an endobronchial blocker. *J Thorac Cardiovasc Surg* 1981; **82**(4): 542–6

39. Karwande SV. A new tube for single lung ventilation. *Chest* 1987; **92**(4): 761–3

40. Arndt GA, Kranner PW, Rusy DA, Love R. Single-lung ventilation in a critically ill patient using a fiberoptically directed wire-guided endobronchial blocker. *Anesthesiology* 1999; **90**(5): 1484–6

41. Cohen E. The Cohen flexitip endobronchial blocker: an alternative to a double lumen tube. *Anesth Analg* 2005; **101**(6): 1877–9

42. Karzai W. Alternative method to deflate the operated lung when using wire-guided endobronchial blockade. *Anesthesiology* 2003; **99**(1): 239–40; author reply 41

43. Campos JH, Kernstine KH. A comparison of a left-sided Broncho-Cath with the torque control blocker univent and the wire-guided blocker. *Anesth Analg* 2003;**96**(1): 283–9, table of contents

44. Narayanaswamy M, McRae K, Slinger P, et al. Choosing a lung isolation device for thoracic surgery: a randomized trial of three bronchial blockers versus double-lumen tubes. *Anesth Analg* 2009; **108**(4): 1097–101

45. Baraka A, Nawfal M, Kawkabani N. Severe hypoxemia after suction of the nonventilated lung via the bronchial blocker lumen of the univent tube. *J Cardiothorac Vasc Anesth* 1996; **10**(5): 694–5

46. Dery R, Pelletier J, Jacques A, Clavet M, Houde J. Alveolar collapse induced by denitrogenation. *Can Anaesth Soc J* 1965; **12**(6): 531–57

47. Campos JH, Kernstine KH. Use of the wire-guided endobronchial blocker for one-lung anesthesia in patients with airway abnormalities. *J Cardiothorac Vasc Anesth* 2003; **17**(3): 352–4

48. Lizuka T, Tanno M, Hamada Y, Shga T, Ohe Y. Uniblocker bronchial bblocker tube to facilitate one-lung ventilation during thoracoscopic surgery. *Anesthesiology* 2007; **108**: A1815

49. Kabon B, Waltl B, Leitgeb J, Kapral S, Zimpfer M. First experience with fiberoptically directed wire-guided endobronchial blockade in severe pulmonary bleeding in an emergency setting. *Chest* 2001; **120**(4):1399–402

50. Slinger P. Sleeve pneumonectomy. *J Cardiothorac Vasc Anesth* 2009; **23**(2): 269–70

51. Bussières JS, Marte F, Somma J, Morin S, Gagné N. A customized stylet for GlideScope insertion of double lumen tubes. *Can J Anaesth* 2012; **59**(4): 424–5

52. Pullerits J, Holzman R. Anaesthesia for patients with mediastinal masses. *Can J Anaesth* 1989; **36**(6): 681–8

53. Greengrass R. Anaesthesia and mediastinal masses. *Can J Anaesth* 1990; **37**(5): 596–7

54. Tinker DT, Crane DL. Safety of anesthesia for patients with anterior mediastinal masses I. *Anesthesiology* 1990; **73**: 1061

55. Zornow MH, Benumof JL. Safety of anesthesia for patients with anterior masses II. *Anesthesiology* 1990; **73**: 1061

56. Bechard P, Letourneau L, Lacasse Y, Cote D, Bussieres JS. Perioperative cardiorespiratory complications in adults with mediastinal mass: incidence and risk factors. *Anesthesiology* 2004; **100**(4): 826–34; discussion 5A

57. Erdos G, Tzanova I. Perioperative anaesthetic management of mediastinal mass in adults. *Eur J Anaesthesiol* 2009; **26**(8): 627–32

58. Blank RS, de Souza DG. Anesthetic management of patients with an anterior mediastinal mass: continuing professional development. *Can J Anaesth* 2011; **58**(9): 853–9, 60–7

59. Azizkhan RG, Dudgeon DL, Buck JR, et al. Life-threatening airway obstruction as a complication to the management of mediastinal masses in children. *J Pediatr Surg* 1985; **20**(6): 816–22

60. John RE, Narang VP. A boy with an anterior mediastinal mass. *Anaesthesia* 1988; **43**(10): 864–6

61. Bray RJ, Fernandes FJ. Mediastinal tumour causing airway obstruction in anaesthetised children. *Anaesthesia* 1982; **37**(5): 571–5

62. Hnatiuk OW, Corcoran PC, Sierra A. Spirometry in surgery for anterior mediastinal masses. *Chest* 2001; **120**(4): 1152–6

63. O'Leary HT, Tracey JA. Mediastinal tumours causing airway obstruction. A case in an adult. *Anaesthesia* 1983; **38**(1): 67

64. Tempe DK, Arya R, Dubey S, et al. Mediastinal mass resection: Femorofemoral cardiopulmonary bypass before induction of anesthesia in the management of airway obstruction. *J Cardiothorac Vasc Anesth* 2001; **15**(2): 233–6

65. Soon JL, Poopalalingam R, Lim CH, Koong HN, Agasthian T. Peripheral cardiopulmonary bypass-assisted thymoma resection. *J Cardiothorac Vasc Anesth.* 2007; **21**(6): 867–9

66. Asai T. Emergency cardiopulmonary bypass in a patient with a mediastinal mass. *Anaesthesia* 2007; **62**(8): 859–60

67. Young-Beyer P, Wilson RS. Anesthetic management for tracheal resection and reconstruction. *J Cardiothorac Anesth* 1988; **2**(6): 821–35

68. Pinsonneault C, Fortier J, Donati F. Tracheal resection and reconstruction. *Can J Anaesth* 1999; **46**(5 Pt 1): 439–55

69. McClish A, Deslauriers J, Beaulieu M, et al. High-flow catheter ventilation during major tracheobronchial reconstruction. *J Thorac Cardiovasc Surg* 1985; **89**(4): 508–12

70. Adelsmayr E, Keller C, Erd G, Brimacombe J. The laryngeal mask and high-frequency jet ventilation for resection of high tracheal stenosis. *Anesth Analg* 1998; **86**(4): 907–8

71. Biro P, Hegi TR, Weder W, Spahn DR. Laryngeal mask airway and high-frequency jet ventilation for the resection of a high-grade upper tracheal stenosis. *J Clin Anesth* 2001; **13**(2): 141–3

72. Beamer WC, Prough DS, Royster RL, Johnston WE, Johnson JC. High-frequency jet ventilation produces auto-PEEP. *Crit Care Med* 1984; **12**(9): 734–7

73. Howland WS, Carlon GC, Goldiner PL, et al. High-frequency jet ventilation during thoracic surgical procedures. *Anesthesiology.* 1987; **67**(6): 1009–12

CHAPTER 34

Anaesthesia for interventional bronchoscopy

Cait P. Searl

Introduction

The first documented interventional bronchoscopic procedure was the removal of a foreign body by Gustav Killien in 1897 (1). Since then the range of applications for bronchoscopy and methods of anaesthesia have evolved as new technology has become available. Bronchoscopy allows visualization of the airways for both diagnostic and interventional purposes. There are two main forms of procedure based around rigid bronchoscopes and flexible fibreoptic bronchoscopes as outlined in table 34.1. The aim of this chapter is review anaesthesia for bronchoscopy in general and then specifically for two important life threatening conditions that it is used to treat.

Rigid bronchoscopes

Around the same time as Killian was performing the first interventional bronchoscopic procedure, an American surgeon, Chevalier Jackson, was developing and promoting the use of endoscopes with distal illumination to examine the oesophagus, trachea, and bronchi (2). The rigid bronchoscopes used today remain of similar design to these originals (figure 34.1a). These consist of tapered stainless steel tubes with a flared bevelled tip and a central opening with side ports to allow ventilation and instrumentation at the other end. A 'telescope' rod with a fibreoptic cable attached to a light source provides the illumination (figure 34.1b). These scopes vary in size from 9 to 14 mm, allowing sizing appropriate to the patient and designed to allow both ventilation and instrumentation of the airway. The most commonly used rigid bronchoscopes are the Storz and Negus.

Although the rigid bronchoscopes have remained largely unchanged over the past 100 years the range of procedures has expanded and the anaesthetic techniques have evolved, from local anaesthesia using topical cocaine paste and intramuscular opiate to the now preferred (by both patient and anaesthetist) general anaesthesia.

Flexible bronchoscopes

Flexible bronchoscopes were first invented in 1966 by Ikeda (3). These consist of a fibreoptic system allowing transmission of an image from its tip to an eyepiece or video camera at the other end. These are long and thin, with an ability to steer using Bowden cables attached to a handle. In contrast to rigid bronchoscopes, flexible bronchoscopes provide improved visualization of the tracheobronchial tree into the peripheral zones of the lung to fifth division bronchi. This gives improved diagnostic and therapeutic yields for biopsy and exploration. With the evolution of endoscopic biopsy under ultrasound, the ability to biopsy lesions has greatly improved. Generally, local anaesthesia, with or without sedation, will suffice for most flexible bronchoscopic indications, although the procedure may be performed under general anaesthesia if deemed necessary. In these circumstances the flexible bronchoscope may be introduced to the airway via a tracheal tube or laryngeal mask airway designed for the purpose.

Preoperative and procedural considerations

Physiological considerations

The Physiological changes associated with bronchoscopy are predominantly cardiovascular and respiratory. These are in general greater with rigid bronchoscopy than with flexible bronchoscopy although both can have significant pathophysiological effects. Increased sympathetic activity secondary to the stimulation of the larynx can result in a substantial rise in both systemic blood pressure and heart rate. These may endanger the patient, in particular risking myocardial ischaemia. Increasing either depth of general anaesthesia often by the addition of an opiate (commonly remifentanil or fentanyl (4)) or ensuring adequacy of local anaesthesia blockade may attenuate this effect. Other methods employed include beta-blockade, sodium nitroprusside, and intravenous lidocaine. Bronchoscopy can also be associated with arrhythmias. These are usual minor and self-limiting without causing major haemodynamic instability.

In awake, spontaneously breathing patients undergoing bronchoscopy, hypoxia may occur even in individuals with normal lung function (5). Pulmonary mechanics may also be similarly affected, including bronchospasm induced by fibreoptic or rigid bronchoscopy.

Assessment of the patient

Assessing the patient prior to bronchoscopy allows planning of any anaesthetic intervention and allows a judgement to be made of the risks likely to be encountered. It also allows consideration of how the airway may need to be managed. Of particular interest are underlying cardiovascular problems, particularly those

Table 34.1 Examples of interventional bronchoscopy

Diagnostic	Therapeutic
Inspection & aspiration	Foreign body retrieval
Bronchial washings	Airway secretion clearance
Bronchoalveolar lavage	Endobronchial tumour destruction
Protected brush for culture	cryotherapy
Cytology brush	laser
Endobronchial biopsy	argon plasma coagulation
Transbronchial needle aspiration	Optimization of airway patency
Transbronchial biopsy	Dilatation
CT & fluoroscopic guided biopsy	Stent placement
Endobronchial ultrasound	Facilitation of:
	Tracheostomy
	Endotracheal intubation
	Bronchial blocker placement

suggesting coronary artery disease, in view of potential haemo-dynamic perturbations.

Using a combination of pulmonary function testing and chest X-ray and tomography imaging any element of obstruction of the airway can be assessed. 3-D reconstruction can be especially useful and guide decisions between operator and anaesthetist as to safely maintain the airway, which is ultimately a shared responsibility. The risks of obtaining such images in terms of patient positioning must be weighed up against the value of the information likely to be obtained.

An explanation of what is to occur is imperative together with an expression of potential risks to gain the patient's consent.

When utilizing local anaesthesia and sedation this is important, so that the patient has foreknowledge of what is likely to occur.

Premedication

Anticholinergic medication has been used as a premedication with the aim of drying airway secretions and to prevent vagotonic bradycardia and bronchoconstriction. Atropine is of questionable benefit relative to placebo (6) and may be associated with potential harm due to tachycardia. Both tachycardia and hypertension are commonly induced by the procedure and can be associated with myocardial ischaemia. Drying of secretions may also not be desirable as airway secretions may become insipissated with resulting bronchial plugs.

Monitoring

For the majority of flexible bronchoscopic procedures under local anaesthesia with or without sedation, non-invasive monitoring of peripheral oxygen saturation, blood pressure and electrocardiograph (ECG) are sufficient. For general anaesthesia, and particularly in those with prior cardiovascular compromise, fuller monitoring may be preferred with the insertion of an arterial line to allow beat-to-beat assessment of haemodynamics. This also allows arterial blood gases to be checked allowing measurement of carbon dioxide tension.

Local anaesthesia and sedation

Local anaesthesia, with or without addition of sedation will suffice for most diagnostic interventions done via flexible bronchoscopy. Although general anaesthesia is the norm for rigid bronchoscopy both local and regional techniques can be utilized and may be necessary in the very sick where preservation of consciousness and spontaneous breathing is paramount. Organe, in 1946 (7), described the experience of undergoing rigid bronchoscopy under local anaesthesia, stating that it was preferable to visiting the dentist.

(a)

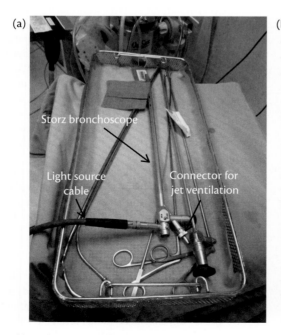

(b)

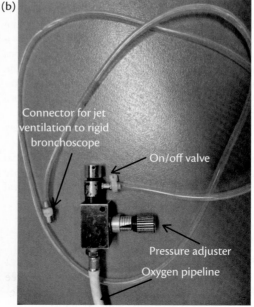

Fig. 34.1 (a) Storz rigid bronchoscope and (b) Sanders venturi jet ventilator.

Local anaesthesia

Topical anaesthesia may be achieved with lidocaine, benzocaine, or cocaine—most commonly lidocaine is used as it has relatively wide margins of safety and a low rate of tissue toxicity. Topical anaesthesia may be produced by spraying lidocaine on to tongue, oropharynx, and pharynx as well as by gargling a 4% lidocaine solution. Commonly, this is supplemented using a 'spray as you go' technique where the local anaesthetic is given through the flexible bronchoscope. The trachea can be anaesthetized using a transtracheal injection of 2% lidocaine at the level of the ligamentum conicum. This can be as effective as using the 'spray as you go' technique (8) and is the preferred method where rigid bronchoscopy is occurring under local anaesthesia. Suppression of the gag reflex can be achieved by the direct application of local anaesthetic to the anterior tonsillar pillar producing a lingual nerve block. This will also blunt the haemodynamic response to manipulation of the larynx. The superior laryngeal nerve can be blocked by injecting local anaesthetic into the thyrohyoid membrane just lateral to the superior cornu of the thyroid cartilage and this achieves anaesthesia of the lower pharynx and laryngeal epiglottis.

Sedation

There have been clinical studies demonstrating that acceptable patient satisfaction and tolerance of the procedure can be achieved with local anaesthesia alone (9). Sedation is however commonly used, as the procedure of bronchoscopy can be unpleasant and may induce considerable anxiety, heightening haemodynamic responses to the stimulus of bronchoscopy.

Various drugs and drug combinations can be used for sedation during bronchoscopy – benzodiazepines, propofol, and opioids being most frequently used. Midazolam is the benzodiazepine most widely used for this purpose. It can be given intravenously or orally, with a dose range of approximately 7 to 15 μg/kg varying with procedural requirements. It reliably produces procedural amnesia as well as sedation. Midazolam has the benefit of being water soluble and short acting, with no significantly active metabolite. Lorazepam and diazepam can also be used but have longer durations of action. They may also be given prior to the procedure. When used alone benzodiazepines will have a limited effect on cardiorespiratory function compared to that when used (as is commonly the case) in combination with opiates, where there is potentiation of respiratory depression.

Propofol can be used as a continuous infusion at a low target-controlled infusion rate. It has the benefit of a rapid offset and quick recovery. However, this form of sedation requires careful monitoring of sedation level as there is a fine line between an adequate depth of sedation and a general anaesthetic. The Ramsay scale (10) can be used to quantify sedation and guide administration, although monitoring ability to rouse and respiratory rate in addition to cardiovascular parameters and oxygen saturation is commonly employed.

Opioids are usually administered in conjunction with either benzodiazepines or propofol. In addition to an analgesic effect they produce synergistic potentiation of sedation and reduce coughing reflexes. Opioids also have numerous unhelpful side-effects including respiratory depression, nausea, vomiting, urinary retention, dysphoria, and pruritus. For most interventions shorter-acting opioids such as alfentanil, fentanyl, and remifentanil, are usually preferred.

Regardless of which drugs are used for sedation, the doses should be adjusted according to the individual's physical status and must also be titrated to the desired effect.

General anaesthesia

For rigid bronchoscopy general anaesthesia is the norm and in some situations it is also used for fibreoptic bronchoscopy. The insertion of a rigid bronchoscope is very stimulating, inducing a pressor response that can be large. The obtunding of this response during anaesthesia is essential as the risks of haemodynamic, cardiac, or cerebral complications are often already high in a patient case-mix that is likely to have considerable cardiac and respiratory co-morbidity.

Anaesthetic agents

The use of virtually every anaesthetic induction agent has been described for use during bronchoscopy. The stimulating effects require an adequate depth of anaesthesia while the nature of the procedures require rapid emergence and recovery of protective airway reflexes. The author's own practice is to use a small dose of midazolam in combination with total intravenous anaesthesia (TIVA) with target-controlled infusions of propofol and remifentanil. Depth of anaesthesia is monitored both through the use of bispectral index (BIS) monitoring, accepting its limitations, and by adequate suppression of haemodynamic reactivity. An opiate in addition to propofol is useful to achieve this effect and the use of remifentanil has the benefit of the relatively rapid offset of effect. Alfentanil or fentanyl may preferentially be used but in small doses.

Neuromuscular blockade

Neuromuscular blockade can be problematic with short and unpredictable length procedures. Rapid reversal again is desirable and must be monitored with the use of peripheral neuromuscular stimulation. Previously, boluses or infusions of suxamethonium were used with the occasional risk of prolonged blockade. A small dose of non-depolarizing neuromuscular blocker may be given first (precurization) to prevent fasciculation. Mivacurium is commonly used, with its rapid offset, although this can be unpredictable. Rocuronium, a short-acting non-depolarizing neuromuscular blocker, is gaining popularity as giving rapid onset blockade when given in adequate dosage (1 mg/kg) and has the added advantage of a rapid reversal agent using sugammadex. With longer procedures, such as laser treatment, most of the shorter-acting neuromuscular blocking drugs may be safely used, provided an adequate dose of neostigmine reversal with atropine or glycopyrrolate is given at the end of the procedure.

Airway management and ventilation during bronchoscopy

Initially during the development of bronchoscopy and continuing into modern-day bronchoscopy under local anaesthetic, ventilation relied on the patient continuing to breathe spontaneously. Room air is generally supplemented with oxygen through nasal cannulae. With the development of bronchoscopy under general anaesthesia, ventilation became part of the technique with various systems of gas delivery being employed.

Apnoeic oxygenation

Apnoeic oxygenation involves the process of denitrogenation of the patient through preoxygenation with 100% oxygen. Neuromuscular blockade is used while oxygen is delivered continuously into the airway either through the bronchoscope or via a catheter. The disadvantage of this method is the inevitable hypercapnia that occurs. Continuous insufflation of oxygen may however permit the bronchoscopist to proceed for significant periods of time (10). This method is now not generally used, apart from the briefest of procedures, as methods of ventilation generally have improved.

Ventilating rigid bronchoscopes

Ventilating bronchoscopes have been available since the mid-1950s (3). These allow ventilation through a side arm of the bronchoscope while the proximal end of the bronchoscope is occluded either by a glass window or the surgeon's thumb. Besides the inevitable intermittent nature of the ventilation, this also requires the cessation of procedures with the temporary removal of instrument during ventilatory periods. The advantages of the system are the ability to give inhalational as well as intravenous anaesthetic agents. The anaesthetic gases can be scavenged from the circuit. End-tidal carbon dioxide can also be measured thus allowing assessment of adequacy of ventilation.

Jet ventilation

Jet ventilation was developed in the 1960s in an attempt to reconcile the demands of a shared airway by facilitating continuous ventilation while maintaining surgical access. High-frequency jet ventilation now provides a generally accepted method of securing ventilation during rigid and interventional bronchoscopy. Its use has also been described via insufflation catheter placed via the nasotracheal route for ventilation during flexible fibreoptic bronchoscopy (12).

Sander's injector

Sanders devised a technique of jet ventilation through a rigid bronchoscope in 1967 (13). He used an adapter connected to the proximal end of the bronchoscope and to the oxygen/ air pipeline via a pressure-regulator (figure 34.1b). Frequency of ventilation is controlled through a hand held on/ off valve. Oxygen is delivered down a narrow lumen nozzle running through the lumen of the bronchoscope. Each jet of gas entrains air through the bronchoscope, according to the Bernoulli effect. Venturi also used this effect, of a high-pressure gas passing through a constriction dropping its pressure such that surrounding gas is entrained with an increase in flow, to develop his injector. The technique is commonly referred to as the Sanders–Venturi technique.

This technique of ventilation relies on passive expiration during the pause between each jet delivery. A hazard of using this system is that the passive ventilation is reliant on either an open glottis or the bronchoscope. If the vocal cords are adducted there is a risk that expiration does not occur with air trapping and a risk of volutrauma and potentially pneumothorax. Adequacy of ventilation is generally assessed through direct observation of chest wall movement and maintenance of oxygen saturation. Arterial blood gases may be necessary during longer procedures to assess carbon dioxide removal as hypercapnia is a potential complication of this method of ventilation. The relative lack of regulation of pressures delivered from pipeline pressure down means relatively high pressures may be generated in the distal airways, with the potential for barotrauma.

Jet ventilation may be further adapted to allow entrainment of volatile anaesthetic agents in addition to air for provision of general anaesthesia. Adequacy of depth of anaesthesia is difficult to assess by conventional volatile monitoring so BIS monitoring or equivalent should be employed in a similar manner to during TIVA. It should also be remembered that these volatile gases are expired, and as this is difficult to scavenge, there may be some risk of the operator inhaling a quantity of the volatile anaesthetic.

Jet ventilators, such as the Monsoon ventilator, have now been developed, which are useful for longer procedures and for procedures requiring use of lasers where the concentration of oxygen needs careful regulation (see later). These ventilators deliver the gas usually an oxygen/air mix, at high frequency and have the advantage of delivering a regular bolus of gas at a rate and a pressure that can be regulated. The risk of barotrauma is significantly reduced as the mean airway pressure is minimal. The technique again allows a delivery of a consistent and predictable concentration of anaesthetic gas.

Ventilation during fibreoptic bronchoscopy

Fibreoptic bronchoscopy is generally performed on awake patients who can easily breathe around the bronchoscope. The bronchoscope generally occupies a fraction of the airway and does not produce undue obstruction. Where general anaesthesia is being used, the patient is generally intubated with an endotracheal tube and the bronchoscope passed through an adapted angle piece. This allows the patient to be ventilated as normal with a standard anaesthesia circuit with both measurement of minute volume and end-tidal carbon dioxide. A tracheal tube of sufficient diameter is required to allow passage of the fibreoptic bronchoscope and allow ventilation without a significant elevation of airway pressure. Jet ventilation can also be used in this situation.

Post-procedure care

Complications following the procedure may relate to the pathophysiology previously described, including hypoxia, respiratory failure, and cardiac dysfunction, or be related to the procedure itself such as acute airway obstruction, bleeding, mucus retention, and pneumothorax. While often an ambulatory procedure, there is a need to include a sufficient period of observation post-procedure to ensure no complications have occurred. If local anaesthetic has been used a continued period of fasting is necessary to ensure full recovery of laryngeal reflexes and to ensure aspiration does not then occur.

Anaesthesia for specific procedures

Rigid bronchoscopy in airway obstruction

Central airway obstruction is a common thoracic anaesthetic emergency. Such obstruction may arise from both intrinsic and extrinsic sources. In the past, patients presenting with central airway obstruction would have been subjected to tracheal surgery with a high level of morbidity or mortality, or would have been regarded as inoperable. Nowadays insertion of a tracheobronchial stent would be normal first-line management. Over the last two decades stents for management of tracheobronchial stenosis and obstruction have evolved from bulky, unwieldy prostheses requiring tracheal resection to small self-expanding devices that can be inserted using fibreoptic techniques. With these developments the variety of anaesthetic management techniques that can be used has also extended.

Early stents were tubes of silicone based on a simplistic cylindrical concept of the trachea. These include the still-used cumbersome Montgomery T-tube that has a tracheostomy tube as its stem of the T. These are awkward to position but once in situ tend not to dislodge. More recent versions are based on the anatomical trachea involving steel rings with silastic membranous portions; metal strut and self or balloon expanding devices including where necessary individually tailored stents (figure 34.2).

Challenges for anaesthetists relate to the management of the underlying condition and often major co-morbidities, coping with central airway obstruction distal to a site suitable for rescue with a surgical airway, and sharing an airway already compromised such that total airway obstruction is a possibility that may occur even if only occasionally. Most practitioners use a rigid bronchoscope as a conduit with use of the flexible bronchoscope through this to manipulate the device (14).

Preoperative management

Prior to managing these critically ill patients a careful assessment by the anaesthetist and operator need to be made of risk versus benefit, and likely or possible complications. Benefit needs to be achievable rapidly—perhaps in terms of early recovery of functioning lung or an immediate increase in the size of the airway—for the risk of procedure and therefore anaesthesia to be justified. The patient must also be aware of these risks.

Before anaesthesia is induced these patients are best managed in an upright sitting position and receiving supplementary inspired

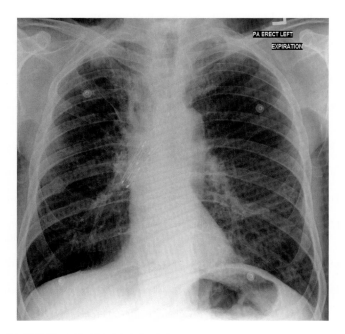

Fig. 34.2 Stents in right main bronchus.

and humidified oxygen. The aim is to prevent severe episodes of coughing which could precipitate further, and critical, airway obstruction. With truly critical obstruction it may be necessary to administer a mixture oxygen 21% and helium 79% (Heliox).

Induction

These patients have an obstruction that is generally below the level at which a surgical airway as rescue might be used. Our normal practice with these patients is to avoid using local anaesthetic approaches to securing the airway as the risk of precipitating a coughing episode and hence critical obstruction outweigh any potential benefits. Similarly, gaseous induction is avoided because of the risk of coughing, even with sevoflurane.

Standard management involves rigid bronchoscopy so in addition to avoidance of coughing it is important to decrease and avoid pressor effects secondary to instrumentation of the airway. Following 1–2 mg of midazolam, a combination of remifentanil and propofol target-controlled infusions are used to achieve TIVA with a small dose of glycopyrrolate (200 μg) available if needed to treat vagotonic effects of remifentanil. This small dose of glycopyrolate is unlikely to greatly increase the viscosity of bronchial secretions. Nevertheless, if its use can be avoided, this potential side effect is also avoided. Once the patient is asleep, ability to ventilate is checked prior to administration of mivacurium, accepting that high pressures may be required to achieve this. When muscle relaxation is achieved, the rigid bronchoscope is inserted thereafter providing a conduit for jet ventilation as described previously and for instrumentation of the more distal airway.

Improvements in stents and particularly the development of self-expanding stents has made placement during flexible bronchoscopy and hence a potentially easier method of managing these patients. Flexible bronchoscopy for these patients can be achieved awake and under local anaesthetic. Our practice remains to avoid this method and to use a rigid bronchoscope as a conduit in most patients. The concern remains around obstruction of the airway with insufficient ability to remove sputum and blood clots during instrumentation. It is equally possible to secure the airway with an intubating laryngeal mask or suitably sized endotracheal tube for manipulation thereafter with a flexible bronchoscope.

Recovery from anaesthesia and the procedure

The main concern following stenting for central airway obstruction is still the risk of complete airway obstruction occurring. The clinical presentation may be mistaken for inadequate reversal of neuromuscular blockade as the jerky shallow pattern of breathing resembles this. A tension pneumothorax should first be excluded, but consider blockage with glutinous secretions from previously obstructed distal airway, stent migration or malfunction, blood clot or other stent blockage.

Our practice is to leave the rigid bronchoscope in until the patient is at the point of coughing it out. Transfer to the recovery room requires the presence of all parts of the cough reflex, including deep inspiration, active glottis closure, and an expiration free of laryngeal spasm with demonstrable clearance of secretions.

Rigid bronchoscopy for management of haemoptysis

Airway haemorrhage is a potentially rapidly fatal condition. Bronchoscopy is central to management but the goals will differ with the circumstances. While the conservative management of haemoptysis is generally preferred with elective exploratory bronchoscopy, in a minority of cases haemoptysis may be massive and life-threatening. Early bronchoscopy in these patients is performed with three goals in mind: lateralization the bleeding site, localization of the bleeding site, and identification of the cause of the bleeding. Various methods of control are described including: endobronchial balloon tamponade, topical application of adrenaline, lavage with cold saline to remove clot, and direct diathermy to the airway. Urgent bronchoscopy is often required in this group of unstable patients. Fibreoptic bronchoscopy on occasion may be more appropriate for more peripherally placed lesions.

The use of bronchoscopy in allowing the location of the bleeding site and guiding further management has the added benefit of providing a protective role of maintaining airway patency. Use of the rigid bronchoscope is generally preferred for this as it offers a greater suctioning ability and maintenance of airway patency—the risk to the patient of asphyxiation is generally as great as of exsanguination. In addition to allowing direct management of the haemoptysis, the rigid bronchoscope may permit the rapid selective intubation of the non-involved lung's main bronchus allowing its protection (15).

The anaesthetist's priorities must be to maintain the airway, optimize oxygenation and to stabilize the haemodynamic status. Nevertheless, haemoptysis is distressing and if consciousness is maintained, this distress must be alleviated commonly with bolus benzodiazepine and opiate in rapid management. With fluid resuscitation the ability to permit a greater depth of anaesthesia may be possible.

Rigid bronchoscopy for foreign bodies

Anything that is small enough may be inhaled most commonly foodstuffs and dentition. The rigid bronchoscope provides the best conduit for instruments to remove the foreign body. This may prove difficult especially if the foreign body has been present for some time. Anaesthesia for this purpose is best achieved with TIVA. It should be remembered if the foreign body is a tooth that the remainder of the dentition may also be at risk being dislodged by the bronchoscope!

Rigid bronchoscopy enabling cryotherapy and laser treatment

Cryoprobes and lasers have evolved such that they can be used via fibreoptic bronchoscopes. The usual practice, however, is to secure the airway and ventilate via a rigid bronchoscope, and treat and apply therapy options secondarily via a fibreoscopy. The laser fibre delivery instruments are small enough to insert through the fibreoptic bronchoscope. This enables laser treatment options further into the airway and the management through using laser of more complicated lesions than previously achievable. The plastic material of the fibreoptic bronchoscope is, however, ignitable by the laser fibre, remaining a potential hazard. The rigid bronchoscope has the advantage over the fibreoptic scope in this respect as its metal construction reduces the fire hazard associated with the use of lasers.

Fire hazard must remain the primary concern for the anaesthetist and operator. During laser treatment it is mandatory that the patient only receive air that is 21% O_2. The easiest way to achieve this is with a jet ventilator such as the Monsoon, which has a LASER setting that only permits the delivery of air. A similar effect can be achieved by having separate air and oxygen Sander's injectors or by having a pipeline adaptor allowing swapping between air and O_2 outlets. This is cumbersome and open to error.

These patients often present with an obstructed airway and anaesthesia should be approached in a similar manner to that described earlier. The necessity for using air during the actual laser treatment may cause difficulties for maintaining acceptable oxygenation. Again, careful planning and discussion with the surgeon before starting maximizes a suitable management plan and reminds all staff to be cognisant of the duration of the laser applications in order to minimize hypoxaemia. We recommend administration of steroids empirically for these procedures usually as a bolus dose of dexamethasone.

Conclusion

Interventional bronchoscopy present a major challenge for the anaesthetist because it requires sharing the airway with the surgeon. However, a sound understanding of how to maintain a patent airway and ventilate patients along with a high level of communication with the surgeon allows the anaesthetist to successfully and safely manage patients during interventional bronchoscopy.

References

1. Kellofrath O. [Removal of a bone fragment from the right bronchus in a natural way and through use of direct laryngoscopy.] *Munchener Medizinishe Wochenschrift* 1897; **38**: 1038–9
2. Jackson C. Bronchoscopy and esophagoscopy: a manual of peroral endoscopy and laryngeal surgery. Philadelphia & London: WB Saunders Company, 1922
3. Folch E. Airway interventions in the tracheobronchial tree. *Semin Respir Care Med* 2008; **29**: 441–52
4. Natalini G, Fassini P, Seramondi V, et al. Remifentanil vs. fentanyl during interventional rigid bronchoscopy under general anaesthetic and spontaneous assisted ventilation. *Eur J Anaesthesiol* 1999; **16**: 605
5. Albertini RE, Harrell JH, Naotsugu K, Moser KM. Arterial hypoxaemia induced by fibreoptic bronchoscopy. *JAMA* 1974; **230**: 1666–7
6. Williams T, Brooks T, Ward C. The role of atropine as premedication in fibreoptic bronchoscopy using midazolam sedation. *Chest* 1998; **113**: 1394–8
7. Organe G. Personal experience of bronchoscopy. *Proc Roy Soc Med* 1946; **39**: 635–6
8. Webb AR, Fernado SS, Dalton HR et al. Local anaesthesia for fibreoptic bronchoscopy: transcricoid injection or the 'spray as you go' technique? *Thorax* 1990; **45**: 474–7
9. Hatton MQ, Allen MB, Vathenen AS et al. Does sedation help in fibreoptic bronchoscopy? *Br Med J* 1994; **309**: 1206–7
10. Ramsay MA, Savege TM, Simpson BR, Goodwin R. Controlled sedation with alphaxolone-alphadone. *Br Med J* 1974; **2**: 656–9.
11. Frumin MJ, Epstein RM, Cohen G. Apneic oxygenation in man. *Anesthesiology* 1959; **20**: 789–98
12. Hautmann H, Gamarra F, Henke M, et al. High frequency Jet ventilation in Interventional bronchoscopy. *Anaesth Analg* 2000; **90**: 1436–40.
13. Sanders RD. Two ventilating attachments for bronchoscopes. *Del Med J* 1967; **39**: 170.
14. Conacher ID. Anaesthesia and tracheobronchial stenting for central airway obstruction in adults. *Br J Anaesth* 2003; **90**: 367–74
15. Karmy-Jones R, Cushieri J, Vallieres E. Role of bronchoscopy in massive hemoptysis. *Chest Surg Clin N Am* 2001; **11**: 873–906

CHAPTER 35

Anaesthesia for lung transplantation

Nandor Marczin, Lakshminarasimhan Kuppurao, I. Gavin Wright, and Andre R. Simon

Introduction

The combination of the recipient's poor underlying condition, surgical stresses and intraoperative complications makes the conduct of anaesthesia for lung transplantation, supremely challenging. Together with surgical advances, utilization of a spectrum of novel monitoring, diagnostic, and therapeutic tools have enhanced anaesthetic management and contributed to improved postoperative outcomes (figure 35.1). However, survival still varies markedly among different patient groups (1) indicating that there are important gaps in our knowledge and management. Therefore, the aim of this chapter is to review the current management of patients undergoing lung transplantation.

Factors influencing outcome from lung transplantation

Although transplantation has become a standard treatment for end-stage lung disease, survival of the listed patient is compromised by donor shortages, low acceptance rate of donor organs, perioperative mortality, and long-term chronic rejection. Moreover, lung transplant surgery has one of the highest mortalities with 12% of patients dying within three months and 21% within one year (1). Surgical complications and cardiovascular failure are each responsible for approximately 10% of the perioperative mortality and infections are responsible for another 20%. However, the leading cause of perioperative mortality is primary graft dysfunction (PGD, figure 35.2) (2).

Donor shortages

Similarly to all other solid organs, the shortage of donor organs has long remained a major problem in lung transplantation, such that 20–30% of patients will die on the waiting list before a donor organ becomes available. In addition to shortage of multi-organ donors, approximately 80% of potential donor lungs in the UK are deemed unusable for clinical lung transplantation due to manifest of presumed lung injury.

Primary graft dysfunction

Histologically PGD is characterized by diffuse alveolar damage (figure 35.3). The principle pathophysiology is increased vascular permeability and alveolar flooding causing the clinical symptoms of pulmonary oedema, impaired gas exchange and altered lung mechanics (figure 35.1).

Such lung injury can be conceptualized as a sequential series of haemodynamic, metabolic and inflammatory insults. It starts with pulmonary manifestations of critical illness and side effects of medical management preceding brain death. The sequence continues with the neurogenic impact of coning followed by suboptimal preservation during the period of ischaemia, and finally, reperfusion injury and early post-implantation management (figure 35.4).

Mechanistically, ischaemic structural and functional damage to the microvascular endothelium and alveolar epithelium, inflammatory activation of alveolar cells, circulating and resident leukocytes, proinflammatory cytokine imbalance and increased oxidative stress all contribute to PGD (3,4) (figure 35.3). There is strong evidence to suggest that inflammatory genetic alterations are already present at the end of the ischaemic period in lungs that subsequently suffer from PGD (5). Furthermore, reperfusion sets into motion programmed cell death cascades with up to 30% lung cells exhibiting signs of apoptosis prior to chest closure (6).

Potentially modifiable intraoperative risk factors include an elevated inspired concentration of oxygen (FiO_2) during allograft reperfusion, pulmonary arterial hypertension, the use of cardiopulmonary bypass (CPB) and the transfusion of large-volumes of blood products (7). Therefore, limiting hydrostatic forces, hyperoxia, and oxidative stress may attenuate degree of PGD. Some centres routinely practice controlled reperfusion, and some routinely administer antioxidants such as vitamin C and N-acetylcysteine.

Severe PGD is strongly associated with increased 90-day and 1-year mortality after lung transplant (7). Early and aggressive treatment with extracorporeal membrane oxygenation (ECMO) for severe PGD is warranted as it offers survival benefits so should no longer be viewed only as a salvage therapy (Chapter 12).

Recipient factors that influence outcome

The registry of the International Society of Heart and Lung Transplantation (ISHLT) reveals that early mortality is influenced by the recipient's age, underlying diagnosis and co-morbidity (1).

Age

Over the age of 55 years, there is an increased early mortality. This risk then rises exponentially with increasing age, and patients

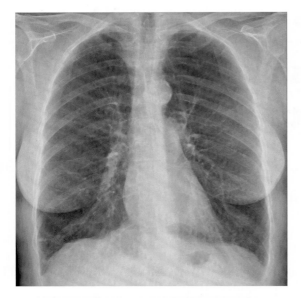

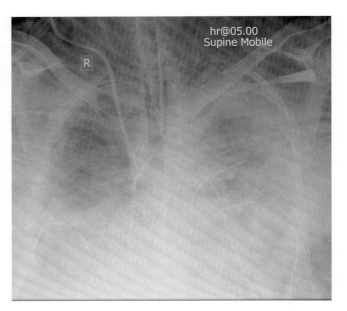

Fig. 35.2 Chest radiograph showing severe primary graft failure.

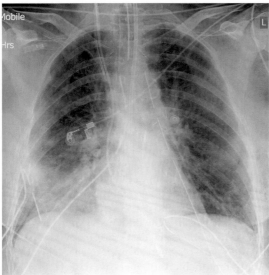

Fig. 35.1 Chest radiographs before (above) and after (below) successful minimally invasive bilateral sequential lung transplantation for emphysema. Note mild degree of infiltrates in the first transplanted right lung.

older than 65 years consistently have a worse survival. This risk factor is increasingly relevant, as the number of lung transplants undertaken in these age categories has nearly doubled in recent years.

Underlying diagnosis

Three-month mortality has been reported to be lowest in patients with chronic obstructive pulmonary disease (COPD; 9%) and highest in those with pulmonary arterial hypertension (PAH; 23%), sarcoidosis (16%), and idiopathic pulmonary fibrosis (IPF;15%) (1). The differences in mortality likely reflect differences in early complication rates between the groups.

Recipient comorbidity

The preoperative comorbidity of the recipient associated with highest early mortality is dialysis dependent renal impairment. A low

cardiac output state and high blood levels of bilirubin are also risk factors. Poor physical status, preoperative hospitalization including prolonged stay in the intensive care unit (ICU), and mechanical ventilation prior to transplant are also associated with higher early postoperative mortality (8). Possible explanations for the increased mortality include poor nutritional status and deconditioning of the patient that results in an inability to sustain the physical challenge of as well as the inflammatory and metabolic responses to, transplant surgery. Indeed, preoperative hypoalbuminaemia and low body weight are both associated with poorer survival and recovery.

Donor factors that influence outcome

Many factors determine the suitability and quality of donor lungs for transplantation including donor history, the circumstances of brain or cardiac death and ICU management prior to retrieval including clinical and physiological parameters.

Age

The outcome of donors aged 55 to 64 years is similar to younger donors. However, donors who were aged 65 years or older had more than a twofold relative risk of mortality in 1- and 3-year follow-ups.

Suboptimal donors

ISHLT criteria exist that donors must meet to be accepted for transplantation. Nevertheless, many centres routinely transplant lungs that do not meet all the criteria for the ideal donor lung. Oto and colleagues have developed a simple lung donor score to assess the overall quality of the donor lung. Components of the score include age, history of smoking, chest X-ray findings, bronchial secretions, and arterial blood gas results (9). The score well differentiated donors who were excluded for lung transplantation. In addition the donor score was significantly associated with post-transplantation gas exchange, grade of PGD and duration of tracheal intubation in bilateral lung transplantation.

The role of smoking history remains controversial (10). Survival seems comparable between donors who were heavy and non-heavy

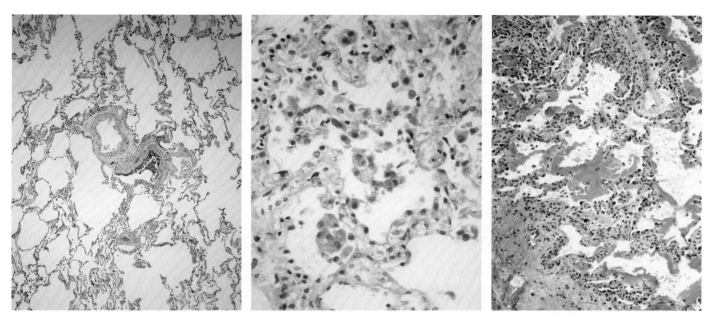

Fig. 35.3 Histology of moderate (b) and severe (c) diffuse alveolar damage and acute lung injury associated with primary graft failure. Panel a shows preserved lung structures.

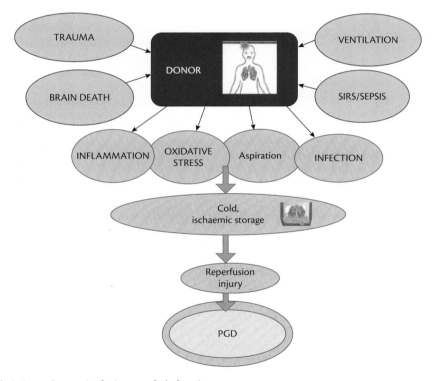

Fig. 35.4 Schematic diagram depicting pathogenesis of primary graft dysfunction.

SIRS, systemic inflammatory response syndrome.

smokers. Donors with diabetes mellitus and cytomegalovirus (CMV) infections are associated with a significantly worse early survival of recipients.

Donor assessment and organ retrieval

The principal aims of the management of the potential lung donor is to minimize donor injury prior to retrieval and to identify irreversible forms of acute lung injury (ALI).

Donors have multiple risk factors for ALI including trauma, prolonged mechanical ventilation, and subclinical aspiration. We have recently observed evidence for both pulmonary and systemic inflammation in patients who required mechanical ventilation for severe head injury (11). Furthermore inappropriate mechanical ventilation causes ventilation induced lung injury (12). Acute inflammation in the donor lung with elevated levels of interleukin-8 (IL-8) in donor bronchoalveolar lavage, or imbalance between pro- and anti-inflammatory cytokine expression has been shown to adversely impact on early outcome from lung transplantation (13).

Assessment of donors with brain death

Brain death causes discharge of the sympathetic nervous system with a massive catecholamine storm that is associated with severe haemodynamic derangement. Such events may result in stress failure of the pulmonary microcirculation leading to neurogenic pulmonary oedema and it is also associated with pulmonary and systemic inflammation (14).

Retrieval teams utilize a structured approach to evaluate the suitability of the donor lungs for donation. This involves reviewing donor history, thorough evaluation of airways, assessment of current ventilation parameters, gas exchange and haemodynamics, and all available imaging. Bronchoscopy should be performed to assess the extent of bronchial secretions and airway inflammation.

However, the internationally accepted selection criteria of the optimal donor are primarily opinion based rather than evidence based, and lung assessments made by retrieval teams are often subjective. Ware and colleagues studied the pathology and function of lungs that had been rejected for clinical transplantation. They found that more than 40% of the rejected lungs might have been suitable for transplantation so emphasizing the need for better scientific assessment of selection of lung donors (15).

Lung donation after circulatory death

Lung donation after circulatory death presents its own problems regarding donor lung injury (16). While the negative impact of brain death and coning are absent in donation after circulatory death donors, the extent of ICU care and resuscitation can be even more intense. There may also be insufficient data available to objectively assess the function of the lungs from donation after circulatory death donors and there is a prolonged warm ischaemic phase after withdrawal of life support, with unpredictable influence on lung biology and function.

Organ retrieval

After sternotomy the retrieval surgeons thoroughly inspect the lungs for any structural anomalies. Significant atelectasis is re-expanded; a deflation test is performed and selective pulmonary vein blood gases are collected to evaluate regional gas exchange. After abdominal dissections, the lungs are re-evaluated and the final acceptance decision is made through discussion with the prospective implanting team.

The principle retrieval technique is based on cold perfusion of the lungs with 4 L Perfadex (Vitrolife, Gothenburg, Sweden) that has been cooled to a temperature of 4°C, generally by using gravity perfusion after aortic cross-clamping. Prior to excision of the lungs they are inflated to mid-expiration with 50% oxygen in air. Once removed from the donor, the lungs are sealed in a plastic bag containing cold Perfadex and transported to the recipient's hospital on ice.

Strategies to improve the donor pool and quality of donor organs

Donor management

Optimizing haemodynamics, employing lung protective ventilation strategies, and advanced routine pulmonary care, have increased both the number of lung donors and the quality of donor organs and this has translated into improved patient outcome (17,18). Many transplant teams have also liberalized their criteria to accept more 'marginal' or 'extended criteria' donors. However, while some centres reported comparable results with standard transplantation, others have observed poorer outcomes (19).

Ex-vivo lung perfusion

Ex-vivo lung perfusion (EVLP) is one of the most significant advances of the last two decades in lung transplantation (18,20) (figure 35.5). Steen and colleagues originally developed EVLP to allow better clinical and physiological assessments of donation after circulatory death lung donors. Subsequently, it has been recognized that EVLP might facilitate better recovery from donor and preservation lung injury and may help recondition lungs that were initially considered unsuitable for transplantation. Clinical experience from Lund, Toronto, Harefield, and others indicate that perioperative and mid-term outcomes of tranplantation of EVLP-reconditioned lungs are comparable to standard lung transplantation (21–25).

The Transmedics group has expanded EVLP evaluation to the donor hospital and to provide continuous machine perfusion during transit between the donor and implanting hospitals. Initial results, using the integrated and portable Organ Care System Lung device (figure 35.5c) suggest that the technology allows favourable organ preservation and transplantation (26,27). Interim results of the INSPIRE multicentre trial that has examined the efficacy and safety of this novel technology, are also promising.

Preoperative assessment and preparation of the lung transplant recipient

Patients presenting for lung transplantation may have been on a waiting list for months to years. During this time, their health may have deteriorated since their original assessment and multidisciplinary evaluation for lung transplant. Acute deterioration in exercise capacity or presence of any new symptoms must be explored. Most patients are very anxious but will poorly tolerate any premedication. So, the value of thorough preanaesthetic interview, with full explanation of events, cannot be overemphasized.

During preanesthetic assessment aggressive measures such as vigorous preoperative bronchodilation and sputum-clearing techniques should be used. Positive inotropes and inhaled and intravenous pulmonary vasodilators are indicated as they may improve the patient's condition so making the induction of anaesthesia smoother and safer (28). A thorough examination of the airway is prudent as some patients may have subglottic stenosis as a consequence of previous prolonged tracheal intubation. In addition, a range of sizes of double-lumen endobronchial tubes (DLTs) and an intubating fiberoptic bronchoscope must be available at induction of anaesthesia.

Monitoring and venous access

Large-bore peripheral venous access is established and an arterial line is placed under local anaesthesia before induction of anaesthesia. They should be performed with meticulous sterile technique in view of the induced immunosuppression. Central venous and pulmonary artery catheters are commonly placed after induction.

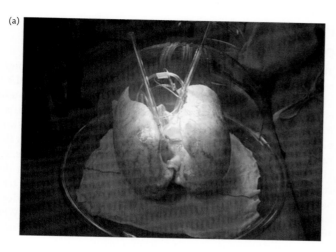

(a)

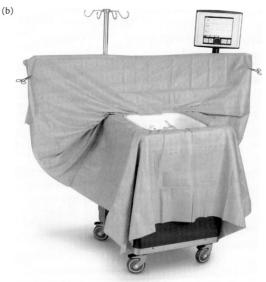

(b)

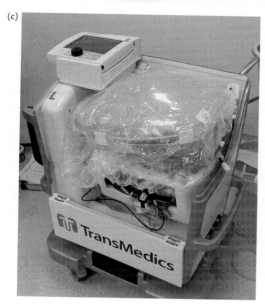

(c)

Fig. 35.5 Various forms of ex vivo lung perfusion setups employed at Harefield Hospital (a) Toronto dome acellular perfusion. (b) Vivoline setup. (c) Transmedics Organ Care Lung System..

However, some centres perform all line placements under local anaesthesia after premedication with anxiolytics and analgesics while administering supplemental oxygen. However, many lung transplant recipients depend on their hypoxic drive to breathe so close monitoring of respiratory status is essential.

Immunosuppresssion

The most common immunosuppressive regimes include steroids, cyclosporin A (CyA), and azathioprine (29). CyA is given in a loading dose of 5 mg/kg by mouth on call of the patient to the operating room. If the patient has renal impairment, the dose is reduced depending on the creatinine clearance. Methylprednisolone is traditionally administered just before lung reperfusion in a dose of between 500 mg–1 g IV. This is changed to oral prednisone once patient's trachea is extubated. Azathioprine and CyA are also continued postoperatively in the ICU and afterwards depending on institutional protocols. A variety of prophylactic antibiotics are given before and after the procedure depending on the local guidelines. These generally include agents directed at bacteria and viral and fungal agents or previous positive cultures.

Team brief

A team brief and World Health Organization checklist prior to surgical preparation of the patient is important to ensure that appropriate prophylactic antibiotic and immunosuppression are administered (Chapter 42). Based on the patient history and actual physical condition, the anesthetic plan should be clearly communicated including the anticipated stability of the patient's haemodynamics and gas exchange during induction of anaesthesia. Potential surgical difficulties with particular reference to the presence of extensive pleural adhesions should be shared with the team. Finally, any donor issues and the expected arrival time of the allograft should be communicated to the team

Induction of anaesthesia

The induction of anaesthesia and transition from spontaneous to mechanical ventilation are critical high-risk events. Multimodal diagnostic approaches should be in place to identify impending cardiovascular collapse. All necessary therapies including vasoactive drugs should be immediately available to aggressively treat haemodynamic compromise. The operating room should be prepared for emergency sternotomy and the surgical team and perfusionist must be ready to initiate cardiopulmonary bypass (CPB). As discussed in the relevant two sections following, dynamic pulmonary hyperinflation and exacerbation of pulmonary hypertension frequently complicate induction of anaesthesia and institution of mechanical ventilation. Older recipients may also have compromised cardiovascular reserve, and patients with emphysema may have smoking-related coronary artery disease that may contribute to haemodynamic instability after induction of anaesthesia.

Dynamic pulmonary hyperinflation

Although it can affect any patient with obstructive physiology, dynamic pulmonary hyperinflation is characteristic of end-stage COPD and results from increased end-expiratory lung volume as bullous or cystic lung units fail to empty during exhalation due to significant airway obstruction (30,31). Progressive increases in the end-expiratory lung volume that are especially likely when high tidal volumes and short expiratory times are used, lead to increased intrapulmonary pressures that is transmitted to the intrathoracic vessels. Consequently, systemic venous return is reduced, right and left ventricular preloads are decreased, and right ventricular afterload is increased, causing dysfunction (32). In addition, the heart is tamponaded with impaired left ventricular relaxation, filling and contractility. These effects combine to decrease cardiac output leading to severe hypotension, myocardial ischemia and finally, cardiovascular collapse.

Temporally stopping mechanical ventilation so allowing a period of apnoea, is both diagnostic and an effective therapeutic measure (32,33). The phenomenon can occur immediately after commencement of mask ventilation in patients with emphysema. Allowing sufficient expiratory time and limiting inspiratory pressures so as to limit tidal volumes can be titrated at this early stage. Additional measures to support the circulation include optimizing patient positioning to facilitate venous return, an intravenous fluid challenge and the administration of vasoconstrictor and positive inotropes. Failure of blood pressure to normalize following an apnoeic period, and these simple support measures, should be treated as an emergency as it may indicate more severe forms of barotrauma such as tension pneumothorax.

Pulmonary hypertension

Anaesthesia for patients with end-stage primary pulmonary hypertension remains most challenging with one of the highest postoperative mortalities. Beyond the idiopathic form, most chronic respiratory disease impact on the pulmonary circulation causing pulmonary hypertension (PH), with subsequent right ventricular remodelling, hypertrophy and dysfunction. Three principal mechanisms contribute to an increased pulmonary vascular resistance (PVR). Alveolar hypoxia induces vasoconstriction of the small, precapillary pulmonary arteries. Chronic hypoxia causes remodelling of the pulmonary vasculature, with intimal and medial hypertrophy of small muscular arteries. Finally, emphysema and to a lesser degree other chronic lung disease, are associated with loss of alveolar lung tissue which may also result in reduction of pulmonary capillary beds. As most of these events progress relatively slowly over the years, the right ventricle responds with chronic adaptive compensation including hypertrophy of individual myocytes, remodeling of the myocardial extracellular matrix and adaptive metabolic alterations ultimately causing concentric hypertrophy of the right ventricle. Despite these changes and significant PH, most patient exhibit preserved right ventricular systolic function and failure is relatively rare.

Importantly, the increased PVR may have a reversible component that may be targeted by oxygen therapy and selective and broad pulmonary vasodilators. In addition, pulmonary vasoconstriction can be further exacerbated by hypercapnia and acidaemia, or by increased sympathetic activity; induction of anaesthesia may compromise a relatively stable pulmonary circulation. Therefore, the principal haemodynamic goals of the induction for lung transplantation are to prevent increases in PVR by hypoxia, excessive hypercarbia and acidosis, and to maintain systemic venous return and adequate preloading of the right and left ventricles and the systolic contractility of the right ventricle (32).

Principles of anaesthesia maintenance

One-lung ventilation

The severe degree of respiratory insufficiency in the recipient requires constant vigilance during one-lung ventilation (OLV). The respiratory goals are to provide pristine lung isolation, and ensure that there is sufficient gas exchange to prevent direct myocardial impairment and systemic haemodynamic disturbance with tissue hypoxia (34). There are wide differences in the responses of individual patients due to their underlying disease. However, the limiting factors appear respiratory acidosis in the range of a pH of 7.15–7.20 and hypoxia at an arterial oxygen tension less than 6 kPa. If these conditions exist then careful attention should be given to DLT positioning, optimization of OLV by recruitment, bronchial toilet, continuous positive airway pressure to the non-dominant lung and titrated positive end-expiratory pressure (PEEP) to the dominant lung, and ensuring that the shunt circulation is minimized. Should acidosis and hypoxia persist then mechanical support needs to be instituted prior to complete respiratory collapse.

Cariovascular monitoring and support

Constant attention to the pulmonary and systemic haemodynamics is also essential. The anesthesiologist should be able to differentiate between transient haemodynamic upset associated with hilar and mediastinal surgical manipulation that can be rapidly and easily reversed by releasing the heart or changing surgical approach, from severe upsets associated with clamping of the pulmonary artery and the slow but intolerable deterioration due to cardiorespiratory interactions during implantation and reperfusion. Again, individual tolerability is variable but controlled institution of mechanical support is preferred to prolonged haemodynamic compromise or circulatory collapse. Many anesthesiologists optimize patients with vasoactive drugs including glyceral trinitrate, nitric oxide and norepinephrine (noradrenaline) and low doses of positive inotropic support with milrinone or adrenaline (28,29). If these pharmacological measures fail and the cardiac index <2.0 L/min/m^2, mean PAP >45 mmHg, mean central venous pressure (CVP) increase >5–10 mm Hg, mean systemic arterial pressure <60 mm Hg, and/or new onset arrhythmias, then conversion to mechanical support is indicated. Information from complementary sources, including direct visualization of the heart, functional imaging by transoesophageal echocardiography (TOE), arrhythmia analysis, and haemodynamic monitoring should be integrated and communicated early and effectively to the surgical team.

Thermal management

Temperature monitoring and prevention of hypothermia by aggressive warming of the patient is mandatory as the adverse effects of hypothermia include exacerbating pulmonary hypertension, promoting arrhythmias and coagulopathy. Application of heating mattresses, lower-body forced-air heating blankets, and warming of intravenous fluids are all valuable and especially required in procedures undertaken without CPB (28).

Awareness

The risk of intraoperative awareness is greater during lung transplantation (34). Commonly used inhalation agents are isoflurane and sevoflurane, but nitrous oxide is usually avoided because of its potential to increase in PVR. Alveolar ventilation is limited in most recipients so the wash-in and diffusion of inhalation agents is compromised. Consequently, the depth of anaesthesia may be unpredictable. In addition, the uptake of inhalational agents may be limited by low cardiac output states. For these reasons, inhalational agents should be supplemented with a modest dose of an intravenous agent such as propofol.

Opioids

To facilitate early tracheal extubation, we restrict the dose of long-acting opioids for example a total dose of fentanyl of less 10 μg/kg, and generally use an intravenous infusion of a short-acting opioid such as remifentanil or alfentanil, during surgery and early postoperatively in the ICU.

Intravenous fluid therapy

Judicious administration of intravenous fluid at induction of anaesthesia is justified. However, the benefits of fluid loading should be balanced with potential detrimental effects of intravascular fluid overload on one-lung perfusion and right ventricular performance, as well as its contribution to interstitial and alveolar oedema following lung reperfusion (34). Evidence of appropriate volume loading of the left and right ventricles should be sought by TOE aiming for adequate renal perfusion but avoiding overload to limit the risk of pulmonary oedema.

Large volumes of intravenous crystalloid infusions should increase pulmonary filtration forces and colloids should reduce fluid filtration by increasing vascular oncotic pressure. However, in the face of increased permeability, the situation may be more complex with colloids contributing to interstitial oedema and reduction of gas exchange. Indeed, single-centre results indicate that increasing volume of intraoperative colloid was associated with impaired gas exchange following transplant, reduced rate of tracheal extubation and a trend for prolonging duration of stay in ICU (35).

Surgery specific anaesthetic considerations

Type of lung transplant

Depending on recipient's condition, single, bilateral lung transplantation or heart and lung transplantation may be indicated. Heart–lung transplantation is now reserved only for patients with irreversible pulmonary disease who have coexisting cardiac failure, and it is performed with decreasing frequency, as more options are now available for managing cardiac failure. Currently, the more commonly used surgical procedure is bilateral sequential lung transplant (figure 35.1), as transplantation of two lungs generally offers longer survival and better quality of life for the patient (1).

Surgical approach

Bilateral sequential lung transplants are commonly performed via a transverse thoracosternotomy popularly called a clamshell incision. For unilateral lung transplant, the recipient can be positioned in full lateral decubitus or supine positions. Generally, for bilateral sequential lung transplantation, the first lung to be transplanted is the one with least perfusion demonstrated by

ventilation perfusion scan, to provide a higher microcirculation surface area during pneumonectomy, less pulmonary hypertension during clamping of the pulmonary artery, and better cardiac performance.

Dissection and pneumonectomy

Commencement of OLV, haemodynamic optimization with management of PH and appropriate volume resuscitations are the most crucial anaesthetic tasks associated with the thoracotomy, hilar dissection, clamping of pulmonary artery and left atrium and surgical haemostasis following pneumonectomy (28,32). It is crucial that surgeon and anesthesiologist maintain close communication during this period.

By strictly monitoring respiratory efficiency and haemodynamic stability, the team has to decide if it is safe to continue without the use of mechanical circulatory support. All measures to optimize OLV should be employed with gas exchange frequently evaluated and all vasoactive support should be in place to reduce PVR and support RV function. The authors regularly commence inhaled NO to provide maximum pulmonary vasodilation in anticipation of PA clamping. A trial PA clamping is routinely performed and stability is assessed by multimodal diagnostic efforts for 5–10 minutes.

Dissection and haemostasis may be prolonged in patients who have extensive pleural adhesions, especially in those who had previous pleurodesis, and significant blood loss may rapidly occur. Differentiation between surgical manipulation, retraction of the heart and hypovolaemia as the cause of hypotension, is essential.

Implantation, deairing and reperfusion

Once the bronchial anastomosis is completed, the anaesthetist should evaluate it by fiberoptic bronchoscopy. Careful bronchial toilet may also be performed, depending on the size of DLT and bronchoscope. During completion of the vascular anastomoses the anaesthetist should be preparing for de-airing and the busy period of reperfusion.

After completion of the atrial anastomoses, the implanted allograft should be gently inflated. TOE is useful to monitor efficacy of deairing at the level of the pulmonary veins, left atrium, and ventricle. TOE examination of ventricular function especially in the right coronary territory, is also important as air may preferentially go down the right coronary artery producing acute myocardial ischemia (28).

Myocardial stunning may occur during reperfusion when the pulmoplegia used for lung preservation washes into the left heart (32). As this solution is cold, acellular, enriched with ischaemic metabolites and supplemented by vasodilators, acute myocardial dysfunction, hypotension, and arrhythmias are frequent at this time. Careful clinical integration of TOE and ECG findings with direct visualization of the heart, is important to correctly diagnose the cause of haemodynamic derangement. Small intravenous boluses of calcium, metaraminol, or epinephrine (adrenaline) usually suffice to restore cardiovascular stability.

Ventilation should improve dramatically as the compliant implanted lung is inflated. However, gas exchange and haemodynamics may also be compromised depending on the PVR of the allograft, the degree of shunt circulation and mismatch of ventilation and perfusion. Sustained elevation of PAP after removal of the pulmonary artery clamp may indicate severe vasoconstriction of the vascular bed of the allograft that may impede perfusion and increase shunt. Differential ventilation may be useful to deliver pulmonary vasodilators to the allograft only and to enable ventilation of the lungs selectively with different FiO_2. One needs to balance potential oxygen toxicity to the allograft with influence of oxygen on pulmonary vasomotor tone and ultimately to provide an acceptable systemic oxygen delivery.

Implantation of the second lung

With bilateral procedures, the implantation of the second lung repeats the sequence of the first one in the contralateral pleural space and the challenges are similar. OLV should be less problematic but there could be severe shunting prior to clamping the PA. In left transplants, the heart needs to be manipulated with consequent haemodynamic compromise. Clamping of the PA may be less or better tolerated depending on the PVR of the first implanted lung. Care must be exercised on pulmonary flow and hydrostatic pressures imposed on the first transplanted lung (figure 35.6). Reduced compliance, progressively worsening gas exchange and requirement for an increased FiO_2 may indicate severe graft dysfunction, which may necessitate converting the procedure to CPB or ECMO.

Minimally invasive lung transplantation

Motivated by reducing the invasiveness of the clamshell incision, there has been a move to using sternum-sparing sequential anterolateral or posterolateral thoracotomies with videoscopic assist (36–38). These incisions achieve better cosmetic results and postoperative wound healing. This surgical approach means that the heart is not directly visible so continuous TOE evaluation of heart function is essential. In addition, surgical manipulations of the hilum and heart are more pronounced requiring the anaesthesiologist to be vigilant and in constant communication with surgeon. Finally, vascular anastomoses need to be secured prior to inflation of lung and there is higher risk for shunt circulation, hypoxia and catastrophic blood loss.

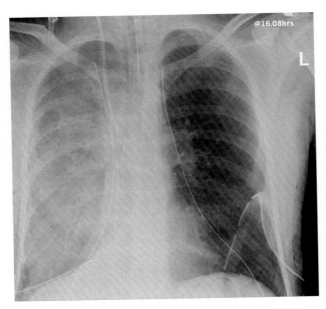

Fig. 35.6 Chest radiograph showing severe selective lung injury in the first implanted lung following bilateral sequential lung transplantation.

Conclusion of surgery

At the end of surgery, the anaesthetist should decide either to resume spontaneous ventilation and extubate the patient's trachea on the table or continue sedation and mechanical ventilation in the ICU. In the latter, the DLT should be changed to single-lumen tracheal tube. Flexible bronchoscopy is performed to examine airway anastomosis, to aspirate blood and secretions, and to evaluate for pulmonary oedema. A nasogastric tube should be inserted but not aspirated so as to retain the cyclosporin that was administered preoperatively. In difficult cases, especially in single lung transplantation for emphysema where there is haemodynamic instability secondary to air trapping in remaining emphysematous lung, differential lung ventilation via DLT should be considered.

Intensive care management

Strategies for lung ventilation and perfusion

Pulmonary recovery is facilitated by measures that reduce graft dysfunction. Measures include lung protective mechanical ventilation and perfusion strategies and prevention of postoperative bacterial and fungal infections and acute rejections (34). The lungs remain prone to develop pulmonary oedema because of delayed reperfusion injury, or pulmonary hyperperfusion. Optimizing haemodynamics, aiming at a low CVP and left ventricular end-diastolic pressure and keeping the lungs reasonably dry, are all important management goals (28). PiCCO® monitoring of extravascular lung water together with global haemodynamic indices may prove helpful to achieve these goals. Hyperoxia should be avoided and FiO_2 should be kept as low as compatible with pulse oximetry reading of more than 90%. As most patients have a degree of ALI, protective ventilation with low tidal volumes, appropriate levels of PEEP and avoidance of high inflation pressures, is indicated.

Haemorrhage

Postoperative bleeding can be significant and the need for early surgical re-exploration is common. Multimodal assessment of coagulation is essential and correction of any coagulopathy with judicious use of factor concentrates rather than large volumes of blood products, is preferred.

Lower respiratory tract infection

Prevention and aggressive treatment of lower respiratory tract infection is a vital component of the postoperative care. Denervation of the lungs and associated absent sensation of retained secretions within the transplanted lungs result in a high risk for lung infection so vigorous chest physiotherapy and postural drainage should be routinely performed. In addition, the donor and recipient could have been colonized or infected with a spectrum of microbes and broad-spectrum antibiotic cover, and specific antimicrobial treatment taking sensitivities into consideration, are essential.

Analgesia

Effective pain control is paramount to facilitate early tracheal extubation and to optimize pulmonary rehabilitation and for these reasons, most institutions utilize thoracic epidural analgesia (29,34). If blood loss was minimal and after ensuring blood clotting is normal, the epidural catheter may be inserted in the operating room after lung implantation. Alternatively, it may be done early postoperatively in the ICU prior to weaning from mechanical ventilation.

Conclusion

The anaesthetic management of patients undergoing lung transplantation is challenging because of underlying condition of the patients, the major degree of surgical trespass and the risk of complications. However, with a sound knowledge of the pathophysiology of lung failure, the potential complications of lung transplantation and sound communication with the surgeon, a good outcome can be achieved for the patient.

References

1. Yusen RD, Christie JD, Edwards LB, et al, International Society for Heart and Lung Transplantation. The Registry of the International Society for Heart and Lung Transplantation: thirtieth adult lung and heart-lung transplant report–2013; focus theme: age. *J Heart Lung Transplant* 2013; **32**: 965–78

2. Christie JD, Carby M, Bag R, Corris P, Hertz M, Weill D, ISHLT Working Group on Primary Lung Graft Dysfunction. Report of the ISHLT Working Group on Primary Lung Graft Dysfunction part II: definition. A consensus statement of the International Society for Heart and Lung Transplantation. *J Heart Lung Transplant* 2005; **24**: 1454–59

3. Shah RJ, Bellamy SL, Localio AR, et al. A panel of lung injury biomarkers enhances the definition of primary graft dysfunction (PGD) after lung transplantation. *J Heart Lung Transplant* 2012; **31**: 942–9

4. Suzuki Y, Cantu E, Christie JD. Primary graft dysfunction. *Semin Respir Crit Care Med* 2013; **34**: 305–19

5. Ray M, Dharmarajan S, Freudenberg J, Zhang W, Patterson GA. Expression profiling of human donor lungs to understand primary graft dysfunction after lung transplantation. *Am J Transplant* 2007; **7**: 2396–405

6. Fischer S, Cassivi SD, Xavier AM, et al. Cell death in human lung transplantation: apoptosis induction in human lungs during ischemia and after transplantation. *Ann Surg* 2000; **231**: 424–31

7. Diamond JM, Lee JC, Kawut SM, et al, Lung Transplant Outcomes Group. Clinical risk factors for primary graft dysfunction after lung transplantation. *Am J Respir Crit Care Med* 2013; **187**: 527–34

8. Christie JD, Edwards LB, Kucheryavaya AY, et al, International Society of Heart and Lung Transplantation. The Registry of the International Society for Heart and Lung Transplantation: 29th adult lung and heart-lung transplant report-2012. *J Heart Lung Transplant* 2012; **31**: 1073–86

9. Oto T, Levvey BJ, Whitford H, et al. Feasibility and utility of a lung donor score: correlation with early post-transplant outcomes. *Ann Thorac Surg* 2007; **83**: 257–63

10. Bonser RS, Taylor R, Collett D, Thomas HL, Dark JH, Neuberger J, Cardiothoracic Advisory Group to NHS Blood and Transplant and the Association of Lung Transplant Physicians (UK). Effect of donor smoking on survival after lung transplantation: a cohort study of a prospective registry. *Lancet* 2012; **380**: 747–55

11. Korovesi I, Papadomichelakis E, Orfanos SE, et al. Exhaled breath condensate in mechanically ventilated brain-injured patients with no lung injury or sepsis. *Anesthesiology* 2011; **114**: 1118–29

12. Mascia L, Pasero D, Slutsky AS, et al. Effect of a lung protective strategy for organ donors on eligibility and availability of lungs for transplantation: a randomized controlled trial. *JAMA* 2010; **304**: 2620–7

13. Fisher AJ, Donnelly SC, Hirani N, et al. Elevated levels of interleukin-8 in donor lungs is associated with early graft failure after lung transplantation. *Am J Respir Crit Care Med* 2001; **163**: 259–65

14. Avlonitis VS, Wigfield CH, Golledge HD, Kirby JA, Dark JH. Early hemodynamic injury during donor brain death determines the severity of primary graft dysfunction after lung transplantation. *Am J Transplant* 2007; **7**: 83–90

15. Ware LB, Wang Y, Fang X, et al. Assessment of lungs rejected for transplantation and implications for donor selection. *Lancet.* 2002; **360**: 619–20

16. Dark JH. Lung transplantation from the non-heart beating donor. *Transplantation* 2008; **86**: 200–1

17. Minambres E, Coll E, Duerto J, et al. Effect of an intensive lung donor-management protocol on lung transplantation outcomes. *J Heart Lung Transplant* 2014; **33**: 178–84

18. Munshi L, Keshavjee S, Cypel M. Donor management and lung preservation for lung transplantation. *Lancet Respir Med* 2013; **1**: 318–28

19. Snell GI, Westall GP, Oto T. Donor risk prediction: how 'extended' is safe? *Curr Opin Organ Transplant* 2013 Aug 29. [Epub ahead of print];

20. Cypel M, Yeung JC, Hirayama S, et al. Technique for prolonged normothermic ex vivo lung perfusion. *J Heart Lung Transplant* 2008; **27**: 1319–25

21. Ingemansson R, Eyjolfsson A, Mared L, et al. Clinical transplantation of initially rejected donor lungs after reconditioning ex vivo. *Ann Thorac Surg* 2009; **87**: 255–60

22. Cypel M, Yeung JC, Liu M, et al. Normothermic ex vivo lung perfusion in clinical lung transplantation. *N Engl J Med* 2011; **364**: 1431–40

23. Zych B, Popov AF, Stavri G, et al. Early outcomes of bilateral sequential single lung transplantation after ex-vivo lung evaluation and reconditioning. *J Heart Lung Transplant* 2012; **31**: 274–81

24. Wallinder A, Ricksten SE, Hansson C, et al. Transplantation of initially rejected donor lungs after ex vivo lung perfusion. *J Thorac Cardiovasc Surg* 2012; **144**: 1222–8

25. Aigner C, Slama A, Hotzenecker K, et al. Clinical ex vivo lung perfusion—pushing the limits. *Am J Transplant* 2012; **12**: 1839–47

26. Warnecke G, Moradiellos J, Tudorache I, et al. Normothermic perfusion of donor lungs for preservation and assessment with the Organ Care System Lung before bilateral transplantation: a pilot study of 12 patients. *Lancet* 2012; **380**: 1851–8

27. Methangkool E, Mahajan A, Gao G, Chua JH. Anesthetic management of bilateral lung transplantation from donor lungs managed by the organ care system. *J Cardiothorac Vasc Anesth* 2013; Oct 16. **pii**: S1053-0770(13)00308-X. doi: 10.1053/j.jvca.2013.05.033. [Epub ahead of print].

28. Haddy SM, Bremner RM. Update on anesthesia for lung transplantation. *Semin Anesth Perioperative Med Pain* 2004; **23**(1): : 34–41

29. Rosenberg AL, Rao M, Benedict PE. Anesthetic implications for lung transplantation. *Anesthesiol Clin N Am* 2004; **22**: 767–88

30. Myles PS. Lessons from lung transplantation for everyday thoracic anesthesia. *Anesthesiol Clin N Am* 2001; **19**: 581–90, vii

31. Myles PS, Ryder IG, Weeks AM, Williams T, Esmore DS. Case 1-1997. Diagnosis and management of dynamic hyperinflation during lung transplantation. *J Cardiothorac Vasc Anesth* 1997; **11**: 100–4

32. Slinger P. Anaesthetic management for lung transplantation. *Tx Med* 2012; **24**: 27–34

33. Myles PS, Weeks AM, Buckland MR, Silvers A, Bujor M, Langley M. Anesthesia for bilateral sequential lung transplantation: experience of 64 cases. *J Cardiothorac Vasc Anesth* 1997; **11**: 177–83

34. Myles PS, Snell GI, Westall GP. Lung transplantation. *Curr Opin Anaesthesiol* 2007; **20**: 21–26.

35. McIlroy DR, Pilcher DV, Snell GI. Does anaesthetic management affect early outcomes after lung transplant? An exploratory analysis. *Br J Anaesth* 2009; **102**: 506–14

36. Bittner HB, Lehmann S, Binner C, Garbade J, Barten M, Mohr FW. Sternum sparing thoracotomy incisions in lung transplantation surgery: a superior technique to the clamshell approach. *Innovations (Phila).* 2011; **6**: 116–21

37. Taghavi S, Birsan T, Pereszlenyi A, et al. Bilateral lung transplantation via two sequential anterolateral thoracotomies. *Eur J Cardiothorac Surg* 1999; **15**: 658–62

38. Fischer S, Struber M, Simon AR, et al. Video-assisted minimally invasive approach in clinical bilateral lung transplantation. *J Thorac Cardiovasc Surg* 2001; **122**: 1196–8

CHAPTER 36

Postoperative thoracic surgical care

Mert Şentürk

Introduction

Among the subspecialities of anaesthesia, thoracic anaesthesia is a prime example where the term perioperative medicine better defines the responsibilities of the anaesthetist. Generally, and especially in Europe, the postoperative care of thoracic surgical patients is under the control of anaesthesiologists either exclusively or as part of a multidisciplinary team with thoracic surgeons and pneumologists. This chapter aims to review the care of patients following thoracic surgery. Complications of, and analgesia for, thoracic surgery, are discussed in Chapters 37 and 38.

Location of postoperative care

Despite improvements in surgery, anaesthesia, and intensive care, thoracic surgery is still associated with a high incidence of postoperative complications, which is most likely because of the ever widening indications for surgery. Patients undergoing thoracic surgery often have several concurrent pulmonary (e.g. emphysema), general (e.g. diabetes mellitus), or cardiovascular (e.g. coronary disease or hypertension) diseases, which can contribute to postoperative complications. Almost all of these comorbidities are associated with impaired postoperative respiratory function and tissue oxygenation. A loss of lung tissue frequently accompanies and worsens, this impairment. Therefore, after thoracotomies, the incidence of pulmonary complications can exceed the cardiovascular ones (e.g. 14.7% versus 11.8%), which is unlike after other types of surgery (1).

Intensive versus postanaesthetic care unit

In the past, patients after thoracotomy were almost routinely sent to an intensive care unit (ICU). However, the increasing quality of the postanaesthetic care unit (PACU) has ensured a cost-effective and reliable alternative for postoperative admission. Unfortunately, there are still no established criteria for deciding whether patients should be managed in ICU or PACU following thoracic surgery. Moreover, whilst elective transfer to the ICU is associated with a reduction in the total morbidity and incidences of complications, it does not change the mortality (7.3% versus 7.3%). However, elective transfer to the ICU is associated with a longer duration of hospital stay (2). Therefore, a standardized preoperative way of predicting whether a patient should be sent to the ICU or the PACU would help to obtain a more effective organization of patient care. Scoring systems and definitions of risk factors have

been reported in different studies and reviews (3). The difference between modifiable and non-modifiable factors is the most clinically relevant information as preoperative interventions on the modifiable factors may decrease the need for treatment in ICU (4).

Risk factors influencing postoperative care

Age

An age of 70 years or older, and in some research 65 years or older, is a non-modifiable risk factor. Decreases in functional residual capacity (FRC) and closing capacity with age impair the lung function (Chapter 4) and there is an increased mortality in older compared to younger patients undergoing the same operation (5).

Pre-existing lung disease

Fibrotic lung disease, in particular, should be an indication for ICU admission (6). The use of preoperative pulmonary rehabilitation programmes, medical and physical therapy, and the cessation of smoking can all improve patient health. However, as such programmes do not eliminate the risk of patients requiring ICU admission, pre-existing lung disease is unmodifiable risk factor. Estimating the predicted postoperative (PPO) pulmonary function and in particular, the PPO forced expiratory volume in the first second ($PPOFEV_1$) can be useful (Chapter 3). Estimating the PPO for carbon monoxide diffusion can also be done but the specificity and sensitivity of this test for predicting the postoperative status is unproven (7). A $PPOFEV_1$ of <40% is associated with major complications, and a $PPOFEV_1$ <30% indicates a likely requirement for postoperative mechanical ventilatory support.

Smoking history

Smoking is a modifiable factor, but smoking cessation less than two months before surgery is not associated with a reduced, and may even be associated with an increased, incidence of perioperative pulmonary complications (8). Pragmatically, a smoking cessation programme of more than 2 months is rarely possible, as postponing surgery to treat lung cancer to implement smoking cessation would be irrational. However, cessation of smoking even 24–72 hours before surgery may be helpful to facilitate the removal of bronchial secretions.

Comorbidity

Some comorbidities are modifiable. A number of cardiovascular diseases, such as hypertension, can be controlled, even if not treated in the short preoperative time. In some cases, the cardiovascular disease, not the operation, may be the indication for ICU admission. Cardiovascular and pulmonary complications are closely related as if one type of complication occurs then this can facilitate the development of the other.

Patients receiving neoadjuvant chemotherapy during the preoperative period are more prone to postoperative complications.

Obesity can be managed with an intensive weight loss programme. Similarly, diabetes mellitus can, and should, be controlled before operation. The physical status of the patient can be changed using rehabilitation programmes, light exercises, and, sometimes, medications. Generally, American Society of Anesthesiologists grades of III or higher should be considered as a reason for elective ICU admission.

Preoperative organisation of the ICU admission benefits patient health, and hospital economics. High-volume centres can successfully predict the patient's postoperative status. However, even in such institutions, a high number of patients unexpectedly become candidates for ICU admission because of intraoperative reasons for example prolonged durations of surgery or one-lung ventilation (OLV), excessive blood loss, and air leak, or postoperative reasons such as respiratory insufficiency, air leak, or atelectasis.

Management of chest tubes

Chest tubes placement is generally mandatory in all the operations with opening of the thoracic cavity. Therefore, the physician should know how to manage drainage of the thorax including diagnosis and treatment of its complications. Chest tubes allow drainage of air (ventral or cranial placement) and/or fluid (dorsal or caudal placement). Thus, the physician's goal is to monitor, prevent, or treat air leaks and excessive pleural drainage (9). A clinician dealing with a patient who has undergone a thoracotomy, should be familiar with the classical three-bottle chest tube drainage system (figure 36.1), which is now commercially available in compact systems. The air from the pleura can be aspirated passively with a water seal or actively by attaching a piped source of vacuum. There are controversial reports regarding the effects of passive and active (or alternating) suction (10,11). A balanced chest drainage system may be the most rational strategy to maintain the mediastinum in a neutral position. In any event, if active aspiration is used then the negative pressure should not exceed 15–20 cmH$_2$O. After pneumonectomy, negative pressure should not be applied to chest tubes because of the risk of causing mediastinal shift and they should never be clamped as for example during patient transport, because of the risk of tension pneumothorax.

The volume of blood draining from chest tubes is important, especially immediately postoperatively. Excessive blood drainage should signal an emergency alarm to recall the surgeons. In later phases, chest tubes are commonly left in situ when drainage is more than 250 mL per day. However, this unproven measure was refuted in a recent study which found that the chest tubes may be removed if the drainage is less than 450 mL per day, as long as there is no air leak and the drainage fluid does not contain cerebrospinal fluid, chyle, or blood (12). Chest X-rays and chest tubes status should be evaluated simultaneously and any discrepancy between them may indicate failing thorax drainage because of tube blockage from kinking or clot, or suction failure.

Monitoring

If the patient is managed in a PACU then no additional monitoring to that used in the operating room is necessary. However, if the patient is transferred to the ICU some additional monitoring might be necessary. Monitoring of fluid balance is mandatory, especially in those patients at risk of acute lung injury (ALI). In recent years, pulmonary artery catheters have been almost entirely replaced by less invasive devices. Among them,

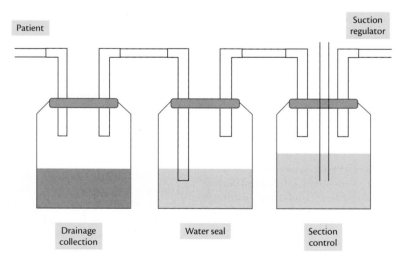

Fig. 36.1 Three-bottle chest drainage system.
Using the first (drainage collection) bottle only would cause an increased resistance to drainage as a result of rising fluid/blood level and/or the foamy mixture of blood and air in the bottle. Adding a second bottle (water seal) allows fluid to drain into the first bottle only and the air into the second, also preventing the foam from forming. However, the added length of the tubing can increase the dead space and add further resistance, causing a reversal of flow back up into the tube and back into the pleural space. Therefore, a third bottle (suction control) allows for active suction to be exerted on the system, preventing the chest tube effluent from going back toward the patient.

the single-indicator thermal dilution method (Pulsion®, Munich, Germany) that can assess the extravascular lung water index and monitor cardiac output using pulse contour analysis of the arterial pressure has been shown to be effective (13,14). Alternative tools use a lithium dilution technique (LiDCO®, LiDCO Ltd, London, UK), or no-calibration methods (FloTrac®, Edwards LifeSciences, Irvine, CA). Pulse-pressure variation analysis can predict the responsiveness to intravenous fluids (15). A recently developed method, called the 'pleth variability index' (Masimo®; Masimo Corporation, Irvine, CA), non-invasively provides information about the volume status using the variations in pulse oximetry (16). Non-invasive or semi-invasive devices to monitor haemoglobin levels (Masimo®), can also be useful in post-thoracotomy patients (17).

Fluid management

Since Zeldin's first definition of 'post-pneumonectomy pulmonary oedema' (PPPO), a series of studies have found fluid overload in the perioperative period to be associated with postoperative respiratory failure and it is considered as one of the probable reasons for PPPO (18). Support for this idea comes from a retrospective study which found that a greater amount of administered intraoperative fluids was a significant predictive factor in patients who develop postoperative respiratory failure (19). Moreover, the lungs have a unique lymphatic drainage system. Lymphatic drainage of the left lung is located on the right, which may explain why PPPO occurs more often after right than left, pneumonectomy. Also, the lungs do not have a third space. Finally, hypotension during and after thoracotomy is rarely caused by hypovolaemia and is more often the result of vasodilation for example from thoracic epidural anaesthesia. Therefore, it is strongly recommended to restrict fluid input both during and after thoracotomies. Slinger and associates have suggested not only to limit the intraoperative period to less than 2 L, but also to limit the whole operation day to less than 3 L (18). A low dose of catecholamines is often more appropriate than administering a large amount of intravenous fluids to treat hypotension.

There are reasons to question that fluid overload is the root cause of PPPO. First, the oedema fluid that occurs in PPPO is an exudate and the onset of the condition is often late after surgery. In addition, PPPO may occur in patients with low central venous pressures. Finally, PPPO can be observed also in patients treated with a restrictive fluid policy. Although the evidence for fluid restriction preventing hypovolaemia is weaker than its reputation, this approach appears to be rational (20). As happens in adult respiratory distress syndrome (ARDS) and ventilator-associated ALI, administering high volumes of intravenous fluids is not the only cause. However, administering excessive intravenous fluids may be a element to worsening symptoms of PPPO (21).

The choice of intravenous fluids used is also controversial. There are no randomized controlled trials (RCTs) in patients undergoing thoracotomy that demonstrate that crystalloids or colloids are any more or less harmful for the post-thoracotomy patient. Fresh frozen plasma, red cell concentrate, and albumin have all been indicated in the pathogenesis of PPPO and a rational strategy or an optimal ratio of different types of intravenous fluids is yet to be determined.

Ventilatory support for the patients after thoracic surgery

Almost all the complications after thoracic surgery result in respiratory failure (figure 36.2). An effective analgesia protocol and adequate physiotherapy help to prevent and treat respiratory failure. However, some patients will require ventilatory support following thoracotomy.

Not only do surgeons remove large parts of the lungs, they often traumatically manipulate some of the remaining healthy lung tissue and damage the respiratory muscles. Also, a thoracotomy is one of the most painful operations which can further impair ventilation. OLV may also cause lung injury (22). In addition, excessive intravenous fluid infusion and blood transfusion can directly harm or exacerbate harm to the lungs. Therefore, even patients who are in good physical status and have no perioperative complications may experience:

- a reduced lung volume because of resection of parenchyma, atelectasis, lung oedema, and thorax restriction from pain
- impaired ventilation because of decreased functional residual and volume capacities, dysfunction of the diaphragm and intercostal muscles, and increased airways resistance
- impaired gas exchange because of ventilation–perfusion mismatch and decreased minute ventilation (23).

Invasive ventilation

Mechanical ventilation in the PACU or ICU should be continued postoperatively only if absolutely necessary, for it can cause a ventilatory-associated or ventilatory-induced lung inury (VALI

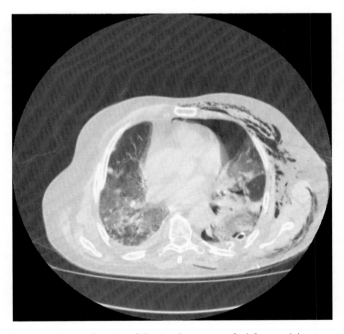

Fig. 36.2 CT scan of a patient following thoracotomy for left upper lobectomy who subsequently developed adult respiratory distress syndrome: There is space where the lung tissue was resected, atelectatic areas in the remaining lung tissue, infiltrations in both lungs without any clinical signs of infection and subcutaneous emphysema. CT scan of a patient who developed adult respiratory distress syndrome after thoracotomy.

or VILI) (24). The possibility of such injuries is higher in patients who have undergone a thoracotomy because the traumatized lungs are more vulnerable to damage. In addition, and although not evidence based, clinical experience would suggest that positive pressure ventilation can injure fresh anastomoses or bronchial stump.

Elective postoperative mechanical ventilation

There are some pragmatic rules that should be followed when deciding to continue mechanical ventilation after thoracotomy. The decision to ventilate should be made intraoperatively, and preoperative predictions should be re-evaluated. If mechanical ventilation needs to be continued, the double lumen tube (DLT) should be replaced with a normal single-lumen tracheal tube at the end of surgery. However, in patients who will be extubated within two hours postoperatively, the DLT may remain although the cuff on the bronchial lumen should be deflated. If a Univent® (LMA North America Inc, San Diego, CA) tube was used then the tube can remain but the blocker should be pulled back into the main lumen. As a rule, spontaneous is better than mechanical ventilation, and assisted is better than controlled ventilation. However, the need for tracheal re-intubation can be the worst case scenario. Finally, weaning from mechanical ventilation is a process that should start on admission of a mechanically ventilated patient to ICU.

Protective lung ventilation

Protective lung ventilation (PLV) becomes even more important in the vulnerable lungs of patients after thoracic surgery. PLV includes using low tidal volumes (TVs) of less than 7 mL/kg, airway pressures less than 30 cmH$_2$O, an appropriate positive end-expiratory pressure (PEEP) and recruitment manoeuvres (RM). Meta-analyses of RCTs have found PLV in a general ICU setting to be effective and protective both in ARDS in the ICU and in OLV (25–27). An intraoperative TV of 6–8 mL/kg has been associated with a decreased frequency of postoperative pulmonary failure (19). Although there is no evidence that the same argument is also valid for the postoperative period, there is clear evidence for using these guidelines in general ICU patients. Moreover, there is already a reduction of functional lung tissue that is similar to the 'baby lung' of the ARDS (22). In this regard, it can also be questionable whether even TV as low as 6 mL/kg is protective enough.

Permissive hypercapnia

Reductions in TV can often be compensated by an increase in frequency to maintain the minute volume. However, the price of shorter inspiration can be high airway pressures, and the price of shorter expiration can be air-trapping and auto-PEEP. More importantly, mild hypercapnia can be permitted in many cases (28) and can even be therapeutic for several hours (29). Permissive hypercapnia may protect the lung and improve the tissue oxygenation as a result of the increased cardiac output and right-shift of the oxygen saturation curve (30). However, because it exacerbates hypoxic pulmonary vasoconstriction, permissive hypercapnia is contraindicated in pulmonary hypertension, which is more frequent in patients after pulmonary resection. In the remaining population, permissive hypercapnia can be considered as a standard part of protective lung ventilation.

Inspired oxygen

The inspiratory fraction of O$_2$ (FiO$_2$) also plays an important role both for patients who are mechanically ventilated and breathing spontaneously. Increased O$_2$ consumption in postoperative patients has led to a routine administration of supplemental O$_2$. However, a recent report has highlighted that this approach could be more harmful than beneficial (31). Although it has not been studied in this setting, the mechanism of the damage from high FiO$_2$ is also valid for patients after thoracic surgery. Hyperoxia causes both coronary and systemic vasoconstriction and results in a decreased stroke volume. Postoperative patients should not be hypoxaemic, but hypoxaemia should be treated with stepwise increases in FiO$_2$, and so hyperoxia should be avoided (31).

Hyperoxia from a high FiO$_2$ is unwarranted in mechanically ventilated patients as even a short period of preoxygenation with a FiO$_2$ of 100% can cause serious atelectasis as a result of collapsed alveoli because of the decreased ratio/absence of nitrogen. However, hyperoxia may help in preventing and treating surgical site infections (32,33), although this potential benefit has not been confirmed in recent larger studies (34).

Ventilation mode

Some studies have shown the benefits of pressure-controlled ventilation in both ALI/ARDS (35) and in OLV (36). However, more recent studies have refuted these findings in both groups of patients (37,38). The most appropriate approach is to avoid high ventilatory pressures especially plateau pressure. Limiting the peak inspiratory pressure in any ventilatory mode to 35, or even to 30 cmH$_2$O, will help prevent lung injury.

Positive end expiratory pressure and recruitment manoeuvres

PEEP has been considered as a questionable treatment for hypoxia during OLV as it may worsen the oxygenation during OLV by diverting pulmonary blood flow to less ventilated regions. However, several studies have showed that PEEP improves the oxygenation (39) and—more importantly—prevents cyclic closing–reopening of the alveoli during ventilation (40,41). In addition, it allows the decrease of FiO$_2$ without compromising the oxygenation. So PEEP should be considered as an important part of protective lung ventilation. However, whilst it can keep the lung open, PEEP is not capable of opening an atelectatic lung. To open collapsed regions, a RM is necessary (42). However, after opening the lung with RM, PEEP is required to prevent re-collapse of the lung. Therefore, both PEEP and RM are obligatory components of the protective lung ventilation. Unfortunately, there are no studies examining the effects of RM in patients who have had a thoracotomy and RM is contraindicated in patients with air leakage. Moreover, the high pressure generated by RM and PEEP may disrupt bronchial stumps and anastomoses so, if used, then they have to be applied with caution.

Differential lung ventilation

Differential lung ventilation (DLV) may be considered as the ICU variation of OLV. Two essential indications of DLV related to thoracic surgery are unilateral lung processes and air leaks (43). The objective is to ventilate both lungs—synchronized or not—with different TVs and/or PEEPs. This method can be used also successfully in bilateral ARDS in the lateral decubitus position (44), but it has only been applied to unilateral processes. Two coupled ventilators ('master' and 'slave') with synchronized inspiration

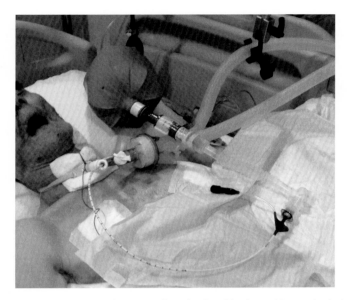

Fig. 36.3 In a patient with persistent bronchopleural fistula requiring mechanical ventilation, the lung (or the lobe) with the fistula can be blocked with a bronchial blocker. The remaining lung can be mechanically ventilated and in the blocked part lung, a low level of continuous positive airway pressure can be applied to prevent a full collapse without exhacerbating a fistula.

and expiration can be used. Two ventilators can also be used in an asynchronized manner but this may cause a mediastinal shift. An easier solution is to ventilate one lung (the 'healthy' one) with the conventional setting, while continuous positive airway pressure (CPAP) or high frequency ventilation (HFV) can be applied to the 'sick' lung (figure 36.3). DLV can protect the healthy lung against the pathological processes of the other lung, including massive unilateral haemoptysis, bronchiectasis, and lung abscesses. In addition, DLV may promote healing in the sick lung, as for example with an air leak or a bronchopleural fistula, whilst compromising less severely oxygenation and gas exchange.

High-frequency ventilation

DLV can be applied with all possible methods of OLV. However the long-term use of these techniques is limited because of the obligatory muscle relaxation required and risk of displacement of the double-lumen tube. Ventilation without high airway pressures can be achieved using HFV. HFV can be varied by adjusting its frequency or pressure, and it can be applied alone or in combination with other methods, such as DLV. A relatively new variant is high frequency percussive ventilation that improves oxygenation, helps to remove produced bronchial secretions, decreases the incidence of pneumonia and reduces the duration of the hospital stay (45).

Non-invasive ventilation

Non-invasive ventilation (NIV) is defined as a partial or complete support of the ventilation without tracheal intubation. Partial NIV involves applying CPAP usually with a tight fitting mask in a spontaneously breathing patient. In complete NIV, full ventilatory support with positive pressure ventilation and PEEP is used. NIV devices also come as nose masks, mouth-nose masks, full-face masks, and helmets. In all these devices even if the device fits well, a leak of the inspired volume is common. However,

many mechanical ventilators can compensate for this leakage by increasing the inspiratory flow. In a hypoxic patient during the immediate postoperative period, CPAP is more logical to use than a high FiO_2 to achieve open alveoli.

The benefits of NIV have been reported mostly in patients who have chronic obstructive pulmonary disease (46). In patients with hypoxic ventilatory failure a NIV is controversial as there is no evidence that it decreases the incidence of pneumonia or the duration of the hospital stay (47). However, several studies have shown the prophylactic and therapeutic beneficial effects of NIV after thoracic surgery (48). NIV is associated with increases in oxygenation and gas exchange, a decrease in the work of breathing that can be of great importance in patients after thoracotomy, and a better management of air leaks (49). Thus, NIV is an alternative for weaning, tracheal reintubation, and for ICU transfer (50). However, during the first hours of its application, continuous visual inspection of ventilation should be undertaken.

NIV should only be applied in cooperative patients who have a pH more than 7.1 and an arterial carbon dioxide tension ($PaCO_2$) of less than 90 mmHg. The contraindications to NIV are shown in box 36.1 (51). If no improvement in oxygenation is observed after 10–15 minutes after initiation of NIV, tracheal intubation and mechanical ventilation should be considered.

Weaning

Weaning from mechanical ventilation should be performed as quickly as possible, but not so fast as to be unsuccessful. Tracheal extubation should be uncomplicated after obtaining normothermia, co-operation, sufficient coughing, reliable spontaneous breathing, and acceptable levels of pH, $PaCO_2$ and arterial oxygen tension. These criteria are also valid for the tracheal extubation of patients who have been intubated and mechanically ventilated for a longer duration.

One of the key points of a successful weaning is to follow a well-defined protocol (52). The weaning protocols should clearly define patients in whom weaning should be tried, the methods and strategies of weaning, and what is successful weaning (figure 36.4).

In 2001, an evidence-based guideline was published for weaning from ventilatory support (53). In every patient who is mechanically

---

Box 36.1 Contraindications to non-invasive ventilation

- Cardiac or respiratory arrest
- Unable to fit mask
- Non-respiratory organ failure
  Severe encephalopathy with a Glasgow coma scale <10
  Severe upper gastrointestinal bleeding
  Haemodynamic instability or unstable cardiac arrhythmia
- Facial surgery, trauma or deformity
- Upper airway obstruction
- Inability to cooperate and/or protect the airways
- Inability to clear the secretions
- High risk of aspiration

Reprinted from *The Lancet*, 374, 9685, Nava S and Hill N, 'Non-invasive ventilation in acute respiratory failure', pp. 250–259, Copyright 2009, with permission from Elsevier

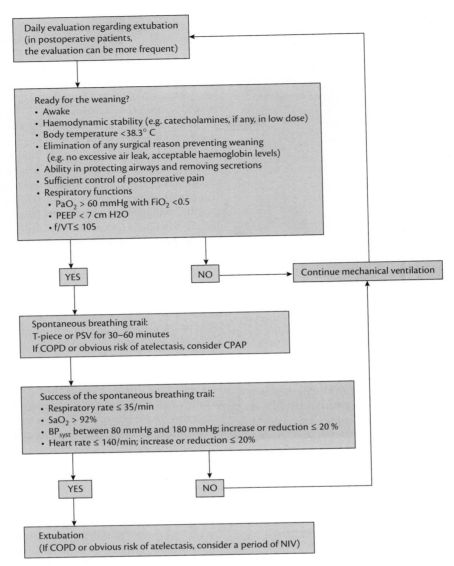

Fig. 36.4 Weaning protocol.
A weaning-protocol for patients with delayed tracheal extubation following surgery including thoracotomy, which is used in the Istanbul Medical Faculty. Note that protocols can differ between centres, but an institutional protocol should exist and be followed.

ventilated more than 24 hr, daily trials of spontaneous breathing should be performed otherwise more than half of the patients will go unrecognized. If patient fails a trial then the underlying reason for the failure should be sought and treated leading back to the protocol of consideration for weaning. There should be a protocol to rationalize and standardize the weaning process that directs a step-down from controlled to supported ventilation or from invasive ventilation to NIV. Similarly, a trial using a T-piece may also be performed. Applying all aspects of a documented algorithm can prevent unpredicted drawbacks such as oversedation, during a trial (54). In every patient, the success of the weaning should also be assessed using a protocol similar to trial of spontaneous ventilation (box 36.2) (52).

Tracheostomy
Prolonged mechanical ventilation of more than 7 days along with unsuccessful weaning trials is associated with additional problems.

In these cases, tracheostomy should be considered. Even when prolonged mechanical ventilation is predicted early in treatment, a tracheostomy may be valuable as the need for sedation is reduced, it eases mobilization and facilitates removal of tracheal secretions.

Extracorporeal ventilatory support

A decade ago, it would have been unnecessary to discuss extracorporeal ventilation for a patient after thoracic surgery. Since then two important developments occurred. We have learnt that mechanical ventilation is a double-edged sword and protecting the lung from injury of positive pressure mechanical ventilation has become as important as achieving adequate oxygenation and gas exchange. Furthermore, systems for extracorporeal ventilation are now less complicated and invasive.

The newly developed Interventional Lung Assist (ILA) device is an extracorporeal membrane ventilator that rests the lung until it

Box 36.2 Criteria for a successful weaning

◆ Oxygenation
(PaO_2 ≥60 mmHg or SaO_2 ≥90% with FiO_2 ≤0.40 or PaO_2/FiO_2 >200 with PEEP ≤5 cmH_2O)

◆ Ventilation
(increase in $PaCO_2$ ≥10 mmHg or reduction of pH≥0.10)

◆ Arterial pressure
(systolic arterial pressure ≥90 mmHg or ≤180 mmHg; increase or reduction ≤20%)

◆ Heart rate
(≥50 or ≤140 beats/min; increase or reduction ≤20%)

◆ Respiratory rate
(≥35 breaths/min)

◆ No signs of excessive work of breathing
(no paradoxical breathing and/or exaggerated use of accessory muscles)

◆ No agitation, exaggerated depression or manifest distress

PaO_2, arterial oxygen tension; SaO_2, arterial oxyhaemoglobin saturation with oxygen; FiO_2, inspired concentration of oxygen; PEEP, positive end expiratory pressure; $PaCO_2$, arterial carbon dioxide tension.

Reprinted by permission of Edizioni Minerva Anestesiologica 2007 Caroleo S et al. Weaning from mechanical ventilation: an open issue. July–August;73(7–8):417–27.

(a)
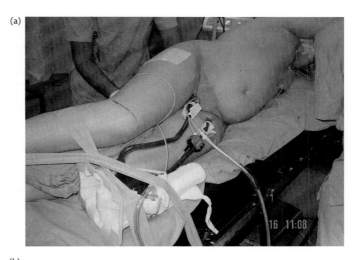

(b)
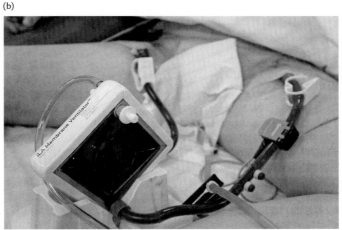

Fig. 36.5 Extracorporeal ventilation.
Use of Novalung (R) ('Interventional Lung Assist') intraoperatively (a) and postoperatively (b).

heals. This device can serve as a bridge to recovery and a bridge to transplantation (55). In six of seven patients with severe ARDS after pulmonary resection, the ILA device allowed them to be successfully weaned (56). The author's own experience is with a child with a previous right pneumonectomy who had to be reoperated because of metastases in the left mediastinum. The ILA was initiated before the operation and continued for 24 hours after the operation, and the device was removed 18 hours after the extubation (figure 36.5A and B).

The ILA device is a membrane artificial lung that allows O_2 and CO_2 gas exchange to occur by simple diffusion and can be used with or without an external pump (55). In the pumpless version, an arteriovenous circle that is often by the femoral artery and vein, is connected to the artificial lung, and the cardiac output drives the circulation. The sustainability of gas exchange is dependent on the stability of the cardiovascular system after initiation. As only 20% of the cardiac output may flow through the artificial lung, the pumpless version is more useful for CO_2 elimination than oxygenation. To improve oxygenation and/ or to correct cardiovascular instability, a venovenous mode with a pump is required.

Conclusion

Most patients who undergo thoracotomy may have tracheal extubation immediately after surgery and managed in a critical care area or PACU although a few will require elective mechanical ventilation in an ICU. A few patients will develop respiratory failure many of whom may be managed with NIV but some will require tracheal re-intubation and mechanical ventilation. Applying a restrictive intravenous fluid management may limit the incidence of respiratory failure. For those patients who require tracheal

intubation and mechanical ventilation, appropriate management applied to ensure early and successful weaning to ensure a good outcome from thoracotomy.

References

1. Licker M, Spiliopoulos A, Frey JG, De Perrot M, Chevalley C, Tschopp JM. Management and outcome of patients undergoing thoracic surgery in a regional chest medical centre. *Eur J Anaesthesiol* 2001; **18**: 540–7
2. Brunelli A, Pieretti P, Al Refai M, et al. Elective intensive care after lung resection: a multicentric propensity-matched comparison of outcome. *Interact Cardiovasc Thorac Surg* 2005; **4**: 609–13
3. Brunelli A, Varela G, Refai M, et al. A scoring system to predict the risk of prolonged air leak after lobectomy. *Ann Thorac Surg* 2009; **90**: 204–9
4. Bryant AS, Cerfolio RJ. The influence of preoperative risk stratification on fast tracking patients after pulmonary resection. *Thorac Surg Clin* 2009; **18**: 113–118
5. Damhuis RA, Schütte PR. Resection rates and postoperative mortality in 7,899 patients with lung cancer. *Eur Respir J* 1996; **9**: 7–10
6. Jordan S, Evans TW. Predicting the need for intensive care following lung resection. *Thorac Surg Clin* 2008; **18**: 61–9
7. Slinger PD, Johnston MR. Preoperative assessment for pulmonary resection. *J Cardiothorac Vasc Anesth* 2000; **14**: 202–11

8. Zwissler B, Reither A. Preoperative abstinence from smoking. An outdated dogma in anaesthesia? *Anaesthesist* 2005; **54**: 550–9

9. Cerfolio RJ, Bryant AS. The management of chest tubes after pulmonary resection. *Thorac Surg Clin* 2010; **20**: 399–405

10. Cerfolio RJ, Bass C, Katholi CR. Prospective randomized trial compares suction versus water seal for air leaks. *Ann Thorac Surg* 2001; **71**: 1613–7

11. Brunelli A, Monteverde M, Borri A, et al. Comparison of water seal and suction after pulmonary lobectomy: a prospective, randomized trial. *Ann Thorac Surg* 2004; **77**: 1932–7

12. Cerfolio RJ, Bryant AS. Results of a prospective algorithm to remove chest tubes after pulmonary resection with high output. *J Thorac Cardiovasc Surg* 2008; **135**: 269–73

13. Katzenelson R, Perel A, Berkenstadt H, et al. Accuracy of transpulmonary thermodilution versus gravimetric measurement of extravascular lung water. *Crit Care Med* 2004; **32**: 1550–4

14. Monnet X, Anguel N, Osman D, Hamzaoui O, Richard C, Teboul JL. Assessing pulmonary permeability by transpulmonary thermodilution allows differentiation of hydrostatic pulmonary edema from ALI/ARDS. *Intensive Care Med* 2007; **33**: 448–53

15. Lee JH, Jeon Y, Bahk JH, et al. Pulse pressure variation as a predictor of fluid responsiveness during one-lung ventilation for lung surgery using thoracotomy: randomised controlled study. *Eur J Anaesthesiol* 2011; **28**: 39–44

16. Loupec T, Nanadoumgar H, Frasca D, et al. Pleth variability index predicts fluid responsiveness in critically ill patients. *Crit Care Med* 2011; **39**: 294–9

17. Colquhoun DA, Forkin KT, Durieux ME, Thiele RHJ. Ability of the Masimo pulse CO-Oximeter to detect changes in hemoglobin. *Clin Monit Comput* 2012; **26**: 69–73

18. Slinger PD. Perioperative fluid management for thoracic surgery: the puzzle of postpneumonectomy pulmonary edema. *J Cardiothorac Vasc Anesth* 1995; **9**: 442–51.

19. Fernández-Pérez ER, Keegan MT, Brown DR, Hubmayr RD, Gajic O. Intraoperative tidal volume as a risk factor for respiratory failure after pneumonectomy. *Anesthesiology* 2006; **105**: 14–8

20. Senturk M. Major key topics concerning one-lung ventilation. Clinical and therapeutic implications, In Molina de Segura AM, Esquinas A, eds. *Yearbook respiratory care clinics and applied technologies*. Pittsburgh: World Federation of Respiratory Care and Applied Technologies, 2008; 221–8

21. Slinger PD. Postpneumonectomy pulmonary edema: good news, bad news. *Anesthesiology* 2006; **105**: 2–5

22. Senturk M. New concepts of the management of one-lung ventilation. *Curr Opin Anaesthesiol*; 2006; **19**: 1–4

23. Kozian A. Management of the thoracic surgery patient in the recovery room, In Hachenberg T, Welte T, Fischer S, eds. *Anaesthesie und Intensivtherapie in der Thoraxchirurgie*. Stuttgart: Georg Thieme Verlag, 2010: 255–65

24. Gothard J. Lung injury after thoracic surgery and one-lung ventilation. *Curr Opin Anaesthesiol* 2006; **19**: 5–10

25. Petrucci N, Iacovelli W. Lung protective ventilation strategy for the acute respiratory distress syndrome. Cochrane Database Syst Rev 2007; **18**(3): CD003844

26. Verbrugge SJ, Lachmann B, Kesecioglu J. Lung protective ventilatory strategies in acute lung injury and acute respiratory distress syndrome: from experimental findings to clinical application. *Clin Physiol Funct Imaging* 2007; **27**: 67–90

27. Kozian A, Schilling T, Schütze H, Senturk M, Hachenberg T, Hedenstierna G. Ventilatory protective strategies during thoracic surgery: effects of alveolar recruitment maneuver and low-tidal volume ventilation on lung density distribution. *Anesthesiology* 2011; **114**: 1025–35

28. Hickling KG, Walsh J, Henderson S, Jackson R. Low mortality rate in adult respiratory distress syndrome using low-volume, pressure-limited ventilation with permissive hypercapnia: a prospective study. *Crit Care Med* 1994; **22**: 1568–78

29. Kavanagh BP, Laffey JG. Hypercapnia: permissive and therapeutic. *Minerva Anestesiol* 2006; **72**: 567–76

30. Akça O. Carbon dioxide and tissue oxygenation: is there sufficient evidence to support application of hypercapnia for hemodynamic stability and better tissue perfusion in sepsis? *Intensive Care Med* 2008; **34**: 1752–4

31. Cornet AD, Kooter AJ, Peters MJL, Smulders YM. Supplemental oxygen therapy in medical emergencies: more harm than benefit? *Arch Intern Med* 2012; **172**: 289–90

32. Belda FJ, Aguilera L, García de la Asunción J, et al. Supplemental perioperative oxygen and the risk of surgical wound infection: A randomized controlled trial. *JAMA* 2005; **294**: 2035–42

33. Greif R, Akça O, Horn EP, Kurz A, Sessler DI, et al. Supplemental perioperative oxygen to reduce the incidence of surgical-wound infection. *N Engl J Med* 2000; **342**: 161–7

34. Meyhoff CS, Wetterslev J, Jorgensen LN, et al. Effect of high perioperative oxygen fraction on surgical site infection and pulmonary complications after abdominal surgery: The PROXI randomized clinical trial. *JAMA* 2009; **302**: 1543–50

35. Prella M, Feihl F, Domenighetti G. Effects of short-term pressure-controlled ventilation on gas exchange, airway pressures, and gas distribution in patients with acute lung injury/ARDS: comparison with volume-controlled ventilation. *Chest* 2002; **122**: 1382–8

36. Tuğrul M, Camci E, Karadeniz H, Sentürk M, Pembeci K, Akpir K. Comparison of volume controlled with pressure controlled ventilation during one-lung anaesthesia. *Br J Anaesth* 1997; **79**: 306–10

37. Dembinski R, Henzler D, Bensberg R, Prüsse B, Rossaint R, Kuhlen R. Ventilation-perfusion distribution related to different inspiratory flow patterns in experimental lung injury. *Anesth Analg* 2004; **98**: 211–9

38. Unzueta MC, Casas JI, Moral MV. Pressure-controlled versus volume-controlled ventilation during one-lung ventilation for thoracic surgery. *Anesth Analg* 2007; **104**: 1029–33

39. Sentürk NM, Dilek A, Camci E, et al. Effects of positive end-expiratory pressure on ventilatory and oxygenation parameters during pressure-controlled one-lung ventilation. *J Cardiothorac Vasc Anesth* 2005; **19**: 71–5

40. Grichnik KP, Shaw A. Update on one-lung ventilation: the use of continuous positive airway pressure ventilation and positive end-expiratory pressure ventilation—clinical application. *Curr Opin Anaesthesiol* 2009; **22**: 23–30

41. Farias LL, Faffe DS, Xisto DG, et al. Positive end-expiratory pressure prevents lung mechanical stress caused by recruitment/derecruitment. *J Appl Physiol* 2005; **98**: 53–61

42. Dyhr T, Nygård E, Laursen N, Larsson A. Both lung recruitment maneuver and PEEP are needed to increase oxygenation and lung volume after cardiac surgery. *Acta Anaesthesiol Scand* 2004; **48**: 187–97

43. Anantham D, Jagadesan R, Tiew PE. Clinical review: Independent lung ventilation in critical care. *Crit Care* 2005; **9**: 594–600

44. Wickerts CJ, Blomqvist H, Baehrendtz S, Klingstedt C, Hedenstierna G, Frostell C. Clinical application of differential ventilation with selective positive end-expiratory pressure in adult respiratory distress syndrome. *Acta Anaesthesiol Scand* 1995; **39**: 307–11

45. Lucangelo U, Antonaglia V, Zin WA. High-frequency percussive ventilation improves perioperatively clinical evolution in pulmonary resection. *Crit Care Med* 2009; **37**: 1663–9

46. Burns KE, Adhikari NK, Keenan SP, Meade M. Use of non-invasive ventilation to wean critically ill adults off invasive ventilation: meta-analysis and systematic review. *Br Med J* 2009; **338**: b1574

47. Berton DC, Kalil AC, Teixeira PJ. Quantitative versus qualitative cultures of respiratory secretions for clinical outcomes in patients with ventilator-associated pneumonia. *Cochrane Database Syst Rev* 2012; **1**: CD006482

48. Chiumello D, Chevallard G, Gregoretti C. Non-invasive ventilation in postoperative patients: a systematic review. *Intensive Care Med* 2011; **37**: 918–29

49. Auriant I, Jallot A, Hervé P, et al. Noninvasive ventilation reduces mortality in acute respiratory failure following lung resection. *Am J Respir Crit Care Med* 2001; **164**: 1231–5

50. Burns KE, Adhikari NK, Keenan SP, Meade MO. Noninvasive positive pressure ventilation as a weaning strategy for intubated adults with respiratory failure. *Cochrane Database Syst Rev* 2010; **8**: CD004127

51. Nava S, Hill N. Non-invasive ventilation in acute respiratory failure. *Lancet* 2009; **374**: 250–9

52. Caroleo S, Agnello F, Abdallah K, Santangelo E, Amantea B. Weaning from mechanical ventilation: an open issue. *Minerva Anestesiol* 2007; **73**: 417–27

53. MacIntyre NR, Cook DJ, Ely EW Jr, et al. Evidence-based guidelines for weaning and discontinuing ventilatory support: a collective task force facilitated by the American College of Chest Physicians; the American Association for Respiratory Care; and the American College of Critical Care Medicine. *Chest* 2001; **120**(6 Suppl): 375S–95S

54. Kress JP, Pohlman AS, O'Connor MF, Hall JB. Daily interruption of sedative infusions in critically ill patients undergoing mechanical ventilation. *N Engl J Med* 2000; **342**: 1471–7

55. Meyer A, Strüber M, Fischer S. Advances in extracorporeal ventilation. *Anesthesiol Clin* 2008; **26**: 381–91

56. Iglesias M, Martinez E, Badia JR, Macchiarini P. Extrapulmonary ventilation for unresponsive severe acute respiratory distress syndrome after pulmonary resection. *Ann Thorac Surg* 2008; **85**: 237–44

CHAPTER 37

Complications of thoracic surgery

Paul S. Myles

Introduction

Thoracic surgical patients typically have co-existent disease, and because of the nature and extent of their surgery are at risk of numerous complications. Common complications include atelectasis, haemorrhage, pulmonary oedema, atrial fibrillation (AF), wound infection, pneumonia, persistent air leak, and respiratory failure. Other, less frequent complications include bronchopleural fistula, empyema, cardiac herniation, pulmonary torsion, chylothorax, thromboembolism, right ventricular (RV) failure, and neurological injury (1–17) (see figure 37.1, box 37.1, and box 37.2).

About 20% of patients undergoing lung resection suffer one or more complications after surgery, of which about 2% die (4–13). These risks are doubled following pneumonectomy (6,10,14), and are far less common after limited wedge resection (4). Risk factors include patient age, current smoking, underlying carcinoma and chronic obstructive pulmonary disease (COPD) (see table 37.1) (4–13,15–17). Periprocedural chemotherapy and radiotherapy pose additional risks (9,18–21).

A thorough preoperative evaluation, smoking cessation, selection of the appropriate surgical procedure, and routine pre- and postoperative physiotherapy, can reduce mortality and major morbidity after lung resection (4,5,7–12,14,22). Clinician and team experience, as suggested by data demonstrating the influence of hospital caseload on patient outcome (23,24) should prevent, detect and treat complications more effectively (24). There is recent evidence to suggest better outcomes with a concentration of major cancer surgeries at higher-volume centres, including a reduction in risk-adjusted mortality (24).

Numerous large case series have identified a consistent set of risk factors associated with mortality after lung resection (5,6,21): older age, COPD, and extent of lung resection are key factors, with greatest risk typically associated with right pneumonectomy. Video-assisted thoracic surgery (VATS) can lower the risk of complications (25–32)—see Chapter 33. Complications add a substantial burden to healthcare costs (33,34), and nearly double hospital stay after thoracic surgery (34).

Pathophysiology of thoracotomy and lung resection

Atelectasis is near-universal after general anaesthesia and mechanical ventilation (2,35). After thoracotomy and pulmonary resection, alveolar capillary leakage, persistent air space, pleural collections, and mediastinal shift may worsen atelectasis. Thoracotomy is associated with an inflammatory response (31,36,37), which can lead to a reperfusion injury in the lung. This is associated with increased vascular permeability, pulmonary oedema and acute lung injury (ALI) (36,38). The aetiology of oedema associated with pulmonary resection was investigated by Mathru and colleagues (39) in seven patients after thoracic surgery. All were found to have X-ray evidence of diffuse pulmonary oedema and other features of ALI within 12 hours of surgery. The calculated shunt fraction exceeded 25%. They also measured the oedema fluid protein to serum protein ratio and found it was at least 0.6, suggestive of substantial permeability changes within the lung (39).

Thoracic surgery is associated with a 30 to 50% reduction in vital capacity and functional residual capacity due to reduced lung compliance, diaphragmatic dysfunction and/or chest wall splinting accompanying postoperative pain (40,41). Some of these changes can take up to six months to recover (42).

Respiratory complications

Respiratory failure

Postoperative respiratory complications after thoracic surgery are the major cause of morbidity and mortality. Failure to clear airway secretions can result in bronchial obstruction, atelectasis and lobar collapse, respiratory insufficiency, and pneumonia. Severe atelectasis occurs in about 5% of patients after lung resection (35). Respiratory failure most often occurs at 24 to 48 hours after surgery (43) (figure 37.2). Left ventricular failure and cardiogenic pulmonary oedema may co-exist. A patent foramen ovale allows right-to-left shunting, exacerbating hypoxaemia, and increasing risk of stroke from paradoxical embolism (44).

Ruffini and colleagues (12) reviewed the frequency and mortality of ALI and adult respiratory distress syndrome (ARDS) in 1221 patients undergoing lung cancer resection. Of these, 27 (2.2%) met the criteria of postoperative ALI/ARDS, though the frequency was highest following right pneumonectomy and other major resections (4.5%). Four patients with ALI (40%) and 10 patients with ARDS (59%) died.

Pulmonary oedema

Pulmonary oedema is not all that uncommon in elderly patients undergoing any type of major surgery. But there are two special

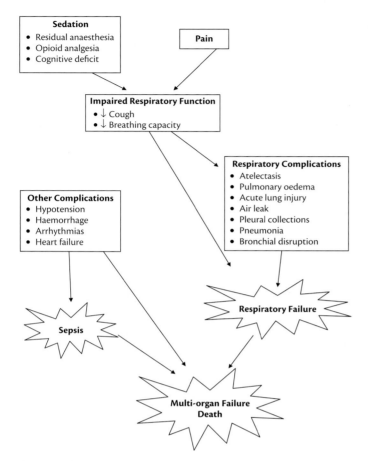

Fig. 37.1 Pathogenesis of respiratory failure and other major complications after pulmonary resection.

Box 37.1 The frequency of complications after lung resection

More common (incidence: 5–15%) complications include:

◆ Hypotension

◆ Postoperative haemorrhage

◆ Arrhythmias (esp. atrial fibrillation)

◆ Atelectasis and pneumonia

◆ Persistent air space, prolonged air leak

◆ Pulmonary oedema (including re-expansion injury)

◆ Acute lung injury

◆ Mediastinal shift

◆ Pleural effusion

◆ Wound infection

◆ Post-thoracotomy pain syndrome

Less common (incidence <2%) complications include:

◆ Empyema

◆ Bronchopleural fistula

◆ Lobar torsion and gangrene

◆ Chylothorax

◆ Diaphragmatic paralysis

◆ Right ventricular failure

◆ Cardiac herniation

◆ Spinal cord injury

Other complications, not specifically related to lung resection

◆ Acute lung injury and adult respiratory distress syndrome

◆ Thromboembolism

◆ Cardiac failure

◆ Myocardial infarction

◆ Acute renal failure

◆ Gastrointestinal haemorrhage

situations that can occur after thoracic surgery and one-lung ventilation (OLV); these are re-expansion and postpneumonectomy pulmonary oedema.

Re-expansion pulmonary oedema

Re-expansion pulmonary oedema can occur when a chronically collapsed lung is rapidly re-inflated, such as following treatment of pneumothorax or pleural effusion (45), but it can also occur after short periods of collapse. Lung isolation and OLV include a period of lung collapse and so re-expansion pulmonary oedema can occur after most types of thoracic surgery, including VATS (46,47).

Factors associated with re-expansion pulmonary oedema include the duration of collapse, technique of re-expansion, increased pulmonary vascular permeability, airway obstruction, and pulmonary artery pressure changes (45). The rate of re-expansion seems to be an important factor (45). There has been some suggestion that loss of surfactant may be an underlying feature, but there are little data to support this conjecture.

Gentle low-pressure manual re-inflations of the collapsed lung should be accompanied by direct inspection of the lung, aiming to avoid hyperinflation and limiting airway pressure below 30 cmH₂O. The key issue is to not aggressively reinflate a collapsed lung. 'Protective' mechanical ventilation should be employed (48–51).

Postpneumonectomy pulmonary oedema

Post-pneumonectomy pulmonary oedema has been attributed to excessive IV fluid administration, damage to lymphatic drainage, inflammatory mediators and endothelial damage, and lung hyperinflation (52). It occurs in about 5% of cases of pneumonectomy and is associated with high mortality of around 50% (6,36). It is most common after right pneumonectomy (36). It usually manifests at about 12 to 24 hours after surgery, and has all the hallmarks of ALI: progressive dyspnoea, hypoxia, and non-cardiogenic pulmonary oedema. The propensity to pulmonary oedema may be increased if there is reduced lymphatic drainage, because of surgical ligation and dependence on flow through channels in the remaining lung. Epidural, compared with paravertebral block, may increase fluid requirements and thus pose greater risk (17,53).

Although some believe that excessive IV fluid administration may be a cause of post-pneumonectomy pulmonary oedema (6,13), the weight of evidence is in favour of there being no direct

Box 37.2 The time onset of postoperative complications after lung resection

1. Early complications (usually within 24 h)
   - Hypotension
   - Postoperative haemorrhage
   - Atelectasis
   - Persistent air space
   - Pulmonary oedema (including re-expansion injury)
   - Mediastinal shift
   - Right ventricular failure
   - Cardiac herniation
   - Spinal cord injury

2. Late complications (usually beyond 48 hr)
   - Prolonged air leak
   - Acute lung injury
   - Pleural effusion
   - Pneumonia
   - Empyema
   - Bronchopleural fistula
   - Lobar torsion and gangrene
   - Chylothorax
   - Diaphragmatic paralysis
   - Wound infection
   - Post-thoracotomy pain syndrome
   - Arrhythmias (esp. atrial fibrillation)
   - Myocardial infarction
   - Thromboembolism
   - Acute renal failure
   - Gastrointestinal haemorrhage

Table 37.1 Risk factors for postoperative complications after lung resection

Risk factors*	Reference(s)	
	Pneumonectomy	Any pulmonary resection
Patient factors	17, 21, 34	4–6, 9, 10, 11, 21
Patient age (esp. >60 years)	5, 8, 20, 63	9, 11
Male gender	8, 13, 21, 34	22
Current smoking	5	7
Nutritional status		4, 9, 11, 15, 16, 20, 56
COPD (esp. FEV_1 <60%)		4, 11, 21
Coexistent medical conditions		6, 7
Cancer		
Surgical factors	5, 14, 21	4–6, 11, 12, 19, 34, 89
Caseload	5, 12, 17, 20, 21, 36, 63, 64	
Extent of lung resection		
Right-sided surgery	14, 39	
Other factors	20, 21	7, 9, 19–21
Adjuvant regimens	6, 8, 13	
Excessive IV fluid therapy (esp >3 L/24 hr)		

*In many cases the risk factor(s) were identified with univariate testing, and so may be spuriously associated because of confounding: for example, excessive IV fluid therapy may be associated with complications because it is used to treat hypotension secondary to underlying heart disease, more extensive resection, postoperative bleeding, and so on.
COPD = chronic obstructive pulmonary disease; FEV_1 = forced expiratory volume in one second; IV = intravenous.

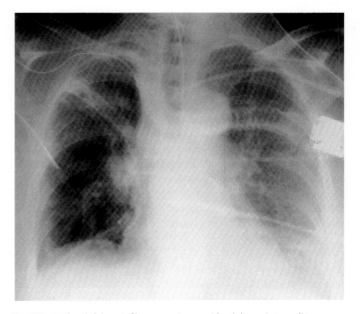

Fig. 37.2 Diffuse left lung infiltrate consistent with adult respiratory distress syndrome, in a patient after right upper lobectomy.
There is a tracheal tube, left-sided pulmonary artery catheter, a right subclavian venous catheter, and right-sided pleural drains in situ.

association (36,37,52). Increased pulmonary vascular permeability seems to be a feature (37,38).

Air spaces and air leak

Persistent air spaces are common, occurring in 15 to 25% of lung resections and most are asymptomatic (54,55). Although the intention of pleural drainage is to avoid such a situation, in major lung resections the remaining thoracic space is not initially filled by fluid or expansion of the remaining lung (figure 37.3). Air spaces usually occur superiorly in the apex and resolve spontaneously over weeks or months. A failure of pleural drainage can also result in subcutaneous or mediastinal emphysema (figure 37.3). This is usually self-limiting and, other than ensuring adequate pleural drainage, no specific treatment is required. Indications for surgery include pain, dyspnoea, haemoptysis, fever, or persistent air leak. Each of these complications may be associated with sepsis.

Small air leaks are relatively common after minor lung resections and lobectomy, usually from raw exposed surfaces of the

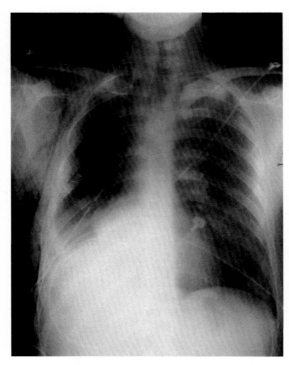

Fig. 37.3 Chest X-ray after right pneumonectomy.
There is extensive chest wall subcutaneous emphysema. The surgical clips project over the right haemothorax, with a pleural drain in situ. A right subclavian central venous catheter tip is directed cephalad into the jugular vein. The right hemithorax is filled with air and fluid, and there is mediastinal shift to the right. The left lung is clear.

lung. Air leak is most common in older patients and those with underlying COPD (55,56), particularly after lung volume reduction surgery (57). Air leak usually presents as persistent bubbling via the pleural drains or as a pneumothorax if pleural drainage is inadequate or absent.

The usual approach to the management of a persistent air leak is to facilitate apposition of lung to parietal pleura to encourage efficient healing. Cerfolio and colleagues (56) tested an algorithm for the management of air leak in 101 consecutive patients undergoing elective pulmonary resection. They found that most air leaks were expiratory only. Cessation of pleural suction was an effective way of sealing the leak in most patients. Intermittent clamping of pleural drains and/or early removal is recommended (56). A persistent air leak (>7 days) can be treated with video-assisted pleurodesis, but more severe air leaks may require lung stapling with the inclusion of a pericardial sleeve (58). In patients undergoing mechanical ventilation, selective bronchial blockade and independent lung ventilation can be used (59,60).

Bronchial disruption

Major pulmonary resections include stapling or ligation of the bronchial stump. Bronchial disruption may occur early after surgery if the staple line or suture slips, or later if there is impaired wound healing. The latter is more common in diabetic patients and those on high-dose steroid therapy, in which case it most commonly occurs 7 to 10 days after surgery. It is also thought to be exacerbated by postoperative mechanical ventilation (61).

Bronchial disruption is associated with massive air leak through the resultant bronchopleural fistula (BPF).

There have been several large cohort studies identifying the incidence and risk factors for BPF. The incidence of BPF is about 3% after pneumonectomy (62,63), and is more common on the right side (63,64). The mortality in those who have a BPF is about 50% (62,63). The belief that early tracheal extubation may prevent the development of BPF is questionable in that the need for mechanical ventilation because of other factors may confound this outcome.

A BPF typically presents with sudden breathlessness, haemoptysis, and air leak, the latter manifest by bubbling via pleural drains, subcutaneous, or mediastinal emphysema, and if a chest tube is not present, pneumothorax. If occurring late, the patient may have signs of sepsis: fever, productive cough and haemoptysis (65). A persistent BPF may lead to empyema. A BPF can be diagnosed with computerized tomography (CT), magnetic resonance imaging (MRI), and nuclear medicine techniques; however, Mulot and colleagues (66) describe a simple and effective method using inhalation of an oxygen:nitrous oxide mixture and sampling the pleural gas via the chest tube. The presence of a BPF was diagnosed by a rapid increase in nitrous oxide concentration, reaching the inspired level within a few minutes.

The emergency treatment of a BPF includes providing oxygen and pleural drainage, and turning the patient into the lateral position with the operated side downwards.

Pneumonia

Pneumonia is the commonest infective respiratory complication after thoracic surgery. It is usually associated with atelectasis. The incidence of pneumonia is about 5% to 10% after lung resection (4,5). The usual organisms are *Staphylococcus* and *Pseudomonas*, but immunosuppressed patients are prone to atypical infections, including a variety of viral and fungal organisms (67). Causative organisms are often resistant to standard antimicrobial drugs.

Pleural collections

Air or fluid may collect in the pleural space after surgery, even if there are pleural drains present. Fluids include blood, interstitial exudate, purulent collections, and lymphatic chyle leakage (figure 37.4, figure 37.5, and figure 37.6).

Pleural effusion

A small pleural effusion is routinely seen after most pulmonary resections, but large collections require reassessment of the pleural drainage in order to avoid atelectasis and empyema (figure 37.4).

Chylothorax

Chylothorax is a rare cause of pleural collection, believed to be due to injury to the thoracic duct or other lymphatic channels and occurring in less than 1% of resections (68–73). The typical presentation is development of a milky pleural drainage. A tension chylothorax can occur (figure 37.6) (70,71).

Chylothorax does not necessarily require surgical re-exploration. Conservative management includes institution of a low-fat diet with medium-chain triglycerides and/or total parenteral nutrition. There have been reports of a beneficial response to octreotide, which inhibits gastric acid and biliary secretions,

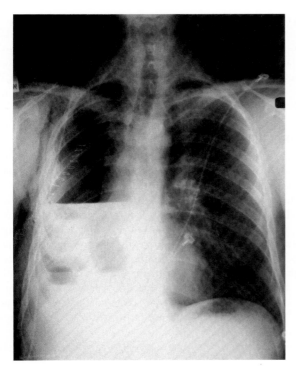

Fig. 37.4 Chest X-ray after right pneumonectomy.
A right-sided loculated pleural collection consistent with empyema.

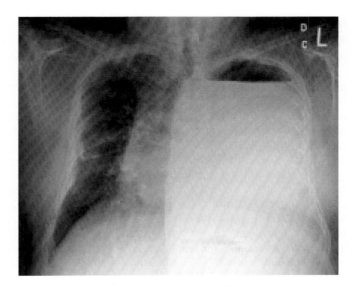

Fig. 37.6 Tension chylothorax, with mediastinal shift, after left pneumonectomy.
Reprinted from Journal of Cardiothoracic Vascular Anaesthesia, 17, Riedel BJCJ and Vaporciyan AA, 'Unusual cause of dyspnea after pneumonectomy', pp. 131–133, Copyright 2003, with permission from Elsevier

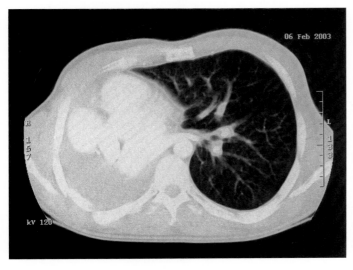

Fig. 37.5 Computerized axial tomography (CAT) scan after right pneumonectomy.
There is marked mediastinal shift to the right and a moderate sized pleural effusion. The left lung is clear.

leading to a reduction in the absorption of fat (72). Surgery is generally required if leakage exceeds 500 mL per day, or if there is no resolution of the mediastinal shift.

Empyema

Postoperative empyema is an uncommon, but serious, infective complication seen in around 2% of thoracic surgical patients. It is more common in patients with malnutrition or underlying immunodeficiency syndromes. It may be associated with persistent pleural effusion, air space or BPF (74). The presence of empyema should be considered if the patient has a pleural collection in association with fever, cough, or haemoptysis. Useful investigations include sputum, blood and pleural fluid cultures, chest X-ray, and CT in which a loculated effusion may be identified (figure 37.4). Serum C-reactive protein (CRP) levels are typically elevated (75).

The two key components of treatment are to drain the infected pleural space and to treat the fistula. Appropriate antibiotic therapy is also required.

Pulmonary torsion

Hilar dissection and lung resection may allow excessive mobility of the lung. This can lead to pulmonary torsion (74–76). This is rare, with a large series reporting an incidence rate of 0.1% (77). The right middle lobe is most at risk because of its adjacent fissures (77,78). It can occur intraoperatively if the surgeon is not attentive during manipulations and closure. The dual blood supply of the lung usually protects the torted lung from ischaemic injury, but infarction and gangrene can occur.

Postoperatively, pulmonary torsion manifests as cough, dyspnoea, haemoptysis, or chest pain (76–78). Respiratory distress may be due to pulmonary collapse, oedema, and/or ischemia. The diagnosis may not be apparent for several days after surgery, with the median time to presentation being about 10 days (77). Chest X-ray may indicate lobar collapse, which may enlarge if repeat X-rays are undertaken. The most useful investigation is fibreoptic bronchoscopy, where an obstructed or markedly compressed bronchus can be seen.

Urgent surgical re-exploration is required to reorient and stabilize the lung, for which lung isolation is required because of the likelihood of subsequent florid pulmonary oedema or intrapulmonary haemorrhage contaminating the non-operative lung. A VATS approach may limit further complications (78).

Mediastinal shift and postpneumonectomy syndrome

All pulmonary and pleural resections have the potential to lead to massive atelectasis and pneumothorax, cardiac herniation or pulmonary torsion. Any of these may lead to mediastinal shift (figure 37.3, figure 37.5, and figure 37.6). The resultant positioning of the mediastinum, particularly after pneumonectomy, is dependent on competing factors: accumulated air and fluid push the mediastinal structures towards the remaining lung, whilst drainage (or removal) or air or fluid, and hyperinflation of the remaining lung, draw the structures towards the operative side. Immediately after chest closure the mediastinal structures are positioned midline, with the empty hemithorax filled with air. As the air is gradually reabsorbed, it creates a negative pressure and facilitates fluid accumulation. This becomes apparent after about 24 hours, and continues for many weeks, being about 90% complete at 1 month (figure 37.3). Needle aspiration of air or, if a pleural drain is present, intermittent unclamping to remove pleural fluid or blood, can centralize the mediastinum. Alternatively, a balanced drainage system can be used (79).

Pneumonectomy can result in persistent mediastinal shift and obstruction to a main bronchus, known as post-pneumonectomy syndrome (80). It mostly affects those recovering from a right pneumonectomy because the aortic arch prevents such an effect on the left side. The extent of mediastinal shift can be monitored with regular chest X-rays, and intermittent unclamping of the pleural drains used to control the amount of pleural fluid removed.

Diaphragmatic paralysis

Hilar dissection during major pulmonary resection may damage phrenic, vagal or recurrent laryngeal nerves (81). A phrenic nerve palsy usually manifests as respiratory insufficiency, and may be suspected on clinical examination if there is poor air entry unilaterally (94). Normally, vital capacity decreases by about 10% in the supine position, and up to 50% after thoracic surgery. In unilateral paralysis, the vital capacity is decreased to 70 to 80% of the predicted level. Blood gas results may be near-normal, indicating no abnormality of gas exchange. The chest X-ray may be normal, but there is usually progressive flattening of the hemidiaphragm over time.

Diaphragmatic paralysis can be diagnosed using fluoroscopy, where a sniff test demonstrates paradoxical elevation of the paralysed diaphragm with inspiration. Diaphragmatic electromyography with skin surface or oesophageal electrode may be helpful if there is some doubt as to its aetiology (neuropathy or myopathy).

Cardiovascular complications

Thoracic surgical patients are at increased risk of a number of cardiovascular complications, some of which can be identified and may be prevented by modifications to their perioperative management (83). Patients with coronary artery disease have a threefold increased risk of death following pneumonectomy (84).

Hypotension

As is seen in all types of major surgery, hypotension is common after thoracic surgery. It is usual to restrict fluid replacement in lung resections because of a concern for pulmonary oedema; this will exacerbate hypovolaemia associated with blood loss and exudation. Other aggravating factors include: myocardial dysfunction associated with arrhythmias or underlying cardiovascular disease, thoracic epidural analgesia, and lung hyperinflation. Rare causes of hypotension include pericardial tamponade and myocardial infarction.

Haemorrhage

Excessive bleeding is one of the commonest complications of thoracic surgery (85). Bleeding usually occurs from lung parenchyma or bronchial vessels, but can also come from the chest wall. The lung and pulmonary vasculature are difficult structures to visualize in their entirety, and incomplete haemostasis may not be apparent, particularly when the operative lung is collapsed. Patients with inflammatory lung disease and/or pleural adhesions, and those undergoing decortication or chest wall resection are particularly at risk. In a retrospective review of 1428 pulmonary resections, postoperative bleeding necessitated emergency thoracotomy in 2.6% of cases (86). Haemorrhage can also occur after VATS (32,87), and because of limited access and exposure this may be profuse.

Many patients with excessive bleeding can be treated conservatively, perhaps only requiring blood transfusion. Reoperation is required if there is a rapid blood loss via pleural drains, or if there is a significant intrapleural collection on chest X-ray, persistent hypovolaemia despite transfusion, or hypoxia due to compression of underlying lung.

Arrhythmias

Postoperative arrhythmias occur frequently after thoracic surgery (19 100), with AF being the most common (5,89). The incidence of symptomatic AF is about 15% (5,17,90,91), but with Holter monitoring episodes of AF can be detected in about 50% of patients after thoracic surgery (89). Most occur within the first 24 hours but may not be symptomatic until the second or third day (89). Risk factors include age (92), extent of resection (89,93), intraoperative hypotension,(94) and postoperative pulmonary oedema (91). Arrhythmias increase hospital length of stay (90,92,93,95). Ventricular arrhythmias can also occur (incidence 15%), but most are transient and do not require treatment (96).

Identification of patients at increased risk of AF after thoracic surgery would allow targeting of those most likely to benefit from prophylactic therapy, and elevations in brain natriuretic peptide may be a very useful biomarker to identify high-risk patients (92). Prophylactic digitalization for major pulmonary resection has been traditionally used but is now considered to be ineffective (89,90,93). There is some evidence to upport the use of diltiazem (93), amiodarone (97), propranolol (98), or verapamil (99). In cardiac surgery, beta-blockers, sotalol, and amiodarone have each been found to reduce the incidence of AF, as well as decreasing hospital length of stay (100). In thoracic surgery, propanolol and verapamil increase the risk of bradycardia and hypotension (98,99), and there is some concern that amiodarone may increase the risk of ALI (97). The comparative role of prophylactic or expectant treatment should be further evaluated.

Right ventricular failure

Thoracic surgical patients commonly have raised pulmonary vascular resistance (PVR) secondary to their underlying lung disease, and this is associated with RV dysfunction (101,102) and an increased incidence of AF (90). Reed and colleagues (102) studied the effect of pulmonary resection on RV performance and its relationship with postoperative complications. Significant RV dysfunction was demonstrated in the postoperative period, with RV end-diastolic volume increased by about 15% on the first two postoperative days. RV ejection fraction was significantly decreased by about 20%. This was despite minimal change in PVR. This suggests that lung resection has a direct adverse effect on RV myocardial contractility. Those with a patent foramen ovale have special risks (44).

Cardiac herniation

Excision of pericardium during major pulmonary resections may be necessary in order to facilitate surgical exposure of the hilum of the lung. This can result in a pericardial defect that can allow herniation of the heart, leading to obstruction to venous return, tracheal obstruction, pulmonary venous congestion and ventricular arrhythmias (see figure 37.7) (103–106). The patient can develop a superior vena cava syndrome (106). Mortality is over 50% if undiagnosed or left untreated.

Cardiac herniation usually occurs in the immediate postoperative period, presenting as severe, acute onset hypotension, cardiac arrest or respiratory distress (104). However, patients may be asymptomatic if there are no immediate effects on venous return or cardiac function (105). It usually occurs following reinstitution of two-lung ventilation, application of negative pressure via the pleural drains, or when the operative side is dependent on turning the patient into the lateral position at any time in the first few days after surgery (104,105). It can also be generated by coughing, and hyperinflation of the remaining lung (such as with positive end-expiratory pressure).

A high index of suspicion at any time when sudden haemodynamic deterioration occurs, particularly if associated with one of the previously mentioned manoeuvres, can identify and reverse the situation. If severe hypotension cannot be corrected by moving the patient into the lateral position, with the herniation uppermost in order to promote venous return, or if cardiac arrest should occur, then immediate thoracotomy and internal cardiac massage will be required. This may have to be undertaken in the surgical ward or intensive care unit.

In less-acute circumstances an X-ray or CT can confirm the diagnosis (figure 37.7). Once the diagnosis has been made, surgical re-exploration is required to reposition the heart and repair the pericardial defect. Induction of anaesthesia and endotracheal intubation should occur in the lateral position (105).

Thromboembolism

Pulmonary embolism occurs in up to 5% of patients after pulmonary resection (21,107). Tumour embolism may also occur (108). Patients undergoing thoracotomy should receive thromboembolism prophylaxis.

Myocardial infarction

Myocardial ischaemia and infarction are relatively uncommon, with an incidence of 3.8% in a series of 598 patients undergoing lung resection for cancer (93).

Other complications

Wound infection

Wound infection occurs in about 2% of patients undergoing thoracotomy or VATS (4,32). Most wound infections are confined to the subcutaneous layers but wound dehiscence can also occur. This will impair ventilation and sputum clearance, and may lead to air leak, thus prolonging hospitalization.

Nerve injury

Most nerve injuries should be avoidable, being dependent on surgical technique and care with patient positioning in order to avoid pressure-induced damage to peripheral nerves (78). Hilar dissection during major pulmonary resection may damage phrenic, vagal or recurrent laryngeal nerves (86). Injury to the phrenic nerve will lead to unilateral diaphragmatic paralysis (see earlier). Injury to the recurrent laryngeal nerve during lung resection most commonly occurs with a left thoracotomy. It will manifest as hoarseness or upper airway obstruction, and places the patient at risk of aspiration. The patient may require tracheal reintubation. Isolated injury to the vagus nerve does not usually cause any problems, other than delayed gastric emptying.

The intercostal nerves are particularly prone to damage due to rib retraction and/or resection (109). This usually manifests as postoperative neuralgia and post-thoracotomy pain syndrome (110,111). Spinal cord injury and paraplegia usually result from surgical haemostasis of an intercostal artery or damage to the anterior spinal artery, leading to a spinal cord ischaemia. Inadequate haemostasis may lead to a spinal haematoma and spinal cord

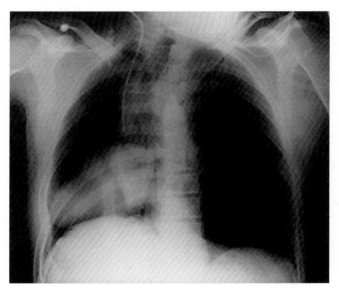

Fig. 37.7 Cardiac herniation.
The heart has shifted into the right hemithorax, having herniated through a deficit in the pericardium.

Reproduced from Self RJ and Vaughan RS, 'Acute cardiac herniation after radical pleuropneumonectomy', Anaesthesia, 54, pp. 564–566, published by Wiley, © 2002 The Association of Anaesthetists of Great Britain and Ireland.

compression. Epidural analgesia is associated with spinal abscess and haematoma formation (112,113).

Attar and colleagues (114) reported five cases of post-thoracotomy paraplegia, and reviewed 35 cases in the literature. The intraoperative factors contributing to the paraplegia were bleeding at the costovertebral angle (n = 9), migration of oxidized cellulose into the spinal canal (n = 9), thrombosis of the anterior spinal artery (n = 4), epidural hematoma (n = 2), direct injury from the epidural catheter (n = 2), metastatic carcinoma (n = 1), and hypotension (n = 1).

Acute renal failure

Renal failure occurs in about 15% of patients undergoing pneumonectomy and is associated with increased mortality (8).

Aggressive treatment should begin at the earliest indication of renal dysfunction. The key considerations are maintenance of intravascular volume status and correction of biochemical abnormalities such as hyperkalaemia and acidosis. Nephrotoxic drugs such as radiocontrast agents, antibiotics such as gentamicin, and non-steroidal anti-inflammatory drugs should be used with great caution.

Conclusion

Thoracic surgical patients are frequently elderly, have substantial coexistent disease, and are particularly prone to respiratory complications. Those undergoing pneumonectomy are at greatest risk. Anaesthetic and surgical techniques that assist early awakening and effective pain control will promote restoration of respiratory function, and this should lead to an uneventful postoperative course. The over-riding determinants, however, are the pre-existing health status of the patient and the quality of the surgery. Some complications can be avoided with prophylactic interventions, and others can be minimized if early diagnosis and treatment are initiated.

References

1. Amar D. Cardiopulmonary complications of esophageal surgery. *Chest Surg Clin N Am* 1997; **7**: 449–56
2. Weissman C. Pulmonary function after cardiac and thoracic surgery. *Anesth Analg* 1999; **88**: 1272–9
3. Whooley BP, Law S, Alexandrou A, et al. Critical appraisal of the significance of intrathoracic anastomotic leakage after esophagectomy for cancer. *Am J Surg* 2001; **181**: 198–203
4. Keagy BA, Lores ME, Starek PJ, et al. Elective pulmonary lobectomy: factors associated with morbidity and operative mortality. *Ann Thorac Surg* 1985; **40**: 349–52
5. Wahi R, McMurtrey MJ, DeCaro LF, et al. Determinants of perioperative morbidity and mortality after pneumonectomy. *Ann Thorac Surg* 1989; **48**: 33–7
6. van Meerbeeck JP, Damhuis RA, Vos de Wael ML. High postoperative risk after pneumonectomy in elderly patients with right-sided lung cancer. *Eur Respir J* 2002; **19**: 141–5
7. Busch E, Verazin G, Antkowiak JG, et al. Pulmonary complications in patients undergoing thoracotomy for lung carcinoma. *Chest* 1994; **105**: 760–6
8. Patel RL, Townsend ER, Fountain SW. Elective pneumonectomy: factors associated with morbidity and operative mortality. *Ann Thorac Surg* 1992; **54**: 84–8
9. Deslauriers J, Ginsberg RJ, Piantadosi S, et al. Prospective assessment of 30-day operative morbidity for surgical resections in lung cancer. *Chest* 1994; **106**: 329S–30S
10. Wada H, Nakamura T, Nakamoto K, et al. Thirty-day operative mortality for thoracotomy in lung cancer. *J Thorac Cardiovasc Surg* 1998; **115**: 70–3
11. Thomas P, Piraux M, Jacques LF, et al. Clinical patterns and trends of outcome of elderly patients with bronchogenic carcinoma. *Eur J Cardiothorac Surg* 1998; **13**: 266–74
12. Ruffini E, Parola A, Papalia E, et al. Frequency and mortality of acute lung injury and acute respiratory distress syndrome after pulmonary resection for bronchogenic carcinoma. *Eur J Cardiothorac Surg* 2001; **20**: 30–6
13. Moller AM, Pedersen T, Svendsen PE, et al. Perioperative risk factors in elective pneumonectomy: the impact of excess fluid balance. *Eur J Anaesthesiol* 2002; **19**: 57–62
14. Vaporciyan AA, Merriman KW, Ece F, et al. Incidence of major pulmonary morbidity after pneumonectomy: association with timing of smoking cessation. *Ann Thorac Surg* 2002; **73**: 420–6
15. Sekine Y, Behnia M, Fujisawa T. Impact of COPD on pulmonary complications and on long-term survival of patients undergoing surgery for NSCLC. *Lung Cancer* 2002; **37**: 95–101
16. Dales RE, Dionne G, Leech JA, et al. Preoperative prediction of pulmonary complications following thoracic surgery. *Chest* 1993; **104**: 155–9
17. Powell ES, Pearce AC, Cook D, et al, UKPOS Co-ordinators. UK pneumonectomy outcome study (UKPOS): a prospective observational study of pneumonectomy outcome. *J Cardiothorac Surg* 2009; **4**: 41. doi: 10.1186/1749–8090-4-41.
18. Cerfolio RJ, Talati A, Bryant AS. Changes in pulmonary function tests after neoadjuvant therapy predict postoperative complications. *Ann Thorac Surg* 2009; **88**: 930–5
19. Doddoli C, Thomas P, Thirion X, et al. Postoperative complications in relation with induction therapy for lung cancer. *Eur J Cardiothorac Surg* 2001; **20**: 385–90
20. Martin J, Ginsberg RJ, Abolhoda A, et al. Morbidity and mortality after neoadjuvant therapy for lung cancer: the risks of right pneumonectomy. *Ann Thorac Surg* 2001; **72**: 1149–54
21. Bernard A, Deschamps C, Allen MS, et al. Pneumonectomy for malignant disease: factors affecting early morbidity and mortality. *J Thorac Cardiovasc Surg* 2001; **121**: 1076–82
22. Nakagawa M, Tanaka H, Tsukuma H, et al. Relationship between the duration of the preoperative smoke-free period and the incidence of postoperative pulmonary complications after pulmonary surgery. *Chest* 2001; **120**: 705–10
23. Finks JF, Osborne NH, Birkmeyer JD. Trends in hospital volume and operative mortality for high-risk surgery. *N Engl J Med* 2011; **364**: 2128–37
24. Shahian DM, Wolf RE, Iezzoni LI, Kirle L, Normand S-LT. Variability in the measurement of hospital-wide mortality rates. *N Engl J Med* 2010; **363**: 2530–39
25. Daniels LJ, Balderson SS, Onaitis MW, et al. Thoracoscopic lobectomy: a safe and effective strategy for patients with stage I lung cancer. *Ann Thorac Surg* 2002; **74**: 860–4
26. Krasna MJ, Deshmukh S, McLaughlin JS. Complications of thoracoscopy. *Ann Thorac Surg* 1996; **61**: 1066–9
27. Plummer S, Hartley M, Vaughan RS. Anaesthesia for telescopic procedures in the thorax. *Br J Anaesth* 1998; **80**: 223–34
28. Nakata M, Saeki H, Yokoyama N, et al. Pulmonary function after lobectomy: video-assisted thoracic surgery versus thoracotomy. *Ann Thorac Surg* 2000; **70**: 938–41
29. Nagahiro I, Andou A, Aoe M, et al. Pulmonary function, postoperative pain, and serum cytokine level after lobectomy: a comparison of VATS and conventional procedure. *Ann Thorac Surg* 2001; **72**: 362–5
30. Jancovici R, Lang-Lazdunski L, Pons F, et al. Complications of video-assisted thoracic surgery: a five-year experience. *Ann Thorac Surg* 1996; **61**: 533–7
31. Allen MS, Deschamps C, Jones DM, et al. Video-assisted thoracic surgical procedures: the Mayo experience. *Mayo Clin Proc* 1996; **71**: 351–9
32. Yim AP, Liu HP. Complications and failures of video-assisted thoracic surgery: experience from two centers in Asia. *Ann Thorac Surg* 1996; **61**: 538–41
33. Dexter F, Tinker JH. The cost efficacy of hypothetically eliminating adverse anesthetic outcomes from high-risk, but neither low- nor moderate-risk, surgical operations. *Anesth Analg* 1995; **81**: 939–44

34. Melendez JA, Carlon VA. Cardiopulmonary risk index does not predict complications after thoracic surgery. *Chest* 1998; **114**: 69–75

35. Korst RJ, Humphrey CB. Complete lobar collapse following pulmonary lobectomy. Its incidence, predisposing factors, and clinical ramifications. *Chest* 1997; **111**: 1285–9

36. Turnage WS, Lunn JJ. Postpneumonectomy pulmonary edema. A retrospective analysis of associated variables. *Chest* 1993; **103**: 1646–50

37. Waller DA, Keavey P, Woodfine L, et al. Pulmonary endothelial permeability changes after major lung resection. *Ann Thorac Surg* 1996; **61**: 1435–40

38. Boujoukis AJ, Martich GD, Vega JD, et al. Reperfusion injury in single-transplant recipients with pulmonary hypertension and emphysema. *J Heart Lung Transplant* 1997; **16**: 439–48

39. Mathru M, Blakeman B, Dries DJ, et al. Permeability pulmonary edema following lung resection. *Chest* 1990; **98**: 1216–8

40. Hansdottir V, Bake B, Nordberg G. The analgesic efficacy and adverse effects of continuous epidural sufentanil and bupivacaine infusion after thoracotomy. *Anesth Analg* 1996; **83**: 394–400

41. Gosselink R, Schrever K, Cops P, et al. Incentive spirometry does not enhance recovery after thoracic surgery. *Crit Care Med* 2000; **28**: 679–83

42. Handy JR Jr, Child AI, Grunkemeier GL, et al. Hospital readmission after pulmonary resection: prevalence, patterns, and predisposing characteristics. *Ann Thorac Surg* 2001; **72**: 1855–9

43. Entwistle MD, Roe PG, Sapsford DJ, et al. Patterns of oxygenation after thoracotomy. *Br J Anaesth* 1991; **67**: 704–11

44. Ng SY, Sugarbaker DJ, Frendl G. Interatrial shunting after major thoracic surgery: a rare but clinically significant event. *Ann Thorac Surg* 2012; **93**: 1647–51

45. Critchley LA, Au HK, Yim AP. Reexpansion pulmonary edema occurring after thoracoscopic drainage of a pleural effusion. *J Clin Anesth* 1996; **8**: 591–4

46. Mahfood S, Hix WR, Aaron BL, et al. Reexpansion pulmonary edema. *Ann Thorac Surg* 1988; **45**: 340–5

47. Iqbal M, Multz AS, Rossoff LJ, et al. Reexpansion pulmonary edema after VATS successfully treated with continuous positive airway pressure. *Ann Thorac Surg* 2000; **70**: 669–71

48. Yanagidate F, Dohi S, Hamaya Y, et al. Reexpansion pulmonary edema after thoracoscopic mediastinal tumor resection. *Anesth Analg* 2001; **92**:m1416–7

49. American Thoracic Society Round Table Conference: acute lung injury. *Am J Resp Crit Care Med* 1998; **158**: 675–9

50. Acute Respiratory Distress Syndrome Network. Ventilation with lower tidal volumes as compared with traditional tidal volumes for acute lung injury and the acute respiratory distress syndrome. *N Engl J Med* 2000; **342**: 1301–8

51. Amato MBP, Barbas CSV, Medeiros DM, et al. Effect of a protective-ventilation strategy on mortality in the acute respiratory distress syndrome. *N Engl J Med* 1998; **338**: 347–54

52. Slinger P. Update on anesthetic management for pneumonectomy. *Curr Opin Anaesthesiol* 2009; **22**: 31–7

53. Slinger PD. Perioperative fluid management for thoracic surgery: the puzzle of postpneumonectomy pulmonary edema. *J Cardiothorac Vasc Anesth* 1995; **9**: 442–51

54. Davies RG, Myles PS, Graham JM. A comparison of the analgesic efficacy and side effects of paravertebral versus epidural blockade—a systematic review and meta-analysis of randomized trials. *Br J Anaesth* 2006; **96**: 418–26

55. Barker WL. Natural history of residual air spaces after pulmonary resection. *Chest Surg Clin N Am* 1996; **6**: 585–613

56. Abolhoda A, Liu D, Brooks A, et al. Prolonged air leak following radical upper lobectomy: an analysis of incidence and possible risk factors. *Chest* 1998; **113**: 1507–10

57. Cerfolio RJ. Recent advances in the treatment of air leaks. *Curr Opin Pulm Med* 2005; **11**: 319–23

58. Buettner A, McRae R, Myles PS, et al. Anaesthesia for bilateral lung volume reduction surgery. *Anaesth Intensive Care* 1999; **27**: 503–8

59. Venuta F, Rendina EA, De Giacomo T, et al. Technique to reduce air leaks after pulmonary lobectomy. *Eur J Cardiothorac Surg* 1998; **13**: 361–4

60. Otruba Z, Oxorn D. Lobar bronchial blockade in bronchopleural fistula. *Can J Anaesth* 1992; **39**: 176–8

61. Tietjen CS, Simon BA, Helfaer MA. Permissive hypercapnia with high-frequency oscillatory ventilation and one-lung isolation for intraoperative management of lung resection in a patient with multiple bronchopleural fistulae. *J Clin Anesth* 1997; **9**: 69–73

62. Baumann MH, Sahn SA. Medical management and therapy of bronchopleural fistulas in the mechanically ventilated patient. *Chest* 1990; **97**: 721–8

63. Algar FJ, Alvarez A, Aranda JL, et al. Prediction of early bronchopleural fistula after pneumonectomy: a multivariate analysis. *Ann Thorac Surg* 2001; **72**: 1662–7

64. Suzuki M, Otsuji M, Baba M, et al. Bronchopleural fistula after lung cancer surgery. Multivariate analysis of risk factors. *J Cardiovasc Surg (Torino)* 2002; **43**: 263–7

65. Ricci ZJ, Haramati LB, Rosenbaum AT, et al. Role of computed tomography in guiding the management of peripheral bronchopleural fistula. *J Thorac Imaging* 2002; **17**: 214–8

66. McCormick BA, Wilson IH, Berrisford RG. Bronchopleural fistula complicating group A beta-haemolytic streptococcal pneumonia. Use of a Fogarty embolectomy catheter for selective bronchial blockade. *Intensive Care Med* 1999; **25**: 535–7

67. Mulot A, Sepulveda S, Haberer JP, et al. Diagnosis of postpneumonectomy bronchopleural fistula using inhalation of oxygen or nitrous oxide. *Anesth Analg* 2002; **95**: 1122–3

68. Camazine B, Antkowiak JG, Nava ME, et al. Herpes simplex viral pneumonia in the postthoracotomy patient. *Chest* 1995; **108**: 876–9

69. Terzi A, Furlan G, Magnanelli G, et al. Chylothorax after pleuro-pulmonary surgery: a rare but unavoidable complication. *Thorac Cardiovasc Surg* 1994; **42**: 81–4

70. Le Pimpec-Barthes F, D'Attellis N, et al. Chylothorax complicating pulmonary resection. *Ann Thorac Surg* 2002; **73**: 1714–9

71. Karwande SV, Wolcott MW, Gay WA Jr. Postpneumonectomy tension chylothorax. *Ann Thorac Surg* 1986; **42**: 585–6

72. Riedel BJCJ, Vaporciyan AA. Unusual cause of dyspnea after pneumonectomy. *J Cardiothorac Vasc Anesth* 2003; **17**: 131–3

73. Buettiker V, Hug MI, Burger R, et al. Somatostatin: a new therapeutic option for the treatment of chylothorax. *Intensive Care Med* 2001; **27**: 1083–6

74. Kelly RF, Shumway SJ. Conservative management of postoperative chylothorax using somatostatin. *Ann Thorac Surg* 2000; **69**: 1944–5

75. Abbas Ael-S, Deschamps C. Postpneumonectomy empyema. *Curr Opin Pulm Med* 2002; **8**: 327–33

76. Icard P, Fleury JP, Regnard JF, et al. Utility of C-reactive protein measurements for empyema diagnosis after pneumonectomy. *Ann Thorac Surg* 1994; **57**: 933–6

77. Moore RA, Forsythe MJ, Niguidula FN, et al. Anesthesia for the patient with pulmonary lobar torsion. *Anesthesiology* 1982; **57**: 129–31

78. Cable DG, Deschamps C, Allen MS, et al. Lobar torsion after pulmonary resection: presentation and outcome. *J Thorac Cardiovasc Surg* 2001; **122**: 1091–3

79. Sung HK, Kim HK, Choi YH. Re-thoracoscopic surgery for middle lobe torsion after right upper lobectomy. *Eur J Cardiothorac Surg* 2012; **42**: 582–3

80. Alvarez JM, Bairstow BM, Tang C, et al. Post-lung resection pulmonary edema: a case for aggressive management. *J Cardiothorac Vasc Anesth* 1998; **12**: 199–205

81. Mehran RJ, Deslauriers J. Late complications. Postpneumonectomy syndrome. *Chest Surg Clin N Am* 1999; **9**: 655–73

82. Feins RH. Neurologic complications in thoracic surgery. *Chest Surg Clin N Am* 1998; **8**: 633–43

83. Gibson GJ. Diaphragmatic paresis: pathophysiology, clinical features, and investigation. *Thorax* 1989; **44**: 960–70

84. Kim MH, Eagle KA. Cardiac risk assessment in noncardiac thoracic surgery. *Semin Thorac Cardiovasc Surg* 2001; **13**: 137–46

85. Licker M, Spiliopoulos A, Frey JG, et al. Risk factors for early mortality and major complications following pneumonectomy for non-small cell carcinoma of the lung. *Chest* 2002; **121**: 1890–7

86. Peterffy A, Henze A. Peterffy A, et al. Haemorrhagic complications during pulmonary resection. A retrospective review of 1428 resections with 113 haemorrhagic episodes. *Scand J Thorac Cardiovasc Surg* 1983; **17**: 283–7

87. Graham DR, Kaplan D, Evans CC, et al. Diaphragmatic plication for unilateral diaphragmatic paralysis: a 10- year experience. *Ann Thorac Surg* 1990; **49**: 248–51

88. Hasegawa S, Isowa N, Bando T, et al. The inadvisability of thoracoscopic lung biopsy on patients with pulmonary hypertension. *Chest* 2002; **122**: 1067–8

89. Sloan SB, Weitz HH. Postoperative arrhythmias and conduction disorders. *Med Clin North Am* 2001; **85**: 1171–89

90. Ritchie AJ, Danton M, Gibbons JR. Prophylactic digitalisation in pulmonary surgery. *Thorax* 1992; **47**: 41–3

91. Amar D, Roistacher N, Burt M, et al. Clinical and echocardiographic correlates of symptomatic tachydysrhythmias after noncardiac thoracic surgery. *Chest* 1995; **108**: 349–54

92. Krowka MJ, Pairolero PC, Trastek VF, et al. Cardiac dysrhythmia following pneumonectomy. Clinical correlates and prognostic significance. *Chest* 1987; **91**: 490–5

93. Amar D, Zhang H, Shi W, et al. Brain natriuretic peptide and risk of atrial fibrillation after thoracic surgery. *J Thorac Cardiovasc Surg* 2012; **144**: 1249–53

94. Amar D, Roistacher N, Burt ME, et al. Effects of diltiazem versus digoxin on dysrhythmias and cardiac function after pneumonectomy. *Ann Thorac Surg* 1997; **63**: 1374–81

95. von Knorring J, Lepantalo M, Lindgren L, et al. Cardiac arrhythmias and myocardial ischemia after thoracotomy for lung cancer. *Ann Thorac Surg* 1992; **53**: 642–7

96. Harpole DH, Liptay MJ, DeCamp MM Jr, et al. Prospective analysis of pneumonectomy: risk factors for major morbidity and cardiac dysrhythmias. *Ann Thorac Surg* 1996; **61**: 977–82

97. Amar D, Zhang H, Roistacher N. The incidence and outcome of ventricular arrhythmias after noncardiac thoracic surgery. *Anesth Analg* 2002; **95**: 537–43

98. Van Mieghem W, Coolen L, Malysse I, et al. Amiodarone and the development of ARDS after lung surgery. *Chest* 1994; **105**: 1642–5

99. Bayliff CD, Massel DR, Inculet RI, et al. Propranolol for the prevention of postoperative arrhythmias in general thoracic surgery. *Ann Thorac Surg* 1999; **67**: 182–6

100. Van Mieghem W, Tits G, Demuynck K, et al. Verapamil as prophylactic treatment for atrial fibrillation after lung operations. *Ann Thorac Surg* 1996; **61**: 1083–5

101. Crystal E, Connolly SJ, Sleik K, et al. Interventions on prevention of postoperative atrial fibrillation in patients undergoing heart surgery: a meta-analysis. *Circulation* 2002; **106**: 75–80

102. MacNee W. Pathophysiology of cor pulmonale in chronic obstructive pulmonary disease. Part One. *Am J Respir Crit Care Med* 1994; **150**: 833–52

103. Reed CE, Spinale FG, Crawford FA Jr. Effect of pulmonary resection on right ventricular function. *Ann Thorac Surg* 1992; **53**: 578–82

104. Baisi A, Cioffi U, Nosotti M, et al. Intrapericardial left pneumonectomy after induction chemotherapy: the risk of cardiac herniation. *J Thorac Cardiovasc Surg* 2002; **123**: 1206–7

105. Baaijens PF, Hasenbos MA, Lacquet LK, et al. Cardiac herniation after pneumonectomy. *Acta Anaesthesiol Scand* 1992; **36**: 842–5

106. Self RJ, Vaughan RS. Acute cardiac herniation after radical pleuro-pneumonectomy. *Anaesthesia* 1999; **54**: 564–6

107. Rodenwaldt J, Lembcke AE, Wiese TH, et al. Postoperative dislocation of the heart after pneumonectomy. *Circulation* 2002; **105**: 49–50

108. Ziomek S, Read RC, Tobler HG et al. Thromboembolism in patients undergoing thoracotomy. *Ann Thorac Surg* 1993; **56**: 223–6

109. Brodsky JB, Brose WG, Cannon WB, et al. Systemic tumor embolism following thoracotomy partially masked by postoperative epidural analgesia. *J Cardiothorac Anesth* 1990; **4**: 95–6

110. Rogers ML, Henderson L, Mahajan RP, et al. Preliminary findings in the neurophysiological assessment of intercostal nerve injury during thoracotomy. *Eur J Cardiothorac Surg* 2002; **21**: 298–301

111. Rogers ML, Duffy JP. Surgical aspects of chronic post-thoracotomy pain. *Eur J Cardiothorac Surg* 2000; **18**: 711–6

112. Ochroch EA, Gottschalk A, Augostides J, et al. Long-term pain and activity during recovery from major thoracotomy using thoracic epidural analgesia. *Anesthesiology* 2002; **97**: 1234–44

113. Wang LP, Hauerberg J, Schmidt JF. Incidence of spinal epidural abscess after epidural analgesia. A national 1-year study. *Anesthesiology* 1999; **91**: 1928–36

114. Attar S, Hankins JR, Turney SZ, et al. Paraplegia after thoracotomy: report of five cases and review of the literature. *Ann Thorac Surg* 1995; **59**: 1410–5

CHAPTER 38

Pain relief after thoracic and cardiac surgery

Desmond P. McGlade and David A. Scott

Thoracic Surgery

Pain after both open thoracotomy and video-assisted thoracoscopic surgery (VATS) can be severe, and threaten recovery after surgery. Effective analgesia is likely to reduce postoperative complications, promote wound healing and limit the progression to chronic pain (1).

Patients undergoing thoracic surgery are often elderly, medically compromised, and predisposed to postoperative complications (2,3). Postoperative pain from the surgical wound, diaphragmatic irritation, and the drain tube site limit the patient's capacity to breathe deeply, cough and mobilize, thereby promoting pulmonary atelectasis and infection. Although thoracic epidural analgesia (TEA) is the standard against which other analgesia techniques are compared (4), concerns regarding potential risks and side-effects have encouraged other options, including thoracic paravertebral block (TPVB) (5,6) (table 38.1).

Nociceptive pathways

Nociceptive signals originating from the chest wall and parietal pleura travel via small myelinated afferents along the intercostal nerves, and are perceived as pain accurately localized to the source, such as a lateral thoracotomy incision, porthole sites for VATS, or drain tubes. Intercostal nerves can be severed during incision, suffer crush injury during rib retraction, or needle penetration (7,8).

Nociceptive afferent transmission from the lungs and the visceral pleura are conducted via unmyelinated C fibres that communicate with the vagus nerve and the thoracic sympathetic chain (T1–T4) via neural plexuses around the hilum of the lung. Pain from these structures is poorly localized. The diaphragm and its associated pleura have a dual nerve supply. Nociception from its peripheral portion is transmitted via the sixth to twelfth intercostal nerves. Nociception from its central portion is via the phrenic nerve, which arises from the third to fifth cervical (C3–C5) nerve roots (9); thus associated pain is somatically referred to dermatomes of the ipsilateral shoulder.

Thoracic epidural analgesia

The optimal level for placement of an epidural catheter to cover a thoracotomy incision is between T4 and T7 (10). Angulation of the vertebral spinous processes is significant at the mid-thoracic level, complicating epidural space location. The paramedian approach avoids negotiating the space between the spinous processes, although in elderly patients osteophyte growth into the lateral aspects of the ligamentum flavum may provide a barrier to paramedian needle access. The paramedian approach may be more uncomfortable for the patient and may have a higher risk of striking the predominantly ventral epidural veins (11).

Hypotension from sympathetic blockade and urinary retention remain significant side effects of TEA (12,13). Local anaesthetics are administered in low dose and concentration (e.g. bupivacaine 1 mg/mL or ropivacaine 2 mg/mL) to minimize side effects such as hypotension and muscle weakness, and opioids, such as morphine, hydromorphone, fentanyl, or sufentanil, are added to improve analgesia (14).

Frequent opioid-related side effects include pruritus and urinary retention. Opioid-induced ventilatory impairment (OIVI), a combination of sedation, respiratory depression, and upper airway obstruction, is less frequent but clinically important (15). This may be caused by systemic absorption of lipophilic opioids (fentanyl, sufentanil) or cephalad spread of hydrophilic opioids (morphine, hydromorphone) within the cerebrospinal fluid (CSF). Other additives to epidural infusions to improve the quality of analgesia include alpha-2 adrenoceptor agonists such as clonidine or adrenaline (epinephrine) at typical concentrations of 2μg/mL (16).

Epidural analgesia is not directly able to reduce the pain associated with diaphragmatic irritation secondary to surgical trauma or drain tube placement.

Respiratory effects

Forced vital capacity (FVC) and functional residual capacity (FRC) decrease by 40% following lateral thoracotomy, and take at least two weeks to recover (17–19). Although dense motor block from TEA impairs intercostal muscle contractility and reduces respiratory capacity, low concentrations of local anaesthetics do not impair respiratory function in those with severe obstructive pulmonary disease (19). Following thoracotomy, TEA preserves tidal volume and vital capacity when compared with systemic analgesia (20).

Cardiovascular effects

An extensive epidural block from T1 to T12 significantly impairs sympathetic outflow resulting in hypotension and a reduction in systemic vascular resistance (12). Major surgery and postoperative

Table 38.1 Summary of analgesia techniques

Regional analgesia techniques	Thoracic epidural analgesia; Thoracic paravertebral block; Lumbar epidural analgesia; Intrathecal opioid analgesia; Intercostal nerve block; Interpleural analgesia
	Phrenic nerve infiltration
Systemic analgesia	Opioids
	Non-opioid (paracetamol, NSAIDs, coxibs, tramadol, gabapentin, ketamine)
Non-pharmacological	Transcutaneous electrical nerve stimulation
	Cryoanalgesia

pain produce a neuroendocrine stress response characterized by increases in sympathetic activity, heart rate and myocardial work, and increases the risk of postoperative myocardial ischaemia and arrhythmias. TEA has beneficial effects on myocardial perfusion (21), and compared with non-epidural techniques is associated with a lower incidence of myocardial infarction (22) and atrial fibrillation after both thoracotomy and VATS (23,24).

Risks of epidural analgesia

Side effects associated with TEA include hypotension and motor block from the local anaesthestic, and opioid-related nausea, pruritis, and sedation, leading to OIVI. Careful and regular patient assessments will identify these problems, which generally respond to adjusting the rate of infusion, administering intravenous fluids, or prescribing naloxone, vasopressors, or antiemetics as indicated. Complications related to the insertion technique are uncommon but potentially serious. The incidence of dural puncture or direct

needle injury to the spinal cord and adjacent neural structures is low at a mid-thoracic level (25). Even so, most clinicians advocate that epidural placement at a level above the termination of the spinal cord should only be performed in conscious patients.

Epidural haematoma

The use of anticoagulant drugs influences the decision and timing of epidural catheter placement and removal. Epidural vessel trauma at the time of instrumentation is not uncommon and usually benign; however, should back pain or neurological signs emerge, early diagnosis and management of an epidural haematoma is critical. The American Society of Regional Anesthesia provides a consensus statement that summarizes current guidelines (26).

Epidural infection

Skin infection at the epidural insertion site and catheter contamination are not uncommon, but usually do not progress to serious deep-seated infection (27). The incidence of epidural abscess in association with epidural analgesia is around 1:10 000 (28), but risk is increased with the duration of TEA, insertion site infection, and patient comorbidity (29). Following thoracic surgery, epidural analgesia is often of benefit for at least 72 hours, or until chest drain removal. Prolonged air leaks and chest drain placement are not uncommon following lung resection and the clinician should make an informed assessment of the risks and benefits justifying a decision for ongoing TEA.

Thoracic paravertebral block

The thoracic paravertebral space is situated adjacent to the thoracic vertebral column (see figure 38.1). The parietal pleura forms the anterolateral boundary, the vertebral body and intervertebral

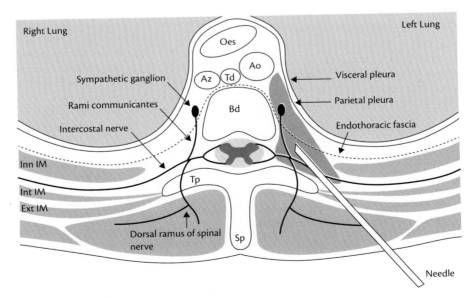

Fig. 38.1 Schematic representation of the paravertebral space with approaching needle and surrounding vertebral body (Bd), transverse process (Tp), and spinous process (Sp). The aorta (Ao), thoracic duct (Td), azygous vein (Az), and oesophagus (Oes) sit anteriorly and innermost (Inn IM), internal (Int IM), and external (Ext IM) intercostal muscles laterally. The blue area represents the paravertebral space and likely extent of spread of anaesthesia. The superior costotransverse ligament is out of view in this cross-section but blends laterally with the external and internal intercostal muscle/membrane complex as they attach to the transverse process. Here, the paravertebral space merges with the intercostal space.

Reproduced from Cowie B, et al., 'Ultrasound-guided thoracic paravertebral blockade: a cadaveric study', Anesthesia Analgesia, 110, pp. 1735–1739, Copyright 2010, with permission from International Anesthesia Research Society.

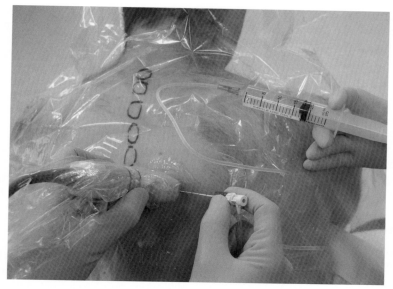

Fig. 38.2 Ultrasound probe and in-plane Tuohy needle angled from lateral to medial at the mid thoracic region for a right paravertebral block.

disc form the medial boundary, and the superior costotransverse ligament forms the posterior boundary (30). This space communicates with the intercostal spaces laterally and with the epidural space via the intervertebral foraminae medially.

The contents of the paravertebral space include the spinal nerves, the grey and white rami communicantes of the sympathetic chain, and the sympathetic ganglia. The endothoracic fascia lines the inside of the thorax and divides the space into two compartments: an anterior 'extrapleural' compartment containing the sympathetic chain, and a posterior compartment containing the spinal nerves. Local anaesthetic deposited into the anterior compartment may not penetrate effectively to the spinal nerves situated within the posterior compartment (31). Cadaveric work has

demonstrated complex spread of injectate within the space, with lateral spread into adjacent intercostal spaces, medial spread into the epidural space, and distal spread between adjacent intercostal spaces. This may explain the variability observed in the clinical response with TPVB (32).

Techniques of thoracic paravertebral block
Percutaneous insertion

A needle is inserted 2.5 cm lateral to the midline in a perpendicular direction to the skin until contact with the transverse process, usually at a depth of 1 cm less than the depth of the thoracic vertebral lamina. The needle is then redirected either

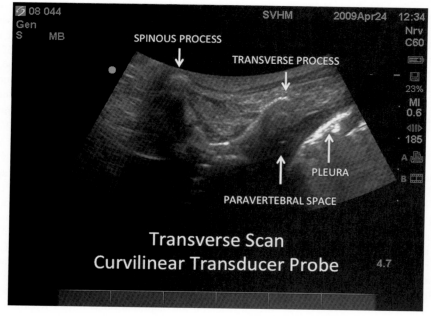

Fig. 38.3 Ultrasound image of the paravertebral space demonstrating the relationships of the spinous process, transverse process, distinct parietal pleura and underlying lung; the paravertebral space lies anterior to the transverse process.

cranially or caudally and inserted a further 1 cm to penetrate the costotransverse ligament. Loss of resistance techniques or the use of a peripheral nerve stimulator have also been described (33,34).

Open insertion

TPVB and catheter placement is possible under direct vision at the time of VATS or thoracotomy, and can be done by the anaesthetist or surgeon. A Tuohy needle is introduced from outside the posterolateral aspect of the chest wall. Without breaching the pleura internally, hydrodissection through the Tuohy needle is used to create an extrapleural pocket along the heads of the ribs at the lateral border of the paravertebral space into which a catheter is positioned (35).

Ultrasound-guided insertion

Several techniques for ultrasound-guided TPVB have been described using both in-plane and out-of-plane approaches (see figure 38.2 and figure 38.3). An advantage of ultrasound is visual confirmation of the hydrodissection (pleural displacement) with injection (36).

Unlike the epidural space, the paravertebral space is not as amenable to catheter threading. Placement more than 3 cm beyond the needle tip can result in the catheter positioning laterally into an intercostal space, medially into the epidural space or anteriorly beyond the paravertebral space (37).

Analgesic drugs used for paravertebral block

In general a 15 mL local anaesthetic bolus will spread to cover at least three dermatomes (33,38). Pharmacokinetic studies show that peak plasma levels are achieved at 25 minutes following a bolus, and plasma levels increase with infusion to reach a maximum level at 48 hours (39). The addition of epinephrine (adrenaline) lowers the peak plasma level achieved after a bolus dose of bupivacaine. There is no evidence that the addition of other adjuvants produce analgesic any benefit in TPVB.

Precautions

Paravertebral blocks do not involve a needle entering the neuraxis, but they are still relatively contraindicated in anticoagulated or coagulopathic patients. Local anaesthetic injected via a paravertebral catheter may also enter the epidural space, resulting in inadvertent epidural block.

Despite the widespread acceptance of TEA, reservations regarding its practice remain. TEA has a significant side effect profile, there is the tendency to manage hypotension primarily with volume replacement, and the potential for neurological complications exists. A meta-analysis comparing TEA with TPVB for thoracotomy showed no difference in pain scores or the consumption of other analgesics, and patients receiving TPVB demonstrated improved postoperative pulmonary function and fewer pulmonary complications (13). Perioperative stress response is reduced with TPVB (40) and the incidence of urinary retention and hypotension is less. The placement of paravertebral catheters may be safer than epidural catheters because they can be placed under direct vision from inside the chest or by ultrasound, which enables real-time needle visualization.

The shift towards VATS has generated interest in analgesia alternatives to TEA. TPVB has excellent analgesia efficacy with low risk and may be the preferred regional analgesia technique following VATS (6), where it has been shown to produce superior analgesia in the immediate postoperative period (41) and reduce postoperative opioid consumption (42,43) when compared with IV morphine alone.

Other regional analgesia techniques

Lumbar epidural opioids

Lumbar epidural opioids are more effective than parenteral opioids following thoracotomy (44,45), and as effective as hydrophilic thoracic epidural opioids (46). But expert opinion does not recommend lumbar epidural opioids as a first choice for pain relief following thoracotomy (47,48).

Intrathecal opioids

Up to 24 hours of postoperative analgesia can be obtained from a single dose of lumbar intrathecal morphine (49), making it a suitable option post-VATS. The finite duration means that transition to another analgesia technique is required at a time when postoperative pain may still be intense. Increasing the dose in order to increase the duration places the patient at risk of OIVI and other side effects like nausea, vomiting, pruritus, thermoregulatory dysfunction, and urinary retention (50).

Intercostal nerve block

Intercostal nerve block will not cover the dorsal ramus of the intercostal nerve and may be inadequate to fully cover a posterolateral thoracotomy incision. Sensory overlap of segmental innervation means that intercostal nerves above and below the level of the incision should also be blocked.

Intercostal blocks provide better analgesia than systemic opioids alone, particularly during the first postoperative day (51). Segmental analgesia can last up to 18 hours following a single injection of 0.5% bupivacaine (52). The finite duration following a single injection necessitates repeated blocks, typically every 12 hours, to maintain analgesia efficacy postoperatively (53). The use of an indwelling catheter inserted prior to chest closure provides an option for prolonged analgesia (54,55). Intercostal blocks may also be used to reduce pain at drain tube sites.

Risks of intercostal blocks include pneumothorax (not usually an issue when performed on an operated chest) and local anaesthetic toxicity from rapid systemic absorption. Maximum dose recommendations should be adhered to.

Interpleural block

A catheter can be placed into the pleural space prior to chest closure and its tip positioned posteriorly in the costovertebral gutter adjacent to the intercostal space at the level of the incision. Bupivacaine with or without epinephrine (adrenaline) has been used by bolus of up to 20 mLor at infusion rates of from 5 to 7 mL/hr, blocking approximately four to five dermatomes (56). The chest tube should be clamped following bolus administration (57). When patients recuperate in the upright position, local anaesthetic may gravitate and preferentially block the lower intercostal nerves, and pooling on the diaphragm may impair respiratory function. For these and other reasons interpleural block is not recommended for thoracotomy (47,48).

Systemic analgesia

Systemic analgesics can be used as the primary analgesia technique or as an adjunct to a regional technique. Systemic analgesics are also needed to maintain pain relief when regional techniques are discontinued or should they prove inadequate.

Opioids

Systemic opioids may be unable to provide satisfactory analgesia without causing OIVI. Opioids are appropriate following VATS, where incisions are small and postoperative pain is less intense. Interindividual variability with opioid responsiveness is best managed with IV patient-controlled analgesia (PCA). Systemic opioids typically provide adequate analgesia at rest but pain scores on movement and indices of function are consistently better with regional analgesia (58–60). Opioid analgesia is not without its side-effects, with up to 1% of patients receiving IV PCA having an adverse event related to OIVI. Therefore appropriate dosing, assessment and monitoring of these patients must be undertaken (15).

Non-steroidal anti-inflammatory drugs (nsaids)

NSAIDs are non-sedating and do not depress respiratory drive. They are suitable analgesic adjuvants following thoracic surgery, where they significantly reduce the use of systemic (61), and epidural (62) opioids, and improve the quality of TEA (63). NSAIDs can also be used to treat referred shoulder pain, which is typically resistant to regional analgesia techniques. The risk of perioperative renal failure is a concern considering the restrictive fluid management that is practiced by many thoracic surgical units. The use of NSAIDs and Cox-2-selective drugs (coxibs) in patients with ischaemic heart disease presents an issue because of their association with arterial thrombosis, although an increased risk with short-term perioperative use in noncardiac surgical patients has not been demonstrated (64,65).

Other analgesics

Following thoracotomy, ketamine produces a 45% decrease in systemic morphine consumption and a reduced incidence of opioid-related side effects (66). IV ketamine can be a useful adjunct to TEA (67) and may decrease long-term pain following thoracotomy (68). When given in low doses, ketamine can reduce morphine consumption and improve analgesia in opioid-tolerant patients (69,70). The potential for confusion, sedation, or hallucinations requires careful observation and dose titration, typically keeping ketamine infusions around 0.1–0.2 mg/kg/hr.

Tramadol, an analgesic with both opioid and non-opioid mechanisms of action, has limited data specifically available for its use thoracic surgery. Tramadol infusions decrease postoperative systemic morphine requirements and may provide comparable analgesia to epidural morphine (71). Side effects include nausea and vomiting, and confusion in the elderly.

Paracetamol (acetaminophen) is a weak analgesic that is well tolerated in conventional doses. Regular (6 hourly) administration following thoracotomy is recommended and can be used to decrease ipsilateral shoulder pain in patients receiving TEA (72).

Gabapentin is ineffective in managing shoulder pain in patients receiving TEA and produces increased sedation (73). In general,

both gabapentin and pregabalin are effective in reducing postoperative opioid requirements and some opioid-related side effects such as vomiting and pruritus (74–76). They may have a role in treating, but not preventing long-term post-thoracotomy pain (68,77). Caution should be used with these drugs in the elderly as they can produce mild sedation, dizziness and ataxia.

Non-pharmacological techniques

Cryoablation

Cryoanalgesia has been largely abandoned with the increasing popularity of regional techniques such as TEA and TPVB. Concerns persist regarding induced neuralgia associated with nerve regrowth, typically beginning at around 6 weeks and lasting six months or longer (78,79). This may be experienced as hyperalgesia and burning or shooting pains in the distribution of the nerve and is typically associated with some persistent numbness.

Shoulder pain

Ipsilateral shoulder pain remains a significant problem affecting most patients following thoracic surgery (72,80). It occurs after both open and thoracoscopic surgery and is more common when a major bronchus has been transected (81). The pain is described as aching in quality, vaguely localized around the shoulder, and is usually unrelated to movement. It is most intense over the first 48 hours following surgery and typically lasts from 2 to 4 days (82). It is resistant to epidural and paravertebral blocks (83), although systemic absorption of epidural opioid may help.

The phrenic nerve is believed to convey most of the nociceptive afferents responsible and its infiltration with local anaesthetic can reduce shoulder pain (80). Diaphragmatic irritation from blood, air or the presence of a chest drain may be the cause, but interpleural local anaesthetic administered to 'pool' on the diaphragm had no effect on the incidence or severity of this pain (84). The role of a chest drain positioned in the apex of the hemithorax has also been suggested and its withdrawal a few centimetres recommended. Local anaesthetic blocks around the neck, such as interscalene brachial plexus block (85) and stellate ganglion block (85), have been used to treat shoulder pain. Both of these blocks can inadvertently block the phrenic nerve, which could explain their efficacy. Most clinicians manage shoulder pain with a multimodal strategy. NSAIDs (83) and paracetamol are effective (72), whereas gabapentin is not (73).

Pre-emptive analgesia and chronic pain states

Chronic post-thoracotomy pain is common, and is defined as pain in the general area of the incision that persists for 2 to 3 months following surgery. It is typically continuous, dysaesthetic, burning, or aching. In one series more than 50% of patients reported painful symptoms one year postoperatively (86), with up to 10% of patients having persistent pain of sufficient severity to impede their activities or require ongoing strong analgesia. Persistent pain can also follow VATS (8,88).

Intercostal nerve damage is implicated in the development of neuropathic pain (7,89). Other possible causes are costochondral and costovertebral disarticulation from extensive rib retraction, and the division of serratus anterior and latissimus dorsi muscles.

Patients who suffer severe acute postoperative pain following thoracotomy are more likely to progress to chronic pain (87). This has stimulated interest in aggressive perioperative pain management in order to minimize long-term pain (88). Although some studies have demonstrated a benefit of pre-emptive analgesia with epidural (89) and paravertebral techniques (93), results have been inconsistent (1,94). Muscle-sparing incisions, such as those not dividing the latissumus dorsi, do not seem to have a benefit (90). Ketamine and pregabalin, which have been shown to be effective in non-thoracic surgical pain (91), may prove to be of benefit (68).

Cardiac surgery and sternotomy

Cardiac surgery is usually performed via a median sternotomy, which is the main source of early postoperative pain. Other sources may include mammary artery and other conduit harvest sites, costochondral disruption produced by sternal retraction, surgical trauma to the pleura and pericardium, and subcostal chest drain sites. Other causes of pain after cardiac surgery must be always considered, such as myocardial ischaemia, early pericarditis, and gastritis or peptic ulceration.

The thoracic intercostal nerves from T2 to T6 innervate the sternum, overlying skin and subcutaneous tissues, and the adjacent parietal pleura. Innervation of the pericardium is via the phrenic and vagus nerves and the sympathetic afferents.

Typically, emergence from anaesthesia following cardiac surgery often takes place over several hours as the residual effects of large-dose opioids gradually diminish. This may add to the perception that the pain from median sternotomy is less intense than that from lateral thoracotomy. Nevertheless, pulmonary function decreases following sternotomy and is associated with impaired mechanics, intrapulmonary shunting, and reduced oxygenation (92). Despite this, evidence that improved perioperative analgesia decreases pulmonary complications following sternotomy is limited (93,94).

An argument for aggressive analgesia in the early postoperative period is to limit the progression to long-term post-sternotomy pain, which is reported at rates of 25% at 2 months (95) and from to 14% to 35% at 1 year (96,97).

Systemic analgesics

Opioid analgesia

Opioid analgesia is widely used following sternotomy and is generally administered by PCA or nurse-administered techniques (98,99), with the latter probably providing better analgesia and reduced pulmonary atelectasis (100). PCA has the advantage of reducing the nursing workload. A comparison between different opioids found little difference in the degree of pain relief each provided and only minor differences in the side effect profiles (101). In opioid-naïve patients, there is no significant benefit with the addition of a background infusion of morphine when used in conjunction with PCA (102).

Non-opioid analgesia

NSAIDs and coxibs are non-sedating analgesics that are effective and produce a significant opioid-sparing effect following cardiac surgery (103–105). However, in the context of cardiac surgery, both classes possess a significant side-effect profile. Both may impair perioperative renal function and NSAIDs can produce gastritis and platelet dysfunction. IV parecoxib, a prodrug of valdecoxib, followed by oral valdecoxib, has been associated with increased sternal wound infection (105) and thrombovascular events following cardiac surgery, including myocardial infarction (106). These drugs should therefore not be used in patients undergoing coronary revascularization. Population studies suggest that even medium-term use of both NSAIDs and coxibs is associated with increased risk of death and recurrent myocardial infarction in patients who have had prior myocardial infarction (107), although analysis of clinical trials of short-term use in noncardiac surgery found no evidence for increased cardiac risk (65).

Regular IV paracetamol can be an effective component of a multimodal analgesia regimen after cardiac surgery (104,108). Ketamine is also effective (109), but it is best reserved for those with chronic pain or opioid tolerance because of its psychotomimetic side effects (110). Tramadol is also efficacious (111,112).

Gabapentin reduces the requirement for tramadol (113) and morphine (114), but not fentanyl (115) after cardiac surgery. Gabapentin, given perioperatively, does not seem to reduce the incidence or degree of post-sternotomy pain at 1 and 3 months (113), but is superior to NSAIDs in the treatment of established chronic post-sternotomy pain after cardiac surgery (116).

Neuraxial analgesia techniques

Thoracic epidural analgesia

High thoracic epidural block can lead to decreased time to tracheal extubation, better pain scores and postoperative respiratory function, decreased risk of supraventricular arrhythmias and improved psychological recovery after cardiac surgery (117). There is no evidence that TEA alters ischaemic outcomes, shortens ICU or hospital stay, or alters the progression to chronic pain (95,118).

The optimal level of epidural insertion is between T1 and T3, and with a preferential spread rostrally (119), the desired dermatomal coverage of T1 and T6 is achieved.

A concern amongst clinicians has been the instrumentation of the epidural space in the context of subsequent high-dose heparinization and the risk of neuraxial haematoma. Many caveats have been placed on the timing of catheter insertion and removal in relation to surgery, the management of difficult or bloody epidural insertions, and the degree of perioperative surveillance required to ensure safety (26). Recent opinion suggests that when meticulously managed, the rate of complications from epidural catheterization in the context of cardiac surgery is no greater than that with non-cardiac surgery (120), although this remains controversial.

Intrathecal opioid analgesia

Intrathecal morphine has the advantage of producing potent, relatively long-acting analgesia following single-dose administration. Although the potential risk of neuraxial haematoma is considered to be less than that following epidural instrumentation, single shot lumbar injection still carries a finite risk of spinal haematoma (121). Intrathecal morphine can result in dose-dependent prolonged postoperative ventilation and difficulty in facilitating fast-track cardiac anaesthesia. Common side effects with intrathecal opioid use include nausea, vomiting, and pruritus, and there is the potential for delayed respiratory depression following extubation. Many units describe extensive and successful experience with this technique using morphine doses up to 500 µg (122).

Other regional analgesia techniques

Large volumes of dilute levobupivacaine injected around the sternotomy wound and into the mediastinal drains at the end of surgery can result in less sedation during the first 4 hours and less morphine consumption during the first 24 hours postoperatively, but no difference in pain scores or time to extubation (123), although oxygenation was improved at the time of extubation (124). Wound catheters placed at the lateral edges of the sternum infusing 0.2% ropivacaine at 4 mL/hr for 48 hours have been shown to reduce morphine consumption postoperatively and improve analgesia (125); however, these must be inserted carefully if done after sternal closure as damage to mediastinal structures can occur, including to the right ventricle (unpublished case data).

Bilateral intercostal nerve blocks from T1 to T12 using 20 mL of 0.2% ropivacaine followed by continuous infusion for 48 hours via a sternal wound catheter was shown to significantly reduce morphine consumption and hospital stay (126).

Progression of analgesia

The stability of the sternal repair, effective physiotherapy, and resumption of bowel function usually means that many patients can transition from parenteral to oral analgesia within 48 hours after surgery. Oral opioids should be minimized, although pain from the leg wounds may require ongoing analgesia to encourage ambulation. Paracetamol should be continued; NSAIDs are best limited to short-term use.

Conclusion

Effective pain relief after cardiothoracic surgery is best achieved with a multimodal analgesic regimen, sometimes including a neuraxial or paravertebral block. This will optimize respiratory function, reduce the need for ventilatory support and enhance a good recovery after surgery.

References

1. Conacher ID. Pre-emptive analgesia and the paravertebral space—an ignis fatuus. *Br J Anaesth* 2006; **96**(5): 667–8
2. McNicol L, Story DA, Leslie K, et al. Postoperative complications and mortality in older patients having non-cardiac surgery at three Melbourne teaching hospitals. *Med J Aust* 2007 ; **186**(9): 447–52
3. Licker M, de Perrot M, Hohn L, et al. Perioperative mortality and major cardio-pulmonary complications after lung surgery for non-small cell carcinoma. *Eur J Cardiothorac Surg* 1999;**15**(3): 314–9
4. Conacher ID. Post-thoracotomy analgesia. *Anesthesiol Clin N Am* 2001; **19**(3): 611–25
5. Conlon NP, Shaw AD, Grichnik KP. Postthoracotomy paravertebral analgesia: will it replace epidural analgesia? *Anesthesiol Clin* 2008; **26**(2): 369–80
6. Daly DJ, Myles PS. Update on the role of paravertebral blocks for thoracic surgery: are they worth it? *Curr Opin Anaesthesiol* 2009; **22**(1): 38–43
7. Rogers ML, Duffy JP. Surgical aspects of chronic post-thoracotomy pain. *Eur J Cardiothorac Surg* 2000; **18**(6): 711–6
8. Landreneau RJ, Mack MJ, Hazelrigg SR, et al. Prevalence of chronic pain after pulmonary resection by thoracotomy or video-assisted thoracic surgery. *J Thorac Cardiovasc Surg* 1994; **107**(4): 1079–85
9. Katz J, Renck, H. *Handbook of Thoraco-Abdominal Nerve Block.* Orlando, FL: Grune and Stratton Inc., 1987
10. Visser WA, Lee RA, Gielen MJ. Factors affecting the distribution of neural blockade by local anesthetics in epidural anesthesia and a comparison of lumbar versus thoracic epidural anesthesia. *Anesth Analg* 2008; **107**(2): 708–21
11. Hogan Q, Toth J. Anatomy of soft tissues of the spinal canal. *Reg Anesth Pain Med* 1999; **24**(4): 303–10
12. Veering BT, Cousins MJ. Cardiovascular and pulmonary effects of epidural anaesthesia. *Anaesth Intensive Care* 2000; **28**(6): 620–35
13. Davies RG, Myles PS, Graham JM. A comparison of the analgesic efficacy and side-effects of paravertebral vs epidural blockade for thoracotomy—a systematic review and meta-analysis of randomized trials. *Br J Anaesth* 2006; **96**(4): 418–26
14. Scott DA, Blake D, Buckland M, et al. A comparison of epidural ropivacaine infusion alone and in combination with 1, 2, and 4 microg/mL fentanyl for seventy-two hours of postoperative analgesia after major abdominal surgery. *Anesth Analg* 1999; **88**(4): 857–64
15. Macintyre PE, Loadsman JA, Scott DA. Opioids, ventilation and acute pain management. *Anaesth Intensive Care* 2011; **39**(4): 545–58
16. Schug SA, Saunders D, Kurowski I, Paech MJ. Neuraxial drug administration: a review of treatment options for anaesthesia and analgesia. *CNS Drugs* 2006; **20**(11): 917–33
17. Slinger PD, McRae K. Regional anesthesia for thoracotomy. In: Chaney MA, ed. *Regional Anesthesia for Cardiothoracic Surgery.* Philadelphia: Lippincott Williams & Wilkins, 2002; 111–38
18. Craig DB. Postoperative recovery of pulmonary function. *Anesth Analg* 1981; **60**(1): 46–52
19. Gruber EM, Tschernko EM, Kritzinger M, et al. The effects of thoracic epidural analgesia with bupivacaine 0.25% on ventilatory mechanics in patients with severe chronic obstructive pulmonary disease. *Anesth Analg* 2001;,**92**(4): 1015–9
20. Fratacci MD, Kimball WR, Wain JC, Kacmarek RM, Polaner DM, Zapol WM. Diaphragmatic shortening after thoracic surgery in humans. Effects of mechanical ventilation and thoracic epidural anesthesia. *Anesthesiology* 1993; **79**(4): 654–65
21. Nygard E, Kofoed KF, Freiberg J, et al. Effects of high thoracic epidural analgesia on myocardial blood flow in patients with ischemic heart disease. *Circulation* 2005; **111**(17): 2165–70
22. Beattie WS, Badner NH, Choi P. Epidural analgesia reduces postoperative myocardial infarction: a meta-analysis. *Anesth Analg* 2001; **93**(4): 853–8
23. Oka T, Ozawa Y, Ohkubo Y. Thoracic epidural bupivacaine attenuates supraventricular tachyarrhythmias after pulmonary resection. *Anesth Analg* 2001; **93**(2): 253–9
24. Neustein SM, Kahn P, Krellenstein DJ, Cohen E. Incidence of arrhythmias after thoracic surgery: thoracotomy versus video-assisted thoracoscopy. *J Cardiothorac Vasc Anesth* 1998; **12**(6): 659–61
25. Giebler RM, Scherer RU, Peters J. Incidence of neurologic complications related to thoracic epidural catheterization. *Anesthesiology* 1997; **86**(1): 55–63
26. Horlocker TT, Wedel DJ, Rowlingson JC, et al. Regional anesthesia in the patient receiving antithrombotic or thrombolytic therapy: American Society of Regional Anesthesia and Pain Medicine Evidence-Based Guidelines (third edition). *Reg Anesth Pain Med* 2010; **35**(1): 64–101
27. Simpson RS, Macintyre PE, Shaw D, Norton A, McCann JR, Tham EJ. Epidural catheter tip cultures: results of a 4-year audit and implications for clinical practice. *Reg Anesth Pain Med.* 2000; **25**(4): 360–7
28. Richman JM, Wu CL. Epidural analgesia for postoperative pain. *Anesthesiol Clin N Am* 2005; **23**(1): 125–40
29. Cameron CM, Scott DA, McDonald WM, Davies MJ. A review of neuraxial epidural morbidity: experience of more than 8,000 cases at a single teaching hospital. *Anesthesiology* 2007; **106**(5): 997–1002
30. Karmakar MK. Thoracic paravertebral block. *Anesthesiology* 2001; **95**(3): 771–80
31. Karmakar MK, Chung DC. Variability of a thoracic paravertebral block. Are we ignoring the endothoracic fascia? *Reg Anesth Pain Med* 2000; **25**(3): 325–7
32. Cowie B, McGlade D, Ivanusic J, Barrington MJ. Ultrasound-guided thoracic paravertebral blockade: a cadaveric study. *Anesth Analg* 2010 1; **110**(6): 1735–9

33. Richardson J, Lonnqvist PA. Thoracic paravertebral block. *Br J Anaesth* 1998; **81**(2)230–8.

34. Lang SA. The use of a nerve stimulator for thoracic paravertebral block. *Anesthesiology* 2002 **97**(2): 521; author reply –2

35. Sabanathan S, Richardson J, Shah R. Continuous intercostal nerve block for pain relief after thoracotomy. Updated in 1995. *Ann Thorac Surg* 1995; **59**(5): 1261–3

36. Renes SH, Bruhn J, Gielen MJ, Scheffer GJ, van Geffen GJ. In-plane ultrasound-guided thoracic paravertebral block: a preliminary report of 36 cases with radiologic confirmation of catheter position. *Reg Anesth Pain Med* 2010; **35**(2): 212–6

37. Luyet C, Herrmann G, Ross S, et al. Ultrasound-guided thoracic paravertebral puncture and placement of catheters in human cadavers: where do catheters go? *Br J Anaesth* 2011; **106**(2): 246–54

38. Casati A, Alessandrini P, Nuzzi M, et al. A prospective, randomized, blinded comparison between continuous thoracic paravertebral and epidural infusion of 0.2% ropivacaine after lung resection surgery. *Eur J Anaesthesiol* 2006; **23**(12): 999–1004

39. Berrisford RG, Sabanathan S, Mearns AJ, Clarke BJ, Hamdi A. Plasma concentrations of bupivacaine and its enantiomers during continuous extrapleural intercostal nerve block. *Br J Anaesth* 1993; **70**(2): 201–4

40. Richardson J, Sabanathan S, Jones J, Shah RD, Cheema S, Mearns AJ. A prospective, randomized comparison of preoperative and continuous balanced epidural or paravertebral bupivacaine on post-thoracotomy pain, pulmonary function and stress responses. *Br J Anaesth* 1999; **83**(3): 387–92

41. Vogt A, Stieger DS, Theurillat C, Curatolo M. Single-injection thoracic paravertebral block for postoperative pain treatment after thoracoscopic surgery. *Br J Anaesth* 2005; **95**(6): 816–21

42. Kaya FN, Turker G, Basagan-Mogol E, Goren S, Bayram S, Gebitekin C. Preoperative multiple-injection thoracic paravertebral blocks reduce postoperative pain and analgesic requirements after video-assisted thoracic surgery. *J Cardiothorac Vasc Anesth* 2006; **20**(5): 639–43

43. Hill SE, Keller RA, Stafford-Smith M, et al. Efficacy of single-dose, multilevel paravertebral nerve blockade for analgesia after thoracoscopic procedures. *Anesthesiology* 2006; **104**(5): 1047–53

44. Baxter AD, Laganiere S, Samson B, Stewart J, Hull K, Goernert L. A comparison of lumbar epidural and intravenous fentanyl infusions for post-thoracotomy analgesia. *Can J Anaesth* 1994; **41**(3): 184–91

45. Grant RP, Dolman JF, Harper JA, et al. Patient-controlled lumbar epidural fentanyl compared with patient-controlled intravenous fentanyl for post-thoracotomy pain. *Can J Anaesth* 1992; **39**(3): 214–9

46. Bouchard F, Drolet P. Thoracic versus lumbar administration of fentanyl using patient-controlled epidural after thoracotomy. *Reg Anesth* 1995; **20**(5): 385–8

47. PROSPECT. Procedure Specific Postoperative Pain Management. Available from: http://www.postoppain.org (accessed 2 June 2014)

48. Joshi GP, Bonnet F, Shah R, et al. A systematic review of randomized trials evaluating regional techniques for postthoracotomy analgesia. *Anesth Analg* 2008; **107**(3): 1026–40

49. Neustein SM, Cohen E. Intrathecal morphine during thoracotomy, Part II: Effect on postoperative meperidine requirements and pulmonary function tests. *J Cardiothorac Vasc Anesth.* 1993; **7**(2): 157–9

50. Gehling M, Tryba M. Risks and side-effects of intrathecal morphine combined with spinal anaesthesia: a meta-analysis. *Anaesthesia* 2009; **64**(6): 643–51

51. Detterbeck FC. Efficacy of methods of intercostal nerve blockade for pain relief after thoracotomy. *Ann Thorac Surg* 2005; **80**(4): 1550–9

52. Perttunen K, Nilsson E, Heinonen J, Hirvisalo EL, Salo JA, Kalso E. Extradural, paravertebral and intercostal nerve blocks for post-thoracotomy pain. *Br J Anaesth* 1995; **75**(5): 541–7

53. Asantila R, Rosenberg PH, Scheinin B. Comparison of different methods of postoperative analgesia after thoracotomy. *Acta Anaesthesiol Scand* 1986; **30**(6): 421–5

54. Dryden CM, McMenemin I, Duthie DJ. Efficacy of continuous intercostal bupivacaine for pain relief after thoracotomy. *Br J Anaesth* 1993; **70**(5): 508–10

55. Luketich JD, Land SR, Sullivan EA, et al. Thoracic epidural versus intercostal nerve catheter plus patient-controlled analgesia: a randomized study. *Ann Thorac Surg* 2005; **79**(6): 1845–9

56. Ferrante FM, Chan VW, Arthur GR, Rocco AG. Interpleural analgesia after thoracotomy. *Anesth Analg* 1991; **72**(1): 105–9

57. Richardson J, Sabanathan S, Shah RD, Clarke BJ, Cheema S, Mearns AJ. Pleural bupivacaine placement for optimal postthoracotomy pulmonary function: a prospective, randomized study. *J Cardiothorac Vasc Anesth* 1998; **12**(2): 166–9

58. Slinger P, Shennib H, Wilson S. Postthoracotomy pulmonary function: a comparison of epidural versus intravenous meperidine infusions. *J Cardiothorac Vasc Anesth* 1995; **9**(2): 128–34

59. Shulman M, Sandler AN, Bradley JW, Young PS, Brebner J. Postthoracotomy pain and pulmonary function following epidural and systemic morphine. *Anesthesiology* 1984; **61**(5): 569–75

60. Boisseau N, Rabary O, Padovani B, et al. Improvement of 'dynamic analgesia' does not decrease atelectasis after thoracotomy. *Br J Anaesth* 2001; **87**(4): 564–9

61. Pavy T, Medley C, Murphy DF. Effect of indomethacin on pain relief after thoracotomy. *Br J Anaesth* 1990; **65**(5): 624–7

62. Singh H, Bossard RF, White PF, Yeatts RW. Effects of ketorolac versus bupivacaine coadministration during patient-controlled hydromorphone epidural analgesia after thoracotomy procedures. *Anesth Analg* 1997; **84**(3): 564–9

63. Senard M, Deflandre EP, Ledoux D, et al. Effect of celecoxib combined with thoracic epidural analgesia on pain after thoracotomy. *Br J Anaesth* 2010; **105**(2): 196–200

64. Nussmeier NA, Whelton AA, Brown MT, et al. Safety and efficacy of the cyclooxygenase-2 inhibitors parecoxib and valdecoxib after non-cardiac surgery. *Anesthesiology* 2006; **104**(3): 518–26

65. Schug SA, Joshi GP, Camu F, Pan S, Cheung R. Cardiovascular safety of the cyclooxygenase-2 selective inhibitors parecoxib and valdecoxib in the postoperative setting: an analysis of integrated data. *Anesth Analg* 2009; **108**(1): 299–307

66. Nesher N, Ekstein MP, Paz Y, Marouani N, Chazan S, Weinbroum AA. Morphine with adjuvant ketamine vs higher dose of morphine alone for immediate postthoracotomy analgesia. *Chest* 2009; **136**(1): 245–52

67. Suzuki M, Haraguti S, Sugimoto K, Kikutani T, Shimada Y, Sakamoto A. Low-dose intravenous ketamine potentiates epidural analgesia after thoracotomy. *Anesthesiology* 2006; **105**(1): 111–9

68. Chaparro LE, Smith SA, Moore RA, Wiffen PJ, Gilron I. Pharmacotherapy for the prevention of chronic pain after surgery in adults. *The Cochrane database of systematic reviews* 2013; 7: CD008307

69. Bell RF, Dahl JB, Moore RA, Kalso E. Peri-operative ketamine for acute post-operative pain: a quantitative and qualitative systematic review (Cochrane review). *Acta Anaesthesiol Scand* 2005; **49**(10): 1405–28

70. Urban MK, Ya Deau JT, Wukovits B, Lipnitsky JY. Ketamine as an adjunct to postoperative pain management in opioid tolerant patients after spinal fusions: a prospective randomized trial. *HSS J* 2008; **4**(1): 62–5

71. Bloch MB, Dyer RA, Heijke SA, James MF. Tramadol infusion for postthoracotomy pain relief: a placebo-controlled comparison with epidural morphine. *Anesth Analg* 2002; **94**(3): 523–8; table of contents

72. Mac TB, Girard F, Chouinard P, et al. Acetaminophen decreases early post-thoracotomy ipsilateral shoulder pain in patients with thoracic epidural analgesia: a double-blind placebo-controlled study. *J Cardiothorac Vasc Anesth* 2005; **19**(4): 475–8

73. Huot MP, Chouinard P, Girard F, Ruel M, Lafontaine ER, Ferraro P. Gabapentin does not reduce post-thoracotomy shoulder pain: a randomized, double-blind placebo-controlled study. *Can J Anaesth* 2008; **55**(6): 337–43

74. Tiippana EM, Hamunen K, Kontinen VK, Kalso E. Do surgical patients benefit from perioperative gabapentin/pregabalin? A systematic review of efficacy and safety. *Anesth Analg* 2007; **104**(6): 1545–56, table of contents

75. Sheen MJ, Ho ST, Lee CH, Tsung YC, Chang FL. Preoperative gabapentin prevents intrathecal morphine-induced pruritus after orthopedic surgery. *Anesth Analg* 2008; **106**(6): 1868–72

76. Zhang J, Ho KY, Wang Y. Efficacy of pregabalin in acute postoperative pain: a meta-analysis. *Br J Anaesth* 2011; **106**(4): 454–62

77. Solak O, Metin M, Esme H, et al. Effectiveness of gabapentin in the treatment of chronic post-thoracotomy pain. *Eur J Cardiothorac Surg* 2007; **32**(1): 9–12

78. Mustola ST, Lempinen J, Saimanen E, Vilkko P. Efficacy of thoracic epidural analgesia with or without intercostal nerve cryoanalgesia for postthoracotomy pain. *Ann Thorac Surg* 2011; **91**(3): 869–73

79. Ju H, Feng Y, Yang BX, Wang J. Comparison of epidural analgesia and intercostal nerve cryoanalgesia for post-thoracotomy pain control. *Eur J Pain* 2008; **12**(3): 378–84

80. Scawn ND, Pennefather SH, Soorae A, Wang JY, Russell GN. Ipsilateral shoulder pain after thoracotomy with epidural analgesia: the influence of phrenic nerve infiltration with lidocaine. *Anesth Analg* 2001; **93**(2): 260–4, 1st contents page

81. Burgess FW, Anderson DM, Colonna D, Sborov MJ, Cavanaugh DG. Ipsilateral shoulder pain following thoracic surgery. *Anesthesiology* 1993; **78**(2): 365–8

82. MacDougall P. Postthoracotomy shoulder pain: diagnosis and management. *Curr Opin Anaesthesiol* 2008; **21**(1): 12–5

83. Barak M, Ziser A, Katz Y. Thoracic epidural local anesthetics are ineffective in alleviating post-thoracotomy ipsilateral shoulder pain. *J Cardiothorac Vasc Anesth* 2004; **18**(4): 458–60

84. Pennefather SH, Akrofi ME, Kendall JB, Russell GN, Scawn ND. Double-blind comparison of intrapleural saline and 0.25% bupivacaine for ipsilateral shoulder pain after thoracotomy in patients receiving thoracic epidural analgesia. *Br J Anaesth* 2005; **94**(2): 234–8

85. Garner L, Coats RR. Ipsilateral stellate ganglion block effective for treating shoulder pain after thoracotomy. *Anesth Analg* 1994; **78**(6): 1195–6

86. Perttunen K, Tasmuth T, Kalso E. Chronic pain after thoracic surgery: a follow-up study. *Acta Anaesthesiol Scand* 1999; **43**(5): 563–7

87. Katz J, Jackson M, Kavanagh BP, Sandler AN. Acute pain after thoracic surgery predicts long-term post-thoracotomy pain. *Clin J Pain* 1996; **12**(1): 50–5

88. Ochroch EA, Gottschalk A, Augostides J, et al. Long-term pain and activity during recovery from major thoracotomy using thoracic epidural analgesia. *Anesthesiology* 2002; **97**(5): 1234–44

89. Senturk M, Ozcan PE, Talu GK, Kiyan E, Camci E, Ozyalcin S, et al. The effects of three different analgesia techniques on long-term postthoracotomy pain. *Anesth Analg* 2002; **94**(1): 11–5, table of contents

90. Athanassiadi K, Kakaris S, Theakos N, Skottis I. Muscle-sparing versus posterolateral thoracotomy: a prospective study. *Eur J Cardiothorac Surg* 2007; **31**(3): 496–9; discussion 9–500

91. Clarke H, Bonin RP, Orser BA, Englesakis M, Wijeysundera DN, Katz J. The prevention of chronic postsurgical pain using gabapentin and pregabalin: a combined systematic review and meta-analysis. *Anesth Analg* 2012; **115**(2): 428–42

92. O'Connor CJ. Pain relief and pulmonary morbidity after cardiac surgery. *Crit Care Med* 1999; **27**(10): 2314–6

93. Baumgarten MC, Garcia GK, Frantzeski MH, Giacomazzi CM, Lagni VB, Dias AS, et al. Pain and pulmonary function in patients submitted to heart surgery via sternotomy. *Rev Bras Cir Cardiovasc* 2009; **24**(4): 497–505

94. Nilsson E, Perttunen K, Kalso E. Intrathecal morphine for post-sternotomy pain in patients with myasthenia gravis: effects on respiratory function. *Acta Anaesthesiol Scand* 1997; **41**(5): 549–56

95. Ho SC, Royse CF, Royse AG, Penberthy A, McRae R. Persistent pain after cardiac surgery: an audit of high thoracic epidural and primary opioid analgesia therapies. *Anesth Analg* 2002; **95**(4): 820–3

96. Lahtinen P, Kokki H, Hynynen M. Pain after cardiac surgery: a prospective cohort study of 1-year incidence and intensity. *Anesthesiology* 2006; **105**(4): 794–800

97. van Gulik L, Janssen LI, Ahlers SJ, et al. Risk factors for chronic thoracic pain after cardiac surgery via sternotomy. *Eur J Cardiothorac Surg* 2011; **40**(6): 1309–13

98. Bainbridge D, Martin JE, Cheng DC. Patient-controlled versus nurse-controlled analgesia after cardiac surgery—a meta-analysis. *Can J Anaesth* 2006; **53**(5): 492–9

99. Pettersson PH, Lindskog EA, Owall A. Patient-controlled versus nurse-controlled pain treatment after coronary artery bypass surgery. *Acta Anaesthesiol Scand* 2000; **44**(1): 43–7

100. Gust R, Pecher S, Gust A, Hoffmann V, Bohrer H, Martin E. Effect of patient-controlled analgesia on pulmonary complications after coronary artery bypass grafting. *Crit Care Med* 1999; **27**(10): 2218–23

101. Gurbet A, Goren S, Sahin S, Uckunkaya N, Korfali G. Comparison of analgesic effects of morphine, fentanyl, and remifentanil with intravenous patient-controlled analgesia after cardiac surgery. *J Cardiothorac Vasc Anesth* 2004; **18**(6): 755–8

102. Dal D, Kanbak M, Caglar M, Aypar U. A background infusion of morphine does not enhance postoperative analgesia after cardiac surgery. *Can J Anaesth* 2003; **50**(5): 476–9

103. Rapanos T, Murphy P, Szalai JP, Burlacoff L, Lam-McCulloch J, Kay J. Rectal indomethacin reduces postoperative pain and morphine use after cardiac surgery. *Can J Anaesth* 1999; **46**(8): 725–30

104. Fayaz MK, Abel RJ, Pugh SC, Hall JE, Djaiani G, Mecklenburgh JS. Opioid-sparing effects of diclofenac and paracetamol lead to improved outcomes after cardiac surgery. *J Cardiothorac Vasc Anesth* 2004; **18**(6): 742–7

105. Ott E, Nussmeier NA, Duke PC, et al. Efficacy and safety of the cyclooxygenase 2 inhibitors parecoxib and valdecoxib in patients undergoing coronary artery bypass surgery. *J Thorac Cardiovasc Surg* 2003; **125**(6): 1481–92

106. Nussmeier NA, Whelton AA, Brown MT, et al. Complications of the COX-2 inhibitors parecoxib and valdecoxib after cardiac surgery. *N Engl J Med* 2005 17; **352**(11): 1081–91

107. Schjerning Olsen AM, Fosbol EL, Lindhardsen J, et al. Duration of treatment with nonsteroidal anti-inflammatory drugs and impact on risk of death and recurrent myocardial infarction in patients with prior myocardial infarction: a nationwide cohort study. *Circulation* 2011 24; **123**(20): 2226–35

108. Cattabriga I, Pacini D, Lamazza G, et al. Intravenous paracetamol as adjunctive treatment for postoperative pain after cardiac surgery: a double blind randomized controlled trial. *Eur J Cardiothorac Surg* 2007; **32**(3): 527–31

109. Lahtinen P, Kokki H, Hakala T, Hynynen M. S(+)-ketamine as an analgesic adjunct reduces opioid consumption after cardiac surgery. *Anesth Analg* 2004; **99**(5): 1295–301

110. Konstantatos A, Silvers AJ, Myles PS. Analgesia best practice after cardiac surgery. *Anesthesiol Clin* 2008; **26**(3): 591–602

111. Rao SM, Netke B, Ponavala T, Kumar S, Dharmarakshak A. Post-operative pain relief by PCA v/s oral tramadol in cardiac surgery. *Ann Card Anaesth* 2001; **4**(1): 13–6

112. But AK, Erdil F, Yucel A, Gedik E, Durmus M, Ersoy MO. The effects of single-dose tramadol on post-operative pain and morphine requirements after coronary artery bypass surgery. *Acta Anaesthesiol Scand* 2007; **51**(5): 601–6

113. Ucak A, Onan B, Sen H, Selcuk I, Turan A, Yilmaz AT. The effects of gabapentin on acute and chronic postoperative pain after coronary artery bypass graft surgery. *J Cardiothorac Vasc Anesth* 2011; (5): 824–9

114. Menda F, Koner O, Sayin M, Ergenoglu M, Kucukaksu S, Aykac B. Effects of single-dose gabapentin on postoperative pain and morphine consumption after cardiac surgery. *J Cardiothorac Vasc Anesth* 2010; **24**(5): 808–13

115. Rapchuk IL, O'Connell L, Liessmann CD, Cornelissen HR, Fraser JF. Effect of gabapentin on pain after cardiac surgery: a randomised,

double-blind, placebo-controlled trial. *Anaesth Intensive Care* 2010; **38**(3): 445–51

116. Biyik I, Gulculer M, Karabiga M, Ergene O, Tayyar N. Efficacy of gabapentin versus diclofenac in the treatment of chest pain and paresthesia in patients with sternotomy. *Anadolu Kardiyol Derg* 2009; **9**(5): 390–6

117. Barrington MJ, Kluger R, Watson R, Scott DA, Harris KJ. Epidural anesthesia for coronary artery bypass surgery compared with general anesthesia alone does not reduce biochemical markers of myocardial damage. *Anesth Analg* 2005; **100**(4): 921–8

118. Jensen MK, Andersen C. Can chronic poststernotomy pain after cardiac valve replacement be reduced using thoracic epidural analgesia? *Acta Anaesthesiol Scand* 2004; **48**(7): 871–4

119. Visser WA, Liem TH, van Egmond J, Gielen MJ. Extension of sensory blockade after thoracic epidural administration of a test dose of lidocaine at three different levels. *Anesth Analg* 1998; **86**(2): 332–5

120. Royse CF. High thoracic epidural anaesthesia for cardiac surgery. *Curr Opin Anaesthesiol* 2009; **22**(1): 84–7

121. Ho AM, Chung DC, Joynt GM. Neuraxial blockade and hematoma in cardiac surgery: estimating the risk of a rare adverse event that has not (yet) occurred. *Chest* 2000; **117**(2): 551–5

122. Roediger L, Larbuisson R, Lamy M. New approaches and old controversies to postoperative pain control following cardiac surgery. *Eur J Anaesthesiol* 2006; **23**(7): 539–50

123. Kocabas S, Yedicocuklu D, Yuksel E, Uysallar E, Askar F. Infiltration of the sternotomy wound and the mediastinal tube sites with 0.25% levobupivacaine as adjunctive treatment for postoperative pain after cardiac surgery. *Eur J Anaesthesiol* 2008; **25**(10): 842–9

124. McDonald SB, Jacobsohn E, Kopacz DJ, et al. Parasternal block and local anesthetic infiltration with levobupivacaine after cardiac surgery with desflurane: the effect on postoperative pain, pulmonary function, and tracheal extubation times. *Anesth Analg* 2005; **100**(1): 25–32

125. Eljezi V, Duale C, Azarnoush K, et al. The analgesic effects of a bilateral sternal infusion of ropivacaine after cardiac surgery. *Reg Anesth Pain Med* 2012; **37**(2): 166–74

126. Dowling R, Thielmeier K, Ghaly A, Barber D, Boice T, Dine A. Improved pain control after cardiac surgery: results of a randomized, double-blind, clinical trial. *J Thorac Cardiovasc Surg* 2003; **126**(5): 1271–8

CHAPTER 39

Chronic pain after cardiothoracic surgery

Lesley Colvin

Epidemiology

Chronic pain poses a major challenge, with evidence from Europe and North America that up to 18% of the population may suffer from chronic pain at some point in their life. There is a direct consequence for patients and their family with a significant impact on quality of life, as well as creating a large burden on society not just in terms of healthcare costs, but also in a much wider context, including loss of employment and associated welfare costs (1). Whereas acute pain may serve a useful biological function, reducing activity and allowing for recovery and wound healing after surgery, chronic pain is disabling and distressing, with no useful function.

While exact definitions of what constitutes chronic pain vary, the International Association for the Study of Pain (IASP) definition: 'Chronic pain is pain without apparent biological value that has persisted beyond the normal tissue healing time (usually taken to be three months)' is generally accepted, although potentially complete wound healing may be longer after major surgery, such as cardiothoracic surgery (2).

Some common types of chronic pain such as back pain and osteoarthritis have a poorly defined onset with many of the causative factors being difficult to modify. In contrast, with chronic post-surgical pain (CPSP) there is a very clear tissue injury (at the time of surgery), that may progress to persistent pain in some individuals. Therefore, the aim of this chapter is to review the mechanisms in the development and maintenance of CPSP and identify modifiable risk factors and effective strategies for the prevention of or early intervention in CPSP.

CPSP can occur after a range of surgical procedures (see table 39.1). Although the precise aetiology is not completely understood, and indeed may vary between types of surgery, what is common to most of these procedures is the risk of nerve damage and often present with marked neuropathic features.

CPSP after thoracic surgery was recognized in the 1990s, with around 70% of patients potentially being affected. The specific surgery, or reason for surgery may be relevant, as a study of CPSP in patients after lung transplantation surgery found that a much lower incidence of patients experienced ongoing problems, with only 18% of patients reporting some pain and 10% reporting moderate to severe pain which is possibly related to immunosuppressant treatment that is required for transplantation. Similarly, CPSP may be lower after video-assisted thoracoscopic surgery (VATS), with around 25% of patients reporting pain (12,13).

CPSP has been less well characterized after cardiac surgery, but post-sternotomy pain is increasingly recognized as a problem, with two large studies from different countries consistently finding around 28% of patients suffered from CPSP (22,23). Other groups have found that prevalence may vary from 11 to 56%, often with at least moderate pain, impacting on quality of life. The pain is most commonly found in the midline or left side, and may have both neuropathic and myofascial features (14,24–27).

Another factor to consider is the severity of CPSP and its impact on quality of life, which can be hard to quantify. In a recent survey of patients 3 months after thoracotomy, 68% had CPSP and overall had worse physical functioning and vitality compared to patients who didn't have pain, with around 15–16% of patients requiring opioid analgesia, or having at least moderate impairment of daily activities (5,6). In the majority of patients with CPSP after thoracotomy, there was at least some impact on activities of daily living (7).

What is chronic post-surgical pain?

It is clear that in many CPSP syndromes, neuropathic pain is one of the key features. Despite this, not all CPSP syndromes are purely neuropathic in nature. Of the 70% of patients who had CPSP 6 months after thoracotomy, just under a half were predominantly neuropathic in nature when assessed using sensory testing and standardized questionnaires (8). Sensory changes that had been perceived by patients were present in 63% of CPSP patients after thoracotomy, whereas only 25% of pain-free patients had long term sensory disturbance (12). Detailed neurophysiological characterization revealed that both pain and pain-free patients had evidence of nerve injury, but that it was likely to be more severe in patients with CPSP after thoracotomy, although this difference was less clear in patients who had VATS (28,29). In a retrospective recall study of patients who had undergone thoracic surgery during childhood or adolescence, the majority of patients had some evidence of sensory dysfunction as assessed by sensory testing, regardless of whether or not they suffered from CPSP (30).

Mechanisms of chronic postsurgical pain after cardiothoracic surgery

A number of preoperative, intraoperative, and postoperative factors may contribute to the development of CPSP. Nerve injury at the time of surgery, with consequent development of neuropathic

Table 39.1 Incidences of chronic post- surgical pain (CPSP)

Surgery	Incidence of patients with reported CPSP (%)	Ref
Amputation	50–75	(3,4)
Thoracotomy	33–69	(5–11)
Video-assisted thoracoscopic surgery	25–47	(9,12)
Lung transplant surgery	5–10	(9,13)
Sternotomy	25–31	(14,15–17)
Mastectomy	30- 50	(18,19)
Hernia repair	10–30	(20,21)

Data from various sources, see reference numbers.

pain plays a major role in many cases, although the presence of chronic sensory dysfunction has been found in both CPSP patients and pain-free patients after surgery. Genetic factors are also likely to play a role in the likelihood of an individual developing CPSP, but as yet, these are not well understood (31).

In response to acute tissue damage, and potentially with associated peripheral nerve injury, a number of changes can occur in both the peripheral and central nervous system that contribute to the development and maintenance of CPSP. The basic pain pathway is outlined in figure 39.1. While this outlines the key anatomical features, the system is highly plastic, with changes occurring in the immediate postoperative period at many points within the system, some of which may contribute to the development of chronic pain.

Peripheral sensitization

In response to surgery and nerve injury a number of changes in pain processing can occur rapidly, with release of inflammatory mediators, peripheral sensitization, and subsequent alterations in neuronal function. A wide variety of cells are recruited in the acute response, with changes in blood vessels and endothelial cells, changes in immune cells (e.g. lymphocytes, macophages, polymorphs, and mast cells) and release of a variety of mediators all contributing to the peripheral sensitization process (32).

Spinal processing

Complex modulation may occur at the first central synapse, in the dorsal horn of the spinal cord, both via intrinsic spinal mechanisms and descending systems from the brain. The second order projection neurones ascend to the brain in specific tracts (33,34).

Neurotransmitters

There are a large number of neurotransmitters in the dorsal horn providing potential sites of action for analgesics (see table 39.2). The main inhibitory amino acids are gamma-aminobutyric acid (GABA) and glycine. A wide range of neuropeptides are produced and released by sensory neurones, as well as by dorsal horn neurones, including opioid peptides.

Supraspinal and cortical processing

The perception of pain is a complex phenomenon, integrating many different components, including peripheral nociceptive input (figure 39.2). Advances in neuroimaging techniques have increased our understanding of the interrelationship between cortical processing of nociceptive input and also the effects of 'top down' regulation from the brain to the spinal cord (35).

Central sensitization

An increase in excitatory activity, or decrease in inhibitory circuits can occur after nerve injury, with persistent amplification of pain messages. There is a resultant hyperexcitability, with wind-up of dorsal horn neurons and changes in neurotransmitters such as glutamate, substance P, neurokinin A, calcitonin gene-related peptide (CGRP) and prostaglandins (36,37). The N-Methyl-D-aspartate (NMDA) receptor plays a key role in this central sensitization and 'wind-up'. With repeated high intensity noxious input (e.g. at the time of surgery), the NMDA receptor block by magnesium ions, is lifted. This persistent increased activation of the NMDA receptor complex may be important in the development of neuropathic pain (38,39).

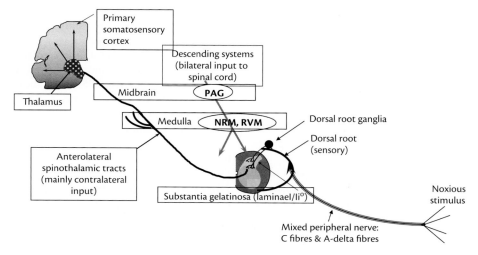

Fig. 39.1 Basic pain pathway.

Table 39.2 Some of the neurotransmitters important in spinal processing of nociceptive information

Neurotransmitter	Receptor (s)	
Glutamate: Ionotropic :	AMPA	Ca^{2+} permeable
	NMDA	Permeable to calcium + sodium; Voltage dependent Mg^{2+} block
	Kainate	On small diameter primary afferent neurons
Glutamate: Metabotropic	Three groups (I, II, III)	Gp I (mGluR1 and 5): superficial dorsal horn
		Gp II (mGlu2 and 3): presynaptic; decrease glutamate release
Substance P	Neurokinin receptors	Mainly excitatory, increased in inflammation, decreased in neuropathic pain
Galanin	Gal Rs	Found in c fibres, low levels, but up regulated in neuropathic pain; inhibitory
Cholecystokinin (CCK)	CCKRs1–8	Excitatory; antagonists have been studied in clinical trials
Calcitonin gene-related peptide (CGRP)	calcitonin *receptor*-like *receptor* (CALCRL)	Excitatory; slows degradation of SP

AMPA, α-amino-3-hydroxyl-5-methyl-4-isoxazole propionic acid; NMDA, *N*-methyl ᴅ-aspartate.

As a component of central sensitization, changes may occur in descending modulation with a shift from inhibitory to facilitatory effects. This is seen particularly in chronic pain states and may help explain persistent pain in the absence of ongoing peripheral tissue damage (40). Changes within cortical processing also occur after nerve injury, with rapid and persistent changes in cortical processing that correlate with pain severity (41).

Risk factors

Identification of the risk factors leading to CPSP is an essential step in reducing the problem (see table 39.3). Some of these risk factors may be directly modifiable in the peri-operative period, whereas others—such as genetic factors may not be, but will at least assist in targeting preventive measures towards those most likely to be at risk. There are fewer studies on post sternotomy pain but there have been a number of potential risk factors for CPSP identified (see table 39.4).

Prevention

The concept of pre-emptive analgesia in order to reduce CPSP was based on evidence from basic science studies, with early clinical studies giving some hope that this might be translated into clinical practice; unfortunately subsequent larger-scale, better quality studies did not bear out the early promise of reducing persistent pain (50,51). What does seem to be clear is that high pain scores in the immediate postoperative period is one of the potentially modifiable risk factors for CPSP. We should therefore try and optimize pain control in the perioperative period.

Regional anaesthesia, whether administered pre-emptively or not, may have some role in reducing CPSP. A systematic review of randomized controlled trials examining long-term pain outcomes after surgery found that epidural anaesthesia may reduce pain 6 months after thoracotomy in about one in four patients, although there were significant shortcomings in study design (52). The timing of the intervention and the type of intraoperative

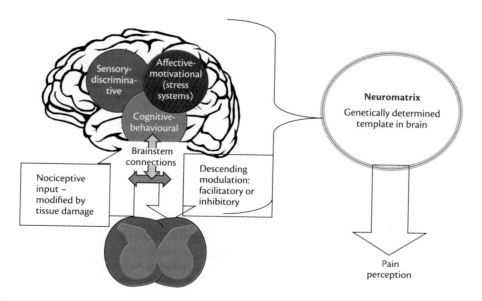

Fig. 39.2 Pain perception.

Table 39.3 Risk factors for chronic post-surgical pain

Risk Factor	Evidence for effect on risk for CPSP	References
Age	Younger age : increased risk	(5)
ASA status	Lower ASA scores: increased risk	(7)
Acute postoperative pain	High pain scores in postoperative period: increased risk	(8,42–44)
	Chance of CPSP nearly doubled per 10 point increase on 0–100 Numerical Rating scale	
	High postoperative opioid consumption: increased risk	
Surgical drains	Long duration in situ; higher number of drains: increased risk	(5,7)
Type of anaesthetic	Sevoflurane higher risk than TIVA with propofol/remifentanil	(45)
Intraoperative nerve function	No increased risk of CPSP if abnormal	(46)
Psychophysical testing	Reduced risk if endogenous inhibitory systems tonically more active	(43,44)
Psychological factors	Emotional numbing: increased risk	(42)

ASA, American Society of Anesthesiologists; CPSP, chronic post surgical pain; TIVA, total intravenous anaesthesia.
Data from various sources, see reference numbers.

Table 39.4 Risk factors for chronic postsurgical pain following sternotomy

Risk Factor	Evidence for effect on risk of CPSP	References
Acute postoperative pain	High pain scores of day 3; high analgesic requirements	(27,47)
Gender	Female > male	(47)
Age	Younger age : increased risk	(48)
Body mass index	BMI >28kgm^{-2}	(27)
Second surgery required	Resternotomy: increased risk	(47)
Anaesthetic technique	Remifentanil during surgery: increased risk	(48)
Surgical technique	Internal mammary artery harvesting: increased risk	(15,49)

CPSP, chronic post surgical pain.
Data from various sources, see reference numbers.

analgesia may also effect long-term outcome, with one study showing a benefit of low-dose remifentanil with preoperative epidural analgesia compared to high-dose remifetanil and postsurgical commencement of epidural analgesia (53). Another study also showed a benefit of beginning epidural analgesia preoperatively, with better postoperative pain control and reduced chronic pain, compared to postoperative epidural analgesia. Patients with the highest risk of CPSP in this study received intravenous patient-controlled morphine (54).

As epidural analgesia may have some disadvantages in terms of requirements for post-operative monitoring, there has been interest in other regional techniques such as paravertebral blocks, with some evidence of a reduction on hospital stay after thoracic surgery, although others have found that it may be less effective than epidural analgesia (55,56).

The use of ketamine perioperatively has also been studied with some evidence of subtle long-term effects on sensory processing when used epidurally for CPSP after amputation, although there was no reduction in CPSP, allodynia, or numbness after thoracotomy (57,58). When ketamine was used intravenously as an adjunct to epidural ropivacaine, there was no major reduction in post-thoracotomy pain 3 months later, nor when used as an adjunct to intercostal analgesia (59,60). Similarly, a 24-hour infusion of ketamine around the time of thoracotomy improved postoperative pain control but had no detectable long-term effects at 4 months after surgery (61). Other adjuvants that have been suggested include the gabapentionoids (gabapentin and pregabalin) (62).

Treatment

Treatment of established CPSP after cardiothoracic surgery can be challenging. After a thorough assessment to determine the characteristics of the pain, and any other contributing factors, there are a number of options.

Pharmacological

There is a wide range of antineuropathic agents available, the majority of which require a period of dose titration to effect, and use may also be limited by unacceptable side effects. Broadly speaking, these can be divided into those from the antidepressant group of medications, anticonvulsants, opioids, and topical agents. There are a number of guidelines giving a suggested framework for treatment. Recommended oral agents include the gabapentinoids or antidepressants such as amitriptyline or duloxetine. Topical therapies include lidocaine patches, with some interest in newer therapies such as a high-dose 8% capsaicin patch. With CPSP, there is often a discrete area around the surgical site that is affected and as such, may be particularly amenable to localized topical treatment (63–65). Combination therapies are often used, and there is some evidence that combining agents may provide better analgesia (66).

Stimulation therapies

This includes simple therapies such as acupuncture and transcutaneous electrical nerve stimulation (TENS) through to more invasive techniques such as spinal cord stimulation. The use of TENS for acute postoperative pain control after thoracotomy has been assessed in a systematic review and meta-analysis where, of the 2489 articles identified, only 11 were suitable for inclusion. There was a benefit in terms of postoperative pain scores by introducing TENS as an adjunct to pharmacological strategies (67). The evidence for use in the chronic setting for postsurgical pain is limited in terms of quality and trial design, but due to its low toxicity and potential for harm a carefully assessed trial of effectiveness would not be unreasonable (68). For more invasive treatments, such as spinal cord stimulation, the evidence is again limited, although there is some evidence of efficacy for neuropathic pain (69,70). Newer and unproven stimulation therapies include different types of peripheral nerve stimulation.

Injection therapies

A number of interventions targeting the regional innervation of the affected surgical area have been used, but good quality evidence for these is limited. A small open-label pilot study of epidural clonidine and steroid found some evidence of benefit after 6 months, but this would need further evaluation (71,72). A retrospective study of 49 patients investigated the effects of pulsed radiofrequency (RF) to intercostal nerves or corresponding dorsal root ganglia. Those receiving dorsal root ganglia pulsed RF demonstrated a greater benefit after 3 months (73).

Multidisciplinary pain management

Most studies have not focussed on CPSP, but in general, chronic pain does demonstrate benefit from focussed pain management input ranging from active rehabilitation to support with coping strategies and use of a range of psychological techniques to address the wider aspects of chronic pain (74).

Conclusion

Chronic pain after cardiothoracic surgery is a major challenge. Despite 'successful' surgery, patients can be left with significant levels of disability and pain. The reasons for this are complex and are likely to include the type of injury or surgery, perioperative management, genetic factors, psychosocial factors and the interaction between these. By improving our understanding of the mechanisms of CPSP, we may be able to develop strategies to prevent, modify or effectively treat CPSP. While some factors may not be amenable to modification, such as genetic influences, it is clear that good pain control in the immediate post-operative period, particularly in those individuals most at risk of CPSP, should reduce the problem. While not all anaesthetists are involved in chronic pain management, we all have a responsibility to provide optimum perioperative analgesia, with potential long-term benefits for our patients.

References

1. Toblin RL, Mack KA, Perveen G, Paulozzi LJ. A population-based survey of chronic pain and its treatment with prescription drugs. *Pain* 2011; **152**: 1249–55
2. IASP Task Force on Taxonomy. Classification of Chronic Pain. Descriptions of Chronic Pain Syndromes and Definitions of Pain Terms. http://www.iasp-pain.org/PublicationsNews/NewsletterArticle.aspx?ItemNumber=2772 second edition Revised, edited by H. Merskey and N. Bogduk:-214
3. Buchheit T, Pyati S. Prevention of chronic pain after surgical nerve injury: amputation and thoracotomy. *Surg Clin N Am* 2012; **92**: 393–407
4. Richardson C, Glenn S, Nurmikko T, et al. Incidence of phantom phenomena including phantom limb pain 6 months after major lower limb amputation in patients with peripheral vascular disease. *Clin J Pain* 2006; **22**: 353–8
5. Wang HT, Liu W, Luo AL, Ma C, Huang YG. Prevalence and risk factors of chronic post-thoracotomy pain in Chinese patients from Peking Union Medical College Hospital. *Chin MedJ* 2012; **125**: 3033–8
6. Kinney MA, Hooten WM, Cassivi SD, et al. Chronic postthoracotomy pain and health-related quality of life. *Ann Thorac Surg* 2012; **93**: 1242–7
7. Mongardon N, Pinton-Gonnet C, Szekely B, Michel-Cherqui M, Dreyfus JF, Fischler M. Assessment of chronic pain after thoracotomy: a 1-year prevalence study. *Clin J Pain* 2011; **27**: 677–81
8. Guastella V, Mick G, Soriano C, et al. A prospective study of neuropathic pain induced by thoracotomy: incidence, clinical description, and diagnosis. *Pain* 201; **152**: 74–81
9. Steegers MA, Snik DM, Verhagen AF, van der Drift MA, Wilder-Smith OH. Only half of the chronic pain after thoracic surgery shows a neuropathic component. *J Pain* 2008; **9**: 955–61
10. Pluijms WA, Steegers MA, Verhagen AF, Scheffer GJ, Wilder-Smith OH. Chronic post-thoracotomy pain: a retrospective study. *Acta Anaesthesiol Scand* 2006; **50**: 804–8
11. Maguire MF, Ravenscroft A, Beggs D, Duffy JP. A questionnaire study investigating the prevalence of the neuropathic component of chronic pain after thoracic surgery. *Eur J Cardiothoracic Surg* 2006; **29**: 800–5
12. Wildgaard K, Ravn J, Nikolajsen L, Jakobsen E, Jensen TS, Kehlet H. Consequences of persistent pain after lung cancer surgery: a nationwide questionnaire study. *Acta Anaesthesiol Scand* 2011; **55**: 60–8
13. Wildgaard K, Iversen M, Kehlet H. Chronic pain after lung transplantation: a nationwide study. *Clin J Pain* 2010; **26**: 217–22
14. Lahtinen P, Kokki H, Hynynen M. Pain after cardiac surgery: a prospective cohort study of 1-year incidence and intensity. *Anesthesiology* 2006; **105**: 794–800.
15. Ho SC, Royse CF, Royse AG, Penberthy A, McRae R. Persistent pain after cardiac surgery: an audit of high thoracic epidural and primary opioid analgesia therapies. *Anesth Analg* 2002; **95**: 820–3
16. Meyerson J, Thelin S, Gordh T, Karlsten R. The incidence of chronic post-sternotomy pain after cardiac surgery—a prospective study. *Acta Anaesthiol Scand* 2001; **45**: 940–4
17. Kalso E, Mennander S, Tasmuth T, Nilsson E. Chronic post-sternotomy pain. *Acta Anaesthiol Scand* 2001; **45**: 935–9
18. Macdonald L, Bruce J, Scott NW, Smith WC, Chambers WA. Long-term follow-up of breast cancer survivors with post-mastectomy pain syndrome. *Br J Cancer* 2005; **92**: 225–30
19. Gärtner R, Jensen M, Nielsen J, Ewertz M, Kroman N, Kehlet H. Prevalence of and factors associated with persistent pain following breast cancer surgery. *JAMA* 2009; **302**(18): 1985–92
20. Franneby U, Sandblom G, Nordin P, et al. Risk factors for long-term pain after hernia surgery. *Ann Surg* 2006; **244**: 212–9
21. Aasvang EK, Gmaehle E, Hansen JB, et al. Predictive risk factors for persistent postherniotomy pain. *Anesthesiology* 2010; **112**: 957–69
22. Kalso E, Mennander S, Tasmuth T, Nilsson E. Chronic post-sternotomy pain. *Acta Anaesthesiol Scand* 2001; **45**: 935–9
23. Mayerson J, Theims S, Gordh T, Karlsten R. The incidence of chronic post-sternotomy pain after cardiac surgery—a prospective study. *Acta Anaesthesiol Scand* 2001; **45**: 940–4
24. Luleci N, Dere K, Akbas M, Aldulkerimov V, Luleci E, Guler M. Myofascial pain at post-sternotomy patients after cardiac surgery: A clinical study in 1226 patients. *J Back Musculoskelet Rehabil* 2008; **21**: 239–43
25. Bruce J, Drury N, Poobalan AS, Jeffrey RR, Smith WC, Chambers WA. The prevalence of chronic chest and leg pain following cardiac surgery: a historical cohort study.[see comment][erratum appears in *Pain* 2004; **112**(3):413. *Pain* 2003; **104**: 265–73
26. Carle C, Ashworth A, Roscoe A. A survey of post-sternotomy chronic pain following cardiac surgery. *Anaesthesia* 2009; **64**: 1387

27. Mazzeffi M, Khelemsky Y. Poststernotomy pain: a clinical review. *J Cardiothorac Vasc Anesth* 2011; **25**: 1163–78

28. Wildgaard K, Ringsted TK, Aasvang EK, Ravn J, Werner MU, Kehlet H. Neurophysiological characterization of persistent postthoracotomy pain. *Clin J Pain* 2012; **28**: 136–42

29. Wildgaard K, Ringsted TK, Hansen HJ, Petersen RH, Werner MU, Kehlet H. Quantitative sensory testing of persistent pain after video-assisted thoracic surgery lobectomy. *Br J Anaesth* 2012; **108**: 126–33

30. Kristensen AD, Pedersen TA, Hjortdal VE, Jensen TS, Nikolajsen L. Chronic pain in adults after thoracotomy in childhood or youth. *Br J Anaesth* 2010; **104**: 75–9

31. Mogil JS. Pain genetics: past, present and future. *Trends Genet* 2012; **28**(6): 258–66

32. Sommer C, Kress M. Recent findings on how proinflammatory cytokines cause pain: peripheral mechanisms in inflammatory and neuropathic hyperalgesia. *Neurosci Lett* 2004; **361**: 184–7

33. Willis WD, Coggeshall RE. *Sensory Mechanisms of the Spinal Cord*, 2nd edn. New York, London: Plenum Press, 1991

34. Morris R, Cheunsuang O, Stewart A, Maxwell D. Spinal dorsal horn neurone targets for nociceptive primary afferents: do single neurone morphological characteristics suggest how nociceptive information is processed at the spinal level. *Brain Res Brain Res Rev* 2004; **46**: 173–90

35. Tracey I. Imaging pain. *Br J Anaesth* 2008; **101**: 32–9

36. Woolf CJ, Salter MW. Neuronal plasticity-increasing the gain in pain. *Science* 2000; **288**: 1765–8

37. Hughes JP, Chessell I, Malamut R,, et al. Understanding chronic inflammatory and neuropathic pain. *Ann N Y Acad Sci* 2012; **1255**: 30–44.

38. Davis SN, Lodge D. Evidence for involvement of N-methyl-d-aspartic acid receptors in 'wind up' of class 2 neurons in the dorsal horn of the rat. *Brain Res* 1987; **424**: 402–6

39. Garry EM, Fleetwood-Walker SM. Organizing pains. *Trends Neurosci* 2004; **27**: 292–4

40. Porreca F, Ossipov MH, Gebhart GF. Chronic pain and medullary descending facilitation. *Trends Neurosci* 2002; **25**: 319–25

41. Flor H. Phantom-limb pain: characteristics, causes, and treatment. *Lancet Neurol* 2002; **1**: 182–9

42. Katz J, Asmundson GJ, McRae K, Halket E. Emotional numbing and pain intensity predict the development of pain disability up to one year after lateral thoracotomy. *Eur J Pain* 2009; **13**: 870–8

43. Yarnitsky D. Conditioned pain modulation the diffuse noxious inhibitory control-like effect: its relevance for acute and chronic pain states. *Curr Opin Anaesthesiol* 2010; **23**: 611–5

44. Yarnitsky D, Crispel Y, Eisenberg E, et al. Prediction of chronic post-operative pain: pre-operative DNIC testing identifies patients at risk. *Pain* 2008; **138**: 22–8

45. Song JG, Shin JW, Lee EH,, et al. Incidence of post-thoracotomy pain: a comparison between total intravenous anaesthesia and inhalation anaesthesia. *Eur J Cardiothorac Surg* 2012; **41**: 1078–82

46. Maguire MF, Latter JA, Mahajan R, et al. A study exploring the role of intercostal nerve damage in chronic pain after thoracic surgery. *Eur J Cardiothoracic Surg* 2006; **29**: 873–9

47. van GL, Janssen LI, Ahlers SJ, et al. Risk factors for chronic thoracic pain after cardiac surgery via sternotomy. *Eur J Cardiothorac Surg* 2011; **40**: 1309–13

48. van GL, Ahlers SJ, van de Garde EM, Bruins P, et al. Remifentanil during cardiac surgery is associated with chronic thoracic pain 1 yr after sternotomy. *Br J Anaesth* 2012; **109**: 616–22

49. Mailis A, Chan J, Basinski A, et al. Chest wall pain after aortocoronary bypass surgery using internal mammary artery graft: a new pain syndrome? *Heart Lung* 1989; **18**: 553–8

50. Bach S, Noreng MF, Tjellden NU. Phantom limb pain in amputees during the first 12 months following limb amputation after preoperative lumbar epidural blockade. *Pain* 1988; **33**: 297–301

51. Nikolajsen L, Ilkjaer S, Christensen JH, Kroner K, Jensen TS. Randomised trial of epidural bupivacaine and morphine in prevention of stump and phantom pain in lower limb amputation. *Lancet* 1997; **350**: 1353–7

52. Andreae MH, Andreae DA. Local anaesthetics and regional anaesthesia for preventing chronic pain after surgery. *Cochrane Database Syst Rev* 2012; **10**: CD007105

53. Salengros JC, Huybrechts I, Ducart A, et al. Different anesthetic techniques associated with different incidences of chronic post-thoracotomy pain: low-dose remifentanil plus presurgical epidural analgesia is preferable to high-dose remifentanil with postsurgical epidural analgesia. *J Cardiothorac Vasc Anesth* 2010; **24**: 608–16

54. Senturk M, Ozcan PE, Talu GK, et al. The effects of three different analgesia techniques on long-term postthoracotomy pain. *Anesth Analg* 2002: **94**: 11–5

55. Elsayed H, McKevith J, McShane J, Scawn N. Thoracic epidural or paravertebral catheter for analgesia after lung resection: is the outcome different? *J Cardiothorac Vasc Anesth* 2012; **26**: 78–82

56. Kanazi GE, Ayoub CM, Aouad M, et al. Subpleural block is less effective than thoracic epidural analgesia for post-thoracotomy pain: a randomised controlled study. *Eur J Anaesthesiol* 2012; **29**: 186–91

57. Wilson JA, Nimmo AF, Fleetwood-Walker SM, Colvin LA. A randomised double blind trial of the effect of pre-emptive epidural ketamine on persistent pain after lower limb amputation. *Pain* 2008; **135**: 108–18

58. Ryu HG, Lee CJ, Kim YT, Bahk JH. Preemptive low-dose epidural ketamine for preventing chronic postthoracotomy pain: a prospective, double-blinded, randomized, clinical trial. *Clin J Pain* 2011; **27**: 304–8

59. Joseph C, Gaillat F, Duponq R, et al. Is there any benefit to adding intravenous ketamine to patient-controlled epidural analgesia after thoracic surgery? A randomized double-blind study. *Eur J Cardiothorac Surg* 2012; **42**: e58–e65

60. Yazigi A, bou-Zeid H, Srouji T, Madi-Jebara S, Haddad F, Jabbour K. The effect of low-dose intravenous ketamine on continuous intercostal analgesia following thoracotomy. *Ann Cardiac Anaesth* 2012; **15**: 32–8

61. Duale C, Sibaud F, Guastella V, et al. Perioperative ketamine does not prevent chronic pain after thoracotomy. *Eur J Pain* 2009; **13**: 497–505

62. Buvanendran A, Kroin JS, la Valle CJ, Kari M, Moric M, Tuman KJ. Perioperative oral pregabalin reduces chronic pain after total knee arthroplasty: a prospective, randomized, controlled trial. *Anesth Analg* 2010; **110**: 199–207

63. Anand P, Bley KR. Topical capsaicin for pain management: therapeutic potential and mechanisms of action of the new high-concentration capsaicin 8% patch. *Br J Anaesth* 2011; **107**(4): 490–502

64. Binder A, Baron R. Postherpetic neuralgia—fighting pain with fire. *Lancet Neurol* 2008; **7**: 1077–8

65. Attal N, Cruccu G, Baron R, et al. EFNS guidelines on the pharmacological treatment of neuropathic pain: 2010 revision. *Eur J Neurol* 2010; **17**: 1113–e88.

66. Chaparro L, Wiffen PJ, Moore RA, Gilron I. Combination pharmacotherapy for the treatment of neuropathic pain in adults. *Cochrane Database Syst Rev* 2012; **7**: CD008943

67. Sbruzzi G, Silveira SA, Silva DV, Coronel CC, Plentz RD. Transcutaneous electrical nerve stimulation after thoracic surgery: systematic review and meta-analysis of 11 randomized trials. *Rev Bras Cir Cardiovasc* 2012; **27**: 75–87

68. Mulvey MR, Bagnall AM, Johnson MI, Marchant PR. Transcutaneous electrical nerve stimulation (TENS) for phantom pain and stump pain following amputation in adults. *Cochrane Database Syst Rev* 2010; **5**: CD007264.-DOI: 10.1002/14651858.CD007264.pub2

69. Mailis A, Taenzer P. Evidence-based guideline for neuropathic pain interventional treatments: spinal cord stimulation, intravenous infusions, epidural injections and nerve blocks. *Pain Res Manage* 2012; **17**: 150–8

70. Graybill J, Conermann T, Kabazie AJ, Chandy S. Spinal cord stimulation for treatment of pain in a patient with post thoracotomy pain syndrome. *Pain Physician* 2011; **14**: 441–5

71. Ayad AE, El MA. Epidural steroid and clonidine for chronic intractable post-thoracotomy pain: a pilot study. *Pain Pract* 2012; **12**: 7–13

72. Goyal GN, Gupta D, Jain R, Kumar S, Mishra S, Bhatnagar S. Peripheral nerve field stimulation for intractable post-thoracotomy scar pain not relieved by conventional treatment. *Pain Pract* 2010; **10**: 366–9

73. Cohen SP, Sireci A, Wu CL, Larkin TM, Williams KA, Hurley RW. Pulsed radiofrequency of the dorsal root ganglia is superior to pharmacotherapy or pulsed radiofrequency of the intercostal nerves in the treatment of chronic postsurgical thoracic pain. *Pain Physician* 2006; **9**: 227–35

74. Scascighini L, Toma V, Dober-Spielmann S, Sprott H. Multidisciplinary treatment for chronic pain: a systematic review of interventions and outcomes. *Rheumatology* 2008; **47**(5): 670–8

CHAPTER 40

Designing state-of-the-art cardiothoracic surgical suites

Bill Rostenberg and D. Kirk Hamilton

Introduction

Of all building types, healthcare facilities are some of the most complex to design (1). In particular, surgical suites, and operating rooms challenge designers to improve patient safety, infection control and clinical throughput while accommodating future changes (2) in care delivery and evolving technology. Similarly, the construction of surgical suites requires constructors to minimize disruption to ongoing services, prevent construction-related infection, and coordinate rapidly changing equipment and systems.

Successful project design and construction requires a highly integrated process in which multiple participants (designers, builders, medical and clinical specialists, patients, and often educators and researchers) must merge their diverse perspectives, languages, and cultures in order to collaboratively create an environment that supports complex processes with a high degree of reliability, efficiency, and longevity. The most successful projects result from active input from key facility users and the skilled facilitation of a process in which divergent needs are resolved equitably for all.

Collaborative input from anaesthesiologists (3), surgeons, nurses, and support staff is of key importance. Each has unique expertise to contribute regarding work flow, safety, operations, and clinical care. Patient input is also invaluable. A common challenge is facilitating a process that does not limit idea generation to that which stems exclusively from individuals' past personal experience. The design of a new or renovated surgical suite is best approached as a catalyst to improve current processes, whether they be clinical, financial, operational, experiential, or all of those. Innovative approaches, successfully used elsewhere, should also be encouraged. Redesign of clinical process that eliminates waste or removes unnecessarily redundant steps will directly affect design decisions (4).

This chapter summarizes important considerations to be addressed while designing a cardiothoracic surgical facility. It begins with suggestions for optimal design of the overall surgical suite and continues with focused design recommendations for specific operating rooms, including evolving configurations of hybrid operating rooms designed for the combined needs of both open and closed surgery and the use of advanced image-guidance equipment.

Evidence-based design

Design decisions related to the development of surgical facilities can be crucially important, and should be made, insofar as possible, on the basis of the best available relevant evidence from credible research and careful evaluation of practice. The implication of evidence-based design is that the design team must seek out the available literature and make careful interpretations of the implications for their specific project, recognizing that new evidence is regularly being generated and published.

Designing surgical suites

Surgical suite design is influenced by several variables: is the project new construction, expansion of an existing facility, or internal renovation (5)? Is it a community hospital or an academic medical centre? Is the suite governed by surgery, anaesthesiology, cardiology, our jointly by all? Are procedures primarily inpatient, outpatient, or both? Are interventional radiology and interventional cardiology integrated with, or separate from, the surgical suite? Each of these variables, as well as financial constraints and personal philosophies will influence design.

Surgical suite location and adjacencies

Regardless of the variables just mentioned, key functional adjacencies typically remain constant. These include, but are not limited to, access to and from emergency services, imaging services, pathology, intensive care and acute surgical beds, helipad, and central sterile instrument processing. The availability of properly sized and configured floor area will determine viable options for the location of new construction or renovation. A space that is relatively unencumbered by 'permanent vertical building components' (such as stairways, elevator shafts, major air handling ducts, utility shafts and large structural elements) will maximize future expansion and renovation opportunities (figure 40.1). A space that is isolated from vibration transmitted from building systems (such as air handlers) will more easily accommodate vibration-sensitive procedures without incurring excessive design and construction cost premiums. Future expansion of surgical services can be a priority for selection of a site. Several potential sites should be evaluated and comparatively ranked in order to determine a preferred location.

Surgical suite configuration and work flow

Operational variables—in addition to the availability of optimal space—will influence the shape and layout of the suite. For example, will the flow of clean and soiled goods be separated in

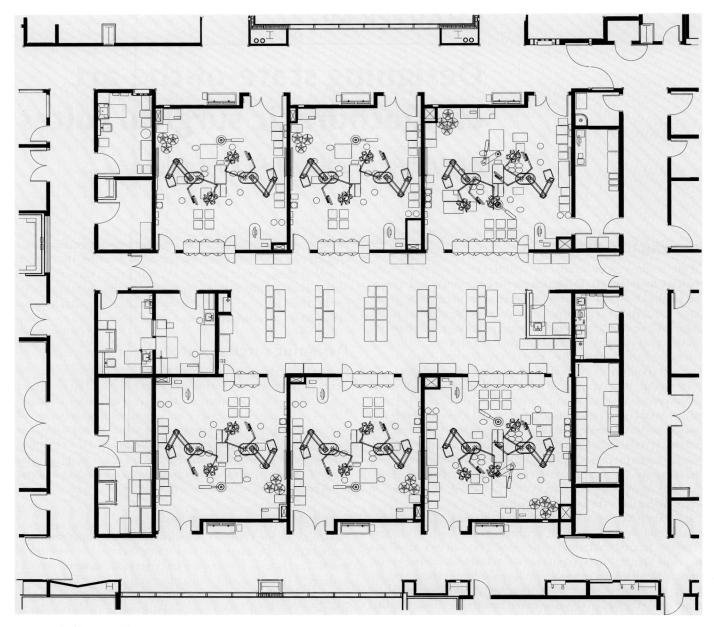

Fig. 40.1 Plan diagram of clean core surgical suite.
Surgical suite layout that is unincumbered by permanent vertical building components provides maximize future flexibility.
Palomar West Medical Center, Escondido, CA; Architect: CO Architects; Associate Architect: Anshen+Allen, a part of Stantec Architecture.© 2012 PPH.

dedicated corridors? Will surgical supplies be transported in closed case carts? Will surgical instruments be processed adjacent to the surgical suite or on a separate floor? A variety of surgical suite typologies—each reflecting different operational approaches—can be abstractly diagrammed (figure 40.2).

A clean core layout segregates clean flow (through the central core) from soiled flow along a perimeter corridor system. In contrast, other configurations separate the flow of patients from the flow of both surgical staff and surgical supplies (figure 40.3). The former approach was once referred to as a 'sterile core', but that term has since been modified to 'clean core' in recognition that while wrapped instruments stored there may be sterile, the space

itself is more accurately described as clean (6). The latter typology is sometimes described as an 'on-stage/off-stage' workflow concept, referring to an innovative design approach developed by the Disney Corporation (7) to segregate customers and services. Applied to surgery, it is often used to improve operational throughput and patient satisfaction, and reflects infection control strategies that optimize the use of closed case cart delivery systems.

Another operational variable that directly influences surgical suite design is the use of anaesthesia induction rooms (figure 40.4) (Chapter 19). This matter is of great interest to anaesthesiologists and surgeons alike. Induction rooms—when utilized—are

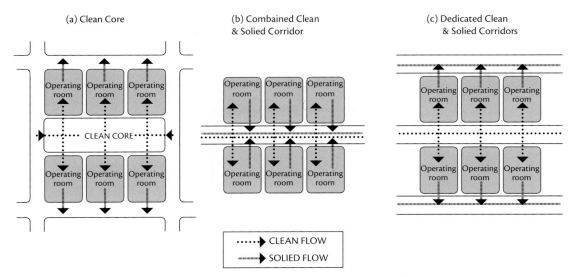

Fig. 40.2 Conceptual diagram of surgical suite typologies.
Surgical suites can be configured (a) around a central clean core with clean goods entering the operating rooms from the clean core and exiting through a perimeter corridor; (b) with soiled and clean goods traveling through a combined corridor; or (c) without a clean core but with dedicated clean and soiled corridors.
© 2012 Stantec Architecture.

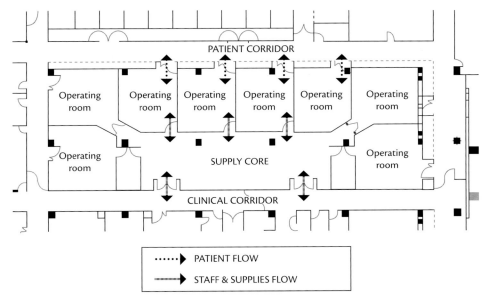

Fig. 40.3 Plan diagram of 'on-stage/off-stage' surgical suite.
This surgical suite separates the flow of patients from the flow of supplies and staff to create an 'on-stage/off-stage' strategy where patients do not cross the flow of clinical traffic.
© 2012 Stantec Architecture.

examples of parallel processing, in which patients are anesthetized outside the operating room while that room is simultaneously being made ready for the patient. Surgical suites with induction rooms adjacent to each operating room require more floor area than suites without induction rooms, but if used effectively they tend to improve the throughput of each operating room and thus reduce overall operating room turn-over time and respectively increase the quantity of procedures per operating room. Induction room work flow has been common in United Kingdom and Commonwealth hospitals while in the United States it has been mostly limited to paediatric surgical facilities (8).

The placement (or the very existence) of flash sterilizers in the surgical suite is another source of debate. Surgeons require sterile instruments be immediately available whenever needed. In recent years, however, The Centers for Disease Control and Prevention (CDC), The Joint Commission (TJC) and the Association of peri-Operative Registered Nurses (AORN) have suggested that flash sterilization of surgical instruments (while safe when performed properly) can lead to surgical site infections (9) when done incorrectly, that improper technique may be related to growing pressure on personnel to work faster, and that flash sterilization should be kept to a minimum and not performed in lieu of having

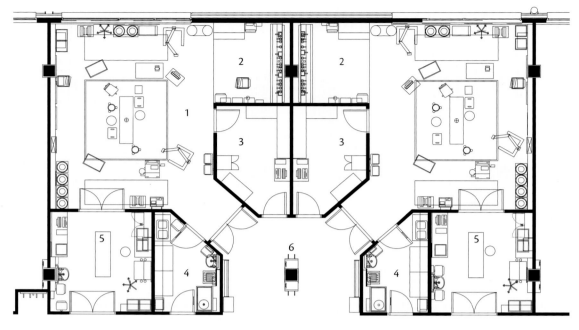

1 Operating room
2 Sterile Set-up
3 Preparation and Storage
4 Dirty Utility
5 Anaesthesia
6 Exit Bay

Fig. 40.4 Plan diagram of surgical suite with anesthetic induction room.
Floor plan showing anaesthesia induction room adjacent to surgical operating room.
© 2012 Stantec Architecture.

backup surgical instruments (10). The growing use of appropriate sealed containers designed for flash sterilization (11) is reducing the need for flash sterilization within the surgical suite when proper central sterile instrument processing operations are in place and appropriately trained personnel are utilized.

General operating room design considerations

Surgical operating room design has evolved over more than a century from simple spaces where procedures were both performed and observed (by a physically present audience) (12,13) within one room into complex technology-driven environments where multifactorial processes take place simultaneously, and the activities therein can be broadcast globally to observers and even to distant participants (14). The earliest operating rooms commonly lacked features to prevent the spread of infection and utilized operable external windows for ventilation. In modern operating rooms both infection control and sophisticated air-handling systems are of critical importance, as is the integration of advanced multimedia image and information communications systems. Key considerations in operating room design include room size, room configuration, internal work flow, lighting, ventilation, and equipment coordination.

Room size

Room size is influenced by the type and complexity of procedures performed within the room as well as variables beyond the

room. One often-overlooked determinant of room size is how much equipment storage is provided (or not provided) within or adjacent to the surgical suite. If adequate equipment storage does not exist, large pieces of surgical equipment are likely to remain within the operating room (or within exit corridors). Both result in safety risks. When inactive surgical equipment resides along the operating room's internal perimeter, an additional 0.91–1.22 m (3–6 lineal feet) of room width may be required in each direction in order to provide an optimal useable floor area. For example, a 56 m^2 (600 square feet) operating room, with 7× 8 m (23 × 26 feet) dimensions would need to be approximately 8 × 9 m (26 × 29 feet), or 70 m^2 (754 net square feet) resulting in a 26% increase in room size.

For many years, recommended general operating room size averaged around 37 m^2 (400 net square feet) of floor area, with minimum room dimensions of 5 m (18 linear feet) and average room dimensions around 6 or 7 m (20 or 22 linear feet). Today it is not uncommon for a sophisticated cardiovascular or cardiothoracic operating room to range in size from 56 to 65 m^2 (600 to 700 square feet) and for hybrid operating rooms to exceed 93 m^2 (1000 square feet) in area.

Room configuration

Most operating rooms tend to be rectangular in shape with a length-to-width proportion of one dimension slightly longer than the other. For example, 7.0 × 8.0 m = 56 m^2; 7.3 × 8.2 m = 60 m^2; 7.6 × 8.5 m =65 m^2 (23 × 26 feet = 598 square feet; 24 × 27 feet = 648 square feet; 25 × 28 feet = 700 square feet). Operating rooms, however, have been designed and built in all permutations of size and shape.

Positioning of the surgical table within the operating room is closely related to room configuration. Similar to other design variables, table position is often driven by personal preference as much as it is by evidence-based science. Many operating rooms are configured with the surgical table perpendicular to the entry corridor and the patient's head on the side of the room farthest from the corridor, because patients are often brought into the room head first. In contrast, in some operating rooms the patient's head is placed closest to the corridor. Other operating room configurations place the surgical table diagonally within the room to better utilize room corners and increase usable space at the sides of the table (figure 40.5).

The advent of image-guided surgery has led to various multi-room operating room configurations. Some arrangements provide dedicated control rooms for the imaging technologist to directly visualize the patient and communicate with the surgical team without having to physically enter the operating room proper and to be protected from radiation scatter (see figure 40.5). Other multi-room configurations provide a space for advanced image-guidance systems to be 'parked' outside the operating

room. In many ways, the surgical operating room of the future will resemble today's cardiac catheterization lab with a dedicated control room and computer electronics room, so the space within the operating room is dedicated to the immediate needs of the surgical procedure.

Charting stations within the operating room should enable staff to visually observe the procedure without having to twist their bodies. The charting station, however, should not extend into circulation space or otherwise obstruct flow within the operating room.

Work flow

A typical clean core layout is intended to create a one-way flow through the operating room, with clean goods entering the operating rooms from the core and soiled goods exiting into the perimeter corridor. Human nature, however, sometimes results in surgical staff taking a 'short-cut' and passing through the clean core to access operating rooms on the other side of the core. This can compromise the intended one-way flow of clean goods from core to operating rooms. In the core design, people (surgical staff, patients, support staff, and so on) enter the operating rooms from the 'soiled' perimeter corridor only after scrubbing in at sinks placed adjacent to the operating room's 'soiled' entrance.

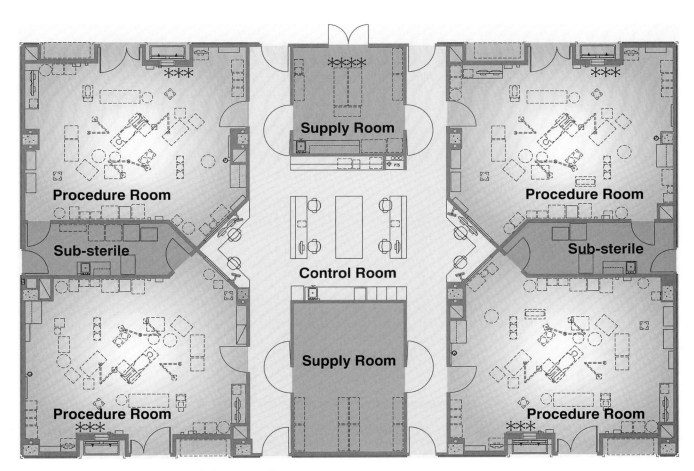

Fig. 40.5 Plan diagram of operating rooms with adjacent control room.
Surgical tables placed diagonally within the operating room provide efficient utilization of the corners of the room and provide good visualization from the adjacent control room. (See also figure in colour plates section)
© 2012 Stantec Architecture.

One variation to the traditional clean core layout places scrub sinks within the core itself to segregate patient flow from staff flow. In such arrangements it is essential that physical barriers protect clean and sterile supplies from water that may splash out of the sink.

Within the operating room, there should be a clear demarcation between circulating, sterile, and anaesthesia zones (figure 40.6) that do not cross each other. In clean core departmental layouts, the sterile zone within the operating room should be separated from circulating activities. The circulating zone should have direct access from the clean core, where sterile supplies and instruments are brought into the operating room and may extend to the perimeter corridor, where scrub sinks are commonly located. The anaesthesia zone—at the patient's head—should be adjacent to the sterile zone. Regardless of how the surgical table is oriented within the operating room, the anaesthesia zone should be protected from all non-anaesthesia related traffic. It is desirable to eliminate potential tripping and connection hazards by providing outlets and connection locations which keep cables, cords, and hoses off the floor.

The zone immediately surrounding the patient on the table, including the surgeon, anaesthetist, anaesthesia work station, surgical assistants, and instrument tables, is often called the 'sterile field', with circulating nurses handing needed items into the field from the perimeter. In some settings the sterile field is marked in a pattern on the floor.

Ventilation

Filtered mechanical ventilation is the current standard for conditioning the environment in an operating room. This usually means cooling the air supply with a high percentage of filtered and humidity controlled fresh air directly from the outside, and smaller amounts of filtered recirculated air. One concept is for the air supply to flow down over the operating field from directly overhead in a laminar-like sheet, across the patient, and on to the floor where it is exhausted at floor level on the diagonally opposite corners of the room. Various opinions exist regarding preferences for the use of laminar flow in the surgical room.

Lighting

Lighting in the operating room has more than one aspect, including specifically the surgical lights intended to support the surgical team's vision in the surgical field, and the general or specific illumination requirements of the room. The highly focused pairs or groups of surgical lights are generally mounted on overhead

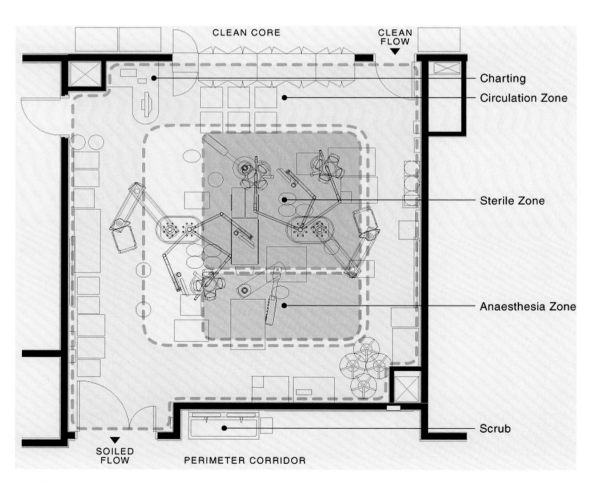

Fig. 40.6 Zoning within the surgical operating room.
Floor plan showing demarcation of circulating, sterile and anesthesia zones. (See also figure in colour plates section)
© 2012 Stantec Architecture.

booms that allow for variable positioning to support the particular procedure underway.

General lighting in the operating room is most often accomplished with banks of fluorescent lights that are configured in a box shape over the table in order to allow for the ventilation system to occupy the central area above the table. Many operating suites have chosen to have the capability for a green lighting option that enhances legibility of monitor images and can reduce glare on monitor surfaces. Applications of LED (light-emitting diode) fixtures—and even LED luminous ceilings—as an alternate approach to surgical lighting are beginning to emerge, although they are currently mostly experimental. It is advisable for task lighting to be associated with the charting area, control stations, or special equipment, such as anaesthesia work stations and intra-aortic pumps. Lighting of hybrid operating rooms poses unique design challenges since typical overhead equipment booms and bridges associated with interventional imaging equipment usually occupy the same ceiling zone, as do surgical lights. Furthermore, ceiling-mounted imaging equipment that travels along overhead bridges will obstruct the light emitted from surgical lights. Special equipment developed for hybrid operating rooms is discussed under 'Hybrid operating rooms.'

Equipment and technology coordination

The technical equipment required for cardiothoracic surgery is complicated and requires coordination in its placement within the room, its connectivity to other devices, and recognition of the requirements for its optimum functionality. Consideration must be given to fixed equipment installed into the room, as well as mobile equipment, which may come and go from the operating room. In contemporary cardiothoracic procedures, coordination between surgical equipment, anaesthesia equipment, information systems, clinical imaging, audio-visual recording systems, and sophisticated communications systems is crucial. Dedicated electronics cabinets adjacent to the operating room enable the growing number of server cabinets to be removed from the operating room proper, allowing the valuable surgical floor space to be dedicated to equipment that must be in the room.

Minimally invasive surgery considerations

The requirements for minimally invasive use of laparoscopic devices include multiple screens upon which images from the inserted cameras can be viewed. The surgical team views the procedure 'indirectly' via these monitors, rather than 'directly' via open incisions. As a result, ambient lighting of minimally invasive operating rooms tends to be darker than in traditional open surgical operating rooms, to enhance monitor visualization. The use of green lighting discussed previously, however, can enable ambient illumination levels to remain relatively high without degrading monitor-displayed images. Ceiling-and wall-mounted monitors (compared to monitors on carts) reduce the need for dangerous loose cables and wires, which can become tripping hazards.

In some cases there may be a need for air-cooled or water-cooled laser devices, and an attendant understanding of the heat loads added to the operating room. Special signage advising of laser use, space for laser storage, and both cooling and heat evacuation capacity should be considered as part of the room design.

Audio-visual equipment

The operating room environment is becoming increasingly sophisticated in terms of audio-visual capabilities. In addition to computerized records and documentation, there is a need to display digital images from previous studies, as well as live images from fluoroscopy, laparoscopy, or catheterization.

Cameras and recording devices can capture the live procedure with time markers. Telemedicine requires high-definition camera and microphone connections. Monitors and screens can be wall mounted, or on booms, which allows positioning for optimum viewing by the surgeon. This requires understanding where the surgeon will stand, and how the monitors can be moved out of the way when not needed.

Many surgeons listen to music while working. In addition, sound systems can be used for voice recordings to accompany film or video. Built-in sound systems can reduce clutter and eliminate system components requiring special cleaning.

Robotic surgery

In instances where robotic surgery is anticipated, the operating room must be sufficiently sized to allow for the robotic device to extend into the space above and around the operating table. The room should ideally be large enough to provide an appropriate area for the console in which the surgeon manipulates the robot. Where this is not possible, the console can be located in a nearby space outside the operating room. In addition, the provision of large wall-mounted monitors should be considered to allow the surgical team to view the procedure in progress. In some instances, an entire wall (or portion thereof) will have multiple monitors affixed to display various types of anatomic, physiological, and alpha-numeric information.

Hybrid operating rooms

As much of surgery has become less invasive and much of imaging has become more interventional, (15) the ever-blurring boundary between surgery and interventional imaging continues to become obscure. As a result, the hybrid surgical operating room—an environment designed for both open and closed surgery—is becoming increasingly popular (figure 40.7).

Hybrid operating rooms are sometimes thought of as surgical operating rooms with advanced imaging capabilities or as advanced interventional procedure laboratories with enhanced infection control standards. In either case, characteristics of a hybrid operating room typically include: (a) the environment is appropriate for both open and closed surgical procedures; (b) it utilizes fixed imaging equipment capable of real-time, or near real-time imaging; (c) it includes dedicated control and electronics equipment rooms; and (d) it adheres to infection control and other surgical protocols typically recommended by AORN and similar professional organizations.

There are several challenges associated with integrating the physical and clinical needs of both surgery and interventional procedures. First, competition for valuable ceiling space abounds. In the surgical environment the ceiling plane is typically needed for surgical lights, equipment and utility booms, air filtration distribution, and so forth. In the interventional environment, the ceiling plane is typically reserved for ceiling-mounted imaging

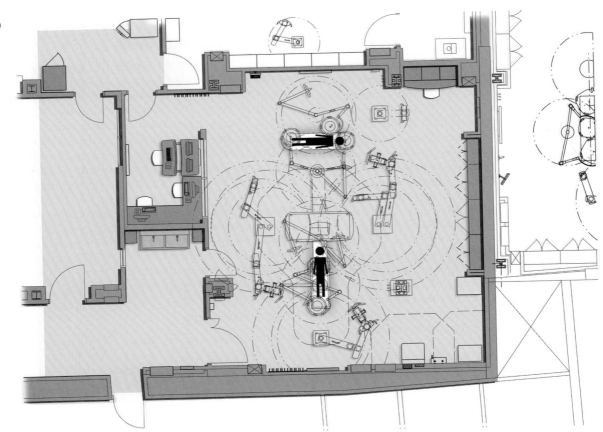

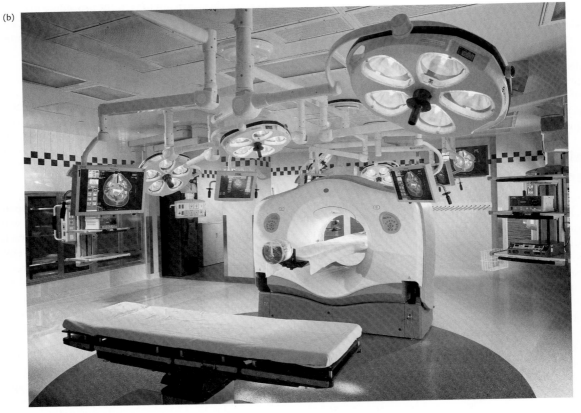

Fig. 40.7 Hybrid surgical operating room.

(a) Floor plan and (b) photograph of hybrid surgical operating room with CT imaging capabilities. (See also figure in colour plates section)

(a) University of Pittsburgh Medical Center Hybrid OR # 12; floor plan, © 2007 Stantec Architecture. (b) Interior photograph of University of Pittsburgh Medical Center Hybrid OR 12, © 2007 Ed Massery.

equipment, such as c-arms, monitors, radiation shielding, and so forth. Recently, equipment vendors have developed some imaging systems designed specifically for use in the surgical environment (16). These systems are attached to the floor and/or ceiling in such a way that they minimize spatial conflicts with most floor- and ceiling-mounted surgical devices.

Second, patient tables associated with most advanced medical imaging systems have traditionally been more monolithic and less flexible than those commonly used in surgical operating rooms. For example, traditional imaging tables are difficult to clean, do not 'break' into the various positions (such as Trendelenburg) that most surgical tables do, and often physically obstruct the surgical team ergonomically from certain postures necessitated by complex procedures. Recently, however, 'breakable' imaging tables designed to be compatible with many surgical procedures have become available.

Various opinions abound regarding the adequacy of currently available surgical tables that are compatible with state-of-the-art interventional imaging systems. In some suites where standard imaging tables are used, additional space for a second surgical table is provided so the room can be scheduled for both minimally invasive and open surgical procedures. Alternatively, some suites equipped with breakable surgical tables integrated into the interventional imaging assembly are designed to accommodate both minimally invasive and open surgical procedures. In such configurations, careful consideration must be given as to how gases and other utilities are conveyed through the floor and table base into the imaging assembly.

First-generation hybrid operating rooms typically were limited to radiographic and fluoroscopic (R/F) imaging, used primarily for endovascular image guidance. Advanced R/F image guidance including rotational angiography soon became desirable, resulting in large floor- and ceiling-mounted c-arms that rotate in place. Later generation R/F rotational angiography capabilities come in the form of enclosed gantry computerized tomography (CT) systems. Most CT image guidance systems are used for neurosurgical, spine and ear, nose, and throat (ENT) procedures.

Intraoperative magnetic resonance imaging (I-MRI) is used increasingly for neurosurgical, ENT, oncological, and other surgical cases. Two basic I-MRI room and equipment configurations are common: either (a) the patient moves between a stationary magnet and surgical zone, or (b) the magnet moves to and from the surgical zone where the patient remains stationary.

In the first configuration, the anaesthetized patient is transported to and from a stationary MRI scanner into a sterile surgical zone to assure that all non-MRI-safe objects (including surgical instruments) remain beyond the magnet's 5-gauss exclusion zone. In a variation to this configuration, both the patient and table move in unison. The surgical table (which is also the scanner table upon which the patient remains) pivots into and out of the non-movable scanner's 5-gauss line during imaging and surgery, respectively. In either case, moving the surgical patient is itself a complex procedure.

In the other I-MRI configuration, the MRI scanner physically moves into and away from the surgical zone while the patient remains stationary on the surgical table (figure 40.8). This approach reduces the need to move the anaesthetized patient, thus reducing the potential for associated clinical complications, but introduces a potentially more complex design and infrastructure challenge.

Some I-MRI hybrid suites provide fluoroscopy in addition to MRI (figure 40.9) for supplementary image navigation that supports particular cardiovascular surgical procedures. Surgical operating rooms where built-in R/F (or CT) imaging systems are installed require environmental radiation protection. Calculations identifying quantities and locations of radiation protection must be determined by a certified medical physicist. Specific radiation protection requirements commonly vary by jurisdiction and geographic location.

I-MRI—regardless of the physical configuration—introduces unique design challenges of both safety and providing a physical environment in which the MR image is not degraded by either electromagnetic or radio-frequency emissions. All MRI rooms require continuous radio-frequency shielding in the walls, ceiling, floor, doors, windows, and any penetrations through any of the above surfaces. Some MRI rooms require magnetic shielding in addition to the radio-frequency shielding to contain the magnet's 5 gauss influence within a specific portion of the operating room, or to compensate for large ferrous masses that would otherwise degrade the magnet's clinical imaging capability.

I-MRI suites must be designed with consideration for MR safety, including restricted access, ferrous metal detection strategies, and prevention of non-MRI-safe devices from approaching areas close to the magnet. All persons involved in the design and use of the I-MRI suite should be familiar with current MRI Safety Guidelines published by the American College of Radiology (ACR) (17). While these guidelines are written primarily for diagnostic MR suites, they include information relevant to general MR safety. Designers and surgical staff should understand that compared to diagnostic MR suites, I-MRI suites are more challenging to design for many reasons, including the need to incorporate both infection control and MR safety, and the realization that procedures performed within the I-MRI suite will likely utilize surgical instruments made of materials that must not be placed near the magnet. (In contrast, diagnostic MR suites are designed to prevent such materials from entering the suite.)

Anaesthetic considerations

Anaesthesia work stations may consist of rolling equipment mounted on antistatic wheels, or apparatus suspended from the ceiling. Continuous flow anaesthesia work stations may be serviced by medical gases in portable cylinders that are mounted on the work station, or from permanent ceiling-mounted pendants. It is recommended practice to provide redundancy in case of a problem with the work station in use. Redundancy generally means duplicate positions for pendant drops of medical gases diagonally off the head and foot of the operating table. If the services at the head become interrupted, the table is rotated to relocate the head at the former foot position, and the duplicate gas pendants are attached to the machine. Dropping pendants from the ceiling contributes to elimination of cords, hoses, and tripping hazards on the floor of the operating room. In the case of self-contained gas systems dependent upon cylinders, redundancy means another work station available close by the operating room.

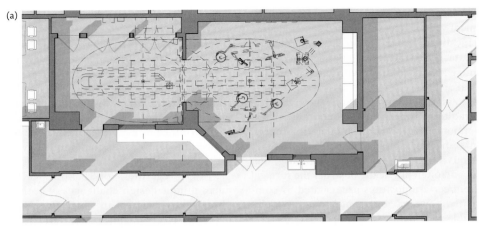

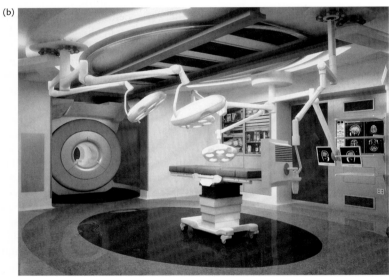

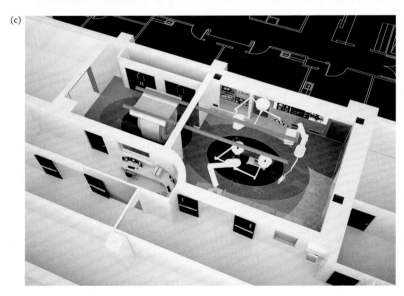

Fig. 40.8 Intraoperative MRI (I-MRI) suite.
Intraoperative MR suite where magnet moves to and from patient (a) floor plan; (b) interior perspective; and (c) axonometric view. (See also figure in colour plates section)
Bostwick Design Partnership, Architect of Record; Anshen+Allen, a part of Stantec Architecture, Consulting Architect.
(a) © 2012 Bostwick Design Partnership. (b) © 2012 Stantec Architecture. (c) © 2012 Stantec Architecture.

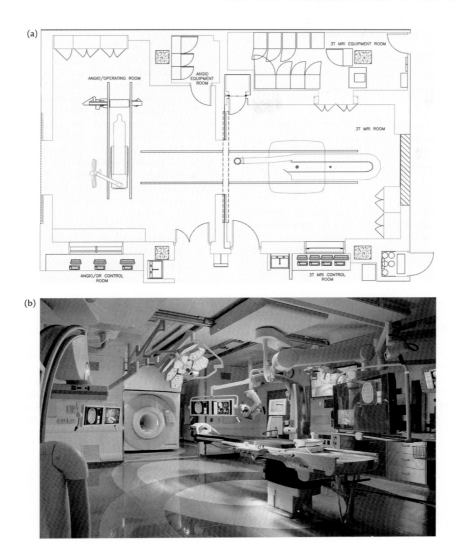

Fig. 40.9 Intra-operative MRI + fluoroscopy suite.
Intraoperative MR suite (with moving magnet) that also provides fluoroscopic image guidance: (a) floor plan and (b) interior photograph.
(a) Floor plan of I-MRI at Brigham and Womens Hospital © 2012 IMRIS. (b) Interior photograph of I-MRI at Brigham and Womens Hospital © 2012 Warren Jaggers Photography.

Regardless of the type of anaesthesia work station, the anaesthetist will be positioned at the head of the table, monitoring the patient's airway, with the work station at his or her side. The principal tasks involve monitoring heart rate, blood pressure, pulse oximetry, and capnography, so convenient views of monitors which display these parameters is important. An anaesthesia cart may also be required to make IV medications available, and to provide ready access to essential anaesthesia supplies. Sufficient space for the anaesthesia functions at the patient's head means provision of sufficient clear space behind the anaesthetist, work station, and cart to allow proper circulation of staff and equipment that may be needed.

Conclusion

Cardiothoracic operating rooms are rooms in which a single patient on an operating table receives a surgical intervention from a skilled multidisciplinary surgical team. Surgery, anaesthesiology, cardiology, and associated clinical specialties all have unique requirements, and the technology continues to advance.

Organizations with a need to plan surgical facilities must be clear about their project's objectives, governance, and budgetary parameters, and all persons involved must understand what happens in a cardiothoracic procedure undertaken by a high-performance team of experts.

Those with upcoming projects should consider touring good examples of recently designed suites that meet similar objectives as their own, and learn from their peers what worked well and what they would do differently. In addition, careful consideration should be given to how both clinical practices and medical technology are changing, and thus how to best accommodate anticipated future developments into the suite's design and construction.

Those undertaking the design and construction of a new cardiothoracic surgical suite should consider the following:

- Begin early. Select a qualified design team. Involve the diverse users of the new facility.
- Research the literature and benchmark successful surgical programmes.

- Base the most important decisions upon solid evidence.

- Test decisions in a full-size mock-up.

- Incorporate design features that accommodate multiple levels of future flexibility as techniques and technology will certainly change.

A properly designed and constructed operating room offers the cardiothoracic surgical team an environment for effective, productive, and safe outcomes, as well as an opportunity to improve upon current work flow, throughput, and operational processes.

References

1. Rostenberg, B. *The architecture of medical imaging: designing healthcare facilities for advanced radiological diagnostic and therapeutic techniques.* Hoboken, NJ: John Wiley & Sons Inc., 2006
2. Beckham, D. The impossibility of predicting the future. Hosp Health Netw Daily. [Internet] 2012 Feb [cited 2012 March 12]; Available at: http://www.hhnmag.com/hhnmag/HHNDaily/HHNDailyDisplay.dhtml?id=5800008207 (accessed 3 June 2014)
3. Tan, TK, Goh J. The anaesthetist's role in setting up of an intraoperative MR imaging facility. *Singapore Med J* 2009; **50**(1): 4–10
4. Stroupe, J. How lean strategies can streamline hospital design. *Health Facil Manage* 2012; **25**(2): 23–7
5. Rostenberg, B, Barach, P. Design of cardiovascular operating rooms for tomorrow's technology and clinical practice—part one. *Prog Pediatr Cardiol* 2011; **32**(2): 121–8
6. Bird BT. Infection control and the central sterile supply department. *Infection Control Today.* [Internet] May 2011 Available at: http://www.infectioncontroltoday.com/articles/2011/05/infection-control-and-the-central-sterile-supply-department.aspx (accessed 3 June 2014]
7. McCullough, C. *Evidence-based design for healthcare facilities [internet].* Indianapolis, IN: Sigma Theta Tau International, 2010
8. Rostenberg, B, Barach, P. Design of cardiovascular operating rooms for tomorrow's technology and clinical practice—part one. *Prog Pediatr Cardiol* 2011; **32**(2): 121–8
9. Mangram, A, Horan, T, Pearson, M, Silver, LC, Jarvis, W. *Guideline for prevention of surgical site infection, 1999 [Internet].* Atlanta, GA: Center for Disease Control; 1999. Available at http://www.cdc.gov/hicpac/pdf/guidelines/SSI_1999.pdf (accessed 3 June 2014)
10. Association of periOperative Registered Nurses. Recommended practices for sterilization in the perioperative setting. In: Standards, Recommended Practices and Guidelines. Denver, CO: AORN, Inc., 2007; p. 673–87
11. Carlo, A. The new era of flash sterilization. *AORN J* 2007; **86**(1): 58–68
12. Rostenberg, B, Barach, P. Design of cardiovascular operating rooms for tomorrow's technology and clinical practice—part two. *Prog Pediatr Cardiol* 2012; **33**(1): 57–65
13. Stevens, EF. *The American hospital of the twentieth century.* New York, NY: Architectural Record Co., 1918
14. Satava, R. Emerging technologies for surgery in the 21st century. *Arch Surg* 1999; **134**: 1197–202
15. Rostenberg B. 'Surgology': the impact on design. *Hosp Manage Int* 2005/06; 13–5
16. Siemens Artis zeego [Internet]. Munich: Siemens Aktiengesellschaft; 2012. Available at: http://usa.healthcare.siemens.com/surgical-c-arms-and-navigation/hybrid-or/artis-zeego (accessed 10 June 2014)
17. Kanal, E. FDA MRI Safety Public Workshop. October 25–26, 2011. Available at: www.fda.gov/downloads/MedicalDevices/.../UCM283560.pdf (accessed 3 June 2014)

CHAPTER 41

Training programmes for cardiothoracic anaesthesia: curricula, administration, and evaluations

Jane Heggie and W. Scott Beattie

Programme introduction

Cardiac (or cardiothoracic) postgraduate educational programmes are essential to both the development and maintenance of anaesthesia as a specialty. These educational programmes can exist as a post-residency specialty programme, as in the US with the Accreditation Council for Graduate Medical Education (ACGME), in Canada a post-specialist qualification Fellowship of the Royal College of Physicians and Surgeons, and in Europe as described by the European Association of Cardiothoracoic Anaesthesiologists (EACTA) (1). In addition, specialized cardiac anaesthesia programmes also exist as an 'in training' year away as a fellowship such as in the UK, Ireland, Australia, and New Zealand.

In our view, dedicated cardiovascular anaesthesia fellowships are an integral component of the expanding scope of practice, not only for the anaesthetist, but also for the varied practitioners that we work with. Previously cardiac anaesthesiology was largely confined to the operating room and a relationship with a surgical team. We now are increasingly viewed as perioperative clinicians working in multiple disciplines of anaesthesia, critical care and echocardiography. Now, we not only work with cardiac, thoracic and vascular surgeons but also interventional radiologists, cardiologists and as, or in conjunction with, critical care physicians.

The mission of the modern training programme is to achieve a set of core competencies, regardless of the candidate's background, and yet be flexible enough to be tailored to the ultimate goals of the individual trainee ('fellow'). The programme should have the ability to train a candidate destined for a leadership role. In addition to teaching the clinical skills of the subspecialty we must also teach them to become educators and possess the ability to critically evaluate aspects of our specialty. Mentorship assumes a key role in the paradigm to allow for the clinical, research and educational aspects for the fellowship (2).

The ACGME curriculum is a prescribed 12-month curriculum with mandatory competencies and case numbers. EACTA has a consensus document with similar benchmarks but allows a maximum of 24 months to achieve these programme requirements. The programme at the University Health Network in Toronto offers a core year as well as enriched training at an advanced level in an optional second year for core graduates as well as international trainees.

It is a crucial requirement of any educational programme that the faculty is committed to funding it. Practice plans that support an academic practice not only for fellows but junior faculty are, in our view, the ideal environment (3). Fellows and junior faculty must be supported with stable salaries that alleviate the strain of delaying a full time practice and payment of student debt (3). The source of funding can be from group billings, sponsoring agencies, the hospital, or from government funding. Deregulation of post-secondary education in many countries in addition to medical school costs has created an unprecedented rise in medical school debt (4). The practice plan will likely be accredited for residency training; however, many tertiary and quaternary care centres that could have fellowship level-only trainees.

EACTA has outlined requirements for physical and educational facilities of the sponsoring institutions for the core rotations of the programme. In North America these requirements would be met by accreditation bodies of the ACGME (USA) and the RCPS (Canada), and programmes must be approved for resident training with these organizations to be considered for fellowship accreditation.

In this chapter we will define clinical curriculum, didactic curriculum, as well as paradigms for the teaching of echocardiography and the conduct of research.

It is obvious that cardiac fellowship programmes be administered by faculty members. The director's role should include the chairing of the selection of candidates, the design and plan of both the clinical and didactic curriculum development, conducting the assessment and feedback of the fellows, while also facilitating mentorship and career planning.

Curriculum

Clinical curriculum

The core clinical competencies are best achieved through the care of patients. Thus, candidates should be exposed to all aspects of the patient experiences. Other educational formats involving didactic lectures, simulation, research and teaching are also important but cannot replace clinical experience. There should be a basic minimum clinical experience in all programmes. The UK, USA, and EACTA have guidelines that mandate a minimum number of cardiac cases (cardiopulmonary (CPB) and off-pump cases) (5). Thus, the number of fellows, in a programme at any time, will be limited by the centre's ability to deliver this caseload. The clinical experience, however, must surpass this operating room 'basic minimum'.

A core curriculum will involve clinical assignments that will include surgical procedures that require CPB. It is the expectation that candidates complete a minimum of number cases per year. The UK, US, and European programmes have guidelines that mandate a minimum number of cardiac cases (CPB and off-pump cases), of which 50% must be valve or revision of congenital repair. The basic number of cases and mix vary from a minimum 100 cases in the EACTA proposal to 110 in the Society of Cardiovascular Anesthesiologists (SCA) guidelines. All programmes have a requirement that the case mix reflect a diverse practice and that less than 50% should comprise routine coronary revascularization but also have exposure to off bypass coronary revascularization, valvular repair and replacement, and cases involving deep hypothermia and circulatory arrest (DHCA). The SCA specifies required competencies in transesophageal echocardiography, transplantation, ventricular assist devices and congenital heart disease whereas the ECATA strongly recommends exposure to these areas, as well as others outlined in subsequent sections, of cardiac practice. The role of critical care training in relation to a cardiac anaesthesia fellowship is under review in North America, Europe, and Australia, with many advocating for a second year of dedicated critical care medicine (CCM) training specific to cardiovascular intensive care.

In addition, candidates should be assigned to other cardiac service lists. There is an expanding role for anaesthesia services in ablation of atrial and ventricular arrhythmias, sedation for outpatient cardiology diagnostic procedures (transoesophageal echocardiography (TOE) and computerized tomography (CT) angiography), and cardioversions (6,7). Interventional cardiology is an expanding commitment, while expanding the utilization of the insertion of aortic stents for coarctation, device closure of atrial septal defects, ventricular septal defects, and perivalvular leak. The advent of newer and better-designed percutaneous valves is expected to increase the need for anaesthesia and echocardiographic evaluation in the operating room for repair and replacement procedures.

Presurgical assessment is a critical component of the cardiac fellowship programme and reflects our increasing role as perioperative physicians. In addition to preoperative cardiac surgery patients, the candidate should be exposed to the planning of care for patients for cardioversions, interventional cardiology procedures, and electrophysiological studies and ablations. Patients with acquired heart disease, congenital heart disease, end-stage heart failure, and who are post transplantation will frequently require non-cardiac surgery. Complex patients presented at multidisciplinary rounds for management discussion should always involve candidates at the initial consultation and subsequent planning meetings.

The majority of patients with congenital (paediatric) heart disease are adults. The number of adults with congenital heart disease has exceeded the number of children and infants with congenital heart disease for over a decade, and will increase significantly over the next decade. In addition to the cardiac surgical cases, these patients will increasingly need non-cardiac surgery and the anaesthetic considerations for these complex patients can be equally if not more challenging and a valuable learning experience for the trainee. Reference centres differ in their delivery of services. Many have a clear delineation at the age of 16–18 when the patient transitions from a paediatric setting to an adult care facility. The pathway for many countries to cardiac anaesthesia for the neonate and young child is via a paediatric anaesthesia fellowship. The inclusion of one month of paediatric congenital heart surgery as an elective in many programmes both in Europe and North America is helpful in providing a context to the adult with congenital heart disease but does not provide sufficient training for the graduate to provide these services at the end of the core year. It may be possible to do a second advanced year or to be recruited to a centre that provides this service and will offer a mentoring role to the recent graduate.

Heart–lung transplantation, and ventricular assist device (VAD) programmes may not be available at some centres; this can, at least in part, be offset with access to each centres cardiology-based heart failure programmes. Ideally the fellow will be exposed to the preoperative assessment and optimization of a heart failure or transplant candidate and learn competencies to provide intraoperative and post-intensive care unit (ICU) management of the VAD or heart transplant recipient. There are specific considerations for a heart transplant or VAD insertion; however, there also many commonalities in complex valve cases. Fellows that become adept at managing pulmonary hypertension or right heart failure in congenital heart disease and end stage left-sided heart disease will have developed competencies to deal with many of the considerations for VAD insertion and heart transplantation. Although direct exposure would be ideal it is possible to train a fellow to become a junior faculty at a centre that does offer these services.

Transoesophageal echocardiography

Dedicated TOE teaching and clinical exposure in compliance with the European and or SCA guidelines is mandatory to a core clinical fellowship. Irrespective of this requirement TOE training should not supersede the development of other core competencies of cardiothoracic anaesthetic practice. We have noticed increasingly that trainees have a disproportionate focus on competency in TOE that is not reflected in a high-volume cardiac practice.

Centres will differ in their TOE training methodology. There are two main philosophies: (i) one staff and one fellow assigned to do all perioperative TOEs in the operating room both pre- and post-bypass, and the ICU; (ii) in centres where all cardiac anaesthesia faculty members are TOE certified it is common for the anaesthetist to provide anaesthetic care and perform the pre- and post-bypass TOE, and to supervise the fellow in each of these activities. There are pros and cons to each method and the choice should be made on what is best for patient care. However, it is our belief that a trainee cannot have the dual responsibility for monitoring the patient while performing, interpreting, and learning the TOE skill set.

Requirements for TOE training are described in the SCA guidelines, and include a minimum of 150 studies in which the fellow personally performs the study and participates in the reporting of the study. In addition there must be a formal reading session in which cases are reviewed to reach a minimum total of 300 studies performed and read. The Australian and New Zealand College of Anaesthetists have similar guidelines, requiring 50 closely supervised studies followed by 50 studies unsupervised, and reviewed by a supervisor who is accredited. A minimum of 100 studies must have a formalized review process. Supervision of theses reviews is expected to be with a certified perioperative TOE clinician or equivalent. The Australian and New Zealand College of Anaesthetists guidelines are explicit; the training should be the equivalent of 50 full-time days or over a minimum of 10 weeks and a maximum of 2 years. They further recommend that early in the training period a fellow have a 2-week period dedicated to TOE to develop a foundation in echo and increase learning opportunities throughout the year (8). The SCA and EACTA guidelines are less explicit. A core number of studies must be attained however they do not dictate the method and distribution of the instruction (9).

Electives

Postoperative cardiac intensive care is a rotation that is mandatory in many programmes and highlights the importance of the anaesthetist as perioperative physician. Decisions that are made intraoperatively impact the patient's recovery. The number of anaesthesia trainees participating in CCM programmes post residency is in steep decline (10). Although many graduates of cardiac anaesthesia fellowships will never go on to practice and recover ICU patients they will gain valuable insights into recovery from a formal rotation in the ICU.

A basic, or limited, transthoracic echocardiography (TTE) examination, as described in the emergency medicine literature as the FOCUS exam (11), is gaining prominence in anaesthesia (12–14). Whether this degree of expertise could be offered in a 1-month elective, or as part of an expanded TOE curriculum, is for individual departments to explore. It will continue to expand and is an important adjunct to the anaesthesiologist's role as perioperative physicians and improving patient safety.

Thoracic surgery exists in most cardiac centres; however, there are some very specialized centres where there is no thoracic service. Ideally, a programme should offer thoracic surgery exposure and exposure to lung transplantation. The ability to provide adequate clinical experience in lung transplantation in addition to the full cardiac core curriculum, described earlier, usually requires training beyond the core year.

Major vascular surgery is another potential elective that in many cases is included in the core curriculum. Anaesthetic exposure to abdominal and thoracic aneurysm repair, for both open and endovascular repair is in our view best managed by anaesthesiologists with core cardiac competencies. Further, this elective should also provide competencies in methods of spinal cord protection. Carotid artery surgery and resection of tumours infiltrating or compressing the cava would enhance the core clinical curriculum.

Didactic curriculum

Core curriculum

The didactic curriculum is designed to include cardiac anatomy, physiology (including electrophysiology), and pharmacology, ideally presented by cardiac anaesthesia faculty. Sessions should include subspecialty seminars on surgical issues, transfusion medicine, infectious disease, and critical care where it may be ideal to include invited faculty. A list of suggested subjects is included in box 41.1.

In addition to faculty, candidates should be encouraged to prepare didactic tutorials on a component of cardiac anesthesia practice, ideally in a formal setting. We also encourage separate sessions dedicated to 'trouble rounds', at regular intervals, where members can present difficult cases and discuss management.

Transoesophageal echocardiography

In our programme, TOE sessions are run as a separate didactic unit. The unit includes review of theory, as well as ongoing review of interesting cases from our library. Candidates also have access to our online teaching simulation to get pre-trained on the 20 basic views, anatomy and probe manipulation (15). Similarly, we encourage the use of TOE simulators at regular intervals. TOE teaching sessions are regularly scheduled. A list of didactic echocardiographic topics is presented in box 41.2. In our institution, all fellows are released from clinical duties to attend these sessions. In our view while TOE is assuming a greater role in our specialty it is still just a tool and no more important than other aspects such as transfusion medicine or pharmacology. Fellows who achieve the core elements of clinical experience should also be reading the associated TOE throughout the year. It is our experience that candidates will learn most when reading about a topic in the context of a challenging case. If possible, members from the corresponding cardiac surgical division should attend these TOE reading sessions. In our experience cardiac surgery fellows can describe intraoperative surgical events and explain the operative

---

Box 41.1 Core didactic topics

- Physics and knobology
- 20 Basic views
- Colour flow and Doppler
- Tricuspid and pulmonary valves
- Left ventricular function
- Right ventricular function
- Mitral valve anatomy
- Mitral valve pathology, repair and replacement
- Aortic valve pathology and replacement
- Valve sparing aortic root surgery and aortic valve repair
- Diseases of the pericardium
- Simple congenital heart disease and septal lesions
- Complex congenital heart disease
- TOE safety

Box 41.2 Core topics for TOE didactic sessions

- ◆ Preoperative assessment of the cardiac surgery patient
- ◆ Induction, cannulation and management of the patient on CPB
- ◆ CPB and extracorporeal membrane oxygenation
- ◆ Management of separation from bypass
- ◆ Common ICU problems immediately following cardiac surgery
- ◆ Heart failure management and surgical therapies
- ◆ Ventricular assist devices
- ◆ Heart, lung, and heart–lung transplantation
- ◆ Aortic root surgery
- ◆ Management of circulatory arrest
- ◆ Congenital heart disease for cardiac surgery
- ◆ Congenital heart disease for non-cardiac surgery
- ◆ Pulmonary hypertension
- ◆ Atrial arrhythmias and current management strategies
- ◆ Ventricular arrhythmias and current management strategies
- ◆ Pacemakers and defibrillators indications and therapies
- ◆ Coagulation disorders and cardiac surgery
- ◆ Heparin induced thrombocytopenia
- ◆ Predictors mortality and increased length of stay in ICU
- ◆ Management of the cardiac patient for non-cardiac surgery
- ◆ Critical appraisal of clinical research

---

repair, which enriches the experience. In addition, early in each cycle, our department hosts a session to perform dissection of a porcine heart, with correlation to TOE images in a lab session, held in conjunction with surgery and cardiology fellows.

Increasingly, programmes are utilizing simulators for instruction in both TOE and transthoracic echocardiography. There are web-based simulation programmes and commercially available manikin simulation; the cost and maintenance and oversight of manikin simulation programmes is substantial (16). The programme at the University Health Network now has both an online training module and a mannequin programme with self-assessments tools that the fellow must utilize prior to their core TOE rotation.

Clinical research

The expectation that a 1- or 2-year cardiac anesthesia fellowship will produce an independent investigator is unrealistic. In our view training programmes should ensure that candidates possess the ability to critically appraise literature, be able to conduct valid quality assurance audits, and participate in trials, conducted by investigators with formalized training in the conduct of clinical research. Thus, trainees should have a basic understanding of trial design, measurement, and evaluation. This mandates that the core didactic curriculum include sessions on methodology, a basic understanding of statistical testing, and understanding the basic reporting requirements for clinical trials. In addition the teaching should include sessions on critical appraisal, understanding bias, and the grading of evidence. The goal is to gain sufficient ability to critique observational, randomized trials, and meta-analyses. We strongly believe that learning these skills are best achieved through active participation and therefore if the department has an active research programme, then participation in ongoing investigations, during training, would be advantageous.

Administration

Selection of candidates

The process of selection must be transparent and uniform for all candidates. Although there is usually a coordinator of the fellowship programme, the programme and the application process should be overseen by a committee to formally review applications.

The fellowship coordinator, or designate, screens applications and those that have met the criteria are presented to the committee to review. The committee should comprise faculty members that represent the varying disciplines of the fellowship programme, which should include research representation. Interviews can occur in person, telephone, or videoconference. Inviting candidates as an elective resident or as a visiting observer are good strategies for selecting candidates that are suitable for the programme. Most programmes have a posted deadline on their website and or that of the website of their accreditation body. The SCA has moved to a national match with agreed application deadlines and dates on which a letter of offer is sent. There is a defined date that a fellow must accept or decline the offer. The SCA recommends interviewing 10 applicants for each position offered.

Governance and evaluations

Governance and the evaluations process for each candidate must be open, transparent, and uniform. The committee, structured similar to that outlined for candidate selection, should oversee the progress of each candidate. Mentorship is a key component to a candidate, as it is for junior faculty progress as well. While each should have an interim mentor, established on starting the core year, invariably candidates will, and should be allowed to gravitate to a 'good fit' mentor (2). A formal orientation should occur at the start of the fellowship to familiarize the fellows to the institution's routines, practice, and processes of care. At the University Health Network a printed manual is available to all fellows. Soon after the orientation each fellow must meet with two faculty members from the committee to review the personal goals and objectives for the year as well to review the institutions expectation of the fellows while in the programme. A provisional orientation or probation period (usually 4 to 8 weeks) should take place where the fellow is supervised closely and assessed for any weaknesses in skills and knowledge. Gaps in skill or knowledge should be identified, and candidates who are deemed to need some remedial training in the basic core competencies should be assigned a clinical mentor to oversee the progress with benchmarks for improvement and regular feedback. With adequate screening and mentoring, candidates failing to achieve core competencies, in the probationary period, are rare. Having completed the evaluation process, a fellow should continue to be supervised with faculty member available at all times, but not necessarily in the immediate clinical environment.

All fellows should be evaluated regularly in an objective and contemporaneous fashion. Web-based links to evaluation tools are easily emailed to the daily supervisor and this process provides for standardized, objective, assessments, with superior compliance than paper-based (mailed) assessments. We also encourage similar email links where the candidate to assesses the faculty, and the ongoing experience.

Programme evaluation should occur separately at regular intervals throughout the core year. The fellows evaluate the format of the programme, clinical and didactic curriculum and faculty specific to each aspect of the programme. An example would be that a faculty member may be a much better ICU teacher than a TOE or cardiac anaesthesia teacher. Ideally they are emailed to the fellow and provide an anonymous response so that fellows can candidly share their impressions of the programme. The responses should be collected and presented to the committee at these regular intervals.

Objective performance feedback for each candidate should occur on a regular basis. It is expedient to link the programme evaluations in timing with a formal meeting with the fellow to review their progress. The fellow should meet with the programme director, and usually at least one other faculty member, for these formalized evaluations. Candidates should be provided with a copy of their evaluations and progress within the programme documented. Furthermore, candidates are encouraged to candidly share which elements of the programme that could be improved.

In addition to the oversight of the committee of the fellowship programme, there must be support and feedback from the cardiac anaesthesia faculty. This can occur in departmental meetings and in scheduled meetings with the division head and or chair of the programme.

Mentorship and career planning

Ideally, career planning should have started before the fellowship has begun. The fellow will have an image or destination of their career in mind at the start of the fellowship and the role of the mentor is to guide the fellow and facilitate their personal goals and objectives. A mentor assigned at the beginning of the fellowship will have knowledge of the faculty's strengths and may recommend that a fellow work closely with a particular faculty member. The mentor should be well appraised of the ultimate goals of the fellow and review these goals informally as well in the feedback session that are scheduled. Career planning should be well on its way at the midpoint of the fellowship. General impressions of a single individual (that is the mentor or the director) are not sufficient and contemporaneous evaluations by the faculty are extremely helpful to the fellow obtaining a junior faculty position. Having all the fellowship candidates complete their personal goals and objectives and secure a junior faculty position post-fellowship should be a core goal of the programme.

Conclusion

Cardiac anaesthesia is a challenging specialty made more rewarding by the teaching and mentoring of fellows and junior faculty. Many departments have the requisite case load and depth of faculty to establish an advanced programme. Planning and a formalized structure will create a robust programme with competent and content graduates and elevate the cardiac anaesthesia community.

References

1. Feneck RO, Consensus Document of the European Society of Anaesthesiology (ESA) and the European Association of Cardiothoracic Anaesthesiology (EACTA) for European Education and Training in Anaesthesia for Cardiothoracic and Major Vascular Surgery. A Proposal for Accreditation of Educational and Training Programmes. Available at: http://mail.eacta.org/pdf/pdf-0091.pdf (accessed 1 June 2014)
2. Flexman AM, Gelb AW. Mentorship in anesthesia: how little we know. *Can J Anaesth* 2012; *59*: 241–5
3. Pagel PS, Hudetz JA. Scholarly productivity of united states academic cardiothoracic anesthesiologists: influence of fellowship accreditation and transesophageal echocardiographic credentials on h-index and other citation bibliometrics. *J Cardiothorac Vasc Anesth* 2011; *25*: 761–5
4. Schwinn DA, Balser JR. Anesthesiology physician scientists in academic medicine: a wake-up call. *Anesthesiology* 2006; *104*: 170–8
5. Society of Cardiovascular Anesthesia. Obtaining ACGME Accreditation Information on ACGME Fellowship Accreditation Application Process. Available at: http://www.acgme.org/acgmeweb/ (accessed 1 June 2014)
6. Gaitan BD, Trentman TL, Fassett SL, Mueller JT, Altemose GT. Sedation and analgesia in the cardiac electrophysiology laboratory: a national survey of electrophysiologists investigating the who, how, and why? *J Cardiothorac Vasc Anesth* 2011; *25*: 647–59
7. Mahajan A, Chua J. Pro: a cardiovascular anesthesiologist should provide services in the catheterization and electrophysiology laboratory. *J Cardiothorac Vasc Anesth* 2011; *25*: 553–6
8. Australian and New Zealand College of Anaesthetists (ANZCA). Guidelines on Training and Practice of Perioperative Cardiac Ultrasound in Adults. Available at: http://www.anzca.edu.au/resources/professional-documents/pdfs/ps46-2013-guidelines-on-training-and-practice-of-perioperative-cardiac-ultrasound-in-adults.pdf (accessed 1 June 2014)
9. Popescu BA, Andrade MJ, Badano LP, et al. European Association of Echocardiography recommendations for training, competence, and quality improvement in echocardiography. *Eur J Echocardiogr* 2009; *10*: 893–905
10. Juve AM, Kirsch JR, Swide C. Training intensivists and clinician-scientists for the 21st century: the Oregon scholars program. *J Grad Med Educ* 2010; *2*: 585–8
11. Labovitz AJ, Noble VE, Bierig M, et al. Focused cardiac ultrasound in the emergent setting: a consensus statement of the American Society of Echocardiography and American College of Emergency Physicians. *J Am Soc Echocardiogr* 2010; *23*: 1225–30
12. Cowie B. Focused cardiovascular ultrasound performed by anesthesiologists in the perioperative period: feasible and alters patient management. *J Cardiothorac Vasc Anesth* 2009; *23*: 450–6
13. Canty DJ, Royse CF, Kilpatrick D, Williams DL, Royse AG. The impact of pre-operative focused transthoracic echocardiography in emergency non-cardiac surgery patients with known or risk of cardiac disease. *Anaesthesia* 2012; *67*: 714–20
14. Canty DJ, Royse CF, Kilpatrick D, Bowyer A, Royse AG. The impact on cardiac diagnosis and mortality of focused transthoracic echocardiography in hip fracture surgery patients with increased risk of cardiac disease: a retrospective cohort study. *Anaesthesia* 2012; *67*: 1202–9
15. Toronto General Hospital, Department of Anesthesia. Perioperative Interactive Education. Available at: http://pie.med.utoronto.ca/TEE (accessed 24 November 2013)
16. Shakil O, Mahmood F, Matyal R. Simulation in echocardiography: an ever-expanding frontier. *J Cardiothorac Vasc Anesth* 2012; *26*: 476–85

CHAPTER 42

Teamwork and minimizing error

Alan F. Merry and Jennifer M. Weller

Introduction

Cardiothoracic surgery is characterized by standardized, but complex and technically demanding procedures, interspersed with non-routine cases that are typically even more demanding. Both categories are associated with substantial risk (1). The clinical pathway extends from primary care to postoperative follow up, and close communication and cooperation between many people is required. In a retrospective study of 4828 incidents involving cardiac surgery in the UK National Reporting and Learning System database (2003–2007), 21% occurred in the operating room (OR) and 79% outside the OR. Harm resulted in 23% of the OR and 34% of the non-OR incidents (2). Thus, outcomes depend on numerous health professionals over extended periods of clinical care.

It is no easy matter to achieve acceptable results for cardiac and thoracic surgery, and any unit doing this must already have highly competent staff functioning as a reasonably effective team. It follows that initiatives to change culture or process should be made with care and measurement to avoid unintended consequences (3) and ensure that improvement truly is achieved. However, evidence suggests room for improvement, at least in those few units that have investigated their own teamwork.

Teams in healthcare are typically transient, with individuals coming together for a particular purpose, and then disbanding. In surgery, geographical and organizational barriers may limit opportunities to establish plans ahead of time and agree on priorities for patient care. A range of skills and knowledge is required to care for surgical patients, and this implies differences in training and capability. Tribalism, in which individuals identify more with their own professional group than with the team as a whole, may lead to stereotypical and potentially unfavourable perceptions of other professional groups. Individuals may differ in their approaches to leadership and teamwork (4), may value and communicate information in different ways, and may have different priorities in patient care (5). Cardiac and thoracic surgery teams are typically more stable than many others, with members working together frequently. This is very helpful in promoting teamwork and overcoming some of these challenges.

Unfortunately, administrators are sometimes sceptical about the benefit of subspecialisation and particularly the loss of the flexibility provided by generalist nurses and anaesthetists able to care for a wide range of cases. Some compromise may be necessary, but the case for requiring subspecialisation increases with the risk and complexity of the work. The move to anaesthesia-provided transoesophageal echocardiography illustrates the point; the skills require time and practice to develop and maintain and are not held by many generalist anaesthetists. Similarly, managing a patient with a failing heart following cardiopulmonary bypass (CPB) or undergoing a complex lung resection is not a setting for occasional team members who have inadequate experience in the field and do not know each other. We think that the primary requirement for establishing effective teamwork and achieving excellent results in cardiothoracic surgery is for practitioners to spend a substantial proportion of their working week in this field in order to build and maintain expertise and skills and to become truly embedded in the team.

In this chapter we start from this premise. We outline the elements of teamwork. We then review the evidence supporting the value of teamwork in healthcare generally and cardiothoracic surgery in particular and evaluate the need for improvement in teamwork in at least some cardiothoracic surgical units. We touch on idiosyncratic variation in clinical practice and its implications for teamwork. We discuss some approaches through which teamwork might be improved and conclude there that the potential to improve outcomes through improving teamwork in cardiothoracic surgery provides an opportunity that should at least be considered by all cardiothoracic units today. We recognize that institutions around the world differ in their configuration and case mix and that some units do only cardiac or thoracic work, but the issues that we will discuss are widely applicable.

Elements of teamwork

Salas et al (6) have proposed a model for teamwork based on empirical evidence from teams across diverse organizations, which could inform interventions to improve teamwork in cardiothoracic surgery. They describe five dimensions of effective teamwork: team orientation, team leadership, mutual performance monitoring, backup behaviour, and adaptability (table 42.1).

Three coordinating factors underpin these five dimensions:

◆ mutual trust

◆ closed loop communication

◆ shared mental models within the team.

Mutual trust, reflecting the belief that members of the team are all doing their best for their patients, encourages sharing of

Table 42.1 Dimensions of teamwork

Dimensions of teamwork	Description
Team orientation	Members take other's views into account, share information, and believe that team goals override individual goals.
Team leadership	A leader directs and co-ordinates, assesses team performance, facilitates team problem solving, assigns tasks, and develops the team.
Mutual performance monitoring	Members identify lapses or mistakes in other team members' performance and provide feedback.
Backup behaviour	Members anticipate other team members' needs through accurate knowledge of their responsibilities.
Adaptability	Members adjust strategies on the basis of new information gathered from the environment and identify new opportunities for team development.

Reproduced from Salas E et al., 'Is there a "Big Five" in teamwork?', *Small Group Research*, 36, 5, pp. 555–599, Copyright © 2005 by SAGE Publications. Reprinted by Permission of SAGE Publications.

information and willingness to admit mistakes. It is linked to respect for one another, demonstrated by style of communication.

Communication skills ensure clear, concise, explicit and directed communication, and the closing of communication loops (7). Closed-loop communication ensures that intended information is received and understood and confirms that the receiver can and will respond appropriately.

A shared mental model implies a common understanding of the situation and the plan and also an understanding by team members of their own roles, capabilities and tasks and those of others. This is self-evidently critical for coordinated teamwork (8). Developing and maintaining a shared mental model requires sharing of information. This enables team members to anticipate and predict each other's needs, identify changes in a situation, and adjust strategies as needed. Team briefings facilitate exchange of information and the development of a shared mental model.

Power gradients, consultative leadership, and teamwork

When things go wrong in surgery, it frequently turns out that someone realized that a mistake was being made but felt unable to say so. A steep power gradient tends to inhibit speaking up and makes mistakes more likely to go unchallenged. Tribalism may further constrain speaking up because team members may tend to focus on their own component of care and feel inhibited by members of other professional groups and disempowered from taking any responsibility for actions of others or for the team's overall mission.

The influence of teamwork on patient outcomes

There is evidence linking teamwork to patient outcomes in healthcare generally, in surgery generally, and in cardiothoracic surgery specifically.

Evidence on teamwork and patient outcomes in healthcare generally

Failures in teamwork and communication have been identified as common preventable factors in the genesis of adverse events in healthcare (9–14). A literature review supported the concept that teamwork and leadership can influence patient safety (15). Mazzocco and colleagues demonstrated an association between positive team behaviours and outcome in surgery (16). A study of 50 patients undergoing major elective gastrointestinal surgery identified many process failures in postoperative care, half of which led directly to patient harm; communication failures were commonly the cause of these (17). Lingard and co-workers (18) classified over 25% of observed communications in the OR as failures, many of which resulted in undesirable effects including inefficiency, tension in the team, waste of resources, delay, or procedural error. Failures were caused by inappropriate timing of communications, inaccurate or missing content, or failure to resolve issues. Curry and colleagues (19) used site visits and in-depth interviews to identify 'what works inside a hospital' to improve outcomes for acute myocardial infarction. There was a substantial difference in organizational values and culture between six high-performing hospitals and four low-performing hospitals. Staff at the high-performing hospitals 'expressed shared organizational values of providing exceptional, high-quality care' reflecting 'a common vision and purpose'. All staff were engaged and valued, in contrast to the low-performing hospitals in which nurses and pharmacists perceived themselves as undervalued and management were less engaged in the commitment to excellence. In the high-performing hospitals, staff recognized their interdependencies and 'repeatedly voiced a shared commitment to ensure effective communication and coordinated, seamless transitions' (19).

There is also evidence that teamwork and communication in healthcare can readily be improved. For example, a meta-analysis of studies of 2650 non-clinical teams attributed nearly 20% of the differences in team processes and outcomes to previous participation of team members in team training (20). Improving teamwork is an explicit objective of the World Health Organization (WHO) Surgical Safety Checklist (the Checklist). Specifically, the Checklist requires introduction of team members and sharing information about important issues or anticipated events (figure 42.1). An important aim of doing this is to activate people: if a person has spoken once, it is much easier for him or her to speak again, and introductions set the tone for participation. Implementation of the Checklist in eight institutions around the world resulted in improved compliance with basic safety processes and a substantial reduction in mortality and other prespecified surgical complications (21). Two further studies in the USA (22) and Europe (23) have demonstrated similar improvements in outcomes through initiatives that included checklists and briefings.

Evidence on teamwork and patient outcomes in cardiac surgery

Many studies have reported high rates of preventable adverse events during acute care hospital admission (24–29). Cardiothoracic surgery is no exception: for example, in a retrospective chart review of 15 000 randomly selected admissions to Colorado and Utah

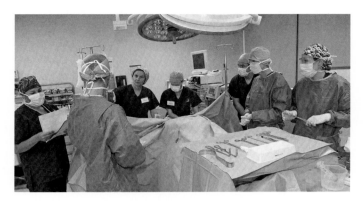

Fig. 42.1 Team-based surgical safety checklist.

hospitals, coronary artery bypass graft/cardiac valve surgery had a higher than average rate of preventable adverse events (29).

In an observational study of 31 cardiac surgical operations, problems with teamwork and communication accounted for 52% of disruptions to flow of care. Surgical errors increased significantly with flow disruptions, and failures in teamwork or communication were the strongest predictor of surgical errors (30).

de Leval and colleagues studied unplanned events in 243 arterial switch operations in 16 UK institutions by 21 surgeons. Nearly 25% of cases were associated with death (6.6%) or a near miss. Major events were significantly related to death and near misses, but the risk of death was reduced by appropriate compensation. Minor events were of little consequence individually, but their total number was closely related to death and near misses (31). de Leval and colleagues subsequently showed that the total number of previous minor events in a case negatively influenced the team's ability to compensate for subsequent major events when they occurred. While major events were readily recognized by the surgical team, minor failures often went unreported in the absence of a trained observer (32). The contribution of minor problems, taken collectively, to poor outcomes has been confirmed (31–33). Errors are multifactorial, and their genesis does not seem to lie in deficiencies in the technical knowledge and skill of clinicians but rather with how these are applied in complex tasks. The overall message is that events whether major or minor, need to be identified, declared, and addressed. This emphasizes the importance of speaking up, clear communication, and collaboration (34).

The Flawless Operative Cardiovascular Unified Systems (FOCUS) project is an initiative of the Society of Cardiovascular Anaesthesiologists and aims for harm-free cardiac surgery. FOCUS started with a systematic review of the literature: of 1438 articles related to errors or safety in cardiac anaesthesia, 55 met the inclusion criteria of addressing cardiac surgery-specific hazards during the intraoperative period. Two key themes emerged: studies were predominantly reactive instead of proactive, and very few tested interventions, suggesting a gap in research; and minor events were predictive of major problems. The main recommendations included promoting a culture of transparency, in which speaking up is the norm, and developing good teamwork and communication (35). The recommendations from a subsequent observational study were somewhat similar and again explicitly included improving communication and teamwork (36).

Interestingly, in an observational study of 40 paediatric cardiac surgical operations by a single team, the hypothesis that effective teamwork can prevent the development of serious situations was not supported. The authors suggested that the team under study exhibited good teamwork behaviours such as explicit communication, more strongly in more challenging cases, thus confounding the study (37). This illustrates the challenge of research in this field and supports our view that elements of effective teamwork are already embedded in many cardiothoracic surgical units. For example, closed-loop communication is explicitly required when administering heparin or protamine at the Green Lane Unit in Auckland Hospital. Also, conversation unrelated to the tasks at hand during critical periods of the procedures is (largely) restricted. This does not necessarily imply that there is no potential for improvement.

It may be easier to embed teamwork during the establishment of a unit than later, when culture and practices have become ingrained. A new cardiac surgery programme based its operation on the principles of the Toyota production system, emphasizing cultural safety for continual improvement. This included daily full-team 10-minute debriefings. Outcomes over the first 28 months were encouraging (38).

Variation and teamwork

Until quite recently, cardiothoracic surgery was a pioneering field with few guidelines and considerable emphasis on the autonomy of senior clinicians to practise as they thought best. Today, operations are increasingly routine, and there is considerable outcome-based evidence to guide practice. Nevertheless, and perhaps understandably, in some units this culture of clinical autonomy persists, and the treatment patients receive may depend more on who provides it than on its appropriateness for them as individuals (39,40). Approaches should vary in response to differences between individual patients, but instead variation often reflects differences in the philosophy and training of individual practitioners for example in relation to protocols for postoperative atrial fibrillation, approaches to cardioplegia, the use of all-arterial grafts or off-pump techniques for coronary surgery, the use of pulmonary artery catheters, and so on (41). Apart from any other consideration, this idiosyncratic variation makes it difficult for nursing staff and junior doctors to know how to treat patients and is contrary to the idea of teamwork. An emphasis on clinical autonomy may be reinforced by reporting individual surgeon's performance rather than the performance of the unit as a whole. Agreed patient care pathways from the selection of patients for routine procedures to their discharge would advance the cause of teamwork and would provide clarity on the treatment plan to all members of the team. Variation from the pathways in response to differences between individual patients would not only be expected, it would also make sense to nurses and junior doctors. In consequence, they may feel that they are contributing to the team effort through rational patient care instead of simply appeasing individual senior clinicians.

Improving teamwork

Skill and expertise are pre-requisites for cardiothoracic surgery; the purpose of improving teamwork is to make these more effective and thereby improve patient outcomes. On the basis of this discussion, several factors emerge that we think would promote effective teamwork in cardiothoracic surgery (box 42.1).

Defining the team

For a team to function its members need to agree that there is a team and that they belong to it. Burford (42) suggested that a culture of belonging to a multidisciplinary team is fostered by increasing the salience of that team so that members identify primarily with the team or unit rather than their professional disciplines. The 2001 report on the inquiry into paediatric cardiac surgery at the Bristol Royal Infirmary (43) supported this concept, recommending specialist units with the relevant disciplines coordinated around their patients—in effect, patient-centred teams.

Who should belong? We believe the aim should be the proper management of patients rather than just productivity with good outcomes measured by the number and mortality rates of specific procedures (see 'Measurement'). That is, the aim should be on doing the right things as well as doing things right. Doing the right things implies meaningful inclusion of patients in the decisions that affect them (44). Percutaneous interventions or simple medical management may at times be more appropriate than surgery, or equally, they may not (39,45). It follows that, in addition to the obvious members who are the surgeons, anaesthetists, nurses, perfusionists, and clinical support staff, cardiologists and respiratory physicians should certainly be included in the unit or team and, given the importance of medications in managing cardiac and thoracic patients, so should pharmacists.

Uniting the tribes with effective leadership

Hospitals operate through a wide range of administrative and leadership models. The situation is very different from that in aeroplane cockpits, where the pilot and copilot belong to the same professional group. Mistrust in the notion of subservience of any one healthcare group to another presents a challenge to effective leadership. The concept of the surgeon as the automatic 'captain of the ship' is no longer tenable either in the OR or more generally. All staff members are held accountable for their actions, and a practitioner from one group cannot often step in and do the clinical work of another group. In the OR, leadership does and must shift according to the most pressing issue at any time. For example, in an airway emergency a surgeon could usefully contribute but not typically assume leadership.

Bleakley (46) advocated democracy in healthcare teams. In an undemocratic team, the 'leader' does all the talking and decision making. A democratic leader engages in open conversations and encourages suggestions from the team. This accesses the full cognitive resources of the team in making decisions and defending against errors. However, in the clinical setting, the ultimate responsibility for decisions clearly lies with the relevant senior clinicians. We suggest that in this context the term 'consultative' is more appropriate. On the other hand we support democracy in the overall leadership of the team.

We therefore propose the establishment of defined multidisciplinary units, or teams, focussed on caring for patients with cardiac disease, thoracic disease, or both. The primary professional identity should be membership of the unit rather than of any professional subgroup. However, we doubt that many clinicians will be comfortable with deserting their tribal affiliations altogether. We therefore advocate an overarching governance structure with representation from the leader of each professional subgroup and a fixed-term chairperson who could come from any subgroup. This would set the tone, facilitate explicit decisions about policy and strategic direction, and provide a forum for the collective resolution of problems. While individual groups would maintain their identities through craft-specific activities, a key feature would be regular combined meetings to discuss clinical, educational, and administrative issues as a team. This would promote shared mental models for policy, direction, and clinical care. Integral to this would be a commitment to standardization within the unit of approaches to common conditions and problems.

Improving communication

A team-wide commitment to effective and respectful communication articulated by its leadership as non-negotiable is essential. This should be supported by training in communication skills. Effective communication should be explicit, clear, and sufficiently comprehensive to avoid misunderstanding. It should also be directed. This implies knowing and using people's names. Names may pose no difficulty for small and stable teams, but larger units often need systems to ensure names are known. The introduction of person and role is a critical aspect of the Checklist and can be reinforced by writing names on a whiteboard and using readable name badges. The role of activation in promoting speaking up has already been mentioned. The concept of graded assertiveness builds on this and should be taught to all (47). Various mnemonics have been designed to assist communication for effectively conveying necessary information in certain contexts (e.g., ISBAR (48), 'what, so what, now what').

Box 42.1 Features facilitating effective teamwork and high performance in cardiothoracic surgery

- A strong focus on patients as central to the unit.

- A clearly defined unit with an explicit and democratic overall governance structure to provide democratic overall leadership.

- High levels of individual skill, knowledge, and commitment to patient care.

- A culture of respect in which effective and respectful communication is fostered and the relentless pursuit of excellence is unequivocally supported by all.

- Committed subspecialization—practitioners should ideally spend a substantial part of their employed time in this field and should strongly identify with the unit (or 'team').

- A commitment to standardization and avoidance of inappropriate variation of care.

- Regular meetings of the whole team (whatever their professional group) for administrative and educational purposes to ensure the same view of how things should be done.

- Outcomes monitored, with an emphasis on making the overall results of the team public rather than those of individuals.

Checklists, briefings, and ward rounds

The value of briefings and checklists has already been discussed. The Checklist should be viewed as the standard of care and used by all surgical units (49). The traditional ward round, attended by all surgical, nursing, and intensive care staff, is a form of team briefing that has been somewhat undermined by shift work and changes in hospital culture. Within the OR, a preoperative briefing and a postoperative debriefing can be very effective in promoting shared mental models, anticipating problems, and learning from what went well and what could have been improved.

Handovers

Handover of patients from team to team is particularly problematic. Catchpole and colleagues conducted a before–after observational study of a handover protocol for infants taken to intensive care after complex heart operations. Clinical observations were supplemented by observation of Formula 1 Racing team pit-stops and input from two aviation captains who observed several handovers. Safety themes were identified, and a protocol was developed through discussions with anaesthetists, surgeons, intensivists, and nurses. Technical errors and information omissions were reduced and the duration of handover was shortened (33).

Simulation

High fidelity, immersive, patient simulation facilitates studying and improving teamwork and performance in health care (figure 42.1) (50–54). Simulators are now available to emulate CPB and extracorporeal membrane oxygenation and for various surgical procedures, as well as for anaesthesia. Integration of surgical and anaesthetic simulators is still at an early stage, but realistic clinical scenarios can already be created to meaningfully engage inter-professional groups. Conditions demanding effective teamwork can be created, manipulated, and repeated with any number of clinical teams. Complex interactions between team members and their environment can be observed, recorded, and rigorously analysed. Opportunities are provided for practice and reflection. Patient safety is not compromised, and participants learn in a safe environment free of potential medicolegal consequences. Gawande's group have developed a simulation-based educational programme to teach teamwork for acute crises in cardiac surgery and have demonstrated that it produces increased appreciation by participants of the value of working as a team and a perceived improvement in speaking up readily and communicating clearly (55).

Monitoring the results of initiatives to improve teamwork

Publicly available outcome data following cardiothoracic surgery often relate to individual surgeons rather than the whole team or unit. Other members of the team, notably anaesthetists, can make substantive differences to the results of cardiac surgery (and probably also thoracic surgery) (56,57). Nevertheless, it is unusual for the results of individual anaesthetists to be published, and it is even more unusual for particular combinations of clinicians to be studied.

If the aim is to improve the overall results of a unit, the futility of this highly individualistic and unidimensional approach becomes apparent. It is statistically inevitable that within any unit the results of one surgeon will be the best, and of another the worst. However, not all patients can be cared for by the best surgeon, and eliminating the worst surgeon simply reassigns those remaining so that the second worst now becomes the worst—repeatedly, ad absurdum! The important thing is that every patient receives excellent care. Furthermore, mortality rates, although important, provide a very incomplete picture of the quality of a cardiothoracic service. It is also worth evaluating the appropriateness of patient selection, the patient's experience and satisfaction, and neurological outcomes.

The effectiveness of teamwork should be measured (58). Nevertheless, it is patient outcomes that matter. We think a combination of case-mix adjusted mortality rates and a rate of formally evaluated strokes reported alongside some measure of patient satisfaction and of teamwork would provide the best indication of progress. The denominator should be based on those patients presenting with particular problems rather than those subsequently selected for particular procedures. In this way the influence of allocating patients between different therapeutic options for example medical management, percutaneous coronary intervention, and surgery, can be understood for the unit as a combined team. This would move the emphasis onto appropriate patient care by the team and away from the numbers of procedures (and their outcomes) undertaken by particular divisions within that team.

Conclusion

Members of highly performing cardiothoracic units must be skilled experts with strong commitment to their patients, but outcomes and efficiency are likely to improve if they work more effectively as a team. This implies a coherent, patient-centred, multiprofessional unit with strong democratic overall leadership, a shared mental model for patient care, mutual respect between professional groups reflected by behaviours and styles of communication, and regular training in skills for effective communication. Some units have investigated communication and teamwork and have found room for improvement. We suspect that all units should at least consider the opportunity that improving teamwork might provide for improving the outcomes of their patients.

References

1. Shahian DM, O'Brien SM, Sheng S, et al. Predictors of long-term survival after coronary artery bypass grafting surgery: results from the Society of Thoracic Surgeons Adult Cardiac Surgery Database (the ASCERT study). *Circulation* 2012; *125*: 1491–500
2. Martinez EA, Shore A, Colantuoni E, et al. Cardiac surgery errors: results from the UK National Reporting and Learning System. *Int J Qual Health Care* 2011; *23*: 151–8
3. Tenner EW. *Why Things Bite Back—Technology and the Revenge of Unintended Consequences.* New York: Vintage Books, 1997
4. Hall P. Interprofessional teamwork: Professional cultures as barriers. *J Interprofessional Care* 2005; *19*: 188–96
5. Weller J. Shedding new light on tribalism in health care. *Med Educ* 2012; *46*: 134–6
6. Salas E, Sims DE, Burke CS. Is there a 'Big Five' in teamwork? *Small Group Research* 2005; *36*: 555–99
7. Gaba D, Fish K, Howard S. *Crisis Management in Anesthesiology,* 1st edn. Edinburgh: Churchill Livingstone, 1994
8. Salas E, Cooke NJ, Rosen MA. On teams, teamwork, and team performance: discoveries and developments. *J Human Factors Ergonomics Soc* 2008; *50*: 540–7

9. Bognor M. *Human Error In Medicine*, 1st edn. New Jersey: Lawrence Erlbaum Association Inc, 1994

10. Helmreich R, ed. Threat and error in aviation and medicine: Similar and different. Special Medical Seminar, Lessons for Health Care: Applied Human Factors Research; 2000 January 2001; NSW. Diana Australian Council of Safety and Quality in Health Care & NSW Ministerial Council for Quality in Health Care

11. Reader TW, Flin R, Cuthbertson BH. Communication skills and error in the intensive care unit. *Curr Opin Crit Care* 2007; **13**: 732–6

12. Reason J. *Human Error*. New York: Cambridge University Press, 1990

13. Manser T, Harrison TK, Gaba DM, Howard SK. Coordination patterns related to high clinical performance in a simulated anesthetic crisis. *Anesth Analg* 2009; **108**: 1606–15

14. Webb RK, Currie M, Morgan CA, et al. The Australian Incident Monitoring Study: An analysis of 2000 incident reports. *Anaesth Intensive Care* 1993; **21**(5): 520–8

15. Kunzle B, Kolbe M, Gudela G. Ensuring patient safety through effective leadership behaviour: A literature review. *Safety Science* 2010; **48**: 1–17

16. Mazzocco K, Petitti DB, Fong KT, Another, Another, Another, et al. Surgical team behaviours and patient outcomes. *Am J Surg* 2009; **197**: 678–85

17. Symons NRA, Wong HWL, Manser T, Sevdalis N, Vincent CA, Moorthy K. An observational study of teamwork skills in shift handover. *Int J Surg* 2012; **10**(7): 355–9

18. Lingard L, Espin S, Whyte S, et al. Communication failures in the operating room: an observational classification of recurrent types and effects. *Qual Safety Health Care* 2004; **13**: 330–4

19. Curry LA, Spatz E, Cherlin E, et al. What distinguishes top-performing hospitals in acute myocardial infarction mortality rates? A qualitative study. *Ann Intern Med* 2011; **154**: 384–90

20. Salas E, DiazGranados D, Klein C, et al. Does Team training improve team performance? A meta-analysis human factors. *J Human Factors Ergonomics Soc* 2008; **50**: 903–33

21. Haynes A, Weiser T, Berry W, et al. A surgical safety checklist to reduce morbidity and mortality in a global population. *N Engl J Med* 2009; **360**: 491–9

22. Neily J, Mills PD, Young-Xu Y, et al. Association between implementation of a medical team training program and surgical mortality. *JAMA* 2010; **304**: 1693–700

23. de Vries EN, Prins HA, Crolla RMPH, et al. Effect of a comprehensive surgical safety system on patient outcomes. *N Engl J Med* 2010; **363**: 1928–37

24. Wilson R. Clinical preceptor conferences as a venue for total quality education. *Optom Educat* 1996; **21**: 85–9

25. Davis P, Lay-Yee R, Briant R, Ali W, Scott A, Schug S. Adverse events in New Zealand public hospitals I: occurrence and impact. *N Z Med J* 2002; **115**:U271

26. Baker GR, Norton PG, Flintoft V, et al. The Canadian Adverse Events Study: the incidence of adverse events among hospital patients in Canada. *CMAJ* 2004 25; **170**: 1678–86

27. Brennan TA, Leape LL, Laird NM, et al. Incidence of adverse events and negligence in hospitalized patients: results of the Harvard Medical Practice Study I. 1991. *Qual Saf Health Care* 2004; **13**: 145–51

28. Vincent C, Neale G, Woloshynowych M. Adverse events in British hospitals: preliminary retrospective record review. *Br Med J* 2001; **322**: 517–9

29. Gawande AA, Thomas EJ, Zinner MJ, Brennan TA. The incidence and nature of surgical adverse events in Colorado and Utah in 1992. *Surgery* 1999; **126**: 66–75

30. Wiegmann DA, ElBardissi AW, Dearani JA, Daly RC, Sundt TM, 3rd. Disruptions in surgical flow and their relationship to surgical errors: an exploratory investigation. *Surgery* 2007; **142**: 658–65

31. de Leval MR, Carthey J, Wright DJ, Farewell VT, Reason JT. Human factors and cardiac surgery: a multicenter study. *J Thorac Cardiovasc Surg* 2000; **119**: 661–72

32. Solis-Trapala IL, Carthey J, Farewell VT, de Leval MR. Dynamic modelling in a study of surgical error management. *Stat Med* 2007; **26**: 5189–202

33. Catchpole KR, de Leval MR, McEwan A, et al. Patient handover from surgery to intensive care: using Formula 1 pit-stop and aviation models to improve safety and quality. *Paediatr Anaesth* 2007; **17**: 470–8

34. Mishra A, Catchpole K, McCulloch P. The Oxford NOTECHS System: reliability and validity of a tool for measuring teamwork behaviour in the operating theatre. *Qual Saf Health Care* 2009; **18**: 104–8

35. Martinez EA, Thompson DA, Errett NA, et al. High stakes and high risk: a focused qualitative review of hazards during cardiac surgery. *Anesth Analg* 2011; **112**: 1061–74

36. Gurses AP, Kim G, Martinez EA, et al. Identifying and categorising patient safety hazards in cardiovascular operating rooms using an interdisciplinary approach: a multisite study. *BMJ Qual Safety* 2012; **21**: 810–8

37. Schraagen JM, Schouten T, Smit M, et al. A prospective study of paediatric cardiac surgical microsystems: assessing the relationships between non-routine events, teamwork and patient outcomes. *BMJ Qual Safety* 2011; **20**: 599–603

38. Culig MH, Kunkle RF, Frndak DC, Grunden N, Maher TD, Jr., Magovern GJ, Jr. Improving patient care in cardiac surgery using Toyota production system based methodology. *Ann Thorac Surg* 2011; **91**: 394–9

39. Van Brabandt H, Neyt M, Hulstaert F. Transcatheter aortic valve implantation (TAVI): risky and costly. *Br Med J* 2012; **345**: e4710

40. Hannan EL, Cozzens K, Samadashvili Z et al. Appropriateness of coronary revascularization for patients without acute coronary syndromes. *J Am Coll Cardiol* 2012; **59**: 1870–6

41. Birkmeyer JD, Sharp SM, Finlayson SR, Fisher ES, Wennberg JE. Variation profiles of common surgical procedures. *Surgery* 1998; **124**: 917–23

42. Burford B. Group processes in medical education: learning from social identity theory. *Med Educ* 2012; **46**: 143–52

43. The Inquiry. The Inquiry into the management of care of children receiving complex heart surgery at the Bristol Royal Infirmary. Bristol 2001

44. Barry MJ, Edgman-Levitan S. Shared decision making—pinnacle of patient-centered care. *N Engl J Med* 2012; **366**: 780–1

45. Farzaneh-Far A, Borges-Neto S. Ischemic burden, treatment allocation, and outcomes in stable coronary artery disease. *Circulation Cardiovasc Imag* 2011; **4**: 746–53

46. Bleakley A. Social comparison, peer learning and democracy in medical education. *Med Teach* 2010; **32**: 878–9

47. Pian-Smith MC, Simon R, Minehart RD, et al. Teaching residents the two-challenge rule: a simulation-based approach to improve education and patient safety. *Simulation in Healthcare* 2009; **4**(2): 84–91

48. Marshall S, Harrison J, Flanagan B. The teaching of a structured tool improves the clarity and content of interprofessional clinical communication. *Qual Safety Health Care* 2009; **18**: 137–40

49. Birkmeyer JD. Strategies for improving surgical quality—checklists and beyond. *N Engl J Med* 2010; **363**: 1963–5

50. Joy BF, Elliott E, Hardy C, Sullivan C, Backer CL, Kane JM. Standardized multidisciplinary protocol improves handover of cardiac surgery patients to the intensive care unit. *Pediatr Crit Care Med* 2011; **12**: 304–8

51. Burtscher MJ, Kolbe M, Wacker J, Manser T. Interactions of team mental models and monitoring behaviors predict team performance in simulated anesthesia inductions. *J Experiment Psych: Appl* 2011; **17**: 257–69

52. Weller J, Frengley R, Torrie J et al. Evaluation of an instrument to measure teamwork in multidisciplinary critical care teams. *Qual Saf Health Care* 2011; **20**(3): 216–22

53. Frengley RW, Weller JM, Torrie J, et al. The effect of a simulation-based training intervention on the performance of established critical care unit teams. *Crit Care Med* 2011; *39*(12): 2605–11

54. Ruel M, Labinaz M. Transcatheter aortic-valve replacement: a cardiac surgeon and cardiologist team perspective. *Curr Opin Cardiol* 2010; *25*: 107–13

55. Stevens L-M, Cooper JB, Raemer DB, et al. Educational program in crisis management for cardiac surgery teams including high realism simulation. *J Thorac Cardiovasc Surg* 2012; *144*: 17–24

56. Merry AF, Ramage MC, Whitlock RML, et al. First-time coronary artery bypass grafting: the anaesthetist as a risk factor. *Br J Anaesth* 1992; *68*: 6–12

57. Slogoff S, Keats AS. Does perioperative myocardial ischemia lead to postoperative myocardial infarction? *Anesthesiology* 1985; *62*: 107–14

58. Weller J, Shulruf B, Torrie J et al. Validation of a measurement tool for self-assessment of teamwork in Intensive Care. *Br J Anaesth* 2013; *111*(3): 460–7.

CHAPTER 43

Audit and research in cardiothoracic anaesthesia

Paul S. Myles

Quality in healthcare: why measure what we do?

Most people want to excel in their chosen careers (1). For many, an opportunity to demonstrate achievement or excellence in their work is a motivating force (2). For those of us working in the healthcare field the strongest motivating factors seems to be a desire to help and heal others, to be intellectually stimulated, being able to demonstrate our skills and to be acknowledged by our peers to have such skills (2). However, it is not sufficient to believe you have done a good job, its needs objective evidence that can be judged by others to represent success.

It is a fundamental human right to have access to healthcare, and there is a strong and growing public expectation that this care should be of an acceptable standard. Furthermore, those who fund healthcare and in turn many in the community want evidence that the care being provided is cost effective (3). Failures of governance and audit in perioperative practices leading to unacceptable and avoidable disability and death, such as occurred with the Patel case in Queensland (4), and in paediatric cardiac surgery in Bristol (5), threaten the public's trust in doctors and healthcare in general. These cases exemplify major failings in audit, medical leadership and quality assurance.

Most advanced countries have established national agencies to oversee quality and safety in healthcare (6–8). But the capacity for such agencies to reliably monitor and encourage quality improvement initiatives is heavily dependent on the quality of the reported data (7). Audit can identify outlier practices (9), and provide useful benchmarking data that eventually lead to improvements in care, and there is evidence that this works (10–12).

Benchmarking is a process of measuring performance, using one or more specific indicators to compare with others. The key features are to identify and agree upon a set of clinical indicators and to collect complete and accurate data. A common aim is to reduce costs whilst at the same time improve process and outcomes of care. Benchmarking is a component of total quality management. For cardiac anaesthesia there are many possible clinical indicators to choose from. For example, process measures such as timely antibiotic administration, rates of blood product transfusion, blood glucose control, and use of aseptic technique for insertion of central venous catheters. Outcome measures can include return to theatre for bleeding, and adverse events such as myocardial infarction (MI), stroke and death. But benchmarking is not limited to performance measures of clinicians: funding and resources are required to deliver good quality care and these are the responsibility of government, funding agencies and hospital administrations. Clinicians can and should demand adequate resources in order for them to deliver the high quality care our patients expect.

A systematic programme for recording adverse events and other measures of performance can reduce error rates and promote a culture of patient safety in anaesthesia and surgery (10,13). More important, however, is to act on the information provided, to make the necessary changes to improve care—quality improvement (14). A good example of this is the Leapfrog Group in the US (11,14).

In cardiac surgery, perhaps more than many other areas of medicine, it is well-known that patient factors affect outcome, and so risk-adjustment is an important process to ensure we are comparing *like with like*. Casemix clearly affects results. Benchmarking exercises need to consider and account for variations in patient demographics, comorbidity, and functional status, as well as complexity of the surgical procedure and the time periods under study [15]. Matching or statistical multivariable adjustment are commonly used for this purpose. Surgical risk scores such as Euroscore (16), or measures of functional status such as the ASA physical function score (17) or NYHA classification, can condense much of the casemix data into simple indices of risk. All validated risk scores begin with audit and identification of risk factors for mortality and major adverse outcomes after surgery (15,16,18–20).

Shroyer and colleagues (21) identified the preoperative risk factors associated with several complications after coronary artery bypass surgery (CABG) surgery, and devised a composite outcome variable that included any major morbidity or death within 30 days of surgery. They used the Society of Thoracic Surgeons (STS) National Adult Cardiac Surgery Database, which included 503 478 CABG procedures, to develop risk-adjusted operative mortality and risk-adjusted morbidity models. The 30-day mortality and major complication rates were 3.1% and 13%, respectively. The latter included stroke (1.6%), renal failure (3.5%), reoperation (5.2%), prolonged ventilation (6.0%), and sternal infection (0.6%). Risk models were developed, for which the predictive utility, based on c-indices, were around 0.70. This indicates moderate clinical usefulness, acceptable for predicting risk of adverse outcomes for groups but not sufficiently reliable for individual patients.

Table 43.1 Observed, predicted and observed to expected (O:E) mortality ratio for each year 1997 to 2005

Year	Observed mortality %	Expected mortality %	O:E ratio
1997–8	2.4	3.0	0.8
1998–9	2.7	3.1	0.87
1999–2000	1.8	3.1	0.58
2000–1	2.1	3.1	0.68
2001–2	1.6	3.3	0.48
2002–3	1.9	3.4	0.56
2003–4	1.9	3.4	0.56
2004–5	1.8	3.5	0.51
P value	0.014	<0.001	<0.05

Reproduced from *Heart*, Bridgewater B et al., 'Has the publication of cardiac surgery outcome data been associated with changes in practice in northwest England: an analysis of 25 730 patients undergoing CABG surgery under 30 surgeons over eight years', 93, 6, pp. 744–748, Copyright 2007, with permission from BMJ Publishing Group Ltd.

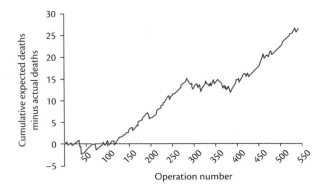

Fig. 43.1 Cumulative summation of performance of one surgeon for 547 consecutive cardiac surgical cases, indicating improved performance after about 120 cases.
Reprinted from The Lancet, 350, 9085, Lovegrove J, et al., 'Monitoring the results of cardiac surgery by variable life-adjusted display' pp. 1128–1130, Copyright 1997, with permission from Elsevier

The Euroscore is the most extensively validated and utilized cardiac surgery risk index around the world (16). In the first instance, patient demographic, perioperative and outcome (mortality) data were collected for over 19 000 cardiac surgical patients in 128 surgical centres in eight European states. The relationship between risk factors and outcome was assessed by univariate and logistic regression analysis. The following risk factors were associated with increased mortality: age, female gender, serum creatinine, extracardiac arteriopathy, chronic airway disease, severe neurological dysfunction, previous cardiac surgery, recent myocardial infarction (MI), left ventricular ejection fraction, chronic congestive cardiac failure, pulmonary hypertension, active endocarditis, unstable angina, procedure urgency, critical preoperative condition ventricular septal rupture, non-coronary surgery, and thoracic aortic surgery (all $p < 0.01$). Additive and logistic models were then developed.

There has been great interest, as well as robust critique, of the role of public reporting of outcomes in cardiac, thoracic and vascular surgery (22–24). The experience of cardiac surgery in New York State (23,25) and the UK (26) are well known (see table 43.1). Some of the concerns include up-scaling of risk indices and denial of surgery for high-risk patients (25,27). Such misuse of risk scores will overestimate the likelihood of morbidity and mortality, and so lead to a spurious conclusion that surgical results are better than predicted. Denial of surgery to those genuinely at high risk is more problematic, in that genuine surgical candidates can be excluded to protect a surgeon's or institution's figures at the expense of optimal medical care.

One particular concern many have when measuring performance in surgical or anaesthetic procedures is to consider and assess the learning curve required to demonstrate an acceptable level of performance. Here cumulative sum (CUSUM) analysis has been used and can be strongly recommended. This is a type of sequential analysis used to monitor performance over time (28,29). Some have included risk-adjustment in such an analysis in order to account for patient comorbidity or other complexity of care (30,31) (see figure 43.1). Non-technical skills are also important; these can be measured in other ways (32).

How best, and what to measure?

Whereas many agree that improving the quality of care is important, few agree on the best way to go about it (33). What this might mean and how it should be measured are the subjects of much debate. What is quality in healthcare? A framework for this was first proposed by Donabedian in 1966, using a paradigm consisting of structure, process, and outcomes of care (34). Although there is ongoing argument about the merits of process and outcome measures in healthcare, it seems obvious that no single measure can suffice. They each measure different things, and none can adequately define good quality care. As with clinical research, a range of measures are needed to properly characterize the benefits or adverse effects of any intervention. Recent efforts have attempted to define a composite of these to provide an overall measure of quality in surgical care (19).

Duration of stay in the intensive care unit (ICU) and/or hospital are commonly measured and reported as part of audit processes or clinical research. They have some value in that they affect the overall costs of care, are surrogate markers of a composite of any of a variety of complications, and have direct value to the patient in that it represents the time denied before their return home. However, they can be limited by other factors affecting discharge time, such as hospital protocols, unavailability of clinical staff to complete paperwork delaying discharge, or limitations of the home environment, when in the fact the patient is quite well (35).

An overall measure of quality of recovery after surgery is useful in that it can provide a global measure of outcome from a patient's perspective (36). A 40-item quality of recovery score (QoR-40) has undergone extensive psychometric evaluation (37,38). and has been used in many perioperative studies (39,40). It has been used after cardiac surgery, and appears to be a better measure of early recovery when compared to a traditional quality of life measure (SF-36), and can predict longer term disability (41). But the QoR-40 is designed to measure outcome up to 30 days after surgery. Other measures of outcome include patient satisfaction and quality of life. There has been some interest in measuring the capacity of patients to return to full functional status, using measures of disability (15,42). However, such measures have yet to be properly validated in surgical patients.

Clinical indicators are another way to define quality of care. They may include process or outcome measures, but the focus is on those that can be reliably collected (and compared) and have been demonstrated to represent quality of care (43). There is some justification in considering unplanned admission to the intensive care unit (ICU) as an ideal measure for most types of surgery (43,44). Another is unplanned reoperation (30,45); this is particularly useful in peripheral arterial bypass surgery (45). Unplanned reoperation is likely to indicate errors in surgical technique (30) and unplanned ICU admission is likely to indicate errors throughout the intraoperative and early postoperative periods, and such analyses can adjust for patient comorbidity (30).

Accurate measurement and monitoring of adverse events is crucial (46). Bruce and colleagues (46) reviewed each step in this process for surgery. They examined the quality of the definition, measurement, reporting and monitoring of selected events that are known to cause significant postoperative morbidity and mortality. Four adverse events were selected on the basis of their frequency of occurrence and usefulness of measurement and monitoring: (i) surgical wound infection, (ii) anastomotic leak, (iii) deep vein thrombosis (DVT), and (iv) mortality. For surgical wound infection there was a total of 41 different definitions and 13 grading scales of surgical wound infection identified from 82 studies. Definitions of wound infection varied from presence of pus to complex definitions such as those proposed by the Centers for Disease Control in the USA (47). For anastomotic leak there were over 40 definitions from 107 studies in gastrointestinal surgery. For surgical mortality, the definition was relatively consistent between monitoring systems, but duration of follow-up varied considerably. Some report in-hospital mortality, others 30-, 60-, or 90-day mortality; others link deaths to national death registries. They concluded that the use of standardized, valid, and reliable definitions is fundamental to the accurate measurement and monitoring of surgical adverse events (47).

Electronic data capture and new analysis tools for large datasets offer great opportunities for audit and quality improvement. A vascular surgical group in the US have used decision analysis with modelling of cohorts with specific characteristics and vascular disease to investigate cost-effectiveness and patient outcome (using quality of life) in vascular surgery (48). This group suggests that such techniques are particularly useful for uncommon operations such as thoracoabdominal aortic aneurysm repair, or when innovative procedures are first being used in clinical practice, such as some new endovascular procedures. They used hospital and surgeon volume as a surrogate marker for quality, and found this was directly correlated with lower morbidity and mortality for many vascular procedures.

Registries

Many surgical and anaesthetic subspecialties report outcome data to local, national or international registries (24,26,49). Some of these publish summaries of this information on publically accessible websites. There are ethical and privacy issues related to use of patient information for a purpose not intended, especially the potential to identify individual clinicians or hospitals. A counter argument is that most hospitals are funded from the public purse

and the public therefore has a right to know how well their money is spent, as well as given an opportunity for patients to consider whether they might want to choose a specific doctor or hospital.

The Society for Cardiothoracic Surgery in the UK and the Society of Thoracic Surgeons registry in the US are probably the largest and most comprehensive databases in cardiothoracic surgery (21,26). Other countries have similar processes (50). There are national or international registries for heart transplantation (51), lung transplantation (52), surgery after coronary stenting (53), cardiac surgery in Malaysia (54), Germany (55), and Australia (50); lung cancer resections in Japan (56), use of recombinant Factor VIIa in cardiac surgery (57), thoracic aortic dissection repair (58), and lung volume reduction surgery in Australia and New Zealand (59). The quality of audit or registry data is affected by reporting rates and the degree to which participating hospitals represent usual practice. It is not uncommon for participating clinicians and/or hospitals to have better performance than those not contributing to the data reporting (60), and so it may not be valid to extrapolate results to practices outside of those providing data.

Public reporting and confidential, collaborative peer education represent distinctly different approaches to surgical quality assessment and improvement (16,27). Shahian and colleagues (27) discussed the controversies regarding their methodology and relative effectiveness in cardiac surgery. There is a belief that mandatory reporting and public access motivate high quality care (61), and that market forces will reward the efforts and results of these improvements (62). Such beliefs have been challenged and there are few supportive data. Despite institutions and healthcare regions reporting significant decreases in risk-adjusted mortality or morbidity (62,63), it is unclear whether this is due to the public disclosure or from ongoing quality improvement occurring within hospitals in any case (see table 43.1). There is also concern for denial of surgery for high-risk cases and up-scaling of risk to over-inflate expected versus observed outcomes (25,27), as outlined earlier. Those with a practical knowledge of these issues argue instead for continuous quality improvement (62).

Volume and performance

Many studies focus on the relationship between hospital caseload or volume and operative mortality rates. No single threshold to define a high volume exists. Instead, it seems that the more cases you do the better you get, better survival with increasing volume (64). Both the surgeon's and the hospital's volume seem to be equally important (34). This has been shown with CABG surgery (65), vascular surgery (55), and thoracic surgery (64). High volume hospitals also have lower costs of care (65).

Nevertheless, some have shown that low volume centres can achieve good results (66). The relationship between volume and outcome may thus be spurious, not so much a reflection of poor care but explained by referral and selection biases (64). For example, high-risk patients may be more likely to undergo CABG at low-volume facilities where their risk of dying is higher (67). Marcin and colleagues (58) used patient-level clinical data collected from two Californian CABG mortality reporting programmes and found higher volume hospitals had significantly lower risk-adjusted in-hospital mortality rates, but after the period of mandatory reporting (2003 and 2004) there was no volume-outcome relationship (2003 odds ratio (OR) = 1.00,

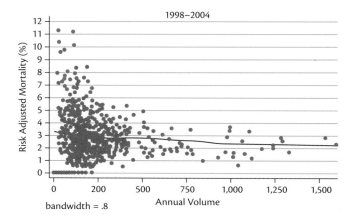

Fig. 43.2 A scatterplot and fitted curve of risk-adjusted mortality and hospital volume, showing no evidence of (non-linear) association between the two.
Reproduced from Marcin JP, et al., 'The CABG surgery volume-outcome relationship: temporal trends and selection effects in California 1998-2004', Health Services Research, 43, 1 Pt 1, pp. 174–192, published by Wiley, © 2008 Health Research & Educational Trust

Table 43.2 Increase in the number of surgical studies using novel designs

	2000	2004	2008	2011	2012
Propensity score	0	5	53	391	433
Equivalence trial	6	13	23	134	36
Non-inferiority trial	0	2	9	76	69

Medline was searched in each year, using terms 'surgery' and each of the designs.

95% confidence interval (CI): 0.94–1.06; 2004 OR = 0.98, 95% CI: 0.92– 1.06)—see figure 43.2. Once again, this supports continuous quality improvement as a means to better care. This begins and ends with audit.

Clinical research

Medical research underpins nearly all advances in healthcare. There is a compelling *beneficence* argument for an obligation to participate in biomedical research (68), and independent, definitive large-outcome studies in particular (69). Biomedical knowledge is a public good, available to any individual, even if that individual does not contribute to it, so both clinicians and patients have a duty to participate (68).

Observational studies

Audit and clinical studies measuring processes and outcomes during routine practice are ideal when wanting to characterize contemporary practice. These are prospective or retrospective cohort studies. The latter are particularly prone to measurement and reporting biases because crucial information is often missing or at least under-reported. A variety of treatments can be compared to determine whether any have an effect on outcome, but because such treatments are provided for specific reasons there is a very real risk of bias and confounding (70–73). Such studies can, however, be valuable in that they are simple to do, can collect key data on many thousands of patients at low cost, and typically represent every day practice without the concerns of exclusion criteria inherent in most clinical trials (74,75).

Administrative databases, often automated, can provide very large-scale datasets, but these are prone to errors (76). There is less ability to check data validity and completeness, and such errors may be directly related to quality or outcomes of care, introducing a systematic bias.

Multivariate techniques can be used to adjust for the range of factors likely to affect the outcome of interest (71,72,77). Propensity score techniques are a relatively new approach to deal with imbalance in observational studies (78)—see table 43.2. They use multivariate analysis to balance all factors that could explain why one treatment was used instead of another and are sometimes therefore referred to as pseudo-randomized trials. One of the earliest uses of propensity score technique was in an analysis of risk with pulmonary artery catheters in the ICU (79), but the technique came to prominence in anaesthesia circles with a non-randomized study of aprotinin for CABG surgery (80).

Clinical trials

Randomized trials are rightly considered the gold standard technique to test the effects of an intervention (81). However, many studies are simply too small to reliably identify clinically important effects; they are underpowered (82). Ideally, a study should have only one nominated primary endpoint and it is this that the sample size calculation should be made. It is reasonable to have a range of secondary endpoints, particularly if they can help the reader interpret the results more fully. Combining study endpoints will increase the number of events and so increase study power, but caution is required when using such composite endpoints (83,84).

Pragmatic trials are those that represent real-world practice, study everyday patients in routine settings, and are sufficiently large to provide reliable results (85,86). Two relatively recent innovations in clinical trials, especially in cardiology, is use of equivalence and non-inferiority designs (87). These address subtly different questions to that most familiar to clinicians: does the treatment being investigated lead to similar outcomes, or outcomes that are no worse, than an existing treatment? These are good designs when considering cheaper, safer, or less complex treatments. To be used properly, there needs to be a determination of what is the minimally clinically important difference. It is this value that defines the boundary of 'equivalence'.

Conclusion

The ultimate goal of medical research is to improve individual and public health by discovering new effective strategies for the maintenance of wellness and for the prevention and treatment of disease (88). Audit and research sit within a broader framework of good quality care. Continuous quality improvement is a repetitive cycle of process and outcomes measurement, design and analysis of interventions to improve the processes of care, and then repeated measurement to determine the impact of such interventions on outcomes (see figure 43.3).

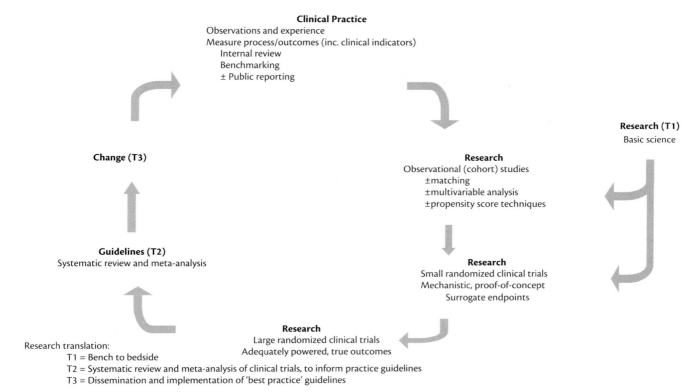

Clinical Practice
Observations and experience
Measure process/outcomes (inc. clinical indicators)
Internal review
Benchmarking
± Public reporting

Research (T1)
Basic science

Change (T3)

Research
Observational (cohort) studies
±matching
±multivariable analysis
±propensity score techniques

Guidelines (T2)
Systematic review and meta-analysis

Research
Small randomized clinical trials
Mechanistic, proof-of-concept
Surrogate endpoints

Research translation:
T1 = Bench to bedside
T2 = Systematic review and meta-analysis of clinical trials, to inform practice guidelines
T3 = Dissemination and implementation of 'best practice' guidelines

Research
Large randomized clinical trials
Adequately powered, true outcomes

Fig. 43.3 Continuous quality improvement, based on an audit cycle of measurement, review and change. Opportunities for improvement in clinical care can be derived from experience and observation, but this is more likely to be reliable if objective measures of process and outcomes of care are used to benchmark against previous results or external providers. Clinical research extends these concepts further. Reliable clinical practice guidelines can then be developed and promulgated. Changes in clinical practice can occur more quickly and widely, providing opportunity for the greatest number of patients to benefit.
Research translation:
T1 = Bench to bedside
T2 = Systematic review and meta-analysis of clinical trials, to inform practice guidelines
T3 = Dissemination and implementation of 'best practice' guidelines.

Advances in medical research ought to be immediately translated into practice, but this is often delayed and incomplete. There are two steps in this translational research agenda, the first being conversion of basic science into clinical studies (T1), the second being conversion of knowledge gained from clinical outcome studies into routine clinical practice (T2) (88). T2 is sometimes divided into a further two components, with T2 including guideline development, meta-analyses, and systematic reviews, whereas T3 including dissemination and implementation research (88). Sadly, the latter steps can take decades—it took more than 10 years for the routine use of beta-blockers after MI to become a guideline, and even today around 30% of such patients do not receive this therapy (89).

The dissemination of up-to-date knowledge should improve patient care. We are then ready to consider the next important question suggested by our clinical observations or laboratory research. It is time to begin the cycle of audit—hypothesis generation—observational studies—and definitive large clinical trials, again.

References

1. Arnold J. *Work Psychology: Understanding Human Behaviour in the Workplace*, 4th edn. Oxford: Pearson Education Ltd, 2005
2. Kinzl JF, Knotzer H, Traweger C, et al. Influence of working conditions on job satisfaction in anaesthetists. *Br J Anaesth* 2005; **94**: 211–5
3. Devlin N, Parkin D. Does NICE have a cost-effectiveness threshold and what other factors influence its decisions? A binary choice analysis. *Health Econ* 2004; **13**: 437–52
4. Queensland Public Hospitals Commission of Inquiry. http://trove.nla.gov.au/work/20106300?q=+&versionId=23693557 (accessed 10 June 2014)
5. The Bristol Royal Infirmary Inquiry. http://webarchive.national-archives.gov.uk/+/www.dh.gov.uk/en/Publicationsandstatistics/Publications/PublicationsPolicyAndGuidance/DH_4005620 (accessed 10 June 2014)
6. Hilborne LH. Setting the stage for the second decade of the era of patient safety: contributions by the Agency for Healthcare Research and Quality and grantees. *Health Serv Res* 2009; **44**: 623–7
7. Greenberg MD, Haviland AM, Yu H, Farley DO. Safety outcomes in the United States: trends and challenges in measurement. *Health Serv Res* 2009; **44**: 739–55
8. Collopy BT, Rodgers L, Woodruff P, Williams J. Early experience with clinical indicators in surgery. *Aust N Z J Surg* 2000; **70**: 448–51
9. Goodnough LT, Johnston MF, Toy PT. The variability of transfusion practice in coronary artery bypass surgery. Transfusion Medicine Academic Award Group. *JAMA* 1991; **265**: 86–90
10. Rebasa P, Mora L, Luna A, Montmany S, Vallverdu H, Navarro S. Continuous monitoring of adverse events: influence on the quality of care and the incidence of errors in general surgery. *World J Surg* 2009; **33**: 191–8
11. Brooke BS, Meguid RA, Makary MA, Perler BA, Pronovost PJ, Pawlik TM. Improving surgical outcomes through adoption of evidence-based

process measures: intervention specific or associated with overall hospital quality? *Surgery* 2010; **147**: 481–90

12. Holman WL, Allman RM, Sansom M, et al. Alabama coronary artery bypass grafting project: results of a statewide quality improvement initiative. *JAMA* 2001; **285**: 3003–10

13. Haller G, Myles PS, Stoelwinder J, et al. Integrating incident reporting into an electronic patient record system. *J Am Med Inform Assoc* 2007; **14**: 175–81

14. Brooke BS, Perler BA, Dominici F, Makary MA, Pronovost PJ. Reduction of in-hospital mortality among California hospitals meeting Leapfrog evidence-based standards for abdominal aortic aneurysm repair. *J Vasc Surg* 2008; **47**: 1155–6; discussion 63–4

15. Khuri S, Daley J, Henderson W, et al. Risk adjustment of the postoperative mortality rate for the comparative assessment of the quality of surgical care: results of the National Veterans Affairs Surgical Risk Study. *J Am Coll Surg* 1997; **185**: 325–38

16. Roques F, Nashef SA, Michel P, et al. Risk factors and outcome in European cardiac surgery: analysis of the EuroSCORE multinational database of 19030 patients. *Eur J Cardiothorac Surg* 1999; **15**: 816–22; discussion 22–3

17. Dripps RD, Lamont A, Eckenhoff JE. The role of anesthesia in surgical mortality. *JAMA* 1961; **178**: 261–6

18. Shapiro M, Swanson SJ, Wright CD, et al. Predictors of major morbidity and mortality after pneumonectomy utilizing the Society for Thoracic Surgeons General Thoracic Surgery Database. *Ann Thorac Surg* 2010; **90**: 927–34; discussion 34–5

19. Shahian DM, Edwards FH, Ferraris VA, et al. Quality measurement in adult cardiac surgery: part 1–Conceptual framework and measure selection. *Ann Thorac Surg* 2007; **83**: S3–12

20. Onaitis M, D'Amico T, Zhao Y, O'Brien S, Harpole D. Risk factors for atrial fibrillation after lung cancer surgery: analysis of the Society of Thoracic Surgeons general thoracic surgery database. *Ann Thorac Surg* 2010; **90**: 368–74

21. Shroyer AL, Coombs LP, Peterson ED, et al. The Society of Thoracic Surgeons: 30-day operative mortality and morbidity risk models. *Ann Thorac Surg* 2003; **75**: 1856–64; discussion 64–5

22. Shroyer AL, McDonald GO, Wagner BD, et al. Improving quality of care in cardiac surgery: evaluating risk factors, processes of care, structures of care, and outcomes. *Semin Cardiothorac Vasc Anesth* 2008; **12**: 140–52

23. Hannan EL, Cozzens K, King SB, 3rd, Walford G, Shah NR. The New York State cardiac registries: history, contributions, limitations, and lessons for future efforts to assess and publicly report healthcare outcomes. *J Am Coll Cardiol* 2012; **59**: 2309–16

24. Paul S, Sedrakyan A, Chiu YL, et al. Outcomes after lobectomy using thoracoscopy vs thoracotomy: a comparative effectiveness analysis utilizing the Nationwide Inpatient Sample database. *Eur J Cardiothorac Surg* 2013; **43**(4): 813–17

25. Burack JH, Impellizzeri P, Homel P, Cunningham JN, Jr. Public reporting of surgical mortality: a survey of New York State cardiothoracic surgeons. *Ann Thorac Surg* 1999; **68**: 1195–200; discussion 201–2

26. Bridgewater B. Cardiac registers: The adult cardiac surgery register. *Heart Failure Rev* 2010; **96**: 1441–3

27. Shahian DM, Normand SL, Torchiana DF, et al. Cardiac surgery report cards: comprehensive review and statistical critique. *Ann Thorac Surg* 2001; **72**: 2155–68

28. Grunkemeier GL, Jin R, Wu Y. Cumulative sum curves and their prediction limits. *Ann Thorac Surg* 2009; **87**: 361–4

29. Wolfe R, Bolsin S, Colson M, Stow P. Monitoring the rate of re-exploration for excessive bleeding after cardiac surgery in adults. *Qual Saf Health Care* 2007; **16**: 192–6

30. Kroon HM, Breslau PJ, Lardenoye JW. Can the incidence of unplanned reoperations be used as an indicator of quality of care in surgery? *Am J Med Qual* 2007; **22**: 198–202

31. Lovegrove J, Valencia O, Treasure T, Sherlaw-Johnson C, Gallivan S. Monitoring the results of cardiac surgery by variable life-adjusted display. *Lancet* 1997; **350**: 1128–30

32. McCulloch P, Mishra A, Handa A, et al. The effects of aviation-style non-technical skills training on technical performance and outcome in the operating theatre. *Qual Saf Health Care* 2009; **18**: 109–15

33. Dimick JB, Upchurch GR, Jr. Measuring and improving the quality of care for abdominal aortic aneurysm surgery. *Circulation* 2008; **117**: 2534–41

34. Birkmeyer JD, Dimick JB, Birkmeyer NJ. Measuring the quality of surgical care: structure, process, or outcomes? *J Am Coll Surg* 2004; **198**: 626–32

35. Farjah F, Lou F, Rusch VW, Rizk NP. The quality metric prolonged length of stay misses clinically important adverse events. *Ann Thorac Surg* 2012

36. Hopkins PM. A shame about the patient? *Br J Anaesth* 2000; **84**: 1–2

37. Myles PS, Weitkamp B, Jones K, Melick J, Hensen S. Validity and reliability of a postoperative quality of recovery score: the QoR-40. *Br J Anaesth* 2000; **84**: 11–5

38. Myles PS, Hunt JO, Fletcher H, et al. Relation between quality of recovery in hospital and quality of life at 3 months after cardiac surgery. *Anesthesiology* 2001; **95**: 862–7

39. Hansdottir V, Philip J, Olsen MF, et al. Thoracic epidural versus intravenous patient-controlled analgesia after cardiac surgery: a randomized controlled trial on length of hospital stay and patient-perceived quality of recovery. *Anesthesiology* 2006; **104**: 142–51

40. Lena P, Balarac N, Lena D, et al. Fast-track anesthesia with remifentanil and spinal analgesia for cardiac surgery: the effect on pain control and quality of recovery. *J Cardiothorac Vasc Anesth* 2008; **22**: 536–42

41. Myles P, Hunt J, Fletcher H, Solly R, Woodward D, Kelly S. Relationship between quality of recovery in hospital and quality of life at three months after cardiac surgery. *Anesthesiology* 2001; **95**: 862–7

42. Guralnik JM, LaCroix AZ, Branch LG, Kasl SV, Wallace RB. Morbidity and disability in older persons in the years prior to death. *Am J Public Health* 1991; **81**: 443–7

43. Haller G, Stoelwinder J, Myles PS, McNeil J. Quality and safety indicators in anesthesia: a systematic review. *Anesthesiology* 2009; **110**: 1158–75

44. Haller G, Myles PS, Wolfe R, et al. Validity of unplanned admission to an intensive care unit as a measure of patient safety in surgical patients. *Anesthesiology* 2005; **103**: 1121–9

45. Ploeg AJ, Lange CP, Lardenoye JW, Breslau PJ. The incidence of unplanned returns to the operating room after peripheral arterial bypass surgery and its value as indicator of quality of care. *Vasc Endovascular Surg* 2008; **42**: 19–24

46. Bruce J, Russell EM, Mollison J, Krukowski ZH. The measurement and monitoring of surgical adverse events. *Health Technol Assess* 2001; **5**: 1–194

47. Horan TC, Andrus M, Dudeck MA. CDC/NHSN surveillance definition of health care-associated infection and criteria for specific types of infections in the acute care setting. *Am J Infect Control* 2008; **36**: 309–32

48. Rectenwald JE, Upchurch GR, Jr. Impact of outcomes research on the management of vascular surgery patients. *J Vasc Surg* 2007; **45**(Suppl A): A131–40

49. Lepantalo M, Venermo M, Laukontaus S, Kantonen I. The role of vascular registries in improving the management of abdominal aortic aneurysm. *Scand J Surg* 2008; **97**: 146–53; discussion 53

50. Reid CM, Brennan AL, Dinh DT, et al. Measuring safety and quality to improve clinical outcomes—current activities and future directions for the Australian Cardiac Procedures Registry. *Med J Aust* 2010; **193**: S107–10

51. Stehlik J, Edwards LB, Kucheryavaya AY, et al. The Registry of the International Society for Heart and Lung Transplantation: twenty-seventh official adult heart transplant report–2010. *J Heart Lung Transplant* 2010; **29**: 1089–103

52. Christie JD, Edwards LB, Kucheryavaya AY, et al. The Registry of the International Society for Heart and Lung Transplantation: twenty-seventh official adult lung and heart-lung transplant report–2010. *J Heart Lung Transplant* 2010; **29**: 1104–18

53. Brilakis ES, Cohen DJ, Kleiman NS, et al. Incidence and clinical outcome of minor surgery in the year after drug-eluting stent implantation: results from the Evaluation of Drug-Eluting Stents and Ischemic Events Registry. *Am Heart J* 2011; **161**: 360–6

54. Anas R, Rahman I, Jahizah H, et al. Malaysian Cardiothoracic Surgery Registry—a patient registry to evaluate the health outcomes of patients undergoing surgery for cardiothoracic diseases in Malaysia. *Med J Malaysia* 2008; **63 Suppl C**: 78–80

55. Gummert JF, Funkat AK, Beckmann A, et al. Cardiac surgery in Germany during 2010: A Report on Behalf of the German Society for Thoracic and Cardiovascular Surgery. *Thorac Cardiovasc Surg* 2011; **59**(5): 259–67

56. Sawabata N, Miyaoka E, Asamura H, et al. Japanese Lung Cancer Registry Study of 11,663 Surgical Cases in 2004: demographic and prognosis changes over decade. *J Thorac Oncol* 2011; **6**(7): 1229–35

57. Dunkley S, Phillips L, McCall P, et al. Recombinant activated factor VII in cardiac surgery: experience from the Australian and New Zealand Haemostasis Registry. *Ann Thorac Surg* 2008; **85**: 836–44

58. Trimarchi S, Nienaber CA, Rampoldi V, et al. Contemporary results of surgery in acute type A aortic dissection: The International Registry of Acute Aortic Dissection experience. *J Thorac Cardiovasc Surg* 2005; **129**: 112–22

59. Munro PE, Bailey MJ, Smith JA, Snell GI. Lung volume reduction surgery in Australia and New Zealand. Six years on: registry report. *Chest* 2003; **124**: 1443–50

60. Lapar DJ, Bhamidipati CM, Lau CL, Jones DR, Kozower BD. The society of thoracic surgeons general thoracic surgery database: establishing generalizability to national lung cancer resection outcomes. *Ann Thorac Surg* 2012; **94**: 216–21

61. Marcin JP, Li Z, Kravitz RL, et al. The CABG surgery volume-outcome relationship: temporal trends and selection effects in California, 1998–2004. *Health Serv Res* 2008; **43**: 174–92

62. Shahian DM, Edwards FH, Jacobs JP, et al. Public Reporting of Cardiac Surgery Performance: Part 1–History, Rationale, Consequences. *Ann Thorac Surg* 2011; **92**: S2–11

63. Bridgewater B, Grayson AD, Brooks N, et al. Has the publication of cardiac surgery outcome data been associated with changes in practice in northwest England: an analysis of 25 730 patients undergoing CABG surgery under 30 surgeons over eight years. *Heart* 2007; **93**: 744–8

64. Romano PS, Mark DH. Patient and hospital characteristics related to in-hospital mortality after lung cancer resection. *Chest* 1992; **101**: 1332–7

65. Auerbach AD, Hilton JF, Maselli J, Pekow PS, Rothberg MB, Lindenauer PK. Case volume, quality of care, and care efficiency in coronary artery bypass surgery. *Arch Intern Med* 2010; **170**: 1202–8

66. Goshima KR, Mills JL, Sr., Awari K, Pike SL, Hughes JD. Measure what matters: institutional outcome data are superior to the use of surrogate markers to define 'center of excellence' for abdominal aortic aneurysm repair. *Ann Vasc Surg* 2008; **22**: 328–34

67. Nallamothu BK, Saint S, Hofer TP, et al. Impact of patient risk on the hospital volume-outcome relationship in coronary artery bypass grafting. *Arch Intern Med* 2005; **165**: 333–7

68. Schaefer GO, Emanuel EJ, Wertheimer A. The obligation to participate in biomedical research. *JAMA* 2009; **302**: 67–72

69. McNeil JJ, Nelson MR, Tonkin AM. Public funding of large-scale clinical trials in Australia. *Med J Aust* 2003; **179**: 519–20

70. Klein-Geltink JE, Rochon PA, Dyer S, Laxer M, Anderson GM. Readers should systematically assess methods used to identify, measure and analyze confounding in observational cohort studies. *J Clin Epidemiol* 2007; **60**: 766–72

71. Normand SL, Sykora K, Li P, et al. Readers guide to critical appraisal of cohort studies: 3. Analytical strategies to reduce confounding. *Br Med J* 2005; **330**: 1021–3

72. Mamdani M, Sykora K, Li P, et al. Reader's guide to critical appraisal of cohort studies: 2. Assessing potential for confounding. *Br Med J* 2005; **330**: 960–2

73. Cleophas TJ, Zwinderman AH. Clinical trials: how to assess confounding and why so. *Curr Clin Pharmacol* 2007; **2**: 129–33

74. Dreyer NA. Making observational studies count: shaping the future of comparative effectiveness research. *Epidemiology* 2011; **22**: 295–7

75. MacMahon S, Collins R. Reliable assessment of the effects of treatment on mortality and major morbidity, II: observational studies. *Lancet* 2001; **357**: 455–62

76. Ray WA. Improving automated database studies. *Epidemiology* 2011; **22**: 302–4

77. Li L, Shen C, Wu AC, Li X. Propensity Score-based Sensitivity Analysis Method for Uncontrolled Confounding. *Am J Epidemiol* 2011; **174**(3): 345–53

78. Adamina M, Guller U, Weber WP, Oertli D. Propensity scores and the surgeon. *Br J Surg* 2006; **93**: 389–94

79. Connors AF, Jr., Speroff T, Dawson NV, et al. The effectiveness of right heart catheterization in the initial care of critically ill patients. SUPPORT Investigators. *JAMA* 1996; **276**: 889–97

80. Mangano DT, Tudor IC, Dietzel C. The risk associated with aprotinin in cardiac surgery. *N Engl J Med* 2006; **354**: 353–65

81. Kunz R, Vist G, Oxman AD. Randomisation to protect against selection bias in healthcare trials. *Cochrane Database Syst Rev* 2007: MR000012

82. Freiman JA, Chalmers TC, Smith H, Jr., Kuebler RR. The importance of beta, the type II error and sample size in the design and interpretation of the randomized control trial. Survey of 71 'negative' trials. *N Engl J Med* 1978; **299**: 690–4

83. Kip KE, Hollabaugh K, Marroquin OC, Williams DO. The problem with composite end points in cardiovascular studies: the story of major adverse cardiac events and percutaneous coronary intervention. *J Am Coll Cardiol* 2008; **51**: 701–7

84. Myles PS, Devereaux PJ. Pros and cons of composite endpoints in anesthesia trials. *Anesthesiology* 2010; **113**: 776–8

85. Tunis SR, Stryer DB, Clancy CM. Practical clinical trials: increasing the value of clinical research for decision making in clinical and health policy. *JAMA* 2003; **290**: 1624–32

86. Yusuf S, Collins R, Peto R. Why do we need some large simple randomized trials? *Statistics in Medicine* 1984; **3**: 409–20

87. Gotzsche PC. Lessons from and cautions about noninferiority and equivalence randomized trials. *JAMA* 2006; **295**: 1172–4

88. Lauer MS, Skarlatos S. Translational research for cardiovascular diseases at the National Heart, Lung, and Blood Institute: moving from bench to bedside and from bedside to community. *Circulation* 2010; **121**: 929–33

89. Ting HH, Shojania KG, Montori VM, Bradley EH. Quality improvement: science and action. *Circulation* 2009; **119**: 1962–74

Index

Note: Page numbers in *italics* refer to boxes, figures, and tables.